Water-Soluble Vitamins							Minerals					
Vitamin C (mg)	Thiamin (mg)	Riboflavin (mg)	Niacin (mg NE)[e]	Vitamin B-6 (mg)	Folacin[f] (μg)	Vitamin B-12 (μg)	Calcium (mg)	Phosphorus (mg)	Magnesium (mg)	Iron (mg)	Zinc (mg)	Iodine (μg)
35	0.3	0.4	6	0.3	30	0.5[g]	360	240	50	10	3	40
35	0.5	0.6	8	0.6	45	1.5	540	360	70	15	5	50
45	0.7	0.8	9	0.9	100	2.0	800	800	150	15	10	70
45	0.9	1.0	11	1.3	200	2.5	800	800	200	10	10	90
45	1.2	1.4	16	1.6	300	3.0	800	800	250	10	10	120
50	1.4	1.6	18	1.8	400	3.0	1200	1200	350	18	15	150
60	1.4	1.7	18	2.0	400	3.0	1200	1200	400	18	15	150
60	1.5	1.7	19	2.2	400	3.0	800	800	350	10	15	150
60	1.4	1.6	18	2.2	400	3.0	800	800	350	10	15	150
60	1.2	1.4	16	2.2	400	3.0	800	800	350	10	15	150
50	1.1	1.3	15	1.8	400	3.0	1200	1200	300	18	15	150
60	1.1	1.3	14	2.0	400	3.0	1200	1200	300	18	15	150
60	1.1	1.3	14	2.0	400	3.0	800	800	300	18	15	150
60	1.0	1.2	13	2.0	400	3.0	800	800	300	18	15	150
60	1.0	1.2	13	2.0	400	3.0	800	800	300	10	15	150
+20	+0.4	+0.3	+2	+0.6	+400	+1.0	+400	+400	+150	*h*	+5	+25
+40	+0.5	+0.5	+5	+0.5	+100	+1.0	+400	+400	+150	*h*	+10	+50

treatment with enzymes (conjugases) to make polyglutamyl forms of the vitamin available to the test organism.

[g]The recommended dietary allowance for vitamin B-12 in infants is based on average concentration of the vitamin in human milk. The allowances after weaning are based on energy intake (as recommended by the American Academy of Pediatrics) and consideration of other factors, such as intestinal absorption; see text.

[h]The increased requirement during pregnancy cannot be met by the iron content of habitual American diets nor by the existing iron stores of many women; therefore the use of 30–60 mg of supplemental iron is recommended. Iron needs during lactation are not substantially different from those of nonpregnant women, but continued supplementation of the mother for 2–3 months after parturition is advisable in order to replenish stores depleted by pregnancy.

Elements[b]			Electrolytes		
Chromium (mg)	Selenium (mg)	Molybdenum (mg)	Sodium (mg)	Potassium (mg)	Chloride (mg)
0.01–0.04	0.01–0.04	0.03–0.06	115–350	350–925	275–700
0.02–0.06	0.02–0.06	0.04–0.08	250–750	425–1275	400–1200
0.02–0.08	0.02–0.08	0.05–0.1	325–975	550–1650	500–1500
0.03–0.12	0.03–0.12	0.06–0.15	450–1350	775–2325	700–2100
0.05–0.2	0.05–0.2	0.1 –0.3	600–1800	1000–3000	925–2775
0.05–0.2	0.05–0.2	0.15–0.5	900–2700	1525–4575	1400–4200
0.05–0.2	0.05–0.2	0.15–0.5	1100–3300	1875–5625	1700–5100

Source: Food and Nutrition Board, National Academy of Sciences-National Research Council, Washington, D.C., 1980.

Normal and Therapeutic Nutrition

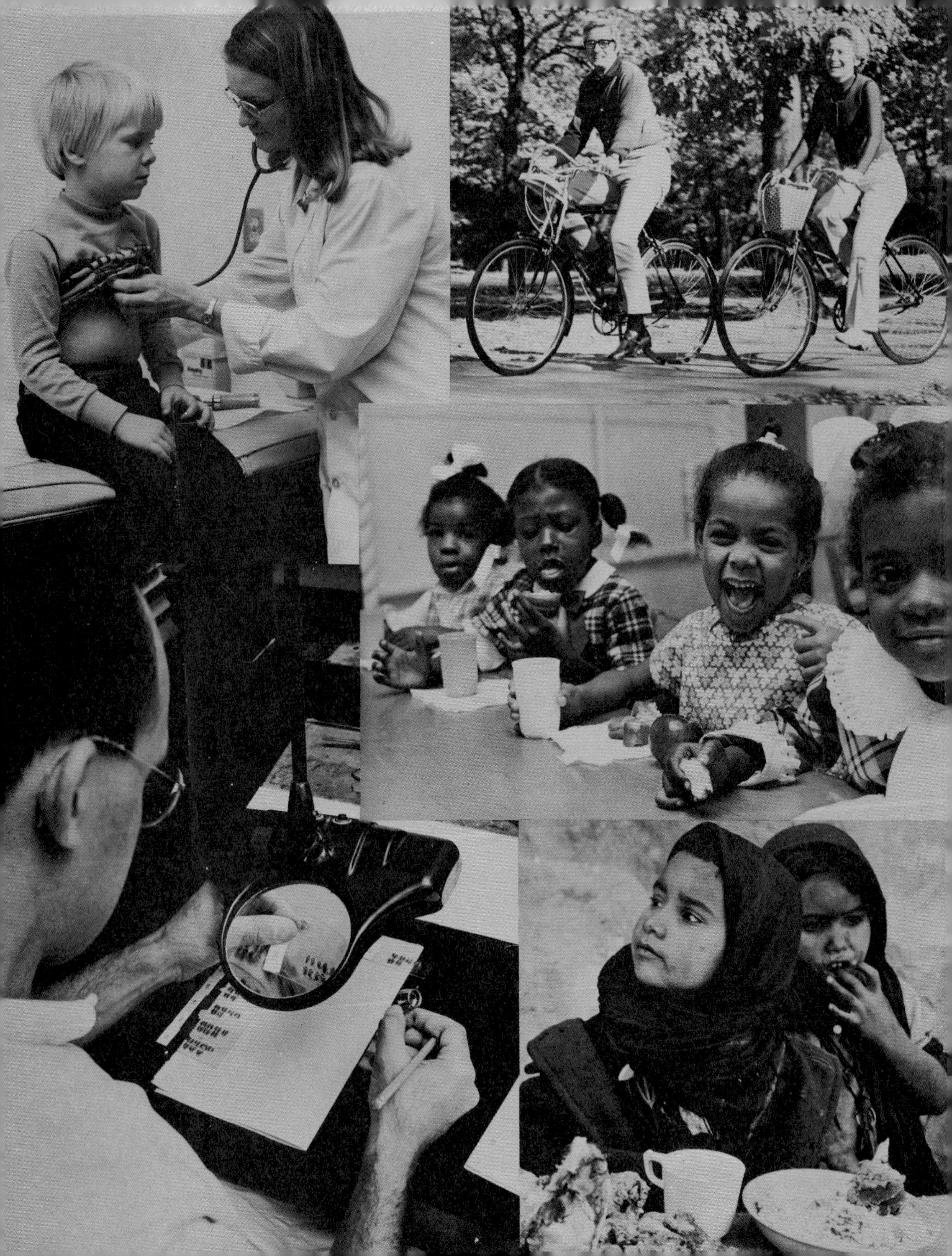

16th Edition

Normal and Therapeutic Nutrition

Corinne H. Robinson

M. S., D. Sc., (Hon.), R. D.
Professor of Nutrition Emeritus. Formerly, Head, Department of Nutrition and Food, Drexel University, Philadelphia

Marilyn R. Lawler

M.S., R.D.
Lecturer, Department of Medicine,
University of Chicago

MACMILLAN PUBLISHING CO., INC.
New York

COLLIER MACMILLAN PUBLISHERS
London

Macmillan Publishing Co., Inc.
866 Third Avenue, New York, New York 10022

Collier Macmillan Canada, Ltd.

Library of Congress Cataloging in Publication Data

Robinson, Corinne Hogden.
Normal and therapeutic nutrition.

Bibliography: p.
Includes index.
1. Diet therapy. 2. Nutrition. 3. Food—Composition—Tables. I. Lawler, Marilyn R., joint author II. Title.
RM216.R6523 1982 613.2 81–6054
ISBN 0–02–402370–1 AACR2
Printing: 1 2 3 4 5 6 7 8 Year: 2 3 4 5 6 7 8

Preface

THE sixteenth edition of *Normal and Therapeutic Nutrition,* as in previous editions, is intended especially for students of nursing and dietetics. It is a useful reference for the practicing nutritionist, dietitian, physician, nurse, and home economist. The text continues to have three objectives: (1) to provide a background in the science of nutrition that individuals can use as the basis for making decisions for dietary planning for themselves or for others in any age group in health or in illness; (2) to show how the principles of nutrition may be integrated with the psychiatric, cultural, and economic factors in the daily selection of meals; and (3) to furnish guidelines for education, dietary counseling, and community services.

The 1980 Recommended Dietary Allowances together with the estimated safe and adequate ranges of intake for other minerals and vitamins recommended by the Food and Nutrition Board are utilized throughout the text. The text has been extensively revised to include reports of recent research in the areas of normal and clinical nutrition. Many new illustrations are included and others have been updated to show current information. References to the literature are as up-to-date as the time span for book publication permits.

The concept of dietary balance to maintain or restore the best possible level of health is emphasized; that is, the diet must furnish sufficient energy and nutrients to meet the metabolic needs at all stages of the life cycle. On the other hand, the excesses that are believed to be etiologic factors in chronic disease ranging from dental caries and obesity to cardiovascular and gastrointestinal disease are to be avoided. The issues that concern so many people are delineated, and the reader is led to the development of responsible positions that can be taken even though final answers are not available.

The text is again divided into two parts. A new chapter "Nutritional Assessment and Dietary Counseling" (Chapter 22) includes a discussion of anthropometric, clinical, dietary, immune response, and biochemical measures together with practical guidelines for dietary counseling. Chapter 3, largely rewritten, includes dietary guides: the *1980 Recommended Dietary Allowances,* the revised five-group *Daily Food Guide* by the U.S. Department of Agriculture; the *Dietary Goals* of the Senate Select Committee on Nutrition and Human Needs; the *Dietary Guidelines for Americans* issued jointly in 1980 by the U.S. Department of Agriculture and the U.S. Department of Health and Human Services; and the recommendations in 1980 by the Food and Nutrition Board in *Toward Healthful Diets.* The practical applications of these guidelines are discussed in the chapters pertaining to the nutrients and to dietary planning throughout the life cycle. Also included in Chapter 3 is a discussion of the index of nutritional quality. The Basic Diet pattern used in the charts of Chapter 4 through 12 has been recalculated to conform to the new Daily Food Guide and new tables of food composition.

Other additions or emphases in Part I include: alcohol, fiber, artificial sweeteners (Chapter 5); the role of dietary lipids in the etiology of chronic disease (Chapter 6); the availability of iron in foods and the calculations of iron availability (Chapter 8); the effects of sodium imbalance (Chapter 9); food habits of native Americans and of Vietnamese (Chapter 15); effects of drug usage on the outcome of pregnancy and the influence of oral contraceptives on the nutritional status of women (Chapter 18); advantages of breast feeding and the later introduction of solid foods in infant feeding (Chapter 19); and diet for athletes (Chapter 20).

Adaptation of the normal diet to meet the needs of individuals with specific pathologic conditions is described in Part II. The introductory chapter, "Comprehensive Nutritional Services" (Chapter 24) describes the process of nutritional care of the hospitalized patient including assessment of nutritional status and food practices; development and implementation of nutritional care plans, including food services and dietary counseling; and provision for follow-up care. Additional criteria for diagnosis, including newer diagnostic tests, have been included in many chapters. Examples are use of breath hydrogen tests in diagnosis of carbohydrate malabsorption (Chapter 33) and revised criteria for diagnosis of diabetes mellitus (Chapter 37). Terminology has been revised to conform to newer usage, and some dietary regimens have been modified (Chapters 36, "Nutrition in Surgical Conditions," and 41, "Diet in Diseases of the Kidney"). Where appropriate the effect of specific drugs on nutrition has been described.

A new chapter, "Nutrition for the Cancer Patient" (Chapter 35) includes a discussion of the role of dietary factors in cancer etiology, the metabolic effects of cancer, the nutritional effects of cancer therapies, and nutritional considerations for the patient with cancer. The National Diabetes Data Group 1979 classification of types of diabetes mellitus and goals for dietary management are presented in chapter 37, "Diabetes Mellitus." The 1979 recommendations by the Committee on Sodium-restricted Diets, Food and Nutrition Board, for levels of sodium restriction in acute and chronic heart disease are listed in Chapter 40. Other additions and revisions of note in Part II include: increased emphasis on the role of exercise in weight control, and expanded discussion of newer approaches to weight reduction, including behavior modification, total starvation, protein-sparing modified fast, and surgical treatment (Chapter 27); description of the immune response and the metabolic consequences of stress due to illness and infection (Chapter 29); and discussion of current controversies over the role of diet in the management of peptic ulcer (Chapter 31); osteoporosis (Chapter 38); and hypertension (Chapter 39).

The Appendix includes many tables for use in nutritional assessment and dietary planning. Table A-1 "Nutritive Values of the Edible Part of Foods" is the 1977 greatly expanded revision of Bulletin 72 by the U.S. Department of Agriculture. Tentative values for the copper content of foods have been added to Table A-2; other values in this table have been revised to include current data on food composition. New to this edition are a table of dietary fiber (A-3); charts showing "Physical Growth NCHS Percentiles" for boys and girls from birth to 18 years (A-6 through A-9); tables stating upper arm circumference and triceps skinfolds together with nomograms for calculating muscle circumference and cross-sectional muscle and fat areas (A-11 through A-14).

Case Studies in Clinical Nutrition: A Workbook and Study Guide for Students of Nursing and Dietetics, second edition, by Corinne H. Robinson, Marilyn R. Lawler, and Ann E. Garwick has been written to accompany this text.

Corinne H. Robinson
Marilyn R. Lawler

Acknowledgments

STUDENTS, faculty, and practicing nutritionists have contributed many suggestions for the development of this edition; for these we are most grateful. Especially we acknowledge the critical evaluation of the 15th edition of this book and the constructive suggestions made for its revision by Dr. Wanda Chenoweth, Associate Professor, Department of Food Science and Human Nutrition, Michigan State University; Dr. P. Vincent J. Hegarty, Professor of Human Nutrition, Department of Food Science and Nutrition, University of Minnesota; Dr. Jacqueline E. Reddick, Associate Professor, Department of Home Economics, Montana State University; and Dr. Eleanor D. Schlenker, Chairperson, Department of Human Nutrition and Foods, The University of Vermont.

Two well-qualified educators in nutrition have contributed to this edition. They are Dr. Jacqueline E. Reddick who revised Chapter 8, Mineral Elements, and Chapter 9, Fluid and Electrolyte Balance; and Dr. Wanda Chenoweth who revised Chapter 10, The Fat-Soluble Vitamins, Chapter 11, The Water-Soluble Vitamins: Ascorbic Acid, and Chapter 12, The Water-Soluble Vitamins: The B-Complex Vitamins. We appreciate their revisions and additions to incorporate recent research. We are also grateful to authors and publishers who have given permission to quote from their publications.

We are indebted to many individuals and organizations for new illustrations. Especially we wish to recognize the contributions made through the courtesy of Mrs. Barbara Pickering, R.D., Clinical Coordinator, Dietary Department, the Metropolitan Medical Center and Hennepin County Medical Center, Minneapolis; Mr. Jeffrey Grosscup, photojournalist, Minneapolis; the Marple-Newtown School District, Newtown Square, Pennsylvania; and many individuals who appeared as models in the photographs. Appreciation is also extended to Leslie M. Klevay, M.D., D.Sc., and Harold H. Sandstead, M.D., USDA Grand Forks Human Nutrition Research Center, and the librarians and staff of the Harley E. French Medical Library, University of North Dakota, Grand Forks.

For about a quarter of a century Miss Joan C. Zulch, Executive Editor, Medical Books Department, Macmillan, guided each edition skillfully throughout its preparation. We learned much from her about books and their making, and we value the many innovative ideas that she contributed. In this long association she has been a good friend and we will treasure this always. With the sixteenth edition, the skillful direction of our new editor, Mr. John J. Beck, Senior Editor, College and Professional Division, Macmillan, is gratefully acknowledged. We look forward to a long association with him.

Contents

part one
Normal Nutrition

part two
Therapeutic Nutrition

Appendixes

Normal and Therapeutic Nutrition

1 Food, Nutrition, and Health

AN INTRODUCTION

NUTRITION is "the science of foods, the nutrients and other substances therein; their action, interaction, and balance in relationship to health and disease; the processes by which the organism ingests, digests, absorbs, transports, and utilizes nutrients and disposes of their end products. In addition, nutrition must be concerned with social, economic, cultural, and psychological implications of food and eating."*

The Meanings of Food, Nutrition, and Nutritional Care

What Does Food Mean to You Food—menu—diet—hunger—nutrition—malnutrition. What images do these words bring to your mind? Are they oriented to your senses? To your social enjoyment? To your concerns about your own well-being? To your emotions? Do they raise questions about the quality of life for your fellow human beings?

When you sit down to your next meal you will have definite ideas—positive or negative—about that meal and the specific foods that are served to you. Through your eyes you will delight in the texture variations and color combinations of the food, the artistic touch of a garnish, and the beautiful table appointments; or perhaps your interest will be diminished because the food lacks color and is carelessly served. Through your nose you will enjoy the tantalizing odors of meat or of freshly baked rolls, or the fragrance of fully ripened fruit; or possibly you will be repelled because of the odor of grease which is too hot or of vegetables which have been cooked too long. Through your sense of taste you will experience countless flavors—the salty, sweet, bitter, and sour and their variations; you will feel the textures of smooth or fibrous, crisp or soft, creamy or oily, moist or dry foods.

But the experiences of your senses alone do not determine what your next meal, or any meal, means to you. Is the meal merely a way of staying alive and keeping in health; an opportunity for fellowship with your family and friends; a way to celebrate an event; an occasion for stimulating conversation; a means of satisfying your feelings when you are hurt and depressed; a display of prestige by which you show that you can afford certain foods others cannot; a token of security and love; a means of asserting your independence; a cause of concern because some foods might make you ill; an occasion of self-denial; something you enjoy leisurely; taken for granted as your right; a precious gift from God for which you are thankful? What other feelings are evoked by the food you eat?

Next to the air you breathe and the water you drink, food has been basic to your existence. In fact, food has been the primary concern of humankind in its physical environment throughout all recorded history. By food, or the lack of it, the destinies of individuals are greatly influenced. People must eat to live, and what they eat will affect in a high degree their ability to keep

* Robinson, W. D.: "Nutrition in Medical Education," in *Proceedings Western Hemisphere Nutrition Congress—1965,* American Medical Association, Chicago, 1966, p. 206.

well, to work, to be happy, and to live long.

Some Important Definitions HEALTH is defined by the World Health organization of the United Nations as the "state of complete physical, mental and social well-being and not merely the absence of disease or infirmity."*

NUTRIENTS are the constituents in food that must be supplied to the body in suitable amounts. These include water, proteins and the amino acids of which they are composed, fats and fatty acids, carbohydrates, minerals, and vitamins.

NUTRITIONAL STATUS is the condition of health of the individual as influenced by the utilization of the nutrients. It can be determined only by the correlation of information obtained through a careful medical and dietary history, a thorough physical examination, and appropriate laboratory investigations.

NUTRITIONAL CARE is "the application of the science and art of human nutrition in helping people select and obtain food for the primary purpose of nourishing their bodies in health or in disease throughout the life cycle. This participation may be in single or combined functions: in feeding groups involving food selection and management; in extending knowledge of food and nutrition principles; in teaching these principles for application according to particular situations; and in dietary counseling."†

MALNUTRITION is an impairment of health resulting from a deficiency, excess, or imbalance of nutrients. It includes UNDERNUTRITION, which refers to a deficiency of calories and/or one or more essential nutrients, and OVERNUTRITION, which is an excess of one or more nutrients and usually of calories.

* *World Health Organization—What It Is, What It Does, How It Works.* Leaflet, Geneva, Switzerland, 1956.

† Committee on Goals of Education for Dietetics, Dietetic Internship Council: "Goals of the Lifetime Education of the Dietitian," *J. Am. Diet. Assoc.*, **54**:92, 1969.

The Science of Nutrition Observations concerning the relationship of food to health have been made throughout recorded history. Occasionally these observations have withstood scientific scrutiny. Others have persisted to this day although their validity has never been established. Knowledge concerning nutrition has its origin in research conducted by chemists, biochemists, microbiologists, molecular biologists, physiologists, pathologists, nutritionists, and others over approximately two centuries.

The science of nutrition had its beginnings in the late eighteenth century with the discovery of the respiratory gases and especially the studies on the nature and the quantification of energy metabolism by Lavoisier, a Frenchman often referred to as the Father of the Science of Nutrition. During the nineteenth century many chemists and physiologists added important information on the need for protein and some minerals such as calcium, phosphorus, and iron. Knowledge of vitamins has been gained in the twentieth century. Indeed, more knowledge concerning nutrition has been gained in this century than in all the preceding centuries combined.

The facts of nutrition are gained by applying the scientific method; that is, setting up an hypothesis, testing the hypothesis under carefully controlled conditions, observing the results, and interpreting them. The research may take place within the borders of a community or within the walls of a laboratory. Epidemiologic studies, surveys, and laboratory investigations are cited frequently in this book. A brief description of each of these will help the reader to understand the several ways by which knowledge of nutrition is obtained.

EPIDEMIOLOGY is the science of epidemic disease. Epidemiologic studies are based on observing the associations that exist between given environmental conditions and the incidence of disease conditions. For example, recent studies have shown that rural Africans who consume a

large amount of fiber have a low incidence of gastrointestinal diseases such as diverticulitis, colon cancer, and others. But in western European countries and the United States the incidence of these diseases is high and the fiber intake is low. These studies establish association, not cause! For example, one might also find that the low incidence of these diseases amongst rural Africans is associated with the presence of few automobiles, and their consequent pollution, or the scarcity of television sets, or the high rate of physical activity of these Africans! Although the epidemiologic study does not establish cause, it is valuable because it suggests hypotheses to be tested. Indeed, much research is now taking place under controlled conditions to determine whether fiber intake is related to gastrointestinal diseases.

Experimental studies. Colleges, universities, the food industry, and governmental agencies such as the U.S. Department of Agriculture, the Food and Drug Administration, the National Institutes of Health, and others are engaged in a wide spectrum of research projects in nutrition. Much research is conducted directly on human beings with their informed consent. For example, under controlled conditions of diet, exercise, and weight maintenance the investigator might study the changes in the blood cholesterol of persons of a given age group when they consume high- or low-fiber diets. Or a carefully selected group of volunteers, often college or medical students, might participate in very exacting balance studies. In a balance study the diets consumed are rigidly controlled in kinds and amounts of foods; analyses are made of the diet for nutrient composition; fecal and urine excretions are collected and analyzed; and changes in blood composition are determined. Such balance studies require weeks or months of participation. Through such studies the requirements for specific nutrients have been determined.

For obvious reasons human beings cannot be used for many studies so the researcher uses animal models. Rats are widely used because their life span is relatively short and they can be studied over the entire life cycle, they are omnivorous as are humans, they can be handled with relative ease, and the costs of studies with them are realistic. The results obtained from animal studies cannot always be directly applied to human beings, but they indicate the direction for further studies that will be appropriate on human beings.

Nutrition surveys. The nutritive quality of diets consumed by a given population and the nutritional status of the people in the sample can be ascertained by using survey techniques. To illustrate, the students in a nutrition course might conduct a survey of the breakfast habits of students living in a dormitory and of those commuting to classes. Or they might survey the snacking habits of normal-weight and overweight students.

Nationwide surveys referred to frequently in this book include the Ten-State Nutrition Survey, 1968–70; the Survey of Preschool Children, 1968–70; the Health and Nutrition Examination Survey (HANES), 1971–72; and the National Food Consumption Survey, 1977–78.[1-4]

Good Nutrition: A Multidisciplinary Effort To meet the nutritional needs of the population of a nation requires a complex system involving many disciplines. Each step in the food chain must provide conditions that ensure retention of maximum nutritive values, safety, and quality. These requirements are met by (1) application of agricultural science and technology to produce sufficient amounts of animal and plant foods; (2) harvesting and transporting of foods to processors; (3) processing and packaging of foods; (4) adequate storage, transportation, and marketing facilities to make foods available at times and places where needed; (5) appropriate governmental controls to ensure wholesomeness and nutritive quality of the food supply; (6) economic conditions that make it possible to procure the necessary foods at a cost within the

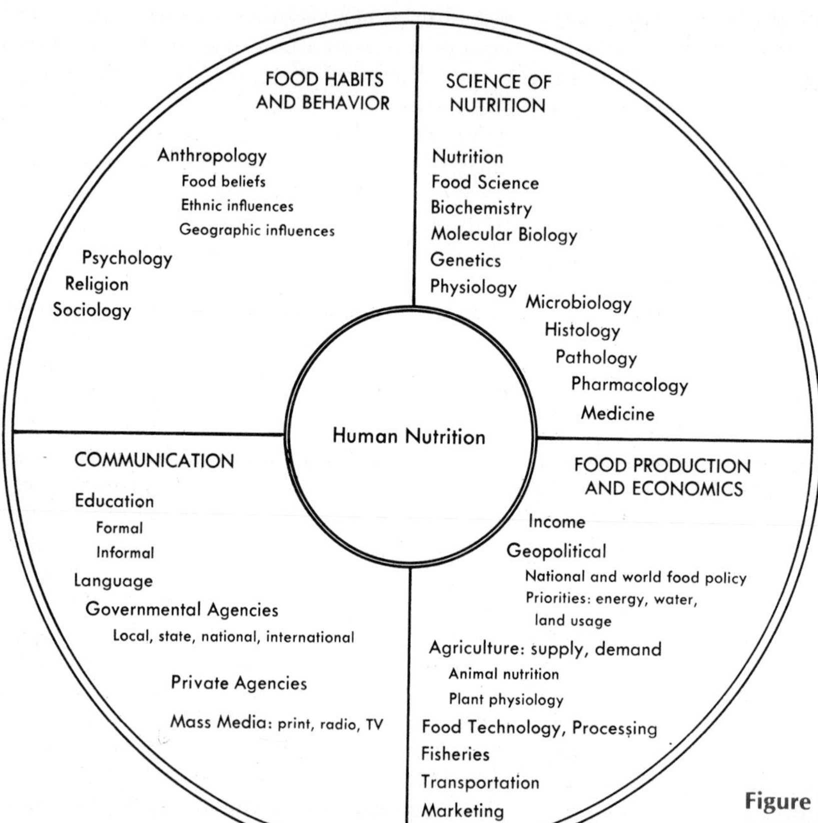

Figure 1–1. Human nutrition encompasses the study and application of many disciplines.

reach of all; (7) educational programs in nutrition within the schools and at the community level; and (8) efficient use of food within the home, public eating place, and institution.

The perspectives of nutrition held by each of the specialists who help to ensure an adequate food supply obviously would be quite different. Thus, the disciplines of the life sciences, human behavior, economics, government, and communications are intertwined in nutrition study. The benefits of good nutrition—health, happiness, efficiency, and longevity—are sought by people all over the world. The achievement of these benefits is like a utopian dream to most of the world's people. (See Figure 1–1.)

Dietary Trends in the United States

Changes in Patterns of Living Since the beginning of this century the population of the United States has shifted from rural to urban areas. Most people must purchase all of their foods, and even on the farm most families purchase a substantial proportion of the foods that they consume. Americans have the benefit of many labor-saving devices in their occupations and in their homes. They work fewer hours in a week, so that the way in which they spend their leisure may be decisive in determining their food needs. Leisure, to many people, means little activity—riding rather than walking, watching television rather than leading an active outdoor life, and so on.

Greater numbers of married women are working away from home than ever before, which means that less time is available for food preparation, more expensive prepared foods are used, and shopping is less frequent. Husbands, as well as wives, are shopping for and preparing foods; sometimes children, especially teenagers, are given too much freedom in their food choices. Marriages occur at an earlier age with pregnancy often presenting an additional stress on the young woman who has not fully matured.

The average American family of today has a higher income and is spending more of it for food. With this higher income, more meals are eaten in restaurants. The growth of the fast-food industry during the last decade has been phenomenal. These restaurants appeal not only to teenagers but to many families who can no longer afford to eat in traditional restaurants. More workers are eating in cafeterias at their place of work rather than carrying lunches, and more children are participating in school breakfast and lunch programs. The family eats fewer meals together, and in far too many families some meals may be skipped by one or more persons. Breakfast is an often neglected meal, although some families have found that this is the one time of the day when they can plan to be together.

The scientific and technologic advances reach into every aspect of daily life, including the quantity, quality, variety, and attractiveness of the foods we eat. Fewer foods are produced from scratch in the home. Frozen foods including complete meals, baked foods of all kinds, mixes, and snacks are commonplace amongst the 10,000 or so items in a supermarket. An increasing number of fabricated foods are replacing conventional foods. The number of brands and the variety are so great that the shopper finds it difficult indeed to make wise selections.

Social changes often have an adverse effect on nutrition: the large number of young as well as elderly persons living alone; the increasing proportion of older people; long periods of unemployment; the breakup of families by divorce or death with the attendant emotional turmoil and also the dual role that must be assumed in maintenance of the home and the supply of the income; and the high incidence of alcoholism and drug addiction.

The Changing American Diet Major changes have taken place in the American diet during the present century. One way to review these changes is to look at the nutrient values of the food supply available for consumption each year. The U.S. Department of Agriculture keeps such records annually. (See Figures 1–2, 1–3, and 1–4.)

Protein in the available food supply has ranged from 88 gm in 1935 to 103 gm in 1945–1946. It is now at 103 gm per capita.[5] In 1909 animal foods supplied about half of the total available protein; today they furnish about two thirds of the total protein. The increasing consumption of meat, espe-

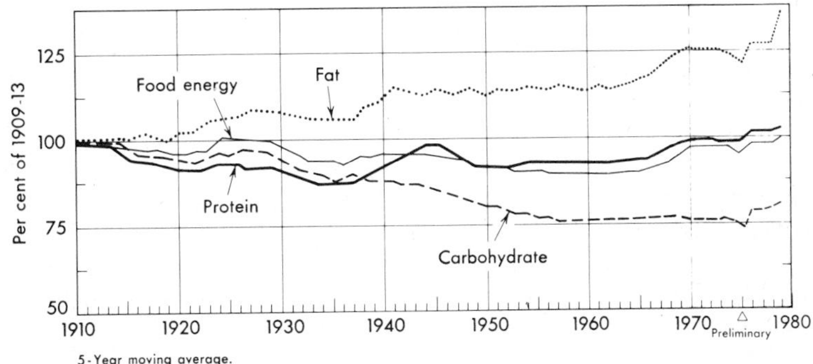

Figure 1–2. Since the beginning of the century there has been a decrease in the consumption of carbohydrate by about one fourth and an increase in fat consumption by about one fourth. (Courtesy, U.S. Department of Agriculture.)

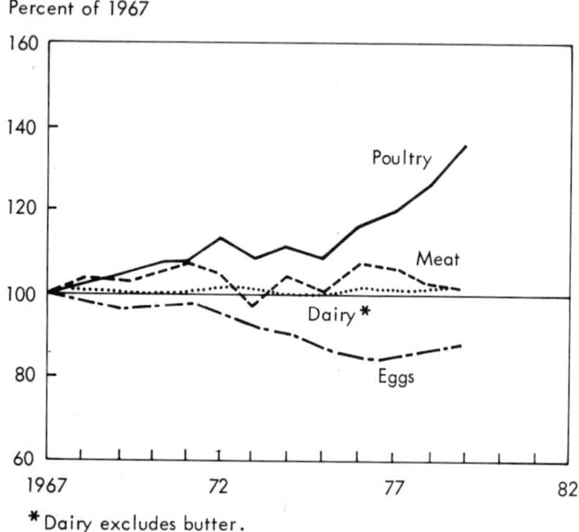

Figure 1–3. Per capita consumption of selected livestock products since 1967. Note the marked increase in poultry consumption and the decline in egg consumption. (U.S. Department of Agriculture.)

cially beef and poultry, together with a substantial decrease in the consumption of grain foods accounts for this shift in the proportion of animal to plant foods. With in-

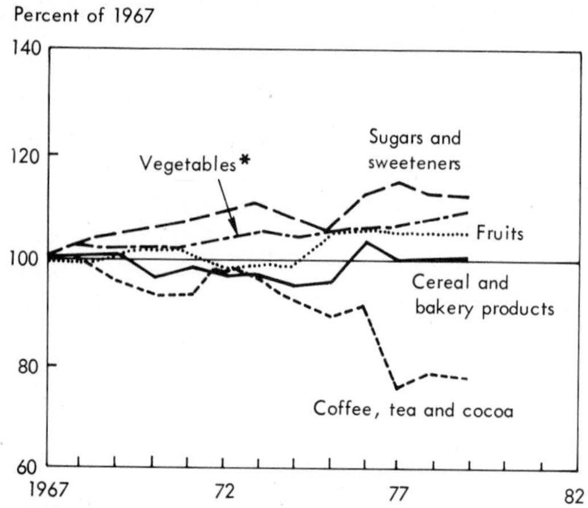

Figure 1–4. Per capita consumption of selected crop products. More fruits, vegetables, and sugars and sweeteners are consumed than in 1967. The increase in sugars and sweeteners has resulted from the greater use of corn sugars and syrups. (Courtesy, U.S. Department of Agriculture.)

creasing affluence Americans and people of other countries consume more animal protein foods and less plant protein foods.

In 1909 carbohydrate represented 56 per cent of the total available calories and now accounts for 46 per cent of the food energy. The consumption of grain foods is about half as high as it was in the beginning of the century, while the sugar available from all sources has increased by about one third—from 157 gm in 1909–1913 to 213 gm in 1979. Sugars now account for 53 per cent of the total available carbohydrate, or about 18 per cent of total available calories.

The amount of fat available in the national food supply has increased from 127 gm in 1909 to 168 gm at present. Fats and oils, including butter, supply about 640 kcal or 18 per cent of the total available calories. Margarine and butter supply some vitamin A, and most vegetable oils are good sources of linoleic acid. Except for these nutrient contributions, fats are poor contributors to the nutritive value of the diet. Thus, sugars and fats and oils together account for more than one third of the available calories in the food supply.

National Food Consumption Survey Since 1936 the U.S. Department of Agriculture has conducted surveys of food consumption at approximately 10-year intervals. The most recent nationwide survey was conducted in 1977–78. It included a survey of foods brought into the home and also the food intake by individuals in the various age-sex categories. Among the preliminary findings are these:[4,6–8]

1. Of the people questioned in this survey, 3 per cent of the entire population but 9 per cent of the lowest income group said they "sometimes or often did not have enough to eat." Translated in terms of the United States population this represents several million people.[4]

2. About 24 per cent of the food dollar was spent away from home, compared with 17 per cent in 1965. This increase is attributed to more women working away from home, higher income, and greater access

to fast-food restaurants. People with higher incomes ate more meals away from home than did those with the lowest income.[4]

3. Diets of people in the lowest income group had improved the most. There was less difference in adequacy of the diet between persons in the several income categories than in 1965. The food assistance programs probably were significant factors in this improvement.[4,7]

4. When compared with 1965, there was an increased intake of meat, poultry, and fish; fruits; soft drinks; and alcoholic beverages. The intake declined for milk, cream, and cheese; grain products; vegetables; eggs, legumes, and nuts; and sugar, syrup, jelly, and candy.[4]

5. Although the energy value of the available food supply is about 3,500 kcal, the caloric value of food actually brought into the household was 2,900 kcal, and the actual intake was 1,800–1,900 kcal. Hegsted[6] raises these questions: Where does all the extra food go? Is it wasted?

6. For all age categories, the average protein intake exceeded the recommended allowances (see Table 3–1). Although the average intake of all vegetables declined, the consumption of dark green vegetables increased, thus improving the vitamin A intake. The consumption of grain products had decreased, but more universal enrichment of all grain foods together with higher fortification levels resulted in improvement of the intake of B-complex vitamins. Ascorbic acid intake was 35 per cent higher than in 1965 owing to increased consumption of citrus fruits and fortified fruit drinks and ades.[7,8]

The calcium intake declined by 4 per cent. The average intake of females over 12 years was about 25 per cent below the recommended allowances. Iron intakes of women 12 to 50 years were 35 to 40 per cent below recommended allowances, and magnesium intakes of this group were about 30 per cent below allowances.[7,8]

7. According to Hegsted, the intakes of vitamin B-6, magnesium, iron, and zinc should be watched more closely. He also states that the survey indicates that the major problem is one of overconsumption—of calories, fat, cholesterol, sugars, salt, and alcohol.[6]

Nutritional Problems in the United States

Public Concerns about Nutrition In recent years the American public has shown increasing interest and concern about food supplies and nutritional needs. This has come about through dramatic, often exaggerated presentations of newscasts, documentaries, and advertising on radio and television and in the print media. Nutritional terms such as protein, saturated and polyunsaturated fats, cholesterol, minerals, and vitamins are familiar, although there are many misconceptions concerning them. This interest provides an excellent opportunity for nutrition education. It also places a responsibility on the professional person in nutrition to provide a sound informational basis for judging the safety of the food supply and for meeting community and world food needs.

What are some of these concerns? Young people especially look upon disruptions in the ecologic balance. Some believe that there is excessive use of pesticides that may harm plant and animal life, and of additives in food processing. They express this concern by selecting foods grown on soils fertilized by manures and without the use of pesticides or chemical fertilizers; they also avoid foods to which additives have been included in food processing. These concerns are exaggerated, as later discussions in the text will show. (See Chapter 16.)

In developing countries people consume an average of 400 pounds of grains per capita annually. In the United States, Canada, and western Europe about 1,500 to 2,000 pounds of grains are consumed per capita, but most of this is fed to animals that are in turn used for food. Most of the world's people consume diets that contain very little animal protein and manage to maintain health when the plant food supply is varied and abundant. Various forms of vegetarianism have been adopted by significant numbers of Americans in the belief that such diets are more healthful and that they represent a more efficient use of world resources since the food is eaten directly rather than consumed by animals first. Some forms of vegetarianism are nutritionally satisfactory; others are not. (See Chapter 15.)

As people approach middle age they are more likely to question whether there are health risks in the present American diet. They are constantly reminded through advertising that some products may reduce one's blood cholesterol and thus lower the risk of cardiovascular disease. More recently the inadequacy of fiber intake has been emphasized through the communications media.

Nutritional Deficiencies An analysis of recent surveys of nutritional status has identified the following deficiencies.[1-3, 9, 10]

1. Some people at all socioeconomic levels fail to obtain a nutritionally satisfactory diet. People at the lowest income level spend as much as 40 per cent of their income for food—yet they remain the most vulnerable. They often have limited access to food, as on Indian reservations, in Appalachia, or in ghetto sections of large cities. Lack of knowledge is a further contributing factor.

2. Although infant mortality has decreased tenfold since the beginning of the century, the present rate (14 per 1,000 births) is still 50 per cent higher than it is in Sweden. Two thirds of all babies who die have low birth weights. The rate is higher for infants born to young women in their teens who are also poor.

3. Anemia occurs frequently in all age categories and is especially prevalent in children under 6 years. The incidence is twice as high in persons below the poverty level.

4. Dental problems affect about nine of every ten persons. These include decayed teeth, missing teeth, and periodontal disease. One in five persons has severe periodontal disease, and one of every six persons over 10 years has trouble in biting or chewing.

5. Retarded growth and retarded bone development have been observed in some children 1 to 3 years of age. Vitamin D deficiency and protein-calorie malnutrition have occasionally been found.

6. Chronic illness is a fact of life for the elderly; about 80 per cent have some chronic condition. Low income, poor nutrition, and social isolation are contributing factors.

Problems of Nutrient Excesses Many Americans consume diets that are excessively high in calories, saturated fat, cholesterol, and sugars, and that are also excessively refined. All of these excesses are believed to increase the risk of chronic diseases. It must be remembered, however, that there are also other factors that relate to the incidence of chronic diseases.

1. Excessive caloric intake leads to obesity, which is highly prevalent in the American population, and which is associated with chronic diseases such as diabetes mellitus, gallbladder disease, gout, cardiovascular diseases, and others.

2. Excessive intake of fats and sugars that are practically devoid of minerals, vitamins, and proteins may result in suboptimal intakes of these essential nutrients. This imbalance may lead to some of the deficiencies described previously.

3. Excessive intakes of saturated fats and cholesterol are believed by many clinicians to be among the important risk factors in the incidence of cardiovascular and cerebrovascular diseases. (See Chapter 39.)

4. Excessive and frequent intake of sugars contributes to an increase in dental caries.

5. Excessive intake of salt has been associated with hypertension.

6. Excessive use of refined foods, on the

part one
Normal Nutrition

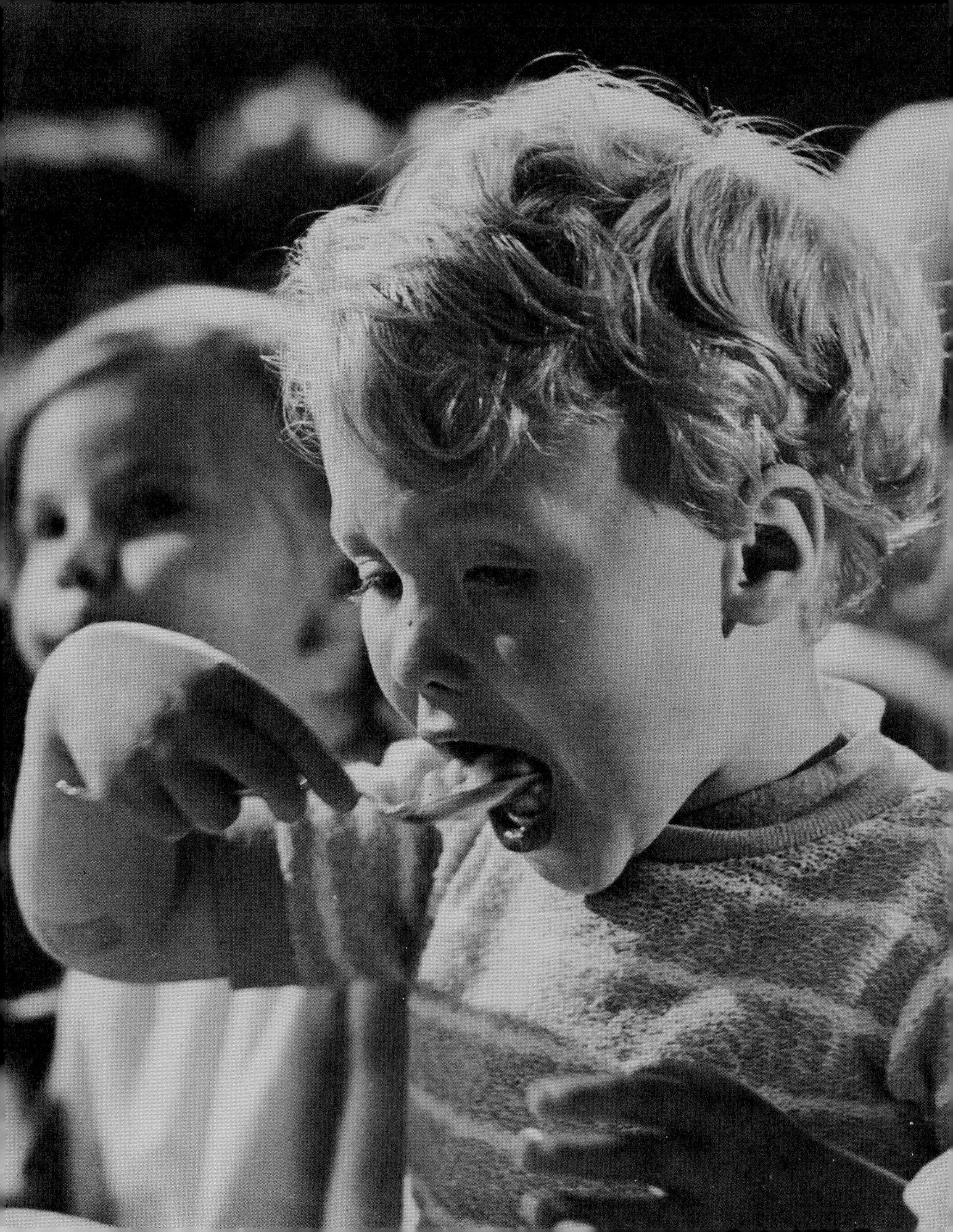

basis of epidemiologic studies, is believed to increase the incidence of gastrointestinal disorders such as diverticulosis, irritable colon, and possibly colon cancer. (See Chapter 32.)

7. Excessive intakes of vitamins A and D are known to be toxic. (See Chapter 10.)

Global Problems in Nutrition

Scope of Malnutrition According to Sol Linowitz, head of the Presidential Commission on World Hunger, "between 15 and 20 million people die each year from starvation and most of them are children under 5."[11] The relentless sequence of poverty, ignorance, malnutrition, disease, and early death are illustrated by the data in Table 1–1.

Although starvation is a problem of tremendous importance, the commission stated that lifelong malnutrition is the major problem in the poor nations. According to the World Bank, more than 1 billion persons are chronically undernourished. Three fourths of the world's undernourished population live on the Indian subcontinent, in Southeast Asia, and in Africa below the Sahara desert. The commission has predicted that in 20 years the global food crisis will be worse than the present energy crisis.[12]

The world population increases by about 200,000 persons each day, with most of the increase occurring in the developing nations. Although these nations have improved their food production, the per capita food supply has not improved. Some nations such as China have succeeded in slowing the rate of population growth, as have a number of Western countries. Other nations have initiated programs of birth control, but there are serious impediments to success: the need for children who will sustain their parents when they are old; the need for child labor in the fields; and religious beliefs.

The energy crisis experienced throughout the world directly affects the food supply. Energy is required for the production

Table 1-1. **The Development Gap, By Groups of Countries**

	Low-income Countries	Lower Middle-income Countries	Upper Middle-income Countries	High-income Countries
Mid-1976 population (millions)	1,341.3	1,145.4	470.6	1,057.0
Average per capita GNP (1974)	$152	$338	$1,091	$4,361
Average PQLI*	39	59	67	95
Average birth rate (per 1000)	40	30	36	17
Average death rate (per 1000)	17	11	10	9
Average life expectancy (years)	48	61	61	71
Average infant mortality rate (per 1,000 live births)	134	70	82	21
Average literacy rate†	33%	34%	65%	97%
Average per capita education expenditures	$3	$10	$28	$217
Average per capita military expenditures	$6	$17	$31	$232

*Each country's physical quality of life index (PQLI) is based on an average of life expectancy, infant mortality, and literacy rates in the mid-1970s.

†Represents proportion of adult population (15 years of age and over) able to read and write.

Note: All averages are weighted by the mid-1976 populations of the countries included in each group. This table defines the low-income countries as those with a per capita GNP under $300; the lower middle-income countries as those with a per capita GNP of $300–699; the upper middle-income countries as those with a per capita GNP of $700–1,999; and the high-income countries as those with a per capita GNP of $2,000 or more.

Source: "WORLD HUNGER and MALNUTRITION: IMPROVING THE U.S. RESPONSE." The White House, Spring 1978, p. 12.

of fertilizers, to run farm machinery, to transport foods, and to process foods. Short supplies of energy together with high costs of energy have affected the poor countries most severely.

The first need is for sufficient food to meet the caloric requirements of the population. Qualitatively, the next need is for sufficient protein to supply the amino acids that are used to build and maintain body structures.

Protein-calorie malnutrition is the single greatest world problem in nutrition. In its severe forms, kwashiorkor and marasmus, it affects millions of preschool children. In fact, in some countries, three children may be dead before one reaches school age. Those children who do survive are physically and mentally retarded—perhaps irreversibly so. (See Chapter 23.)

Anemia (especially in mothers and young children), blindness resulting from vitamin A deficiency, and riboflavin deficiency are especially frequent. Rickets, scurvy, pellagra, beriberi, and endemic goiter occur in severe forms in some parts of the world. The characteristics of these deficiencies will be described in the chapters related to the specific nutrients involved.

Responsibility for World Nutrition No thinking man or woman can afford to avoid the fact that so many of the world's people simply do not have enough to eat, nor can he or she, even in self-interest, evade the responsibility for alleviating hunger. In chronic starvation lie the frustration, tension, and envy of masses of people who will ultimately resort to violence.

World peace cannot be guaranteed by supplying adequate food alone, but one road to world peace is surely through a better-fed world population. Beyond this, charity and brotherhood are at the root of the Judeo-Christian religions and indeed of all ethical systems, and to practice them should be on the conscience of mankind.

A number of groups under the United Nations are directly concerned with global problems of nutrition, namely the Food and Agriculture Organization (FAO); World Health Organization (WHO); United Nations Children's Fund (UNICEF); United Nations Educational, Scientific and Cultural Organization (UNESCO). (See Chapter 23.)

The Presidential Commission on Hunger has pointed out that the United States, based on its gross national product (GNP), ranked thirteenth among donor nations to world food aid. It has recommended that the United States aid be tripled from 0.23 per cent of GNP, or about $4.85 billion, to 0.70 per cent of GNP, or about $16 billion.[12]

Achieving Nutritional Balance

Nutritional Balance From the preceding discussion it becomes evident that the concept of nutritional balance is important. A good diet must fulfill these criteria: (1) it must furnish the appropriate levels of all nutrients to meet the physiologic and biochemical needs of the body at all stages of the life cycle; and (2) it must avoid the excesses of calories, fat, sugar, salt, and alcohol that are associated with increased risk of diet-related diseases. Giving more attention to avoiding excesses does not mean that one gives less attention to dietary adequacy. The key words in achieving the two criteria are *moderation* and *prudence.* (See Figure 1–5.)

Nutrition and Disease Prevention Traditionally, health care has been concerned primarily with healing the sick and helping them to maintain health. Today prevention is described as a "unifying theme" among public health professionals, consumers, employers, workers, physicians, nurses, nutritionists, legislators, and policy makers.[9] Of ten health problems that have been given high priority for prevention research, five are related in some degree to nutrition: alcohol-related problems, cancers of medium and high prevalence, cardiovascular disease, dental disease, and infant mortality.[13]

The preventive measures described in

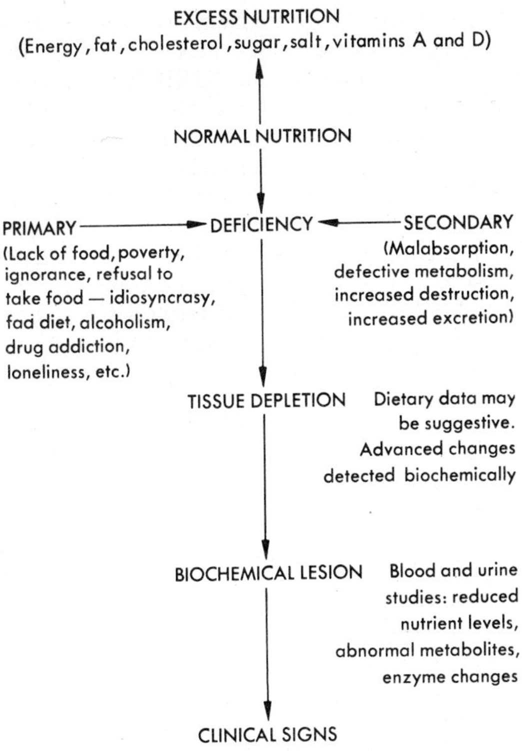

Figure 1–5. Normal nutrition implies a balance that avoids deficiency of intake, on one hand, and excessive intake, on the other hand.

this book are related to nutrition. However, it must be emphasized that the etiology of chronic disease is complex and that there are many other risk factors such as cigarette smoking, alcohol and drug abuse, stress, lack of exercise, heredity, poverty, age, sex, and occupation. One cannot change one's heredity, age, or sex, but one can control most of the environmental factors.

In assessing the value of preventive measures one must differentiate between that which has been proven and that for which final proof is not yet available. To illustrate, the following measures are of proven value: the adequate intake of specific vitamins to prevent scurvy, pellagra, beriberi, rickets, and other deficiency diseases; adequate prenatal diets to reduce infant mortality; iodinization of salt to prevent endemic goiter; fluoridation of water supplies to reduce dental decay; and many others.

There is much evidence to support some widely recommended measures, but final proof is not yet forthcoming. Thus, lowering the intake of saturated fat and cholesterol is associated with a lower serum cholesterol, but it has not been proven that premature heart attacks are less frequent. High salt intake is associated with hypertension, but it has not been proven that reducing the salt intake over the life span will reduce the occurrence of hypertension.

Since moderation of fat, cholesterol, and salt intake carries no health risks, and since a reduced intake of fats and sugars is likely to improve the nutrient quality of the diet, it seems prudent to adopt such measures even though final proof is not yet available. Indeed, it seems irresponsible to wait for final proofs or to wait for disease signs to appear before making any modifications in diet.

The case for prevention of breast and colon cancer by changes in diet is on much more tenuous grounds. Epidemiologic studies have shown an association between lack of dietary fiber and colon cancer and between a high fat intake and breast cancer. Much research will be required before these relationships can be proven. Although an increase in fiber intake and a reduction in fat intake is prudent, the health professional should be cautious about making firm claims when evidence is still lacking.

Nutrition Issues and Research Priorities At every level of government, food and nutrition are important issues. Legislation imposes controls on food production, marketing, distribution, safety, and assistance to the needy of this nation and to food-deficit countries. Nutritional guidelines have been developed by governmental and voluntary agencies. (See Chapter 3.) Many chapters in this book identify important issues that concern the consumer and the health professional.

Research workers throughout the world

are continually adding to nutrition knowledge. But there is urgent need to extend knowledge by basic and applied research. The U.S. Department of Agriculture has identified seven priorities for nutrition research:

1. What do people need nutritionally for optimum growth, functional performance, and continued well-being?
2. What are people actually eating, and how do their eating habits affect their nutritional health?
3. What factors shape people's eating habits?
4. What happens to our food from its origin on the farm to our tables and how does this affect the safety, quality, and nutritional value of our diets?
5. How do Government intervention and nutrition education programs affect people's health, nutritional status and performance?
6. What are the nutritional effects of Government policies and regulatory programs?
7. What special considerations must we take into account in helping to meet the dietary needs of people in other countries?*

Some Objectives in the Study of Nutrition

You bring to the study of nutrition your lifetime experience with food that may serve you well in further improving your nutritional status and the nutritional health of others. But it may also be that you have many incorrect ideas and such strong feelings about food that it will take much patience and perseverance on your part to change your attitudes and motivations. As you enter upon this study it is a good idea for you to examine carefully your present feelings about food, as well as your current knowledge of nutrition, so that you can build upon what is good in your dietary pattern and correct that which is undesirable.

* *Food and Nutrition for the 1980's: Moving Ahead.* U.S. Department of Agriculture, Washington, D.C., April 1979, p. 3.

Personal and Family Nutrition Regardless of one's future career plans, the study of nutrition should first be directed to oneself. Many young men and women today live alone and are solely responsible for their own nutritional well-being. Physical and mental health are essential assets to meet the exciting and sometimes arduous requirements of one's life work. Those who expect to help other people to achieve better health through nutrition must themselves be enthusiastic living examples of the benefits of the application of nutrition knowledge.

Nutrition education applied to the individual also reaches the family. This is especially important for young men and women as they establish their own families. In most families the wife and mother is still the principal decision maker concerning the family's food. She plans the menus, purchases the food, and prepares the meals. In some families men are assuming more responsibility for meal planning, food purchasing, and preparation. Thus, the prevailing attitudes and practices of both parents are significant in helping children to form good food habits.

Professional Opportunities in Nutrition Professional people in any discipline related to health are engaged in activities related to education, prevention, and therapy.

Nutrition education in schools. Education of the population holds promise of long-range benefits to the greatest numbers. Teachers, nurses, nutritionists, dietitians, home economists, and physicians assume varying responsibilities for individual and group education. The elementary and secondary schools afford the single best opportunity for helping the child to establish attitudes and practices concerning food selection that will lead to a more healthful, productive life. Nutrition education must begin in the kindergarten and continue through the twelfth grade if it is to achieve maximum effectiveness. It is the responsibility of the elementary teacher as well as teachers of home economics, health, and physical education.

The school nurse, physician, and dentist have many opportunities to note defects in health that suggest the need for improved nutrition; they can influence children in changing their food habits, provide experiences in the classroom, and lend their support to school food service and nutrition education programs.

The school breakfasts and lunches demonstrate that good nutrition and good food are, in fact, partners. School dietitians serve as teachers and also as consultants to teachers and also as consultants to teachers.

Nutrition programs for the public. Voluntary and governmental agencies together with industry are accepting responsibility for nutrition programs. The focus of nutrition programs is on maintaining *wellness* by avoiding excesses as well as protecting against deficiencies. The researcher in nutrition and food sciences is equally at home in the laboratories of a food company, a university, a hospital, or in the public health field. Nutritionists, dietitians, and home economists, depending upon their education and particular interests, are the experts who interpret a product for a company; develop new uses for a food; advise mothers and children concerning their diets in a clinic; serve as consultants to a public health team; supervise food service in a college dormitory, industrial cafeteria, or hospital; assist individuals and groups in dietary selection; and teach in nursing schools, colleges, and universities.

Nutrition and health care. The concern of today's health worker is for the maintenance as well as the restoration of health. Traditionally, health care has been directed to the patient—that is, the horizontal individual. Today, health care includes the concept of continuity of care. The health worker soon learns that there must be concern for the patient who makes the transition from the hospital to the home. To implement continuity of care with respect to nutritional needs, the patient may require counseling in the proper choice of foods in the market, assistance in planning for the best use of food money, and practical suggestions for food preparation with meager facilities or in the face of physical handicaps. Some of the assistance required by the patient may be provided by the nurse, but more often a team effort—nurse, dietitian, social worker—is needed. (See also Chapter 24.)

In the community the nurse is often the coordinator of services. The nurse encounters a legion of problems and needs related to nutrition; perhaps a mother needs to know how to prepare an infant formula; another person would like some help in budgeting her limited income so that she can feed her family adequately; another needs instruction in preparing food for an ill member of the family; and another needs counseling so that the diet conforms to religious beliefs. In some of these situations the nurse can use nutrition knowledge to assist the client. For more complex problems she or he may need to consult a nutritionist or refer the client to the nutritionist.

Some Guidelines for Nutrition Study
It is often said that one can judge a worker by the way in which he or she uses tools. This is also true of the use a student makes of the study tools available. First, one must become acquainted with a tool and gain some practice in using it before it becomes comfortable to use. With your text, for example, look through the table of contents to learn something of the topics that are covered and the sequence of their presentation. Then browse through the book to become aware of the kinds of study aids that are provided.

Terminology in any study is basic to understanding, and the time used in developing the ability to use nutrition terms with accuracy and ease is well spent. Terms with which you should be familiar are set in small capital letters and are defined at the point of their first use. Terms that are used frequently throughout the text have also been listed in the Glossary in the Appendix.

Many tables, diagrams, charts, and photographs emphasize and summarize important points made in the discussion. If you study these, you will find that they reinforce the reading of the text itself. The tables of food composition in the Appendix contain a gold mine of information. Perhaps half of all the questions people will pose to you are concerned with nutritive values, and in these tables you can find the answers. But to use them with confidence means that you must consult them often.

Review questions at the end of each chapter will help you to focus on the important points that have been made. The suggested problems are examples of situations that may be encountered in making applications of the principles of nutrition. You will soon learn to find answers to problems that come within your own daily experiences.

Any student of nutrition should be aware of the current issues before the public. You will find that your interest will be deeper if you try to relate your course of study to some of the reporting in newspapers and magazines, for example. Try to evaluate what you read in the popular publications with what you learn in your study.

Additional references have been included for each chapter to enable you to read more extensively on selected topics, to familiarize you with reliable publications in nutrition, to foster the habit of consulting the literature, and perhaps even to provide the starting point for a paper you may wish to develop. The references included are at a reading level comparable to this text.

In your reading you need to begin to become critical of the contents. Has there been scientific testing of the issue? Are the authors recognized practitioners in the field about which they are writing? Are there explanations for contradictory findings? Is there bias in the article in favor of a product, device, or belief? Has the information been gained through repeated research, or is it based on a single study?

Problems and Review

1. What is your understanding of the following terms: nutrition, malnutrition, foodstuff, nutrient, health, food, nutritional care, primary prevention?
2. Industrial and economic developments have been a powerful factor in the changing of our food habits. List several of these which have had an influence on our dietary habits within your lifetime.
3. Within your experience give an example of a situation in which the community has fostered better nutrition.
4. Select an article related to food from the daily newspaper or a popular magazine and discuss its merits.
5. In what ways is a knowledge of the following sciences helpful in the study of nutrition: bacteriology, chemistry, sociology, psychology, anthropology?
6. What is the difference between a dietary survey and a nutritional status study?
7. *Problem.* Start a list of resources for the study of nutrition and dietetics. Add to this list as you continue in your study. Include only those books and journals which you have examined. Include the names of official and voluntary agencies in your own community and at state, federal, and international levels as you become familiar with the work they do in the area of nutrition.
8. *Problem.* Compile a list of characteristics which describe a person who is in good nutritional status. How do you measure up with this?
9. *Problem.* Review the suggested objectives for study in this chapter. Then prepare a statement in your own words which best describes the goals you think are most important. Limit your statement to 300 words; be concise but specific.

Cited References

1. U.S. Department of Health, Education and Welfare: *Ten State Nutrition Survey, 1968–70.* Pub. No. (HSM) 72–813–8134, Government Printing Office, Washington, D.C., 1972.
2. Owen, G., et al.: "A Study of Nutritional Status of Preschool Children in the United States, 1968–70," *Pediatrics,* 53 (Suppl.): 597–646, 1974.
3. U.S. Department of Health, Education and Welfare: *Preliminary Findings of the First Health and Nutrition Examination Survey, 1971–72.* Pub. No. (HRA) 74–1219–1, Government Printing Office, Washington, D.C., 1973.
4. Hama, M. Y.: "Household Food Consumption, 1977 and 1965," *Family Econ. Rev.,* Winter 1980, pp. 4–9.
5. Marston, R. M., and Welsh, S. O.: "Nutrient Content of the National Food Supply," *National Food Rev.,* Winter 1981, pp. 19–22.
6. Hegsted, D. M.: "Nationwide Food Consumption Survey—Implications," *Family Econ. Rev.,* Winter 1980, pp. 20–22.
7. Cronin, F. J.: "Nutrient Levels and Food Used by Households, 1977 and 1965," *Family Econ. Rev.,* Winter 1980, pp. 10–15.
8. Pao, E. M.: "Nutrient Consumption Patterns of Individuals, 1977 and 1965," *Family Econ. Rev.,* Winter 1980, pp. 16–20.
9. U.S. Public Health Service: *Healthy People. The Surgeon General's Report on Health Promotion and Disease Prevention.* DHEW (PHS) Pub. No. 79–55071A, Government Printing Office, Washington, D.C., 1979.
10. Boehm, W. T. et al.: *Progress Toward Eliminating Hunger in America.* Ag. Econ. Rep. No. 446, U.S. Department of Agriculture, Washington, D.C., 1980.
11. Roberts, T.: "The Presidential Commission on World Hunger," *Nat. Food Rev.,* Winter 1979, p. 39.
12. "Global Food Crisis Predicted: More Aid from U.S. Urged," *The Bulletin* (Philadelphia), 11 December 1979.
13. Ruby, G.: "Increasing the Knowledge Base for Prevention," in *Healthy People,* U.S. Department of Health, Education and Welfare, Washington, D.C., 1979, pp. 459–70.

Additional References

American Medical Association: "Concepts of Nutrition and Health," *Nutr. News* (National Dairy Council), November/December 1979.

Comptroller General of the United States: *What Foods Should Americans Eat? Better Information Needed on Nutritional Quality of Foods.* U.S. General Accounting Office, CED-80–68, 30 April 1980.

Connor, W. E.: "Too Little or Too Much: The Case for Preventive Nutrition," *Am. J. Clin. Nutr.,* **32**:1975–78, 1979.

Dwyer, J. T., and Mayer, J.: "Beyond Economics and Nutrition: The Complex Basis of Nutrition Policy," *Science,* **188**:566–70, 1975.

Economics, Statistics, and Cooperative Service: *Agricultural-Food Policy Review.* U.S. Department of Agriculture, Washington, D.C., February 1980.

Hegsted, D. M.: "Food and Nutrition Policy: Probability and Practicality," *J. Am. Diet. Assoc.,* **74**:534–38, 1978.

McGinnis, J.: "Prevention—Today's Dietary Challenge," *J. Am. Diet. Assoc.,* **77**:129–32, 1980.

Meekhof, R. L., and Miller, T. A.: "Food and Agricultural Policy: The Legacy of the Past and the Needs of the Future," in *Agricultural-Food Policy Review,* U.S. Department of Agriculture, Washington, D.C., February 1980, pp. 73–85.

National Nutrition Consortium: "Official Statements of Guidelines for a National Nutrition Policy," *Nutr. Today,* 9:33–35, March/April 1974.

OLSON, R. E.: "Are Professionals Jumping the Gun in the Fight Against Chronic Disease," *J. Am. Diet. Assoc.,* **74**:543–50, 1979.

STAMLER, J.: "Lifestyles, Major Risk Factors, Proof and Public Policy," *Circulation,* **58**:3–19, 1978.

WINIKOFF, B.: "Nutrition, Population, and Health: Some Implications for Policy," *Science,* **200**:895–902, 1978.

2 Introduction to the Study of the Nutritive Processes

Digestion, Absorption, and Metabolism

NUTRITIONAL processes of the organism as a whole are the sum total of the physical and chemical activities that take place within the cell and the relationships that exist between the cells and the surrounding environment. Thus, cellular biology, physiology, and biochemistry are the sciences that describe these processes. The purpose of this chapter is to present an overview of some basic concepts from these sciences so that they can be integrated into the study of nutrition. The discussion in the chapters pertaining to each nutrient will provide further details.

Composition of the Body The predominating chemical elements in the body are oxygen, 65 per cent; carbon, 18 per cent; hydrogen, 10 per cent; and nitrogen, 3 per cent. Together they represent about 96 per cent of body weight and account for the principal body constituents, namely, water, proteins, fats, and a small amount of glycogen. The remaining 4 per cent of body weight is made up of mineral elements, of which calcium and phosphorus account for three fourths. (See page 132 for details of mineral composition.)

Water is present in all body tissues and accounts for 55 to 70 per cent of body weight. The water content varies inversely with the amount of fat in the body. Infant bodies have a low fat content and a high water content. Lean adults have a higher body water content than obese adults.

About three fourths of the body water is in the INTRACELLULAR compartment (fluid within the cells), and one fourth is in the EXTRACELLULAR compartment, which includes the blood circulation, the lymph, and the interstitial fluids that bathe all cells. Tissues vary considerably in their water content, with bones, teeth, and adipose tissue, for example, containing appreciably less water than muscle and nervous tissue.

Proteins account for about 18 per cent of body weight. The normal body fat content is 7 to 15 per cent for men and is 12 to 25 per cent for women.[1] Body fat content in excess of 20 per cent for men and 30 per cent for women is generally regarded as obesity. A gradual increase in body fat content occurs in both sexes with aging.

Only about 300 gm carbohydrate in the form of glycogen is present in the body, with very small additional amounts involved in the structure of various tissues. Many of the most important body constituents such as vitamins, hormones, and enzymes are present in such small amounts that they have no significant effect on total body weight.

Functions of Food "You are what you eat" is, in a sense, true inasmuch as the nutrients derived from food supply the *energy* for the activity of the body, the *structural materials* for every cell of the body, and the thousands of *regulatory substances* that are essential for all body processes.

Energy is supplied by carbohydrates, fats, and proteins. Minerals and vitamins are not sources of energy, but they are required in many steps of the release of energy.

Amino acids and mineral elements are constantly required for the growth and maintenance of body tissues. Carbohydrates and lipids enter into specialized tissues—often at very low but vital concentrations. All of the structural elements contain water.

Regulatory activities of the body require innumerable substances that are composed of water, amino acids, fatty acids, sugars, mineral elements, and vitamins.

The Nature of Metabolism

Metabolic Processes METABOLISM is a broad term that includes the series of processes pertaining to the release of nutrients from foods, transformations required for energy, and synthesis of structural and regulatory materials. These processes are anabolic or catabolic.

ANABOLISM refers to those processes by which new substances are synthesized from simpler compounds; for example, enzymes, hormones, and tissue proteins from amino acids, glycogen from glucose, and cholesterol from two-carbon units. CATABOLISM refers to the breakdown of complex substances to simpler compounds, for example, the oxidation of glucose to yield energy, carbon dioxide, and water, and the hydrolysis of fats to yield glycerol and fatty acids.

To study metabolism the pathway of a single nutrient may be traced. For example, one can trace the digestion, absorption, and intermediary metabolism of a given carbohydrate. This oversimplifies the complex manner by which the body utilizes nutrients since the metabolism of each nutrient never occurs in isolation but is always interlinked with a multitude of metabolic events. Each of these events is affected by other events that preceded it or occurred at the same moment.

In the broad usage of the term metabolism, the coordination of these processes is implied.

1. Ingestion: the intake of food.
2. Digestion, which breaks up foods into their constituent nutrients.
3. Absorption of nutrients from the gastrointestinal tract into the circulation.
4. Transportation of nutrients by the circulatory system to the sites for their use, and of wastes to the points of excretion.
5. Respiration, which supplies oxygen to the tissues for the oxidation of food, and which removes waste carbon dioxide. The circulatory system is again responsible for transportation of these gases.
6. Use of nutrients: oxidation to create heat and energy; incorporation into new cells and tissues.
7. Excretion of wastes: undigested food wastes and certain body wastes from the bowel; carbon dioxide by the lungs; nitrogenous, mineral salt, and other wastes from metabolism by the kidneys and by the skin.

Numerous physical and chemical methods have been developed for measuring the metabolic changes that occur with variations in nutrition. Analyses of blood, of urine, and, somewhat less frequently, of feces for various constituents are utilized in nutrition research. Part of the study of nutrition is concerned with a knowledge of such changes and an interpretation of their significance in assessing the quality of nutrition.

Enzymes All living tissues, plant and animal, produce thousands of enzymes without which the myriad chemical reactions could not take place. ENZYMES are organic catalysts of a protein nature which remarkably increase the rate of reactions without becoming a part of the reaction products. When protein is denatured (as by heating), the enzyme activity is lost. A small amount of enzyme will accomplish a chemical change on a great deal of substance, sometimes as much as 4,000,000 times its own weight. Enzymes, like all organic materials, are gradually used up, and therefore they must be continuously synthesized by the living cell.

Some enzymes are simple proteins, whereas others consist of a protein and another grouping which is loosely or firmly bound to the protein molecule. In an enzyme system the protein molecule is called the APOENZYME; its attached grouping is called the PROSTHETIC GROUP. For many enzyme systems the prosthetic group is comprised of COENZYMES, which are organic compounds, including several of the vitamins. The same coenzyme, it should be noted, may be used in different enzyme systems; it is the protein molecule that gives an enzyme its particular specificity. Some enzymes may require the presence of a COFACTOR (e.g., a mineral element) for their proper functioning.

Some enzymes are produced in an inactive form known as PROENZYME or ZYMOGEN and require some other substance to activate them. For example:

$$\text{Trypsinogen (proenzyme or zymogen)} \xrightarrow[\text{(activator)}]{\text{enterokinase}} \text{Trypsin (active enzyme)}$$

$$\text{Protein + water (substrate)} \xrightarrow{\text{trypsin}} \text{Proteoses, peptones, polypeptides}$$

Most enzymes participate in only one chemical reaction on a single substance, although some act on a class of compounds. They are named for the substances upon which they act, for example, *proteases* for proteins, *lipases* for fats, and so on. Thus, a single cell contains hundreds to thousands of enzymes that are responsible for as many different actions. An enzyme, such as *lactase,* will split only the sugar lactose; it has no action on the sugar sucrose, or on any other sugar, protein, or fat.

Enzymes are classified broadly by the functions they perform. Among the many important functions are hydrolysis, oxidation, dehydrogenation, and transfer of chemical groupings—thus, hydrolases, oxidases, dehydrogenases, and transferases.

Each enzyme has optimum activity at a specific pH. Pepsin, which digests proteins in the stomach, is one of the few enzymes active in the very acid reaction of the stomach, whereas the enzymes found in the small intestine are active at a slightly alkaline pH.

Enzyme activity depends on the amount of exposed surface. For example, much more activity by oxidases occurs if a potato is cut up into small pieces than if it is left whole. Likewise, in digestion, enzyme activity is great because the muscular movements of the tract have reduced the food mass to minute particles with thousands of exposed surfaces.

Enzymes are inactivated but not destroyed at freezing temperatures. When a frozen food or other substance is thawed, the enzyme activity proceeds normally. On the other hand, enzymes are destroyed at temperatures that coagulate proteins.

Homeostasis Cellular materials are constantly being broken down and equally rapidly synthesized. The rate of cellular turnover is exceedingly high, especially in the most active organs such as the intestinal wall. In spite of the remarkable rate of turnover, the body tends to maintain a state of equilibrium, often referred to as DYNAMIC EQUILIBRIUM or HOMEOSTASIS; that is, the removal of cells is accompanied by an equal replacement. Likewise, there are checks and balances for the biochemical reactions that take place at each level. The maintenance of equilibrium is governed by an adequate supply of nutrients, a balance between the nutrients, a normal complement of enzyme systems, the secretion of hormones that regulate metabolic rates, and controls by the nervous system.

Cells as Functioning Units

The simplest living organism consists of a single cell such as a bacterium or yeast cell that is capable of respiration, ingestion, digestion, absorption, circulation, synthesis of new materials, breakdown of materials for energy, response to the environment, excretion, and reproduction. Survival of the cell is dependent upon a favorable external environment. The cells of complex organisms such as those in the human being carry out these multiple activities but cannot exist independently; they function through intricate coordination with other cells. Cells are so tiny that they can be seen only with a light microscope. Many structures within cells have been identified by means of the electron microscope that permits magnification of 100,000 times or more. Cells are of infinite variety in size, shape, and specialized functions. They also possess some structures and functions in common so that it is possible to diagram and describe a so-called typical cell. (See Figure 2–1.)

The CELL MEMBRANE surrounds the protoplasm, maintains the constancy of the internal environment, and establishes dynamic equilibrium with the external environment by its highly selective ability to regulate the kinds and amounts of materials that enter and leave the cell.

The NUCLEUS of the cell is the storehouse for deoxyribonucleic acid (DNA), the genetic plan for the construction of proteins that enable new cells to have the characteristics of the parent cell.

The CYTOPLASMIC MATRIX is the continuous phase extending from the cell membrane throughout the cell and surrounding the ORGANELLES, or living structures, as well as certain lifeless materials known as INCLUSIONS. The organelles include the mitochondria, lysosomes, and endoplasmic reticulum.

MITOCHONDRIA are rod-shaped or round structures that vary in size and shape depending upon their activity. Within the mi-

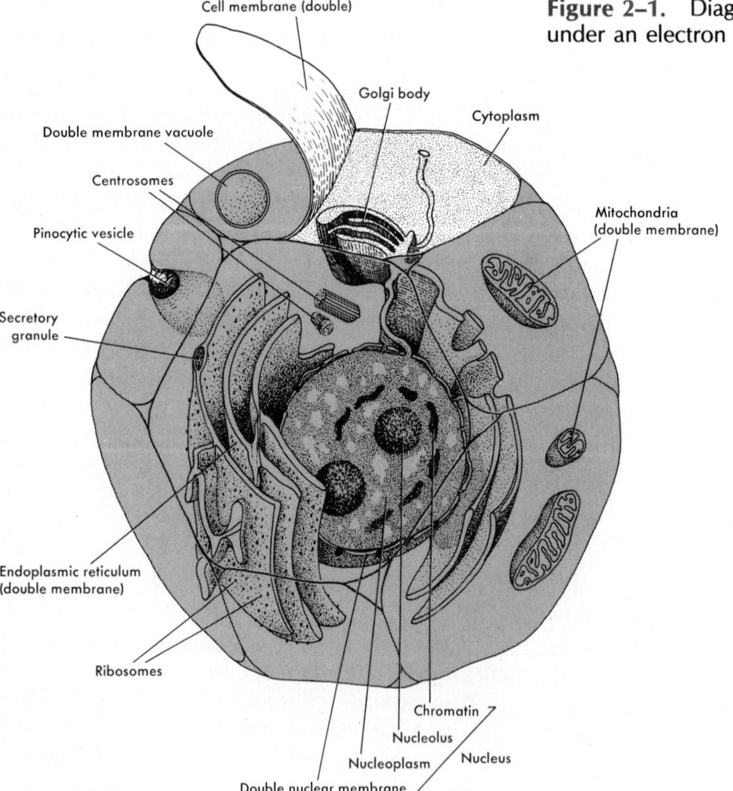

Figure 2–1. Diagram of a cell as it would appear under an electron microscope.

tochondria are hundreds to thousands of oxidative enzymes that are responsible for carrying on the reactions that yield the high-energy compound adenosine triphosphate (ATP). ATP supplies the energy needed by the cell to carry on its activities.

LYSOSOMES are membranes, or bags, that contain digestive enzymes. When the membrane bursts, the cell itself is digested, this being normal as worn-out cells are replaced by new. Lysosomes also release amino acids from proteins and are able to engulf bacteria and other substances. The phagocytic activity is a special property of the white blood cells.

The ENDOPLASMIC RETICULUM is the system of channels that allows flow of materials to and from the various parts of the cell as well as to the extracellular environment. The endoplasmic reticulum is associated with several special structures that vary considerably according to the type of cell. RIBOSOMES are the site of protein synthesis according to the genetic information supplied by the nucleus. They are abundant in cells where protein synthesis is great, but are lacking in some cells, such as red blood cells, where protein synthesis does not take place. The GOLGI COMPLEX appears as flattened bags and is well developed in secretory cells. It stores and concentrates enzymes and secretes them on demand.

Digestion

Purposes Only a few substances contained in foods are suitable for use by the body without change, namely, water, simple sugars, and some mineral salts and vitamins. DIGESTION includes the mechanical and chemical processes whereby complex food materials are hydrolyzed to forms that are suitable in size and composition for absorption into the mucosal wall and for utilization by the body. The nutrients that are absorbed include amino acids, fatty acids, glycerol, simple sugars, minerals, and vitamins.

In addition to its hydrolytic activities the gastrointestinal tract controls the amounts of certain substances that will be absorbed, for example, calcium and iron; prevents the absorption of unwanted molecules; synthesizes enzymes and hormones that are required for the digestive process; eliminates the wastes remaining from the digestion of food as well as certain endogenous wastes; and renews its own structure every 24 to 48 hours.

The Digestive Organs The gastrointestinal tract is a tube about 7.5 to 9 meters (25 to 30 feet) long in the adult and includes the mouth, esophagus, stomach, small intestine (duodenum, jejunum, and ileum), and large intestine (cecum, colon, rectum, and anal canal). The liver and pancreas, although situated apart from the tract itself, are important for the secretions that they contribute to the digestive process. (See Figure 2–2.)

The wall consists of the following layers:[2]

1. The mucosal lining has a layer of surface epithelium and glands which lie in loose connective tissue known as the LAMINA PROPRIA. It is richly supplied with blood and lymph vessels. A thin layer of muscle facilitates the constant increase and decrease of the mucosal folds. The mucosal layer secretes hormones and enzymes, brings about absorption, and is the first line of defense against infection.
2. The submucosa is a dense layer of connective tissue with blood and lymph vessels.
3. The muscular layer includes muscle fibers arranged in circular and longitudinal bands and also supplied with blood and lymph vessels. This layer regulates the size of the intestinal lumen and the movements of the intestinal wall.
4. The serosa is the outer covering of the wall, which is supplied with blood and lymph vessels and nerve branches.

Muscular controls are in effect at several

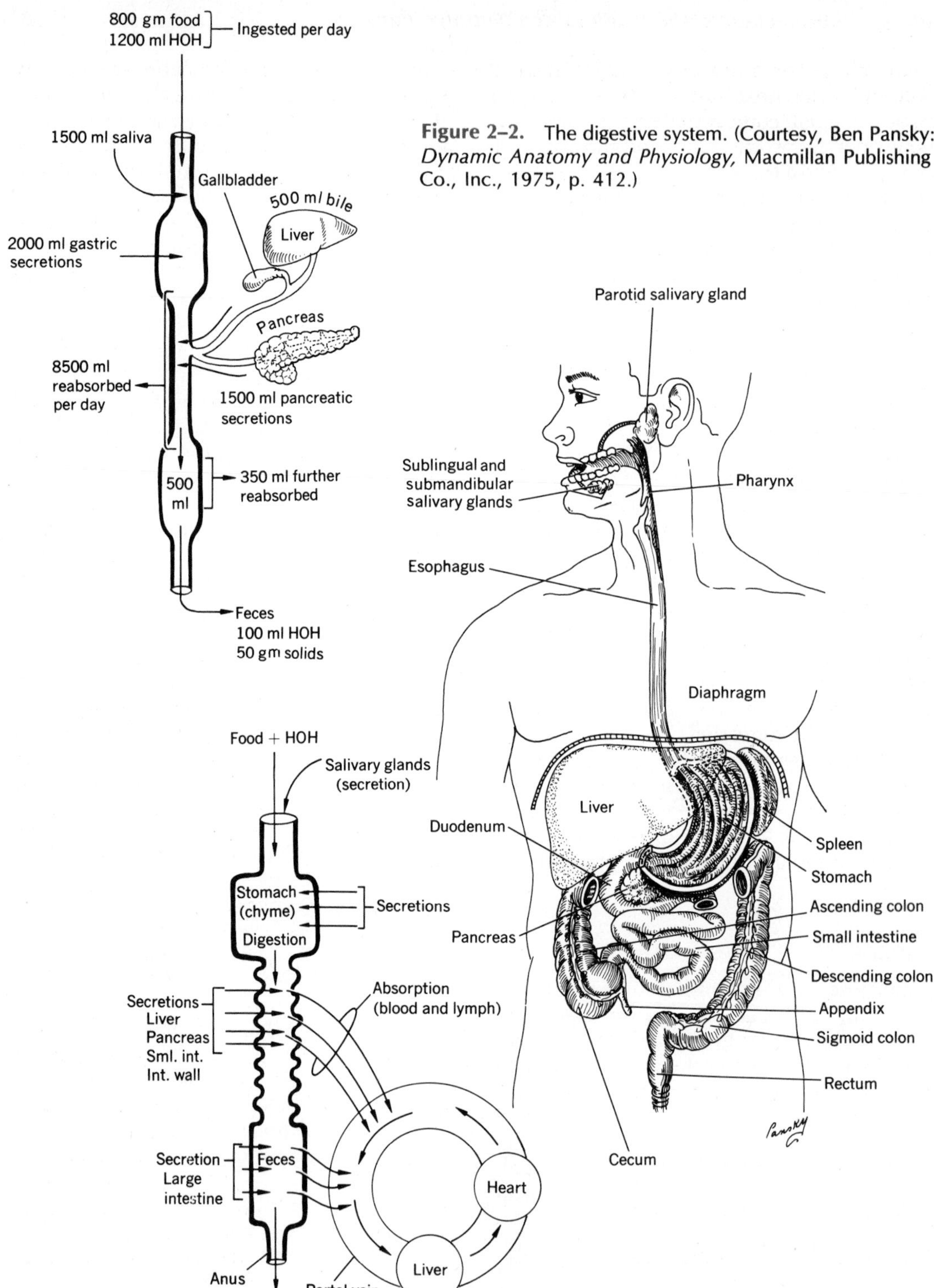

Figure 2–2. The digestive system. (Courtesy, Ben Pansky: *Dynamic Anatomy and Physiology,* Macmillan Publishing Co., Inc., 1975, p. 412.)

points along the tract to permit the influx of food to the next site for digestion and, under normal conditions, to prevent the backward flow of food (regurgitation). These are the cardiac opening from the esophagus to the stomach; the pyloric sphincter at the gastric-duodenal juncture; and the ileocecal valve, which regulates the passage of material from the ileum into the large intestine.

Controls for Activity of the Digestive Tract The secretion of digestive juices and the motor activity of the tract, and hence the speed and completeness of digestion, are regulated by nervous, chemical, and physical factors.

Everyone is familiar with the fact that the thought, sight, or smell of foods creates the desire for food and increases the flow of saliva and gastric juices. On the other hand, an unpleasant environment or worry and fear are likely to depress the secretion of digestive juices and thus delay digestion. Strong emotions such as anger often increase gastric secretion, but sometimes depress it.

Of the many digestive processes, the only activities under voluntary control are mastication and defecation. The central nervous system and local nerve circuits exercise control over the secretory and motor activity throughout the entire tract. One example of the feedback mechanism pertains to the regulation of stomach acid. The pressure of food against the mucosal walls of the stomach or specific substances such as alcohol or caffeine stimulates the release of the hormone gastrin, which in turn stimulates the flow of acid. Once there is a sufficient amount of acid in the stomach, the secretion of gastrin is turned off and no more acid is produced.

Hormones are the chemical messengers produced at a given site as a result of specific stimulation. Table 2–1 summarizes the hormones that affect secretory and motor activity.

Mechanical Digestion Rhythmic coordinated muscle activity causes foods to be reduced to minute particles and intimately mixed with digestive juices so as to facilitate movement throughout the tract and to provide for maximum exposure to the hydrolyzing enzymes and contact with the absorbing surfaces of the mucosal wall.

By mastication solid foods are cut, ground, mixed with saliva, and prepared for swallowing. Within seconds rhythmic contractions of the muscles of the esophagus force the food particles into the fundus of the stomach, which serves as a reservoir. Each addition of food expands the stomach walls just enough to hold the contents and pushes the mass preceding it forward to-

Table 2-1. **Hormones That Regulate Secretory and Motor Activity of the Digestive Tract**

Hormone	Where Produced	Stimulus to Secretion	Action
Gastrin	Pyloric and duodenal mucosa	Food in the stomach, especially proteins, caffeine, spices, alcohol	Stimulates flow of gastric juice; increases gastric motility
Enterogastrone	Duodenum	Acid chyme, fats	Inhibits secretion of gastric juice; reduced motility
Cholecystokinin	Duodenum	Fat in duodenum	Contraction of gallbladder and flow of bile to duodenum
Secretin	Duodenum	Acid chyme; polypeptides	Secretion of thin, alkaline, enzyme-poor pancreatic juice
Pancreozymin	Duodenum; jejunum	Acid chyme; polypeptides	Secretion of thick, enzyme-rich pancreatic juice
Enterocrinin	Upper small intestine	Chyme	Secretion by glands of intestinal mucosa

ward the central part of the organ. Because there is little motor or secretory activity in the fundus, food may remain there for an hour or more, thus allowing salivary digestion of carbohydrates to continue for a while. Small, regular contractions in the middle region of the stomach gradually increase in rate and intensity. The food is mixed with gastric juice, broken up further, and finally reduced to a thin, souplike consistency called CHYME.

The principal digestive activity is in the small intestine. Because the stomach has considerable storage capacity and because of the controls exerted by the pyloric valve, only small amounts of chyme enter the duodenum at a given time. The rhythmic movements of the intestine are known as PERISTALSIS. In the small intestine the circular muscle fibers have a constricting and squeezing action so that the chyme is constantly mixed with the digestive enzymes and given maximum exposure to the absorbing surfaces. This motion of the circular muscles is referred to as segmentation. As the longitudinal muscle fibers contract, a wavelike motion is produced that gradually moves the food mass forward. The muscular activity of the tract also serves as a stimulus to the secretion of the digestive juices and increases the blood supply to the digestive organs.

Motility through the tract. The rate at which foods move through the digestive tract depends upon the consistency, composition, and amount of food eaten. Liquids begin to leave the stomach from 15 minutes to ½ hour after ingestion, a fact that explains why liquid diets do not have great satiety value. Carbohydrates, when eaten alone, leave the stomach more rapidly than do proteins. Fats check the secretion of gastric juices and retard peristaltic activity so that their presence in the diet delays the emptying of the stomach. Normally, the stomach empties in 2 to 6 hours.

The unabsorbed food residue from the small intestine begins to pass through the ileocecal valve into the large intestine in from 2 to 5½ hours, but 9 hours or more from the time of eating may be required for the last of a large meal to pass this point. The length of time required to eliminate food residues as feces varies widely; a range of 20 to 36 hours after the consumption of the meal is typical.

Chemical Digestion A complex mixture of substances is presented to the various sites of the tract for hydrolysis. Depending upon the location, these include food materials in various stages of hydrolysis, secretions of digestive fluids containing enzymes and hormones, cellular materials from the desquamating mucosa, bile, bacteria, and various products of metabolism within the body that have entered the tract.

About 8 to 9 liters of digestive juices are produced daily by the secretory cells of the digestive tract and by the pancreas and liver. These juices are 98 to 99 per cent water and contain varying proportions of inorganic and organic compounds. One of the organic compounds of importance is MUCIN, a glycoprotein that lends the slippery quality to mucus and thus facilitates the smooth movement of food throughout the tract. Mucus also furnishes a protective coating to the gastric and duodenal mucosa against the corrosive action of hydrochloric acid. Except for bile, the digestive juices contain enzymes that are appropriate for a particular stage of hydrolysis. The final stages of hydrolysis for some nutrients, for example, the disaccharides, occurs within the mucosal cell itself and not in the lumen. Table 2–2 presents a summary of the digestive juices, their components, and the results of enzyme activity. See Chapters 4 to 6 for details of digestion of proteins, fats, and carbohydrates.

Functions of the Large Intestine By the time chyme reaches the large intestine practically all of the nutrients and water have been absorbed and the volume has been reduced to about 500 ml. The cecum fills slowly, and the peristaltic waves forcing the residues forward together with antiperistaltic waves forcing them back enable additional amounts of water to be absorbed. The large intestine secretes alkaline juices with a large amount of mucus but no hydrolytic enzymes so that there is practically no hydrolysis or absorption of nutrients at this point. The activity of the large intestine is greatest after meals and after exercise.

The daily excretion of feces is about 100 to 200 gm. The fecal material consists of small amounts of food residues, especially indigestible fiber, billions of bacteria, yeasts, and fungi, wastes from desquamated cells, bile pigments, cholesterol, and unabsorbed minerals such as calcium and iron.

The predominant bacteria in the large intestine are *Escherichia coli*. Bacteria that are fermentative are favored by a high carbohydrate intake, and those that are putrefactive by a high protein intake. Bacterial action in the large intestine releases (1) gases including ammonia, methane, carbon dioxide, and hydrogen, (2) lactic and acetic acids, and (3) certain substances such as indole and phenol that may have toxic properties.

Physicians and clinicians are reemphasizing the importance of ample amounts of fiber in the diet in order to reduce the time fecal residues remain in the large intestine.[3] The reasons for this emphasis are (1) diverticula, present in large proportions of the population by middle age, are less likely to form if the transit time through the colon is shortened, and (2) a more rapid elimination reduces the length of time a potentially toxic substance has contact with the mucosa. (See also pages 88 to 91.)

Absorption

The Nature of Absorption The process whereby nutrients are moved from the intestinal lumen into the blood or lymph circulation is known as ABSORPTION and results in a net gain of nutrients to the body. It is an *active process* in that substances are moved into the body against forces that would normally cause a flow in the opposite direction. It is also a *selective process* by which some materials, such as glucose, are transported in their entirety across the cell; others, for example, calcium and iron, are absorbed only according to body need; and still others, such as intact proteins, are held back.

Absorption requires that the nutrient penetrate the cell wall, cross the cell, exit from the cell into the lamina propria, and cross the epithelium of the blood or lymph vessels. In some instances absorption includes a metabolic change within the cell before it is transferred to the circulation. The absorption of specific nutrients will be discussed in Chapters 4 to 12.

Sites and Rates of Absorption Absorption appears to take place primarily from the duodenum and jejunum.[4] A notable exception is vitamin B-12, which has a specific absorption site in the lower ileum. Bile is reabsorbed from the distal part of the intestine. Most, if not all, substances that are proximally absorbed can also be absorbed by the ileum; thus, those substances that escaped absorption proximally are absorbed distally.

Normally, 98 per cent of the carbohydrate, 95 per cent of the fat, and 92 per cent of the protein in the diet is hydrolyzed and the end products are absorbed. These percentages are sometimes referred to as COEFFICIENTS OF DIGESTIBILITY.

Malabsorption can occur under a variety of circumstances: a reduction in the number of functioning villi; an increase in motility so that the time of exposure to absorptive surfaces is inadequate; a lack of specific enzymes or of bile; an interference by insoluble compounds or of an excess of one nutrient over another; and removal of part of the intestine by surgery.

The Absorptive Surface The small intestine provides an absorbing surface that is probably 600 times as great as its external surface area.[5] This is possible because of the arrangement of the mucosal wall in numerous folds, the 4 to 5 million villi that constitute the mucosal lining, and the 500 to 600

Table 2-2. **Digestive Juices and Their Actions**

Site of Secretion	Stimuli to Secretion	Daily Volume and pH	Important Constituents	Action
Mouth: saliva Salivary glands Submaxillary Sublingual Parotid	Psychic: thought, sight, smell, taste Mechanical: Presence of food in mouth Chemical: contact of sugar, salt, spices, etc., on taste buds	1,000–1,500 ml pH 5.9–6.8	Mucin *Amylase** (ptyalin)	Lubrication Cooked starch → dextrins, maltose Enzyme activity in the mouth is not extensive
Stomach: gastric juice Parietal cells	Psychic: as above Mechanical: contact with mucosa; distension Hormonal: gastrin increases flow; enterogastrone inhibits	1,500–2,500 ml pH 2.0–2.5	HCl	Pepsinogen → pepsin Bactericidal Reduces ferric iron to ferrous iron
Chief cells			*Pepsinogen* *Pepsin*	Inactive form of pepsin Proteins → proteoses, peptones, polypeptides
Columnar epithelium			Mucin	Lubrication; protects gastric and duodenal lining
			?*Lipase*	Emulsified fats → fatty acids + glycerol (action is negligible)
			?*Rennin* (infants only)	Casein → paracasein
			Intrinsic factor	Enables absorption of vitamin B-12
Liver: bile	Cholecystokinin contracts gallbladder and releases bile to duodenum	500–1,100 ml pH 6.9–8.6	Bile salts Bile acids Bile pigments Cholesterol Mucin	Neutralizes acid chyme Emulsifies fats for action of lipase Facilitates absorption of fats and fat-soluble vitamins Path of cholesterol excretion

Pancreas: pancreatic juice	Secretin	600–800 ml pH 7–8	Thin, watery, alkaline, enzyme-poor juice	Neutralizes acid chyme
	Pancreozymin		*Amylase*	Starch → dextrins, maltose
			Chymotrypsinogen	Inactive form of enzyme
			Chymotrypsin	Proteins → proteoses, peptones, polypeptides
			Trypsinogen	Inactive enzyme
			Trypsin	Proteins → proteoses, peptones, polypeptides
			Lipase	Fats → monoglycerides, fatty acids, glycerol
			Carboxypeptidase	Splits off amino acid with free COOH group
Small intestine: Intestinal juice (succus entericus)	Enterocrinin Presence of food in small intestine	2,000–3,000 ml pH 7–8	*Enterokinase*	Trypsinogen → trypsin
			Aminopeptidase	Splits off amino acid having free amino group
			Dipeptidase	Dipeptides → amino acids
			Nucleinase	Nucleic acid → nucleotides
			Nucleotidase	Nucleotides → nucleosides + phosphoric acid
			Nucleosidase	Nucleosides → purine or pyrimidine base + pentose
			Lecithinase	Lecithin → diglycerides + choline phosphate
Within mucosal cells			*Sucrase* (invertase)	Sucrose → glucose + fructose
			Maltase	Maltose → glucose + glucose
			Lactase	Lactose → glucose + galactose

*Constituents in italics are enzymes.

MICROVILLI that form the "brush border" of each epithelial cell of the villus.

VILLI are visible by a light microscope. They are tiny fingerlike projections of the mucosa and consist of a single layer of epithelial cells resting on the lamina propria, which is a bed of supporting connective tissue supplied by arterial and venous blood vessels and lacteals or lymph channels. (See Figure 2–3.)

At the base of each villus is the *crypt of Lieberkühn.* This is where the epithelial cells are formed. As new cells are formed they migrate up the sides of the villus. When they reach the tip of the villus, about one to three days later, they are extruded into the intestinal lumen and are constantly replaced by newly functioning cells.

Microvilli can be seen only by means of an electron microscope. They elaborate some of the hydrolytic enzymes, and the final stages for hydrolysis of some substances such as disaccharides are completed here and not in the lumen of the intestine.

Mechanisms for Absorption Four mechanisms have been postulated to explain absorption, although it must be emphasized that the pores, carriers, and pumps that are hypothesized have not been seen.[5]

1. SIMPLE DIFFUSION THROUGH PORES OR CHANNELS. Substances of very low molecular weight (probably 100 or lower), such as water and some electrolytes, appear to move freely across the membrane from the side of higher concentration to the side of lower concentration. This mechanism would operate in the direction of the circulation after meals when the concentration of

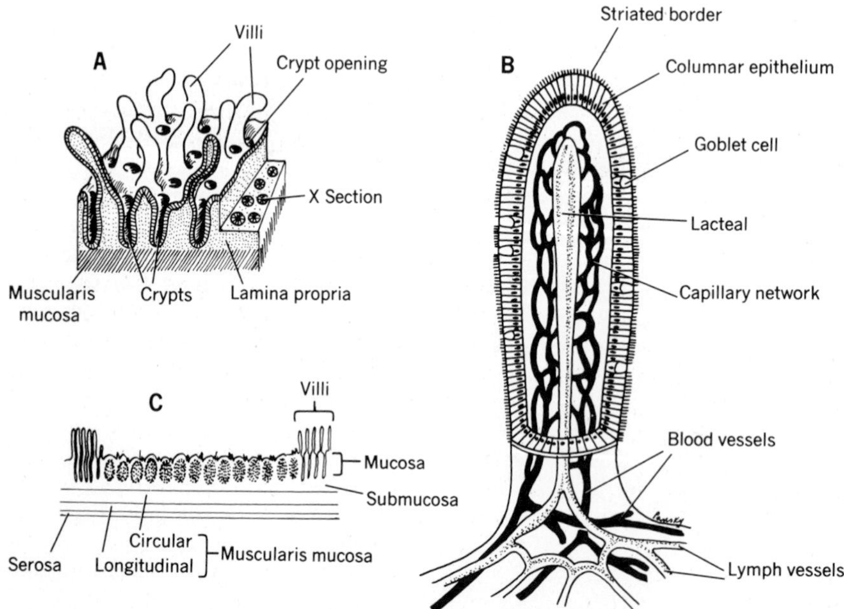

Figure 2–3. Intestinal villus. *(A)* Lining of the small intestine; villi with cores of the lamina propria that extend into the lumen. Note that crypts (of Lieberkuhn) are glands that dip down into the lamina propria. *(B)* An enlarged view of a typical villus. (Courtesy, Ben Pansky: *Dynamic Anatomy and Physiology,* Macmillan Publishing Co., Inc., 1975, p. 427.)

these small molecules in the intestinal lumen is higher than that in the blood and lymph. Being a two-way channel, this mechanism is effective in maintaining osmotic equilibrium. The molecular size of most nutrients is too great for diffusion by pores.

2. CARRIER-FACILITATED PASSIVE DIFFUSION. Water-soluble nutrients cannot penetrate the lipid-rich membrane of the cell. Therefore, they are attached to "carriers" or "ferries" that facilitate crossing the cell membrane. This is known as *facilitated diffusion.* In passive diffusion the nutrients move downhill, that is, from an area of higher concentration to one of lower concentration; no energy is required for this mechanism. When the concentration of nutrients in the circulation is equal to or exceeds that in the lumen, nutrients can no longer passively diffuse. They remain in the intestinal tract until excreted in the feces, which represents a large wastage of essential nutrients.
3. ACTIVE TRANSPORT. The absorption of most nutrients is accounted for by active transport. As in passive diffusion, carriers are necessary for the penetration of the cell membrane. Active transport involves the uphill pumping of nutrients from the lumen into the circulation; that is, the nutrient is moved from a site of lower concentration to one of higher concentration. Energy is required for active transport and is supplied by ATP from the metabolism of glucose within the cell. Sodium plays an essential role in the active transport of water, sugars, and amino acids. The metabolic energy required for the operation of the sodium pump also serves for the transport of these other nutrients, and is thus an energy-saving device.
4. PINOCYTOSIS. In some instances the cell appears to "drink up" or surround a substance and to extrude it into the interior of the cell. Some fats appear to be absorbed by this process. Occasionally, intact proteins may be absorbed in this fashion, which helps to explain the incidence of allergy.

Intermediary Metabolism

INTERMEDIARY METABOLISM refers to the physical and chemical changes that take place in the internal environment. As pointed out earlier, these changes are the sum of the activities occurring within each and every cell. The nutrients diffuse from arterial capillary blood into the interstitial fluids surrounding the cells and thence are absorbed by processes such as those described in the preceding section. Likewise, the cells dispose of waste materials to the interstitial fluid and in turn to the venous circulation.

The enzyme systems of a given cell determine the specific functioning of that cell. A compound—for example, glucose—that is to be utilized by the cell is attacked by one enzyme after another in assembly-line fashion until the desired end product has been achieved. If a single enzyme in the cell is missing, there is a breakdown in the assembly line and all sorts of problems arise. During the last 30 years a better understanding of enzyme activities has led to the identification, and in some cases effective treatment, of the so-called inborn errors of metabolism seen in far too many infants. The condition *galactosemia* results from the lack of a specific enzyme needed for using galactose; *phenylketonuria,* likewise, results from an enzyme defect that leads to failure to utilize the amino acid phenylalanine. (See Chapter 44.)

The Metabolic Pool The term METABOLIC POOL is often used to refer to the total supply of a given nutrient that is momentarily available for metabolic purposes.

It is the environment surrounding and within the cells and tissues from which nutrients are drawn. For example, the metabolic pool of amino acids at any given moment would include those available from absorption into the circulation from the digestive tract and also those available from cellular breakdown. From this mixture of amino acids the cells withdraw those needed for the synthesis of a specific protein.

Common Pathways Carbohydrate, fat, and protein are metabolized in an interdependent fashion. Glucose, fatty acids, glycerol, and amino acids can enter a common pathway that yields energy. (See Figure 2–4.) Glucose can also be metabolized to fatty acids and cholesterol, and some oxidative products of glucose can combine with amino groups to form amino acids. Amino acids are potential sources of both glucose and fatty acids, and so on. Not only are these major nutrients intertwined in their utilization, but they are dependent upon the correct concentrations of electrolytes and vitamins for making these changes take place. Further details of the metabolic pathways will be presented in Chapters 4, 5, and 6.

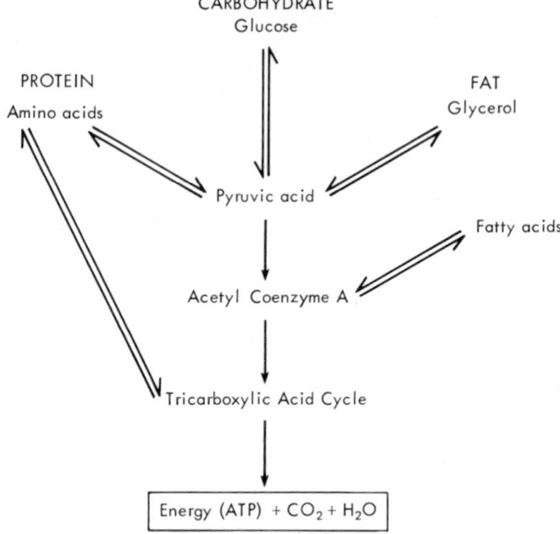

Figure 2–4. Glucose, amino acids, glycerol, and fatty acids enter into a common pathway to yield energy. Details of these pathways are shown in Figures 4–5, 5–5, and 6–5.

Problems and Review

1. Key terms: absorption; active transport; anabolism; catabolism; coefficient of digestibility; coenzyme; diffusion; digestion; enzyme; homeostasis; hormone; intermediary metabolism; metabolism; pinocytosis; prosthetic group; selective absorption; villus.
2. Name five characteristics of enzymes.
3. In what way does the chewing of food facilitate digestion?
4. What is the influence of attractive service of food on digestion?
5. Differentiate between pepsin and pepsinogen. What is the substrate on which pepsin acts?
6. A meal consisted of 25 gm protein, 35 gm fat, and 50 gm carbohydrate. Using coefficients of digestibility of typical American diets, calculate the amounts that actually would be absorbed.
7. What is meant by a feedback mechanism?
8. Explain the differences between passive diffusion, active transport, and pinocytosis.

Cited References

1. Fox, E. L.: *Sports Physiology.* W. B. Saunders Company, Philadelphia, 1975.
2. Pansky, B.: *Dynamic Anatomy and Physiology.* Macmillan Publishing Co., Inc., New York, 1975, ch. 12.

3. Burkitt, D. P., and Walker, A. R. P.: "Dietary Fiber and Disease," *JAMA,* **229**:1068–74, 1974.
4. Booth, C. C.: "Sites of Absorption in the Small Intestine," *Fed. Proc.,* **26**:1583–88, 1967.
5. Ingelfinger, F. J.: "Gastrointestinal Absorption," *Nutr. Today,* **2**:2–10, 1967.

Additional References

ASIMOV, I.: *The Chemicals of Life.* The New American Library of World Literature, New York, 1962.

BAYLESS, T. M., ed.: "Symposium: Structure and Function of the Gut," *Am. J. Clin. Nutr.,* **24**:44–167, 1971.

CRANE, R. K.: "A Perspective of Digestive-Absorptive Function," *Am. J. Clin. Nutr.,* **22**:242–49, 1969.

FLOCH, M. H., ed.: "Symposium: Current Concepts in Intestinal Absorption and Malabsorption," *Am. J. Clin. Nutr.,* **22**:239–351, 1969.

GUYTON, A. C.: *Textbook of Medical Physiology,* 4th ed. W. B. Saunders Company, Philadelphia, 1971.

MASON, M., et al.: *Nutrition and the Cell. The Inside Story.* Year Book Medical Publishers, Chicago, 1973.

MILLER, M. A., and LEAVELL, L. C.: *Kimber-Gray-Stackpole's Anatomy and Physiology,* 16th ed. Macmillan Publishing Co., Inc., New York, 1972.

NASSET, E. S.: "Role of Digestive System in Protein Metabolism," *Fed. Proc.,* **24**:953–58, 1965.

PIKE, R. L., and BROWN, M. L.: *Nutrition: An Integrated Approach.* 2nd ed., John Wiley & Sons, Inc., New York, 1975.

Review: "Gastric Emptying, Pancreatic and Biliary Secretion During Digestion," *Nutr. Rev.,* **33**:169, 1975.

Review: "Fat Absorption Physiology and Biochemistry," *Nutr. Rev.,* **26**:168–70, 1968.

ROSENSWEIG, N. S.: "Dietary Sugars and Intestinal Enzymes," *J. Am. Diet. Assoc.,* **60**:483–86, 1972.

SPENCER, R. P.: "Intestinal Absorption of Amino Acids. Current Concepts," *Am. J. Clin. Nutr.,* **22**:292–99, 1969.

3 *Dietary Guides and Their Uses*

THE Recommended Dietary Allowances and tables of food composition are two of the most important tools for professionals in the nutrition field. On the basis of food composition the allowances can be translated into practical food guides that the consumer can use to achieve nutritionally adequate diets under a variety of cultural and socioeconomic circumstances.

Controversial Issues

Although tremendous progress has been made in defining the nutritional needs of people, full agreement on the answers to questions such as the following is not yet forthcoming.

1. What are the best guidelines for dietary planning for a healthy population? A discussion of the recommended dietary allowances and of several practical guidelines will provide a background of information upon which to base one's choices.
2. What is meant by "nutritious"? What criteria should be applied to describe a food as nutritious? The determination of nutrient density is one approach to defining nutritional quality.

Recommended Dietary Allowances

Development of Dietary Allowances Humans have always been concerned about the kinds and amounts of foods that would keep them physically fit. Nevertheless, significant progress in identifying the nutrients needed by the body and the amounts required under varying circumstances has come about principally in this century as a result of thousands of investigations in research laboratories. Periodically, summaries of such research have been made in order to recommend the levels of intake desirable for various categories of the population. The first national effort in the United States came about late in 1940 when the Food and Nutrition Board of the National Research Council was organized to guide the government in its wartime nutrition program. One of the first activities of this board was the careful review of research on human requirements for the various nutrients. This led to the publication of the *Recommended Dietary Allowances* (RDAs) in 1943. Since that time the board has evaluated new research and has published revisions of the standards every 4 to 6 years.

The 1980 RDAs, listed in Table 3–1, include 17 age-sex categories. Each category is described in terms of height and weight. For example, the "reference" man weighs 70 kg (154 lb) and is 178 cm (70 in.) tall; the "reference" woman weighs 55 kg (120 lb) and is 163 cm (64 in.) tall. Adjustments for variations in body size within a given category are sometimes indicated.

In the current revision the requirements for energy are listed separately. (See Table 7–3.) Unlike the nutrient allowances that are intended to meet the needs of most of the population, the energy levels are average requirements that will maintain

Table 3-1. Food and Nutrition Board, National Academy of Sciences–National Research Council Recommended Daily Dietary Allowances,* Revised 1980
Designed for the Maintenance of Good Nutrition of Practically all Healthy People in the U.S.A.

	Age (years)	Weight (kg)	Weight (lbs)	Height (cm)	Height (in)	Protein (g)	Fat-Soluble Vitamins: Vitamin A (μg RE)†	Vitamin D (μg)‡	Vitamin E (mg α TE)§	Water-Soluble Vitamins: Vitamin C (mg)	Thiamin (mg)	Riboflavin (mg)	Niacin (mg NE)**	Vitamin B6 (mg)	Folacin †† (μg)	Vitamin B12 (μg)	Minerals: Calcium (mg)	Phosphorus (mg)	Magnesium (mg)	Iron (mg)	Zinc (mg)	Iodine (μg)
Infants	0.0–0.5	6	13	60	24	kg × 2.2	420	10	3	35	0.3	0.4	6	0.3	30	0.5‡‡	360	240	50	10	3	40
	0.5–1.0	9	20	71	28	kg × 2.0	400	10	4	35	0.5	0.6	8	0.6	45	1.5	540	360	70	15	5	50
Children	1–3	13	29	90	35	23	400	10	5	45	0.7	0.8	9	0.9	100	2.0	800	800	150	15	10	70
	4–6	20	44	112	44	30	500	10	6	45	0.9	1.0	11	1.3	200	2.5	800	800	200	10	10	90
	7–10	28	62	132	52	34	700	10	7	45	1.2	1.4	16	1.6	300	3.0	800	800	250	10	10	120
Males	11–14	45	99	157	62	45	1000	10	8	50	1.4	1.6	18	1.8	400	3.0	1200	1200	350	18	15	150
	15–18	66	145	176	69	56	1000	10	10	60	1.4	1.7	18	2.0	400	3.0	1200	1200	400	18	15	150
	19–22	70	154	177	70	56	1000	7.5	10	60	1.5	1.7	19	2.2	400	3.0	800	800	350	10	15	150
	23–50	70	154	178	70	56	1000	5	10	60	1.4	1.6	18	2.2	400	3.0	800	800	350	10	15	150
	51+	70	154	178	70	56	1000	5	10	60	1.2	1.4	16	2.2	400	3.0	800	800	350	10	15	150
Females	11–14	46	101	157	62	46	800	10	8	50	1.1	1.3	15	1.8	400	3.0	1200	1200	300	18	15	150
	15–18	55	120	163	64	46	800	10	8	60	1.1	1.3	14	2.0	400	3.0	1200	1200	300	18	15	150
	19–22	55	120	163	64	44	800	7.5	8	60	1.1	1.3	14	2.0	400	3.0	800	800	300	18	15	150
	23–50	55	120	163	64	44	800	5	8	60	1.0	1.2	13	2.0	400	3.0	800	800	300	18	15	150
	51+	55	120	163	64	44	800	5	8	60	1.0	1.2	13	2.0	400	3.0	800	800	300	10	15	150
Pregnant						+30	+200	+5	+2	+20	+0.4	+0.3	+2	+0.6	+400	+1.0	+400	+400	+150	§§	+5	+25
Lactating						+20	+400	+5	+3	+40	+0.5	+0.5	+5	+0.5	+100	+1.0	+400	+400	+150	§§	+10	+50

*The allowances are intended to provide for individual variations among most normal persons as they live in the United States under usual environmental stresses. Diets should be based on a variety of common foods in order to provide other nutrients for which human requirements have been less well defined. See text for detailed discussion of allowances and of nutrients not tabulated. See Table 7-3 for suggested average energy intakes.

†Retinol equivalents. 1 retinol equivalent = 1 μg retinol or 6 μg β-carotene. See text for calculation of vitamin A activity of diets as retinol equivalents.

‡As cholecalciferol, 10μg cholecalciferol = 400 I.U. vitamin D.

§α tocopherol equivalents. 1 mg d-α-tocopherol = 1 α TE. See text for variation in allowances and calculation of vitamin E activity of the diet as α tocopherol equivalents.

**1 NE (niacin equivalent) is equal to 1 mg of niacin or 60 mg of dietary tryptophan.

††The folacin allowances refer to dietary sources as determined by *Lactobacillus casei* assay after treatment with enzymes ("conjugases") to make polyglutamyl forms of the vitamin available to the test organism.

‡‡The RDA for vitamin B-12 in infants is based on average concentration of the vitamin in human milk. The allowances after weaning are based on energy intake (as recommended by the American Academy of Pediatrics) and consideration of other factors such as intestinal absorption; see text.

§§The increased requirement during pregnancy cannot be met by the iron content of habitual American diets nor by the existing iron stores of many women; therefore the use of 30–60 mg of supplemental iron is recommended. Iron needs during lactation are not substantially different from those of nonpregnant women, but continued supplementation of the mother for 2–3 months after parturition is advisable in order to replenish stores depleted by pregnancy.

Table 3-2. **Estimated Safe and Adequate Daily Dietary Intakes of Additional Selected Vitamins and Minerals***

		Vitamins			Trace Elements†						Electrolytes		
	Age (years)	Vitamin K (μg)	Biotin (μg)	Pantothenic Acid (mg)	Copper (mg)	Manganese (mg)	Fluoride (mg)	Chromium (mg)	Selenium (mg)	Molybdenum (mg)	Sodium (mg)	Potassium (mg)	Chloride (mg)
Infants	0–0.5	12	35	2	0.5–0.7	0.5–0.7	0.1–0.5	0.01–0.04	0.01–0.04	0.03–0.06	115–350	350–925	275–700
	0.5–1	10–20	50	3	0.7–1.0	0.7–1.0	0.2–1.0	0.02–0.06	0.02–0.06	0.04–0.08	250–750	425–1275	400–1200
Children and Adolescents	1–3	15–30	65	3	1.0–1.5	1.0–1.5	0.5–1.5	0.02–0.08	0.02–0.08	0.05–0.1	325–975	550–1650	500–1500
	4–6	20–40	85	3–4	1.5–2.0	1.5–2.0	1.0–2.5	0.03–0.12	0.03–0.12	0.06–0.15	450–1350	775–2325	700–2100
	7–10	30–60	120	4–5	2.0–2.5	2.0–3.0	1.5–2.5	0.05–0.2	0.05–0.2	0.1 –0.3	600–1800	1000–3000	925–2775
	11+	50–100	100–200	4–7	2.0–3.0	2.5–5.0	1.5–2.5	0.05–0.2	0.05–0.2	0.15–0.5	900–2700	1525–4575	1400–4200
Adults		70–140	100–200	4–7	2.0–3.0	2.5–5.0	1.5–4.0	0.05–0.2	0.05–0.2	0.15–0.5	1100–3300	1875–5625	1700–5100

*Because there is less information on which to base allowances, these figures are not given in the main table of the RDA and are provided here in the form of ranges of recommended intakes.

†Since the toxic levels for many trace elements may be only several times the usual intakes, the upper levels for the trace elements given in this table should not be habitually exceeded.

Food and Nutrition Board: *Recommended Dietary Allowances,* 9th ed. National Research Council–National Academy of Sciences, Washington, D.C., 1980.

health and normal weight in adults and support growth in children. The requirements for energy vary widely from one individual to another.

An important addition to the 1980 revision is the inclusion of a table of estimated allowances for twelve nutrients for which data, as yet, are limited. (See Table 3–2.) Because some trace elements can be toxic, safe ranges of intake are listed. Habitual intakes that exceed the maximum level could lead to signs of toxicity.

In addition to the tables of allowances, the Food and Nutrition Board has described the basis for establishing each nutrient allowance.[1] It also provides some recommendations for water, fat, essential fatty acids, carbohydrate, and fiber in the diet. The allowances for specific nutrients and the factors that influence their needs are covered in more detail in Chapters 4 through 12.

Interpretation of the RDA The Food and Nutrition Board defines the RDA thus:

> Recommended Dietary Allowances (RDA) are the levels of intake of essential nutrients considered, in the judgment of the Committee on Dietary Allowances of the Food and Nutrition Board on the basis of available scientific knowledge, to be adequate to meet the nutritional needs of practically all healthy persons.*

The word "allowance" should not be confused with the word "requirement." An individual's requirement for nutrients is influenced by numerous interdependent physical, environmental, social, and dietary characteristics. Thus, people vary widely in their needs. Since it is not practical to determine each individual's exact needs, the allowances have been set high enough to take care of almost all healthy people. (See Figure 3–1.)

The allowances are the amounts of nutrients to be actually consumed. The food supply brought into the kitchen for a given group must be sufficient to allow for waste in preparation, losses of nutrients in cooking, and plate waste.

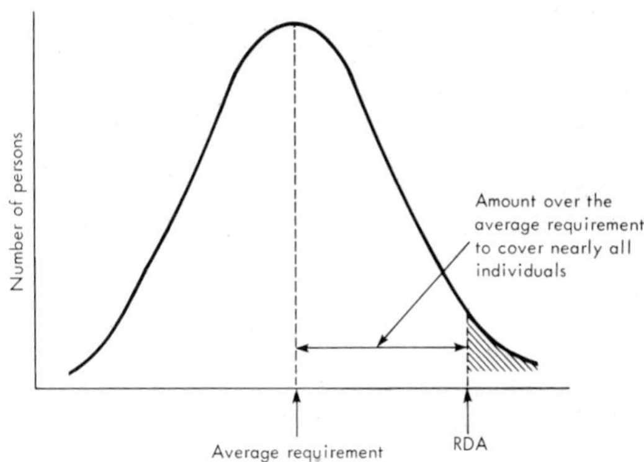

Figure 3–1. Normal distribution curve of the variation of requirements among individuals. Relatively small numbers of people have either low or high requirements. Most have needs that are near the average. The RDAs are set high enough so that most people with high needs are also protected. Conversely, a given allowance will be higher than most people actually need.

In the practice of dietetics the allowances are frequently used to determine the adequacy of the food intake of an individual. When the nutrient intake of a healthy individual is equal to, or exceeds, the recommended allowances, it is highly likely that the diet is meeting the needs of that person to achieve his or her full potential for growth or productivity. An intake below the recommended allowances for a prolonged period of time increases the possibility of nutritional deficiency.

Uses for the RDA The dietary allowances are a professional tool that is appropriately used in the following ways:

Evaluating the adequacy of the national food supply; setting goals for food production.
Setting standards for menu planning for publicly funded nutrition programs such as school food services, day-care centers, programs for the elderly, and others.
Establishing nutrition policy for public assistance, nursing homes, and institutions such

* Food and Nutrition Board. *Recommended Dietary Allowances*, 9th ed. National Research Council—National Academy of Sciences, Washington, D.C., 1980, p. 1.

as children's homes, mental institutions, and prisons.

Interpreting the adequacy of diets in food consumption studies. The Household Food Consumption Survey, the Health and Nutrition Examination Survey, and the Ten-State Survey have evaluated diets on the basis of the RDA or some modification of it.

Developing materials for nutrition education. The RDA are used to develop food guides and other educational materials for the public.

Setting the pattern for the normal diet used in hospitals. Although modified diets may require increased or decreased amounts of nutrients, the normal diet is the reference point for making these modifications.

Establishing labeling regulations. The USRDA labeling standard is an adaptation of the RDA.

Setting guidelines for the formulation of new food products or the fortification of specific foods.

Limitations and Misuse of the RDA Those who use the RDAs should also understand their limitations.[1,2]

They are too complex for direct use by consumers.

They do not state *ideal* or *optimal* levels of intake. These are concepts that cannot be realized.

The allowances for some age categories such as adolescents and the elderly are based on limited data.

Data on the food content of some nutrients such as trace minerals are limited. Therefore, reliable evaluation of diets against the RDAs cannot always be achieved.

The RDAs do not evaluate nutritional status. Because the allowances are higher than the requirements of most people, failure to achieve the recommended allowance for one or more nutrients does not mean that nutritional deficiency is present. However, the risk of nutritional deficiency increases the further below the RDA a given nutrient intake habitually falls. Nutritional status can be determined only by physical, clinical, and biochemical examination of the individual. (See Chapter 22.)

The RDAs do not apply to people who are ill and who require increased or decreased levels of nutrients because of pathology or because of the use of medications.

Other Standards

Canadian Dietary Standard Since 1938 the Canadian Council on Nutrition has published recommendations for nutrient levels for age and sex categories. The most recent revision was published in 1975.[3] (See Table A-18 in the Appendix.)

The purpose of the Canadian standard is essentially the same as that of the Food and Nutrition Board, namely, to recommend nutrient intakes at levels adequate for good health for most Canadians. The standards are above minimum levels and take individual variations into account. The data are derived from essentially the same base lines. The standards are to be used for "planning of diets and food supplies for individuals" and are not to be used as a measure of nutritional status.

An examination of the two tables shows that there are some differences in the recommended levels for nutrients, for example, iron, zinc, and ascorbic acid among others. These differences emphasize that there still exists a good deal of ignorance regarding the criteria for optimum health, the desirable margin of safety, and so on. The assigned levels for each nutrient represent the best judgment of the committees that set up each table.

Dietary Guides in Other Countries Dietary allowances have been established for populations of many countries. In addition, the Food and Agriculture Organization and the World Health Organization have adopted recommendations for allowances for many nutrients. The aim of the various standards is essentially to provide a level of nutrition that maintains good health for substantially all of the population.[4] The allowances are not minimum requirements, nor are they average needs.

The allowances in various countries differ because they are intended for the population of a given environment—for example, climate, occupation and activity, dietary practices—and therefore they are not interchangeable. For example, more calories would be allowed for men and women in a country where considerable physical activity is involved in daily work than in a country where work is mechanized and activity is sedentary. The increased calorie allowances in turn necessitate increased allowances for some of the B-complex vitamins such as thiamin. The allowances in the various countries also differ because of varying interpretations of data by committees who set up the allowances.[4] As research becomes more extensive these differences are narrowing somewhat. A comparison of allowances set up for men and women for several groups is shown in Table 3–3.

Labeling The U.S. Recommended Daily Allowances (USRDA) was established by the Food and Drug Administration as a standard for labeling the numerous packaged foods in the marketplace. (See page 34.) This standard should not be used in place of the RDAs for planning diets.

Food Guides

A Daily Food Guide The RDAs should be translated into diets consisting of a wide variety of foods. On a given day a diet may not always furnish all nutrients at recommended levels. However, the body has sufficient adaptability that an average intake over a 5-to-8-day period that meets the allowance is satisfactory.

The RDAs have been translated into food guides such as the "Basic Seven" and later the "Basic Four," also known as the "Four Food Groups."[5] Recently the U.S. Department of Agriculture issued a revision of the Daily Food Guide.[6] The revised guide retains the four food groups but adds a fifth group—fats, sweets, and alcohol. (See Table 3–4.) Daily selections from these groups can be adjusted to comply with the dietary guidelines described on page 42.

Limitations of the Daily Food Guide The Daily Food Guide is intended primarily for consumers. Its limitations should also be recognized.

1. A food guide appropriate for one group of people is not necessarily applicable to another group; for example, guides based on the food supplies in the United States would not be suitable for nations in Africa or the Far East.
2. Some new foods, mixtures of foods, and many convenience foods are not

Table 3–3. **Dietary Allowances for Adults by Four Standards**

	United States 1980*	Canada 1974*	Food and Agriculture Organization*†	United Kingdom*‡
Body weight, kg	70, 55	70, 56	65, 55	65, 55
Energy, kcal	2,700, 2,000	3,000, 2,100	3,000, 2,200	3,000, 2,200
Protein, gm	56, 44	56, 41	37, 29	75, 55
Calcium, mg	800	800, 700	400–500**	500
Iron, mg	10, 18	10, 14	5–9, 14–28	10, 12
Vitamin A, RE	1,000, 800	1,000, 800	750	750
Thiamin, mg	1.4, 1.0	1.5, 1.1	1.3, 0.9	1.2, 0.9
Riboflavin, mg	1.6, 1.2	1.8, 1.3	1.8, 1.3	1.7, 1.3
Niacin, mg	18, 13	20, 14	21.1, 15.2	18, 15
Ascorbic acid, mg	60	30	30	30

*The first figure in each column refers to men, and the second to women. Where the allowance for men and women is the same, only one figure is given.

†Passmore, R., et al.: *Handbook on Human Nutritional Requirements.* WHO Monogram Ser. No. 61, World Health Organization, Geneva, 1974.

‡Davidson, S., et al.: *Human Nutrition and Dietetics,* 6th ed. Churchill Livingstone, Edinburgh, 1975, p. 184.

**This allowance for calcium represents a range for men and women.

Table 3-4. **A Daily Food Guide***

Vegetable-Fruit Group: 4 basic servings daily.
One serving is ½ cup or a typical portion such as one orange, half a medium grapefruit, a medium potato, or a bowl of salad.
Include one good vitamin C source daily.
Include deep yellow or dark green vegetables frequently.
Include unpeeled fruits and vegetables and those with edible seeds for fiber.

Bread-Cereal Group: 4 basic servings whole-grain and enriched or fortified products.
One serving is 1 slice bread or ½ to ¾ cup cooked cereal, cornmeal, grits, macaroni, noodles, rice, or spaghetti; or 1 ounce ready-to-eat cereal.
Include some whole-grain breads and cereals for fiber.

Milk-Cheese Group: children under 9—2-3 servings
children, 9 to 12—3 servings
teenagers—4 servings
pregnant women—3 servings
nursing mothers—4 servings

One serving is one 8-ounce cup of milk: whole, skim, low fat, evaporated, buttermilk, or nonfat dry milk may be used.

Equivalents for calcium are

1 cup plain yogurt	= 1 cup milk
1 ounce Cheddar or Swiss cheese	= ¾ cup milk
1-inch cube Cheddar or Swiss cheese (natural or processed)	= ½ cup milk
1 ounce processed cheese food	= ½ cup milk
½ cup ice cream or ice milk	= ⅓ cup milk
1 tablespoon or ½ ounce processed cheese spread; or 1 tablespoon grated Parmesan cheese	= ¼ cup milk
½ cup cottage cheese	= ¼cup milk

Meat, Fish, Poultry, and Beans Group: 2 basic servings daily.
One serving is 2 to 3 ounces of lean, cooked meat, poultry, or fish without bone.
Count as 1 ounce of meat, poultry, or fish:
1 egg
½ to ¾ cup cooked dry beans, dry peas, soybeans, or lentils
2 tablespoons peanut butter
¼ to ½ cup nuts, sesame seeds, sunflower seeds

Fats, Sweets, Alcohol Group: no basic servings suggested.
Includes butter, margarine, salad dressings, mayonnaise, fats, oils; candy, sugar, jams, jellies, syrups, sweet toppings; soft drinks and other highly sugared beverages; wine, beer, and liquor; also unenriched breads, pastries, and flour products.

**Food.* HG228. U.S. Department of Agriculture, Washington, D.C. 1980.

easily classified according to the food groups.

3. Foods within a group vary widely in their caloric content. There are also wide variations of nutrient levels within each group. Some fruits and vegetables are outstanding for their content of ascorbic acid and vitamin A, whereas others supply only small amounts. Thus, the user must become acquainted with these variations.
4. Adherence to a food guide does not guarantee nutritive adequacy. The nutrient needs are more likely to be met when a wide variety of foods is selected from each group.

A Basic Diet A diet that includes the minimum number of servings for the adult from each of the four food groups is used in this text as a basis for dietary planning. (See Table 13–2 for calculations of the basic diet.) The plan substantially furnishes the recommended nutrient levels and approximately 1,200 kcal. Additional selections from the four food groups that make up the diet will significantly increase the nutrient intake. If additional calories are selected from the fats, sweets, and alcohol group there will be little increase in nutrient intake.

Dietary Guidelines With the ever-increasing costs of health care and the high incidence of chronic diseases such as coronary heart disease, stroke, and cancer, professional and public interest has increased rapidly concerning the possible role that diet may play in preventing these diseases. For many years the American Heart Association has recommended that the general public modify food intake to maintain desirable weight and to consume less saturated fat, cholesterol, sugar, and salt. With much fanfare by the media, three guidelines have been published in recent years. Each has been subjected to much criticism by nutrition scientists, clinicians, politicians, the food industry, and advocates for the public. None of the guidelines is considered a substitute for the Daily Food Guide, but each of them can be adapted to use with the guide.

Dietary Goals for the United States In February 1977 the Senate Select Committee on Nutrition and Human Needs published a report on the Dietary Goals. Based on suggestions made by nutrition and medical scientists the report was revised in December 1977.[7] The revised goals are as follows:

1. To avoid overweight, consume only as much energy (calories) as is expended; if overweight, decrease energy intake and increase energy expenditure.
2. Increase the consumption of complex carbohydrates and naturally occurring sugars from about 28 per cent of energy intake to about 48 per cent of energy intake.
3. Reduce the consumption of refined and processed sugars by about 45 per cent to account for about 10 per cent of total energy intake.
4. Reduce overall fat consumption from approximately 40 per cent to about 30 per cent of energy intake.
5. Reduce saturated fat consumption to account for about 10 per cent of total energy intake; and balance that with polyunsaturated and monounsaturated fats, which should account for about 10 per cent of energy intake each.
6. Reduce cholesterol consumption to about 300 mg a day.
7. Limit the intake of sodium by reducing the intake of salt to about 5 grams a day.

The following changes in food selection and preparation are suggested to implement the Goals:

1. Increase consumption of fruits and vegetables and whole grains.
2. Decrease consumption of foods high in total fat and partially substitute polyunsaturated fat for saturated fat.
3. Decrease consumption of animal fats. Choose meat, poultry, and fish that are low in saturated fat.
4. Except for young children, substitute low-fat or nonfat milk for whole milk, and low-fat dairy products for high-fat dairy products.
5. Decrease consumption of butterfat, eggs, and other high cholesterol sources.
6. Decrease consumption of sugar and foods high in sugar content.
7. Decrease consumption of salt and foods high in salt content.

No issue in nutrition in recent years has provoked as much controversy as these Goals. Those who support the Goals believe that the scientific evidence supports the hypothesis that present eating habits are contributing to disease. They agree that the overall adoption of the Goals will improve public health, although not everyone will necessarily benefit because of genetic and individual variability. They view the Goals as applicable to the general population, and not modifications intended only for persons who are at risk or who are ill. They maintain that there is no evidence that consuming the diet lower in saturated fat, cholesterol, sugar, and salt will cause harm to the population. Finally, they regard the Goals as being a first step in a national nutrition policy, which are subject to revision with new research findings.

Those who oppose the Goals state that the evidence supporting them is limited and often confusing. The Goals do not provide guidelines for a nutritionally adequate diet, but place emphasis on the prevention of disease. It is maintained that the Goals promise too much and that this can only lead to disillusionment of the public. By themselves, the Goals are too simplistic an approach to the prevention of diseases that are known to have multiple risk factors. Finally, the present American diet is believed to be a good one that should not be tampered with until more research has been accomplished.

Dietary Guidelines for Americans. In a joint publication by the U.S. Department of Agriculture and the U.S. Department of Health, Education, and Welfare, the following seven guidelines have been identified:

1. Eat a variety of foods.
2. Maintain ideal weight.
3. Avoid too much fat, saturated fat, and cholesterol.
4. Eat foods with adequate starch and fiber.
5. Avoid too much sugar.
6. Avoid too much sodium.
7. If you drink alcohol, do so in moderation.[8]

These Guidelines resemble the Dietary Goals in the overall recommendations, but no quantitative levels of restriction for fat, cholesterol, sugar, and sodium are indicated. Although the consumer is cautioned to "avoid too much . . ." there is no indication what is meant by "too much." However, the bulletin that accompanies these Guidelines describes food selections that should be avoided.

Toward Healthful Diets. In developing recommendations for diets for Americans, the Food and Nutrition Board has stated:

A fundamental element of any national nutrition policy, inherent in the recommendations of the Board, is to ensure the provision of a supply of diverse, safe, and attractive foods that will meet nutritional requirements of the population at reasonable cost.[9]

The Board has expressed concern about excessive hopes and fears resulting from some present claims for food and nutrition. Nutritionists will recognize the following recommendations of the Board for the diet of adult Americans as important concepts that have governed their efforts in nutrition education for many years.

Select a nutritionally adequate diet from the foods available, by consuming each day appropriate servings of dairy products, meats or legumes, vegetables and fruits, and cereal and breads.

Select as wide a variety of foods in each of the major food groups as is practicable in order to ensure a high probability of consuming adequate quantities of all essential nutrients.

Adjust dietary energy intake and energy expenditure so as to maintain appropriate weight for height; if overweight, achieve appropriate weight reduction by decreasing total food and fat intake and by increasing physical activity.

If the requirement for energy is low (e.g., reducing diet), reduce consumption of foods such as alcohol, sugars, fats, and oils, which provide calories but few essential nutrients.

Use salt in moderation; adequate but safe intakes are considered to range between 3 and 8 grams of sodium chloride daily.[9]

The Nutritive Value of Foods

Factors Affecting Food Composition The composition of foods of plant or animal origin is influenced by genetic origin and environment. Thus, plant variety, animal species, soil, geographic area, climate, season, processing techniques, storage facilities, and preparation procedures are among the factors that influence food composition.

The composition of the soil influences some of the nutritive values of foods grown on it. It has long been known that a low iodine content of the soil produces foods with a low iodine content. More recently it has been shown that some soils are depleted of trace minerals, which results in mineral-deficient foods. For example, livestock suffer severe disease when the food they eat contains either a deficiency or an excess of selenium because of soil deficiency or excess.

The variety of plants and the climate are important determinants of nutritive value. The latter cannot be controlled, but much progress has been made in developing plant varieties that have superior nutritive qualities. For example, strains of corn and wheat are helping to improve the food supply in many of the developing countries.

The conditions of storage—length of time, temperature, light—are known to modify the nutritive value of foods. Some nutrients such as ascorbic acid are rapidly lost when the temperature is high or when foods are bruised. Other nutrients may be lost to a varying degree but not quite so readily as ascorbic acid.

Processing techniques enhance or interfere with the nutritive value of foods. Dehydration, canning, and freezing yield foods of high nutritive value, but each process, in certain ways, modifies somewhat the nutrient contribution of a given food.

Divergent procedures in food preparation are major factors that affect the nutritive value of a food as it is consumed. Losses in food preparation may be brought about through solubility of the nutrient in water, or through destruction of the nutrient. The latter is increased with high temperature and is also dependent upon the pH of the medium in which it is cooked. The amount of peelings removed, the size of pieces subjected to cooking, the temperature used, the length of time for cooking, the amount of water used, the length of time food is held after cooking—as on a steam table—are but a few of the many variables which may result in wide differences between two foods that were identical in nutritive value at the start of the cooking procedure.

Tables of Food Composition Through research in laboratories of universities, food industries, and the U.S. Department of Agriculture data on the nutritive composition of foods are continually being expanded. Tables A-1 and A-2 in the Appendix illustrate the kinds of data that are available. With thousands of products in markets and with some 50 or so nutrients needed for good nutrition, the task of accumulating data is indeed enormous. The USDA now maintains a computer data bank that facilitates the dissemination of information on nutritive composition.

For the most part, nutritive analyses are based on chemical methods. In some instances, such as the evaluation of protein quality, or the determination of the presence of vitamin D, animal feeding (BIOASSAY) is used. Certain of the B vitamins and some of the amino acids are best determined by measuring the rate of reproduction, or selected metabolic processes, of microorganisms (MICROBIOLOGIC ASSAY).

At least four uses for tables of food composition can be cited:

1. To compare the nutritive value of one food with another. For example, an examination of the calcium content of many foods clearly indicates that milk is an outstanding source. Although every medium-size orange could not be expected to yield exactly the same number of milligrams of ascorbic acid, the tables give information on the relative amount of ascorbic acid in an orange as compared with an apple.
2. To calculate the nutritive value of any diet, and to compare that diet with the RDA.
3. To plan diets that must meet specific requirements such as 500 mg sodium, or 100 gm protein, and so on.
4. To provide a ready reference to answer hundreds of questions that people ask about foods. Proper use of the tables can counteract much nutritional misinformation.

Tables of food composition also have their limitations. Only limited data are yet available for some nutrients such as amino acids, vitamin B-6, vitamin B-12, folacin, copper, zinc, and a number of other trace elements. For some foods there are no data, and for others the values must be regarded as tentative until more analyses have been made. Tables of food composition give no indication of the BIOAVAILABILITY of a nutrient, that is, the amount of a nutrient that is actually absorbed and available for body use. The bioavailability of nutrients such as iron and zinc depends upon the chemical form in which the nutrient is present in food, the interactions that can occur in the intestinal tract between two or more foods eaten at the same time, the pH of the intestinal tract, and so on.

What is Meant by a "Nutritious" Food All foods are nourishing depending upon the circumstances. Even fats and sugars are important when the primary need is energy, although it is generally agreed that these foods have a low concentration (low density) of nutrients.

The nutritive quality of foods may be expressed in a variety of ways. By consulting tables of food composition, one can arrange foods in arbitrary groupings such as excellent, good, fair, poor. The boundaries that might be used to place foods in one grouping or another are subjectively chosen, and the differing lists become confusing to the public.

The comparative values of foods can be expressed by listing the data for various foods. For example, from such data one quickly learns that cantaloupe and strawberries are far better sources of vitamin C than are bananas and peaches.

But for many people who have low caloric requirements because of a sedentary life-style, it is important that each 100 kcal supplied by the food eaten also "carry its weight" in terms of nutrients. Many years ago Dr. Mary Schwartz Rose, one of the pioneers in nutrition education, devised a "share system" that showed the nutritive contribution of food in relation to its caloric content.[10] A recent graphic modification of this method has been developed by the National Dairy Council, using the USRDA to show nutritive values.[11]

Nutrient Density The relationship of the nutrient content of a food to its caloric contribution is known as NUTRIENT DENSITY. This relationship can be expressed by the following equation:[12]

$$\text{INDEX OF NUTRITIONAL QUALITY (INQ)} = \frac{\text{Per cent of nutrient allowance}}{\text{Per cent of energy requirement}}$$

Such an index shows the extent to which a human nutrient allowance is met in proportion to the energy requirement. Thus an index of 1.0 indicates that the food supplies the nutrient in the same proportion to need as the calories it contains. Indexes above 1.0 indicate increasingly high nutrient density.

Before any calculations can be made one must agree upon the standards to be used. One such standard could be the RDA. But since the caloric requirements and the nutrient allowances differ for the various age-sex categories, it becomes obvious that there would be differences in the INQ for these several groups. A practical approach is to use the USRDA (see Table 17–1). Although this standard does not specify a caloric level, an appropriate energy level of 2,300 kcal has been suggested.[12] A sample calculation follows for the protein in peanut butter:

2 tablespoons peanut butter contain 190 kcal and 8 gm protein
The USRDA for protein is 65 gm.

$$\frac{190 \text{ kcal}}{2{,}300 \text{ kcal}} \times 100 = 8.3\ \%\ \text{of standard caloric allowance}$$

$$\frac{8 \text{ gm}}{65 \text{ gm}} \times 100 = 12.3\ \%\ \text{of USRDA for protein}$$

$$\text{INQ} = \frac{12.3\ \%}{8.3\ \%} = 1.5$$

		Per Cent of USRDA	Index of Nutritional Quality
Energy, kcal	190	8.3	1.0
Protein, gm	8	12.3	1.5
Calcium, mg	18	1.8	0.2
Iron, mg	0.6	3.3	0.4
Thiamin, mg	0.04	2.7	0.3
Riboflavin, mg	0.04	2.3	0.3
Niacin, mg	4.8	24.0	2.8

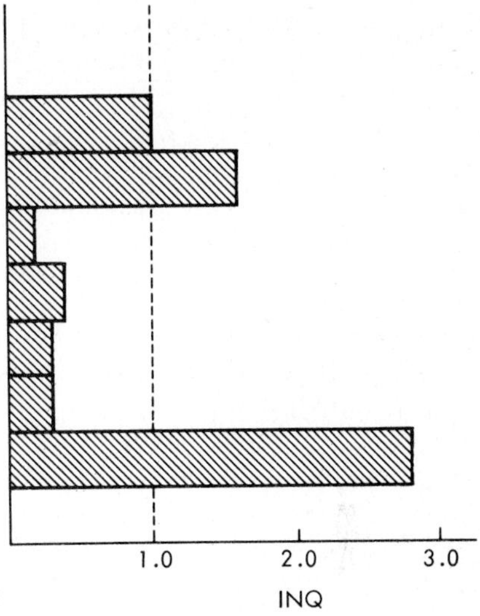

Figure 3–2. Index of nutritional quality for peanut butter. Protein and niacin indexes above 1.0 indicate that peanut butter is a good source of these nutrients in relation to the caloric content. Note that 2 tablespoons peanut butter is listed in the Daily Food Guide as equivalent to 1 ounce meat.

Figure 3–2 illustrates the profile for 2 tablespoons peanut butter. With computer programs nutritionists have been able to arrive at indexes for numerous foods, and also to obtain printouts of the nutrient profiles.

Problems and Review

1. Key terms: basic diet; bioassay; bioavailability; Daily Food Guide; dietary guidelines; Food and Nutrition Board; index of nutritional quality; microbiologic assay; nutrient density; Recommended Dietary Allowances; Safe and Adequate Intakes; U.S. Recommended Daily Allowances.
2. List the Recommended Allowances for yourself. If a dietary calculation indicated that you were getting less than these allowances in one or more respects, how should you interpret this?
3. List five reasons that two oranges may differ in ascorbic acid content.
4. Two students had hamburgers for lunch, each raw hamburger weighing 4 ounces. One student received more calories in her hamburger than did the other. Explain.
5. Examine the tables in the Appendix to become familiar with the information they provide.
6. *Problem.* Using Table A–1, list five fresh fruits that are the most outstanding sources of vitamin A. In your community, which of these, if any, are not practical for dietary planning?
7. *Problem.* Use Table A–1 to find answers to the following questions:
   a. A woman asks whether whole-wheat bread is more nutritious than enriched white bread.
   b. A teenager wants to know if potatoes are more fattening than ice cream.
   c. A mother asks if she can substitute tomato juice for orange juice in her child's diet.

d. A man asks if beefsteak is richer in protein than Swiss cheese.

8. *Problem.* Keep a careful record of your own food intake for three days. See above for directions.
   a. Score your diet according to the Daily Food Guide. What food group, if any, requires more emphasis in order to improve your diet?
   b. Select one of the three days that is most typical of your usual practice. Calculate the nutritive values using Table A–1. Compare your intake with your recommended allowances.
   c. Keep this evaluation for reference as you study the nutrients in chapters that follow.
9. List the similarities and the differences between the dietary guidelines of the Senate Select Committee on Nutrition, the USDA and the USDHEW, and the Food and Nutrition Board.
10. *Problem.* Calculate the index of nutritional quality for the nutrients listed in Table A–1 for whole-wheat bread. For your calculations assume a base of 2,300 kcal and the USRDA, page 325.

Cited References

1. Food and Nutrition Board: *Recommended Dietary Allowances,* 9th ed. National Research Council—National Academy of Sciences, Washington, D.C., 1980.
2. Report by the Comptroller General of the United States: *Recommended Dietary Allowances: More Research and Better Food Guides Needed.* U.S. General Accounting Office, Washington, D.C., 1978.
3. Nutrition Bureau, Health and Welfare: *The Canadian Dietary Standard, Revised 1975.* Canada Health Protection Branch, Ottawa, Canada.
4. Patwardhan, V. A.: "Dietary Allowances—An International Point of View," *J. Am. Diet. Assoc.,* **56**:191–94, 1970.
5. Hertzler, A. A., and Anderson, H. L.: "Food Guides in the United States," *J. Am. Diet. Assoc.,* **64**:19–28, 1974.
6. *Food.* HG 228. Science and Education Administration, U.S. Department of Agriculture, Washington, D.C., 1980.
7. U.S. Senate Select Committee on Nutrition and Human Needs: *Dietary Goals for the United States,* rev. Government Printing Office, Washington, D.C., December 1977.
8. *Nutrition and Your Health: Dietary Guidelines for Americans.* U.S. Department of Agriculture and U.S. Department of Health, Education, and Welfare, Washington, D.C., 1980.
9. Food and Nutrition Board: *Toward Healthful Diets.* National Research Council—National Academy of Sciences, Washington, D.C., 1980.
10. Rose, M. S.: *A Laboratory Handbook for Dietetics.* Macmillan Company, New York, 1929.
11. *U.S. RDA Comparison Charts.* National Dairy Council, Chicago, 1974.
12. Sorenson, A.W. et al.: "An Index of Nutritional Quality for a Balanced Diet," *J. Am. Diet. Assoc.,* **68**:236–42, 1976.

Additional References

ABDEL-GHANY, M.: "Evaluation of Household Diets by the Index of Nutritional Quality," *J. Nutr. Educ.,* **10**:79–81, 1978.

American Dietetic Association: "Position Paper on a National Nutrition Policy," *J. Am. Diet. Assoc.,* **76**:596–97, 1980.

BIERI, J. G.: "An Overview of the RDAs for Vitamins," *J. Am. Diet. Assoc.,* **76**:134–36, 1980.

CONNOR, W. E.: "Too Little or Too Much: The Case for Preventive Nutrition," *Am. J. Clin. Nutr.,* **32**:1975–78, 1979.

Handbook of Human Nutritional Requirements. Nutritional Series No. 28. Food and Agriculture Organization of the United Nations, Rome, 1974.

HANSEN, R. G., and WYSE, B. W.: "Expression of Nutrient Allowances per 1000 Kilocalories," *J. Am. Diet. Assoc.,* **76**:223–27, 1980.

HARPER, A. E.: "Dietary Goals—A Skeptical View," *Am. J. Clin. Nutr.,* **31**:310–21, 1978.

HARPER, A. E.: "Recommended Dietary Allowances—1980," *Nutr. Rev.,* **38**:290–94, 1980.

HEGSTED, D. M.: "Dietary Goals—A Progressive View," *Am. J. Clin. Nutr.,* **31**:1504–09, 1978.

HEGSTED, D. M.: "On Dietary Standards," *Nutr. Rev.,* **36**:33–36, 1978.

MCNUTT, K.: "Dietary Advice to the Public: 1957 to 1980," *Nutr. Rev.,* **38**:353–60, 1980.

MERTZ, W.:" The New RDAs: Estimated Adequate and Safe Intake of Trace Elements and Calculation of Available Iron," *J. Am. Diet. Assoc.,* **76**:128–33, 1980.

MUNRO, H. N.: "Major Gaps in Nutrient Allowances. The Status of the Elderly," *J. Am. Diet. Assoc.,* **76**:137–41, 1980.

PASSMORE, R., et al.: "RDAs, Part II: Prescription for a Better British Diet," *Nutr. Today,* **14**:23–27, September/October 1979.

PETERKIN, B. B., et al.: "Some Diets that Meet the Dietary Goals for the United States," *J. Am. Diet. Assoc.,* **74**:423–30, 1979.

ROBINSON, C. H.: "Dietitian's Use of the RDAs," *J. Am. Diet. Assoc.,* **73**:434–37, 1978.

Symposium: "Report of the Task Force on the Evidence Relating Six Dietary Factors to the Nation's Health," *Am. J. Clin. Nutr.,* **32** (Suppl.): 2621–2748, 1979.

4 *Proteins and Amino Acids*

In 1838 a Dutch chemist, Mulder, described certain organic material which is "unquestionably the most important of all known substances in the organic kingdom. Without it no life appears possible on our planet. Through its means the chief phenomena of life are produced."* Berzelius, a contemporary of Mulder, suggested that this complex nitrogen-bearing substance be called *protein* from the Greek word meaning to "take the first place."[1]

Important Issues

Proteins are abundantly supplied in the diets of most people living in the Western world, but protein shortages are second only to energy deficits for people living in the developing nations. The plight of hungry, malnourished children is especially sad. The contrast between the diets of the affluent and the economically deprived is indeed great. On one hand is the abundance of high-quality protein available from animal foods, and on the other a food supply consisting chiefly of plant foods that furnish inadequate amounts as well as quality of protein. That the protein content of the diet has attracted the attention of the public is not surprising. This has led to a number of ambiguous, misleading, or even erroneous ideas.

—People have been encouraged to consume more and more animal foods. To be sure, these foods are excellent sources of high-quality proteins and of other nutrients as well. But how much protein do we really need? What factors influence the need for protein? Are there any dangers attached to the overconsumption of protein-rich foods?

—In the United States vegetarianism is applauded by many and criticized by others. Since most of the world's population consumes diets that are largely, if not completely, made up of plant foods, what are some ways by which the quality of the protein in the diet can be ensured?

—Protein supplements are advertised as aids to increased vitality and well-being. Athletes have been led to believe that their performance will improve if they use such products. Others are convinced that these supplements are needed to replace worn-out tissues. Although patients with some disease states may require protein supplementation of their diets, do healthy people really need them? Do athletes and laborers engaged in vigorous physical activity have an increased need for protein?

—Some advocates of "health foods" proclaim the exceptional nutritional attri-

* Mulder, G. J.: *The Chemistry of Animal and Vegetable Physiology.* Quoted in Mendel, L. B.: *Nutrition: The Chemistry of Life.* Yale University Press, New Haven, Conn., 1923, p. 16.

butes of specific foods: for example, foods rich in nucleoproteins such as organ meats, "red meats", seeds and sprouts, and so on. Based upon the body's metabolism of protein, are such claims valid?

Composition, Structure, and Classification

PROTEIN is now retained as a group name to designate the principal nitrogenous constituents of the protoplasm of all plant and animal tissues; proteins are necessary for the synthesis of all body tissues and for innumerable regulatory functions. To say that proteins are more important than other nutrients is not appropriate, however, for we shall see in the study of nutrition that an inadequate dietary supply or an interference with the utilization of any nutrient can have serious consequences.

Composition Proteins are extremely complex nitrogenous organic compounds in which amino acids are the units of structure. They contain the elements carbon, hydrogen, oxygen, nitrogen, and, with few exceptions, sulfur. Most proteins also contain phosphorus, and some specialized proteins contain very small amounts of iron, copper, and other inorganic elements.

The presence of nitrogen distinguishes protein from carbohydrate and fat. Proteins contain an average of 16 per cent nitrogen and have a molecular weight that varies from 13,000 or less to many millions. Thus, the protein molecule is much larger than those of carbohydrates and lipids. The large protein molecules form colloidal solutions that do not readily diffuse through membranes.

Structure AMINO ACIDS are organic compounds possessing an amino (NH_2) group and an acid or carboxyl (COOH) group. All the amino acids obtained by hydrolysis from native proteins are α-amino acids; that is, the amino group is attached to the carbon adjacent to the acid group. The structure of an amino acid may be represented thus:

$$
\begin{array}{c}
NH_2 \\
| \\
R-C-COOH \\
| \\
H
\end{array}
$$

By varying the grouping (R) that is attached to the carbon containing the amino group, many different amino acids are possible. The R grouping might contain a straight or a branched chain; an aromatic or heterocyclic ring structure; or a sulfur grouping.

Most amino acids are neutral in reaction; that is, they have one amino and one carboxyl group. Amino acids with two carboxyl groups and one amino group are acid in reaction, whereas those with two amino and one carboxyl group are basic in reaction. (See Table 4–1 and Figure 4–1.)

Twenty-two amino acids are widely distributed in proteins, and small amounts of four or five additional amino acids have been isolated from one or more proteins. Some amino acids—ornithine and citrulline—are important intermediates in metabolism but are not constituents of intact proteins. See page 62.

Proteins consist of chains of amino acids joined to each other by the PEPTIDE LINKAGE; that is, the amino group of one amino acid is linked to the carboxyl group of another amino acid by the removal of water. (See Figure 4–2.) Thus, two amino acids form a dipeptide, three amino acids form a tripeptide, and so on. Proteins consist of hundreds of such linkages.

The PRIMARY STRUCTURE of the protein molecule is determined by the chain of amino acids. Chains vary from one another according to (1) the number and kinds of amino acids, (2) the number of times each

Table 4-1. **Classification of Amino Acids**

Classification	Essential Amino Acids	Nonessential Amino Acids
Aliphatic amino acids		
Monoamino-monocarboxylic (neutral reaction)	Threonine Valine* Leucine* Isoleucine*	Glycine Alanine Serine
Sulfur-containing	Methionine	Cysteine
Diamino-dicarboxylic (Sulfur-containing, neutral reaction)		Cystine†
Monoamino-dicarboxylic (acid reaction)		Aspartic acid Glutamic acid
Diamino-monocarboxylic (basic reaction)	Lysine	Arginine Hydroxylysine
Aromatic amino acids		
Monoamino-monocarboxylic (neutral reaction)	Phenylalanine	Tyrosine†
Heterocyclic amino acids		
Monoamino-monocarboxylic (neutral reaction)	Tryptophan Histidine (slightly basic)	Proline Hydroxyproline

*Also referred to as *branched-chain amino acids.*
†Sometimes classed as semiessential. See page 53.

amino acid might appear in the chain, and (3) the length of the chain. A tripeptide consisting of only three amino acids could vary in six ways. With twenty or more amino acids occurring in protein molecules, it becomes evident that almost innumerable combinations are possible.

The SECONDARY STRUCTURE of the protein pertains to bonds such as hydrogen and sulfur that occur between amino acids in the chain that are near, but not adjacent to, each other. The TERTIARY STRUCTURE of the protein refers to the manner in which the amino acid chains are bound together to give the shape and characteristics of performance needed by the protein.

Some estimates place the number of functioning proteins in the human body at more than 100,000. Each protein is synthesized to perform a specific function, and that function cannot be assumed by another. Hemoglobin, insulin, albumin, myosin, keratin, collagen, retinene, and carboxylase are only a few examples of proteins that differ widely in their structure, properties, and functions. Moreover, proteins of one species differ from those of another, for example, pig, horse, and sheep insulin. The latter differences are sometimes the result of substitution of one or two amino acids for another in the peptide chain.

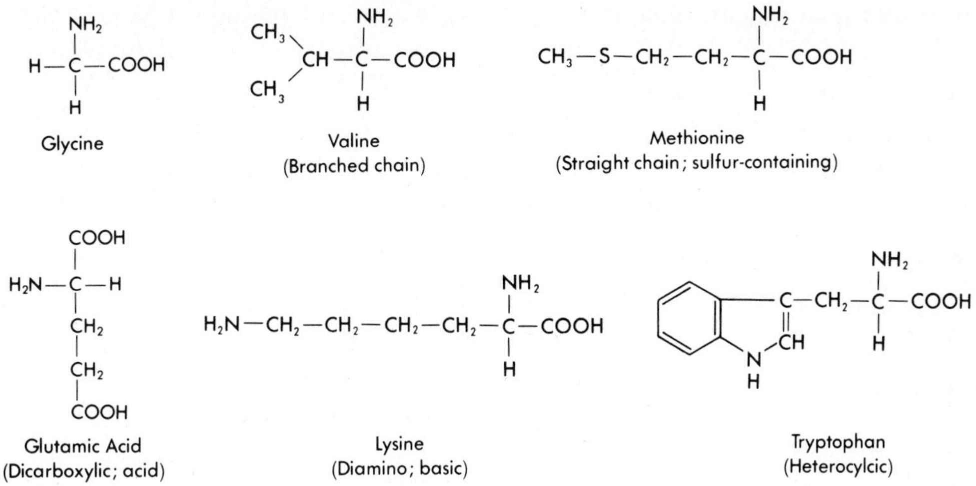

$$\mathrm{H{-}\overset{\displaystyle NH_2}{\underset{\displaystyle H}{C}}{-}COOH}$$

Glycine

$$\mathrm{(CH_3)_2CH{-}\overset{\displaystyle NH_2}{\underset{\displaystyle H}{C}}{-}COOH}$$

Valine
(Branched chain)

$$\mathrm{CH_3{-}S{-}CH_2{-}CH_2{-}\overset{\displaystyle NH_2}{\underset{\displaystyle H}{C}}{-}COOH}$$

Methionine
(Straight chain; sulfur-containing)

$$\mathrm{HOOC{-}CH_2{-}CH_2{-}\overset{\displaystyle COOH}{\underset{\displaystyle H}{C}}{-}NH_2}$$

Glutamic Acid
(Dicarboxylic; acid)

$$\mathrm{H_2N{-}CH_2{-}CH_2{-}CH_2{-}CH_2{-}\overset{\displaystyle NH_2}{\underset{\displaystyle H}{C}}{-}COOH}$$

Lysine
(Diamino; basic)

$$\mathrm{(indolyl)\;C{-}CH_2{-}\overset{\displaystyle NH_2}{\underset{\displaystyle H}{C}}{-}COOH}$$

Tryptophan
(Heterocylcic)

Figure 4–1. Amino acids with different groupings attached to the carbon that holds the amino group.

Classification Proteins may be classified in a number of ways including physical and chemical properties, physical shape, and nutritional properties.

Physical-chemical properties. Each of the three groups within this classification may be subdivided into a number of classes according to solubility.

1. SIMPLE PROTEINS upon hydrolysis by acids, alkalies, or enzymes yield only amino acids or their derivatives. Examples of this group are albumins and globulins found within all body cells and in the blood serum; keratin, collagen, and elastin in supportive tissues of the body and in hair and nails; globin in hemoglobin and myoglobin; and zein in corn, gliadin and glutenin in wheat, legumin in peas, and lactalbumin and lactoglobulin in milk.

2. CONJUGATED PROTEINS are composed of simple proteins combined with a nonprotein substance. This group includes *lipoproteins,* the vehicles for the transport of fats in the blood; *nucleoproteins,* the proteins of the cell nuclei; *phosphoproteins,* such as casein in milk and ovovitellin in eggs; *metalloproteins,* such as the enzymes that contain mineral elements; *mucoproteins,* found in connective tissues, mucin, and gonadotropic hormones; *chromoproteins,* such as

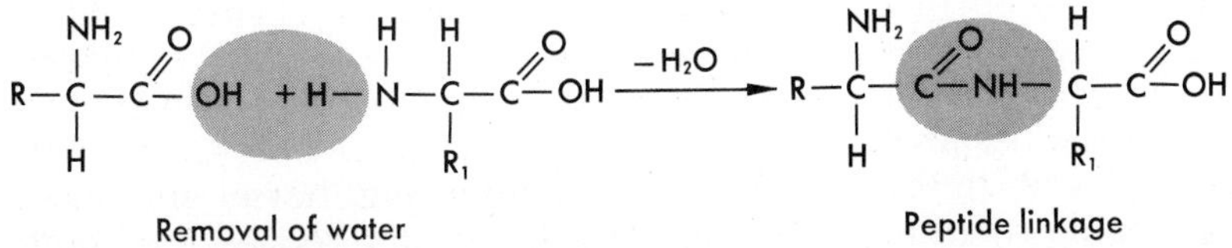

$$\mathrm{R{-}\overset{\displaystyle NH_2}{\underset{\displaystyle H}{C}}{-}\overset{\displaystyle O}{C}{-}OH + H{-}\overset{\displaystyle H}{N}{-}\overset{\displaystyle H}{\underset{\displaystyle R_1}{C}}{-}\overset{\displaystyle O}{C}{-}OH \xrightarrow{-H_2O} R{-}\overset{\displaystyle NH_2}{\underset{\displaystyle H}{C}}{-}\overset{\displaystyle O}{C}{-}NH{-}\overset{\displaystyle H}{\underset{\displaystyle R_1}{C}}{-}\overset{\displaystyle O}{C}{-}OH}$$

Removal of water — Peptide linkage

Figure 4–2. Peptide linkage (CONH). The carboxyl group of one amino acid is linked to the amino group of another amino acid by the removal of water. This reaction is reversed by hydrolysis as in the digestion of proteins.

hemoglobin and visual purple; and *flavoproteins,* which are enzymes that contain the vitamin riboflavin.

3. DERIVED PROTEINS are substances resulting from the decomposition of simple and conjugated proteins. These include rearrangements within the molecule without breaking the peptide bond, such as that occurring with coagulation, and also substances formed by hydrolysis of the protein to smaller fragments.

Physical shape. FIBROUS PROTEINS consist of long polypeptide chains bound together in more or less parallel fashion to form a linear shape. They are generally insoluble in body fluids and give strength to tissues in which they appear. Keratin in hair and nails, collagen in tendons and bone matrices, and elastin in the blood vessel walls are a few examples.

GLOBULAR PROTEINS are chains of amino acids that are coiled and tightly packed together in a round or ellipsoidal shape. They are generally soluble in body fluids and include such proteins as hemoglobin, insulin, enzymes, albumin, and others.

Nutritional properties. The body requires twenty or so amino acids for the synthesis of its proteins. In 1915 Osborne and Mendel observed that rats failed to grow or even survive if some amino acids were omitted from the diet but that the elimination of other amino acids had no such harmful effects. Later work by others, especially Dr. William C. Rose,[2] established that this was also true for human beings. Thus, amino acids came to be classified as *essential or indispensable* and *nonessential or dispensable.* (See Table 4–1.)

ESSENTIAL AMINO ACIDS are those that cannot be synthesized in the body at a rate sufficient to meet body needs. Histidine, for which the requirement by adults has long been uncertain, is now believed to be essential.[3] Thus, the human being requires nine essential amino acids.

Methionine, an essential amino acid, can be converted to cystine, but cystine cannot be converted to methionine. Likewise, phenylalanine can be converted to tyrosine, but tyrosine cannot be converted to phenylalanine. When cystine and tyrosine are present in the diet, the requirements for methionine and phenylalanine are reduced. Thus, cystine and tyrosine are sometimes classified as *semiessential.*

NONESSENTIAL or DISPENSABLE AMINO ACIDS are those that the body can synthesize from an available source of nitrogen and a carbon skeleton. Typical mixed diets contain ample amounts of both essential and nonessential amino acids.

Based upon their content of amino acids, foods are often classified as sources of *complete, partially complete,* or *incomplete proteins.* A COMPLETE PROTEIN contains enough of the essential amino acids to maintain body tissues and to promote a normal rate of growth and is sometimes referred to as having a HIGH-BIOLOGIC VALUE. Egg, milk, and meat (including poultry and fish) proteins are all complete but are not necessarily identical in quality. Wheat germ and dried yeast have a biologic value approaching that of animal sources.

PARTIALLY COMPLETE PROTEINS will maintain life, but they lack sufficient amounts of some of the amino acids necessary for growth. Gliadin, which is one of a number of proteins found in wheat, is a notable example of proteins of this class. Adults under no physiologic stress can maintain satisfactory nutrition for indefinite periods when consuming sufficient amounts of protein from certain cereals or legumes.

Totally INCOMPLETE PROTEINS are incapable of replacing or building new tissue, and hence cannot support life, let alone promote growth. Zein, one of the proteins found in corn, and gelatin are classic examples of proteins that are incapable of even permitting life to continue. This is an inexact and sometimes misleading classification since single foods are rarely eaten alone.

We shall see in the discussion that follows that one food can effectively make up for the lack in another.

Functions

Maintenance and Growth Proteins constitute the chief solid matter of muscles, organs, and endocrine glands. They are major constituents of the matrix of bones and teeth; skin, nails, and hair; and blood cells and serum. In fact, every living cell and all body fluids, except bile and urine, contain protein. The first need for amino acids, then, is to supply the materials for the building and the continuous replacement of the cell proteins throughout life.

Regulation of Body Processes Body proteins have highly specialized functions in the regulation of body processes. Some of these can be classified as follows:

Nucleoproteins contain the blueprint for the synthesis of all body proteins.

Catalytic proteins, that is, the enzymes, number in the thousands to facilitate each step of digestion, absorption, anabolism, and catabolism.

Hormonal proteins set or release the brakes that control metabolic processes.

Immune proteins maintain the body's resistance to disease.

Contractile proteins (myosin, actin) regulate muscle contraction.

Blood proteins include a wide variety of functions. The *transport* proteins ferry nutrients to the tissues; for example, hemoglobin, lipoproteins, transferrin (iron transport), retinol-binding protein (vitamin-A transport), and others. Hemoglobin is involved not only in the transport of oxygen and carbon dioxide but contributes to acid-base balance. The serum proteins, especially serum albumin, are of fundamental importance in the regulation of osmotic pressure and in the maintenance of fluid balance.

Individual amino acids also have specific functions in metabolism. Tryptophan serves as a precursor for niacin and also for serotonin, a vasoconstrictor; methionine supplies labile methyl groups for the synthesis of choline, a compound that helps to prevent storage of fat in the liver; glycine contributes to the formation of the porphyrin ring in the hemoglobin molecule and is also an important constituent of the purines and pyrimidines in nucleic acid.

Energy Proteins are a potential source of energy, each gram of protein yielding on the average 4 kcal. The energy needs of the body take priority over other needs, and if the diet does not furnish sufficient calories from carbohydrate and fat, the protein of the diet as well as tissue proteins will be catabolized for energy. When amino acids are used for energy, they are then lost for synthetic purposes. Conversely, when amino acids are incorporated into the protein molecule, they are not furnishing energy until such time as the tissue proteins are again being catabolized.

Digestion and Absorption

Digestion The purposes of digestion are to hydrolyze proteins to amino acids so that they can be absorbed and to destroy the biologic specificity of the proteins by such hydrolysis. (See also Chapter 2.) The protein to be digested in the intestinal tract includes that provided by food (exogenous source) and also that available from worn-out cells of the mucosa and of the digestive enzymes (endogenous source). The total protein requiring digestion could be as much as 160 gm or so (90 to 100 gm from food and 70 gm from endogenous sources).[4] Within the digestive tract the endogenous and exogenous sources are indistinguishable.

Saliva contains no proteolytic enzyme, and thus the only action in the mouth is an increase in the surface area of the food mass as a result of the chewing of food. Most of the hydrolysis of protein occurs in the stomach, duodenum, and jejunum. The protein molecule is split into smaller fragments by the proteases with final cleavage by the peptidases. The enzymes are secreted in their inactive form and are activated when they are needed for protein hydrolysis. Each enzyme is highly specific and is capable of splitting only one type of peptide linkage. For example, pepsin attacks only those peptide linkages where phenylalanine or tyrosine provides the amino group. The rate of hydrolysis appears to be regulated to the rate of absorption so that there is never a large excess of amino acids in the intestinal lumen. Table 4–2 summarizes the important enzymes in protein digestion and the linkages with which they react.

Table 4-2. **Enzyme Activity in Protein Digestion**

Enzyme and Its Location	Action
Stomach	
Pepsinogen	Activated to pepsin by hydrochloric acid
Pepsin	Splits peptide chain where phenylalanine or tyrosine furnishes amino group
Small intestine	
Trypsinogen*	Activated to trypsin by enterokinase
Trypsin	Splits peptide chain where lysine or arginine furnishes carboxyl group
Chymotrypsinogen*	Activated to chymotrypsin by trypsin
Chymotrypsin	Splits peptide chain where carboxyl group is furnished by tryptophan, methionine, tyrosine, or phenylalanine
Intestinal mucosa	
Aminopeptidase	Splits peptide linkage next to a terminal amino group
Carboxypeptidase*	Splits peptide linkage next to a terminal carboxyl group

*These enzymes are secreted by the pancreas.

Effect of protein denaturation. Proteolytic enzymes not only bring about the splitting of the peptide linkages but they also split the crosslinks that connect the peptide chains. During moderate heating of proteins some of the cross-linkages are split, thereby facilitating digestion. On the other hand, excessive heating results in the formation of linkages that are resistant to the digestive enzymes. As a consequence the amino acids so linked may not be available at a rate that is necessary for incorporation into new proteins.

One resistant linkage known as the *Maillard* or *browning reaction* is that of lysine with carbohydrate as a result of high, usually prolonged heat. Some breakfast cereals processed at high temperatures are subject to such losses. These changes assume some importance when the diet supplies limited amounts of low-quality proteins.

Effect of enzyme inhibitors. Some foods such as navy beans and soybeans contain substances that inhibit the activity of enzymes such as trypsin. Heating inactivates these inhibitors, thereby improving the digestibility of the protein.

Coefficient of digestibility. The digestibility of a protein is the percentage of protein intake that is available for absorption. Since nitrogen from endogenous sources is excreted even when no protein is eaten, a correction must be made to determine the true digestibility of a protein. The determination requires nitrogen analysis of food and of feces. The calculation is as follows:

$$CD = \frac{\text{N intake} - (\text{fecal N} - \text{fecal N on protein-free diet})}{\text{N intake}} \times 100$$

Milk and eggs have a coefficient of digestibility of about 97, meat, fish, and poultry slightly less than that, and plant proteins about 75 to 85. Thus, diets containing substantial amounts of animal foods will have

a higher digestibility than those consisting primarily of plant foods. Typical mixed American diets have a digestibility of about 92 per cent.

Absorption Amino acids are absorbed from the proximal intestine into the portal circulation. The rates of absorption are regulated by complex mechanisms not fully understood. These rates are dependent upon (1) the total load of amino acids released through digestion, (2) the proportions of the various amino acids present in the mixture to be absorbed, (3) the availability of carriers to ferry the amino acids into the mucosal cells, and (4) the uptake of amino acids by tissues. Because the liberation of amino acids through digestion is coordinated with the rate of absorption, there is a minimal loss of amino acids in the feces. The rate of absorption also appears to be controlled by the levels existing in the blood. Amino acids are rapidly removed from the circulation, and the concentration in the blood at any given time is relatively low.

Active transport and specific carriers. Amino acids are absorbed by active transport, but some diffusion of amino acids also occurs. The amino acids are in competition for the carriers, some amino acids being absorbed much more rapidly than others. In one study an essential amino acid mixture in amounts usually present in a protein meal was administered into the jejunum of normal adults, and the rates of absorption were measured.[5] Methionine, leucine, isoleucine, and valine had the highest rates of absorption, and these were two to three times as rapid as that for threonine, which was the lowest. Whether these same rates apply to a protein meal fed intact is not known. If they do, as is strongly suspected, a protein that might contain an excess of a rapidly absorbed amino acid such as leucine would be less effective than a more balanced protein inasmuch as carriers would be less available for the amino acids with the lower rates of absorption.

Metabolism

Strictly speaking, the metabolism of proteins is the metabolism of the amino acids. Each cell within the body utilizes the available amino acids to synthesize all the numerous proteins required for its own functions and also makes use of amino acids to furnish energy. In addition, some specialized cells, such as those of the liver, also synthesize proteins and nonprotein nitrogenous substances that are required for the functioning of the body as a whole. Whether the fate of an amino acid, at any given moment, is that of anabolism or catabolism is determined by a number of interrelated factors.

Methods for Study of Protein Metabolism The biochemist and the nutrition scientist use many techniques for the study of protein metabolism. The nitrogen balance technique described in more detail on page 62 is a classic method for determining the amino acid and protein requirements of human beings under varying conditions. The quality of food proteins has been assayed by animal growth studies, by nitrogen balance studies on animals, and by analyses for amino acid content (see page 64).

Biochemical methods are available for evaluating nutritional status with respect to protein and also for tracing metabolic pathways of amino acids. The determination of hemoglobin, total serum protein, serum albumin, and gamma globulins provides information on the ability to fulfill such diverse functions as supplying oxygen to the tissues, maintaining water balance, and resisting infections. Measurement of the nonprotein nitrogenous constituents of the blood—total nonprotein nitrogen, urea, creatinine, and uric acid—gives clues to renal function. (See Tables A-11 and A-12.) The researcher in cellular nutrition uses highly sophisticated procedures for tracing the pathways of metabolism of individual acids. Many of these studies are possible

today because of automated techniques and the application of computer science.

Dynamic Equilibrium The liver is the key organ in the metabolism of protein. As amino acids are absorbed, the concentration in the portal circulation rises considerably. The liver rapidly removes the amino acids from the portal circulation for the synthesis of its own proteins and for many of the specialized proteins such as lipoproteins, plasma albumins, globulins, and fibrinogen as well as nonprotein nitrogenous substances such as creatine. The liver is also the principal organ for the synthesis of urea.

Amino acids are transported throughout the body by the systemic circulation and are rapidly removed from the circulation by the various tissue cells. Likewise, amino acids and products of amino acid metabolism are constantly added to the circulation by the tissues. The AMINO ACID POOL available to any given tissue at any given moment thus includes dietary sources (exogenous) and tissue breakdown (endogenous sources). These sources are indistinguishable. Body proteins are not static structures, but there is a continuous taking up and release of amino acids. In the adult the gains and losses are about equal, and the state is known as *dynamic equilibrium*. (See Figure 4–3.)

The rate of turnover varies widely in body tissues. The intestinal mucosa, for example, renews itself every one to three days—a fantastic rate of repletion! The liver also has a high rate of turnover. Muscle proteins have a much slower rate of turnover, but the size of the muscle mass in the body is so great that the turnover of muscle protein alone had been estimated to be about 75 gm daily.[4] The turnover rate of collagen is very slow and that of the brain cells is negligible.

Protein reserves. Although the body

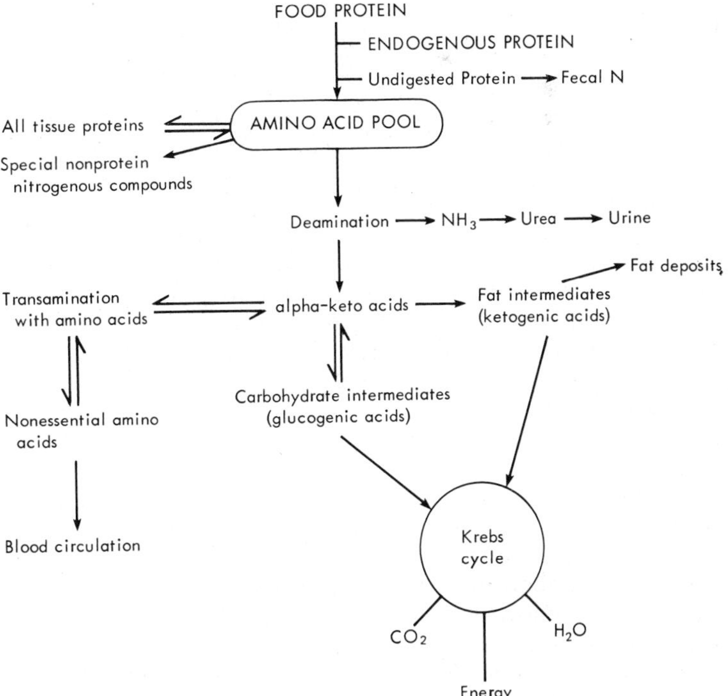

Figure 4–3. Amino acids may be synthesized to body proteins or may be deaminized to yield carbon skeletons that lead to formation of carbohydrates or fats or to the production of energy. By transamination these carbon skeletons can also be used to form nonessential amino acids.

does not store protein in the sense that it stores fat, or glycogen, or vitamin A, certain "reserves" are available from practically all body tissues for use in an emergency. Based upon animal studies, about one fourth of the body protein can be depleted and repleted.[6] Thus, the vital functions of the organism may be protected for 30 to 50 days of total starvation or for much longer periods of partial starvation. It should be apparent that the use of these reserves eventually requires restoration of tissue to their normal protein composition.

Anabolism or Catabolism Whether an amino acid is utilized for the synthesis of new proteins or is deaminized and used for energy depends upon a number of factors.

1. The "all-or-none" law. All the amino acids needed for the synthesis of a given protein must be simultaneously present in sufficient amounts. If a single amino acid is missing, the protein cannot be constructed. If a given amino acid is present only to a limited extent, the protein can be formed only as long as the supply of that amino acid lasts. The amino acid in short supply is known as the LIMITING AMINO ACID. If one or more amino acids are missing from the pool, the remaining amino acids are unavailable for later synthesis and will be catabolized for energy.

2. Adequacy of calorie intake. For protein synthesis to proceed at an optimum rate, the calorie intake must be sufficient to supply the energy needs. A deficiency of calories necessitates the use of some dietary and tissue proteins for energy.

3. The nutritional and physiologic state of the individual. The rate of synthesis is high during growth and in tissue repletion following illness or injury. In the adult synthesis just balances tissue depletion when the calorie intake is adequate.

Protein catabolism is greatly increased immediately following an injury, burns, and immobilization because of illness. It is also increased as a result of fear, anxiety, or anger. For example, unmarried pregnant girls who are worried about their future often have a negative nitrogen balance in spite of diets that appear to be adequate.

4. Development of specific tissues. Some tissues may be synthesized even though the overall nitrogen balance might be negative. Thus, the fetus and maternal tissues may be developed at the expense of the mother when her diet is inadequate. Another example of specific tissue development is that of rapidly growing tumors that use amino acids at the expense of normal tissues.

5. Hormonal controls. The pituitary growth hormone has an anabolic effect during infancy and childhood, and the estrogens and androgens exert an anabolic effect during preadolescent and adolescent years. By bringing about normal carbohydrate metabolism insulin has an indirect anabolic effect by reducing the breakdown of proteins to supply glucose. Insulin probably facilitates the transport of amino acids into the cell. In normal amounts thyroid hormone also stimulates growth.

Among the hormones that increase the catabolism of body tissues are adrenocortical hormones, which stimulate the breakdown of tissue proteins to yield glucose. An excessive production of thyroxine also increases the breakdown of proteins.

Synthesis of Proteins Each cell is capable of synthesizing an enormous number of proteins. Some of these proteins remain with the cell to carry out cellular functions. Other proteins, for example pancreatic enzymes and insulin, leave the cell to carry out specialized functions.

For the synthesis of each protein there must be (1) a source of information or a pattern, (2) a "transcription" of that pattern to the site of synthesis, and (3) a "translation" of that pattern into a new protein. (See Figure 4–4.)

The source of information. The pattern for each protein exists within the nucleus of the cell in giant molecules known as DEOXYRIBONUCLEIC ACID (DNA). The backbone of the molecule consists of two

intertwining chains containing five carbon sugar (deoxyribose) and phosphate groupings to form the long double-helix molecule. Four nitrogenous bases (nucleotides) are joined in pairs and attached by hydrogen bonds to the sugar-phosphate chain to give a firm structure that resembles a spiral staircase. Adenine forms bonds only with thymine; guanine forms bonds only with cytosine. The sequence of the nucleotides in the DNA is the code for the synthesis of new proteins. The coding unit (codon) consists of a combination of three nucleotides.

Transcription. Since the DNA is within the nucleus and protein synthesis takes place in the cytoplasm, how is the code transferred to the site of synthesis? A special type of ribonucleic acid (RNA) called *messenger RNA (mRNA)* brings this about. RNA is very similar to DNA in its structure except that (1) it contains the sugar ribose instead of deoxyribose, (2) the nucleotide uracil replaces thymine, and (3) RNA consists of one strand instead of two. The information from DNA is copied in the nucleus by mRNA which then moves into the cytoplasm to the ribosomes that are the site of protein synthesis.

Translation. Some of the amino acids in the cytoplasm have crossed the cell membrane from the amino acid pool, and other nonessential amino acids may have been synthesized within the cell. Now, let us see how these amino acids are brought to the ribosomes to match up with the pattern brought by mRNA. Each amino acid is activated by a reaction that requires a specific activating enzyme and a source of energy, ATP. The activated amino acid is attached to another kind of RNA, known as *transfer RNA (tRNA).* The amino acid-

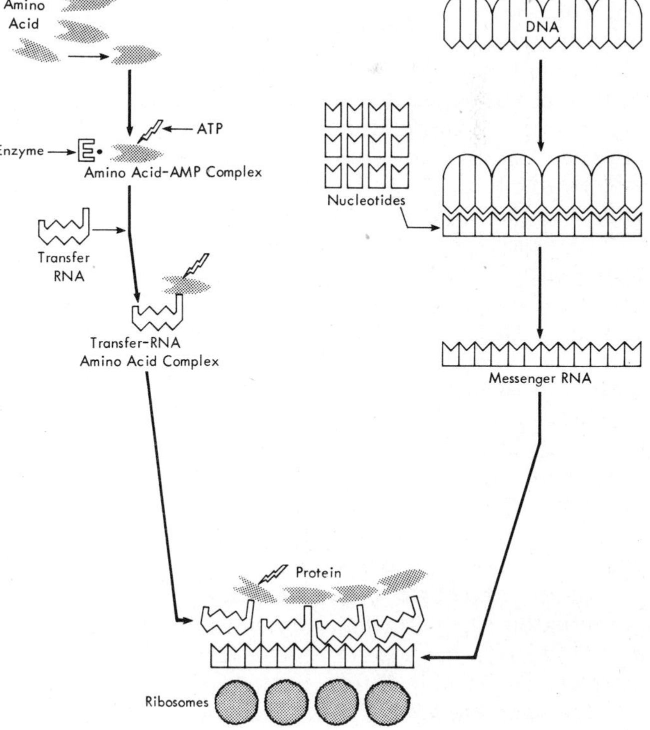

Figure 4–4. (This page) Schematic representation of protein synthesis. The transfer of amino acids by transfer RNA causes the two halves to line up according to the pattern brought from the nucleus by messenger RNA. (Courtesy, Dr. J. Paul Burnett and Eli Lilly and Company.) (Facing page) The Watson-Crick DNA model. Shown here are only a few of the thousands of turns in the double-helix structure of the molecule. The two outer ribbons are the backbone of the molecule, consisting of the sugar *(S)* deoxyribose and phosphate *(P)*. Cross-links between the two ribbons are pairs of bases: adenine *(A)* with thymine *(T)* and guanine *(G)* with cytosine *(C)*. (Courtesy, World Health Organization.)

tRNA complex moves to the ribosomal-mRNA site and is positioned into the peptide linkage in exactly the sequence of the mRNA pattern. When the peptide bond has been formed the tRNA is released so that it can again combine with another activated amino acid to repeat its function.

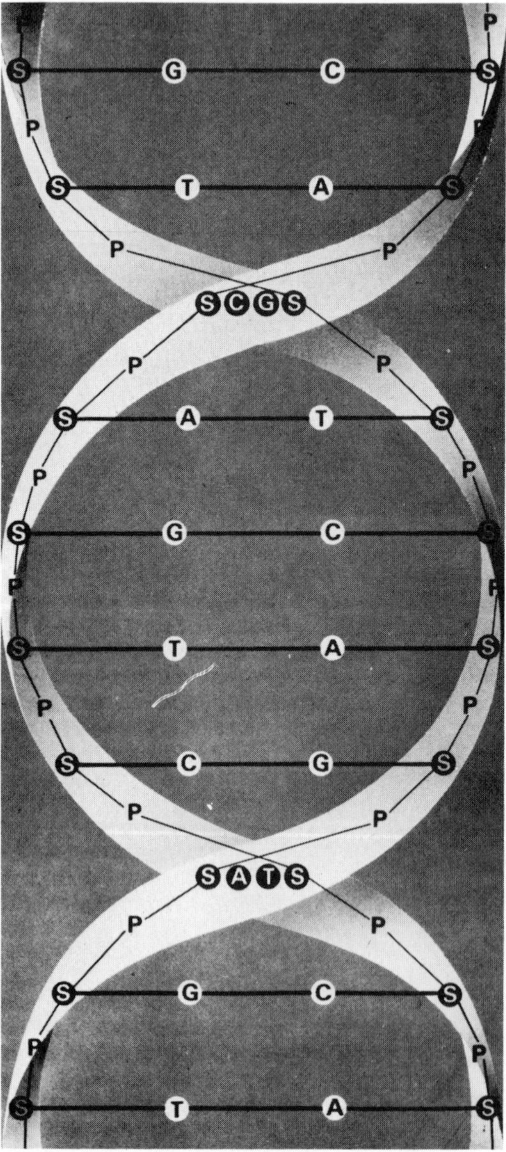

When the new protein molecule is complete, it is released from the template.

The daily protein synthesis in the body has been estimated to be about 300 gm by the adult, an amount that is three to four times the daily intake of protein.[4]

Synthesis of Nonessential Amino Acids The materials for the formation of the nonessential amino acids are keto acids such as pyruvic and α-ketoglutaric acid formed in the metabolism of carbohydrates (see Figure 5–5) and ammonia that is released through deamination of amino acids. The synthesis involves a process known as TRANSAMINATION in which an amino group is transferred to a keto acid. Enzymes known as *transaminases* and pyridoxal phosphate, a coenzyme containing vitamin B-6, are involved. By this mechanism a new amino acid is formed without the appearance of ammonia in the free state. Glutamic acid often serves as a donor of nitrogen in this reaction. The general reaction is as follows:

$$\underset{\text{Amino acid}_1}{R_1CHNH_2COOH} + \underset{\text{Keto acid}_2}{R_2COCOOH} \rightleftarrows \underset{\text{Amino Acid}_2}{R_2CHNH_2COOH} + \underset{\text{Keto acid}_1}{R_1COCOOH}$$

Catabolism When amino acids are used for energy, the amino group is removed and a keto acid remains. Most of the deamination of amino acids occurs in the liver, but some also occurs in the kidney. Ammonia is liberated from the amino acids by oxidative enzymes according to the following general reaction:

$$\underset{\text{Amino acid}}{RCHNH_2COOH} + \tfrac{1}{2}O_2 \rightarrow \underset{\text{Keto acid}}{RCOCOOH} + \underset{\text{Ammonia}}{NH_3}$$

The two fractions resulting from the deamination of the amino acids are disposed of in the following ways.

Keto acids. The keto-acid fractions enter the common pathway for energy metabolism at various points of the cycle depending upon the amino acids from which they were derived. There they may be completely oxidized to yield energy, carbon dioxide, and water. The common pathway for the release of energy is described in Chapter 5 (page 81). (See also Figure 4–5.)

Some of the amino acids, accounting for about 58 per cent of the molecule, are said to be GLUCOGENIC; that is, after deamination they can be synthesized to glucose. Other amino acids, slightly less than half of the protein molecule, are potentially KETOGENIC; that is, they can be synthesized to fat. These distinctions are not fully valid. For example, in Figure 4–5 it may be noted that a number of amino acids are converted to pyruvic acid, which, in turn, can form glucose or can combine with coenzyme A and proceed to form fatty acids.

Disposal of ammonia. Most of the ammonia released through deamination is synthesized to urea. A small amount of ammonia may be used in the formation of new amino acids or purines, pyrimidines, creatine, and other important nonprotein nitrogenous substances. The transfer of amino groups by transamination has been described on page 60.

The liver is the primary organ for the synthesis of urea. This is an essential mechanism for the disposal of ammonia, which is highly toxic if it enters the systemic circulation. When the function of the liver is seriously impaired, ammonia enters the circulation and produces harmful effects on the central nervous system.

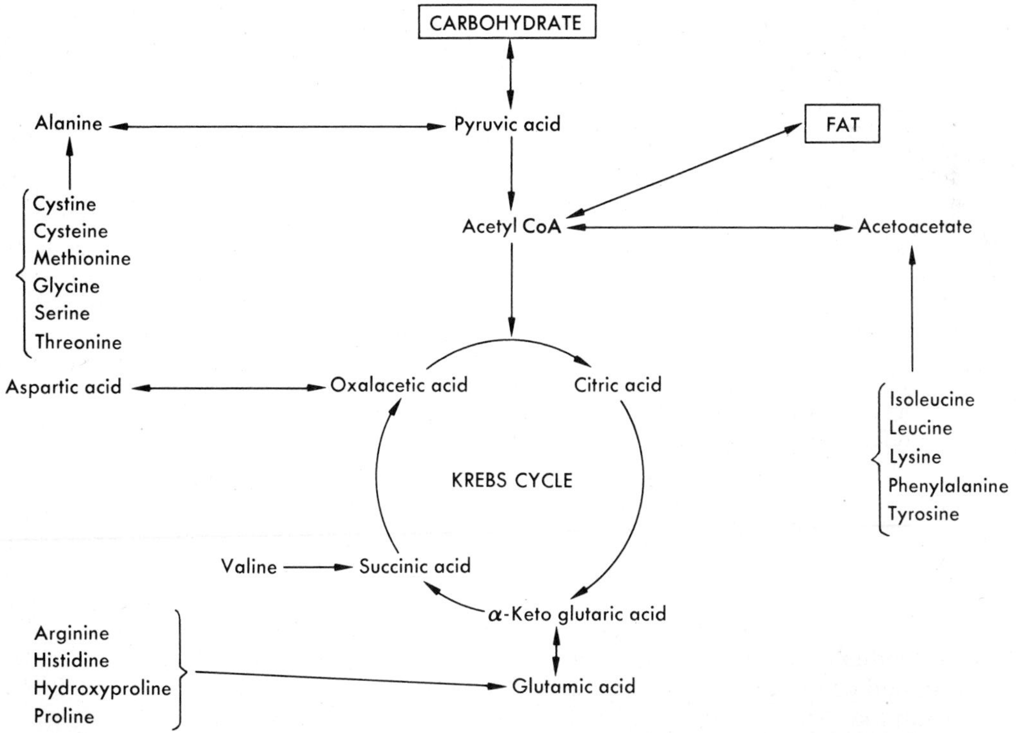

Figure 4–5. Amino acids enter the pathways common to carbohydrate and fat metabolism. Most amino acids are glucogenic; some are ketogenic; and a few may be either ketogenic or glucogenic.

The KREBS-HENSELEIT CYCLE is a mechanism that explains the formation of urea. (See Figure 4–6.) This is an energy-requiring process. The ammonia combines with carbon dioxide (available from oxidation in the Krebs cycle) and ATP to form a carbamyl phosphate. This compound combines with ornithine—an amino acid—to initiate the urea cycle. A second molecule of ammonia is contributed to the cycle from aspartic acid. In the presence of arginase, an enzyme, and magnesium, arginine yields one molecule of urea and of ornithine. Thus, one turn of the cycle has effected the release of ammonia in the form of urea and is able to recycle again.

The excretion of urea and other nitrogenous products in the urine entails an obligatory excretion of fluid as well. In the absence of sufficient fluid the work of the kidney will be increased.

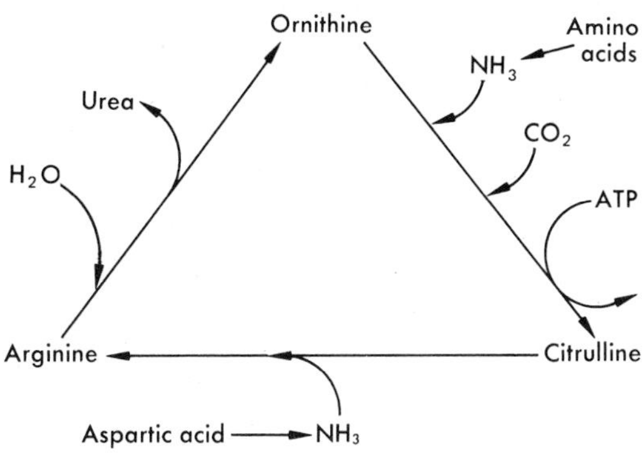

Figure 4–6. The Krebs-Henseleit cycle. A mechanism for disposing of ammonia by urea synthesis.

Dietary Protein Requirements and Allowances

Nitrogen Balance The protein requirement of individuals of varying ages has been determined primarily by the nitrogen balance technique. Nitrogen balance studies are based on the fact that protein, on the average, contains 16 per cent nitrogen; thus, 1 gm nitrogen is equivalent to 6.25 gm protein. The balance may be expressed thus:

Nitrogen balance = Nitrogen intake − nitrogen excretion (urine + feces + skin)

Nitrogen excretion. The fecal nitrogen includes that from undigested dietary protein and also nitrogen from undigested endogenous sources. The latter are composed of the undigested protein fractions of desquamated cells of the intestinal mucosa, the used-up enzymes from the digestive juices, and bacterial cells. The daily fecal excretion of nitrogen by the adult is approximately 1 gm, but this varies with the quality of the protein fed, the gastrointestinal motility, and so on. The difference between the amount of nitrogen in the diet and the fecal nitrogen is the amount of nitrogen absorbed and available for tissue use.

More than 90 per cent of the urinary nitrogen results from the deamination of the amino acids in the body and is excreted chiefly as urea with small amounts of ammonia. Nonprotein nitrogenous end products include creatinine, uric acid, and a number of others. When the calorie intake is fully adequate and the protein intake is just sufficient to cover the repletion of body tissues, the urinary nitrogen is at its lowest level. As the protein intake increases above the tissue maintenance requirement, the excess amino acids are not stored but are deaminized and used for energy or stored as fat, thereby increasing the amount of urinary nitrogen. Therefore, in studies of the minimum protein requirement by the nitrogen balance technique it is always necessary to determine the balance at gradually decreasing levels of intake until the point of negative balance is reached. That level just above negative balance that is just sufficient for tissue replacement represents the *minimum* protein requirement under the conditions of the experiment.

Nitrogen is also lost through perspiration and from the desquamated cells of the skin surfaces, the hair, and the nails. Such losses are extremely difficult to measure. A few studies have shown that the average daily losses by the adult male are about 1.4 gm nitrogen. When people live and work at high environmental temperatures so that sweating is profuse, the losses from the skin have been found to be as high as 3.75 gm nitrogen (equivalent to 23 gm protein) in 24 hours.[7]

States of balance. NITROGEN EQUILIBRIUM is that state of balance when the intake of nitrogen is equal to that which is excreted. A state of equilibrium is normal for the healthy adult. It is established at any level of protein intake that exceeds the minimum requirement, provided that the calorie intake is also adequate.

POSITIVE NITROGEN BALANCE is that state in which the intake of nitrogen exceeds the excretion. It indicates that new protein tissues are being synthesized, as in growing children or during pregnancy. Positive nitrogen balance also occurs when tissues depleted of protein during illness or injury are being replenished, or when muscles are being developed, as in athletic training. Positive nitrogen balance should not be interpreted as storage in the usual sense of the word. There is no further addition of protein to already well-nourished cells.

NEGATIVE NITROGEN BALANCE is that condition in which the excretion of nitrogen exceeds the intake. An individual with a negative nitrogen balance is losing nitrogen from tissues more rapidly than it is being replaced—an undesirable state of affairs. It may occur because (1) the calorie content of the diet is inadequate and therefore tissues are being broken down to supply energy; (2) the quality of the protein is poor and/or the amount fed is inadequate for tissue replacement; or (3) injury, immobilization, or disease are causing excessive breakdown of tissues.

Factors Affecting the Protein Requirement The following list summarizes the factors that determine the protein requirement of a given individual:

1. Sufficient protein for adults is needed to cover daily nitrogen losses in the urine, feces, desquamated skin, hair, nails, perspiration, and other secretions.
2. Essential amino acids must be present in sufficient amounts to meet needs for tissue regeneration.
3. Sufficient calories must be furnished to meet energy needs so that protein is not preferentially used for energy. Thus, carbohydrate and fat "spare" protein for its synthetic functions.
4. Growth needs of infants and children increase the protein requirements per kilogram of body weight.
5. Development of maternal tissues and the fetus during pregnancy increases the protein need.
6. Milk production by the mother increases the protein need.
7. A poor state of nutrition necessitates additional protein for repletion.
8. Infections, immobilization, surgery, burns, and other injuries increase protein catabolism and hence the protein requirement.
9. Emotional stress increases protein catabolism.
10. Diseases of malabsorption can seriously interfere with digestion and absorption, thus increasing the amount of protein needed or the manner of its feeding or both.

Essential amino acid requirements Dr. Rose[8] has determined the quantitative requirements of the essential amino acids for healthy young men by feeding a controlled diet which included a mixture of pure amino acids flavored with lemon juice and sugar, and wafers made of cornstarch, sucrose, centrifuged butterfat, corn oil, and vitamins. Similar studies have been reported for young women and for infants.[9,10] The requirements on the basis of these studies are summarized in Table 4–3; they suffice only when the diet provides enough nitrogen for the synthesis of the nonessen-

Table 4-3. **Estimated Amino Acid Requirements of Man***

Amino Acid	Requirement (per kg of body weight) mg per day Infants§ (4-6 mo)	Child (10-12 yr)	Adult	Amino Acid Pattern for High-Quality Proteins mg/gm of Protein
Histidine	33	?	?	17
Isoleucine	83	28	12	42
Leucine	135	42	16	70
Lysine	99	44	12	51
Total S-containing amino acids†	49	22	10	26
Total aromatic amino acids‡	141	22	16	73
Threonine	68	28	8	35
Tryptophan	21	4	3	11
Valine	92	25	14	48

*Food and Nutrition Board: *Recommended Dietary Allowances,* 9th ed. National Academy of Sciences-National Research Council, Washington, D.C., 1980, p. 43.

†Methionine plus cystine.

‡Phenylalanine plus tyrosine.

§Two grams of protein per kilogram of body weight per day of the quality listed in column 4 would meet the amino acid needs of the infant.

tial amino acids so that the essential amino acids will not be used for this purpose. On a weight basis, it will be noted that the infant requirements are several times higher—a fact that one would expect in view of the high rate of tissue synthesis during infancy. For adults, only 20 per cent of the total nitrogen requirement need be supplied by essential amino acids. For infants, essential amino acids should furnish about 35 per cent of the total nitrogen requirement.[11]

Recommended Protein Allowance On a protein-free diet adequate in calories, the daily nitrogen losses for the adult are as follows:[11]

	mg per kg
Urine	37
Feces	12
Sweat	3
Minor losses through saliva, sputum, menstruation, seminal ejaculation	2
	54

The protein equivalent for this nitrogen loss is 0.34 gm per kilogram (0.054 × 6.25). To allow for individual variability, an intake of 0.45 gm protein per kilogram should cover the daily nitrogen losses, assuming the intake of protein of maximum biologic availability. Although a protein such as egg is almost perfectly utilized at submaintenance levels, there is a loss of efficiency of about 30 per cent as the maintenance level is approached. In addition, allowances must also be made for the efficiency of protein in typical mixed diets. This is estimated to be about 75 per cent of that of egg protein. Thus, one arrives at an allowance of 0.8 gm protein per kg body weight for adults according to the following calculation:

	Protein, gm per kg
Minimum protein requirement using dietary protein of maximum biologic value	0.45
Allowance for loss of efficiency at maintenance level, 30 per cent	0.135
	0.585
Adjustment for 75 percent efficiency in typical mixed diet (0.6 ÷ 0.75)	0.8

The recommended allowance for the 70 kg man is 56 gm protein and, for the 55 kg woman, 44 gm.

Allowances for growth. The allowances for infants are based upon human milk as the source of protein. The allowance decreases from 2.2 gm per kilogram during the first 6 months to 2.0 gm per kilogram for the second half year. For children from 1 to 10 years the daily allowances range from 23 to 34 gm. On the basis of body weight, these are equivalent to 1.8 to 1.2 gm per kilogram, the higher level being given during the second and third years and gradually decreasing with age.

An additional 30 gm protein per day during pregnancy will take care of the growth of the fetus and of the maternal tissues. During lactation, an increase in the protein allowance of 20 gm is satisfactory for the production of an upper limit of 1,200 ml milk.

Quality of Food Proteins

Measurement of Protein Quality The *protein efficiency ratio (PER)* is one of the simplest techniques for determining protein quality. The growth of young rats is observed over 28 days while they are fed an adequate diet which contains the test protein. The ratio is calculated thus:

$$\text{PER} = \frac{\text{grams weight gain}}{\text{grams protein consumed}}$$

Animal foods, except gelatin, yield high ratios, and plant foods have lower, widely varying ratios.

The PER is used as the basis for the USRDA labeling standard (see page 325). The standard is 45 gm for foods that have a PER equal to or greater than that of casein (PER = 2.5). The standard is 65 gm for foods that have a PER less than casein.

Amino acid score (chemical score). The protein quality of a food can be determined by comparing its amino acid composition with the amino acid pattern of a reference protein such as the high-quality protein listed in the right column of Table 4–3. The calculation of the score for each amino acid is as follows:

$$\text{AA score} = \frac{\text{milligrams of amino acid in 1 gm test protein}}{\text{milligrams of amino acid in 1 gm high-quality protein}} \times 100$$

The amino acid that has the lowest score for any of the nine essential amino acids is the limiting amino acid for that protein. Amino acid scores do not take the absorption of amino acids into account, and thus the actual utilization from a given food might differ.

Table 4–4 shows a comparison of the scores for the three limiting amino acids in beans and rice. Note that methionine plus cystine is most limiting in beans, while lysine is most limiting in rice. But when beans and rice are eaten together, the two foods are *complementary*, or each may be said to *supplement* the other.

Biologic value (BV). The biologic value is the percentage of absorbed nitrogen that is retained by the body. This determination requires measurement of the nitrogen content of food ingested and of the urinary and fecal excretions by the test animal under controlled conditions with the protein intake set below the requirement level.[11] In order to arrive at the true biologic value it is also necessary to take into account the urinary and fecal nitrogen excretion (N_0) that would occur when a protein-free diet is fed. The following equation shows the calculation:

$$\text{BV} = \frac{\text{Food N} - [(\text{urine N} - N_0) + (\text{fecal N} - N_0)]}{\text{Food N} - (\text{fecal N} - N_0)} \times 100$$

Table 4-4. **Comparison of the Content of Three Limiting Amino Acids in Beans and Rice with a High-Quality Protein**

	Lysine	Methionine +Cystine	Tryptophan
Amino acid pattern for high-quality protein,*			
Milligrams per gram protein	51	26	11
Beans			
Milligrams per gram protein	74	20	9
Amino acid score	145	77†	82
Rice			
Milligrams per gram protein	39	32	11
Amino acid score	77†	123	100
Average, rice and beans			
Milligrams per gram protein	57	26	10
Amino acid score	112	100	90†

*See Table 4-3 for pattern for high-quality protein.
†Limiting amino acid.

A protein that has a biologic value of 70 or more is capable of supporting growth provided that sufficient calories are also ingested. Biologic values of typical protein sources are as follows: egg, 100; milk, 93; rice, 86; casein, fish, and beef, 75; corn, 72; peanut flour, 56; and wheat gluten, 44.

Net protein utilization (NPU). This is the proportion of nitrogen consumed that is retained by the body under standard conditions. It takes into account the digestibility of food proteins. When food proteins are completely digested, the NPU and BV would be the same. When foods contain much fiber and have a lower digestibility, the NPU would be lower than the BV.

Like the biologic value, the intake of nitrogen and the urinary and fecal nitrogen must be determined. A correction must also be made for the nitrogen excretion on a protein-free diet.

$$NPU = \frac{\text{Food N} - [(\text{urine N} - N_0) + (\text{fecal N} - N_0)]}{\text{Food N}} \times 100$$

Improving Protein Quality of Foods Most of the world's people consume diets in which the protein is derived principally or solely from plant foods. When foods are combined so that they supply sufficient amounts of all essential amino acids satisfactory protein nutrition is possible. This state is more readily achieved for adults than for infants and children. The principle of complementarity provides several possibilities for improving the protein quality of foods.

The vegetarian way. In the United States millions of people have adopted vegetarian diets for religious, ecologic, or economic reasons. (See pages 286–288 for fuller description.)

Lactovegetarians consume milk and cheese along with a variety of plant foods. Lacto-ovo-vegetarians eat eggs as well as milk and cheese. When appreciable amounts of plant proteins are fed with a small amount of animal protein foods, the quality of the mixture is as effective as if only animal proteins had been fed. For example, small amounts of milk, cheese, or egg will supply the lysine that is limiting in cereal foods. Thus, macaroni and cheese, cereal and milk, and bread and milk are complementary.

Legumes, whole grains, nuts, and vegetables provide a satisfactory combination of amino acids for pure vegetarians.[12] A recent study on preschool children has shown that smallness, lightness, and leanness was characteristic of vegetarian children. These characteristics were more pronounced in the older children who had not been breast-fed and who had a limited variety of foods.[13]

In order for plant foods to supply all essential amino acids simultaneously, food combinations must be consumed at the same meal. The amino acid composition of foods within each category varies considerably; thus, selections should be made from a variety within each category.

Legumes (low in methionine plus cystine; good sources of lysine): peas, chickpeas (garbanzos), black-eyed peas, white beans, red beans, Lima beans, soybeans, peanuts, lentils

Cereal grains, nuts, seeds (low in lysine; good sources of methionine plus cystine): whole wheat, cracked wheat, bulgur, oatmeal, millet, rye, barley, cornmeal; almonds, Brazil nuts, cashews, filberts, pecans, walnuts; pumpkin, sesame, and sunflower seeds

Vegetarian diets that offer little variety can be extremely dangerous. One example is the Zen macrobiotic diet in which the final stage consists principally of brown rice.[14] It is true that rice can meet the protein needs of the healthy adult when sufficient amounts are consumed to also meet caloric requirements. But rice alone cannot meet the protein needs of infants, children, pregnant women, and protein-depleted persons. Moreover, a diet consisting principally of rice fails to supply essential minerals and vitamins, and metabolic de-

Table 4–5. **Average Protein Content of Foods in Four Food Groups***

Food	Average Serving	Protein gm	Protein Quality Limiting Amino Acids
Milk Group			
Milk, whole or skim	1 cup	8	Complete
Nonfat dry milk	0.8 ounce (3–5 tablespoons)	8	Complete
Cottage cheese	2 ounces	8	Complete
American cheese	1 ounce	7	Complete
Ice cream	1/8 quart	3	Complete
Meat Group			
Meat, fish, poultry	3 ounces, cooked	15–25	Complete; higher protein for lean cuts
Egg	1 whole	6	Complete
Dried beans or peas	1/2 cup cooked	7–8	Incomplete; methionine
Peanut butter	1 tablespoon	4	Incomplete; several amino acids borderline
Seeds (sunflower; sesame)	1/4 cup	9	Incomplete; lysine
Vegetable-Fruit Group			
Vegetables	1/2 cup	1–3	Incomplete
Fruits	1/2 cup	1–2	Incomplete
Bread-Cereals Group			
Breakfast cereals, wheat	1/2 cup cooked 3/4 cup dry	2–3	Incomplete; lysine
Bread, wheat	1 slice	2–3	Incomplete; lysine
Macaroni, noodles, spaghetti	1/2 cup cooked	2–3	Incomplete; lysine
Rice	1/2 cup cooked	2	Incomplete; lysine and threonine
Cornmeal and cereals	1/2 cup cooked	2	Incomplete; lysine and tryptophan

*These values represent approximate group averages. For specific food items, consult Table A–1, in the Appendix.

rangements occur, including interference with protein metabolism.

Amino acid supplementation. Lysine and methionine can be produced at costs sufficiently low to make it practical to add them to foods in which they are limiting. Thus, the addition of lysine to white bread improves the biologic value of the bread. Amino acid supplementation is not yet employed in food processing because the possibility exists that the addition of one or more amino acids could create an imbalance of amino acids in low-protein diets which would actually retard growth.

Plant food mixtures. In many developing countries animal protein sources are scarce and expensive. For children a protein supply of satisfactory quality is particularly critical. A number of mixtures using locally available plant foods have been developed that are comparable to milk in their biologic value. *Incaparina,* a mixture of cottonseed and corn flours, torula yeast, vitamins, and minerals has been used successfully in Central America. (See also page 433.)

Food Sources of Protein

Protein Content of Foods The average protein composition of common foods is shown in Table 4–5. The protein concentration is high in dry milk, meat, poultry, fish, cheese, and nuts; intermediate in eggs, legumes, flours, cereals, and liquid milk; and low in most fruits and vegetables. One pint of liquid milk furnishes one fourth to one third of the recommended allowance for most age categories. Breads and cereals supply an appreciable amount of protein by virtue of the amounts consumed in a day.

The protein contribution made by the recommended number of servings from each food group in the Basic Diet is shown in Figure 4–7. About three fourths of this pro-

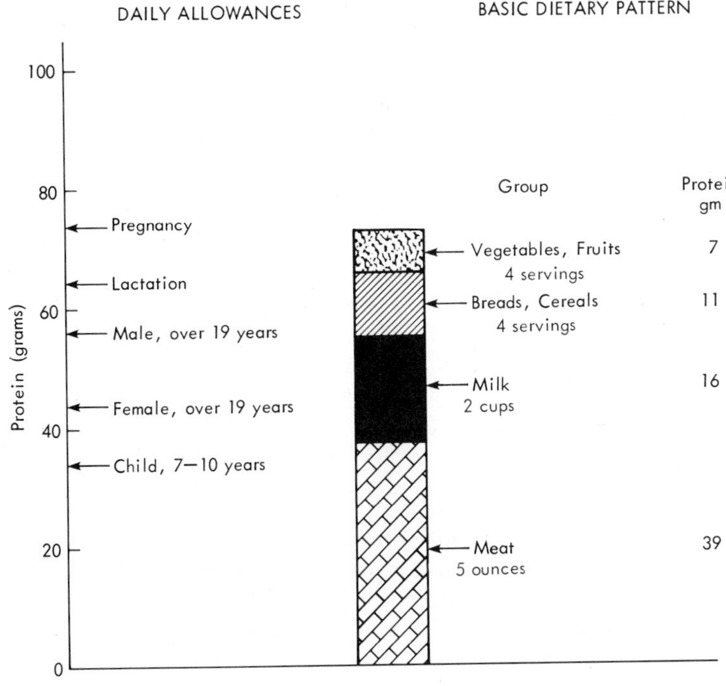

Figure 4–7. The Basic Diet furnishes sufficient protein to meet the recommended dietary allowances for most categories of the population. The addition of 1 cup of milk or 1 ounce of meat will fulfill the increased needs of the pregnant woman. Note that the milk and meat groups supply about three fourths of the total protein in this pattern. See Table 13–2 for complete calculations.

tein is supplied by high-quality protein from animal sources. Inasmuch as some of the foods added to this Basic Diet would contain some protein, the daily intake would be more than sufficient to meet the needs of healthy people of all ages.

The Basic Diet pattern and typical American diets furnish substantially more protein than is recommended by the Food and Nutrition Board. A protein-rich diet is also likely to supply much of the requirement for some minerals such as iron and other trace minerals as well as the B-complex vitamins. Indeed, if the protein intake were to be kept at recommended levels, good dietary planning would become difficult.

Protein in the United States Food Supply Since 1910 the available food supply has furnished 88 to 103 gm protein per capita daily. This corresponds to approximately 12 per cent of the calories available in the food supply. Although the total protein available in the food supply has not varied greatly from year to year, the sources of this protein have changed significantly. In 1910 just over half of the protein was derived from animal sources and more than a third was obtained from flour and cereal foods. Gradually the consumption of animal foods has increased and that of flour-cereal foods decreased until presently more than two thirds of the protein is derived from animal sources and about one sixth from flour-cereal foods. (See Table 4–6.)

Table 4-6. **Sources of Protein in the American Food Supply**

Food Group	Percentage Contribution to the Total Protein Supply		
	1909–1913	1957–1959	1980
Meat, poultry, fish	29.9	35.7	42.9
Dairy, excluding butter	16.4	24.5	20.2
Eggs	5.2	6.8	4.9
Total—animal sources	51.5	67.0	68.0
Flour, cereals	35.8	19.9	18.8
Dry beans, peas, nuts	4.5	5.2	5.5
Potatoes, sweet potatoes	4.2	2.4	2.3
Other vegetables, and fruits	3.7	5.0	5.0
Total—plant sources	48.2	32.5	31.6

U.S. Food Consumption: Sources of Data and Trends, 1909–63. Statistical Bulletin No. 364, U.S. Department of Agriculture, Washington, D.C., 1965.

Marston, R. M., and Peterkin, B. B.: "Nutrient Content of the National Food Supply," *National Food Review,* U.S. Department of Agriculture, Washington, D.C., Winter 1980.

Marston, R. M., and Welsh, S. O.: "Nutrient Content of the National Food Supply" National Food Review, U.S. Department of Agriculture, Washington, D.C., Winter 1981.

Effects of Protein Excess or Deficiency

Liberal Protein Intakes Although protein intakes by most people in the United States far exceed the recommended allowances, there is no evidence that such intakes by healthy persons are harmful. Arctic explorers who consumed diets consisting mainly of meats for several years showed no pathologic effects. Consumption of a high-protein diet is wasteful, however. Since the body does not store protein in the sense that it stores other nutrients, the excess amino acids are deaminized and then enter the common pathway of metabolism for fat and carbohydrate. Protein foods thus entail more work for the liver and kidney and also cost more in the marketplace.

High-protein diets are undesirable in some circumstances. As the protein intake increases, calcium absorption is reduced. (See Chapter 8.) With an increase in nitrogenous wastes there is an increased need for water to excrete them. Premature and very young infants do not have the ability to excrete the additional nitrogenous wastes incurred from high-protein formulas. Persons who have chronic renal failure also have less ability to excrete nitrogenous wastes, and blood urea levels are elevated when protein is fed in excess of synthetic needs.

Diets that provide a high proportion of protein from animal sources also furnish considerable amounts of saturated fats and cholesterol, two factors that can lead to elevation of serum cholesterol and low-density lipoproteins. The intake of saturated fats and cholesterol can be effectively reduced in the following ways without affecting the nutritive quality of the diet.

1. Substitute low-fat or skim milk for whole milk and low-fat cheeses for whole-milk cheeses.
2. Select only lean cuts of meat; trim off visible fat.
3. Use more poultry, fish, and legumes, and less beef.
4. Restrict the size of portions of meat, poultry, and fish to the recommended 4 to 5 ounces daily.

Protein Deficiency The Household Food Consumption Survey, the Ten-State Nutrition Study, and the Health and Nutrition Examination Survey (HANES) showed that the mean intakes of protein for each age-sex category exceeded the recommended allowances.[15] Within each group, however, some individuals had protein intakes below standard. For example in the Ten-State Survey, limited primarily to low-income groups, one third of 12- to 16-year-old girls had lower protein intakes, probably because of calorie and weight consciousness. The HANES data showed that protein intakes were below standard for 12 per cent of children 1 to 5 years, 32 per cent of women 18 to 44 years, and 27 per cent of persons over 60 years. The protein intake per 1,000 kcal was 38 to 40 gm and varied little regardless of income. Thus, the failure to ingest the recommended amount of protein appeared to be related to the inadequate quantity of food. The lower intakes of protein were not correlated with lower blood protein levels. In fact, not a single case of severe protein deficiency showing clinical signs and a serum albumin below 2.5 gm was found in the HANES survey.

Clinicians sometimes do encounter persons with protein deficiency. Among these are young children who have had diets grossly deficient in protein and calories because of parental abuse or ignorance. Pregnant women who are ignorant of the essentials of a good diet or who place emphasis on a low-calorie diet are more likely to have anemia, miscarriages, and premature births. (See Chapter 18.) Some elderly people show signs of protein deficiency because their incomes are too small to purchase enough food, they have insufficient understanding of their nutritional needs, they lack the incentive to cook and eat, and they have little appetite because of poor health.

A protein intake that fails to meet the individual requirements leads first to depletion of tissue reserves and then to a lowering of the blood protein levels. Nutritional edema is a clinical sign but it does not appear until substantial depletion of tissue reserves has taken place and the serum albumin level is decreased. It must be differentiated from the edema that is caused by fluid-electrolyte imbalance in cardiac failure. Protein deficiency sometimes becomes abruptly evident when an infection, injury, or surgery occur.

Protein-Calorie Malnutrition (PCM) On a worldwide basis the shortage of protein is second only to the shortage of calories. Protein-calorie malnutrition, also known as protein-energy malnutrition (PEM), is a broad term that encompasses kwashiorkor and marasmus together with milder stages of these diseases. Literally millions of infants and young children are victims of these diseases in Asia, Africa, Central America, the West Indies, and South America. Many of the children who survive are unable to achieve their full physical growth and development. Even more serious is the threat that the most severely malnourished may be retarded in their mental development, and that this retardation may be irreversible.

KWASHIORKOR (meaning "the displaced child") occurs in children shortly after weaning, usually between the ages 1 and 4 years, and is characterized by growth failure, skin lesions, edema, and changes in hair color. The liver is extensively infiltrated with fat. The principal dietary defect is a lack of good quality protein in the foods available to the child when he or she is weaned. (See Figure 4–8.)

MARASMUS (from a Greek word meaning "withering") is usually seen at a somewhat earlier age than kwashiorkor and is caused by a deficiency of both protein and calories. Growth failure is even more severe than in kwashiorkor, but edema is usually absent. Not infrequently the deficiency has resulted because the mother has substituted inadequate quantities of a formula for breast milk. (See also Chapter 23.)

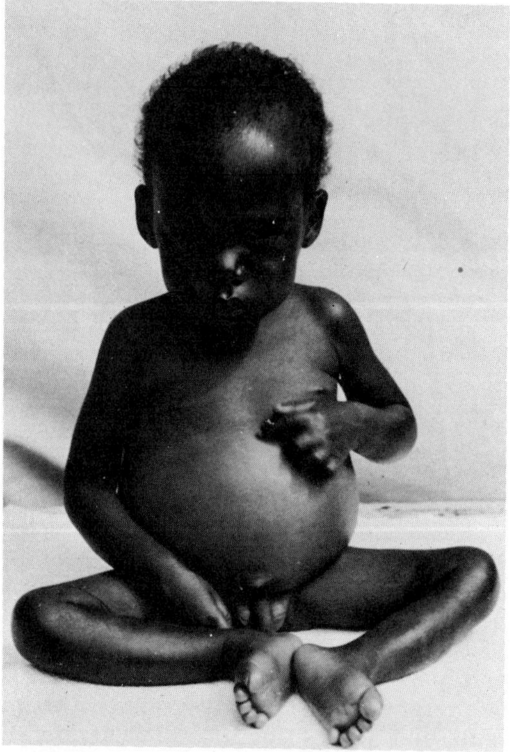

Figure 4–8. Child suffering from kwashiorkor—Africa. (Courtesy, M. Autret and the Food and Agriculture Organization.)

Some Points for Emphasis in Nutrition Education

1. Proteins are made up of building units called amino acids. They are required by people of all ages to replace the tissues that are constantly being broken down. Children and pregnant and lactating women need additional protein for synthesis of new proteins.
2. Proteins, like carbohydrates and fats, contribute calories to the diet. If too few calories are included in the diet, protein will be used for energy. Then it cannot also be used for building tissues.
3. Muscular work does not increase the requirement for protein.
4. Nine amino acids, called essential, must be supplied in the diet because the body cannot make them.
5. Animal protein foods, except gelatin, are complete because they contain balanced proportions of the essential amino acids. Include some good-quality protein at each meal.
6. About one seventh to one sixth of the day's allowance for protein for the adult will be supplied by 1 ounce meat, fish, or poultry, or 1 cup milk, or 1 egg, or 1 ounce cheese.
7. Proteins from plant foods are incomplete but they are useful in reducing the amount of expensive animal protein that is needed. Breads, cereals, dry beans and peas, and peanut butter when combined with small amounts of eggs, cheese, meat, fish, and poultry give just as good an assortment of amino acids as a large amount of animal foods.

8. In vegetarian diets a variety of plant proteins can provide the amounts and kinds of essential amino acids required. Thus, cereal grains and legumes when consumed together provide satisfactory biologic value. Since the protein concentration in plant foods is lower than that in flesh foods, the bulk of the diet is greater.

Problems and Review

1. Key terms: amino acid; amino acid pool; biologic value; browning reaction; coefficient of digestibility; complete protein; deoxyribonucleic acid; essential amino acid; glucogenic acid; incomplete protein; ketogenic acid; kwashiorkor; marasmus; net protein utlization; nitrogen balance; nonessential amino acid; peptide linkage; protein complementarity; protein efficiency ratio; ribonucleic acid; urea cycle.
2. Describe the synthesis of tissue proteins. Under what circumstances would synthesis be accelerated?
3. List four ways in which proteins are used in the regulation of body functions.
4. Explain why proteins are considered to be a wasteful source of energy.
5. *Problem.* Prepare an outline or diagram that shows the steps in the digestion of protein.
6. Under what circumstances does positive nitrogen balance occur? negative nitrogen balance?
7. How can you explain the fact that a person on a low-protein, high-calorie diet is less likely to go into negative nitrogen balance than one who is on a low-calorie diet of the same protein level?
8. How can you explain the fact that some vegetarians maintain good protein nutrition while others do not?
9. *Problem.* Plan a diet for a woman that provides 44 gm of protein, of which not more than one third is in the form of animal protein. What foods are especially important in such a diet plan?
10. What happens to protein that is eaten in excess of body requirements? Why is it important to provide a margin of safety in planning for the daily protein allowance?
11. What foods would you include in your own diet to ensure an adequate protein intake? How would you modify this plan for a growing child?
12. *Problem.* A diet contains 3,000 kcal and 150 gm of protein. What percentage of the calories is supplied by protein?
13. *Problem.* One pint of milk supplies 18 gm of protein. What amounts of these foods would be required to replace the protein of the milk: nonfat dry milk; ice cream; Cheddar cheese; eggs; halibut; beef liver; sirloin steak; peanut butter; dry navy beans; oatmeal? How does the quality of protein in the various foods listed compare?
14. *Problem.* On the basis of current market prices, calculate the cost for the amounts of foods which were needed to replace the protein of 1 pint milk (problem 13). What conclusions can you draw from this calculation?
15. A friend asks you whether she should buy lysine-enriched bread in preference to the usual enriched loaf of bread. How would you reply?
16. What are the effects of insufficient protein in the diet?

Cited References

1. Vickery, H. B.: "The Origin of the Word Protein," *Yale J. Biol. Med.*, **22**:387–93, 1950.
2. Rose, W. C., et al.: "Further Experiments on the Role of Amino Acids in Human Nutrition," *J. Biol. Chem.*, **148**:457–58, 1943.

3. Kopple, J. D., and Swendseid, M. E.: "Evidence That Histidine Is an Essential Amino Acid in Normal and Chronically Uremic Man," *J. Clin. Invest.*, **55**:881–91, 1975.
4. Crim, M. C., and Munro, H. N.: "Protein," in *Present Knowledge in Nutrition*, 4th ed., The Nutrition Foundation, Inc., Washington, D.C., 1976.
5. Adibi, S. A., and Gray, S. J.: "Intestinal Absorption of Essential Amino Acids in Man," *Gastroenterology*, **52**:837–45, 1967.
6. Allison, J. B., and Wannamacher, R. N., Jr.: "The Concept and Significance of Labile and Over-all Protein Reserves of the Body," *Am. J. Clin. Nutr.*, **16**:445–52, 1965.
7. Consolazio, C. F.: "Comparison of Nitrogen, Calcium, and Iodine Excretion in Arm and Total Body Sweat," *Am. J. Clin. Nutr.*, **18**:443–48, 1966.
8. Rose, W. C., et al.: "The Amino Acid Requirements of Man. XV. The Valine Requirements: Summary and Final Observations," *J. Biol. Chem.*, **217**:987–95, 1955.
9. Leverton, R. M., et al.: "The Quantitative Amino Acid Requirements of Young Women," *J. Nutr.*, **58**:59, 83, 219, 341, 355, 1956.
10. Holt, L. E., and Snyderman, S. E.: "The Amino Acid Requirements of Children," in Cole, W. H., ed.: *Some Aspects of Amino Acid Supplementation.* Rutgers University Press, New Brunswick, N.J., 1956, pp. 60–68.
11. Food and Nutrition Board: *Recommended Dietary Allowances*, 9th ed. National Academy of Sciences–National Research Council, Washington, D.C., 1980.
12. Hardinge, M. G., et al.: "Nutritional Studies of Vegetarians. V. Proteins and Essential Amino Acids," *J. Am. Diet. Assoc.*, **48**:25–28, 1966.
13. Dwyer, J. T., et al.: "Preschoolers on Alternate Life-style Diets," *J. Am. Diet. Assoc.*, **72**:264–70, 1978.
14. Council on Foods and Nutrition: "Zen Macrobiotic Diets," *JAMA.*, **218**:397, 1971.
15. Chopra, J. G., et al.: "Protein in the U.S. Diet," *J. Am. Diet. Assoc.*, **72**:253–58, 1978.

Additional References

CLARK, H. E., et al.: "Ability of 6 grams of Nitrogen from a Combination of Rice, Wheat, and Milk to Meet Protein Requirements of Young Men for 4 weeks," *Am. J. Clin. Nutr.*, **31**:585–91, 1978.

CONSOLAZIO, C. F., et al.: "Protein Metabolism during Intensive Physical Training in the Young Adult," *Am. J. Clin. Nutr.*, **28**:29–35, 1975.

Expert Committee, FAO–WHO: *Energy and Protein Requirements.* WHO Tech. Rep. 522, World Health Organization, Geneva, 1973.

HEGSTED, D. M.: "Assessment of Nitrogen Requirements," *Am. J. Clin. Nutr.*, **31**:1669–71, 1978.

HUANG, P-C., et al.: "Protein Requirements of Men in a Hot Climate. Decreased Urinary Losses Concomitant with Increased Sweat Nitrogen Losses during Exposure to High Environmental Temperature," *Am. J. Clin. Nutr.*, **28**:494–501, 1975.

MILLER, J., et al.: "Protein Component of Several Multi-component Commercially Prepared Foods," *J. Am. Diet. Assoc.*, **75**:262–64, 1979.

RAO, C. N., et al.: "Influence of Varying Energy Intake on Nitrogen Balance in Men on Two Levels of Protein Intake," *Am. J. Clin. Nutr.*, **28**:1116–21, 1975.

Review: "Human Protein Deficiency—Biochemical Changes and Functional Implications," *Nutr. Rev.*, **35**:294–96, 1977.

RICHARDSON, D. P., et al.: "The Effect of Dietary Sucrose on Protein Utilization in Healthy Young Men," *Am. J. Clin. Nutr.*, **33**:264–72, 1980.

SCRIMSHAW, N. S.: "Through a Glass Darkly: Discerning the Practical Implications of Human Dietary Protein-Energy Interrelationships," *Nutr. Rev.*, **35**:321–37, 1977.
WILLIAMS, C. D.: "The Story of Kwashiorkor," *Nutr. Rev.*, **31**:334–40, 1973.
ZANNI, E., et al.: "Protein Requirements of Elderly Men," *J. Nutr.*, **109**:513–24, 1979.

5 *Carbohydrates*

THE ability of plants to harness solar energy in usable form is basic to the continuance of life by all species. All energy and inorganic nutrients for human use are first processed by microorganisms, plants, and animals. Starches and sugars stored in the leaves, stems, fruits, seeds, and roots of plants supply from 45 to 80 per cent of the energy requirements of people throughout the world. The human body has remarkably efficient although complex mechanisms for the conversion of plant energy to meet the moment-by-moment needs for all involuntary and voluntary activities.

Current Issues

Two aspects of carbohydrate nutrition are of particular concern to the public at the present time.

1. Sugars account for 24 per cent of the caloric composition of the American diet. According to the Dietary Goals (see page 42) an intake of 10 per cent of calories as refined sugar is preferable. What are the effects of a high sugar intake on nutritive adequacy? What advantages would be gained by substituting starchy foods for part of the sugar? What evidence exists that a high sugar intake contributes to disease? What dietary adjustments can be made to reduce sugar intake?
2. High-fiber diets are a current fashion with many consumers and health professionals alike. Are the claims that a liberal intake of fiber will reduce the risks of gastrointestinal disorders, cancer of the colon, coronary heart disease, and many other disease conditions justified? What are the characteristics of dietary fiber? How does fiber react within the intestinal environment? We shall see that there are some answers for these concerns, but there are also theories that remain to be proven.

Photosynthesis An exceedingly complex process known as PHOTOSYNTHESIS is used by plants to synthesize the carbohydrate that is unique for each plant. Sunlight is absorbed by several pigments in the plant, the most important of which is the green pigment, CHLOROPHYLL. The absorbed solar energy is used by the plant to bring about a complicated sequence of chemical reactions that essentially transfer two atoms of hydrogen from a molecule of water to a molecule of carbon dioxide. As a result there is the release of oxygen to the air and the fixation of carbon as carbohydrate.

$$6\ CO_2 + 6\ H_2O + \text{light energy} \xrightarrow[\text{plant enzymes}]{\text{chlorophyll}} \underset{\text{chemical energy}}{C_6H_{12}O_6} + 6\ O_2$$

The plant uses some of the carbohydrate to meet its own metabolic needs such as the synthesis of the amino acids that make up its proteins. The rest is stored in the form of polysaccharides. Carbohydrates are the most abundant compounds in the universe. Cellulose, which makes up the structural parts of plants, accounts for about half of the carbon in vegetation. Plants are valued as food for their large stores of starches and sugars.

Composition CARBOHYDRATES are simple sugars or polymers of sugars such as starch that can be hydrolyzed to simple sugars by the action of digestive enzymes or by heating with dilute acids. Like thousands of organic compounds, they contain carbon, hydrogen, and oxygen. Generally, but not always, the hydrogen and oxygen are in the proportions to form water; hence the term *carbohydrate*. However, many compounds such as acetic acid ($C_2H_4O_2$) and lactic acid ($C_3H_6O_3$) that are not carbohydrate also contain hydrogen and oxygen in the same proportions as water.

Classification, Distribution, and Characteristics

Carbohydrates are classified as monosaccharides, or simple sugars, disaccharides, or double sugars, and polysaccharides, which include many molecules of simple sugars.

MONOSACCHARIDES are compounds that cannot be hydrolyzed to simpler compounds. Although naturally occurring simple sugars may contain three to seven carbon atoms, only the hexoses (6-carbon atoms) are of dietary importance.

Glucose, galactose, fructose, and mannose have the same empiric formula, $C_6H_{12}O_6$. They differ in the arrangement of the groupings about the carbon atoms (see Figure 5–1) and are distinctive in their physical properties, such as solubility and sweetness. Glucose, galactose, and mannose possess an aldehyde grouping (CHO) and are known as aldohexoses. Fructose possesses a ketone grouping (CO) and is known as a ketohexose.

Glucose, also known as dextrose, grape sugar, or corn sugar, is somewhat less sweet than cane sugar and is soluble in hot or cold water. It is found in sweet fruits such as grapes, berries, and oranges and in some vegetables such as sweet corn and carrots. It is prepared commercially as corn syrup or in its crystalline form by the hydrolysis of starch with acids. Glucose is the chief end product of the digestion of the di- and polysaccharides, is the form of carbohydrate circulating in the blood, and is the carbohydrate utilized by the cell for energy.

Fructose (levulose or fruit sugar) is a highly soluble sugar that does not readily crystallize. It is much sweeter than cane sugar and is found in honey, ripe fruits, and

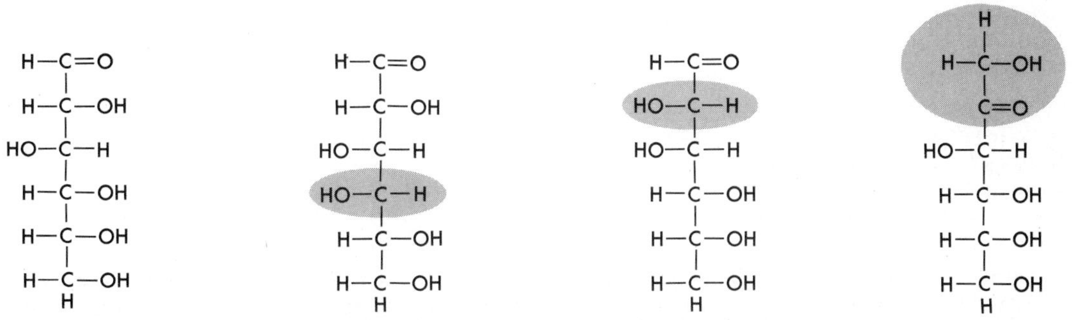

D-Glucose	D-Galactose	D-Mannose	D-Fructose
			H
H—C=O	H—C=O	H—C=O	H—C—OH
H—C—OH	H—C—OH	HO—C—H	C=O
HO—C—H	HO—C—H	HO—C—H	HO—C—H
H—C—OH	HO—C—H	H—C—OH	H—C—OH
H—C—OH	H—C—OH	H—C—OH	H—C—OH
H—C—OH	H—C—OH	H—C—OH	H—C—OH
H	H	H	H

Figure 5–1. These hexoses differ in the arrangement of the groupings about the carbon atoms. The encircled grouping shows how the sugar differs from glucose in its structure. Fructose is a ketose; the others are aldoses.

some vegetables. It is also a product of the hydrolysis of sucrose.

Galactose is not found free in nature, its only source being from the hydrolysis of lactose. *Mannose* is of limited distribution in foods, is poorly absorbed, and is of little consequence in nutrition.

Ribose, xylose, and *arabinose* are three pentoses (5-carbon sugars) that are of little dietary significance. Xylose and arabinose are widely distributed in many root vegetables and fruits. Ribose is of great physiologic importance as a constituent of riboflavin, a B-complex vitamin, and of ribonucleic acid (RNA) and deoxyribonucleic acid (DNA). It is rapidly synthesized by the body and is not a dietary essential.

DISACCHARIDES or double sugars, result when two hexoses are combined with the loss of one molecule of water, the empiric formula being $C_{12}H_{22}O_{11}$. They are water soluble, diffusible, and crystallizable and vary widely in their sweetness. They are split to simple sugars by acid hydrolysis or by digestive enzymes.

Sucrose is the table sugar with which we are familiar and is found in cane or beet sugar, brown sugar, sorghum, molasses, and maple sugar. Many fruits and some vegetables contain small amounts of sucrose.

Lactose, or milk sugar, is produced by mammals and is the only carbohydrate of animal origin of significance in the diet. It is about one sixth as sweet as sucrose and dissolves poorly in cold water. The concentration of lactose in milk varies from 2 to 8 per cent, depending upon the species of animal.

Maltose, or malt sugar, does not occur to any appreciable extent in foods. It is an intermediate product in the hydrolysis of starch. Maltose is produced in the malting and fermentation of grains and is present in beer and malted breakfast cereals. It is also used with dextrins as the source of carbohydrate for some infant formulas.

POLYSACCHARIDES, $(C_6H_{10}O_5)_n$, are complex compounds with a relatively high molecular weight. They are amorphous rather than crystalline, are not sweet, are insoluble in water, and are digested with varying degrees of completeness. Starches, dextrins, glycogen, and several indigestible carbohydrates are of nutritional interest.

Starch is the storage form of carbohydrate in the plant and a valuable contributor to the energy content of the diet. The starch granules are encased in a cellulose-type wall and are distinctive in size and shape for each source. The characteristics of the starch molecule depend upon the way in which the 2,000 or so glucose units that make up the molecule are linked. Two types of glucose chains are present: (1) *amylose,* consisting of long straight chains of glucose, accounts for 10 to 20 per cent of the molecule; and (2) *amylopectin,* consisting of short branched chains of glucose units, accounts for the major part of the molecule. (See Figure 5–2.)

When starch is cooked in moist heat, the granules absorb water and swell, and the walls of the cell are ruptured, thus permitting more ready access to the digestive enzymes. Amylopectin has colloidal prop-

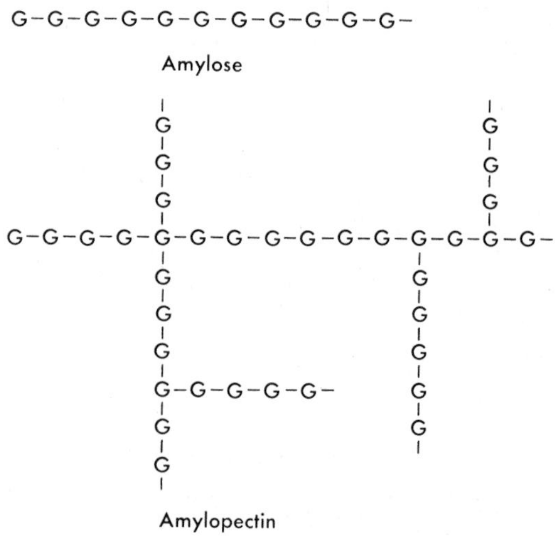

Figure 5–2. The starch molecule is composed of (1) amylose, with straight chains of glucose units, and (2) amylopectin, with branched chains of glucose units.

erties so that thickening of a starch-water mixture occurs when heat is applied.

Dextrins are intermediate products in the hydrolysis of starch and consist of shorter chains of glucose units. Some dextrins are produced when flour is browned or bread is toasted.

Glycogen, the so-called "animal starch," is similar in structure to the amylopectin of starch but contains many more branched chains of glucose. It is rapidly synthesized from glucose in the liver and muscle.

Indigestible polysaccharides include cellulose, hemicellulose, pectins, gums, and mucilages. They will be discussed fully under the heading Dietary Fiber in this chapter (see page 88).

Carbohydrate Derivatives Sugars react chemically to form sugar alcohols, amino sugars, glycosides, uronic acids, and many complex compounds with lipids and proteins. *Glycerol* is the 3-carbon alcohol that is a component of glycerides. *Sorbitol,* a sugar alcohol, is sweet, is water soluble, and is found in cherries, plums, and berries. *Inositol* is an alcohol related to the hexoses. It occurs in the bran of cereal grains. When combined with phosphate it forms phytic acid, a compound that interferes with the absorption of minerals such as calcium, iron, and zinc.

Ascorbic acid, one of the water-soluble vitamins, is a hexose derivative that can be synthesized by plants and by some animals but not by the human being. Numerous carbohydrate derivatives are constituents of connective, nervous, and other tissues and are involved in many metabolic functions.

Functions

Body Distribution The amount of carbohydrate in the adult body is about 300 to 350 gm. Of this, 100 gm is stored as glycogen in the liver, another 200 to 250 gm is present as glycogen in cardiac, smooth, and skeletal muscles, and about 15 gm makes up the glucose in the blood and extracellular fluid. Carbohydrates provide the carbon skeletons for the synthesis of the nonessential amino acids by the body (see page 60). Very small amounts of carbohydrate are constituents of numerous essential body compounds such as the following:

Glucuronic acid, which occurs in the liver and is also a constituent of a number of mucopolysaccharides. Glucuronic acid in the liver combines with toxic chemicals and bacterial byproducts and is thus a detoxifying agent.
Hyaluronic acid, a viscous substance that forms the matrix of connective tissue.
Heparin, a mucopolysaccharide, a substance that prevents the clotting of blood.
Chondroitin sulfates found in skin, tendons, cartilage, bone, and heart valves.
Immunopolysaccharides as part of the body's mechanism to resist infections.
Deoxyribonucleic acid (DNA) and ribonucleic acid (RNA), the compounds that possess and transfer the genetic characteristics of the cell.
Galactolipins as constituents of nervous tissue.
Glycosides as components of steroid and adrenal hormones.

Energy Carbohydrates are the least expensive source of energy to the body. Each gram of carbohydrate when oxidized yields, on the average, 4 kcal. Glucose is the primary source of energy for the nervous system and the lungs. Following absorption from the intestinal tract, the carbohydrate meets these principal fates: (1) immediate use to meet energy needs of tissue cells; (2) conversion to glycogen and storage in the liver or muscle for later release to meet energy needs; and (3) conversion to fat as a larger reserve for energy. The total glycogen reserves in the body would meet about half of one day's energy needs of the adult. Glycogen stored in the liver can be converted to glucose to maintain the sugar level of the blood. Glycogen in muscle can be used to supply energy needs of muscle cells but is not available for regulation of the blood sugar level. The amount of energy stored as fat can be large and is a ready and continuing supply to meet energy needs when glycogen stores are depleted.

Protein-sparing action. The body will use carbohydrate preferentially as a source of energy when it is adequately supplied in the diet, thus sparing protein for tissue building. Since meeting energy needs of the body takes priority over other functions, any deficiency of calories in the diet will be made up by using adipose and protein tissues.

Regulation of Fat Metabolism Some carbohydrate is necessary in the diet so that the oxidation of fats can proceed normally. When carbohydrate is severely restricted in the diet, fats will be metabolized faster than the body can take care of the intermediate products. The accumulation of these incompletely oxidized products leads to dehydration, loss of body sodium, and ketosis. As little as 50 gm carbohydrate in the diet will prevent ketosis under normal conditions. In uncontrolled diabetes mellitus, ketosis is often present.

Role in Gastrointestinal Function Lactose has several functions in the gastrointestinal tract. It promotes the growth of desirable bacteria, some of which are useful in the synthesis of B-complex vitamins. Lactose also enhances the absorption of calcium. It is undoubtedly no accident of nature that milk, which is the outstanding source of calcium, is also the only source of lactose.

Dietary fiber yields no nutrients to the body, but aids in the stimulation of peristaltic movements of the gastrointestinal tract, gives bulk to the intestinal contents, and reduces the length of time that food wastes remain in the colon. (See page 90.)

Digestion and Absorption

Digestion The purpose of carbohydrate digestion is to hydrolyze the di- and polysaccharides of the diet to their constituent simple sugars. This is accomplished by enzymes of the digestive juices and yields these end products:

$$\text{Starch} \xrightarrow{\text{amylase}} \text{Glucose}$$

$$\text{Sucrose} \xrightarrow{\text{sucrase}} \text{Glucose} + \text{fructose}$$

$$\text{Maltose} \xrightarrow{\text{maltase}} \text{Glucose} + \text{glucose}$$

$$\text{Lactose} \xrightarrow{\text{lactase}} \text{Glucose} + \text{galactose}$$

Although some hydrolysis of starch to maltose occurs in the mouth by the action of salivary amylase and continues in the stomach until the food mass is acidified, the principal site of digestion of carbohydrate is in the small intestine. Salivary amylase does not act upon raw starch but pancreatic amylase hydrolyzes both raw and cooked starch to dextrins and, in turn, to maltose. Cooked starch is more rapidly hydrolyzed because the cell walls have been ruptured and the enzymes have more ready access to the starch granules.

Disaccharidases are produced within the mucosal cell and are not secreted into the lumen of the intestine. Sucrose, lactose, and maltose are hydrolyzed within the brush border of the epithelial cell. The behavior of dietary fiber in the intestinal tract is described on page 89.

Absorption The process by which the monosaccharides are absorbed is by no means simple. The single sugars must enter the epithelial cell, be transported across the cell, enter the interstitial fluid, and then pass through the walls of the blood capillaries for transport to the portal circulation and the liver, and be dispensed according to need to the systemic circulation.

Glucose and galactose can be absorbed by passive diffusion with a carrier as an intermediary only as long as the concentration at the luminal surface is greater than that in the circulation. Passive diffusion accounts for only a small amount of the total glucose that is absorbed. Fructose apparently is absorbed only by passive diffusion.

When the concentration in the circulation exceeds that at the luminal surfaces of the intestine, active transport is required.

Active transport accounts for most of the absorption of glucose and galactose. It is effected by the sodium pump and a mobile carrier system. The same energy that is required to pump sodium out of the cell also serves to transport glucose and galactose. The energy required to operate the sodium pump is provided by ATP that has been generated from a supply of glucose within the cell.

Most absorption occurs from the jejunum. When the concentration of sugar in the intestine is great, the need for carriers to ferry sugars across the epithelial cells may exceed the numbers present; hence, some sugars will move along the tract to carrier sites in the ileum.

The rate of absorption is about equal for galactose and glucose, whereas fructose is absorbed about half as rapidly. Mannose and xylose are poorly absorbed, indicating a high level of selectivity at the absorption sites.

About 97 to 98 per cent of the carbohydrate in diversified American diets is digested and absorbed. The fuel factor of 4 kcal (17 kJ) per gram is based upon this level of absorption. In countries where plant foods comprise most of the diet, the percentage of carbohydrate absorbed is lower, and the energy value per gram of dietary carbohydrate is somewhat lower.

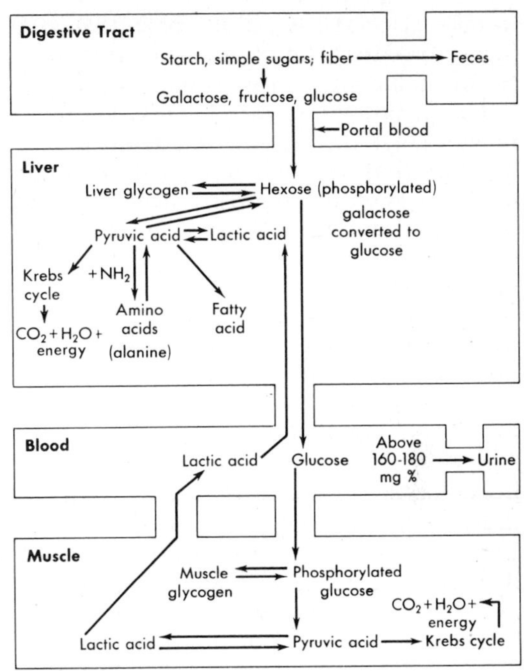

Figure 5–3. Pathways of carbohydrate metabolism.

Intermediary Metabolism

Glucose is quantitatively the most important carbohydrate available to the body whether it be by absorption from the diet or by synthesis within the body. Galactose and fructose from the diet or from endogenous sources are rapidly synthesized to glucose in the liver. Therefore, any discussion of carbohydrate metabolism is essentially that of glucose. (See Figure 5–3.)

Interrelation with Other Nutrients Glucose metabolism consists of an interrelated series of biochemical reactions that are facilitated by enzymatic activity. Glucose metabolism cannot be completely separated from the metabolism of fats and proteins. On the one hand, proteins and fats are potential sources of glucose, and on the other, glucose can be converted to fatty acids, glycerol, and certain amino acids. A number of points in the sequence of glucose metabolism are also the crossroads for amino acid and fatty acid metabolism, and in some respects one nutrient can substitute for another. For example, a decrease in carbohydrate metabolism is accompanied by an increase in fatty acid oxidation.

Trace amounts of magnesium, iron, and other mineral elements and several of the B-complex vitamins are essential for enzyme activity. Thus, the metabolism of the nutrients is interdependent, and the lack of any one of them affects the total metabolism of the organism. For example, when there is a deficiency of any one of the vitamins, the result is a failure of the reaction to take place at the point where that vitamin is essential. Any reactions subsequent to this point, therefore, cannot occur.

The details of these elegant metabolic mechanisms are beyond the scope of this text, but they are well described in a number of texts on biochemistry. Nevertheless, the nurse and nutritionist frequently encounter patients with some defect in carbohydrate metabolism. The following paragraphs will furnish a general understanding of the mechanisms for the regulation of the blood glucose and a broad outline of the anaerobic and aerobic phases of glucose metabolism.

The Liver in Carbohydrate Metabolism Following absorption from the small intestine, the monosaccharides are carried by the portal vein to the liver. Just as the control tower in an airport regulates the flow of traffic in the air, so the liver exercises the principal control of the pathways that glucose (and other nutrients) shall take. The liver converts galactose and fructose to glucose. It synthesizes glycogen (GLYCOGENESIS) from glucose, stores it, and reconverts it to glucose (GLYCOGENOLYSIS) according to need. It deaminizes amino acids so that the carbon skeletons can be used for the synthesis of glucose (GLUCONEOGENESIS) if the glycogen stores are depleted. It can transform excess glucose into fatty acids (LIPOGENESIS) and can also use the glycerol fraction of lipids to form glucose. Many carbohydrate compounds that have a regulatory function throughout the body are synthesized by the liver. (See page 77.) From carbon skeletons donated by carbohydrate, the liver can also synthesize nonessential amino acids.

These many chemical transformations are facilitated by enzymes that are specific for each reaction and that are under the influence of hormones secreted by the pancreas and the adrenal, pituitary, and thyroid glands.

The Blood Glucose By means of the blood circulation glucose is made continuously available to each and every cell of the body as a source of energy and for the synthesis of a variety of substances. The glucose taken from the circulation by the cells is constantly replaced by the liver so that the blood glucose level is maintained within relatively narrow limits.

In the fasting state the blood glucose concentration is normally 60 to 85 mg per 100 ml. Shortly after a meal it rises to about 140 to 150 mg per 100 ml, but within a few hours the concentration will have returned to the fasting level. Should the blood sugar level reach 160 to 180 mg per 100 ml some glucose will be excreted in the urine (GLUCOSURIA). This level, varying somewhat from one individual to another, is known as the RENAL THRESHOLD FOR GLUCOSE. The regulation of the blood sugar level by the liver is so efficient that glucosuria does not normally occur. Occasionally, an individual who has a lower renal threshold for glucose but who has no other abnormalities will excrete some glucose following meals that are especially rich in carbohydrate.

A blood sugar concentration in excess of normal levels is known as HYPERGLYCEMIA; this is characteristic of diabetes mellitus. A glucose concentration below normal levels is known as HYPOGLYCEMIA and may occur in certain abnormalities of liver function or when insulin is produced in excessive amounts by the pancreas.

Regulation of the Blood Sugar Level The liver is the only organ able to supply glucose to the circulation, and it also participates in the removal of glucose not immediately needed. The sources of glucose to the blood and the avenues of its removal are shown in Figure 5–4. Glucose is made available to the circulation by (1) the absorbed sugars from the diet, (2) glycogenolysis, (3) gluconeogenesis, and, (4) to a lesser extent, the reconversion of pyruvic and lactic acids formed in the glycolytic pathway.

Several hormones bring about an increased supply of glucose to the blood. *Thyroid hormone* increases the rate of absorption from the gastrointestinal tract.

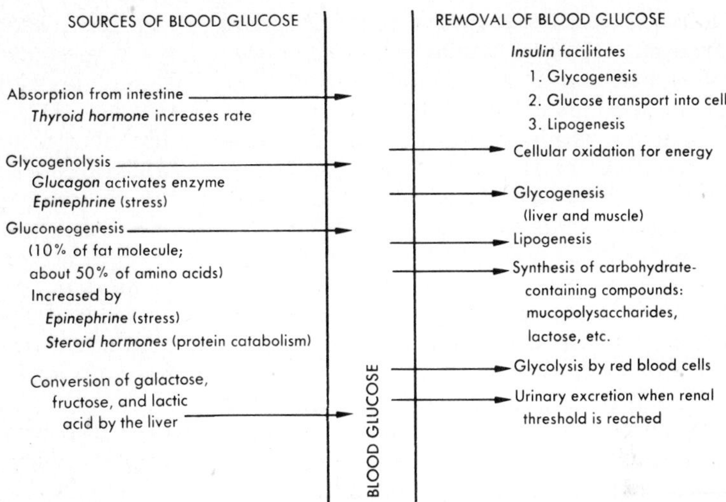

Figure 5–4. The blood glucose is maintained within physiologic limits by replacement as rapidly as it is removed to meet metabolic needs. Glycogenesis and lipogenesis are mechanisms that prevent hyperglycemia in the normal individual. The renal threshold is rarely exceeded in the healthy person.

Glucagon, a hormone secreted by the cells of the pancreas, is believed to activate phosphorylase, thus initiating glycogenolysis. *Epinephrine,* produced by the adrenal gland under conditions of stress, increases the rate of glycogen breakdown. *Steroid hormones* accelerate the catabolism of proteins, thus bringing about gluconeogenesis. *Adrenocorticotropic hormone* is antagonistic to the action of insulin and thus prevents the blood sugar level from dropping.

Removal of glucose from the blood. Six pathways are available for the removal of glucose from the blood: (1) the continuous uptake of glucose by every cell in the body and its oxidation for energy; (2) the conversion of glucose to glycogen by the liver (GLYCOGENESIS); (3) the synthesis of fats from glucose (LIPOGENESIS); (4) the synthesis of numerous carbohydrate derivatives (see page 77); (5) glycolysis in the red blood cells; and (6) elimination of glucose in the urine when the renal threshold is exceeded.[1]

The amount of glycogen that can be formed is limited, but there is no limit to the amount of fat that is formed. Glycogen reserves are maintained at their maximum level by diets high in carbohydrate. A diet high in protein and relatively low in carbohydrate will result in moderate glycogen reserves, but a diet high in fat and low in carbohydrate and protein will result in poor glycogen reserves.

Insulin. Only one hormone is known to lower the blood sugar. An increase in the concentration of blood glucose stimulates the release of INSULIN, the hormone produced by the beta cells of the islands of Langerhans. Insulin lowers the blood glucose by several actions: (1) facilitation of the synthesis of glycogen in the liver; (2) the active transport of glucose across cell membranes; and (3) the conversion of glucose to fatty acids.

Oxidation of Glucose Within each of the billions of cells of the body the oxidation of glucose is continuously taking place. The end products of this oxidation are carbon dioxide, water, and energy. If the potential energy of glucose, fatty acids, and amino acids were released in an explosive reaction, much of it would be lost and wasted as heat. The cell utilizes energy efficiently by releasing a small amount of it at the time in a series of steps that occur in the mitochondria of the cell. The energy liberated in these steps is trapped in the form of ADENOSINE TRIPHOSPHATE (ATP). This is a compound consisting of adenine (a nitrogenous base), ribose, and three phosphate groupings, two of which are high-energy phosphate bonds, designated thus ~. One of these bonds is broken to release energy whenever required for the innumerable transactions of the cell (ATP → ADP). As energy is liberated in the catabolism of glucose, fatty acids, or amino acids, ATP is again formed (ADP → ATP). ATP is sometimes called the "currency" or the "legal tender" for energy of the living organism, because, like coins of money, it is the convenient form for small bursts of energy.

The first step in glucose catabolism is GLYCOLYSIS, principally an anaerobic phase that results in the formation of two molecules of pyruvic acid from each molecule of glucose. The second phase of glucose catabolism is an aerobic phase that includes the decarboxylation of pyruvic acid to acetic acid, the condensation of acetic acid with coenzyme A, and the transfers through the CITRIC ACID CYCLE to yield hydrogen and electrons, carbon dioxide, and water. This is the common pathway for the oxidation of deaminized amino acids and fatty acids as well as for glucose. The final step in the release of energy is the immediate trapping of the energy in ATP through the ELECTRON TRANSPORT SYSTEM. Each of these phases involves many reactions, a broad outline of which is described in the paragraphs that follow. (See Figure 5–5.)

Glycolysis The chemical reactions that constitute glycolysis, also known as the *Embden-Meyerhof pathway* for the men who first described them, take place in the cytoplasmic matrix of the cell. These reactions degrade glucose to pyruvic acid in preparation for entrance into the mitochondria. They are catalyzed by a specific enzyme in each case, some of which require the presence of inorganic phosphate, inorganic ions, nicotinamide adenine dinucleotide (NAD), and nicotinamide adenine dinucleotide phosphate (NADP). The reactions do not require oxygen. Almost all of the glucose catabolized in the body undergoes breakdown through these steps.

The entrance of glucose into the cell is facilitated by insulin. Within the cell the first step in glycolysis is the phosphorylation of glucose with ATP in the presence of glucokinase and magnesium to form glucose-6-phosphate and ADP. The phosphorylated glucose then proceeds through the glycolytic pathway to pyruvic acid and lactic acid, or to the synthesis of glycogen, or, to a lesser extent, through an alternative oxidative pathway known as the *pentose shunt.*

Conversion to trioses. The hexose molecule is split into trioses, which undergo a series of changes until pyruvic acid ($CH_3COCOOH$) is formed. One of the trioses—glyceraldehyde-3-phosphate—instead of proceeding to pyruvic acid may be sidetracked to form α-glycerophosphate, which furnishes the glycerol molecule for the synthesis of neutral fats. (See page 108.)

Lactic acid. Pyruvic acid can proceed anaerobically to form lactic acid, which is utilized for muscle contraction under conditions when the energy need exceeds the supply of oxygen. Thus, the runner in a race can continue beyond his or her capacity to supply oxygen to muscles. Under normal conditions only a small amount of lactic acid is formed. About one fifth of the lactic acid produced in the muscle is further oxidized through the citric acid cycle; the rest enters the blood circulation and is synthesized to glycogen by the liver.

Figure 5–5. Glucose is oxidized anaerobically to pyruvic and lactic acids—the Embden-Meyerhof pathway. Glucose may also be oxidized through the pentose shunt. Pyruvic acid is decarboxylated to form acetate. Active acetate condenses with oxalacetic acid, and each turn of the Krebs cycle releases two molecules of CO_2 and eight hydrogen ions and uses up two molecules of water.

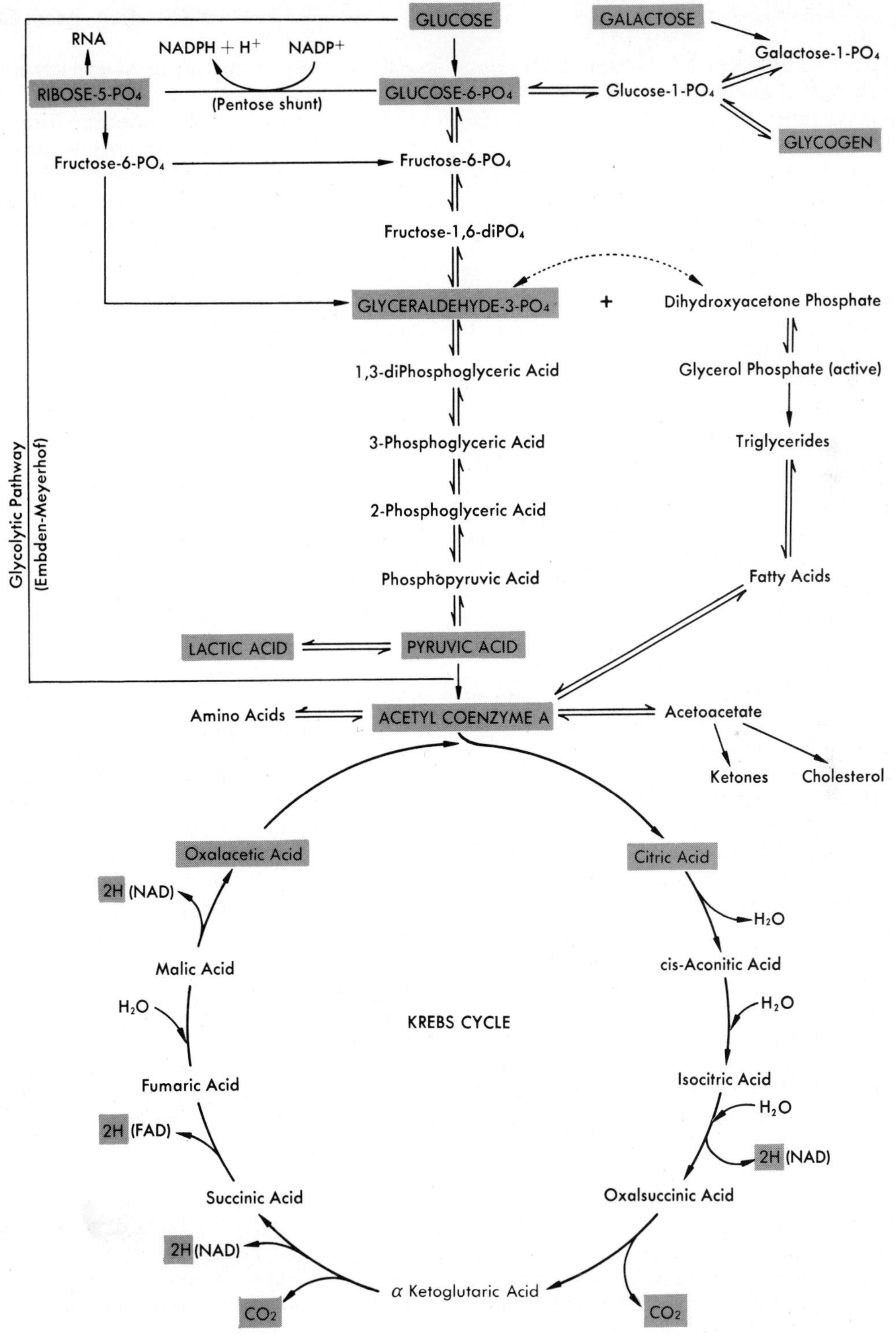

GLUCOSE
GALACTOSE
RNA
NADPH + H+
NADP+
Galactose-1-PO4
RIBOSE-5-PO4
(Pentose shunt)
GLUCOSE-6-PO4
Glucose-1-PO4
GLYCOGEN
Fructose-6-PO4
Fructose-6-PO4
Fructose-1,6-diPO4
GLYCERALDEHYDE-3-PO4
+
Dihydroxyacetone Phosphate
1,3-diPhosphoglyceric Acid
Glycerol Phosphate (active)
3-Phosphoglyceric Acid
Triglycerides
Glycolytic Pathway
(Embden-Meyerhof)
2-Phosphoglyceric Acid
Phosphopyruvic Acid
Fatty Acids
LACTIC ACID
PYRUVIC ACID
Amino Acids
ACETYL COENZYME A
Acetoacetate
Ketones
Cholesterol
Oxalacetic Acid
Citric Acid
2H (NAD)
H2O
cis-Aconitic Acid
Malic Acid
H2O
KREBS CYCLE
H2O
Fumaric Acid
Isocitric Acid
H2O
2H (FAD)
2H (NAD)
Succinic Acid
Oxalsuccinic Acid
2H (NAD)
α Ketoglutaric Acid
CO2
CO2

The Pentose Shunt An aerobic bypass for glycolysis may be utilized especially by the liver and adipose tissue. This is also known as the *hexose monophosphate shunt* or the *oxidative shunt.* Through the reactions occurring in this pathway, ribose, which is a constituent of RNA, is synthesized. Also, NADPH is produced, which is essential for the synthesis of fatty acids and for the utilization of lactic acid in muscular work.

Aerobic Metabolism Most of the pyruvic acid formed in the glycolytic pathway enters the mitochondria of the cells where it is oxidized. By a complex series of steps pyruvic acid is decarboxylated to a 2-carbon fragment (acetate), which reacts with coenzyme A to form ACETYL COENZYME A also known as ACTIVE ACETATE. These reactions require NAD, thiamin, pyrophosphate, lipoic acid, magnesium, coenzyme A, and a series of enzymes. In this conversion 3 moles of ATP are formed, or 6 moles for each glucose molecule.

COENZYME A is a complex molecule of which pantothenic acid, a B-complex vitamin, is a constituent. Acetyl coenzyme A is derived not only from pyruvic acid but also from the oxidation of fatty acids (see page 108) and from certain amino acids (see page 61). Acetyl coenzyme A is something like the hub of a wheel in that it can proceed in a number of directions, namely, through the citric acid cycle to yield energy or to form a number of new compounds.

Citric acid cycle. This is also known as the *tricarboxylic acid cycle* (because the acids involved contain three carboxyl groups) or the *Krebs cycle* (for the man who first formulated the sequence). Through this cycle about 90 per cent of the energy of the body is produced.

The citric acid cycle is initiated by the condensation of acetyl coenzyme A with oxalacetic acid to form citric acid. In one turn of the cycle two molecules of carbon dioxide and four pairs of hydrogens and electrons are produced. The overall reaction is

$$CH_3COOH + 2\,H_2O \rightarrow 2\,CO_2 + 8\,H^+$$

One molecule of carbon dioxide is released in the formation of α-ketoglutaric acid and one in the formation of succinyl coenzyme A. (See Figure 5–5). A full turn of the cycle again yields one molecule of oxalacetic acid, which then combines with a new molecule of acetyl coenzyme A for another cycle.

Electron Transport System The hydrogens released in the catabolism of glucose are never in the free state but are accepted by dehydrogenases NAD and flavin adenine dinucleotide (FAD). These enzymes exist in the oxidized or reduced form ($NAD \leftrightarrow NADH_2$ and $FAD \leftrightarrow FADH_2$). The hydrogen is transported through the *cytochrome system,* also known as the *respiratory chain* or the *electron transport system.* In this transport the oxidation of hydrogen to water and phosphorylation are coupled; hence, this is referred to as OXIDATIVE PHOSPHORYLATION.

The CYTOCHROMES are a series of iron-containing enzymes. They accept hydrogens from the dehydrogenases and transfer them step by step from one cytochrome to another until they react with oxygen to form water. The acceptance of hydrogen by the dehydrogenases and the transfer along the respiratory chain yields three molecules of ATP for each pair of hydrogens. (See Figure 5–6.)

The amount of energy converted to ATP from glucose and fat is, at a maximum, 38 to 40 per cent of the potential energy. The remainder is dissipated as heat. Each molecule of glucose can yield 38 molecules of ATP: 8 through the glycolytic pathway, 6 in the conversion of pyruvic acid to acetyl coenzyme A, and 24 in the TCA cycle. Hegsted[2] has described several ways by which the yield of 38 molecules of ATP from glucose is not likely to be realized. First, the coupling in the respiratory chain is not always complete so that three molecules of ATP are not always obtained. Second, the abundance of phosphatases may result in the wasteful removal of high-en-

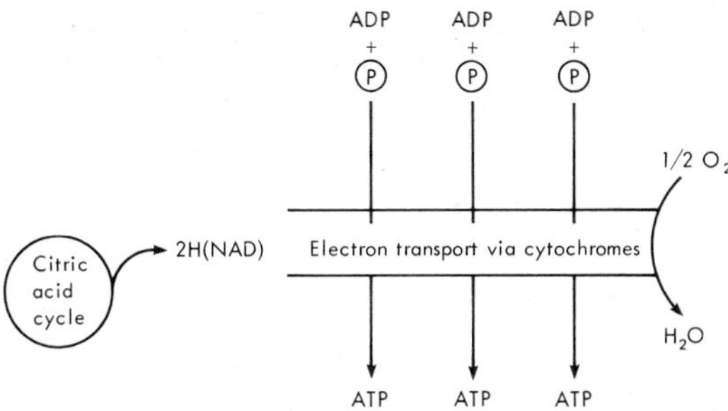

Figure 5–6. Each pair of hydrogens generated in glucose catabolism is carried by niacin- or riboflavin-containing enzymes and transferred step by step through a series of cytochromes in the electron transport system. The oxidation of hydrogen is coupled with the phosphorylation of ADP to ATP. Each pair of hydrogens yields three ATP molecules.

ergy bonds from ATP. Third, the energy cost of producing new tissue is high. These and other variations emphasize how complex the maintenance of energy balance becomes.

Carbohydrate in the Diet

Dietary Allowance The low-carbohydrate diet of the Eskimos and the high-carbohydrate diet of many people in Far Eastern countries indicate that humans can be healthy with wide variations in carbohydrate intake. This wide variation is compatible with health because of the interrelations with fatty acids and amino acids in meeting the energy needs of the body.

The minimum requirement for carbohydrate is not known, but at least 50 to 100 gm carbohydrate daily is desirable to prevent ketosis.[3] Intakes considerably above this level are customary and desirable.

The revised Dietary Goals recommend that complex carbohydrates and naturally occurring sugars provide about 48 per cent of the total caloric intake and that refined sugars provide no more than 10 per cent of the energy requirement.[4]

Dietary Sources The carbohydrate composition of typical foods is shown in Table 5–1. Pure sugars are 100 per cent carbohydrate, and syrups, jellies, and jams contain 65 to 80 per cent. Cereal foods, flours, and crackers contain 65 to 85 per cent carbohydrate on a dry weight basis, chiefly in the form of starch.

Fruits and vegetables vary widely in their carbohydrate concentration. Those with a high water content such as spinach, cabbage, other leafy vegetables, and melons contain 6 per cent or less of carbohydrate and are correspondingly low in calories. Potatoes, sweet potatoes, Lima beans, corn, and bananas are somewhat lower in water content and furnish approximately 20 per cent carbohydrate or more. Dried beans and peas and dried fruits have a carbohydrate content in excess of 60 per cent. For convenience in dietary planning, fruits and vegetables have been grouped according to their carbohydrate content. (See Table A–4.)

The degree of ripeness determines the relative proportions of sugars and starches in fruits and vegetables. Green bananas are high in starch and low in sugar, whereas ripe bananas have little starch and consist primarily of sugars. On the other hand, freshly picked and immature vegetables, for example, sweet corn, tender peas, and young carrots, contain more sugar and less starch than mature vegetables.

Milk is the only animal food that contributes to the daily carbohydrate intake. Freshly opened oysters and scallops contain some glycogen, but the amount is of no practical significance. The glycogen in liver is rapidly converted to lactic and pyruvic acids when the animal is slaughtered.

Carbohydrate in the United States Diet In 1979 the national available food supply furnished about 400 gm carbohydrate.[5] Of this total, sugars furnished 53.3 per cent and starches 46.7 per cent. This represents a significant shift in the consumption when compared with that early in this century when sugars accounted for less than one

Table 5-1. **Carbohydrate Content of Some Typical Foods**

Food	Per 100 gm of Food gm	Per Serving Portion: Measure	Weight gm	Carbohydrate gm
*Complex Carbohydrates**				
Bread, all kinds	50–56	1 slice	25	13
Cereals, breakfast, dry	68–84	1 cup wheat flakes	30	24
Crackers, all kinds	67–73	4 saltines	11	8
Flour, all kinds	71–80	2 tablespoons	14	11
Legumes, dry	60–63	½ cup navy beans, cooked	95	20
Macaroni, spaghetti, dry	75	½ cup cooked	70	16
Nuts	15–20	¼ cup peanuts	36	7
Pie crust, baked	44	⅙ shell	30	13
Potatoes, white, raw	17	1 boiled	135	20
Rice, dry	80	½ cup cooked	105	25
Complex and Simple Carbohydrates (½ and ½)				
Cake, plain and iced	52–68	1 piece layer, iced	71	45
Cookies	51–80	1 chocolate chip	10	6
Simple Carbohydrates				
Beverages, carbonated	8–12	8 ounces cola	246	24
Candy (without nuts)	75–95	1 ounce milk chocolate	28	16
Fruit, dried	59–69	4 prunes	32	18
Fruit, fresh	6–22	1 apple	138	20
		1 orange	180	16
Fruit, sweetened, canned or frozen	16–28	½ cup peaches	128	26
		3 ounces frozen strawberries	85	24
Ice cream	18–21	½ cup	67	16
Milk	5	1 cup	244	12
Pudding	16–26	½ cup vanilla	128	21
Sugar, all kinds	96–100	1 tablespoon white	12	12
Syrups, molasses, honey	65–82	1 tablespoon molasses	20	13
Vegetables	4–18	½ cup green beans	63	4
		½ cup peas	80	10

*Foods are grouped according to the predominating type of carboyhdrate present.

third of the total carbohydrate. (See Figure 5–7.) This shift has occurred with an increase in the consumption of sugar together with a steady decline in the consumption of foods supplied by cereal grains and potatoes.

From 1909–13 to 1925–29 the proportion of carbohydrate from sugar increased by 10 percentage points. Although sugar now accounts for more than half of the dietary carbohydrate, the proportion has increased by less than 3 percentage points since the period from 1957 to 1959.

The total sugar in the diet in 1979 was 213 gm, which accounts for 24.4 per cent of the available calories. The caloric contribution from each category of sugars was as follows:[5]

	per cent
Naturally occurring sugars (sucrose, fructose, glucose in fruits and vegetables; lactose in milk)	6.7
Refined cane and beet sugars	12.2
Other caloric sweeteners (syrups, high-fructose corn syrup, corn sugar, molasses, honey)	5.5
	24.4

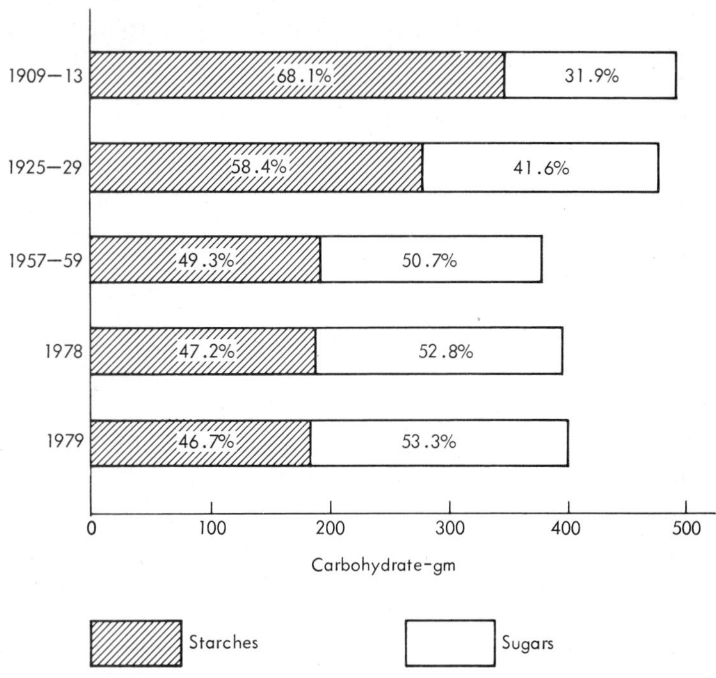

Figure 5-7. Sugars account for over half of the carbohydrate in today's diets. Early in the century starchy foods accounted for about two thirds of the carbohydrate intake. (Data from "Nutritional Review" by B. Friend and R. Marston, *National Food Situation,* November 1974, p. 29; and R. Marston and B. B. Peterkin, *National Food Review,* Winter 1980, p. 22.)

Today's consumer has less control of the use of sugar in foods. Prior to World War II most baking, canning, pickling, and jelly-making took place in the home and accounted for about two thirds of the refined sugar used. For the last 40 years most sugar is used by the food industry: baked foods and mixes, sugar-coated cereals, candy, fruits canned in syrups, sweetened juices and fruit drinks, sweetened beverage mixes, jellies, jams, pickles, ice cream, and soft drinks. The consumer is less aware of the sugar included in numerous products such as nondairy creamers, catsup, breading mixtures for meats, peanut butter, and others. By reading labels the consumer soon becomes aware of the uses of refined sugars and other caloric sweeteners. Thus, a single label might indicate the presence of not only cane sugar but also corn syrup and honey!

Soft drink consumption has more than doubled since 1960 and was equivalent to 384 12-ounce cans per capita per year by 1978.[5] Soft drinks alone account for about 25 pounds of refined sugar per capita annually. In addition, about 40 per cent of all high-fructose corn syrup is used by the beverage industry.

Adjustments to Conform to the Dietary Goals In view of the high proportion of sugars and also of fats in typical American diets, the following substantial modifications would be required if the Dietary Goals were applied:

Substantially increase the proportion of calories provided by breads, cereals, pastas, rice, and so on.
Increase the amounts of potatoes, legumes, fruits, and vegetables.
Decrease the consumption of sugar, sugar-containing beverages, cakes, cookies, candy, sugared cereals, and so on.

One way to adjust the Basic diet (page 262) for the woman who requires 2,000 kcal so that it furnishes 48 per cent of the calories from complex carbohydrates and naturally occurring sugars is shown in Table 5-2. This plan suggests the addition of 9 teaspoons of fat as an accompaniment for the bread equivalents and 1 ounce sugar that could be consumed as such or in some sugar-containing food. As you can see, the nine slices of bread or its equivalent as rice, pastas, or other source and the two potatoes are more than most women are accustomed to eating.

Artificial Sweeteners Saccharin and aspartame are the only noncaloric sweeteners that are presently approved for use. Aspartame is a dipeptide of phenylalanine and aspartic acid and is 200 times as sweet as sugar.

Saccharin is 350 times as sweet as sugar and has been extensively used during this century in foods for special dietary use and more recently in sugar-free soft drinks. Persons with diabetes mellitus, those who are trying to correct obesity, and others who are carbohydrate-sensitive have long used saccharin as substitute sweeteners. Whether its use promotes dietary adherence is not certain.

In 1977 a Canadian study was reported that showed the occurrence of bladder cancer in male rats that had been fed a diet containing 5 per cent saccharin over a 2-year period. Based on the requirement of the 1958 Delaney Amendment (see page 318) that the use of a substance must be prohitited if it is carcinogenic in any degree, the Food and Drug Administration moved to ban the use of saccharin. But there was great consumer resistance to this ban. It was argued that, based on body size, the dosages used to produce the cancers in the rats far exceeded the amounts that humans could ingest day by day over a lifetime. Also, many maintained that substituting sugar for saccharin could be a greater risk to health. In November 1977 Congress passed a law that placed a moratorium on the ban for 18 months; this moratorium has been extended again.

In the meantime, saccharin exists under a cloud as a possibly harmful substance.[6] Based on the animal studies it is a weak carcinogen. Epidemiologic studies on diabetic persons have not shown a correlation between saccharin and bladder cancer. Further studies are now in progress. Individuals make their own choices—whether to smoke, to remain obese, or to use saccharin! For those who are diabetic or who are carbohydrate sensitive, the slight risk of cancer may be preferred to the inability to adhere to their diets or even to enjoy sweet-tasting foods. But the wide use of saccharin-sweetened soft drinks and of many foods that are somewhat lower in calories because saccharin has been used instead of sugar is inadvisable–especially by children and youth.

A number of nonnutritive sweeteners are being studied.[6] One of these, cyclamate, was widely used for a number of years until Canadian studies on rats in the 1960s showed it to be mildly carcinogenic. Cyclamate was banned in 1970, but on the basis of recent investigation the question of its use is being reopened. Others that are being studied include *monellin*, a protein from a tropical fruit that is about 3,000 times as sweet as sugar.

Table 5-2. **Carbohydrate Adjustment of the Basic Diet**

	Carbohydrate gm	Energy kcal
Basic Diet (page 41)	144	1106
Potato, 1	20	90
Bread, 6 slices	76	380
	240	1576
Fat, 9 teaspoons		300
Sugar, 1 ounce	30	120
	270	1996
Complex carbohydrate, per cent of calories		48
Sugars, per cent of calories		6

Dietary Fibers

"Roughage," "bulk," "residue," "cellulose," and "fiber" are imprecise terms that have long been applied to the indigestible substances of plant foods. The value of fiber in maintaining normal elimination of feces has been recognized for centuries.

Since the early 1970s there has been renewed interest in the role of fibers in the diet. This has come about because of the reports by some British clinicians that showed a correlation between fiber intake and the incidence of disease. Their epidemiologic studies showed that rural Africans who had a high-fiber intake had a low incidence of diverticulitis, irritable colon, hiatus hernia, hemorrhoids, cancer of the colon, coronary heart disease, obesity, diabetes, dental caries, and gallstones.[7,8] People in the Western world whose diets are low in fiber have a high incidence of these diseases. But it is important to keep in mind that fiber is only one of many environmental factors that differ in the two groups, such as climate, pollutants, physical activity, fat and cholesterol intake, sugar intake, quality and amount of protein intake, and so on. Nonetheless, the British investigations have provided attractive hypotheses that require further testing. Although hundreds of reports have been published within the past decade, the results are often contradictory and confusing.

What is Dietary Fiber DIETARY FIBERS include a number of polysaccharides and lignin that are not digested by the enzymes of the gastrointestinal tract. These nonnutritive substances have specific chemical structures with varying physical and chemical properties. Their quantitative determination in foods is difficult, and the isolation of their effects on gastrointestinal function presents even greater problems to the investigator.

Cellulose is the most abundant molecule in nature and is the principal structure of cell walls. It is insoluble in water and is found abundantly in the bran of cereal grains.

Lignin, though classified with dietary fibers, is not a polysaccharide since it contains no sugar units. It is a water-insoluble component that makes up the woody part of plants. Legumes and fruits with seeds and the lignified cells of pears are important sources. Whole-grain cereals are moderate in lignin content, whereas most vegetables are low.

Hemicelluloses are found in the cell walls of many plants. Some investigators include pectins, gums, and mucilages under this heading. The hemicelluloses are soluble in hot water and occur in a variety of plant foods: carrots, cabbage, celery, leafy vegetables, apples, melons, peaches, pears, and whole-grain cereals.

Pectin, unlike cellulose and lignin, does not have true fiber or threadlike characteristics. Nonetheless, it is an important structural material found in cell walls and functions as an intercellular cement. It is soluble in hot water and has the capacity to hold water and to form gels. Apples and citrus fruits are important sources, while cereals contain very little.

Mucilages and gums are nonstructural components of plant cells that are soluble in hot water.

Several indigestible polysaccharides are used in the food industry. Pectins are used in making fruit jellies. *Agar* obtained from seaweed is also useful for its gelling properties. *Carrageen* (Irish moss) and *alginates* from seaweed are often used to enhance the smoothness of foods such as ice cream and evaporated milk.

Effect of Fiber on Intestinal Physiology The effect of fiber on the gastrointestinal tract is influenced by the characteristics of the fiber itself, the particle size of the ingested fibers, the interaction between fibers, other dietary components, and bacterial flora. The following effects have been postulated. Some are well recognized while others remain speculative.[9]

1. Dietary fiber holds water so that stools are soft, bulky, and readily eliminated. Coarse bran is effective but fine bran has little effect. It is generally agreed that a high-fiber intake prevents or relieves constipation. The large, bulky stool also represents a dilution of colon contents so that any potentially toxic substances such as car-

cinogens that might be present would thus be less harmful.

2. Fiber generally increases motility of the small intestine and colon and decreases transit time. This could result from the stimulation of the mucosa by mechanical effect or perhaps by the by-products of bacterial fermentation. If transit time is shortened, then there could be less time for exposure of the mucosa to harmful toxicants. Also, there could be less time for bacteria to produce harmful substances. Transit time, however, is individually variable and unpredictable.

3. Pectins, mucilages, and gums retard gastric emptying. This can have two benefits: increased satiety so that less food is eaten, thus helping to keep energy intake within the requirement; and a smoother response by the blood circulation to glucose and hence lesser insulin secretion. This effect is one explanation for the lower insulin requirement observed in diabetic patients who consume a high-carbohydrate high-fiber diet.

4. High-fiber diets have been found to reduce intraluminal pressure in the colon of some persons who have diverticulitis or irritable colon. Yet, there is no evidence that low-fiber diets cause diverticulosis.

5. High-fiber diets, such as vegetarian diets, have somewhat lower coefficients of digestibility. Thus, the net energy realized to the body is a little less than that from diets containing high proportions of animal foods.

Cellulose and lignin have the capacity to bind minerals such as calcium, magnesium, phosphorus, zinc, and others. This poses a possiblity of nutritional deficiency, especially when diets contain marginal levels of mineral elements. For example, growth failure has been observed in Iranian boys who consumed a very high-fiber diet but with a low dietary intake of zinc.[10] Such diets also contain high levels of phytic acid which also has the ability to bind mineral elements.

6. Pectins, mucilages, and gums chelate with bile acids and steroid materials. The chelating effect helps to explain the reduction in blood cholesterol levels. But it must also be recognized that the lipid-lowering effect could be associated with the reduced level of fats that is characteristic of many high-fiber diets. Rolled oats and some legumes have been found effective in bringing about modest lowering of the blood cholesterol but the bran of wheat has had no such result.[11]

7. Pectins, hemicelluloses, gums, and mucilages are partially fermented by intestinal bacteria to volatile fatty acids, carbon dioxide, and methane. The caloric yield to the body by this fermentation accounts for only about 5 per cent of the caloric equivalent of the total fiber ingested and is of no practical significance.

Whether the action of bacteria on fiber, or the effects of fiber can alter bacterial metabolism is not known. Thus, it is speculative that fiber can modify intestinal flora so that less harmful substances are being produced.

Fiber Content of the Diet Many tables of food composition give data on "crude fiber" content of foods. By definition, CRUDE FIBER is the residue that remains after a food sample has been subjected to treatment by acid and then by alkali under standard conditions. The method excludes about 80 per cent of the hemicelluloses, 50 to 90 per cent of the lignin, and even up to 50 per cent of the cellulose.[9] Because the proportions of fiber components vary from one food source to another, there is no practical way to convert crude fiber values to meaningful values of dietary fiber. In recent years more precise methods have been developed for identifying the various dietary fibers. Table A–3 gives values for fiber contents of foods.

The amount of fiber that should be present in the diet is not known. Most American diets could be improved by (1) substituting whole-grain for refined breads and cereals and (2) increasing the intake of fruits, vegetables, nuts, and legumes. Raw vegetables and fruits, including skins and seeds, are especially high in fiber.

Any increase in the fiber intake should be accomplished gradually. This is especially important for those persons who choose to use bran daily for its extra fiber content (1 to 2 tablespoons is usually sufficient, starting with teaspoonful amounts). Initially many persons experience distention, cramping, and even diarrhea when the fiber intake is increased rapidly.

Excessive fiber intake should be avoided, not only because of the interference with absorption of mineral elements but also because it occasionally leads to intestinal obstruction.

Problems Related to Carbohydrate Intake

Low-Carbohydrate Diets From time to time claims are made for the effectiveness of low-carbohydrate, high-protein, high-fat diets in bringing about weight loss. Such diets can be dangerous since they lead to ketosis with the associated clinical findings of excessive fatigue, dehydration, water loss, and electrolyte deficits. In susceptible individuals there is retention of uric acid which sometimes leads to symptoms of gout. The increased supply of fat, especially saturated fat, results in elevated blood lipids and increased risk of coronary heart disease. Low-carbohydrate diets are also low in fiber content. (See page 89.)

Hypoglycemia. Contrary to popular opinion, nonfasting reactive hypoglycemia is not common. The symptoms of hypoglycemia are hunger, weakness, trembling, sweating, headache, and, if severe, coma. People sometimes make a self-diagnosis based on what they have read or heard from a pseudo-scientist and attempt to treat themselves with a low-carbohydrate diet. The diagnosis, however, can be made only by a physician who relies not only on the presenting symptoms but also on the glucose tolerance test.

High-Carbohydrate Diet A high proportion of calories from carbohydrate is generally desirable provided that most of the carbohydrate is furnished by complex carbohydrates. Such diets furnish liberal intakes of minerals, vitamins, and fiber. By virtue of their lower fat content the risk of coronary heart disease is also reduced.

Some concern about high intakes of sugar is justified. Nonetheless, many people regard all refined sugar as harmful while regarding other forms of sugar—honey, raw sugar, molasses, maple syrup—as satisfactory substitutes. Although the substituted sweeteners may furnish some mineral elements, the amounts are too small to be of significance in the diet.

Sugar is useful as a concentrated source of energy and is valuable for contributing to diet palatability. But the recommendation that sugars furnish no more than 10 per cent of the daily calories is sound.[4]

Nutritional adequacy. An excessive intake of sugars, candies, cakes, cookies, pastries, and sugar-containing soft drinks is likely to crowd out essential foods, thereby contributing to nutrient deficiencies as well as to problems of overweight. For example, the increasing use of soft drinks tends to reduce the intake of milk. The establishment early in life of habits of judicious consumption of sweets can scarcely be overemphasized.

Dental caries. The causes of tooth decay are many and complex. Yet, dentists agree that sugar is one of the important etiologic agents. Sugars provide the energy for bacterial growth, which leads to gradual buildup of plaque, a sticky carbohydrate-bacterial matrix that adheres firmly to the teeth. The acids formed by the bacteria from the sugar substrate gradually erode the tooth enamel and bring about decay. Two conditions accelerate the process: sticky carbohydrates that adhere to tooth surfaces for a long time; and frequent exposure of tooth surfaces to sugar. For example, sticky caramels are likely to be more harmful than a soft drink providing the same amount of sugar since the latter is less likely to adhere to the tooth for a long period of time. But also, eating five caramels at five intervals during the day results in five exposures, while eating the five caramels at one time would reduce the total time of exposure.

Lactose intolerance. Orientals, Latin Americans, Alaskan Indians, and blacks often are unable to tolerate milk because they have an intestinal deficiency of lactase. As lactose accumulates in the intestinal tract, fermentation produces distention, cramping, and diarrhea. Although adults may be unable to drink milk, infants are usually lactose tolerant and can be raised on milk formulas. Children and teenagers can drink sufficient milk to meet their calcium requirements if the intake is well spaced throughout the day. To eliminate milk from the diets of all children belonging to these groups is a nutritional disservice. When there is indication of some intolerance in children, a determination should be made of what levels of milk can be tolerated.

Sugar and chronic disease. High-carbohydrate diets, per se, do not cause diabetes, nor is there convincing evidence that sugar will cause it. But there is a high association between obesity and maturity-onset diabetes mellitus. Thus, caloric control rather than limitation of carbohydrate alone is the more important factor in delaying onset in susceptible individuals.

The claims that a high-carbohydrate intake contributes to the elevation of blood triglycerides are not convincing.[12] Again, persons who are obese are more likely to have elevated blood triglycerides. Some persons are genetically predisposed to hypertriglyceridemia and usually need to restrict their intake of sugar and also alcohol.

Alcohol

Alcoholic beverages have been used throughout history. In the United States the consumption continues to increase, with wine especially gaining tremendously in popularity. On one hand is the social enjoyment and relief from tension that some people experience by consuming a cocktail, a tankard of beer, or a glass of wine. At the other extreme is the problem of the alcoholic and the consequences of malnutrition and illness. Parents and educators are especially concerned about the increasing use of alcohol by teenagers.

Metabolism Alcohol is rapidly absorbed from the stomach and small intestine and is promptly dispersed throughout the body fluids. There is no upper limit of absorption but the rate of absorption is reduced when foods, especially those containing fat, are taken with the beverage.

Alcohol is oxidized almost exclusively by the liver to acetaldehyde, then to acetic acid. Because the muscles do not contain the enzymes necessary for the conversion to acetaldehyde, exercise is of no value in hastening the return to sobriety. The acetic acid formed is condensed with coenzyme A, and through the citric acid cycle yields energy to the peripheral tissues as well as the liver.

Two pathways for the oxidation of alcohol to acetaldehyde by the liver have been described.[13] The first of these is the conversion to acetaldehyde in the presence of alcohol dehydrogenase and NAD^+, a niacin-containing coenzyme.

$$\underset{\text{ethanol}}{CH_3CH_2OH} + NAD^+ \xrightarrow{\text{alcohol dehydrogenase}} \underset{\text{acetaldehyde}}{CH_3CHO} + NADH + H^+$$

This is the primary pathway when the concentration of alcohol in the circulation is low. The availability of NAD^+ is the rate-limiting factor. About 0.1 gm alcohol is metabolized per kilogram body weight per hour. Thus, it would require about 5 hours for a 70 kg man to completely metabolize the alcohol from 100 ml 86 proof (43 per cent alcohol) whiskey.

The second pathway is accomplished by

mixed function oxidase, a system that requires two cytochrome enzymes.

$$CH_3CH_2OH + NADPH + H^+ \xrightarrow{\text{mixed function oxidase}} CH_3CHO + NADP^+ + 2\,H_2O$$

This pathway is active when the ethanol concentration in the circulation is high. With chronic exposure to alcohol the amount and catalytic activity of this pathway increases, which helps to explain the tolerance shown by alcoholics.

This pathway is called the mixed function oxidase system because it also is responsible for the detoxification of various substances such as barbiturates. But the presence and interaction with one substance also reduces the activity toward the other. Obviously, barbiturates and alcohol become a dangerous mix!

Alcohol and Nutrition Beer, wine, and distilled liquors contribute calories and these must be accounted for in maintaining caloric equilibrium. Each gram of alcohol yields 7.1 kcal (5.6 kcal per ml). Thus, 100 ml 86 proof whiskey would yield 241 kcal (43 ml alcohol × 5.6). Calories in excess of needs, regardless of source, will contribute to weight gain. Beer and wine contain minimal amounts of nutrients, and distilled liquors contain none. Alcoholic beverages consumed in moderate amounts need not adversely affect nutritional status provided that foods are selected in recommended amounts from the essential food groups.

Generalized malnutrition, gastritis, fatty infiltration of the liver and iron overload are among the effects of chronic alcoholism. Often alcohol replaces essential foods in the diet because of reduced appetite or because the individual does not have enough money to purchase both food and alcohol. With the reduced intake of nutrients the stage is set for nutritional deficiency. Moreover, the metabolism of alcohol requires thiamin, niacin, and pantothenic acid, and the lack of these nutrients helps to explain the neuropathy that is sometimes present in alcoholism.

When alcohol is consumed there is increased synthesis of fatty acids as well as a reduced production of lipoproteins, leading to deposition of fat in the liver. Fatty infiltration can lead to hepatitis and, in some persons, eventually to cirrhosis of the liver.

Iron overload is manifested by the appearance of iron in the plasma cells from the bone marrow.[14] The mechanism is not clear, but it is suggested that chronic alcoholics probably should not eat iron-fortified foods.

An alcoholic binge accompanied by failure to eat for several days and followed by several hours of vomiting sometimes leads to metabolic acidosis, which is often life threatening. The acidosis must be distinguished from diabetic acidosis since the treatments differ. Treatment with 5 per cent dextrose in water dramatically reverses the condition.[14]

When alcohol is consumed regularly in large amounts it has been observed that there is less weight gain than there would be with an equivalent excess of carbohydrate. Thus, it seems that some calories don't count. This is explained by the lesser production of energy by the mixed oxidase system and a greater production of heat. By the alcohol dehydrogenase route, one molecule of alcohol yields 16 molecules of ATP; but the mixed function oxidase system yields only 10 ATP per molecule alcohol.

Some Points for Emphasis in Nutrition Education

1. Carbohydrates include sugars, starches, and fiber from plant foods. Milk, which contains lactose, is the only important source of carbohydrate from animal foods.
2. The principal function of carbohydrate is to furnish energy to the body. In the United States most diets furnish less than half of the energy value of the diet from carbohydrate.

3. Only a small amount of carbohydrate is stored in the body in the form of glycogen. If there is an excess of carbohydrate beyond the body's immediate need, it is stored as fat.
4. The nutritive value of typical diets in the United States would be improved by including more complex carbohydrates and by reducing the intake of sugars.
5. Weight for weight, fresh fruits and vegetables contain much less carbohydrate than breads and cereals. But breads and cereals furnish energy at low cost, and if selections are made from whole-grain or enriched products the contribution of B-complex vitamins and iron is good.
6. Raw fruits and vegetables, legumes, nuts, and whole-grain breads and cereals should be emphasized for their fiber content.
7. Sugars and sweets should be used with discretion lest they replace essential foods in the diet. The nutritional contribution of brown sugar, honey, raw sugar, and maple syrup is of little significance. Palatable diets are possible when sugars are restricted to less than 10 per cent of the caloric requirement.

Problems and Review

1. Key terms: adenosine triphosphate (ATP); aerobic metabolism; anaerobic metabolism; cellulose; citric acid cycle; coenzyme A; cytochrome; dietary fiber; disaccharide; electron transport; gluconeogenesis; glycogenesis; glycolysis; hemicellulose; lignin; lipogenesis; monosaccharide; oxidative phosphorylation; pectin; pentose shunt; polysaccharide; renal threshold.
2. What are the important differences between the three classes of carbohydrates?
3. What advantages might be realized by increasing the intake of complex carbohydrates?
4. Drinking a glass of fruit juice removes feelings of hunger quickly but for a relatively short period of time. Explain this on the basis of physiologic and biochemical reactions that take place.
5. Even though you eat a diet that is high in carbohydrate the blood glucose will usually not reach the renal threshold. Explain the mechanisms whereby the blood sugar is maintained within such narrow limits.
6. If an individual is not eating, what mechanisms provide for the maintenance of a supply of glucose to the tissues?
7. If carbohydrate is eaten in excess of the energy requirement, what happens to it?
8. What are some effects on gastrointestinal physiology of a high-fiber intake?
9. *Problem.* Calculate the carbohydrate and caloric content of your diet for one day. What percentage of calories are furnished by complex carbohydrates? By sugars? What steps could you take to increase the proportion of complex carbohydrate? the amount of fiber?
10. When counseling a client about his or her diet, why is it useful to know about the individual's consumption of alcohol?

Cited References

1. West, E. S., et al.: *Textbook of Biochemistry,* 4th ed. Macmillan Publishing Co., Inc., New York, 1966, p. 1039.
2. Hegsted, D. M.: "Energy Needs and Energy Utilization," *Nutr. Rev.,* **32**:33–38, 1974.
3. Food and Nutrition Board: *Recommended Dietary Allowances,* 9th ed. National Academy of Sciences–National Research Council, Washington, D.C., 1980.

4. U.S. Senate Select Committee on Nutrition and Human Needs: *Dietary Goals for the United States,* rev. Government Printing Office, Washington, D.C., December 1977.
5. Marston, R. M., and Peterkin, B. B.: "Nutrient Content of the National Food Supply," *National Food Review* (USDA), Winter 1980, pp. 21–25.
6. American Dietetic Association: "The Saccharin Question Re-examined: An A.D.A. Statement," *J. Am. Diet. Assoc.,* **74**:574–81, 1979.
7. Burkitt, D. P., et al.: "Dietary Fiber and Disease," *JAMA,* **229**:1068–74, 1974.
8. Trowell, H.: "Ischemic Heart Disease and Dietary Fiber," *Am. J. Clin. Nutr.,* **25**:926–32, 1972.
9. Mendeloff, A. I.: "Dietary Fiber and Health. An Introduction," *Nutrition in Disease* (Ross Laboratories), 1978, pp. 5–15.
10. Prasad, A. D., et al.: "Zinc and Iron Deficiencies in Male Subjects with Dwarfism and Hypogonadism but Without Ancylostomiasis, Schistosomiasis, or Severe Anemia," *Am. J. Clin. Nutr.,* **12**:437–44, 1963.
11. Truswell, A. S.: "Food Fibre and Blood Lipids," *Nutr. Rev.,* **35**:51–54, March 1977.
12. Connor, W. E., and Connor, S. L.: "Sucrose and Carbohydrate," in *Present Knowledge in Nutrition,* 4th ed. The Nutrition Foundation, New York, 1976, pp. 33–42.
13. Boeker, E. A.: "Metabolism of Ethanol," *J. Am. Diet. Assoc.,* **76**:550–54, 1980.
14. Review: "Dextrose, Phosphorus and Iron Metabolism in Alcoholism," *Nutr. Rev.,* **36**:142–44, 1978.

Additional References

AHRENS, R. A.: "Sucrose, Hypertension, and Heart Disease," *Am. J. Clin. Nutr.,* **27**:403–22, 1974.

American Diabetes Association, Select Committee on Sugar Substitutes: "Position Statement on Saccharin," *Diabetes Forecast,* **31**:6, July 1978.

American Dietetic Association: "Position Paper on Food and Nutrition Misinformation," *J. Am. Diet. Assoc.,* **66**:277–79, 1975.

ANDERSON, J. W., and CHEN, W. J. L.: "Plant Fiber. Carbohydrate and Lipid Metabolism," *Am. J. Clin. Nutr.,* **32**:346–63, 1979.

Anon. "Too Much Sugar," *Consumer Reports,* March 1978, pp. 136–42.

BIERMAN, E. L.: "Carbohydrate and Sucrose Intake in the Causation of Atherosclerotic Heart Disease, Diabetes Mellitus, and Dental Caries," *Am. J. Clin. Nutr.,* **32**:2644–47, 1979.

BING, F. C.: "Dietary Fiber—in Historical Perspective," *J. Am. Diet. Assoc.,* **69**:498–505, 1976.

BOHANNON, N. V., et al.: "Endocrine Responses to Sugar Ingestion in Man," *J. Am. Diet. Assoc.,* **76**:555–60, 1980.

Committee on Nutrition, American Academy of Pediatrics: "Should Milk Drinking by Children Be Discouraged?" *Nutr. Rev.,* **32**:363–69, 1974.

EASTWOOD, M. A., and KAY, R. M.: "An Hypothesis for the Action of Dietary Fiber Along the Gastrointestinal Tract," *Am. J. Clin. Nutr.,* **32**:364–67, 1979.

Editorial: "Statement on Hypoglycemia," *JAMA,* **223**:682, 1973.

HARDINGE, M. G., et al.: "Carbohydrates in Foods," *J. Am. Diet. Assoc.,* **46**:197–204, 1965.

MCNUTT, K. W.: "Perspective—Fiber," *J. Nutr. Educ.,* **8**:150–52, 1976.

Review: "Nutritional Significance of Lactose Intolerance," *Nutr. Rev.,* **36**:133–34, 1978.

STEVENS, H. A., and OHLSON, M. A.: "Estimated Intake of Simple and Complex Carbohydrates," *J. Am. Diet. Assoc.,* **48**:294–96, 1966.

SOUTHGATE, D. A. T., et al.: "A Guide to Calculating Intakes of Dietary Fiber," *J. Human Nutr.,* **30**:303–13, 1976.

6 *Lipids*

FATS are the most concentrated source of energy, and supply as much as two fifths of the total caloric intake in typical American diets. They provide the body's chief reserve of energy and are essential for diverse functions such as insulation and padding, cell membrane integrity, synthesis of some hormones, and carriers of fat-soluble vitamins. They are valued for the enhancement of food palatability.

Controversial Issues

Few issues in nutrition have created as much controversy as the fat content of the diet. Nutrition scientists, physicians, nutritionists, public health workers, politicians, and consumers have taken sides. Some segments of the food industry are aligned on one side and some on the other. Many years, perhaps decades, may be needed to fully resolve the controversy. In the meantime Americans continue to ask:

Should we reduce our fat intake? Should we omit whole milk and eggs because they are high in saturated fats and cholesterol? What changes should we make in our consumption of meat?

What are the possible benefits of substituting special margarines and cooking oils for regular margarine, butter, and solid fats? Are there any adverse effects on nutritional status and health by such dietary adjustments?

Although final answers to these questions obviously cannot be provided, the reader of this chapter should be able to achieve an overall perspective and to provide responsible guidance to the public.

Composition, Classification, and Characteristics

Composition *Lipids* include fats, oils, and fatlike substances that have a greasy feel and that are insoluble in water but soluble in certain organic solvents such as ether, alcohol, and benzene. They are composed of fatty acids and glycerol. Like carbohydrates, fats are organic compounds of carbon, hydrogen, and oxygen, but the resemblance ends there. Fats have a much smaller proportion of oxygen than do carhohydrates and differ in important ways in their structure and properties. Some lipids also contain carbohydrates, phosphates, or nitrogenous compounds.

Fatty Acids The main constituents of all lipids are fatty acids. They consist of chains of carbon atoms with a methyl (CH_3) group at one end and a carboxyl (COOH) group at the other end.

Most fatty acids in foods and in the body are straight, even-numbered carbon chains, which contain as few as four or as many as twenty-four carbon atoms. Short-chain fatty acids contain four and six carbon atoms, medium-chain fatty acids contain eight to twelve carbon atoms, and long-chain fatty acids contain more than twelve carbon atoms.

Fatty acids are "saturated" or "unsaturated." A fatty acid in which each of the carbon atoms in the chain has two hydrogen atoms attached to it is saturated:

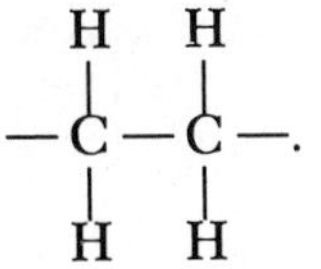

$-\overset{H}{\underset{H}{C}}-\overset{H}{\underset{H}{C}}-$. An unsaturated fatty acid is one in which a hydrogen atom is missing from each of two adjoining carbon atom-thus necessitating a double bond between the two carbon atoms: $-\overset{H}{C}=\overset{H}{C}-$. A MONOUNSATURATED FATTY ACID has one double bond; oleic acid is widely distributed in food and body fats. A POLYUNSATURATED FATTY ACID (PUFA) contains two or more double bonds; linoleic, linolenic, and arachidonic acids are nutritionally important examples of this group. The formulas for four fatty acids that contain eighteen carbon atoms but that differ in their saturation are shown in Figure 6–1.

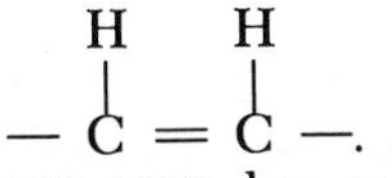

Unsaturated fatty acids can exist as geometric isomers. In the *cis* form the molecule folds back upon itself at each double bond. In the *trans* from the molecule extends to its maximum length.

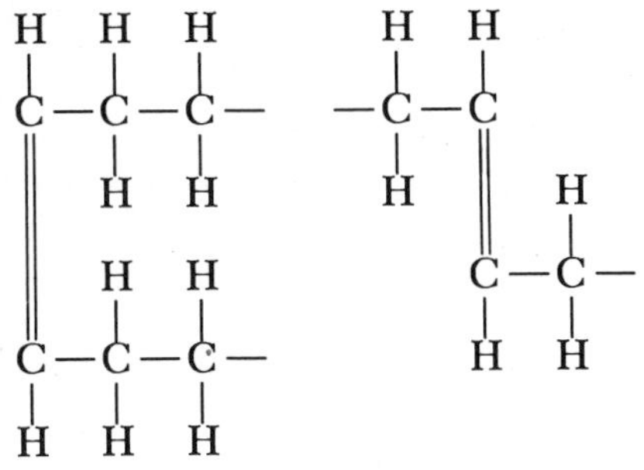

$$\begin{array}{ccccc} H & & H & & H \\ | & & | & & | \\ C & - & C & - & C - \\ \| & & | & & | \\ \| & & H & & H \\ \| & & H & & H \\ \| & & | & & | \\ C & - & C & - & C - \\ | & & | & & | \\ H & & H & & H \end{array} \qquad \begin{array}{ccccc} H & & H & & \\ | & & | & & \\ -C & - & C & & \\ | & & \| & & H \\ H & & \| & & | \\ & & C & - & C - \\ & & | & & | \\ & & H & & H \end{array}$$

The form in which a fatty acid occurs markedly influences the melting point and other properties of the fat. Food and body fats exist principally in the *cis* form.

Classification Lipids are usually classified in three groups:

1. *Simple lipids* are esters of glycerol and fatty acids. GLYCEROL is a 3-carbon alcohol with three hydroxyl groups, each of which can combine with a fatty acid. A MONOGLYCERIDE is formed by combining a fatty acid with one of the hydroxyl groups of the glycerol molecule; DIGLYCERIDES contain two fatty acids; TRIGLYCERIDES, also referred to as *neutral fats,* contain three fatty acids.

A *simple triglyceride* is one in which the three fatty acids are the same. A *mixed triglyceride* is one in which at least two fatty acids are different. Mixed triglycerides account for 98 per cent of fats in foods and over 90 per cent of fat in the body. (See Figure 6–2.)

Waxes are esters of fatty acids and long-chain or cyclic alcohols. This group includes the esters of cholesterol, vitamin A, and vitamin D.

2. *Compound lipids.* These are esters of glycerol and fatty acids, with substitution of other components such as carbohydrate, phosphate, and/or nitrogenous groupings. PHOSPHOLIPIDS such as lecithin and cephalin contain a phosphate and nitrogen grouping replacing one of the fatty acids in the molecule. (See Figure 6–3.) GLYCOLIPIDS such as the cerebrosides contain a molecule of glucose or galactose. LIPOPROTEINS in-

$CH_3(CH_2)_{16}COOH$ Stearic acid (saturated) 18:0

$CH_3(CH_2)_7$ $CH{=}CH$ $(CH_2)_7COOH$ Oleic acid (monounsaturated) 18:1

$CH_3(CH_2)_4$ $CH{=}CH$ CH_2 $CH{=}CH$ $(CH_2)_7COOH$ Linoleic acid (2 double bonds; polyunsaturated) 18:2

CH_3CH_2 $CH{=}CH$ CH_2 $CH{=}CH$ CH_2 $CH{=}CH$ $(CH_2)_7COOH$ Linolenic acid (3 double bonds; polyunsaturated) 18:3

Figure 6–1. These fatty acids contain eighteen carbon atoms but differ in the level of saturation, having one, two, and three double bonds.

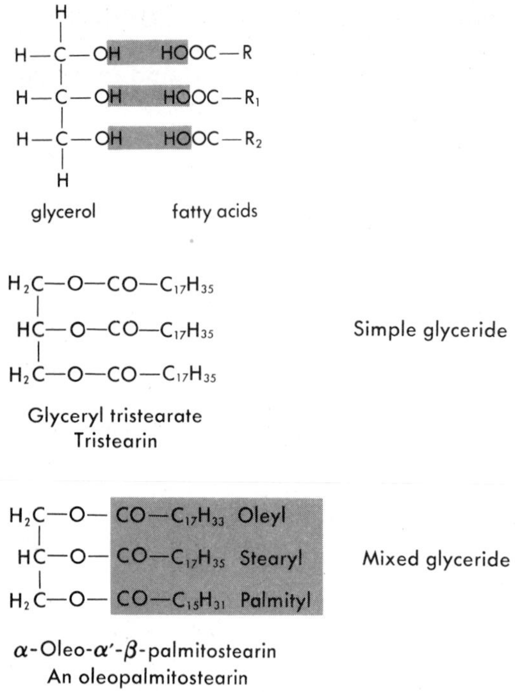

H
H—C—OH HOOC—R
H—C—OH HOOC—R_1
H—C—OH HOOC—R_2
H
glycerol fatty acids

$H_2C—O—CO—C_{17}H_{35}$
$HC—O—CO—C_{17}H_{35}$ Simple glyceride
$H_2C—O—CO—C_{17}H_{35}$

Glyceryl tristearate
Tristearin

$H_2C—O—CO—C_{17}H_{33}$ Oleyl
$HC—O—CO—C_{17}H_{35}$ Stearyl Mixed glyceride
$H_2C—O—CO—C_{15}H_{31}$ Palmityl

α-Oleo-α′-β-palmitostearin
An oleopalmitostearin

Figure 6–2. Formation of a triglyceride by condensation of three fatty acids and glycerol. Simple and mixed triglyceride.

clude a variety of lipid molecules bound to protein molecules in order to facilitate transport in the aqueous medium of the blood.

3. *Derived lipids.* These include fatty acids; alcohols (glycerol and sterols); carotenoids; and the fat-soluble vitamins, A, D, E, and K.

Characteristics of Fats The nature of fats—their hardness, melting point, and flavor—is determined by the length of the carbon chain and the level of saturation of the fatty acids as well as the order in which the fatty acids are attached to the glycerol molecule. Although pure triglycerides are practically tasteless, they have the ability to hold flavors and aromas. A tremendous number of fats exist in nature. Each food fat—beef, lamb, chicken, olive oil, for example—has its distinctive flavor and hardness.

Hardness. The hardness of a fat is determined by its fatty acid composition. In turn, the fatty acid composition of body fat, and hence its hardness, can be modified by the diet. Fatty acids containing twelve carbon atoms or fewer and unsaturated fatty acids are liquid at room temperature. Saturated fatty acids containing fourteen carbon atoms or more are solid at room temperature. Food and body fats contain mixtures of short- and long-chain fatty acids and of satu-

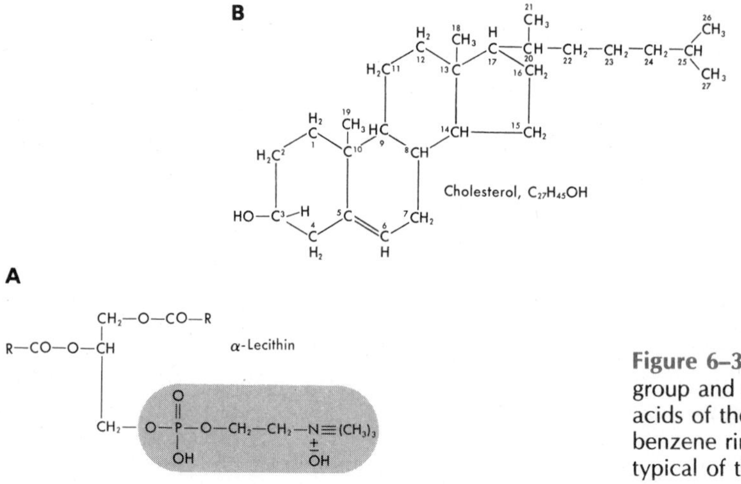

B

Cholesterol, $C_{27}H_{45}OH$

A

$CH_2—O—CO—R$
$R—CO—O—CH$ α-Lecithin
$CH_2—O—P(=O)(OH)—O—CH_2—CH_2—N\equiv(CH_3)_3$ $\overset{+}{O}H$

Figure 6–3. *(A)* In lecithin a phosphate group and choline replace one of the fatty acids of the glyceride. *(B)* The composite benzene ring structure of cholesterol is typical of the structure of many steroids.

rated and unsaturated fatty acids. No natural fat is made up completely of either saturated or unsaturated fatty acids.

The distribution of fatty acids in a number of fats is shown in Table 6–1. Only about 5 per cent of fatty acids in food and body fats contain fewer than fourteen carbon atoms, coconut oil being an exception.

Animal fats, often classified as "saturated," contain 30 to 60 per cent saturated fatty acids, of which palmitic and stearic acids predominate. Also, they contain about 30 to 50 per cent oleic acid and small amounts of polyunsaturated fatty acids. In general, herbivora have harder fats than carnivora, and land animals have harder fats than aquatic animals. Lamb and beef fat, with their high content of palmitic and stearic acids, are much harder than pork and chicken fat, which contain somewhat more of the unsaturated fatty acids. Fats from fish have a high proportion of polyunsaturated fatty acids containing twenty to twenty-four carbon atoms. The proportion of saturated fatty acids is high in milk fat, but this fat is soft because of the presence of many short-chain fatty acids.

Oleic and linoleic acids predominate in vegetable fats, except for coconut oil. Safflower, corn, cottonseed, and soybean oils are very rich in linoleic acid, whereas peanut and olive oils are rich in oleic acid and correspondingly lower in linoleic acid. Of the vegetable fats, coconut oil is unique in that it is composed largely of the 12-carbon lauric acid, which is liquid at room temperature. Coconut oil is classified as a "saturated" fat and other vegetable fats as "unsaturated." Those fats that have a high proportion of fatty acids with two or more double bonds are referred to as "polyunsaturated."

Hydrogenation. In the presence of a catalyst such as nickel, liquid fats can be changed to solid fats by HYDROGENATION; this consists of the addition of hydrogen at the double bonds of the carbon chain. In the manufacture of vegetable shortenings and margarines, some, but not all, of the double bonds in the oils are hydrogenated, thereby forming fats that are somewhat soft and plastic. During hydrogenation some of the fatty acids are changed from the *cis* to the *trans* form, but both forms are utilized by the body. Hydrogenation reduces the linoleic acid content of the fat.

Emulsification. Fats are capable of forming emulsions with liquids; that is, the fats can be dispersed into minute globules, thus increasing the surface area and reducing the surface tension so that there is less tendency for the globules to coalesce. Bile salts and lecithin are essential biochemical emulsifiers in digestion and absorption. The property of emulsification is also utilized in the homogenization of milk and in the preparation of mayonnaise. Lecithin and other emulsifiers are widely used by the food industry.

Saponification. The combination of a fatty acid with a cation to form a soap is known as SAPONIFICATION. In the alkaline medium of the intestine, for example, free fatty acid may combine with calcium to form an insoluble compound that is excreted in the feces. In certain diseases characterized by poor fat absorption—sprue, for example—the loss of calcium in this manner could be significant.

Rancidity. Air at room temperature can induce oxidation of fats, resulting in the changes in odor and flavor commonly known as rancidity. These changes are accelerated upon exposure to light and in the presence of traces of certain minerals. The oxygen attacks the double bonds of fatty acids to form *peroxides.* Hence, peroxidation occurs more readily in fats that have a high proportion of unsaturated fatty acids. Some fats are naturally protected by the presence of antioxidants, one of which is vitamin E. But in the process of preventing oxidation, the activity of vitamin E is lost. Commercially processed fats and oils are usually protected by the addition of small amounts of antioxidants.

Effect of heat. Excessive heating of fats leads to the breakdown of glycerol, produc-

Table 6-1. **Typical Major Fatty Acid Analyses of Some Fats of Animal and Plant Origin*†**

		Saturated								Unsaturated				
		Capric	Lauric	Myristic	Palmitic	Stearic	Arach-idic	Behemic	Palmit-oleic	Oleic	Linoleic	Linolenic	Arachi-donic	Other Polyenoic Acids
	4-8	10.0	12.0	14.0	16.0	18.0	20.0	22.0	16.1	18.1	18.2	18.3	20.4	
Animal														
Lard				1.5	27.0	13.5			3.0	43.5	10.5	0.5		
Chicken			2.0	7.0	25.0	6.0			8.0	36.0	14.0			
Egg					25.0	10.0				50.0	10.0	2.0	3.0	
Beef				3.0	29.0	21.0	0.5		3.0	41.0	2.0	0.5	0.5	
Butter	5.5	3.0	3.5	12.0	28.0	13.0			3.0	28.5	1.0			
Human milk		1.5	7.0	8.5	21.0	7.0	1.0		2.5	36.0	7.0	1.0	0.5	
Menhaden				9.0	19.0	5.5			16.0					48.5
Human adipose‡			0.1-2	2-6	21-25	2-8			3-7	39-47	4-25			2-8
Vegetable														
Corn					12.5	2.5	0.5			29.0	55.0	0.5		
Peanut					11.5	3.0	1.5	2.5		53.0	26.0			
Cottonseed				1.0	26.0	3.0			1.0	17.5	51.5			
Soybean					11.5	4.0				24.5	53.0	7.0		
Olive					13.0	2.5			1.0	74.0	9.0	0.5		
Coconut	7.0	6.0	49.5	19.5	8.5	2.0				6.0	1.5			

*Food and Nutrition Board: *Dietary Fat and Human Health.* Pub. 1147, National Academy of Sciences–National Research Council, Washington, D.C., 1966, p. 6.

†Composition is given in weight percentages of the component fatty acids (rounded to nearest 0.5) as determined by gas chromatography. The number of carbon atoms and the number of double bonds is indicated under the common name of the fatty acid. These data were derived from a variety of sources. They are representative determinations rather than averages, and considerable variation is to be expected in individual samples from other sources.

‡Adapted from West, E. S., et al.: *Textbook of Biochemistry*, 4th ed. Macmillan Publishing Co., Inc., New York, 1966, p. 134.

ing a pungent compound (acrolein) which is especially irritating to the gastrointestinal mucosa. Fatty acids are also oxidized by prolonged heating at high temperatures. Under ordinary conditions of home or commercial frying no adverse effects on nutritional properties have been found.

Functions

Body Composition All body cells contain some fat. In healthy nonobese women fat comprises about 18 to 25 per cent of body weight, and in healthy nonobese men about 15 to 20 per cent. With aging the proportion of fat in the body generally increases as that of protoplasmic tissue decreases.

Adipose tissue which consists principally of triglycerides is stored in the subcutaneous tissues and in the abdominal cavity. It also surrounds the organs and is laced throughout muscle tissue.

Cell membranes contain lipids that facilitate the transfer of nutrients. Cerebrosides, galactose-containing lipids, are components of the myelin sheath of nerves and the white matter of the brain. Gangliosides, glucose- and galactose-containing lipids, are constituents of brain tissue and of the synaptic membranes.

Energy The primary function of fat is to supply energy. Each gram of fat when oxidized yields approximately 9 kcal (37.8 kJ), or more than twice as much energy as a gram of carbohydrate or protein. The high density and low solubility of fats make them an ideal form in which to store energy. In fact, not only are fats as such stored in adipose tissue but any glucose and amino acids not promptly utilized are also synthesized into fats and stored.

A woman who weighs 55 kg, of which 20 per cent is fat, has a store of about 85,000 kcal (7,700 kcal per kilogram of fat). Many examples could be cited of individuals who have survived starvation for 30 or 40 days or partial starvation for much longer periods of time. Their survival was possible only because of the energy available from the adipose tissue.

Satiety Function Closely related to the provision of energy is the satiety value of fats. Because fats reduce gastric motility, and remain in the stomach longer, the onset of hunger sensations is delayed. Diets that contain generous amounts of fat are sometimes described as "sticking to the ribs," "rich," or "satisfying"; that is, they have high satiety value.

Palatability How much food we eat, and the kind of food we eat, depends in part on our enjoyment of it. Fats lend palatability to the diet, whether it be as butter or margarine on bread, seasoning for vegetables, dressings on salads, or an ingredient of cakes, cookies, pastries, and other desserts. The fats in meats, poultry, and fish and the oils in fruits lend the characteristic flavors that we enjoy. If most fat is eliminated from the diet, as is necessary for some patients with disturbances of fat metabolism, the diet becomes very bulky and it is often difficult to ingest sufficient food to meet energy requirements.

Carriers of Fat-Soluble Vitamins Dietary fat is a carrier of the fat-soluble vitamins; A, D, E, and K. Some fat is also necessary for the absorption of vitamin A and its precursor, carotene.

Insulation and Padding The subcutaneous layer of fat is an effective insulator and reduces losses of body heat in cold weather. Excessive layers of subcutaneous fat, as in obesity, interfere with heat loss during warm weather, thus increasing discomfort. The vital organs such as the kidney are protected against physical injury by a padding of fat. Fats and oils also have some value as a lubricant for the gastrointestinal tract.

Essential Fatty Acids LINOLEIC ACID, the 18-carbon acid with two double bonds, is an essential fatty acid; that is, it cannot be synthesized in the body and must be present in the diet. In the body linoleic acid is rapidly converted to ARACHIDONIC ACID, the physiologically functioning polyunsaturated fatty acid. LINOLENIC ACID, another of the polyunsaturated fatty acids, promotes normal growth in animals but it does not cure the dermatitis that occurs from fatty acid deficiency. It is, therefore, not an essential fatty acid and is not a substitute for linoleic acid.

The polyunsaturated fatty acids are constituents of phospholipids and thus have a role in regulating cell permeability. Arachidonic acid is a precursor of PROSTAGLANDINS, a group of hormonelike compounds that stimulate contraction of smooth muscle. Prostaglandins appear to have a role in the regulation of blood pressure, transmission of the nerve impulse, and inhibition of gastric secretion and lipolysis.

In the absence of linoleic acid in the diet of animals there is growth retardation, skin lesions, and liver degeneration. Dryness and scaling of the skin has been observed in infants who received formulas lacking linoleic acid.[1] The eczemalike symptoms disappeared when a source of linoleic acid was provided. (See Figure 6–4.)

Phospholipids All cells contain phospholipids, but brain, nervous tissue, and liver are especially rich in them. The phospholipid level in the body is not reduced even in starvation, which suggests the vital role that they must play in metabolism. Phospholipids are powerful emulsifying agents and have an affinity for water. Hence, they are essential to the digestion and absorption of fats and they facilitate the uptake of fatty acids by the cells.

Phospholipids comprise a significant proportion of the blood lipoproteins but their function in lipid transport is not clearly understood. They are manufactured and removed by the liver and apparently do not enter the tissue cells, which readily synthesize their own supply of phospholipid. Because of the ease with which the body synthesizes phospholipids there is no need for them in the diet.

Cholesterol The concentration of cholesterol is high in the liver, the adrenal, the white and gray matter of the brain, and the peripheral nerves. It is present in small amounts in almost all body tissues and constitutes an important fraction of the blood

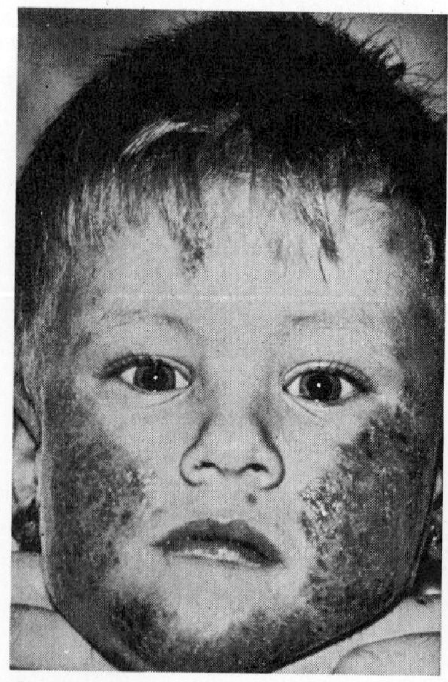

A

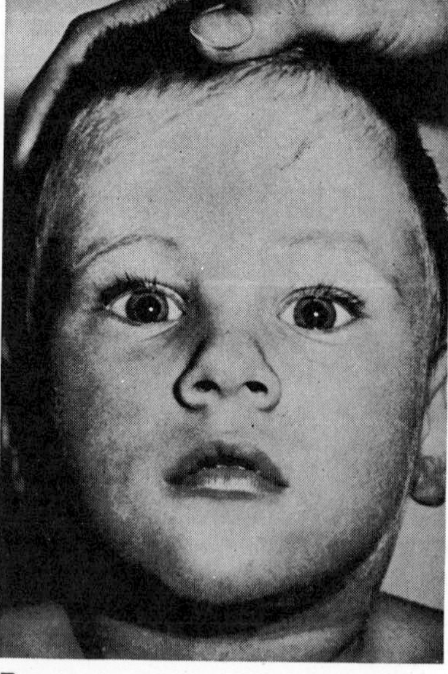

B

Figure 6–4. Child 2½ years old showing *(A)* eczema present since 2 months of age; *(B)* 1 month after adding a source of linoleic acid to the diet. (Courtesy, Dr. A. E. Hansen, Galveston, Texas.)

lipoproteins. It is synthesized by the liver to meet body needs regardless of dietary intake.

Cholesterol is a component of cell membranes and furnishes the nucleus for the synthesis of provitamin D, adrenocortical hormones, steroid sex hormones, and bile salts.

Digestion and Absorption

Digestion Almost all the fats presented to the digestive tract for hydrolysis are triglycerides. Only a small fraction of dietary fat consists of cholesterol esters and phospholipids. Fats are hydrolyzed primarily in the small intestine. Although gastric lipase brings about some hydrolysis of finely divided fats from foods such as egg yolk and cream, the action is not important.

As the chyme enters the duodenum, the presence of fat stimulates the release of the hormone *enterogastrone.* This hormone reduces motility and regulates the flow of chyme to correspond to the availability of the pancreatic secretions. The presence of fat in the duodenum also stimulates the intestinal wall to secrete CHOLECYSTOKININ, a hormone that is carried to the gallbladder by the bloodstream. Cholecystokinin stimulates the contraction of the gallbladder, thereby forcing bile into the common duct and thence into the small intestine.

Bile has several important functions in fat digestion and absorption: (1) it stimulates peristalsis; (2) it neutralizes the acid chyme so as to provide the optimum hydrogen ion concentration for enzyme activity; (3) it emulsifies fats, thereby increasing the surface area exposed to enzyme action; and (4) it lowers the surface tension so that intimate contact between the fat droplets and the enzymes is possible.

The triglycerides are hydrolyzed stepwise by lipase; that is, one of the end fatty acids is removed at the time, yielding in turn a diglyceride and then a monoglyceride, with the fatty acid attached in the middle or number 2 position. Only about one fourth to one half of the triglycerides are completely hydrolyzed to glycerol and fatty acids. Some of the phospholipids are hydrolyzed by phospholipases that can attack several linkages of the molecule. Cholesterol esters are hydrolyzed by *cholesterol esterase* to cholesterol and fatty acids. The end products of lipid hydrolysis that are presented for absorption include fatty acids, glycerol, monoglycerides, some di- and triglycerides, cholesterol, and phospholipids. (See Figure 6–5.)

Speed of Digestion Fats reduce the motility of the gastrointestinal tract, and hence any diet containing fat remains in the stomach longer than one that is low in fat. Fats that are liquid at body temperature are hydrolyzed more rapidly than those that are solid at body temperature. Typical mixed diets contain complex mixtures of fats including short- and long-chain as well as saturated and unsaturated fatty acids. Adults normally experience no difficulty in digesting fats from any source. Infants and young children, as well as some elderly persons, seem to have somewhat better tolerance for the softer, more highly emulsified fats such as those in dairy products. They also may experience some discomfort following meals that are high in fat.

Fried foods are digested somewhat more slowly than foods prepared by other methods of cookery because the food particles coated with fat must be broken up before they can be acted upon by enzymes. Properly fried foods do not normally cause digestive difficulties, even for persons who require therapeutic diets. When the frying temperature is too low, foods absorb excessive amounts of fat, thus lengthening the time required for digestion. On the other hand, if foods are fried at too high a temperature the resulting decomposition products may be irritating to the intestinal mucosa.

Absorption In the lumen of the small intestine the free fatty acids, monoglycerides, some diglycerides and triglycerides,

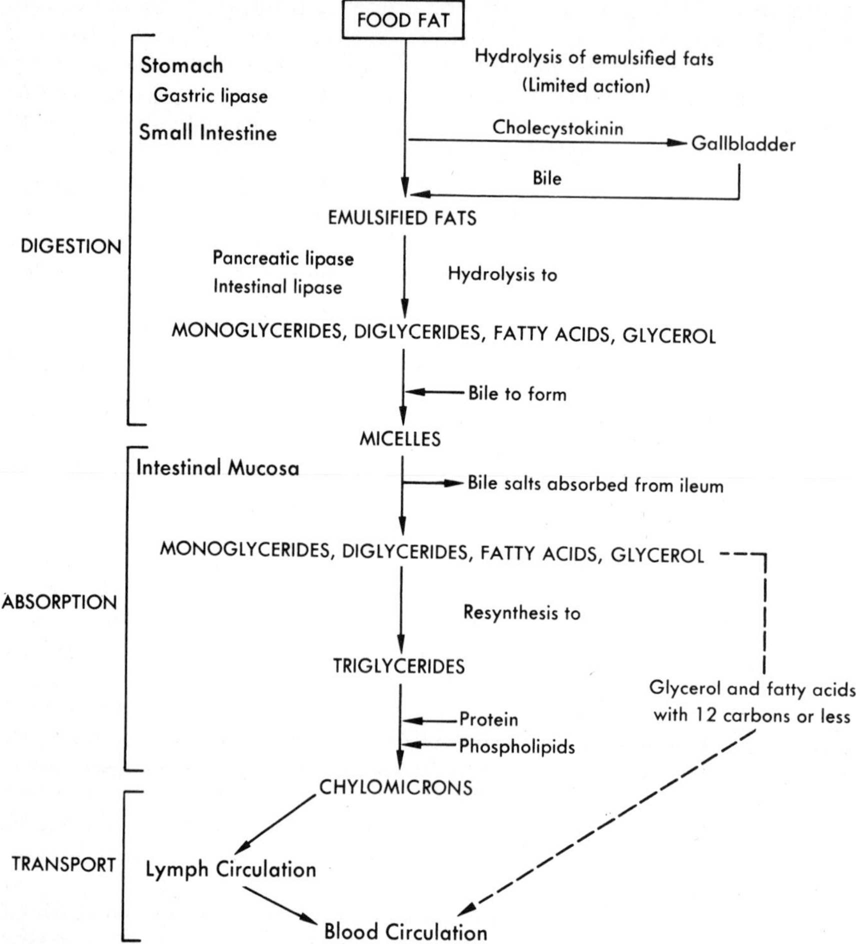

Figure 6–5. The digestion, absorption, and transport of fat.

and cholesterol are complexed with bile salts to form MICELLES, which are water-soluble microscopic particles that can penetrate the mucosal membrane. At the point of contact of the micelle with the brush border of the epithelial cell, the lipids are apparently released from the complex and enter the cell by mechanisms not fully understood. *Pinocytosis,* that is, engulfing the fat and subsequently releasing it to the interior of the cell, is believed to be one of the operative mechanisms. When the lipids are released from the micelle, new products of hydrolysis of fats can again combine with the bile salts. Most of the absorption of fats occurs from the jejunum.

Fatty acids that contain twelve carbon atoms or fewer are absorbed into the portal circulation without reesterification in the mucosal cell. They are attached to albumin for their transportation, and they may be used within the liver or released to other tissues in the body. The glycerol resulting from fat hydrolysis is also carried by the portal circulation.

Fatty acids that contain fourteen carbon

atoms or more are resynthesized to new triglycerides within the epithelial cell of the mucosa before they are extruded into the lymph circulation. The new fats are formed by the addition of two fatty acids to a monoglyceride molecule or by esterification of glycerol with three fatty acids. This is an energy-requiring process. Cholesterol is also reesterified within the epithelial cell. See page 108 for a further discussion of fat synthesis.

Chylomicrons. In order to penetrate the lipoprotein membrane of the epithelial cell for entrance to the lymph circulation, the newly formed fats are made soluble by surrounding them with a lipoprotein envelope consisting chiefly of phospholipids and a very small amount of protein. These particles are known as CHYLOMICRONS, having first been identified in chyle (lymph). They are of very low density and give the lymph a milky appearance. The chylomicrons enter the lymph circulation, which empties into the thoracic duct.

Enterohepatic circulation. Bile salts are utilized over and over again through the cycle known as the *enterohepatic circulation.* This consists of (1) the secretion of bile into the duodenum, (2) the complexing of bile with fat particles to form micelles, (3) the release of bile salts from the micelles at the brush border, (4) the reabsorption of bile salts by active transport from the ileum, (5) the entrance of the salts into the hepatic circulation, and (6) the secretion of bile once again into the duodenum. The total body pool of bile salts is estimated to be about 3 gm, but this pool can be recirculated as much as ten times in a day. This results in the effectiveness of 30 gm bile salts daily. The liver normally synthesizes approximately 0.5 gm bile salts daily, an amount that just about covers the excretion in the feces.

Completeness of Digestion and Absorption Normally about 95 per cent of dietary fats and 10 to 50 per cent of dietary cholesterol are absorbed.

A number of factors reduce the amount of fat that is digested and absorbed. Among these are increased motility so that food is moved along the tract too rapidly for complete enzyme action; disease of the biliary tract so that the secretion of bile is deficient or does not reach the small intestine; disease of the pancreas so that lipase is not secreted; and reduction in the absorbing surfaces as in celiac disease or following surgery on the small intestine. When fat absorption is decreased, large amounts of fat are excreted in the feces (steatorrhea) with a consequent serious loss of calories. (See Chapter 33.)

Metabolism

The blood is the means of transportation of lipids from one site to another, and the liver and adipose tissues are the specialized organs that control lipid metabolism. The synthesis of new lipids (LIPOGENESIS) and the catabolism of lipids (LIPOLYSIS) are taking place continuously. These reactions are catalyzed by specific enzymes under the control of nervous and hormonal mechanisms. (See Figure 6–6.)

Blood Lipids The levels of cholesterol and of triglycerides in blood serum are frequently determined in the clinical laboratory, and provide clues to the presence or absence of hyperlipidemia. In normal adults the serum cholesterol concentration ranges from 150 to 250 mg per 100 ml. Many clinicians believe that a level below 250 mg and preferably at about 200 mg per 100 ml reduces the risk of coronary disease.

The normal triglyceride level after a 12- to 14-hour fast is 140 mg per 100 ml or less. Triglyceride levels vary widely during the day. They are increased when chylomicrons and very low density lipoproteins are being transported following a meal. The levels increase with lipolysis by adipose tissue as during weight loss. They decrease when fat is being synthesized by the adipose tissue or liver. The triglyceride levels

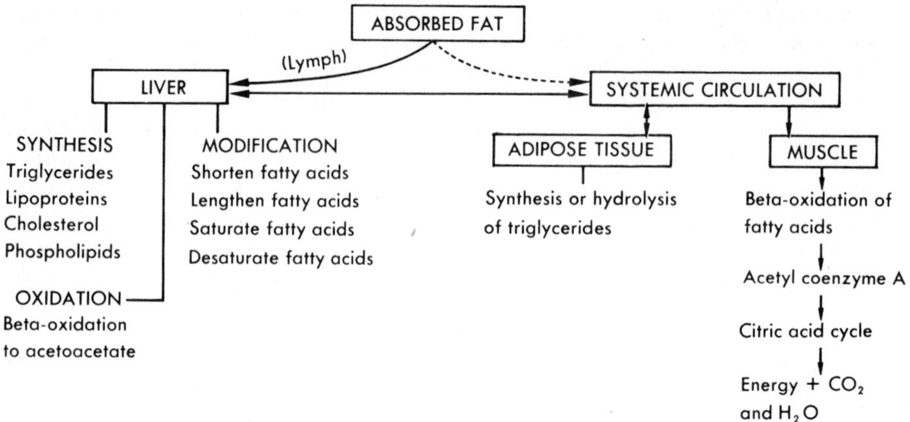

Figure 6–6. The liver and adipose tissue are the principal organs of fat metabolism.

increase gradually with age, but such an increase is not necessarily desirable.

However, cholesterol and triglycerides do not exist in the free state in the circulation. Since fats are insoluble in water, proteins provide the mechanism for their transport in the aqueous medium of the blood. These protein-lipid complexes are known as lipoproteins. (See Table 6–2.) The chylomicrons synthesized in the intestinal mucosa (see page 105) are large particles consisting principally of triglycerides. They give a milky appearance to blood serum shortly after a fat-rich meal, but they are rapidly hydrolyzed by lipoprotein lipase and the released fats are used by the tissues. The blood serum is thus "cleared."

Low-density or beta lipoproteins. Two broad classes have been described. Very low density lipoproteins (VLDL) contain a high proportion of triglycerides and a small amount of protein. When this class is elevated, there is a presumption of carbohydrate-induced hyperlipidemia. Low-density lipoproteins (LDL) are the chief carriers of cholesterol and are relatively low in triglycerides. The concentration of this group increases with age and when diets are rich in saturated fatty acids, and to a lesser extent when diets contain substantial

Table 6-2. **Approximate Composition of Lipoproteins***

	Protein	Lipids			
		Triglycerides	Cholesterol	Phospholipids	Total
	per cent	per cent			
Chylomicrons	0.5-1.0	>85	2-5	3-6	99
Very low density lipoproteins (VLDL)	5-15	50-70	10-20	10-20	95
Low-density lipoproteins (LDL)	25	5-10	40-45	20-25	75
High-density lipoproteins (HDL)	45-55	2	18	30	50

*Adapted from Herrera, G., and Nicolosi, R. J.: "A Clinician's Guide to Lipid Metabolism," in *Atherosclerosis,* MEDCOM, Inc., New York, 1974, p. 27.

amounts of cholesterol. Patients who have had a myocardial infarction, those who have angina pectoris, and those individuals who are considered to be high risks for cardiovascular disease usually show increased concentrations of the β-lipoprotein group (HYPERLIPOPROTEINEMIA). Other pathologic conditions in which this group is often elevated include diabetes mellitus, nephrosis, hypothyroidism, and xanthomatosis.[2]

High-density or alpha lipoproteins. Until recently little was known about the high-density lipoproteins (HDL), except that they consisted of about 50 per cent protein and 20 per cent cholesterol. Now this group has been found to have a protective effect; that is, it reduces the risk of coronary heart disease. The influence of diet on this group does not appear to be great, but persons who exercise regularly, who do not smoke, and who are of normal weight have higher levels than do those who are sedentary and obese.

Free fatty acids (FFA), also designated as nonesterified fatty acids (NEFA), are the principal source of fatty acids made available to the cells for energy. They enter the circulation as the result of the hydrolysis of triglycerides, chiefly by adipose tissue. The fatty acids are attached rather tightly to plasma albumin and do not circulate in their free state. At the cell surfaces the fatty acid is released with ease from its carrier. The concentration of FFA in the blood at any given time is quite low, but the rate of turnover is so rapid that several thousand calories are transported daily in the circulation in this way. The concentration of free fatty acids is somewhat higher in the circulation during fasting, thus indicating more rapid release from adipose tissue. It is somewhat lower when carbohydrate is being absorbed, which indicates that carbohydrate is being used for energy as well as synthesized to fat.

Adipose Tissue and Fat Metabolism The adipose cell is a specialized cell that provides for the synthesis, storage, and release of fats. It contains less water than protoplasmic cells, and as the cell size increases with the storage of fat the water content decreases. It is endowed with enzymes that bring about lipogenesis and lipolysis. Fat synthesis and breakdown take place continuously, but they are in equilibrium when the energy needs of the body are exactly met.

Several studies have shown that the number of adipose cells increases rapidly during infancy and childhood. The number usually remains constant during adult life, regardless of weight status, although some investigators have observed further hyperplasia. If the energy supplied to the body exceeds the body's needs, lipogenesis takes place and the cells enlarge (weight is gained) regardless of whether the calories were derived from fats, carbohydrates, or proteins.[3] For the synthesis of fat, insulin is required.

When a calorie deficit exists, the adipose tissue will be catabolized more rapidly than it is being synthesized (weight is lost). The release of fatty acids from adipose tissue is accelerated by the same hormones that increase glucose breakdown: epinephrine, norepinephrine, glucagon, growth hormone, adrenocorticotropic hormone, and thyrotropic hormone.

The Liver and Fat Metabolism The liver is the key organ in the regulation of fat metabolism. It is able to accomplish the shortening or lengthening of the carbon chain of the fatty acids and to introduce double bonds into fatty acids. For example, a double bond can be introduced into stearic acid to yield oleic acid. On the other hand, a second double bond cannot be introduced into oleic acid to yield linoleic acid. With a dietary supply of linoleic acid, this essential fatty acid can be converted to arachidonic acid by adding a 2-carbon unit and by introducing two additional double bonds.

The liver hydrolyzes the triglycerides brought to it, re-forms new triglycerides, and again releases them to the circulation. It also synthesizes triglycerides from free fatty acids, glucose, or the carbon skeletons of amino acids. Phospholipids and lipoproteins are synthesized and released to the circulation or removed from the circulation, thus maintaining control over blood levels.

The liver is probably the chief regulator of the total body content of cholesterol and of the circulating blood cholesterol. It governs the endogenous synthesis of cholesterol, the removal of cholesterol from the circulation, the production of bile acids, and the excretion of cholesterol and bile acids by way of the bile into the intestine.

Certain LIPOTROPIC SUBSTANCES must be present to prevent the accumulation of fat in the liver. They include choline, vitamin B-12, betaine, and possibly inositol. Methionine, one of the essential amino acids, donates methyl groups for the synthesis of choline and is therefore a lipotropic substance.

Synthesis of Fats Triglycerides are synthesized by the epithelial cells of the intestinal mucosa, by the adipose tissue, and by the liver. In order to synthesize triglycerides, a source of α-glycerophosphate is essential. This is furnished by the normal oxidation of glucose that occurs in each of these tissues through the Embden-Meyerhof pathway (see page 82). A second source of α-glycerophosphate is available from the glycerol released from fat hydrolysis in the intestinal mucosa and in the liver.[4] The glycerol so released combines with ATP in the presence of glycerokinase to form α-glycerophosphate. Adipose tissue does not contain glycerokinase and cannot convert glycerol to the active form.

The fatty acids for the triglyceride molecule are available from the hydrolysis of fats and also through synthesis from acetyl coenzyme A derived through the oxidation of fats, glucose, and some amino acids.

The synthesis of fats from acetyl coenzyme A is accomplished essentially by building up the carbon chain by successive additions of 2-carbon fragments. NADPH, a niacin-containing coenzyme, is required for this synthesis. It is made available through the pentose shunt of the glycolytic pathway (see page 84). The synthesis of fatty acids from acetyl coenzyme A is thus seen to be dependent upon normal carbohydrate metabolism and to require insulin. Free fatty acids are not esterified directly with glycerophosphate but must first be converted to fatty acyl coenzyme A. They are then attached stepwise to glycerophosphate to form the triglyceride.

Oxidation of Fatty Acids All cells of the body except those of the central nervous system and red blood cells can oxidize fatty acids to yield energy. Although glucose is normally the only source of energy for the central nervous system, the brain cells after a period of total starvation can adapt to the utilization of ketone bodies derived from fat and amino acids.[6]

The oxidation of fatty acids takes place in the cell mitochondria. BETA OXIDATION is the major pathway for oxidation. By this process oxidation occurs at the carbon that is beta from the carboxyl group. To prime the reaction ATP is required. The oxidation is accomplished in five steps, the end result of which is a fatty acid that is two carbons shorter plus a molecule of acetyl coenzyme. A. Thus, the complete breakdown of an 18-carbon fatty acid requires 45 reactions.

$$\underset{\text{Stearic acid}}{CH_3(CH_2)_{16}COOH} + \text{Coenzyme A} \rightarrow$$

$$\underset{\text{Palmityl coenzyme A}}{CH_3(CH_2)_{14}COOCoA} + \underset{\text{Acetyl coenzyme A}}{CH_3COOCoA}$$

Each molecule of acetyl coenzyme A can (1) enter the Krebs cycle for oxidation to energy, carbon dioxide, and water, or (2) be used for the synthesis of new fatty acids, cholesterol, and other compounds. (See Figure 5–5.)

The glycerol made available from the hydrolysis of fatty acids enters the glycolytic pathway by combining with ATP to form glycerophosphate. Thus, it is a potential source of glucose, glycogen, and energy or may be the backbone for the new glyceride molecule.

Ketogenesis Within the liver two molecules of acetyl coenzyme A can condense to form acetoacetyl coenzyme A, which in turn yields acetoacetic acid, beta-hydroxybutyric acid, and acetone. These compounds are known as KETONE BODIES and the process as KETOGENESIS. The ketone bodies are normally produced in small amounts by the liver. Although the liver cells do not possess the enzymes necessary for their further oxidation, muscle and other cells can utilize them to yield energy.

During rapid weight reduction using a starvation regimen or a low-calorie diet consisting of protein and fat but little if any carbohydrate, ketones are produced more rapidly than the tissues can utilize them. The carbohydrate metabolism is greatly reduced while the production of acetyl coenzyme A is sharply increased. The reduction in carbohydrate metabolism means that the amount of oxalacetate available to combine with acetyl coenzyme A in the Krebs cycle is also reduced. The liver synthesizes vastly increased amounts of the ketones—far beyond the ability of the tissues to oxidize them. The principal effect of the increased production is a disturbance of the acid-base balance. Acetoacetic acid and β-hydroxybutyric acid are fairly strong acids and combine with the available base. They are excreted (KETONURIA) and the alkali reserve is reduced. Acetone, being volatile, is excreted by the lungs. In normal persons small intakes of carbohydrate (50 gm or less) are sufficient to reverse the ketosis.

In uncontrolled diabetes mellitus, ketosis occurs because of lack of insulin for the metabolism of carbohydrate. It is a serious complication that can lead to coma and even death, and prompt measures are required to correct the acidosis and to restore normal carbohydrate metabolism.

Cholesterol Metabolism The liver and intestine are the chief sites of cholesterol synthesis, but all cells are able to produce some cholesterol. The endogenous production of cholesterol has been variously estimated at 800 to 1,500 mg daily and is apparently independent of the dietary supply. Acetyl coenzyme A is the direct precursor of cholesterol, and thus any donor of acetyl coenzyme A—fatty acids, glucose, and some amino acids—is a potential source of cholesterol.

Cholesterol is transported in the blood in the various classes of lipoproteins. (See Table 6–2.) The body is unable to break down the cholesterol nucleus, but the liver converts it by enzyme action to bile acids. This is apparently rate limited.[5] and therefore any excess supply poses problems of disposal. Cholesterol as such and bile acids are constituents of bile, and excretion occurs from the intestine.

Fat in the Diet

Dietary Allowance People of the Orient consume diets that provide around 10 per cent or less of the calories from fat, whereas Americans derive about 40 per cent of their calories from fat. These extremes of intake cannot be described categorically as being damaging to health or as affording promise of good health.

The Food and Nutrition Board has not set precise recommendations for either the quantity or type of fat that should be included in the diet. Since the energy value of the diet is derived mainly from fat and carbohydrate, any drastic restriction in the one means that the other must be increased in order to maintain caloric equilibrium.

The Dietary Goals for the United States recommend the following

Reduce overall fat consumption from approximately 40 per cent to about 30 per cent of energy intake.

Reduce saturated fat consumption to account for about 10 per cent of total energy intake; and balance that with polyunsaturated and monounsaturated fats, which should account for about 10 per cent of energy intake each.

Reduce cholesterol consumption to about 300 mg a day.[6]

The recommendation presented in the Dietary Guidelines is less specific: "Avoid too much fat, saturated fat, and cholesterol."[7]

Essential fatty acid requirement. Each diet must provide some linoleic acid. The signs of deficiency are prevented when 1 to 2 per cent of dietary calories are provided by linoleic acid. For infants, a formula that supplies 3 per cent of calories as linoleic acid is recommended. This level of linoleic acid is also satisfactory for persons who have a relatively low fat intake (less than 25 per cent of calories). Most people in the United States consume diets in which the fat intake is 35 to 40 per cent of calories and would benefit by a higher intake of linoleic acid.[8] Some persons at high risk for coronary disease often require a fat-controlled diet with fat restricted to 35 per cent of calories or less. Of this fat intake, one fourth to one third, or 8 to 10 per cent of total calories, should be supplied by polyunsaturated (essential) fatty acids.

Food Sources In the United States the fat available for consumption in 1980 was 168 gm.[9] The percentages contributed by each food group were: fats and oils, including butter, 43.0; meat, poultry and fish, 36.1; dairy products excluding butter, 11.2; legumes, 3.7; eggs, 2.7; flour and cereals, 1.3; and fruits and vegetables, 0.9.

The so-called "visible" fats include oils, lard, hydrogenated shortening, butter, margarine, fat back of pork, bacon, and salad dressings, and are concentrated sources of fat. A small amount of them contribute importantly to the caloric level of the diet.

"Invisible" fats include meat, poultry, fish, eggs, whole milk, cream, cheese, and baked products. Meats, poultry, and fish vary widely in their fat content. The amount of fat ingested from meat will depend upon the cut that was used, whether fat was carefully trimmed, whether fat drippings were used, and what the method of preparation was. Lean cuts of beef, pork, lamb, and veal differ little in their fat content. Fish is somewhat lower in fat than is meat. Fish that have a colored flesh are somewhat higher in fat than those with white flesh.

All of the fat in the egg is in the yolk, about one third of this being in the form of phospholipid. Whole milk, cream, ice cream, and whole-milk cheeses furnish appreciable amounts of fat. Fruits, vegetables, legumes, cereals, and flours are low in fat. On the other hand, nuts contain an appreciable amount of fat.

Linoleic acid. Corn, cottonseed, safflower, and soy oils are good sources of linoleic acid. Some special margarines now available in food markets are processed by adding hydrogenated fat to oils, thereby retaining a greater proportion of linoleic acid. These margarines are much softer than regular margarines. In the labeling of such margarines the words *liquid oil* appear first, followed by a listing of hydrogenated oil as well as other ingredients. Fish and poultry furnish small amounts of linoleic acid.

Cholesterol. Only animal foods furnish cholesterol. Liver, egg yolk, kidney, brains, sweetbreads, and fish roe are rich sources. Much smaller concentrations are found in whole milk, cream, butter, cheese, and meat. (See Table A-5.)

An individual who eats no eggs or organ meats probably ingests not more than 200 mg cholesterol daily; if, in addition, he or she uses skim milk and substitutes vegetable margarine for butter, the intake will be further reduced to 100 to 150 mg daily. Each egg yolk adds about 250 mg cholesterol.

Fat Content of the Basic Diet The contributions of the food groups to the fat content of the basic diet pattern is shown in Table 6–3. Note that the basic diet supplies approximately equal amounts of saturated and oleic acids, a proportion that is quite characteristic of American diets. The choice of additional foods to supply the

Table 6-3. **Fat Content of the Basic Diet***

		Total Fat	Fatty Acids			Cholesterol
			Saturated	Oleic	Linoleic	
		gm	gm	gm	gm	mg
Vetetable-fruit group	4 servings	tr	tr	tr	tr	0
Bread-cereal group	4 servings	4	0.5	1.3	1.0	0
Milk, 2 per cent	2 cups	10	5.8	2.4	0.2	44
Meat group	5 ounces	18	5.2	6.6	2.5	292
Total		32	11.5	10.3	3.7	336
Typical additions of fat to Basic Diet						
Margarine, soft	1 tablespoon	12	2.0	4.5	4.1	0
French dressing	1 tablespoon	6	1.1	1.3	3.2	0
Chocolate pudding	½ cup	6	3.8	1.7	0.2	30
Corn oil in cooked foods	1 tablespoon	14	1.7	3.3	7.8	0
Total additions		38	8.6	10.8	15.3	30
Total		70	20.1	21.1	19.0	366
Alternative additions to Basic Diet						
Butter for table and cooking	2 tablespoons	24	14.4	5.8	0.6	70
Mayonnaise	1 tablespoon	11	2.0	2.4	5.6	10
Ice cream	½ cup	7	4.5	1.8	0.2	27
Total additions		42	20.9	10.0	6.4	107
Total fat		74	32.4	20.3	10.1	443

*See Table 13-2 for details of calculations.

needed energy requirements affords a wide range of possibilities for modifying the kind as well as the amount of fat that is included. In the two examples given, there are important differences in the amounts of linoleic acid that are provided.

The Dietary-Fat Health Controversy

Fat in the U.S. Diet Any consideration of the relationship of fat intake to health must begin with a review of the changing pattern of fat intake in the United States. The total fat content of the available food supply in the United States has increased from 124.8 gm in 1909–1913 to 159.1 gm in 1978. (See Table 6–4) In 1909–1913 fat accounted for 32 per cent of the total calories in the food supply. By 1978 this had risen to 42 per cent of total calories. The cholesterol content of the diet has remained about the same since 1909–1913—about 500 mg per capita daily.[10]

Animal sources continue to predominate as sources of fat, although the ratio of animal to vegetable sources has declined. Meat, poultry, and fish contribute gradually increasing amounts of fat, but butter, lard, and beef fat now account for only two fifths as much animal fat as in 1909–1913.

The gradual decline in fat from animal sources has been more than compensated for by a threefold increase in fats from plant sources. Most of this increase has been occasioned by the far greater use of salad and cooking oils in the home, by food processors, and by fast-food outlets. This has led to an increase in the linoleic acid content from 2.3 per cent in 1909–1913 to 6.7 per cent of calories in 1978.

It must be emphasized that data pertaining to available food supplies describe

Table 6-4. **Fat in the U.S. Diet from Animal and Vegetable Sources (per capita daily)**

	Animal Sources					Plant Sources			
	Meat, Poultry, Fish	Eggs	Dairy Products Excluding Butter	Butter, Lard, Edible Beef Fat	Total	Other Fats and Oils	Other Plant Foods	Total	Total All Fats
	grams								
1909–13	46.4	4.8	18.6	33.8	103.5	12.3	9.0	21.3	124.8
1947–49	46.8	6.0	24.5	27.4	104.8	25.1	10.6	35.8	140.5
1967	52.2	5.2	20.2	19.6	97.3	41.6	10.9	52.5	149.7
1978	53.5	4.4	19.8	13.4	91.2	55.5	12.5	67.9	159.1

Adapted from Marston, R., and Page, L.: "Nutrient Content of the National Food Supply," *National Food Review,* U.S. Department of Agriculture, December 1978, p. 30.

trends in consumption, but do not indicate the actual amounts consumed. According to preliminary data from the 1977 Household Food Consumption Survey, the average fat intake for all age groups had declined since 1965—by as much as 20 per cent for half of the age-sex groups.[11] Even so, fat continued to account for two fifths or more of the total energy intake.

Fat and Nutritive Quality of the Diet Although meat, poultry, fish, eggs, and dairy products furnish significant amounts of fat to the diet, these foods also supply many nutrients. On the other hand, visible fats and oils that contribute about 18 per cent of the total available calories in the American food supply are of rather limited nutritive value. Butter and margarine provide about 9 per cent of the vitamin A value of the food supply. Vegetable oils supply most of the linoleic acid and substantial amounts of vitamin E. The other nutrient contributions made by fats and oils are negligible. It was noted in Chapter 5 that sweets and sugars also make low nutrient contributions. Consequently, as the intake of fats and oils and sugars and sweets increases, the likelihood of meeting recommended allowances for nutrients decreases if the caloric intake is in balance with requirements.

Obesity This widely prevalent form of malnutrition results from a caloric intake that exceeds requirements, regardless of the source of the calories. Because fat contains more than twice as many calories per gram as carbohydrate and protein, it is easy to exceed one's caloric intake by consuming fat-rich foods. Moreover, many of the fats that add so much to palatability come in concentrated forms so that their addition does not appreciably affect dietary bulk. A few examples of day-to-day uses of fat illustrate how easy it is to increase caloric intake.

	kcal
Baked potato, medium	145
Butter, 1 tablespoon	100
Lettuce and tomato salad	25
Mayonnaise, 2 teaspoons	65
Fresh peach, medium	40
Ice cream, ½ cup	135
Bread, whole-wheat, 1 slice	65
Margarine, 2 teaspoons	65
Milk, skim, 1 cup	85
Milk, 2 per cent, 1 cup	120
Milk, whole, 1 cup	150
Half milk, half cream, 1 cup	315

The Diet-Heart Disease Controversy Because cardiovascular diseases account for more than half of all deaths in the United States and also affect millions of others, it is not surprising that any factor that appears to reduce the risks will be widely acclaimed by the public.

Since 1960 the age-adjusted mortality

rate from heart disease has declined about 20 per cent.[12] How can this decline be explained: better medical supervision? more control of hypertension? reduced intake of saturated fat? increased intake of polyunsaturated fat? reduced intake of cholesterol? less cigarette smoking? weight reduction? more exercise? less stressful life-style? The answers are not known, but it is likely that a number of these factors rather than a single factor may have contributed.

The diet-heart disease controversy has existed for about a quarter of a century and is destined to continue for many more years. Prominent nutrition scientists and clinicians have examined the evidence for and against the diet-heart disease hypothesis.[13-17]

Atherosclerosis is a disease process that begins early in life with the formation of cholesterol-containing plaques on the inner walls of the arteries. Smooth muscle fibers and connective tissue infiltrate these plaques (called hardening of the arteries). Gradually the lumen through which the blood flows is narrowed, and the heart must work harder to pump the blood through the arteries. When the condition is severe, the lumen may close thus depriving a given tissue of its blood supply (ischemia). If the heart vessels are affected, the individual has a heart attack (myocardial infarction); if any of the vessels of the brain are affected, the person has a stroke or cerebrovascular accident.

All children and young adults have fatty streaks in the walls of the aorta. Under some circumstances not yet fully understood, these fatty streaks progress to form the disease lesions. Many studies have shown that persons with a serum cholesterol level above 225 mg per 100 ml are at increased risk for coronary heart disease. As the hypercholesterolemia increases, so does the probability of a coronary event. Therefore, it is hypothesized that measures to reduce the serum cholesterol levels will also reduce risk. A number of measures will bring about lowering of the serum cholesterol: loss of weight by the obese; increased activity; reduced intake of total fat and of saturated fat; and increased intake of polyunsaturated fat. Dietary cholesterol, in the usual range of intake, appears to have a minimal effect on serum cholesterol levels. Thus, healthy men who consumed two eggs daily over a period of two to three months did not show serum cholesterol levels in excess of those who ate no eggs.[18,19]

Dietary modification has been widely used for patients who have been identified as being at high risk or who have had a heart attack. The results have not always been as successful as anticipated. But one may argue that dietary adjustments, if they are to be effective, must begin early in life—not after pathologic changes have occurred.

One of the perplexing questions is this: When serum cholesterol levels are lowered, what happens to the cholesterol that has been removed from the circulation? Has it been excreted? The answer is not known since few studies have been made of fecal excretion of cholesterol and its metabolites.[20]

The Diet-Cancer Hypothesis The role of fat in the incidence of cancer is even less understood than its role in heart disease. Based on epidemiologic studies an association with colon cancer has been reported.[21] The theory holds that bacterial flora can produce metabolites that are potential carcinogens. A high-fat diet might contribute by modifying the intestinal flora or by furnishing the substrate for formation of carcinogens. At the present, there are no proofs that support or destroy this theory.

An association between overweight and a high-fat diet and the incidence of cancer of the breasts and uterus has also been suggested. Although epidemiologic studies suggest that a high-fat intake may increase the risks for women, again there are no proofs that this is so.

Toward Moderation in Diet Although it is important to avoid making exaggerated claims about the preventive aspects of diet, there is sufficient evidence to justify modifying the diet to provide not more than 35 per cent of calories from fat. Such an adjustment can reduce the likelihood of excessive caloric ingestion, may improve the nutritional quality of the diet, and may be helpful as a preventive measure. In no way is such adjustment harmful. The diet is palatable, affordable, and available from the American food supply. These changes in food selection are designed to keep fat intake within 35 per cent of calories.

1. Select lean cuts of meat. Use poultry and fish more often instead of meat. Limit daily intake to 5 ounces per day. Trim off visible fat. Cook by broiling, roasting, or stewing rather than frying. Do not use fat drippings.
2. Use low-fat milk (2 per cent, 1 per cent, or skim) instead of whole milk. Use less cream, sour cream, ice cream, and full-fat cheese.
3. Reduce the intake of visible fats. Substitute soft margarines for regular margarines and butter. Use oils for cooking instead of lard or solid shortenings.

Some Points for Nutrition Education

1. Fats are essential constituents of all body cells and the principal source of energy stores within the body.
2. Fats are the most concentrated source of energy in the diet and furnish more than twice as many calories, gram for gram, as do carbohydrates and proteins. Consequently, a small volume of fatty food will increase the calorie intake considerably, and excessive intakes of fats and oils can rapidly contribute to obesity.
3. Linoleic acid is an essential fatty acid abundantly supplied by corn, cottonseed, soy, and safflower oils.
4. Lecithin and other phospholipids are essential constituents of nervous tissue and important for the transport of fats. The liver readily synthesizes the phospholipids so that their presence in the diet is not essential. An additional intake of lecithin does not convey unique benefits to health and is not necessary.
5. Cholesterol is an essential constituent of body tissues and is required for the regulation of important body functions. The liver synthesizes cholesterol so that body needs are not dependent upon the dietary cholesterol. Daily intakes of 300 to 500 mg cholesterol do not appear to adversely affect serum cholesterol levels.
6. A diet that furnishes 30 to 35 per cent of the calories as fat, and that is also designed to maintain normal weight contributes to maintaining a serum cholesterol level within desirable limits.

Problems and Review

1. Key terms: arachidonic acid; beta oxidation; cholesterol; chylomicrons; enterohepatic circulation; high-density lipoprotein; ketones; ketogenesis; lecithin; linoleic acid; lipogenesis; lipolysis; low-density lipoproteins; micelles; peroxidation; phospholipid; polyunsaturated fatty acids; prostaglandins; triglyceride.
2. Prepare an outline that shows the digestion, absorption, and metabolic fate of triglycerides supplied by the diet.
3. Give several reasons why fat is a useful constituent of the diet.
4. What is a hydrogenated fat? Give several examples. How does it compare in nutritional value with the fat from which it was made?
5. What effect will the inclusion of fatty foods such as fried potatoes and pork chops have on the digestion of the meal as a whole?

6. *Problem.* Compare the fat and calorie values of ½ cup ice cream; 1 tablespoon mayonnaise; 1 ounce cream cheese; 2 teaspoons butter; 1 cup milk.
7. *Problem.* Calculate your own fat intake for one day. Which of the foods you ate are good sources of linoleic acid? What percentage of the total calories in your diet was derived from fat?
8. A margarine may be manufactured from 100 per cent vegetable oil but may still be a poor source of linoleic acid. Explain why this might be true.
9. *Problem.* Examine the labels of three or four brands of special types of margarine. What information do they give you about their value as sources of linoleic acid? How do these margarines compare with regular margarines in cost?
10. A patient tells you that he has not been eating butter, eggs, or whole milk because he read in a magazine that cholesterol causes heart disease. How would you respond to this?

Cited References

1. Hansen, A. F.: "Essential Fatty Acids in Infant Feeding," *J. Am. Diet. Assoc.*, **34**:239–41, 1958.
2. Fredrickson, D. S., et al.: *The Dietary Management of Hyperlipoproteinemia. A Handbook for Physicians.* National Institutes of Health, U.S. Department of Health, Education and Welfare, Washington, D.C., 1970.
3. Stern, J. S., and Greenwood, M. R. C.: "A Review of Development of Adipose Cellularity in Man and Animals," *Fed. Proc.*, **33**:1952–55, 1974.
4. Isselbacher, K. J.: "Metabolism and Transport of Lipid by Intestinal Mucosa," *Fed. Proc.*, **24**:16–22, 1965.
5. Connor, W. E., et al.: "Cholesterol Balance and Fecal Neutral Steroid and Bile Acid Excretion in Normal Men Fed Dietary Fats of Different Fatty Acid Composition," *J. Clin. Invest.*, **48**:1363–75, 1969.
6. U.S. Senate Select Committee on Nutrition and Human Needs: *Dietary Goals for the United States*, rev. Government Printing Office, Washington, D.C., December 1977.
7. *Nutrition and Your Health: Dietary Guidelines for Americans.* U.S. Department of Agriculture and U.S. Department of Health, Education and Welfare, Washington, D.C., 1980.
8. Food and Nutrition Board: *Recommended Dietary Allowances*, 9th ed. National Research Council–National Academy of Sciences, Washington, D.C., 1980.
9. Marston, R. M., and Welsh, S. O.: "Nutrient Content of the National Food Supply," *National Food Review*, U.S. Department of Agriculture, Winter, 1981, pp. 19–22.
10. Marston, R., and Page, L.: "Nutrient Content of the National Food Supply," *National Food Review*, U.S. Department of Agriculture, December 1978, pp. 28–33.
11. Pao, E. M.: "Nutrient Consumption Patterns of Individuals, 1977 and 1965," *Family Economics Review*, U.S. Department of Agriculture, Spring 1980, pp. 16–20.
12. Food and Nutrition Board: *Toward Healthful Diets.* National Research Council–National Academy of Sciences, Washington, D.C., 1980.
13. Ahrens, E. H., and Connor, W. I., Chairmen, Task Force of the American Society for Clinical Nutrition: "The Evidence Relating Six Dietary Factors to the Nation's Health," *Am. J. Clin. Nutr.*, **32**:2621–2748, 1979.
14. Gotto, A. M.: "Is Atherosclerosis Reversible?" *J. Am. Diet. Assoc.*, **74**:551–57, 1979.
15. Glueck, C. J.: "Appraisal of Dietary Fat as a Causative Factor in Atherogenesis," *Am. J. Clin. Nutr.*, **32**:2637–43, 1979.
16. McGill, H. C., Jr.: "Appraisal of Cholesterol as a Causative Factor in Atherogenesis," *Am. J. Clin. Nutr.*, **32**:2632–36, 1979.

17. Olson, R. E.: "Statement to the House Agriculture Subcommittee on Domestic Marketing, Consumer Relations, and Nutrition," *Nutr. Today,* **15**:12–19, May/June 1980.
18. Kummerow, F. A., et al.: "The Influence of Egg Consumption on the Serum Cholesterol Level in Human Subjects," *Am. J. Clin. Nutr.,* **30**:664–73, 1977.
19. Flynn, M. A., et al.: "Effect of Dietary Egg on Human Serum Cholesterol and Triglycerides," *Am. J. Clin. Nutr.,* **32**:1051–57, 1979.
20. Hill, P., et al.: "Effect of Unsaturated Fats and Cholesterol on Serum and Fecal Lipids," *J. Am. Diet. Assoc.,* **75**:414–20, 1079.
21. Wynder, E. L.: "Personal Habits," *N. Y. Acad. Med.,* **54**:397–412, 1978.

Additional References

BROWN, H. B.: *Current Focus on Fat in the Diet.* The American Dietetic Association, 1977.

LEVY, R. I.: "The Meaning of Lipid Profiles," *Postgrad. Med.,* **57**:34–38, April 1975.

MANN, G. V.: "Current Concepts, Diet-Heart: End of an Era," *New Engl. J. Med.,* **297**:644–49, 1977.

MATTER, S., et al.: "Body Fat Content and Serum Lipid Levels," *J. Am. Diet. Assoc.,* **77**:149–52, 1980.

SHOREY, R. L., et al.: "Efficacy of Diet and Exercise in the Reduction of Serum Cholesterol and Triglycerides in Free-living Adult Males," *Am. J. Clin. Nutr.,* **29**:512–21, 1976.

TALL, A. R., and SMALL, D. M.: "Current Concepts: Plasma High-Density Lipoproteins," *New Engl. J. Med.,* **299**:1232–36, 1978.

VERGROESEN, A. J.: "Physiological Effects of Dietary Linoleic Acid," *Nutr. Rev.,* **35**:1–5, 1977.

WELTMAN, A., et al.: "Caloric Restriction and/or Mild Exercise: Effects on Serum Lipids and Body Composition," *Am. J. Clin. Nutr.,* **33**:1002–1009, 1980.

Energy Metabolism 7

THE amount of available energy has become a crucial issue in our times, whether it be the oil, gas, coal, or electrical power to heat, air-condition, or light our homes, drive our automobiles, run our factories, and so on; or whether, in direct human terms, it be the amount of available food to yield the energy required to accomplish the involuntary and voluntary activities of the body. Sufficient food to meet the energy needs is the first nutritional priority. When the supply of calories is moderately reduced, the capacity to work is also reduced, and in children growth is retarded or ceases. As the energy available to the body continues to decrease, the body's own substance will be utilized until eventually no more of the body mass can be sacrified. In the United States excess energy intake leading to obesity is far more frequent than energy deficit.

Energy Transformation

Energy is the capacity to do work. The sun is the original source of all energy, arising from nuclear reactions. Through the action of chlorophyll with sunlight, by the process known as photosynthesis, plants synthesize carbohydrates from carbon dioxide and water. The carbohydrates stored by the plants are then available as energy to animals and to humans. All of an individual's energy is derived from the plant and animal food she or he eats. Carbohydrates, fats, and proteins are the energy-yielding substances. In a typical American diet carbohydrate furnishes 45 to 55 per cent of the calories, fats, 35 to 45 per cent, and proteins about 15 per cent.

Forms of Energy Potential (storage) energy is continuously available in the body from the small amounts of glycogen in muscle and liver, the sizable fat depots, and the cellular mass itself. The potential energy is transformed to other forms to accomplish the work of the body: for example, *mechanical* energy for muscle contraction; *osmotic* energy to maintain the transport of fluids and nutrients; *electrical* energy for the transmission of nerve impulses; *chemical* energy as in the synthesis of new compounds; and *thermal* energy for heat regulation.

Whenever one form of energy is produced, another form is reduced by exactly the same amount. This is known as the law of CONSERVATION OF ENERGY, which states that energy can be neither created nor destroyed. When foods supply more energy than is needed for the work of the body, the excess is stored as fat; the result is weight gain. This store of energy is available at such a time as the food supply might furnish too few calories for the body's activities.

ATP, the Currency for Energy ATP is used for all the work of the body: the synthesis of all cellular materials, the secretion of hormones and enzymes, the transport of nutrients and wastes in the circulation and across cell membranes, the contraction of muscles, and so on.

The formation of ATP occurs in the metabolic pathways described in the preceding chapters on carbohydrates, fats, and proteins. Initially these nutrients are oxidized independently to the "common denominators," namely, pyruvic acid, acetyl coenzyme A, and alpha-ketoglutaric acid. In this first phase some of the reactions require ATP for their initiation; other reactions release small amounts of energy so that ATP is regenerated from ADP, but the net yield is not great.

The common denominators enter the tricarboxylic acid (TCA) cycle, which is the common pathway for the oxidation of glucose, fatty acids, and amino acids. About 90 per cent of the energy liberated from food occurs by this pathway. (See page 82 and Figure 5–5.) Oxidative phosphorylation is the mechanism whereby the hydrogens yielded by the TCA cycle are passed along the respiratory chain and energy is trapped as ATP. (See page 84 and Figure 5–6.)

Measurement

Kilocalories The potential energy value of foods and the energy exchange of the body are expressed in terms of the calorie, which is a heat unit. By definition, a KILOCALORIE (kcal) is the amount of heat required to raise the temperature of 1 kg water 1°C (from 15 to 16°C). In the nutrition literature the kilocalorie is intended whether it is expressed as calorie, Calorie, or kilocalorie. The unit is 1,000 times as large as the small calorie used in the sciences of chemistry and energy.

Joules The joule (J) is the unit of energy used in the metric system. By definition, 1 J is the amount of energy expended when 1 kg is moved a distance of 1 m by a force of 1 newton; it is equal to 10^7 ergs. It is energy expressed in mechanical equivalents, not heat equivalents.

The eighth International Congress of Nutrition in Prague in 1969 and the Committee on Nomenclature of the American Institute of Nutrition in 1970 have recommended the adoption of the joule in place of the calorie as the unit of energy. The conversion of energy values in food composition tables to joules will require some time. But, also, students and practitioners in nutrition must begin to think in terms of joules. To facilitate this, the joule equivalents in this chapter have been placed in parentheses whenever caloric values are given.

The following factors apply for the interconversion of calories and joules:

1 calorie (the unit used in physics) = 4.184 J
1 Kcal = 4.184 kilojoules (kJ)
1,000 Kcal = 4.184 megajoules (MJ)
1 kJ = 0.240 kcal
1 MJ = 240 kcal

Thus, a dietary allowance of 2,000 kcal is 8368 kJ or 8.368 MJ. For approximate calcuations the factor 4.2 may be used instead of 4.184.

Bomb Calorimeter The fuel values of foods are readily determined by means of an instrument known as a BOMB CALORIMETER. (See Figure 7–1.) A weighed sample of dried food is placed in a heavy steel container called a "bomb." The bomb is held in place in a well-insulated vessel and is surrounded by a known volume of water. After the bomb is charged with oxygen, the sample is ignited and the heat is dissipated into the water. By noting the change in the temperature of the water, one can calculate the energy value of the food by applying the definition for a calorie. The HEAT OF COMBUSTION for the energy-yielding nutrients is shown in the first column of Table 7–1.

Physiologic Fuel Factors Certain small losses occur in digestion so that it is necessary to reduce the values obtained in the bomb calorimeter to those that are physiologically available. For the typical American diet the coefficient of digestibility is 98 per cent for carbohydrate, 95 per cent for fat, and 92 per cent for protein. In addition, the end products of protein metabolism such as urea and other nitrogenous products are combustible; their loss in the urine is equivalent to about 1.25 kcal per gram

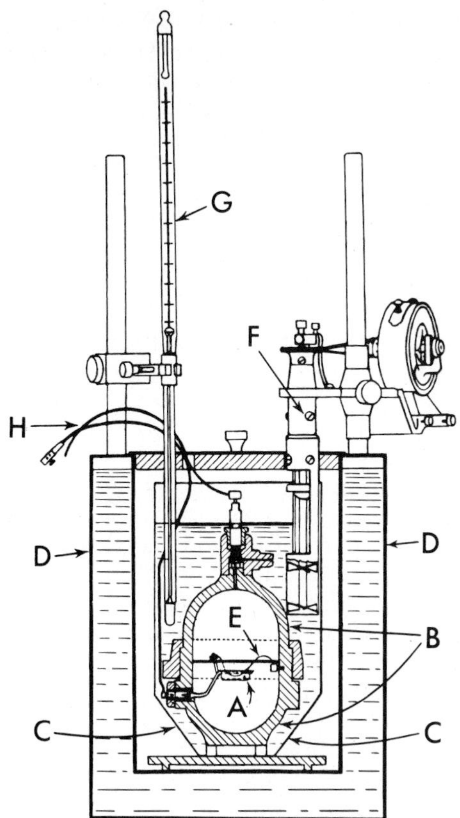

Figure 7–1. Diagram of bomb calorimeter with bomb in position. (Courtesy, the Emerson Apparatus Company.) *(A)* Platinum dish holding weighed food sample. *(B)* Bomb filled with pure oxygen enclosing food sample. *(C)* Can holding water of known weight in which the bomb is submerged. *(D)* Outer double-walled insulating jacket. *(E)* Fuse, which is ignited by an electric current. *(F)* Motor-driven water stirrer. *(G)* Thermometer calibrated to 1/1000°C. *(H)* Electric wires to send current through fuse.

protein. By applying these corrections, as shown in Table 7–1, the PHYSIOLOGIC FUEL FACTORS, first derived by Atwater are carbohydrate and protein, per gram, 4 kcal (17 kJ); fat, per gram, 9 kcal (38 kJ); and alcohol, per gram, 7 kcal (29 kJ).

Specific Fuel Factors Each food has a specific coefficient of digestibility, and thus the fuel value likewise would be specific for each given food. For example, the coefficient of digestibility for the protein in milk, eggs, and meat is 97 per cent, but for the protein of whole ground cornmeal it is only 60 per cent; the coefficient of digestibility for the carbohydrate of wheat is 98 per cent when white flour (70 to 74 per cent extraction) is used, but is 90 per cent when whole-wheat flour (97 to 100 per cent extraction) is used. Specific fuel factors, rather than the average fuel factors, have been used for the caloric values stated in tables of food composition. Thus, students may find that their calculations using the physiologic fuel factors do not always agree exactly with caloric values given in the food tables. The error introduced by using the average values is small for typical mixed diets used in the United States.

Measurement of Energy Exchange of the Body

Direct and Indirect Calorimetry DIRECT CALORIMETRY is the measurement of the amount of heat produced by the body. By this method the individual is placed in a specially constructed chamber called a

Table 7–1. **Conversion of Bomb Calorimeter Values to Physiologic Values**

	Heat of Combustion kcal	Digestibility per cent	Absorbed Energy Value kcal/gm	Urinary Loss kcal/gm	Physiologic Fuel Value kcal	kJ
Carbohydrate	4.1	98	4.02		4.0	17
Fat	9.45	95	8.98		9.0	38
Protein	5.65	92	5.20	1.25	4.0	17
Alcohol	7.1	100	7.1 (5.6/ml)	0.1 (lungs)	7.0	29

respiration calorimeter. The chamber is so well insulated that no heat can enter into or escape through the walls. The heat given off by the individual is picked up by water flowing through coils in the chamber. Measurements are made of the temperature of the water at the beginning of the study, at intervals, and at the termination of the study. The volume of water flowing through the coils is also measured, and the calories expended can be calculated from these data. These calorimeters are very expensive to construct and require careful attention to many details of measurement. They are used only in a few research centers.

The respiration calorimeter is so designed that the oxygen consumption and the carbon dioxide excretion can be measured at the same time as the heat production. The volume of oxygen consumed and the carbon dioxide expelled permit the calculation of the RESPIRATORY QUOTIENT (RQ) as follows:

$$RQ = \frac{CO_2}{O_2}$$

The RQ varies with the type of food being oxidized. For example, for pure glucose

$$C_6H_{12}O_6 + 6\ O_2 = 6\ CO_2 + 6\ H_2O$$

$$RQ = \frac{6\ CO_2}{6\ O_2} = 1.0$$

For a fatty acid such as palmitic acid

$$CH_3(CH_2)_{14}COOH + 23\ O_2 = 16\ CO_2 + 16\ H_2O$$

$$RQ = \frac{16\ CO_2}{23\ O_2} = 0.7$$

Proteins give an average RQ of 0.8. Under resting conditions with no food for 12 to 14 hours, the RQ is 0.82.

Numerous studies using the respiration calorimeter have established that each RQ has a caloric equivalent that can be used to determine the energy expenditure under given conditions. Thus, it becomes possible to determine the level of energy metabolism by the less time-consuming and far less costly procedures of indirect calorimetery.

INDIRECT CALORIMETRY measures the amount of oxygen consumed in a given time period and, in other than basal conditions, the amount of carbon dioxide excreted. Numerous experiments on people of all ages have shown that 1 liter of oxygen is equal to 4.825 kcal when the conditions for a basal metabolism test, described later, are met.

The energy expenditure at varying levels of activity can be measured by a respirometer under controlled conditions when the subject walks on a treadmill or rides on a stationary bicycle. (See Figure 7–2.) In other situations such as mountain climbing, or typing, or ironing, a portable apparatus is used. This lightweight piece of equipment consists of a meter for measuring the volume of expired air and a bag for collecting the sample of expired air. The air samples are analyzed for their amounts of oxygen and carbon dioxide, and from the data it is possible to determine caloric equivalents.

Basal Metabolism Test The amount of energy required to carry on the involuntary work of the body is known as the *basal metabolic rate.* It includes the functional activities of the various organs such as the brain, heart, liver, kidneys, and lungs, the secretory activities of the glands, the peristaltic movements of the gastrointestinal tract, the oxidations occurring in resting tissues, and the maintenance of muscle tone and body temperature. The brain and nervous tissue account for about one fifth of the energy utilized in the basal state, and the liver, kidneys, lungs, and heart for an additional three fifths.

The basal metabolic rate is measured by indirect calorimetry under the following specific conditions.

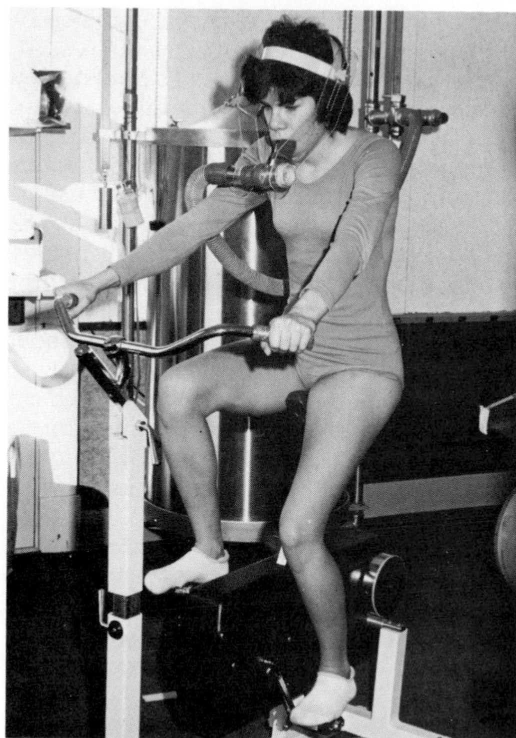

Figure 7–2. This student's energy expenditure while bicycling is being measured by using a respirometer under controlled conditions. (Courtesy, Department of Nutrition and Food Sciences, Texas Woman's University, Denton.)

1. Postabsorptive state: 12 to 16 hours after the last meal; usually performed in the morning.
2. Reclining, but awake: one-half to one hour of rest before the test is necessary if there has been any activity in the morning.
3. Relaxed and free from emotional upsets or fear of the test itself.
4. Normal body temperature.
5. Comfortable room temperature and humidity: about 21° to 24°C.

Under these conditions, normal individuals fall within ± 15 per cent of standards established for their body size, sex, and age. Suppose a young woman consumes 1,200 cc oxygen in a 6-minute test period; in a 24-hour period her basal heat expenditure is calculated as follows:

$$\frac{10 \times 1{,}200 \times 24}{1{,}000} = \begin{array}{l}\text{288 liters oxygen}\\ \text{in 24 hours}\end{array}$$

$$288 \times 4.825 \text{ kcal} = 1{,}390 \text{ kcal}$$

Factors Influencing the Basal Metabolic Rate The adult basal metabolic rate is approximately 1 kcal (4.2 kJ) per kilogram per hour for men and about 0.9 kcal (3.8 kJ) per kilogram per hour for women. Thus, the range of basal metabolism for normal adults is about 1,300 to 1,700 kcal (5,439 to 7,113 kJ). This accounts for the largest proportion of the total energy requirement for most people. The rate of basal metabolism is influenced by size, shape, and weight of the individual, sex, age, rate of growth, the activity of the endocrine glands, sleep, body temperature, and state of nutrition.

Surface area. About 80 per cent of the energy from glucose and fat is lost as heat, all but 15 per cent of heat loss being from the skin. The remaining heat loss occurs from the lungs and through the excreta. Since the heat loss is proportional to the skin surface, the basal heat production is directly proportional to the surface area. A tall, thin person has a greater surface area than an individual of the same weight who is short and fat, and the former therefore will have a higher basal metabolism.

In clinical practice the caloric expenditure is expressed as kilocalories per square meter of body surface per hour. For convenience, charts have been developed by which surface area can be determined for any given height and weight.

The metabolic rate also has a linear relationship to metabolic body size, which is expressed as body weight to the three fourths power ($W^{0.75}$). For research purposes this is the preferred relationship. For practical purposes the calculations using surface area and those using metabolic size are comparable.

Sex. Women have a metabolic rate about 6 to 10 per cent lower than that of men. Formerly this was attributed to the fact that women had relatively higher portions of adipose tissue, believed to be metabolically inert. However, this explanation is not fully satisfactory inasmuch as adipose tissue is now known to be metabolically active. The influence of the sex hormones may account for some of the difference.

Age. Per unit of surface area the basal metabolic rate is at its highest during the first 2 years of life. It declines gradually throughout childhood and accelerates slightly in adolescence. Thereafter the decline continues throughout life and averages about 2 per cent per decade after age 21. The rapid growth rate explains the high metabolic rate in early childhood. In the later years the lessened muscle tone and the reduction in muscle mass account for the lower rate.

Sleep. During the sleeping hours the basal metabolism is about 10 per cent lower than in the waking state. However, this is quite variable depending upon the amount of motion of the individual while asleep.

Body temperature. An elevation of the body temperature above 37°C (98.6°F) increases the basal metabolism by 13 per cent for each degree Celsius (7 per cent for each degree Fahrenheit).

Endocrine glands. The thyroid gland regulates the rate of energy metabolism, and any change in thyroid activity is reflected in the metabolic rate. If the thyroid is overactive (HYPERTHYROIDISM), the metabolism may be speeded up as much as 75 to 100 per cent; if the activity of the gland is decreased (HYPOTHYROIDISM), the metabolism may be reduced by 30 to 40 per cent.

The measurement of *protein-bound iodine* has now largely replaced the basal metabolism test as a measure of thyroid activity. This test is based upon the fact that the level of protein-bound iodine circulating in the blood is proportional to the degree of thyroid activity. The basal metabolism test is still the method of choice for nutritional studies.

The growth hormones that stimulate new tissue formation are responsible for the higher metabolism that is observed in infants, children, and teenagers. Other endocrine secretions have a more transitory effect on the basal metabolism. An increased excretion of epinephrine during excitement or fear temporarily raises the metabolic rate. Disturbances of the pituitary gland may also modify the metabolic rate. Just prior to the onset of the menstrual period the metabolism is increased slightly, but it is a little lower than normal during the period. These slight changes are of no overall significance in determining the energy requirement.

State of nutrition. In starvation the rate of oxidation by active lean tissue mass is similar to that occurring normally. Some underweight schoolchildren appear to have a higher-than-normal metabolic rate because the proportion of active lean tissue is higher. When undernutrition is severe, the destruction of body tissues lowers the rate.

Pregnancy. During the last trimester of pregnancy the basal metabolism increases from 15 to 25 per cent. This increase can be accounted for almost entirely by the increase in weight of the woman and the high rate of metabolism of the fetus.

Resting Metabolism The term RESTING METABOLISM should be differentiated from basal metabolism. It applies to energy expenditure under normal life conditions while at rest. It includes the specific dynamic effect of foods (see page 124) and takes into account the minimum metabolism at night and the metabolism during the day when there is no exercise and no exposure to cold.

Total Energy Requirement

Factors Influencing the Total Energy Requirement Superimposed upon the energy expenditure for maintaining the involuntary activities of the body are such factors as voluntary muscular activity, the effect of food, and the maintenance of the body temperature.

Muscular activity. Next to the basal metabolism, activity accounts for the largest energy expenditure; in fact, for some persons who are vigorously active, the energy needs for activity may exceed those for the basal metabolism. Sedentary work, which includes office work, bookkeeping, typing, teaching, and so forth, calls for less energy than more active and strenuous occupations such as nursing, homemaking, or gardening. A still greater amount of energy is required by those individuals who do hard manual labor such as ditch digging, shifting freight, and lumbering.

The energy expenditure for many activities has been measured in adults and children,[1,2] and the data serve as a guide in setting standards for various groups of people. A wide range of activities has been classified in five groups in Table 7–2. The calorie expenditures listed for each category include the basal metabolism and are representative for adults of average body size. The lower figure for each category would apply to women, and the higher figure to men. Of course, it must be realized that these vary from one individual to another not only on the basis of body size but especially because of variations of intensity of effort expended.

The figures in Table 7–2 illustrate the value of exercise in weight control, for it is quite evident that the student who sits quietly watching television, for example, is expending only half as many calories as one who is walking leisurely, and only one fourth as many calories as one who swims for an hour.

Not infrequently the question is raised as to the reason for the differing caloric needs of two people of the same build and body weight who are doing the same kind

Table 7–2. **Calorie Expenditure for Various Kinds of Activity***

Type of Activity	Kilocalories per Hour†
Sedentary Reading; writing; eating; watching television or movies; lstening to the radio; sewing; playing cards; typing; and miscellaneous office work and other activities done while sitting that require little or no arm movement	80 to 100
Light Preparing and cooking food; doing dishes; dusting; hand washing small articles of clothing; ironing; walking slowly; personal care; miscellaneous office work and other activities done while standing that require some arm movement; and rapid typing and other activities done while sitting that are more strenuous	110 to 160
Moderate Making beds; mopping and scrubbing; sweeping; light polishing and waxing; laundering by machine; light gardening and carpentry work; walking moderately fast; other activities done while standing that require moderate arm movement; and activities done while sitting that require more vigorous arm movement	170 to 240
Vigorous Heavy scrubbing and waxing; hand washing large articles of clothing; hanging out clothes; stripping beds; other heavy work; walking fast; bowling; golfing; and gardening	250 to 350
Strenuous Swimming; playing tennis; running; bicycling; dancing; skiing; and playing football	350 and more

*Adapted from Page, L., and Fincher, L. J.: *Food and Your Weight.* Home and Garden Bulletin No. 74, U.S. Department of Agriculture, 1960, p. 4.

†Lower figures apply to w nen, higher figures to men. The figures include the metabolism at rest as well as for the activity.

of work. The energy needs will be greater for the person who wastes many motions in the performance of a piece of work, who works under greater muscle tension, or who finds it difficult to relax completely even when at rest.

Mental effort. The nervous system is continuously active, and its energy requirement is about 20 per cent of the basal rate. However, the energy expenditure beyond the basal rate for intense mental effort as in problem solving or writing examinations does not add appreciably to the caloric requirement. Some students become tense and restless while solving problems, but the increased expenditure of energy in such a situation is not primarily that of mental work.

Calorigenic effect of food. The ingestion of food results in increased heat production known as the *calorigenic effect* or SPECIFIC DYNAMIC ACTION OF FOOD. It represents the energy required for digestion and absorption and also the stimulating effect of nutrients upon metabolism. Protein when eaten alone has been shown to increase the metabolic rate by 30 per cent, whereas carbohydrates and fats will produce much smaller increases in metabolism. On the basis of the mixed diets usually eaten, the specific dynamic action is approximately 6 per cent of the energy requirement.[3]

Maintenance of body temperature. Under normal conditions the temperature of the body is controlled by the amount of blood brought to the skin. Vasodilation of the blood vessels occurs when the environmental temperature is high and vasoconstriction occurs when the temperature is low. When the surrounding temperature is low, most of the heat is lost by radiation and convection, but when the environmental temperature is high, the body heat is lost chiefly through evaporation. It is a well-known fact that more heat is lost by evaporation when the air is dry than when it is humid.

During cold weather, excessive heat losses from the body are avoided by the use of suitable clothing and the heating of the home or place of work. Moreover, body heat is conserved if there is a layer of adipose tissue under the skin. The subcutaneous fat serves to keep heat in the body rather than allowing it to be dissipated through the skin—an advantage in cold weather, but a disadvantage in warm weather. Infants and young children have a relatively large surface area and lose much heat from the body when they are exposed.

When the body is subjected to extreme cold, the body temperature is maintained by an increase in involuntary and often voluntary activity. The blood vessels constrict so that there is less blood reaching the skin surface, the muscles become tense, and shivering follows. These involuntary activities result in a considerable increase in the metabolic rate. As anyone knows who has been exposed to a cold winter day, one is not likely to stand still. In addition, then, to the increased energy expenditure occasioned by the involuntary activities, the individual increases voluntary activity.

Growth. The building of new tissue represents a storage of energy in one form or another; for example, every gram of protein in body tissue represents about 4 kcal. When growth is rapid, as during the first year of life, the energy allowance must be high. In fact, the caloric need is greater per unit of body weight than at any other time in life. In pregnancy, likewise, the energy needs are increased to cover the building of new tissues. These needs are discussed in more detail in Chapters 18, 19, and 20.

Energy Allowances

Estimating Energy Requirements One method for estimating the energy requirement of an individual is to keep a record of the amount of time spent for each activity during the day and calculate the energy equivalent. The calculation can be made by using the data from Table 7–2 or by referring to more precise tables of energy expenditure for given activities per kilogram of body weight.[2] An example of a woman's daily activities grouped according to the categories in Table 7–2 follows:

	Hours	Kilocalories per Hour	Total kcal
Sleep	8	50	400
Sedentary	10	80	800
Light	3	110	330
Moderate	2	170	340
Vigorous	1	250	250
	24		2120

Keeping a detailed record of activities is tedious, and at best becomes only an approximation of actual caloric requirement inasmuch as wide variations occur from one individual to another within each category.

Another method widely used in clinical practice is to estimate an individual's activity to be sedentary, moderately active, or active. The approximate energy expenditure per kilogram of body weight is as follows:

Sedentary	30–35 kcal (126–147 kJ)
Moderately active	35–40 kcal (147–168 kJ)
Active	40–45 kcal (168–189 kJ)

Using these factors, a moderately active woman weighing 55 kg would require 1,925 to 2,200 kcal (8.1 to 9.2 MJ). Although these are only approximations, they provide a starting point for planning diets.

Recommended Allowances The energy intake recommended by the Food and Nutrition Board[4] for males and females of all ages is shown in Table 7–3. The bases for these allowances are described in the footnotes of the table.

Several adjustments may be required to take into account factors that increase or decrease an individual's energy requirement. The range of ± 400 kcal for adults indicates customary variation in activity. For children, this range is greater. The declining requirement for adults over 50 years takes into account the reduction in basal metabolism and also in activity.

Body size influences the energy requirement. People who are active and who are larger than the weight stated in the table will require more calories; those who are smaller will require less. Any activity that requires movement of the whole body such as walking entails more energy expenditure by an 80 kg person than by a 60 kg person. The differences are small with activities that involve only parts of the body—such as reading, typing, and so on.

Activity is the greatest variable in the energy requirement. Today the average work week is 35 to 40 hours; sleep accounts for 50 to 60 hours; eating and travel to and from work consumes 20 hours, more or less; and leisure time amounts to 50 or 60 hours in a given week. The leisure activities may range from reading, watching television or movies, or stamp collecting, on the one hand, to such vigorous activities as tennis, gardening, golf, and swimming, on the other hand. Obviously, to set up a caloric allowance in terms of one's activity at work alone is to ignore a large part of one's day.

For persons who are moderately active the allowances should be increased by about 300 kcal (1.26 MJ). Very active individuals such as athletes, military recruits, and construction workers may require 600 to 900 kcal (2.52 to 3.78 MJ) above the recommended allowances.

Adjustment for climate. In summer and winter most Americans live in an environmental temperature of 20 to 25°C. In winter they wear warm clothing, live and work in well-heated buildings, and travel by heated means of transportation. Likewise, in summer many of them live and work in air-conditioned buildings. Therefore, adjustments for temperature are not usually necessary.

Table 7-3. **Mean Heights and Weights and Recommended Energy Intake***

Category	Age years	Weight kg	Weight lb	Height cm	Height in	Energy Needs (with range) kcal	MJ
Infants	0.0–0.5	6	13	60	24	kg X 115 (95–145)	kg X 0.48
	0.5–1.0	9	20	71	28	kg X 105 (80–135)	kg X 0.44
Children	1–3	13	29	90	35	1,300 (900–1,800)	5.5
	4–6	20	44	112	44	1,700 (1,300–2,300)	7.1
	7–10	28	62	132	52	2,400 (1,650–3,300)	10.1
Males	11–14	45	99	157	62	2,700 (2,000–3,700)	11.3
	15–18	66	145	176	69	2,800 (2,100–3,900)	11.8
	19–22	70	154	177	70	2,900 (2,500–3,300)	12.2
	23–50	70	154	178	70	2,700 (2,300–3,100)	11.3
	51–75	70	154	178	70	2,400 (2,000–2,800)	10.1
	76+	70	154	178	70	2,050 (1,650–2,450)	8.6
Females	11–14	46	101	157	62	2,200 (1,500–3,000)	9.2
	15–18	55	120	163	64	2,100 (1,200–3,000)	8.8
	19–22	55	120	163	64	2,100 (1,700–2,500)	8.8
	23–50	55	120	163	64	2,000 (1,600–2,400)	8.4
	51–75	55	120	163	64	1,800 (1,400–2,200)	7.6
	76+	55	120	163	64	1,600 (1,200–2,000)	6.7
Pregnancy						+300	
Lactation						+500	

*The data in this table have been assembled from the observed median heights and weights of children, together with desirable weights for adults for the mean heights of men (70 inches) and women (64 inches) between the ages of 18 and 34 years as surveyed in the U.S. population (HEW/NCHS data).

The energy allowances for the young adults are for men and women doing light work. The allowances for the two older age groups represent mean energy needs over these age spans, allowing for a 2 percent decrease in basal (resting) metabolic rate per decade and a reduction in activity of 200 kcal/day for men and women between 51 and 75 years, 500 kcal for men over 75 years, and 400 kcal for women over 75. The customary range of daily energy output is shown for adults in parentheses, and is based on a variation in energy needs of ±400 kcal at any one age, emphasizing the wide range of energy intakes appropriate for any group of people.

Energy allowances for children through age 18 are based on median energy intakes of children of these ages followed in longitudinal growth studies. The values in parentheses are 10th and 90th percentiles of energy intake, to indicate the range of energy consumption among children of these ages.

Food and Nutrition Board: *Recommended Dietary Allowances,* 9th ed. National Academy of Sciences–National Research Council, Washington, D.C. 1980.

During work at temperatures below 14°C the energy expenditure is about 5 per cent greater than in a warm environment. A small increase in calories (2 to 5 per cent) may be necessary in winter for the person carrying a weight of heavy clothing. When a person is inadequately clothed, the calorie expenditure increases considerably.

When people are physically active at high environmental temperatures, an increase in the calorie allowance of 0.5 per cent for each degree above 30°C is indicated. This increase is necessary to cover the slight increase that occurs in the metabolic rate and in the extra energy expenditure to maintain normal body temperature. In warm climates, most individuals tend to reduce their activity and thus their caloric needs.

Body Weight and Energy Requirement The best guide to the adequacy of the caloric intake lies in the maintenance of desirable weight by adults and the normal rate of growth by children. When there is weight gain despite adherence to a diet that furnishes the recommended levels of calories, the amount of activity should be increased rather than relying on a low-calorie diet alone.

Foods for Energy The caloric value of the Basic Diet is shown in Table 7–4. This includes the recommended number of servings from the four essential food groups of the Daily Food Guide. The plan is suitable for a low-calorie diet for those who are overweight.

Typical additions for women and men of normal weight and whose energy requirement is 2,000 and 2,700 kcal, respectively, are also shown in Table 7–4. It should be especially noted that some of the typical additions are not high in nutrient density. To improve the nutrient density, additional servings of vegetables and fruits, breads and cereals, and low-fat milk would be preferable.

Foods that are high in fat, sugar, or starch content but low in water are concentrated sources of calories. By contrast, foods high in water content are low in calories. For example, a teaspoon of margarine contains 35 kcal, a tablespoon of sugar 45 kcal, and ½ cup tomatoes 25 kcal. Thus, the addition of small amounts of concentrated foods to the diet increases the calorie intake rapidly, and vegetables and fruits can be eaten in appreciable amounts without great increases in caloric intake.

Persons who use alcoholic beverages daily may derive 5 to 10 per cent of their caloric intake from this source.[4] It has been reported that some individuals consume up to 1,800 kcal from this source on a daily

Table 7–4. **Energy Values of the Basic Diet with Typical Additions***

Food Groups	Servings	Energy kcal
Vegetable-fruit	4	240
Bread-cereal	4	290
Milk, 2 per cent	2 cups	240
Meat, lean	5 ounces	335
Total, Basic Diet		1,105
Typical additions by a woman		
Cream of mushroom soup	1 cup	135
Saltines	4	50
Margarine or butter	1 tablespoon	100
French dressing	2 tablespoons	130
Sugar, jam, jelly	1 tablespoon	45
Peanut butter	1 tablespoon	95
Blueberry pie	1 piece	325
Total for the day		1,985
RDA, woman, 55 kg, 23–50 years		2,000
Further additions by a man		
Bread	2 slices	145
Margarine or butter	1 tablespoon	100
Meat group	2 ounces	135
French fried potatoes	10 strips	135
Whisky, 86 proof	2 jiggers	210
Total for the day		2,710
RDA, man, 23–50 years, 70 kg		2,700

*See Table 13–2 for complete calculations of the Basic Diet. Refer to Table A–1 for caloric values of specific foods.

basis. Such consumption has an adverse effect on the nutritive adequacy of the diet since alcohol provides no nutrients.

Problems Related to Energy Intake

Nutritive Quality of the Diet It has been emphasized in preceding chapters that sugars and sweets, fats and oils, and alcohol contribute substantial energy value to the diet but have limited if any nutrient content. Numerous attractive snack foods that are high in calories but of low nutrient density are available in today's market. By reading labels on nutritional information the consumer can learn to make wiser choices.

Healthy people can use foods of low nutrient density in moderation, and indeed some of these foods enhance diet palatability. However, when they are eaten in excessive amounts the result may be (1) a caloric intake greater than energy output, which results in obesity, or (2) a reduced intake of essential nutrient-rich foods, which impairs nutritional status, or (3) both.

Weight Control The primary problem of malnutrition in the United States is obesity. Its prevention requires balance of energy intake and energy output. Such prevention must begin early in life when good food habits are being formed.

When the caloric expenditure is less than 1,800–2,000 kcal, it is difficult to include all nutrients at recommended levels—especially for some of the trace elements. Thus, it is more appropriate to increase exercise than it is to decrease caloric intake below 2,000 if the goal is weight maintenance. For those who are obese, low-calorie diets ranging from 1,000 kcal to 1,800 kcal are used, depending upon individual needs. (See Chapter 27 for full discussion of obesity.)

Some Points for Emphasis in Nutrition Education

1. Energy values in nutrition are expressed as kilocalories or kilojoules. The kilocalorie (1,000 times the small calorie) expresses energy in heat units. The kilojoule expresses energy in mechanical units. One kilocalorie equals 4.184 kilojoules.
2. A calorie is the same whether it comes from carbohydrates, fats, or proteins. Carbohydrates and proteins furnish 4 kcal (17 kJ) per gram and fats 9 kcal (38 kJ) per gram.
3. Weight for weight, foods that are dry or greasy are relatively high in calories: for example, cereals, cookies, cakes, pastries, sweets, butter, fatty meats. Foods that have a high concentration of water are much lower in calories: for example, fruits and vegetables.
4. The basal metabolism is the amount of energy the body uses at rest. It ranges from about 1,300 to 1,700 kcal (5.4 to 7.1 MJ) for adults and accounts for about half or more of the total calories needed by the average American.
5. The amount of activity is the important factor determining the number of calories needed above the basal metabolism. For the average young woman in America about 2,000 kcal (8.4 MJ) are needed daily; the average young man needs about 2,700 kcal (11.3 MJ). Sedentary young adults require less than this, and older persons require considerably fewer calories.
6. In addition to furnishing most of the needed amounts of protein, minerals, and vitamins, the Daily Food Guide in the recommended amounts provides 1,100 to 1,200 kcal. Thus, a young woman can use a reasonable amount of desserts, fats, and sugars without exceeding her energy requirement, but the older woman has very little leeway in using these foods if she is also going to meet her nutritional requirements.
7. The body is in energy balance when the calories supplied by food are exactly equal to the energy needed for all the involuntary and voluntary activities of the body. Weight is neither gained nor lost.
8. If the calorie intake is greater than the body needs, weight is gained, and if the calorie intake is less than the body needs, weight is lost.

Problems and Review

1. Define or explain what is meant by calorie; joule; calorimetry; bomb calorimeter; respiration calorimeter; indirect calorimetry; heat of combustion; physiologic fuel factor; basal metabolism; resting metabolism.
2. *Problem.* Using data from Table A–1, calculate the number of grams of each of the following foods to furnish 100 kcal: butter, whole milk, cheese, egg, potato, apple, banana, orange, sugar, bread, pork chop, cooked rice, chocolate cake.
3. What are the standard conditions for performing a basal metabolism test? What factors might make the basal metabolism of two adult individuals of the same age vary? How does age itself affect the basal metabolism?
4. Explain how the following factors affect the total energy requirement: muscular activity; food; climate; clothing; growth; muscle tension; endocrine secretions. Which of these has the greatest effect?
5. *Problem.* Calculate your own calorie intake for one day. What percentage of your calories was derived from each of the four food groups? What percentage from sweets, fats, desserts, and snack foods?
6. Why would you expect the caloric requirement of many poor people to be higher during cold weather than that of people in better economic circumstances?
7. What is the best indication of adequate caloric intake?

Cited References

1. Taylor, C. M., and MacLeod, G.: *Rose's Laboratory Handbook of Dietetics,* 5th ed. The Macmillan Company, New York, 1949, p. 73.
2. Passmore, R., and Durnin, J. V. G. A.: "Human Energy Expenditure," *Physiol. Rev.,* **34**:801–40, 1955.
3. Swift, R. W., et al.: "The Effect of High Versus Low Protein Equicaloric Diets on the Heat Production of Human Subjects," *J. Nutr.,* **65**:89–102, 1958.
4. Food and Nutrition Board: *Recommended Dietary Allowances,* 9th ed. National Academy of Sciences–National Research Council, Washington, D.C., 1980.

Additional References

American Dietetic Association: "Nutrition and Physical Fitness, An A.D.A. Statement," *J. Am. Diet. Assoc.,* **76**:437–43, 1980.

AMES, S. R.: "The Joule—Unit of Energy," *J. Am. Diet. Assoc.,* **57**:415–16, 1970.

BRAY, G. A., et al.: "The Acute Effects of Food Intake on Energy During Cycle Ergometry," *Am. J. Clin. Nutr.,* **27**:254–59, 1974.

BUSKIRK, E. R., and MENDEZ, J.: "Nutrition, Environment and Work Performance with Special Reference to Altitude," *Fed. Proc.,* **26**:1760–67, 1967.

Energy and Protein Requirements, FAO Nutrition Meetings Report Series 52, Geneva, 1973.

FLATT, J.-P., and BLACKBURN, G. L.: "The Metabolic Fuel Regulatory System. Implications for Protein-sparing Therapies During Caloric Deprivation and Disease," *Am. J. Clin, Nutr.,* **27**:175–87, 1974.

FREINKEL, N.: "The Role of Nutrition in Medicine. Recent Developments in Fuel Metabolism," *JAMA,* **239**:1868–72, 1978.

GROEN, J. J.: "An Indirect Method for Approximating Caloric Expenditure of Physical Activity. A Recommendation for Dietary Surveys," *J. Am. Diet. Assoc.,* **52**:313–17, 1968.

HAVEL, R. L.: "Caloric Homeostasis and Disorders of Fuel Transport," *N. Engl. J. Med.*, **287**:1186–92, 1972.
HAWKINS, W. W.: "The Calorie, the Joule," *J. Nutr.*, **102**:1553–54, 1972.
HEGSTED, D. M.: "Energy Needs and Energy Utilization," *Nutr. Rev.*, **32**:33–38, 1974.
KONISHI, F.: "Food Energy Equivalents of Various Activities," *J. Am. Diet. Assoc.*, **46**:186–88, 1965.
KONISHI, F., and HARRISON, S. L.: "Body Weight Gain Equivalents of Selected Foods," *J. Am. Diet. Assoc.*, **70**:365–68, 1977.
LEHNINGER, A. L.: "Energy Transformation in the Cell," *Sci. Am.*, **202**:102–14, 1960.
LEON, A. S., et al.: "Effects of a Vigorous Walking Program on Body Composition, and Carbohydrate and Lipid Metabolism of Obese Young Men," *Am. J. Clin. Nutr.*, **32**:1776–87, 1979.
MAHALKO, J. R., and JOHNSON, L. K.: "Accuracy of Prediction of Long-term Energy Needs," *J. Am. Diet. Assoc.*, **77**:557–61, 1980.
SWINDELLS, Y. E.: "The Influence of Activity and Size of Meals on Caloric Response in Women," *Br. J. Nutr.*, **27**:65–73, 1972.
WILDER, R. M.: "Calorimetry, the Basis of the Science of Nutrition," *Arch. Intern. Med.*, **103**:146–54, 1959.

Mineral Elements 8

THE story of each mineral element required by the human being is every bit as dramatic as that of proteins, or vitamins, or the energy-yielding components. With new developments in laboratory technology it is now possible to trace minute amounts of mineral elements in living tissues, and many an element formerly considered to be a contaminant in foods has joined the ranks of the essential nutrients.

This chapter is concerned with calcium, phosphorus, sulfur, magnesium, iron, iodine, and zinc. A brief discussion is presented of several trace minerals for which recommended allowances have not been set. Of these copper, manganese, fluorine, chromium, selenium, and molybdenum have had an "estimated safe and adequate daily dietary intake" suggested.[1] Sodium, potassium, and chlorine together with water balance and acid-base balance are discussed in Chapter 9.

The setting of estimated safe and adequate intakes emphasizes the requirement for these minerals and the lack of data available to establish traditional recommended daily allowances[1] Thus the safe and adequate intakes are more tentative and suggested ranges of intakes for maintaining health. The upper limit set on these ranges emphasizes the risk of possible toxicity for these nutrients. For many minerals the range between what is necessary and what becomes toxic is quite narrow. Although this danger is not widespread, it can become very real through the use of highly fortified products and supplements.

Mineral Composition of the Body MINERALS are those elements that remain largely as ash when plant or animal tissues are burned. About 4 per cent of the body weight consists of mineral matter. Seven MACRONUTRIENTS—that is, those occurring in appreciable amounts—account for most of the body content of minerals. Calcium and phosphorus account for three fourths of all mineral matter.

Some fifteen to twenty elements are present in such minute amounts that they are generally referred to as TRACE ELEMENTS or MICRONUTRIENTS. In recent years some elements such as chromium and selenium, long considered to be contaminants, have been found to be essential. It is altogether possible that functions will be found for lead, mercury, gold, and others; no such evidence presently exists. Certainly the ecologic balance is important. On the one hand, there is a critical need for some trace elements; on the other hand, excesses of these same elements are toxic. Table 8–1 summarizes the mineral composition of the body, including approximate concentrations of some minerals.

General Functions Mineral elements are present in organic compounds such as phosphoproteins, phospholipids, hemoglobin, and thyroxine; as inorganic compounds such as sodium chloride and calcium phosphate; and as free ions. They enter into the structure of every cell of the body. Hard skeletal structures contain the greater proportions of some elements such as calcium, phosphorus, and magnesium, and soft tissues contain relatively higher proportions of potassium.

Mineral elements are constituents of enzymes such as iron in the catalases and cytochromes; of hormones such as iodine in

Table 8-1. **Mineral Composition of the Body**

	Approximate Amount in Adult Body	
	per cent	per 70 kg
Minerals for which an RDA has been set		
Calcium	1.75	1,200 gm
Phosphorus	1.10	750 gm
Magnesium	0.04	24 gm
Iron	0.006	4 gm
Zinc	0.002	1.7 gm
Iodine	0.00004	28 mg
Minerals for which an Estimated Safe and Adequate Intake has been set		
Potassium	0.35	245 gm
Sodium	0.15	105 gm
Chlorine	0.15	105 gm
Molybdenum	0.004	2.5 gm
Selenium	0.003	1.8 gm
Fluorine	0.001	1 gm
Manganese	0.0002	150 mg
Copper	0.0002	150 mg
Chromium	trace	5 mg
Required minerals as constituents of other nutrients		
Sulfur	0.25	175 mg
Cobalt	trace	5 mg
Possibly essential (needed by some animals)		
Arsenic		
Cadmium		
Nickel		
Silicon		
Tin		
Vanadium		
No known function		
Aluminum		
Barium		
Boron		
Bromine		
Gold		
Lead		
Mercury		
Strontium		

thyroxine; and of vitamins such as cobalt in vitamin B-12 and sulfur in thiamin. Their presence in body fluids regulates the permeability of cell membranes; the osmotic pressure and water balance between intracellular and extracellular compartments; the response of nerves to stimuli; the contraction of muscles; and the maintenance of acid-base equilibrium.

The amount of an element present gives no clue to its importance in body functions. For example, the approximately 1,200 gm of calcium in the body is just as critical to health as the few milligrams of iodine present.

Dynamic Equilibrium For the normal adult a balance usually exists between the intake of an element and its excretion. On the one hand, absorption and excretion are constantly adjusted to guard against an overload that might produce toxic effects. On the other hand, precise mechanisms carefully conserve needed amounts of mineral elements.

Homeostasis is maintained in spite of the fact that a continuous flow of nutrients into the cell and away from the cell is taking place. For example, bone, often thought of as being inert, is an exceedingly active tissue in its constant uptake and release of mineral constituents. Nevertheless, a state of balance or dynamic equilibrium is maintained provided that the supply of nutrients is adequate.

Foods as Sources of Mineral Elements When selecting foods for their mineral content, these factors must be considered: (1) the concentration of the mineral in the food; (2) how much of a given food is ordinarily consumed; (3) whether the food has lost some of its minerals through refinement or in cooking processes; and (4) whether the food contains the mineral in available form.

The best assurance that the diet will supply sufficient amounts of the essential mineral elements is to select a wide variety of foods, using the Basic Diet pattern (Table 13–2) as the basis. Fats and sugars are practically devoid of mineral elements, and highly refined cereals and flours are poor sources of most of them. Fabricated foods may lack important trace minerals for which no recommended allowances have been set. Many adolescent girls and women are unable to obtain sufficient iron even from a good diet and still keep within their caloric requirement.

Calcium

Distribution and Functions Of the approximately 1,200 gm of calcium in the adult body, 99 per cent is combined as the salts that give hardness to the bones and teeth. The bones not only provide the rigid framework for the body, but they also furnish the reserves of calcium to the circulation so that the concentration in the plasma can be kept constant at all times.

The remaining 1 per cent of the calcium in the adult—about 10 to 12 gm—is distributed throughout the extracellular and intracellular fluids of the body. It fulfills important functions such as these:

1. Activates a number of enzymes including pancreatic lipase, adenosine triphosphatase, and some proteolytic enzymes.
2. Is required for the synthesis of ACETYLCHOLINE, a substance necessary for transmission of nerve impulses.
3. Increases the permeability of cell membranes, thus aiding in the absorptive processes.
4. Aids in the absorption of vitamin B-12 from the ileum.
5. Regulates the contraction and relaxation of muscles, including the heartbeat.
6. Catalyzes two steps in the clotting of blood. When tissue cells are injured the following sequence takes place:

Cell injury:

$$\text{blood platelets} \xrightarrow{Ca^{++}} \text{thromboplastin}$$

$$\text{Thromboplastin} + \text{prothrombin} \longrightarrow \text{thrombin}$$

$$\text{Thrombin} + \text{fibrinogen} \xrightarrow{Ca^{++}} \text{fibrin (the clot)}$$

Absorption Calcium is absorbed by active transport, an energy-requiring process, chiefly from the duodenum. Passive diffusion of calcium across the intestinal mucosa also occurs from the jejunum and ileum. (See Figure 8–1.)

Factors favoring absorption. Body need is the major factor governing the amount of calcium that is absorbed. Healthy adults receiving a diet that meets the recommended allowances absorb approximately 20 to 30 per cent of their dietary calcium. At higher levels of intake the proportion that is absorbed is lower but the absolute amount that crosses the intestinal membranes depends upon need. In many areas of the world, the diet supplies low amounts of calcium. People in these areas have adapted to these low levels and absorb a high proportion of the intake. During growth the absorption is increased to take care of increase in size and hardness of the skeleton. Thus children absorb proportionally more calcium than adults. Pregnancy and lactation are also two physiological states which trigger an increased absorption. It has also been found that men have a more efficient absorption rate than nonpregnant women.

Several mechanisms control the amount

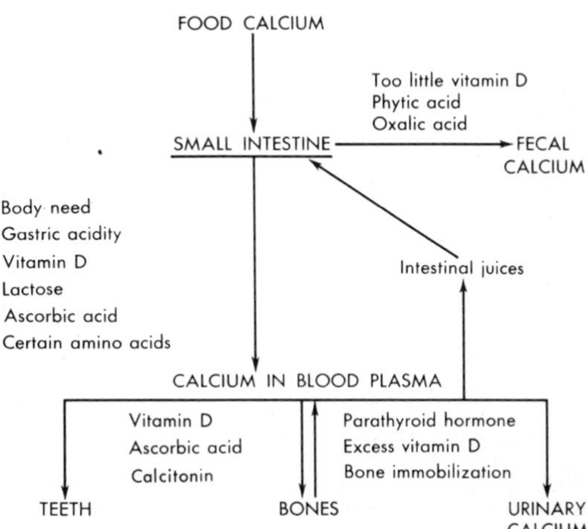

Figure 8–1. The utilization of calcium.

of calcium that is absorbed. Two of these are the hormone secreted by the parathyroid gland, PARATHORMONE, and vitamin D. Parathormone is secreted when the blood calcium level is lowered. One of its functions is to stimulate the kidney to synthesize vitamin D hormone. This metabolically active vitamin D functions with parathormone to stimulate increased absorption from the intestine. (See vitamin D, Chapter 10.)

An acid reaction aids in the absorption of calcium since calcium salts are then more soluble. Once bile and pancreatic juice have mixed with the chyme, the reaction becomes strongly alkaline and the solubility of the calcium salts is reduced. The presence of ascorbic acid and some amino acids facilitates absorption by increasing the solubility of the calcium salts.

The ability of lactose to increase absorption has long been recognized. Being slowly absorbed, lactose favors the growth of intestinal microorganisms that increase the acidity of the intestinal contents.

Factors interfering with absorption. The lack of vitamin D seriously impairs the absorption of calcium. Such lack may arise from inadequate exposure to sunlight or failure to ingest vitamin D in some form. A reduction in the amount of acid, sometimes found in elderly persons, reduces the solubility of the calcium salts. A marked increase in gastrointestinal motility reduces the length of time that calcium remains in contact with the intestinal mucosa. Emotional stress also reduces the utilization of calcium.

The presence of oxalic acid or phytic acid in foods and an abnormal calcium-to-phosphorus ratio are known to result in the formation of insoluble calcium complexes and thus interfere with calcium absorption. These effects can be clearly demonstrated on experimental animals when a decidedly abnormal diet is fed. None of these factors are of sufficient magnitude to be of practical importance in typical American diets.

Oxalic acid is found in spinach, Swiss chard, beet tops, cocoa, and rhubarb. Spinach, for example, contains sufficient calcium to bind the oxalic acid, and none of the calcium in other foods eaten at the same meal would be adversely affected.[2] The amount of cocoa that is ingested at a time is too small to reduce the absorption of calcium significantly; thus, one would expect chocolate-flavored milk to supply about the same amounts of calcium for absorption as plain milk.

PHYTIC ACID is an organic phosphorus compound found in the outer layers of cereal grains. It binds calcium into insoluble complexes, but the effect would be important only when whole-grain cereals comprised a major part of the diet and when the calcium intake was also low, as is true in some vegetarian diets in which unleavened bread or whole-grain cereals are a major part of the caloric intake. Yeast fermentation in a bread sponge destroys much of the phytate present in whole meals, and therefore leavened bread should be recommended.[3]

The effect of high intakes of dietary fiber has been suspected of reducing calcium absorption. A recent study has shown that in human volunteers, a high-fiber diet increases the dietary calcium requirement slightly.[4] The fibers used in this study were from natural sources such as cereal bran and vegetable powder rather than a purified fiber such as cellulose; thus, the increased calcium requirement could in part be due to the higher phytate intake as well as the high fiber intake.

The amount of phosphorus consumed along with the calcium influences the availability of the calcium. For adults a 1:1 calcium to phosphorus ratio is recommended, although slight deviations from this ratio do not have a significant effect. Within the acceptable ratio, an increase in phosphorus intake tends to increase the efficiency of calcium absorption.

Similarly, dietary protein levels influence calcium availability. When high protein diets (100 gm or more) are consumed, calcium needs increase in order to maintain calcium balance. Approximately 100 gm protein per day are consumed by many persons in the United States. As the protein level is decreased to the RDA levels, calcium needs are similarly lowered. The effect of higher protein levels on calcium needs is greater with a diet high in dietary fiber.

The effect of fats on absorption is reported variously by different investigators. On the one hand, fats reduce intestinal motility so that there is longer contact with the absorbing surfaces. On the other hand, free fatty acids combine with calcium to form insoluble soaps that are excreted. Foods high in unsaturated fatty acids have little effect, whereas those high in saturated fatty acids are more likely to yield some soaps.

Within the ranges of these nutrients usually consumed by people in the United States, the RDA can be used as a guide for nutritional adequacy. These factors influencing calcium availability may pose a problem of calcium nutrition in people with marginal calcium intakes and high protein and cereal intakes. By following a varied diet such as in Table 13–2, the average person should have little concern about these influences.

Metabolism The concentration of calcium in the plasma is kept within the narrow range of 9 to 11 mg per 100 ml (4.5 to 5.5 mEq per liter). About 40 per cent of the calcium is bound to plasma protein and 60 per cent is diffusible. The plasma level is regulated by (1) vitamin D hormone synthesized by the kidney, (2) parathormone, and (3) CALCITONIN, a hormone secreted by the thyroid gland.

When the blood calcium level is lowered, parathormone is secreted. The kidney is stimulated to synthesize active vitamin D either by the action of parathormone or by the flow of the blood with its lower calcium content through the kidney. The calcium level of the blood is increased by three actions: (1) increased absorption from the intestinal tract; (2) release of calcium from the bone (RESORPTION); and (3) increased reabsorption of calcium by the renal tubules. The excretion of phosphate in the urine is also increased, thereby maintaining a normal calcium-to-phosphorus ratio in the blood.

Calcitonin is antagonistic to parathormone and lowers the blood calcium when it becomes abnormally high. It does this by inhibiting bone resorption.

Bone. Bone consists of organic and inorganic substances. The principal organic substance is the protein COLLAGEN, and the ground substance consists of small amounts of mucoproteins and mucopolysaccharides, especially chondroitin sulfate. The formation of bone is initiated early in fetal life with the development of the cartilagenous matrix. During the latter part of pregnancy some mineralization of the fetal skeleton takes place so that the infant at birth has a body calcium content of about 28 gm.

During growth the addition of mineral to bone exceeds the amounts that are removed. The bone hardness consists of a gradual addition of minerals by the process referred to as MINERALIZATION or OSSIFICATION. During fetal development and the first few months after birth the bones achieve sufficient mineralization so that the skeleton can support the weight of the baby when he or she walks. Throughout childhood and adolescence the bones increase in length and diameter. This increase in size is dependent upon adequate protein as well as mineral elements. The hardness of bones increases throughout the first 20 years—sometimes longer. About 165 mg calcium are added to the skeleton daily during the early growing years. At adolescence the retention is as high as 300 mg a day, with a yearly increase as high as 90 gm.

The complex mineral substance in bone consists of an amorphous phase and a crystalline phase that is similar to HYDROXYAPATITE—$Ca_{10}(PO_4)_6(OH)_2$. Small amounts of calcium can be replaced by magnesium, sodium, potassium, lead, or strontium. Likewise, the anions sulfate, fluoride, citrate, carbonate, and chloride can enter the structure.

Bone is the principal reserve of calcium and phosphorus in the body. Contrary to popular belief, bones are continuously remodeled and reshaped by OSTEOBLASTS (bone-forming cells) and OSTEOCLASTS (bone-destroying cells). About 700 mg calcium enter and leave the bone each day in the adult.[5] Because of the turnover of calcium within the bone, widely varying intakes of calcium have no direct effect on the blood calcium.

In the well-nourished individual the readily available stores of calcium are in the ends of the long bones, and are known as TRABECULAE. In the absence of trabeculae calcium is withdrawn from the shaft of the long bone.

Teeth. Like bones, teeth are complex structures consisting of a protein matrix (keratin in the enamel, and collagen in the dentin) and mineral salts, principally calcium and phosphorus as hydroxyapatite. In the fetus the development of teeth begins by the fourth month and calcification proceeds during the growth of the fetus. Prenatally and during infancy and childhood tooth development requires adequate supplies of many diet factors including not only calcium and phosphorus, but also vitamins A and D, and protein. The deciduous teeth of the infant are fully mineralized by the end of the first year of life, but the calcification of permanent teeth is completed at various times during childhood and adolescence; for some teeth the mineralization is not completed until early adult years.

The turnover of calcium in teeth is very slow, but, unlike calcium in bone, once the calcium in teeth is lost it cannot be replaced. Thus, any factor that increases the solubility of mineral salts at the tooth surfaces will lead to decay: for example, the acids produced by microbial activity when sugars stick to the teeth. On the other hand, the presence of fluoride in the salts of tooth enamel increases the hardness, thereby reducing their decay. (See page 152.) Because of the slow rate of turnover of calcium in teeth, the fetus does not take much calcium from the mother's teeth, and the popular notion of the loss of "a tooth for every child" is false. (See Chapter 18.)

Excretion The urinary excretion for a given individual remains relatively constant regardless of calcium intake, but varies widely from one individual to another. The calcium excretion is increased as the protein intakes is increases.[6–8] In one investigation adults were fed a diet containing 800 mg calcium and 47, 95, and 142 gm protein.[6] The urinary calcium excretion on the three levels of protein were 217, 303, and 426 mg, respectively. The calcium balances were +12, +1, and −85 mg, respectively. Thus, high protein diets used in osteoporosis, weight reduction, and other clinical situations could lead to negative calcium balances.

Fecal calcium includes endogenous calcium that is not reabsorbed from the digestive juices and dietary calcium. The fecal calcium varies directly with the dietary calcium. Under normal conditions the skin losses are small. When people work strenuously at very high temperatures and perspire profusely, the calcium losses could be considerable.

Daily Allowances The recommended allowance for calcium is 800 mg for adults and for children 1 to 10 years; 1,200 mg for boys and girls 11 to 18 years and for pregnant and lactating women; and 360 to 540 mg during the first year of life.[1] The allowance for adults is based upon replacement of daily losses including 175 mg in the urine, 125 mg as endogenous loss from digestive juices in the feces, and 20 mg from the skin. Assuming absorption to be 40 per cent, this daily loss of 320 mg would necessitate an allowance of 800 mg.

A great deal of controversy exists concerning the requirement for calcium. The calcium balance technique for determining the calcium requirement has been criticized by many. People who ingest high levels of calcium are in negative balance if they suddenly shift to a lower intake, but in time most of them adjust to the lower level of intake. Adults throughout the world consume diets that often provide 400 mg or less of calcium, yet they do not show any adverse effects.

The FAO/WHO committee has recommended 400 to 500 mg calcium as a "practical allowance" for adults.[9] Such levels can be realized in most countries for the entire population, whereas higher levels would be impractical in terms of available food supplies. The Canadian allowance is 800 mg for men and 700 mg for women, with an additional 500 mg allowance for pregnancy and lactation.

Food Sources of Calcium The calcium content of some typical foods is shown in Table 8–2, and the calcium contribution of the basic diet pattern is charted in Figure 8–2. Milk is the outstanding source of calcium in the diet; without it, a satisfactory intake of calcium is extremely difficult. Whole or skimmed, homogenized or nonhomogenized, plain or chocolate-flavored, sweet or sour milks are equally good. For the adult 2 to 3 cups milk daily and for the child 3 to 4 cups daily will ensure adequate calcium intake. Cheddar cheese is an excellent source of calcium. Cottage cheese and ice cream are good sources but will not adequately substitute for milk. The dairy products, excluding butter, account for three fourths of the calcium in the American dietary.

All foods other than dairy products when considered together contribute not more than 200 to 300 mg calcium daily. Certain green leafy vegetables such as mustard greens, turnip greens, kale, and collards are important sources of calcium when they are eaten frequently. Canned salmon with the bones, clams, oysters, and shrimp are like-

Table 8–2. **Calcium Content of Some Typical Foods**

	Household Measure	Calcium mg	Per Cent of Adult Daily Allowance*
Milk, fresh, whole	1 cup	291	36
Milk, nonfat dry, low-density	1/3 cup	279	35
Cheese, American processed	1 ounce	174	22
Salmon, pink, canned	3 ounces	167†	21
Collards, cooked from frozen	1/2 cup	150	18
Turnip greens, cooked	1/2 cup	126	16
Clams or oysters	1/2 cup	113	14
Mustard greens, cooked	1/2 cup	97	12
Shrimp	3 ounces	98	12
Ice cream	1/8 quart	87	11
Kale, cooked	1/2 cup	78	10
Soybeans, mature, cooked	1/2 cup	73	9
Cottage cheese, creamed	1/2 cup	68	9
Broccoli, cooked	1/2 cup	68	9
Orange, whole	1 medium	54	7
Sweet potato, boiled	1 medium	48	6
Molasses, light	1 tablespoon	33	4
Egg, whole	1 medium	28	3
Cabbage, raw, shredded	1/2 cup	22	3
Carrots, cooked	1/2 cup	26	3
Bread, soft crumb type	1 slice	13	2

*Recommended Dietary Allowance of calcium for the adult is 800 mg.
†Includes bones packed with salmon.

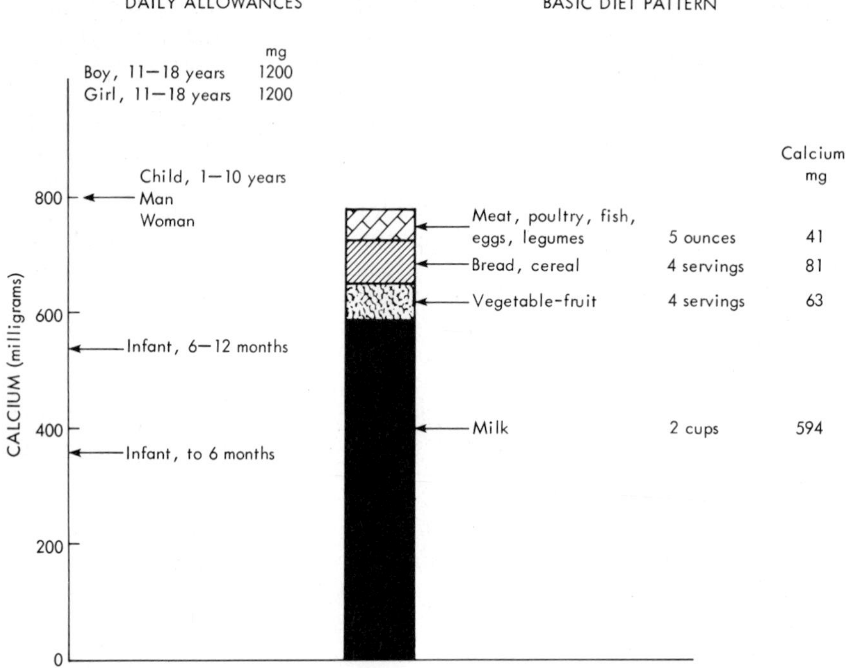

Figure 8–2. The milk group furnishes almost three fourths of the calcium allowance of the adult. The addition of 1 to 2 cups milk ensures sufficient calcium during periods of growth, in pregnancy, and in lactation. See Table 13–2 for complete calculation.

wise good sources, but they are not eaten with frequency. Meats and cereal grains are poor sources. The use of nonfat dry milk, dough conditioners, and mold inhibitors in bread enhances the calcium value of the diet. Calcium is also an optional enrichment ingredient in flours and breads.

Calcium Deficiency The evidence regarding the effect of a low intake of calcium on deficiency symptoms is contradictory. If a low calcium intake alone could cause deficiency, one would expect to see much more deficiency throughout the world than actually exists. There are, however, a number of disturbances of calcium metabolism that have serious consequences.

Bone resorption is increased during immobilization from illness or injury. The loss of calcium from bone occurs almost immediately, as demonstrated in the space flights by the astronauts.[10] The release of calcium from the bones of those who are bedfast for long periods of time sometimes leads to calcium deposits in soft tissues and the formation of renal calculi.

Failure to provide vitamin D by exposure to sunshine or in the diet reduces the absorption and utilization of calcium. Eventually this leads to rickets in the young or osteomalacia in adults. (See also Chapter 10.) OSTEOMALACIA is a reduction in the mineral content of the bone without reduction in bone size. In a report describing osteomalacia, a Bedouin woman had a calcium intake of less than 500 mg daily, but apparently an adequate source of vitamin D.[11] More than half of the calories in her diet were furnished by whole-grain unleavened bread. The phytate content of the unleavened bread was sufficient to combine with all of the calcium in the diet.

OSTEOPOROSIS is a reduction in the total

bone mass. It occurs in millions of American women after age 50 and to a somewhat lesser extent in men. According to Lutwak, a low-calcium diet for 20 to 40 years is an important etiologic factor in periodontal disease and 5 to 10 years later in osteoporosis.[12] The loss of mineral from bone is not detected by radiography until 30 to 40 per cent has disappeared. Lutwak believes that a daily intake of 800 to 1,000 mg calcium would reduce the incidence of osteoporosis. Hegsted, on the other hand, has presented evidence that low calcium intakes are not necessarily causative nor are high intakes preventive.[13] Data are accumulating that adequate fluoride intake is protective against osteoporosis.

In malabsorption diseases such as sprue large amounts of fat are excreted. The fat combines with calcium in the intestinal lumen to form soaps and the absorption of calcium as well as fat-soluble vitamins is greatly decreased. Hypocalcemia, tetany, and osteoporosis are frequently seen in these cases.

Chronic renal disease has long been recognized as contributing to hypocalcemia, osteitis, and osteomalacia. The cause of the metabolic disorder is the failure of the malfunctioning kidney to synthesize the metabolically active vitamin D-3. When the synthetic hormone is given, the calcium absorption and utilization are improved.

TETANY is a condition characterized by a low blood calcium, increased excitability of the nerves, and uncontrolled contractions of the muscles. It is not caused by a dietary lack of calcium, but is the consequence of lowered parathyroid function. Administration of parathormone brings the blood calcium back to normal.

Hypercalcemia A number of conditions can cause HYPERCALCEMIA, or increase in the blood calcium. It is accompanied by increased deposition of calcium in the soft tissues and increased calcium excretion in the urine. A high intake of calcium is not, in itself, a causative factor.

One of the situations in which hypercalcemia occasionally occurs is the milk-alkali syndrome in which patients with peptic ulcer have used excessive amounts of readily absorbed alkalies together with large amounts of milk over a period of years. The hypercalcemia in these patients was accompanied by vomiting, gastrointestinal bleeding, and increase in blood pressure.

Hypercalcemia occurs in infants who are given an excess of vitamin D. Gastrointestinal upsets are noted and growth is retarded. The condition is corrected by the removal of the excess vitamin from the diet.

Phosphorus

Distribution Phosphorus accounts for about 1 per cent of body weight or one fourth of the total mineral matter in the body. About 85 per cent of the phosphorus is in inorganic combination with calcium as the insoluble apatite of bones and teeth. In bones the proportion of calcium to phosphorus is about 2 to 1. Soft tissues contain much higher amounts of phosphorus than of calcium. Most of this phosphorus is in organic combinations.

Functions Perhaps no mineral element has as many widely differing functions as does phosphorus. In fact, reference has been made to phosphorus compounds at many points in preceding chapters of the text, and some of the many roles are listed here for review purposes.

1. Phosphorus is a constituent of the sugar-phosphate linkage in the structures of DNA and RNA, the substances that control heredity (see page 59).
2. Phospholipids are constituents of cell membranes, thus regulating the transport of solutes into and out of the cell. The phosphorus-containing lipoproteins facilitate the transport of fats in the circulation.
3. Phosphorylation is a key reaction in many metabolic processes: for example, the phosphorylation of glucose for

absorption from the intestine, the uptake of glucose by the cell, and the reabsorption of glucose by the renal tubules. Likewise, monosaccharides are phosphorylated in the initial stages of metabolism to yield energy (see page 81).

4. Phosphorus compounds are essential for the storage and controlled release of energy—the ADP-ATP system (see page 82); in the niacin-containing coenzymes required for oxidation-reduction reactions—NADP-NADPH (see page 226); and for the active form of thiamin for decarboxylation reactions—TPP (see page 219).
5. Inorganic phosphates in the body fluids constitute an important buffer system in the regulation of body neutrality (see page 178).

Metabolism Much of the phosphorus in foods is in organic combinations that are split by intestinal phosphatases to free the phosphate. The phosphorus is absorbed as inorganic salts. About 70 per cent of dietary phosphorus is normally absorbed.

The inorganic phosphorus content of blood serum ranges from 2.5 to 4.5 mg per cent and is slightly higher in children. The level is kept constant through regulation by the kidney. All of the plasma inorganic phosphate is filtered through the renal glomeruli but most of it is reabsorbed. Vitamin D increases the rate of reabsorption by the tubules, and parathormone decreases the reabsorption.

Daily Allowances The phosphorus allowances recommended by the Food and Nutrition Board[1] are the same as those for calcium, except for infants. With ordinary diets, the phosphorus intake exceeds the calcium intake, but within a relatively wide range of calcium-to-phosphorus ratios there are no adverse effects in children and adults.

During the first 6 months of life the phosphorus allowance is 240 mg, and during the remainder of the first year the allowance is 400 mg. By keeping the phosphorus allowance below that of calcium during the first weeks of life, hypocalcemic tetany is avoided.

Food Sources Phosphorus is widely distributed in foods, the milk and meat groups being important contributors. Thus, a diet that furnishes enough protein and calcium will normally provide sufficient phosphorus. Whole-grain cereals and flours contain much more phosphorus than refined cereals and flours; however, much of this occurs in phytic acid, which combines with calcium to form an insoluble salt that is not absorbed. Vegetables and fruits contain only small amounts of phosphorus. Consumption of excessive amounts of phosphorus can change the Ca:P ratio so as to decrease calcium availability. Large amounts of phosphorus without a balanced consumption of calcium can be obtained by consuming diets containing excessive amounts of meat, soft drinks and foods containing phosphorus additives. (See Table A–1.)

Magnesium

Distribution The amount of magnesium in the body is much smaller than that of calcium and phosphorus. Of the 20 to 35 gm in the adult body, about 60 per cent is present at phosphates and carbonates chiefly at the surfaces of the bones. Most of the remaining magnesium is within the cells where it ranks next to potassium in magnitude.

Extracellular fluids account for about 2 per cent of the body's magnesium. The normal concentration of magnesium in blood serum is 2 to 3 mg per cent, about 80 per cent of this being ionized; the remainder is bound to protein.

Functions Magnesium is essential for all living cells. In plants magnesium is present in chlorophyll in a chemical structure similar to the iron in hemoglobin. In addition to its function in the skeletal structures, magnesium is a catalyst in numerous metabolic reactions. It is involved in protein synthesis through its action on the aggregation of ribosomes. It is an activator for the enzymes involved in the oxidative phosphorylation of ADP to ATP (see page 82), and also for all enzymes that bring about the conversion of ATP to cyclic-AMP which in turn regulates parathormone secretion. These reactions are essential whenever energy is expended, as in active transport across cell membranes, and the accomplishment of physical work.

Magnesium, together with calcium, sodium, and potassium, must be in balance in the extracellular fluids so that transmission of nerve impulses and the consequent muscle contraction can be regulated.

Metabolism Magnesium is absorbed by active transport and competes with calcium for carrier sites. Thus, a high intake of either element interferes with absorption of the other. Many of the factors that enhance calcium absorption such as acidity, or that interfere with calcium absorption such as oxalic and phytic acids, also affect the absorption of magnesium. Neither vitamin D nor parathyroid hormone is believed to influence magnesium absorption. The absorption of magnesium varies inversely with the intake; at low levels of intake it is as high as 75 per cent, and at high levels of intake it may be as low as 25 per cent. The absorption on typical intakes in America is about 45 per cent.[14]

In magnesium deficiency the kidneys and the intestinal mucosa have a marked ability to retain magnesium. Thus, homeostasis can be maintained over a wide range of intake. The urinary excretion of magnesium in adults normally ranges between 100 and 200 mg. Almost all of the magnesium in the feces represents unabsorbed dietary magnesium.

Daily Allowances The Food and Nutrition Board has recommended a daily allowance of magnesium for men at 350 mg and for women at 300 mg.[1] During pregnancy and lactation a daily allowance of 450 mg is recommended. The allowances range from 50 to 70 mg during the first year of life and thereafter gradually increase from 150 mg for the toddler to 250 mg for the child of 7 to 10 years.

Food Sources The food supply available for consumption in the United States supplies 343 mg magnesium daily per capita. The per cent of this magnesium supplied by each food group is as follows; dairy products excluding butter, 19.8; vegetables, 19.8; grain products, 19.1; meat, poultry, and fish, 14.0; dry beans, peas, soybeans, and nuts, 12.3; fruits, 7.1; and miscellanous foods, 7.0. (See Table 13–3 for calculations of the Basic Diet.) Green leafy vegetables are especially good sources as are also dry beans and peas, soybeans, nuts, and whole grains. High losses of magnesium occur in the refinement of foods, and some losses are sustained when cooking waters are discarded. (See Table A–2 for magnesium content of foods.)

The average mixed American diet supplies about 120 mg magnesium per 1000 kcal.[1] Thus, if girls and women stay within their caloric requirements it would appear that they could not easily meet the recommended allowances. There is no evidence, however, that magnesium deficiency occurs except under conditions described in the following

Effects of Imbalance Under normal conditions of health and food intake, magnesium deficiency is not likely to occur. Unlike calcium, magnesium is only slowly mobilized from bone. Therefore, a generally poor intake of magnesium, if it is also accompanied by increased excretion, leads to rapid lowering of the plasma magnesium. The ionic imbalance thus produced in the extracellular fluid upsets the regulation of nervous irritability and muscle contraction. Characteristic symptoms of magnesium deficiency include muscle tremor, paresthesias, and sometimes convulsive seizures and delirium. Since these symptoms are similar to hypocalcemic tetany, a differentiation can usually be made by determining the blood levels of the two cations.

Among the circumstances under which magnesium deficiency is encountered are these: chronic alcoholism, cirrhosis of the liver, malabsorption syndromes such as sprue, kwashiorkor, severe vomiting, prolonged use of magnesium-free parenteral fluids, diabetic acidosis, and diuretic therapy. In most of these instances the deficiency has occurred because of curtailment of food intake or lowered absorption or both. The loss of magnesium from the body is increased during diuretic therapy, and also in diabetic acidosis.

High blood magnesium levels are sometimes encountered when there is an unusual increase in absorption or a marked reduction in urinary excretion. The symptoms of such excess include extreme thirst, a feeling of excessive warmth, marked drowsiness, a decrease in muscle and nerve irritability, and atrial fibrillation. The early stages of hypermagnesemia are readily corrected by giving calcium gluconate.

Sulfur

Distribution Sulfur accounts for about 0.25 per cent of body weight, or 175 mg in the adult male. It is present in all body cells, chiefly as the sulfur-containing amino acids methionine, cystine, and cysteine. Sulfur is a constituent of thiamin and biotin, two vitamins that must be present in the diet. Connective tissue, skin, nails, and hair are especially rich in sulfur.

Functions and Metabolism Sulfur is an essential element for all animal species inasmuch as they all require the sulfur-containing amino acid methionine. Almost all of the sulfur absorbed from the intestinal tract is in organic form, principally as the sulfur amino acids. Inorganic sulfates, present in only small amounts in foods, are poorly absorbed.

Sulfur is a structurally important constituent of mucopolysaccharides such as chondroitin sulfate found in cartilage, tendons, bones, skin, and the heart valves. Sulfolipids are abundant in such tissues as liver, kidney, the salivary glands, and the white matter of the brain. Other important sulfur-containing compounds are insulin (page 81) and heparin, an anticoagulant.

Sulfur compounds are essential in many oxidation-reduction reactions. Included among these compounds are a number of coenzymes discussed elsewhere in this text: thiamin (page 218); biotin (page 232); coenzyme A (page 84); and lipoic acid (page 231). Glutathione, an important compound in oxidation-reduction reactions, is a tripeptide of glutamic acid, cysteine, and glycine. The concentration of glutathione is especially high in the red blood cells.

The metabolism of the sulfur amino acids within the cells yields sulfuric acid, which is immediately neutralized and excreted as the inorganic salts. One of the important reactions of sulfuric acid is the conjugation with phenols, cresols, and the steroid sex hormones, which thereby detoxifies compounds that would otherwise be harmful.

Excretion About 85 to 90 per cent of the sulfur excreted in the urine is in the inorganic form, being derived almost entirely from the metabolism of the sulfur amino acids. The ratio of nitrogen to sulfur excreted in the urine is about 13 to 1. The range of excretion by the adult is 1 to 2 gm. On a low-protein diet the excretion would be much less than on a high-protein diet.

From 5 to 10 per cent of the sulfur excreted is in the form of organic esters produced in the detoxification reactions. The fecal excretion of sulfur is about equal to the inorganic sulfur content of the diet.

Cystinuria is a relatively rare hereditary defect in which large amounts of cystine as well as lysine, arginine, and ornithine are excreted because of a failure of renal reabsorption. Being somewhat insoluble, the cystine forms renal calculi.

Requirements and Sources The daily requirement for sulfur has not been determined. A diet that is adequate in methionine and cystine is considered to meet the body's sulfur needs.

The sulfur content of foods depends upon the concentration of methionine and cystine. Food proteins vary from 0.4 to 1.6 per cent in their sulfur content, with an average of 1 per cent for a typical mixed diet. Thus, meat, poultry, milk, and eggs may be considered to be important sources.

Trace Elements or Micronutrients

Iron

Distribution The amount of iron in the body of the adult male is about 50 mg per kilogram, or a total of 3.5 gm; in the woman it is about 35 mg per kilogram, or a total of 2.3 gm. All body cells contain some iron. Approximately 75 per cent of the iron is in the hemoglobin, 5 per cent is held as myoglobin, 5 per cent is present in cellular constituents including the iron-containing enzymes, and 20 per cent is stored as FERRITIN or HEMOSIDERIN by the liver, spleen, and bone marrow. In healthy men the iron reserve is about 1,000 mg, but in menstruating women it is not more than 200 to 400 mg.

Iron circulates in the plasma bound to a β-globulin, TRANSFERRIN—also known as SIDEROPHILIN. The concentration of iron in the serum for men ranges from 80 to 165 μg per 100 ml, and for women from 65 to 130 μg per 100 ml. Normally, the saturation of transferrin with iron ranges from 20 to 40 per cent.

Functions Hemoglobin is the principal component of the red blood cells and accounts for most of the iron in the body. It acts as a carrier of oxygen from the lungs to the tissues and indirectly aids in the return of carbon dioxide to the lungs.

MYOGLOBIN is an iron-protein complex in the muscle which stores some oxygen for immediate use by the cell. Enzymes such as the catalases, the cytochromes in hydrogen ion transport (see page 84), and xanthine oxidase contain iron as an integral part of the molecule. Iron is required as a cofactor for other enzymes.

Metabolism The amount of iron that will be absorbed from the intestinal tract is governed by (1) the body's need for iron, (2) the conditions existing in the intestinal lumen, and (3) the food mixture that is fed. (See Figure 8–3). Iron is absorbed into the mucosal cells as (1) nonheme iron from inorganic salts in foods, and (2) as heme iron. In the latter the porphyrin ring is split open in the cell and the iron is released into the blood circulation.

The absorption of iron is meticulously regulated by the intestinal mucosa according to body need. An increase in erythropoiesis leads to withdrawal of iron from the iron-transferrin complex in the circulation, and the lowering of transferrin saturation in turn brings about an increase in the amount of iron that is absorbed. Thus, growing children, pregnant women, and anemic individuals will have a higher rate of absorption than healthy males. The absorptive mechanism in normal individuals is also highly effective in preventing an overload of iron entering the body and causing toxic reactions. Although excess iron can be absorbed, extremely large intakes would be necessary for a long period of time before toxic reactions would result.

In the acid medium of the stomach and upper duodenum ferric iron is reduced to ferrous iron, a more soluble form that is readily absorbed. Achlorhydria, observed in many elderly persons and present in pernicious anemia, reduces the absorption of iron. Likewise, the surgical removal of the portion of the stomach that produces acid will result in lower absorption of iron. The alkaline reaction of pancreatic juice reduces the solubility of iron so that little absorption takes place from the jejunum and ileum. Absorption of iron is also hindered

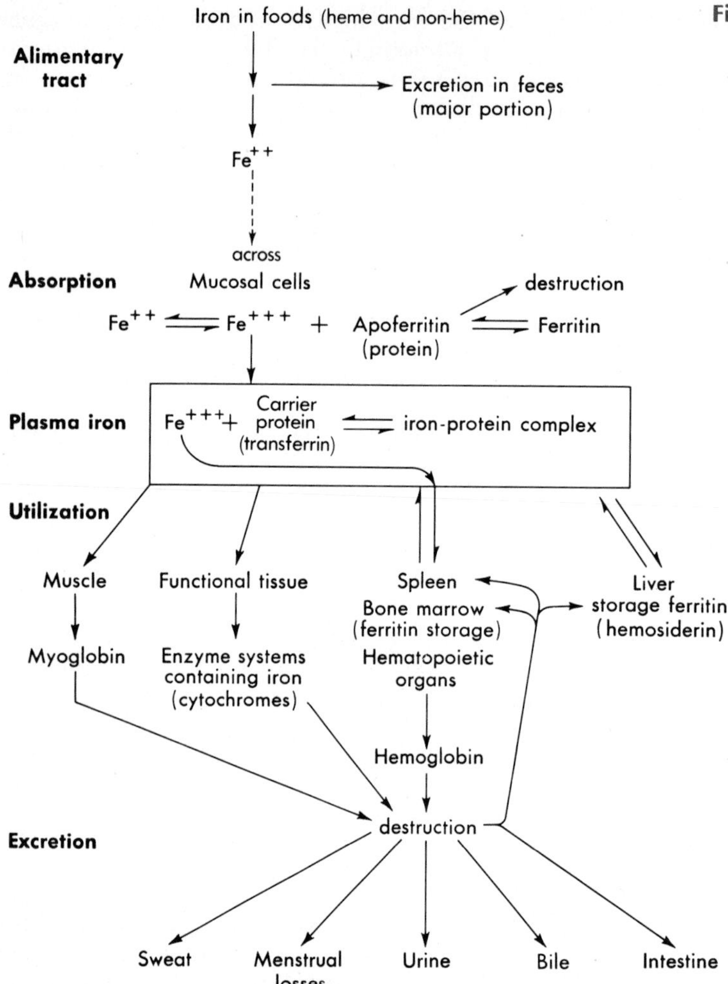

Figure 8–3. The utilization of iron.

in malabsorption syndromes, and in the presence of excess phytates.

The absorption of iron from foods varies depending on whether HEME or NONHEME IRON is consumed.[16] The composition of the rest of the meal and the status of the individual's iron stores are also major influences on iron absorption (see Table 8–3). An individual with moderate iron stores would be expected to absorb about 23 per cent of the heme iron consumed in a meal. Nonheme iron absorption can vary from 3 per cent to 8 per cent in the individual with moderate iron stores depending on the presence of absorption enhancing factors. The most important absorption enhancing factors are storage iron status, the amount of vitamin C consumed with the meal, and the amount of meat, poultry, or fish consumed. Inhibitory factors present with the meal such as tannins from tea, phytates from cereals, and antacids are recognized but inadequate data are available to include these factors in absorption calculations.

Transport and utilization. Iron in the plasma is made available from three

Table 8-3. **Available Nonheme and Heme Iron in Different Meals***

Meal Description	Per Cent of Iron Available for Absorption at Each Meal† Nonheme Iron	Heme Iron
Low availability of nonheme iron a. <30 gm (1 oz) lean, raw weight, of meat, poultry, or fish OR b. <25 mg ascorbic acid	3	23
Medium availability of nonheme iron a. 30–90 gm (1–3 oz) lean, raw weight, of meat, poultry, or fish OR b. 25–75 mg ascorbic acid	5	23
High availability of nonheme iron a. >90 gm (3 oz) lean, raw weight, of meat, poultry, or fish OR b. >75 mg ascorbic acid OR c. 30–90 gm lean meat, poultry, or fish *plus* 25–75 mg ascorbic acid	8	23

*Adapted from Monsen, E. R., et al.: "Estimation of Available Dietary Iron," *Am. J. Clin. Nutr.*, 31:134–41, 1978.

†The factors cited here assume that a woman has a 500 mg store of iron. It is recommended that these factors be used for dietary calculations. For men with larger iron stores, the per cent of iron absorbed is lower; for women with iron stores below 500 mg the per cent of iron absorbed is higher. For appropriate factors when iron stores are known, see cited publication.

sources: (1) absorption from the intestinal tract, (2) release from body reserves, and (3) release from the breakdown of hemoglobin that takes place constantly. Within a 24-hour period the turnover of iron is about 27 to 28 mg.[17] Only 1 to 1.5 mg of this has been available from absorption.

Iron is withdrawn from the plasma into the bone marrow for the synthesis of HEMOGLOBIN, which is a complex substance composed of a basic protein, GLOBIN, linked to a prosthetic group, HEME. The heme molecule consists of protoporphyrin with reduced iron at its center; four heme molecules together with globin make up the hemoglobin. Copper and pyridoxine play a catalytic role in the incorporation of iron into the protoporphyrin molecule.

The body exercises amazing economy in the use of iron. When the red blood cell has fulfilled its life cycle of about 120 days, the cell is destroyed within the reticuloendothelial system. The amino acids of the stroma and the globin, and the lipids, are utilized again. Heme is disintegrated to release iron once again to the circulation and the bile pigments are synthesized from the remainder of the molecule.

Excretion. The daily excretion of body iron by adults is about 0.1 mg from the urine and 0.3 to 0.5 mg into the intestinal lumen. Small amounts of iron are also lost in the perspiration and by exfoliation of the skin. The iron losses through menstruation range from 0.3 to 1.0 mg on a daily basis, but about 5 per cent of women have losses in excess of 1.4 mg daily.[1] Thus, the total iron losses by women are 1 to 2 mg daily.

Most of the iron in the feces represents the unabsorbed iron from the diet. A small amount of fecal iron is of endogenous origin, namely, that derived from the sloughing off of mucosal cells, bile pigments, and other digestive juices.

Daily Allowances Dietary iron is required for (1) replacement of the daily losses of all individuals; (2) an expanding blood volume and increasing amounts of hemoglobin in growing children; (3) replacement of the varying losses through menstruation; (4) development of the fetus and to avoid anemia in pregnant and lactating women; and (5) a reserve of iron that is available when blood loss occurs from any cause whatsoever.

Table 8–4 lists the amount of iron that must be absorbed to replace losses and to meet the synthetic requirements of various age groups and the recommended allowances of the Food and Nutrition Board.

Food Sources Of all nutrients, the iron allowance is the most difficult to provide in the diet. The iron content of typical diets adequate in other respects is estimated to be 6 mg per 100 kcal[1] but the amount of absorbed iron varies. (See Table 8–3).[1] Thus, men and boys with their caloric requirements can easily meet their iron needs, but girls and women with their lower caloric requirements cannot supply their needs even with a good selection of diet.

Table 8-4. **Daily Iron Requirements***

	Absorbed Iron Requirement mg/day	Recommended Dietary Allowance† mg/day
Men and nonmenstruating women	0.5–1	10
Menstruating women	0.7–2	18
Pregnant women	2 –4.8	18+‡
Adolescents	1 –2	18
Children	0.4–1	10–15
Infants	0.5–1.5	10–15

*Adapted from: Committee on Iron Deficiency, Council on Foods and Nutrition: "Iron Deficiency in the United States," *JAMA*, 203:407–14, February 5, 1968; and Food and Nutrition Board: *Recommended Dietary Allowances*, 9th ed. National Academy of Sciences–National Research Council, Washington, D.C., 1980.

†Assuming an absorption of 10 per cent.

‡This amount of iron cannot be derived from diet and should be met by iron supplementation during pregnancy.

Much more research is required to determine the availability of iron from various food sources and the conditions that enhance or detract from that availability. Lean meats, poultry, and fish contain about 40 per cent of their iron as heme iron which is absorbed intact. Nonheme iron is found in the remaining 60 per cent of the iron in animal tissues as well as the iron in other foods. Of these, legumes, dried fruit, and cereals are good sources. Even though the absorption of nonheme iron is lower than heme iron, the amount of nonheme iron consumed is much greater. Thus, nonheme iron usually makes the larger contribution to available iron in the average diet.

Cooking procedures are an important determinant in the amount of iron that is actually ingested. Some mineral salts are leached out when large amounts of water are used and subsequently discarded. Cast-iron cookware was widely used many years ago, and the uptake of iron from such cooking vessels added appreciably to the daily intake. Today, iron skillets are about the only such cookware used frequently. There are substantial differences between the iron content of foods cooked in cast-iron ware and the same foods cooked in glass or aluminum.[18]

Calculation of Available Dietary Iron Absorption availability of iron can be estimated by the computation of five variables for *each meal*:[16]

1. Total iron consumed from each food item in the meal (from food composition table);
2. Estimating heme iron (40 per cent of total iron in animal tissues, that is, meat, poultry, and fish);

3. Estimating nonheme iron (variable 1 minus variable 2);
4. Estimating total amount of vitamin C in the meal as consumed (estimated from food composition table);
5. Estimating total amount of meat, poultry, and fish consumed. Each meal can then be determined to have high, medium, or low nonheme iron availability and the total iron for the meal can be calculated. (See Tables 8–3 and 8–5.) For these estimation purposes, moderate iron stores are assumed. At these storage levels it is assumed that 23 per cent of the heme iron is absorbed. The heme iron absorption does not vary as it is not influenced by the composition of the meal.

Effects of Imbalance The characteristics of iron-deficiency anemia are a low serum level of iron, high iron-binding capacity, low hemoglobin, low red cell volume, and low mean corpuscular hemoglobin. The serum ferritin is a good indicator of iron stores.[19] However, inflammation, liver disease, and increased red cell turnover as in hemolytic anemia raise serum ferritin levels to a degree disproportionate to stores. Iron-deficiency anemia is characterized by reduced red cell and hemoglobin levels in the blood and by small, pale cells (microcytic, hypochromic). It is widely prevalent in the United States and throughout the world, but the exact incidence is not known. Infants, preschool children, adolescent girls, and pregnant women are especially susceptible. See Chapter 30 for discussion of anemias.

HEMOSIDEROSIS is a disorder of iron metabolism in which large deposits of iron are made especially in the liver and in the reticuloendothelial system. The transferrin of the circulation becomes saturated and is unable to bind all of the iron that is absorbed. This disorder affects a high proportion of the adult Bantu population in South Africa and is believed to be caused by an overload of dietary iron.[20] Bantu men commonly ingest 30 mg iron daily and frequently as much as 100 mg per day. The beer that they drink is fermented in iron pots, and likewise the acid-fermented cereal foods and sour porridge are cooked in these pots. The resulting foods have a high iron content.

Hemosiderosis also occurs when there is abnormal destruction of the red blood cells as in hemolytic anemia. It may also occur following prolonged iron therapy when it

Table 8–5. **Sample Calculation of Iron Availability from a Meal**

Food	Weight gm	Ascorbic Acid mg	Total Iron mg	Heme Factor	Heme Iron mg	Nonheme Iron mg
Roast pork, 2 ounces	56	0	2.2	0.4	0.9	1.3
Mashed potato, ½ cup	105	10.5	0.4			0.4
Buttered carrots, ½ cup	78	4.5	0.45			0.45
Dinner roll, 1	26		0.5			0.5
Milk, 2 per cent, 1 cup	244	2	0.1			0.1
Cantaloupe, ⅓ 5-in. melon	180	60	0.7			0.7
		77	4.35		0.9	3.45
High Availability of Iron*						
Per cent of iron absorbed					23	8
Amount of iron absorbed					0.21	0.28
Total available for absorption (0.21 + 0.28)					0.49	

*If a fruit low in ascorbic acid were substituted for the cantaloupe in this example, the rating would be medium availability.

is not needed. The iron overload leads to deposits of iron in the liver cells, following which typical symptoms of cirrhosis develop. The excess iron may also be deposited in the lungs, pancreas, and heart.

In the United States, increased iron fortification of cereals has been proposed to help alleviate the widespread incidence of iron deficiency. The proposals, first made in 1971, have not yet been adopted because of debate about whether the target population, namely women during their reproductive years, would be reached by this measure. The unknown possible incidence of hemosiderosis among adult men is another factor hindering acceptance of higher fortification levels. The maximum safe level of iron intake for adults is unknown, but daily intake levels of 25 to 75 mg are unlikely to cause problems.[21]

Iodine

Distribution and Function About one third of the iodine in the adult body, variously estimated from 25 to 50 mg, is found in the thyroid gland where it is stored in the form of THYROGLOBULIN. The concentration of iodine in the thyroid gland is about 2,500 times as great as that in any other tissues.

The only known function of iodine is as a constituent of the thyroid hormones, THYROXINE and TRIIODOTHYRONINE. Tyrosine, one of the amino acids, incorporates four atoms of iodine to form thyroxine. The thyroid hormones regulate the rate of oxidation within the cells and in so doing influence physical and mental growth, the functioning of the nervous and muscle tissues, circulatory activity, and the metabolism of all nutrients.

Metabolism Iodine is ingested in foods as inorganic iodides and as organic compounds. In the digestive tract iodine is split from organic compounds and is rapidly absorbed as inorganic iodide. The degree of absorption is dependent upon the level of circulating thyroid hormone.

Iodine is transported by the circultion as free iodide and as PROTEIN-BOUND IODINE. The protein-bound fraction (PBI) is sensitive to changes in the level of thyroid activity; it rises during pregnancy and with hypertrophy of the gland and falls with hypofunction of the gland. The measurement of PBI, therefore, is a specific diagnostic tool for thyroid activity and has largely replaced the basal metabolism test as a study of thyroid function.

Another measure of thyroid activity is the uptake of radioactive iodine 24 hours after a measured dose of ^{131}I has been given. Normally, the thyroid gland takes up about 40 to 50 per cent of the dose given; this is increased in hyperthyroidism, and decreased in hypothyroidism.

Thyroid activity is controlled by the thyroid-stimulating hormone (TSH) secreted by the anterior lobe of the pituitary. When the blood level of the thyroid hormone is low, the activity of the thyroid is increased by TSH. By this action the thyroid gland withdraws iodide from the circulation, concentrates it, oxidizes it to iodine, and incorporates it into tyrosine to form diiodotyrosine, triiodothyronine, and thyroxine. These iodine-containing amino acids then become part of the thyroglobulin complex.

When thyroid hormone is utilized for cellular oxidation, iodine is released into the circulation. About one third of the released iodine is again incorporated into thyroid hormone and the remainder is excreted in the urine.

Daily Allowances The recommended allowance for men and women over the age of 11 is 150 μg. Infants should receive 40 to 50 μg during the first year, and children up to 10 years, 70 to 120 μg. The allowances in pregnancy and lactation are 175 and 200 μg, respectively.[1]

Sources The most important dietary source of iodine is iodized salt. The concentration of iodine used in salt is 1 part sodium or potassium iodide per 10,000 parts of salt.

One gram of salt would furnish about 76 μg iodine. About half of the table salt sold in the United States is iodized. Recent changes in labeling requirements have required iodized salt to be more conspicuously labeled as much. Salt used in the processing of food and bulk salt for institutional use is not likely to be iodized.[1]

Seaweed, saltwater fish, and shellfish contain important amounts of iodine for people who consume these foods on a regular basis. The iodine content of eggs, dairy products, and meats depends upon the iodine content of the animal's diet. Vegetables grown on iodine-rich soils near the seacoast are good sources of iodine; those grown on iodine-poor soils, generally inland, contain little iodine. Because of widespread food distribution, the geographic source of most foods is unknown. Thus, the iodine content of foods purchased in stores cannot be determined without analysis. Unless it is known that the foods consumed come from an iodine-rich area, another source of dietary iodine, such as iodized salt, should be used.

Effects of Deficiency ENDEMIC GOITER, the iodine-deficiency disease, occurs in those areas where the iodine content of the soil is so low that insufficient iodine is obtained through food and water, and when no provision is made for supplying iodized salt. Among the areas of iodine-poor soils are the Great Lakes region, the Pacific Northwest, Switzerland, Central American countries, mountainous areas of South America, New Zealand, and the Himalayas. The World Health Organization has estimated that up to 200 million people throughout the world may be affected. The iodine intake in the United States is generally adequate, and deficiency is no longer considered to be a problem.

Lack of iodine leads to an increase in the size and number of epithelial cells in the thyroid gland and thus an enlargement of the gland. This condition known as simple or endemic goiter, presents no other abnormal physical findings. The basal metabolism remains normal. The deficiency is more prevalent in females than males and is more frequent during adolescence and pregnancy.

The most urgent reason for stressing iodine as a preventive measure is not the goiter itself but the cretinism which is its ultimate sequel in areas severely deficient in iodine. Cretinism occurs in the infant when the pregnant woman is so severely depleted that she cannot supply iodine for the development of the fetus. CRETINISM is characterized by a low basal metabolism, muscular flabbiness and weakness, dry skin, enlarged tongue, thick lips, arrest of skeletal development, and severe mental retardation. Desiccated thyroid given early enough to the infant results in marked improvement of physical development; mental retardation may be less severe, but any damage which has occurred to the central nervous sytem cannot be reversed. Endemic cretinism is rare or nonexistent in the United States today.

Goitrogens Certain substances called GOITROGENS are known to interfere with the use of thyroxine and will produce goiters, at least in experimental animals, even though the iodine intake would normally be adequate. Goitrogens are present in the *Brassica* family which includes a number of widely used vegetables—cabbage, turnips, rutabagas, radishes, cauliflower, and Brussels sprouts. Goitrogens are also present in peanuts and oilseeds, such as rape seed. Oilseed proteins may become more important in our food supply as these products are developed as alternative protein sources. The substances are inactivated by cooking, and there is currently no evidence that goiters in endemic regions are caused by them.

Zinc

Distribution in the Body About 2 to 3 gm zinc is present in the adult body. It is distributed widely in all tissues but not evenly. High concentrations are found in the eye, especially the iris and retina, in the liver, bone, prostate and prostatic secretions, and in the hair. In the blood about 85 per cent of the zinc is in the red blood cells; however, each leukocyte contains about 25 times as much zinc as each red blood cell.

Functions Zinc is essential for all living organisms. Its numerous functions include the following:

1. As an integral part of at least 20 enzymes that belong to a large group known as metalloenzymes. Among these are

CARBONIC ANHYDRASE, an enzyme isolated and purified in 1940 and found to contain zinc. Carbonic anhydrase is as essential to the transport of carbon dioxide to the lungs as hemoglobin is to the transport of oxygen.

LACTIC DEHYDROGENASE involved in the interconversion of pyruvic and lactic acid in the glycolytic pathway.

ALKALINE PHOSPHATASE required in bone metabolism. The concentration is especially high in white blood cells.

CARBOXYPEPTIDASE and AMINOPEPTIDASE, which bring about removal of the terminal carboxyl and amino groups in the digestion of proteins.

ALCOHOL DEHYDROGENASE in the liver which oxidizes not only ethanol but other primary and secondary alcohols as well, including methanol and ethylene glycol, thus serving as a major detoxifying mechanism.

2. As a cofactor in the syntheis of DNA and RNA, and thus proteins. In this role it is especially important in cellular systems that undergo rapid turnover, as in the gastrointestinal tract including the taste buds. Thus, zinc plays a role in the sensory systems that control food intake.[22]
3. The mobilization of vitamin A from the liver to maintain normal concentrations in the blood circulation.
4. Enhancement of the action of follicle-stimulating hormone and luteinizing hormone.

Metabolism Most of the zinc is absorbed primarily from the duodenum and jejunum. Although absorption ranges widely, the usual uptake by the intestinal mucosa is probably less than 50 per cent. Large intakes of calcium, vitamin D, and phytate interfere with absorption.

Upon absorption zinc combines with a protein for transport. The rate of turnover in the liver, pancreas, kidney, and pituitary is rapid. The normal serum concentration of zinc is about 100 to 140 μg per 100 ml. There is little day-to-day variation in plasma concentrations and no increase in the blood level after meals. Unlike iron, the body stores of zinc are not readily utilized, thus regular daily intake is needed.

Zinc is excreted primarily by pancreatic and intestinal juices. The normal urinary loss is about 500 μg daily. For the very young infant, prior to the development of intestinal zinc absorption mechanisms, a recently discovered zinc-protein carrier in breast milk may be very important.[23]

Recommended Allowances Only a limited amount of research has been conducted on the requirements for zinc. The recommended allowances are 15 mg for adults; 3 to 5 mg for infants; 10 mg for children; 20 mg during pregnancy; and 25 mg for the lactating woman.[1]

Food Sources Data on food composition are sparse, and there is little information on the variability from sample to sample. Rich sources include oysters, liver, high-protein foods, and whole-grain cereals, Beef, lamb, and pork contain three to four times as much as fish; and dark meat of chicken furnishes about three times as much as light meat. Legumes, peanuts, and peanut butter are good sources, but fruits and most vegetables are poor sources. The zinc in plant proteins is less available than that in animal proteins. Vegetarian diets and low-protein diets are likely to be deficient in zinc. (See Table A–2.)

Deficiency The first description of human deficiency of zinc was reported from Iran and Egypt.[24-26] Dwarfs in those countries were observed to consume a diet in which more than half of the calories were furnished by unleavened whole-grain bread. Although the whole-grain cereals are good sources of zinc, practically all of the mineral is tied up by the high concentration of phytate in the unleavened bread. In addition to growth failure, there were hypogonadism, enlarged liver, and severe anemia. Serum zinc levels were about 50 μg per 100 ml. With the addition of zinc to the diet there was considerable improvement in growth and development of the sexual organs.

As research on zinc status is accumulated, reports of marginal zinc status in the United States are becoming more frequent. Based on hair assays for zinc studies in children show that some have a history of poor zinc nutrition. These children show symptoms consistent with mild zinc deficiency but without exhibiting the clinical deficiency state.[27]

Impaired taste and odor acuity is a consequence of zinc deficiency. HYPOGEUSIA is a decrease in taste acuity; DYSGEUSIA is an unpleasant, perverted, and obnoxious taste. HYPOSMIA is a decrease in odor acuity; DYSOSMIA is a disagreeable odor sensation. Patients often complain of persistent foul odor in the nasopharynx, metallic taste in the absence of food; or saltiness, sweetness, sourness, or bitterness.[28, 29] Studies by electron microscope have shown the taste buds to be fewer in number, smaller, and with a number of histologic changes.

In some patients, with severe burns serum zinc levels are about two thirds of normal, urinary excretions are doubled, and anorexia is severe. Therapy with zinc has improved the appetite so that food intake begins to approximate the high protein and caloric needs for recovery.[30] Hyposmia, dysosmia, and hypogeusia are often severe in acute viral hepatitis, cirrhosis of the liver, hepatic coma, kwashiorkor, and malabsorption syndrome.

Toxicity Zinc salts are relatively nontoxic. About 60 to 120 times the recommended allowance will induce vomiting, cramps, and diarrhea in 3 to 12 hours, but the symptoms subside shortly. Intake of excessive zinc has been reported when acid foods or beverages such as lemonade were prepared and stored in galvanized containers. The acidity of the food dissolves enough zinc to produce the toxic symptoms.

Copper

Distribution The presence of copper in blood was first recognized in 1875, but the nutritional significance was not established until Hart and Elvehjem at the University of Wisconsin found that traces of copper were essential for the formation of hemoglobin. The body of the human adult contains about 100 to 150 mg of copper. Traces of copper are found in all tissues, but by far the highest concentrations are found in the liver, brain, heart, and kidney. In the fetus and at birth the levels in these organs are several times higher, and they decrease during the first year.

Metabolism and Function Copper is absorbed from the stomach and from the upper gastrointestinal tract. About 95 per cent of the copper in blood plasma is firmly bound to a protein complex, CERULOPLASMIN, and 5 per cent is loosely bound to albumin. Molybdenum, zinc, and cadmium are antagonistic to copper; thus, an increased intake of these trace elements increases the requirement for copper. Vitamin C can also decrease the absorption of copper by decreasing its ability to bind one of the carrier proteins needed for absorption. Almost all of the excretion of copper is in the feces, chiefly through the excretion of bile.

The copper-containing ceruloplasmin has a role in the transport of iron in transferrin for hemoglobin synthesis. Thus metabolic deficiency of copper can result in anemia. Other diverse functions requiring copper are taste sensitivity, melanin pigment formation, electron transport, integrity of the myelin sheath, maturation of collagen, elastin formation, phospholipid synthesis, bone development, and hemoglobin formation. Copper has been identified as a constituent of a number of enzymes: butyryl coenzyme A dehydrogenase required for the oxidation of fatty acids; tyrosinase required for melanin pigment formation; uricase in purine metabolism; and in the cytochrome oxidation system for energy production. Several copper-containing proteins such as hepatocuprein and erythrocuprein help protect against the toxic effects of oxygen.

Estimated Safe and Adequate Intake The intake of copper considered adequate and safe for adults is 2 to 3 mg per day. For infants an intake of 0.5 to 1 mg is considered satisfactory. One to 3 mg per day is the suggested intake for children, increasing with age.[1]

Food Sources Typical diets furnish from less than 1 to 5 mg copper. The copper content of foods is somewhat dependent upon the copper content of soil. Among rich sources are organ meats, shellfish, whole-grain cereals, legumes, and nuts. Milk is a poor source. (See Table A–2.)

Effects of Imbalance Dietary deficiency of copper is not common in humans. Low blood levels of copper have been observed in kwashiorkor, the nephrotic syndrome, and sprue, and occasionally in patients with iron-deficiency anemia or with total parenteral nutrition.

In excessive amounts copper is toxic. A rare hereditary disorder known as Wilson's disease is characterized by a marked reduction of blood ceruloplasmin and greatly increased deposits of copper in the liver, brain, and other organs. The excess copper in these tissues leads to hepatitis, lenticular degeneration, renal malfunction, and neurologic disorders.

Recent epidemiological data have indicated that a high zinc-to-copper ratio may be a factor in the development of cardiovascular diseases, particularly elevated cholesterol levels in the blood. Further research is needed to clarify whether the interrelationship of these minerals is a causative agent.[31]

Fluorine

Distribution and Function Fluoride occurs normally in the body primarily as a calcium salt in the bones and teeth. Small amounts of fluoride bring about striking reductions in tooth decay, probably because the tooth enamel is made more resistant to the action of acids produced in the mouth by bacteria.

Carefully controlled studies in a number of cities for more than 10 years have established that fluoridation of the water supplies at a level of 1 part fluoride per million (1 ppm or 1 mg/liter) may be expected to reduce the incidence of dental caries in children by approximately 50 to 60 per cent. Several thousand communities in the United States have now initiated water fluoridation as an effective public health measure. Children who have been drinking fluoridated water since infancy show the greatest benefits; those who begin the ingestion of fluoridated water in later school years are helped to a lesser extent.

Fluorides may be involved in some way in the maintenance of bone structure. Some studies have shown that osteoporosis occurs less frequently in elderly persons who live in areas supplied with fluoridated water.[32] The fluoride salts of calcium are less readily lost from bone during immobilization or following the menopause.

Metabolism Fluorides are absorbed readily from the gastrointestinal tract. They replace the hydroxyl groups in the calcium-phosphorus salts of bones and teeth to form fluoroapatite. The fluoride crystals are less readily resorbed than are crystals of hydroxyapatite. Most of the fluoride ingested is excreted in the urine. An average daily excretion is about 3 mg.

Estimated Safe and Adequate Intake The intake of fluorine considered adequate and safe for adults is 1.5 to 4.0 mg per day. For children and adolscents a range of 0.5 to 2.5 mg per day is recommended, depending on age. Infants should have a daily intake of 0.1 to 1.0 mg.[1] For breast-fed infants, supplementation may be considered.

Food Sources Fluoride occurs in all soils, water supplies, plants, and animals, and is a normal constituent of the diet. The amounts present are in direct correlation with the fluoride concentration of water and soils. In low-fluoride areas the daily diet furnishes only 0.3 mg; in high-fluoride areas the daily intake from food is about 3.1 mg.[1] Six glasses of water containing 1 ppm will provide an additional 1.2 mg.

Effects of Excess Chronic dental FLUOROSIS results when the concentration of fluoride in drinking water is in excess of 2.0 ppm. The teeth become MOTTLED; that is, the tooth enamel becomes dull and unglazed with some pitting. At higher concentrations of fluoride some dark-brown stains appear. Although aesthetically undesirable, such teeth are surprisingly free of dental caries.

Large excesses of fluorine—20 to 80 mg daily for several years—lead to bone fluorosis with symptoms resembling arthritis.

Other Trace Elements

Manganese, molybdenum, selenium, chromium, and cobalt are essential trace elements. Their principal functions are as integral constituents of enzymes or as activators of enzymes.

For these minerals, estimated safe and adequate daily intake ranges have been recommended because of sparse experimental data on the human requirements. Data on the distribution and the availability of these elements in foods are also sparse. A diet that is adequate in other nutrients, and that does not contain a high proportion of refined foods, is considered to satisfy the needs for these trace elements. Dietary deficiency is not likely in human beings.

Experimental studies on animals have shown that the mineral elements are closely interrelated. Thus, an excess of one element may increase the need for another. Excessive amounts of trace elements produce symptoms of toxicity in animals.

Manganese About 2.5 to 7 mg manganese are supplied in the daily diet of the adult.[1] Seeds of plants—nuts, legumes, and whole-grain cereals—are good sources, but animal foods are much lower in their content.

The intake of manganese considered adequate and safe for people over 11 years is 2.5 to 5.0 mg per day. Recommendations range from 0.5 to 3.0 mg per day for infants and younger children.[1]

Manganese is rather poorly absorbed from the small intestine by a mechanism similar to that for the absorption of iron. It is loosely bound to a protein and transported as TRANSMANGANIN. Tissues that are rich in mitochondria take up manganese readily from the blood. A dynamic equilibrium exists between intracellular and extracellular manganese. Most of the metabolic manganese is excreted into the intestine as a constituent of bile, but much of this is again reabsorbed, indicating an effective body conservation. Very little manganese is excreted in the urine.

Studies on experimental animals have shown that manganese is required for normal bone growth and development, normal lipid metabolism, reproduction, and regulation of nervous irritability. Manganese is an activator for a number of enzymes including arginase, which is required for the formation of urea, and a number of peptidases that bring about the hydrolysis of proteins in the intestine. Manganese can substitute for magnesium in a number of enzymes required for oxidative phosphorylation.

Molybdenum A precise balance of molybdenum is essential for plant and animal life. Nitrogen-fixing bacteria require this metal for their growth, and thus the synthesis of proteins and ultimately animal life are affected. A deficiency of molybdenum will adversely affect the growth of legumes. Also, in molybdenum deficiency the growth of certain fungi that produce mycotoxins is favored. These mycotoxins have been shown to be carcinogenic in animals. (See also Chapter 16.)

The concentration of molybdenum in food is highly variable but considered adequate in mixed diets in the United States. Intake has been estimated at between 0.1 and 0.46 mg.[1] Molybdenum is found especially in legumes, whole-grain cereals, and organ meats. It is absorbed as molybdate and is concentrated especially in the liver, adrenal, and kidney. It is a cofactor for a number of flavoprotein enzymes and is found in XANTHINE OXIDASE, an enzyme that brings about the oxidation of xanthine to uric acid. High molybdenum intakes have been linked to goutlike symptoms in a human population.[1] The estimated safe and adequate intake for people over 7 years is 0.1 to 0.5 mg with 0.03 to 0.15 mg suggested for infants and younger children.[1]

Molybdenum competes with copper for the same metabolic sites, and an excess of molybdenum will result in symptoms of copper deficiency. Cattle grazing on lands that have a high molybdenum content develop a condition known as *teart* and characterized by diarrhea, brittle bones, loss of pigmentation, and weight loss. When the sulfate content of the diet is increased, the symptoms of toxicity are avoided inasmuch as the excretion of molybdenum is increased. This affords an interesting example of the interrelationship of sulfur, copper, and molybdenum.

Selenium Some selenium is present in all tissues, with the highest concentrations in kidney, liver, spleen, pancreas, and testes. In whole blood the average concentration of selenium is about 25 μg per 100 ml. Values as low as 11 μg per cent have been found in children with protein-calorie malnutrition, and as high as 81.3 μg per cent in Venezuelan children living in seleniferous areas.[33]

For many years it has been known that selenium and vitamin E could spare each other. Both nutrients can behave as antioxidants and have a role in preventing cellular damage by lipid peroxidases. Lipid peroxides are strong oxidizing agents which can injure cell membranes. Selenium is an integral component of the enzyme GLUTATHIONE PEROXIDASE which is believed to deactivate lipid peroxides. It is hypothesized that vitamin E functions to prevent the formation of these peroxides. Selenium also functions in the oxidative phosphorylation of energy compounds.

Meats and seafoods are rich sources of selenium. Cereals contribute varying amounts depending upon the soil concentration. Unlike some elements there is relatively little loss in the milling of grains. Vegetables and fruits are poor sources. Frozen foods and some baby foods were found to contain marginal amounts of selenium.[33] The concentration of selenium in foods correlates closely with the protein content.

The estimated safe and adequate intake ranges from 0.05 to 0.2 mg selenium per day for people over the age of 7 years. For infants and younger children, an intake of 0.01 to 0.12 mg is suggested. Diets in the United States provide a range of 0.05 to 0.2 mg per day without difficulty.[1]

The effects of selenium deficiency in humans are not known. Animals consuming a selenium-deficient diet show a variety of symptoms: faulty development of the vascular system, cataracts, and alopecia in rats; degeneration of the pancreas in chicks. Many attempts have been made to correlate selenium deficiency with specific diseases, but none has been successful.

Excess selenium is toxic. Many cattle grazing in areas where the soil has a high selenium content suffer from "alkali disease" characterized by stiffness, blindness, deformity of the hooves, loss of hair, and sometimes death. An increase in dental caries in Oregon schoolchildren who lived in seleniferous areas has been reported.[34]

Chromium The adult body contains about 5 mg chromium. There are high concentrations in the hair, spleen, kidney, and testes, and lower concentrations in the heart, pancreas, lungs, and brain. The plasma chromium is about 3 parts per billion.[35] With age there is a decline in body chromium, possibly caused by an accumulated dietary deficit.[33] One usable form of chromium is the GLUCOSE TOLERANCE FACTOR (GTF), an organic compound containing glycine, glutamic acid, cysteine, and niacin. The absorption of the trivalent chromium in GTF is about 10 to 25 per cent; only 1 per cent of inorganic chromium is absorbed.

Glucose tolerance factor is essential for the efficient use of insulin. It enhances the removal of glucose from the blood. Its action appears to increase the uptake of glucose by the cells, the oxidation of glucose to carbon dioxide, and the stimulation of fatty acid and cholesterol synthesis. It has been found to be associated with RNA and is believed to have a role in protein synthesis. Chromium is also an activator of several enzymes.

The estimated safe and adequate intake ranges from 0.05 to 0.2 mg chromium per day for people over the age of 7 years. For infants and younger children, an intake of 0.01 to 0.12 mg is suggested.[1]

Diets in the United States furnish about 50 to 100 μg chromium,[1] a level that is lower than in Italy, Egypt, South Africa, and India. Yeast, beer, liver, whole-grain cereals and breads, meat, and cheese are good sources. The milling of grains removes up to 83 per cent of chromium.[33] Milk, white flour and bread, chicken breast, fish, and vegetables are low in chromium. Even diets that are considered to be adequate in other respects may be marginal in chromium.

Chromium deficiency is believed to occur in the United States and may be manifested by impaired glucose tolerance. It is seen especially in older persons, in maturity-onset diabetes, and in infants with protein-calorie malnutrition. Supplements with chromium have been found to improve the glucose tolerance in some diabetic patients and in persons with impaired glucose tolerance.

Cobalt This element is an essential constituent of vitamin B-12 and must be ingested in the form of the vitamin molecule inasmuch as humans cannot synthesize the vitamin. No other function of cobalt has been established.

Other Minerals Deficiencies of nickel, vanadium, and silicon have been produced in experimental animals. This suggests that they are essential for some animals but to date, this cannot be established for humans. Experimental data on the need for tin, arsenic, and cadmium is even more sparse. Further research is necessary before it can be determined if they are needed by humans.

A summary of mineral elements and review questions appear at the end of Chapter 9.

Cited References

1. Food and Nutrition Board: *Recommended Dietary Allowances,* 9th ed. National Academy of Sciences, Washington, D.C., 1980.
2. Johnston, F. A.: "Calcium Retained by Young Women Before and After Adding Spinach to the Diet," *J. Am. Diet. Assoc.,* **28**:933–38, 1952.
3. Reinhold, J. C.: "Phytate Destruction by Yeast Fermentation in Whole Wheat Meals," *J. Am. Diet. Assoc.,* **66**:38–41, 1975.
4. Sandstead, H. H., et al.: "Effects of Dietary Fiber and Protein Level on Mineral

Element Metabolism," in Inglett, G. E., and Falkehag, S. I., eds.: *Dietary Fibers: Chemistry and Nutrition,* Academic Press, New York, 1979.

5. Whedon, G. D.: "The Combined Use of Balance and Isotopic Studies in the Study of Calcium Metabolism," in Mills, C. F., and Passmore, R., eds.: *Proceedings VI International Congress of Nutrition,* E. & S. Livingstone, Ltd., Edinburgh, 1964, pp. 425–38.
6. Walker, R. M., and Linkswiler, H. M.: "Calcium Retention in the Adult Human Male as Affected by Protein Intake," *J. Nutr.,* **102:**1297–1302, 1972.
7. Anand, C. R., and Linkswiler, H. M.: "Effect of Protein Intake on Calcium Balance of Young Men Given 500 mg Calcium Daily," *J. Nutr.,* **104:**695–700, 1974.
8. Margen, S., et al.: "Studies in Calcium Metabolism. I. The Calciuretic Effect of Dietary Protein," *Am. J. Clin. Nutr.,* **27:**584–89, 1974.
9. FAO: *Handbook on Human Nutritional Requirements.* FAO Nutritional Studies Report No. 28, FAO, Rome, 1974.
10. Mack, P. B., and LaChance, P. A.: "Effects of Recumbency and Space Flight on Bone Density," *Am. J. Clin. Nutr.,* **20:**1194–1205, 1967.
11. Berlyne, G. M., et al.: "Bedouin Osteomalacia Due to Calcium Deprivation Caused by High Phytic Acid Content of Unleavened Bread," *Am J. Clin. Nutr.,* **26:**910–11, 1973.
12. Lutwak, L.: "Continuing Need for Dietary Calcium Throughout Life," *Geriatrics,* **29:**171–78, 1974.
13. Hegsted, D. M.: "Calcium and Phosphorus," in Goodhart, R. S., and Shils, M. E., eds.: *Modern Nutrition in Health and Disease,* 5th ed. Lea & Febiger, Philadelphia, 1973, pp. 268–86.
14. Shils, M. E.: "Magnesium," in Goodhart, R. S., and Shils, M. E., eds.: *Modern Nutrition in Health and Disease,* 5th ed. Lea & Febiger, Philadelphia, 1973, pp. 287–96.
15. Marston, R. M., and Peterkin, B. B.: "Nutrient Content of the National Food Supply," *National Food Rev.,* Winter 1980, pp. 21–25.
16. Monsen, E. R., et al.: "Estimation of Available Dietary Iron," *Am. J. Clin. Nutr.,* **31:**134–41, 1978.
17. Gubler, C. J.: "Absorption and Metabolism of Iron," *Science,* **123:**87–90, 1956.
18. White, H. S.: "Current Use and Changes in Use of Cast-Iron Cookware," *J. Home Econ.,* **60:**724–27, 1968.
19. Lipschitz, D. A., et al.: "A Clinical Evaluation of Serum Ferritin as an Index of Iron Stores," *N. Engl. J. Med.,* **290:**1213–16, 1974.
20. deBruin E. J. P., et al.: "Iron Absorption in the Bantu," *J. Am. Diet. Assoc.,* **57:**129–31, 1970.
21. Finch, C. A., and Monsen, E. R., "Iron Nutrition and the Fortification of Food with Iron," *JAMA,* **219:**1462–5, 1972.
22. McConnell, S. D., and Henkin, R. I.: "Altered Preference for Sodium Chloride, Anorexia, and Changes in Plasma and Urinary Zinc in Rats Fed a Zinc-Deficient Diet," *J. Nutr.,* **104:**1108–14, 1974.
23. Hurley, L. S., et al., "Zinc binding Ligands in Milk and Intestine: A Role in Neonatal Nutrition," *Proc. Natl. Acad. Sci, U.S.A.,* **74:**3547, 1977.
24. Prasad, A. D., et al.: "Zinc and Iron Deficiencies in Male Subjects with Dwarfism and Hypogonadism but Without Ancylostomiasis, Schistosomiasis, or Severe Anemia," *Am. J. Clin. Nutr.,* **12:**437–44, 1963.
25. Halsted, J. A., et al.: "A Conspectus of Research on Zinc Requirements of Man (Monograph)," *J. Nutr.,* **104:**345–78, 1974.
26. Ronaghy, H. A., et al.: "Zinc Supplementation of Malnourished Schoolboys in Iran: Increased Growth and Other Effects," *Am. J. Clin. Nutr.,* **27:**112–21, 1974.
27. Hambidge, K. M., et al., "Zinc Nutrition of Preschool Children in the Denver Head Start Program," *Am. J. Clin. Nutr.,* **29:**734–38, 1976.

28. Henkin, R. I., et al.: "Idiopathic Hypogeusia, Hyposmia and Dysosmia: A New Syndrome," *JAMA*, **217**:434–40, 1971.
29. Hussey, H. H.: "Taste and Smell Deviations: Importance of Zinc," *JAMA*, **228**:1669–70, 1974.
30. Cohen, I. K., et al.: "Hypogeusia, Anorexia, and Altered Zinc Metabolism Following Thermal Burn," *JAMA*, **223**:914–16, 1973.
31. Klevay, L. M., "Coronary Heart Disease: The Zinc/Copper Hypothesis," *Am. J. Clin. Nutr.*, **28**:764–68, 1975.
32. Rich, C., and Ensinck, J.: "Effect of Sodium Fluoride on Calcium Metabolism of Human Beings," *Nature*, **191**:184–85, 1961.
33. Levander, O. A.: "Selenium and Chromium in Human Nutrition," *J. Am. Diet. Assoc.*, **66**:338–44, 1975.
34. Tank, G., and Storvick, C. A.: "Effect of Naturally Occurring Selenium and Vanadium on Dental Caries," *J. Dent. Res.*, **39**:473–88, 1960.
35. Hambidge, K. M.: "Chromium Nutrition in Man," *Am. J. Clin. Nutr.*, **27**:505–14, 1974.

Additional References

Calcium and Phosphorus

De Luca, H. F.: "The Vitamin D System in the Regulation of Calcium and Phosphorus Metabolism," *Nutr. Rev.*, **37**:161–93, 1979.

Hankin, J. H., et al.: "Contribution of Hard Water to Calcium and Magnesium Intakes of Adults," *J. Am. Diet. Assoc.*, **56**:212–24, 1970.

Irwin, M. I., and Kienholz, E. W.: "Monograph: A Conspectus of Research on Calcium Requirements of Man," *J. Nutr.*, **103**:1019–95, 1973.

Lotz, M. E., et al.: "Evidence for a Phosphorus-Depletion Syndrome in Man," *N. Engl. J. Med.*, **278**:409–15, 1968.

McBean, L. D., and Speckman, E. W.: "A Recognition of the Interrelationship of Calcium with Various Dietary Components," *Am. J. Clin. Nutr.*, **27**:603–609, 1974.

Moon, Wan-Hee, et al.: "Phosphorus Balances of Adults Consuming Several Food Combinations," *J. Am. Diet. Assoc.*, **64**:386–90, 1974.

Review: "Calcium Transport in the Ileum," *Nutr. Rev.*, **33**:84–85, 1975.

Spencer, H. J., et al.: "Effect of High Phosphorus Intake on Calcium and Phosphorus Metabolism in Man," *J. Nutr.*, **86**:125–32, 1965.

Tewell, J. T., et al.: "Phosphorus Balances of Adults Fed Rice, Milk, and Wheat Flour Mixtures," *J. Am. Diet. Assoc.*, **63**:530–35, 1973.

Chromium

Mayer, J.: "Chromium in Medicine," *Postgrad. Med.*, **49**:235–36, January 1971.

Mertz, W.: "Effects and Metabolism of Glucose Tolerance Factor," *Nutr. Rev.*, **33**:129–35, 1975.

Mertz, W., et al.: "Present Knowledge of the Role of Chromium," *Fed. Proc.*, **33**:2275–80, 1974.

Mitman, F. W., et al.: "Urinary Chromium Levels of Nine Young Women Eating Freely Chosen Diets," *J. Nutr.*, **105**:64–68, 1975.

Morgan, J. M.: "Hepatic Chromium Content in Diabetic Subjects," *Metabolism*, **21**:313–16, 1972.

Copper

Butler, L. C., and Daniel, J. M.: "Copper Metabolism in Young Women Fed Two Levels of Copper and Two Protein Sources," *Am. J. Clin. Nutr.*, **26**:744–49, 1973.

Dowdy, R. P.: "Copper Metabolism," *Am. J. Clin. Nutr.*, **22**:887–92, 1969.

FRIEDEN, E.: "Ceruloplasmin, a Link Between Copper and iron Metabolism," *Nutr. Rev.*, **28**:87–91, 1970.

HILL, C. H.: "A Role of Copper in Elastin Formation," *Nutr. Rev.*, **27**:99–102, 1969.

KLEVAY, L. M., et al.: "The Human Requirement for Copper, I. Healthy Men Fed Conventional, American Diets," *Am. J. Clin. Nutr.*, **33**:45–50, 1980.

KRISHNAMACHARI, K. A. V. R.: "Some Aspects of Copper Metabolism in Pellagra," *Am. J. Clin. Nutr.*, **27**:108–11, 1974.

Review: "Copper and Taste Sensitivity," *Nutr. Rev.*, **26**:175–77, 1968.

Review: "Copper and the Aorta," *Nutr. Rev.*, **27**:325–28, 1969.

Review: "Copper Toxicity, Rats and Wilson's Disease," *Nutr. Rev.*, **33**:51–53, 1975.

SOLOMONS, N. W.: "On the Assessment of Zinc and Copper Nutriture in Man," *Am. J. Clin. Nutr.*, **32**:856–71, 1979.

TAPER, L. J., et al.: "Effects of Zinc Intake on Copper Balance in Adult Females," *Am. J. Clin. Nutr.*, **33**:1077–82. 1980.

FLUORIDE

American Dietetic Association: "Policy Statement on Fluoridation," *J. Am. Diet. Assoc.*, **64**:68, 1974.

BERNSTEIN, D. S., et al.: "Prevalence of Osteoporosis in High- and Low-Fluoride Areas in North Dakota," *JAMA*, **198**:499–504, 1966.

KRAMER, L., et al.: "Dietary Fluoride in Different Areas in the United States," *Am. J. Clin. Nutr.*, **27**:590–94, 1974.

Review: "Daily Fluoride Supplements and Dental Caries," *Nutr. Rev.*, **36**:329–31, 1978.

Review: "Skeletal Fluorosis and Dietary Calcium, Vitamin C, and Protein," *Nutr. Rev.*, **32**:13–15, 1974.

SMITH, E. H.: "Fluoridation of Water Supply," *JAMA*, **230**:1569, 1974.

IODINE

FIERRO-BENITEZ, R., et al.: "Endemic Goiter and Endemic Cretinism in the Andean Region," *N. Engl. J. Med.*, **280**:296–302, 1969.

Food and Nutrition Board: *Iodine Nutriture in the United States.* National Academy of Sciences–National Research Council, Washington, D.C., 1970.

KIDD, P. S., et al.: "Sources of Dietary Iodine," *J. Am. Diet. Assoc.*, **65**:420–22, 1974.

MATOVINOVIC, J., et al.: "Goiter and Other Thyroid Diseases in Tecumseh, Michigan," *JAMA*, **192**:234–40, 1965.

Review: "Endemic Goiter and Antithyroid Agents," *Nutr. Rev.*, **33**:171–72, 1975.

Review: "The Etiology of Endemic Cretinism," *Nutr. Rev.*, **29**:227–30, 1971.

Staff Report: "Iodized Salt," *Nutr. Today,* **4**:22–25, Spring 1969.

TROWBRIDGE, F. L., et al.: "Findings Relating to Goiter and Iodine in the Ten-State Nutrition Survey," *Am. J. Clin. Nutr.*, **28**:712–16, 1975.

IRON

AMINE, E. K., and HEGSTED, D. M.: "Biological Assessment of Available Iron in Food Products," *J. Agr. Food Chem.*, **22**:470–76, 1974.

COOK, J. D., et al.: "Absorption of Fortification Iron in Bread," *Am J. Clin. Nutr.*, **26**:861–72, 1973.

Council on Foods and Nutrition: "Fortification of Flour and Bread with Iron," *JAMA*, **223**:322, 1973.

CROSBY, W. H.: "Bureaucratic Clout and a Parable. Commentary," *JAMA*, **228**:1651–52, 1974.

GAINES, E. G., and DANIEL, W. A., Jr.: "Dietary Iron Intakes of Adolescents," *J. Am. Diet. Assoc.*, **65**:275–80, 1974.

LAYRISSE, M., et al.: "Measurement of the Total Daily Dietary Iron Absorption by the Extrinsic Tag Model," *Am. J. Clin. Nutr.*, **27**:152–62, 1974.

LEIBEL, R. L.: "Behavioral and Biochemical Correlates of Iron Deficiency," *J. Am. Diet. Assoc.*, **71**:398–404, 1977.
NORMAN, C.: "Iron Enrichment," *Nutr. Today*, **8**:16–17, November 1973.
Review: "Problems in Iron Enrichment and Fortification of Foods," *Nutr. Rev.*, **33**:46–47. 1975.
RUNDELS, J. C.: "Iron Deficiency in Children," *Nurs. Care*, **6**:16–18, September 1973.
VAGHEFI, S. B., et al.: "Availability of Iron in an Enrichment Mixture Added to Bread," *J. Am. Diet. Assoc.*, **64**:275–80, 1974.
WADDELL, J.: "The Bioavailability of Iron Sources and Their Utilization in Food Enrichment," *Fed. Proc.*, **33**:1779–83, 1974.
WALLACK, M. K., and WINKELSTEIN, A.: "Acute Iron Intoxication in an Adult," *JAMA*, **229**:1333–34, 1974.
WINTROBE, M. W.: "The Proposed Increase in the Iron Fortification of Wheat Products," *Nutr. Today*, **8**:18–20, November 1973.

MAGNESIUM
FLINK, E. B.: "Magnesium Deficiency Syndrome in Man," *JAMA*, **160**:1406–1409, 1956.
HATHAWAY, M. L.: *Magnesium in Human Nutrition.* Home Econ. Res. Rept. 19, U.S. Department of Agriculture, Washington, D.C., 1962.
HUNT, S. M., and SCHOFIELD, F. A.: "Magnesium Balance and Protein Intake Level in Adult Human Female," *Am. J. Clin, Nutr.*, **22**:367–73, 1969.
JONES, J. E., et al.: "Magnesium Requirements in Adults," *Am. J. Clin. Nutr.*, **20**:632–35, 1967.
Review: "Clinical Signs of Magnesium Deficiency," *Nutr. Rev.*, **37**:6–8, 1979.
Review: "Hypermagnesemia," *Nutr. Rev.*, **26**:12–15, 1968.
Review: "Hypomagnesemia in Protein-Calorie Malnutrition," *Nutr. Rev.*, **29**:89–90, 1971.
Review: "Magnesium Toxicity in the Newborn," *Nutr. Rev.*, **26**:139–40, 1968.
SHILS, M. E.: "Experimental Human Magnesium Depletion. I. Clinical Observations and Blood Chemistry Alterations," *Am. J. Clin. Nutr.*, **15**:133–43, 1964.
WACKER, W. E. C., and PARISI, A. F.: "Magnesium Metabolism," *N. Engl. J. Med.*, **278**:658–63; 712–17; 772–76, 1968.

ZINC
COUSINS, R. J.: "Regulation of Zinc Absorption: Role of Intracellular Ligands," *Am. J. Clin. Nutr.*, **32**:339–45, 1979.
EVANS, G. W.: "Normal and Abnormal Zinc Absorption in Man and Animals: The Tryptophan Connection," *Nutr. Rev.*, **38**:137–41, 1980.
HENKIN, R. I.: "Zinc in Wound Healing," *N. Engl. J. Med.*, **291**:675–76, 1974.
MILLS, C. F., et al.: "Metabolic Role of Zinc," *Am. J. Clin. Nutr.*, **22**:1240–49, 1969.
MURPHY, E. W., et al.: "Provisional Tables on the Zinc Content of Foods," *J. Am. Diet. Assoc.*, **66**:345–55, 1975.
PRASAD, A. S., ed.: *Zinc Metabolism.* Charles C Thomas, Springfield, Ill., 1966.
Review: "Growth and Zinc Deficiency," *Nutr. Rev.*, **31**:145–46, 1973.
Review: "Zinc Availability in Leavened and Unleavened Bread," *Nutr. Rev.*, **33**:18–19, 1975.
Review: "Zinc in Hair as a Measure of the Zinc Nutriture of Human Beings," *Nutr. Rev.*, **28**:209–11, 1970.
SANDSTEAD, H. H.: "Zinc Nutrition in the United States," *Am. J. Clin. Nutr.*, **26**:1251–60, 1973.
SMITH, J. C., et al.: "Zinc: A Trace Element Essential in Vitamin A Metabolism," *Science*, **181**:954–55, 1973.
SWANSON, C. A. and KING, J. C.: "Human Zinc Nutrition," *J. Nutr. Educ.*, **11**:181–83, 1979.

Other Trace Elements

CARLISLE, E. M.: "Silicon as an Essential Element," *Fed. Proc.*, **33**:1758–66, 1974.

COHEN, N. L., and BRIGGS, G. M.: "Trace Minerals in Nutrition," *Am. J. Nurs.*, **68**:807–11, 1968.

Food and Nutrition Board: "Are Selenium Supplements Needed (by the General Public)?," *J. Am. Diet. Assoc.*, **70**:249–50, 1977.

HARLAND, B. F., et al.: "Calcium, Phosphorus, Iron, Iodine and Zinc in the 'Total Diet,'" *J. Am. Diet. Assoc.*, **77**:16–20, 1980.

HOPKINS, L. L., JR., and MOHR, H. E.: "Vanadium as an Essential Nutrient," *Fed. Proc.*, **33**:1773–75, 1974.

KREHL, W. A.: "Mercury, the Slippery Metal," *Nutr. Today*, **7**:4–15, Nov. 1972.

KREHL, W. A.: "Selenium—The Maddening Mineral," *Nutr. Today*, **5**:26–32, Winter 1970.

MARGEN, S., and KING, J. C.: "Effect of Oral Contraceptive Agents on the Metabolism of Some Trace Elements," *Am. J. Clin. Nutr.*, **28**:392–402, 1975.

MERTZ, W.: "Mineral Elements: New Perspectives," *J. Am. Diet. Assoc.*, **77**:258–63, 1980.

MERTZ, W.: "The New RDAs: Estimated Adequate and Safe Intake of Trace Elements and Calculation of Available Iron," *J. Am. Diet. Assoc.*, **76**:128–33, 1980.

MORRIS, V. C., and LEVANDER, O. A.: "Selenium Content of Foods," *J. Nutr.*, **100**:1383–88, 1970.

NIELSEN, F. H., and OLLERICH, D. A.: "Nickel: A New Essential Trace Element," *Fed. Proc.*, **33**:1767–72, 1974.

NIELSEN, F. H., and SANDSTEAD, H. H.: "Are Nickel, Vanadium, Silicon, Fluorine, and Tin Essential for Man? A Review," *Am. J. Clin. Nutr.*, **27**:515–20, 1974.

Review: "Does Lead Make Children Hyperactive?" *Nutr. Rev.*, **31**:88–90, 1973.

Review: "Silicon and Bone Formation," *Nutr. Rev.*, **38**:194–95, 1980.

SCHROEDER, H. A., et al.: "Essential Trace Elements in Man: Molybdenum," *J. Chron. Dis.*, **23**:481–99, 1970.

SCHROEDER, H. A., et al.: "Essential Trace Metals in Man: Manganese. A Study in Homeostasis," *J. Chron. Dis.*, **19**:545–71, 1966.

SCHWARTZ, K.: "Recent Dietary Trace Element Research Exemplified by Tin, Fluorine, and Silicon," *Fed. Proc.*, **33**:1748–57, 1974.

SCOTT, M. L.: "The Selenium Dilemma," *J. Nutr.*, **103**:803–10, 1973.

TSONGAS, T. A., et al.: "Molybdenum in the Diet: An Estimate of Average Daily Intake in the United States," *Am. J. Clin. Nutr.*, **33**:1103–07, 1980.

UNDERWOOD, E. J.: "Cobalt," *Nutr. Rev.*, **33**:65–69, 1975.

UNDERWOOD, E. J.: "Trace Element Imbalances of Interest to the Dietitian," *J. Am. Diet. Assoc.*, **72**:177–79, 1978.

UNDERWOOD, E. J.: *Trace Elements in Human and Animal Nutrition*, 3rd ed. Academic Press, New York, 1971.

9 Fluid and Electrolyte Balance

THE interchange that constantly takes place between the body and its external environment, and within the body between cells, tissues, and organs and their environment, is dependent upon the fluid medium that is precisely regulated in its volume, composition, and concentration. The electrolytes and nonelectrolytes held in solution in this aqueous medium maintain normal osmotic pressure relationships, control nervous irritability and muscle contraction, regulate acid-base balance, and facilitate movement of nutrients into cells and removal of wastes from cells.

Water is the main solvent in the body. It has been called the "forgotten nutrient" because it is generally overlooked until it becomes a problem such as during scarcity. Consideration of water needs becomes imperative whenever humans are in a confined area under environmental control. Perhaps the ultimate such environment is in space travel.

This chapter includes a discussion of the role of water; the electrolyte composition of body fluids; three important electrolytes, namely, sodium, potassium, and chloride; the role of the kidney; mechanisms for fluid-electrolyte balance; and acid-base balance.

Water

The body's need for water is second only to that for oxygen. One can live for weeks without food but death is likely to follow a deprivation of water for more than a few days. A 10 per cent loss of body water is a serious hazard, and death usually follows a 20 per cent loss.

Distribution Water makes up 50 to 70 per cent of the weight of the human body. Lean individuals have a higher percentage of body water than do obese individuals. Men have a higher proportion of body water than women inasmuch as even women of normal weight have more adipose tissue. The young have a higher ratio of water than older individuals.

All body tissues contain water, but the variations in tissue contents are wide. For example, the approximate percentage of water in teeth is 5; fat and bone, 25; and striated muscle, 80.

Fluid compartments. Body fluids exist in two so-called compartments that are disseminated throughout the entire body. The INTRACELLULAR FLUID is that which exists within the cells. It accounts for about 45 per cent of body weight. The EXTRACELLULAR FLUID is subdivided as follows: (1) the plasma fluid, accounting for 5 per cent of body weight, which contains protein as well as numerous substances that easily penetrate the capillary membrane; and (2) the interstitial fluid, representing about 15 per cent of body weight, which is similar to plasma fluid except in its much lower concentration of protein. Also included in the extracellular fluids are the lymph circulation and secretions such as those of the lacrimal glands, pancreas, liver, and gastrointestinal mucosa. (See Figure 9–1.)

Function Most of the many functions of water are self-evident. Water is a structural component and a cushion of all cells. Each gram of protein holds about 4 gm water, and each gram of fat is associated with about 0.2 gm water. In some instances, as in bone, water is tightly bound, but in most

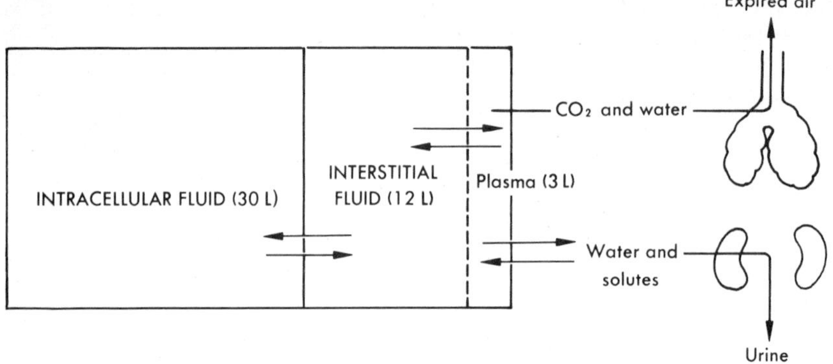

Figure 9–1. Fluid compartments of the body and interchanges from one compartment to another.

tissues there is a constant interchange between intracellular and extracellular fluid in order to maintain osmotic pressure relationships.

Water is the medium of all body fluids including digestive juices, lymph, blood, urine, and perspiration. All the physiochemical changes that occur in the cells of the body take place in the precisely regulated environment of the body fluids. Water enters into many essential reactions, such as hydrolysis that occurs in digestion. In oxidation-reduction reactions water is often the end product as in the oxidation of glucose.

Water is a solvent for the products of digestion, holding them in solution and permitting them to pass through the absorbing walls of the intestinal tract into the bloodstream. Because nutrients and cellular wastes are soluble in water, it is the means whereby nutrients are carried to the cells and wastes are removed to the lungs, kidney, gut, and skin. The metabolic wastes are diluted by water, thereby preventing cellular injury.

Water regulates body temperature by taking up the heat produced in cellular reactions and distributing it throughout the body. About 25 per cent of the heat lost from the body occurs by evaporation from the lungs and skin. Each liter of water lost in perspiration represents a heat loss of about 600 kcal. When there is an increase in body temperature, centers in the hypothalamus stimulate increased sweating and hence greater evaporation and loss of body heat.

Water is essential as a body lubricant: the saliva that makes possible the swallowing of food; the mucous secretions of the gastrointestinal, respiratory, and genitourinary tracts; the fluids that bathe the joints; and so on.

Sources of Water to the Body Water to meet the body's needs is supplied by (1) the ingestion of water and beverages, (2) the preformed water in foods, and (3) the water resulting from the oxidation of foodstuffs.

As may be seen in the following list, water is the principal constituent by weight of almost all foods, pure sugars and fats being the important exceptions.

	Per Cent Water
Milk	87
Eggs	75
Meat, well done	40
Meat, rare	75
Fruits, vegetables	70–95
Cereals, ready to eat	1–5
Cereals, cooked	80–88
Breads	35

The oxidation of glucose, fatty acids, and amino acids yields water; for example:

$$C_6H_{12}O_6 + 6\ O_2 \rightarrow 6\ H_2O + 6\ CO_2$$

The following amounts of water are produced in the oxidation of foodstuffs:

	ml Water
100 gm fat	107
100 gm carbohydrate	56
100 gm protein	41

Using these equivalents, the water of oxidation for a 2,000-kcal diet consisting of 80 gm protein, 80 gm fat, and 240 gm carbohydrate is approximately 253 ml.

Daily Losses of Water The daily losses of water include

	ml
Feces	100–200
Urine	1000–1500
Lungs	250–400
Insensible perspiration	400–600
Visible perspiration	None to 10,000

Some losses of water are OBLIGATORY, that is, they are essential for the maintenance of physicochemical equilibrium. The losses in the feces, through the lungs, and in insensible perspiration occur regardless of intake.

Renal losses. The amount of water loss from the kidney that is obligatory depends upon the amount of wastes that must be dissolved. Under normal circumstances it is about 600 ml. Urea and sodium chloride are the principal solids that are excreted, and thus any reduction in their production will correspondingly reduce the obligatory loss of water in the urine. A diet that is high in carbohydrate to minimize tissue catabolism and low in protein is one that reduces the formation of urea and thus will spare body water. FACULTATIVE WATER EXCRETION by the kidney is in addition to the obligatory losses, and varies according to body needs and water intake.

Skin. Insensible perspiration accounts for a relatively constant amount of water loss that is proportional to the surface area of the body. It is so called because the evaporation takes place from the skin immediately and the water loss is not noticeable. This evaporation is an important means by which body temperature is maintained. An infant weighing 10 pounds or so has a surface area that is about one third that of the adult, and thus the infant is much more vulnerable to water losses from the skin and rapid changes in body temperature.

The water losses by visible perspiration are highly variable, ranging from zero in cool weather to several liters during very warm weather under conditions of strenuous activity. Whenever a great deal of water is lost by perspiration, body water is conserved by the elimination of a much more concentrated urine.

Lungs. Air expired from the lungs also contains water. Any condition that would increase the rate of respiration—for example, fever—likewise increases the water loss by this route. The individual engaged in vigorous activity will lose more water by this route than the one who is sedentary.

Requirement The 24-hour water requirement is that amount that replaces the losses by the kidneys, lungs, skin, and bowel. Ordinarily, thirst is an accurate guide to supplying the necessary amounts of water. Under ideal conditions including a low-solute diet, a minimum of physical activity, and absence of sweating, the water need for the adult is about 1.5 liters from beverages, food, and water of oxidation. Although conditions are variable, the daily requirement is about 1 ml per kilocalorie for adults and 1.5 ml per kilocalorie for infants.[1]

Table 9–1 illustrates a typical balance between water intake and water losses from the body. The mechanisms for the regulation of fluid balance and some of the problems of imbalance are discussed on pages 173 through 176.

Table 9-1. **Normal Water Balance for an Adult***

Available Water	gm	Excreted Water	gm
Water, coffee, tea, etc.	1,200	In urine	1,350
Water in foods, including milk	900	In stool	200
Water of oxidation	250	In vapor from lungs	400
		From skin	400
Total	2,350		
		Total	2,350

*Assumes light activity and no visible sweating.

Electrolytes

Definitions and Measurement An ION is an atom or group of atoms that carries an electrical charge. CATIONS (Na^+, K^+, Ca^{++}, Mg^{++}) carry positive electrical charges; they are electron donors. ANIONS (Cl^-, HCO_3^-, HPO_4^{--}, SO_4^{--}) carry negative electrical charges; they are electron acceptors. In any solution the total cations are exactly equal to the total anions.

An ELECTROLYTE is any substance that dissociates into its component ions when dissolved in water. It is so named because an electrical current can be transmitted by a solution containing any one of these substances. The dissociation for a given substance is constant, but the degree of dissociation varies widely from one substance to another. Strong electrolytes are those substances such as inorganic acids or bases that dissociate almost completely.

The concentrations of physiologic solutions are expressed, and most easily compared, in milliequivalents (mEq) rather than in weights per 100 ml or per liter. A MILLIEQUIVALENT is the weight in milligrams of an element that combines with or replaces 1 mg of hydrogen. Snively and Brown[2] used a dance analogy to describe this concept. For a dance one would invite equal numbers of boys and girls—not 1,400 pounds of boys and 1,400 pounds of girls. It is the number of boys to pair off with girls that is important, not their weight. With an equal number of boys and girls, any boy could dance with any girl.

Likewise, with cations and anions; any cation can pair off with any anion. For example, 1 mEq of sodium combines with 1 mEq of chloride. Expressed in weight, 23 mg sodium have combined with 35 mg chloride. But 1 mEq of potassium can also combine with 1 mEq of chloride; in this instance, 39 mg potassium have combined with 35 mg chloride. Another example: calcium, with two positive charges, can pair off with two chloride ions; it can, instead, pair off with one phosphate ion, since phosphate carries two negative charges. Thus, it is the *chemical combining power* rather than the weights of the substances that is most convenient in measuring electrolyte concentrations. The calculation of milliequivalents of an electrolyte, when the concentration in milligrams is known, may be expressed as follows:

$$\text{Milliequivalents/liter} = \frac{\text{milligrams per liter}}{\text{Equivalent weight}}$$

$$\text{Equivalent weight} = \frac{\text{Atomic weight}}{\text{Valence of the element}}$$

Suppose the concentration of calcium in blood serum is 9.5 mg per 100 ml. Since the atomic weight of calcium is 40 and the valence is 2, the equivalent weight is $40 \div 2 = 20$.

$$\text{Milliequivalents/liter} = \frac{9.5 \times 10}{20} = 4.75$$

Electrolyte Composition of Body Fluids The electrolyte balance of the body is studied principally by determining the electrolyte concentrations in blood plasma. The electrolyte compositions of plasma and of cellular fluid are compared in Table 9–2. The electrolyte patterns for plasma and interstitial fluid are almost identical except for the much greater concentration of protein in the plasma. Note that within each fluid compartment the total milliequivalents of cations exactly balance the total milliequivalents of anions. There are remarkable differences in the electrolyte composition of plasma and intracellular fluid, yet the concentrations are such that osmotic balance is maintained. Because of the higher protein within the cell, the total of all electrolytes is higher than that in extracellular fluid. Each protein molecule carries eight negative charges thus combining with eight potassium ions; the protein molecule and the eight potassium ions would thus yield only nine osmotically active particles.

Extracellular fluid. Sodium accounts for over 90 per cent of the cations in plasma and interstitial fluid; potassium, magnesium, and calcium are found in very small, though physiologically important, concentrations. The principal anion of plasma is chloride; there are smaller concentrations of bicarbonate and proteinate and very small amounts of phosphate, sulfate, and organic acids.

Wide variations in electrolyte concentrations are found in the digestive juices. For example, in the acid gastric juice, the concentration of sodium is low, and that of chloride is high and is balanced by hydrogen ions. Intestinal juice and bile compare with plasma in their principal electrolytes.

Intracellular fluid. By contrast, potassium is the principal cation in intracellular fluid, with magnesium, sodium, and calcium accounting for the remainder. Phosphate as the organic phosphate in adenosine triphosphate, creatine phosphate, and sugar phosphate as well as inorganic phosphate is the principal balancing anion. Proteinate accounts for about one fourth of the anions in intracellular fluid,

Table 9–2. Electrolyte Composition of Body Fluids*

	Blood Plasma		Cellular Fluid
	mg per 100 ml	mEq per liter	mEq per liter
Cations			
Sodium (Na^+)	327	142	10
Potassium (K^+)	19	5	148
Calcium (Ca^{++})	10	5	2
Magnesium (Mg^{++})	3.6	3	40
Total cations		155	200
Anions			
Chloride (Cl^-)	365	103	
Bicarbonate (HCO_3^-)	165	27	8
Phosphate (HPO_4^{--})	9.6	2	
including other nonprotein ions			136
Sulfate (SO_4^{--})	4.8	1	
Organic acids$^-$		6	
Proteinate$^-$		16	56
Total anions		155	200

*Adapted from Tables 17-3 and 17-4 in West, E. S., et al.: *Textbook of Biochemistry,* 4th ed. Macmillan Publishing Co., Inc., New York, 1966, pp. 689, 690.

and the amounts of bicarbonate, chloride, and sulfate are small.

Sodium

Throughout human history salt has occupied a unique position. Mosaic law prescribed the use of salt with offerings made to Jehovah, and there are frequent biblical references to the purifying and flavoring effects of salt. Greek slaves were bought and sold with salt, and a good slave was said to be "worth his weight in salt." Because salt was scarce and greatly prized, the Via Salaria of Rome was a carefully guarded artery for the transport of salt. Salt served as a medium of exchange; thus the word *salary* from the Latin *salaria.* To own salt was a privilege, and royal banquet halls had imposing salt cellars. Important persons were invited to "sit above the salt" and those of lesser importance were seated "below the salt." Today salt is so commonplace that only those who are denied its free use give more than casual thought to it.

Distribution About 50 per cent of the body's sodium is present in the extracellular fluid, 40 per cent in bone, and 10 per cent or less in intracellular fluid. Much of the sodium in bone is readily interchangeable with extracellular fluid, but some of it is located deeply in dense long bones. In terms of concentration, the sodium content of blood plasma is about fourteen times that of intracellular fluid. (See Table 9–2.)

Functions Sodium is the principal electrolyte in extracellular fluid for the maintenance of normal osmotic pressure and water balance. It is the largest component of the extracellular total base and supplies the alkalinity of the gastrointestinal secretions. It functions mutually with some and antagonistically with other ions in maintaining the normal irritability of nerve cells and the contraction of muscles, and in regulating the permeability of the cell membrane. The sodium "pump" maintains electrolyte differences between intracellular and extracellular fluid compartments. (See page 174.)

Metabolism Most of the sodium in the diet is in the form of inorganic salts, principally sodium chloride. The absorption of sodium from the gastrointestinal tract is rapid and practically complete, there being only small amounts of sodium in the feces. The kidneys regulate the sodium level in the body. When the intake of sodium is high, the excretion is likewise high. But if the intake of sodium is low, the excretion of sodium is likewise decreased. An analysis of a 24-hour collection of urine is a good measure of the level of intake in the normal individual. When sodium is drastically restricted in the diet, the excretion of sodium by the normal kidney practically reaches the vanishing point, and sodium is almost completely conserved. The mechanisms for these controls will be discussed further on page 175.

The losses of sodium in perspiration depend upon the concentration and the total volume of sweat. In very warm weather the initial losses may be so high that the sodium depletion syndrome occurs unless compensation is made by increasing salt and fluid intake. With acclimatization there is a gradual reduction in the concentration of sodium in perspiration and hence the amount of sodium that will be lost through the skin. Concentrations of sodium in sweat ranging from 12 to 120 mEq per liter have been reported.[3]

Requirements The exact requirement for sodium is not known, but in the absence of visible perspiration the need is very low. Patients who have consumed diets restricted to 500 mg sodium daily, or even less, have been able to maintain sodium balance.

Estimated safe and adequate intake. For adults the estimated safe and adequate intake of sodium is 1,100 to 3,300 (48 to 144 mEq) per day. The range for infants is 115 to 350 mg (5 to 15 mEq); for adolescents it is 900 to 2,700 mg (39 to 117 mEq).[1] (See also Table 3–2.)

Guidelines for the public. Several recently published guidelines for good nutrition (see Chapter 3) make these recommendations:

Senate Select Committee on Nutrition and Human Needs: "Limit the intake of sodium by reducing the intake of salt to about 5 gm a day."[4] Senator McGovern later issued a clarification of this goal, stating that the limit of 5 gm sodium chloride referred to the salt added to raw foods, whether in commercial processing, home preparation, or at the table. This is in addition to the sodium occurring naturally in foods equivalent to about 3 gm sodium chloride.[5]

U.S. Department of Agriculture: "Avoid too much sodium."[6]

Food and Nutrition Board: "Use salt in moderation; adequate but safe intakes are considered to range between 3 to 8 gm of sodium chloride daily."[7]

Average sodium intakes. From 6 to 15 gm salt is consumed daily by Americans. This is equivalent to 2,500 to 6,000 mg sodium (108 to 260 mEq). Such intakes are more than twice the estimated safe and adequate intake and are far in excess of physiologic requirements. They reflect an acquired taste for salt. Some people desire so much salt that they add salt to food without tasting it, whereas others prefer only a light salting of food.

Food Sources The principal source of sodium in the diet is sodium chloride by virtue of its universal use in food preservation, in cookery, and at the table. One teaspoon of salt contains almost 2,000 mg sodium. The basic diet pattern (Table 13–3) furnishes about 400 mg sodium if all foods are prepared and cooked without the addition of salt or other sodium-containing compounds. Naturally occurring sources of sodium are milk, egg white, meat, poultry, fish, and certain salt-loving vegetables such as spinach, beets, celery, and chard. Most vegetables, fruits, cereals, and legumes are naturally low in sodium. Most drinking waters contain less than 20 mg sodium per liter, but in some areas the sodium content is considerably higher, particularly if home-softened water is used. (See also Table A-2.)

Many sodium-containing compounds are used in processed foods. These may be ingredients or additives. The sodium content of processed foods is frequently listed on the label. In the absence of this labeling information, the user should look for the word "sodium" in the ingredient listing. Commonly used sodium compounds in prepared foods are baking soda, baking powder, monosodium glutamate, sodium citrate, and sodium propionate. (See also Chapter 40.)

Reducing sodium intake. To keep sodium intakes within the recommended safe and adequate range, the following changes are compatible with a palatable diet:

1. Use no salt at the table.
2. Reduce the amount of salt used in food preparation; for example, ½ to ¾ teaspoon salt instead of a full teaspoon stated in a recipe is satisfactory for most foods. In some recipes salt can be omitted without significant effect on taste acceptance—cakes and cookies.
3. Use herbs and spices for flavoring foods.
4. Use salty foods sparingly; for example, pickles, relishes, potato chips, salted meats, and many snack items.
5. Read labels for information on sodium and salt content.

Sodium Imbalance Hypertension (high blood pressure) is a sign that may be present because of a number of factors, including genetic predisposition, obesity, smoking, type A stress, cardiovascular and renal pathology, and a lifetime history of high sodium intake. Epidemiologic studies have shown that hypertension occurs frequently in populations such as the Japanese who have a salt intake of 20 to 25 gm daily.[8,9]

On the other hand, hypertension is absent among people who consume about 2 gm salt daily in some nonindustrialized areas such as the Coco Islands in Polynesia, the Solomon Islands, and the Amazon basin.[7]

It is strongly suggested that the risk of high sodium intakes is genetically determined. If animal models hold true for humans, the consumption of high sodium levels from infancy in genetically susceptible individuals can increase the risk of hypertension. An imbalance of the sodium-to-potassium ratio can also affect blood pressure. It should be noted that the ranges for safe, adequate intakes for sodium, potassium, and chloride are on an equimolar basis—in each case, 48 to 144 mEq for the adult.

Lower intakes of salt over a lifetime may benefit about 20 per cent of the population believed to be genetically predisposed. Unfortunately, it is not yet practical to identify early in life those 40 million or so persons who are so predisposed. Although moderation of salt intake by the rest of the population may not be of value, there is no known harm resulting from reduced intakes, nor is there any known benefit of excessive intakes.

Sodium retention. When sodium excretion is reduced, water accumulates as excess extracellular fluid, a condition known as *edema.* The acid-base balance is also disrupted. Neither excessive sodium or fluid intake is the primary cause, and restricting either the water or sodium intake will not solve the underlying problem. Cardiac and renal failure are among the principal causes of reduced sodium excretion. An excessive secretion of cortical hormones, as by adrenal tumors, leads to increased retention of sodium. Likewise, adrenocorticotropic hormone used therapeutically in a variety of conditions also increases the retention of sodium.

Sodium depletion. Athletes and persons at heavy labor lose significant amounts of sodium in sweat, and these sodium and fluid losses must be replaced. Salt tablets are not recommended. The individual who experiences these losses should be advised to increase salt intake at meals by using salt at the table and by eating more salty foods. Weight before and after an athletic event indicates the amount of fluid that should be replaced.[10]

A deficiency of adrenocorticotropic hormone that is characteristic of Addison's disease leads to such large losses of sodium that the patient hungers for salt. With persistent vomiting and diarrhea, sodium is drawn into the gastrointestinal tract, and ultimately the extracellular fluid is depleted of its normal sodium content.

The symptoms of sodium depletion include weakness, giddiness, nausea, lethargy, muscle cramps, and in severe depletion, circulatory failure.

Potassium

Distribution The total potassium content of the adult body is about 250 gm. Of this, about 97 per cent is within the tissue cells with the remainder being distributed in the extracellular fluid compartment. From Table 9–2 it may be seen that the concentration of potassium in cellular fluid is about thirty times that in the plasma.

Functions Potassium is an obligatory component of all cells and increases in proportion to the increase in the body's cell mass. Because a fixed proportion of potassium is bound to protein, the measurement of body potassium is often used to determine the total lean body mass.

Within the cell potassium is the principal cation for the maintenance of osmotic pressure and fluid balance, just as sodium is the principal cation in extracellular fluid.

Potassium is required for enzymatic reactions taking place within the cell. Some potassium is bound to phosphate and is required for the conversion of glucose to glycogen; this potassium is released during glycogenolysis.

The small concentration of potassium in

extracellular fluid is essential, together with other ions, for the transmission of the nerve impulse and for concentration of muscle fibers.

Metabolism Potassium is readily absorbed from the gastrointestinal tract. Although the digestive juices contain relatively large amounts of potassium, most of this is reabsorbed and the losses in the feces are small.

Under conditions of protein synthesis, glycogen formation, and cellular hydration, potassium is rapidly removed from the circulation. With the removal of sodium from the cell to the extracellular fluid by the sodium pump, potassium ions move in, thus balancing the cations between the fluid compartments. Potassium leaves the cell during protein catabolism, dehydration, or glycogenolysis.

Excess potassium is excreted by the kidney. Aldosterone secretion increases potassium excretion. Although the normal kidney readily excretes excess potassium, the ability to conserve potassium in the face of a deficit is much less rigid than that for sodium. Even in the absence of any potassium intake and with low tissue levels, the urinary losses may be 15 to 30 mEq per day.[11]

Requirements For the adult the suggested range of intake of potassium is between 1,875 and 5,625 mg (48 to 144 mEq) per day. For infants less than 1 year, 350 to 1,275 mg are suggested. Children 1 year old to adulthood should consume between 550 and 4,575 mg depending on their age.[1] (See Table 3–2.)

Food Sources Because potassium is widely distributed in foods, the daily intake increases as the caloric intake increases. Typical diets furnish 50 to 150 mEq (2 to 6 gm) daily.[1] Meats, poultry, and fish are good sources. Fruits, vegetables, and whole-grain cereals are especially high in potassium. Bananas, potatoes, tomatoes, carrots, celery, oranges, and grapefruit are rich sources. (See Table A–2 for potassium values in foods.)

Potassium Deficiency Potassium deficiency is not primarily of dietary origin, but there are numerous circumstances under which it can occur. One of these is defective food intake such as that in severe malnutrition, chronic alcoholism, anorexia nervosa, low carbohydrate diets for weight reduction, or some illness that seriously interferes with the appetite. Any condition that reduces the availability of nutrients for absorption can lead to potassium depletion: for example, prolonged vomiting, gastric drainage, and diarrhea. Adrenal tumors that increase aldosterone secretion lead to potassium loss. Losses may exceed replacement in severe tissue injury, following surgery, in burns, and during prolonged fevers. Some therapeutic measures may also initiate potassium deficiency: for example, prolonged parenteral feeding without potassium in the parenteral fluids; excessive adrenocortical steroid therapy; or some diuretics used in the treatment of hypertension and edema. Rapid infusions of glucose and insulin in diabetic acidosis bring about such rapid shifts of potassium into the cell that the plasma potassium levels may be reduced to levels that could bring about cardiac failure.

Potassium deficiency is characterized by low plasma levels of potassium (hypopotassemia or hypokalemia). The symptoms of deficiency include nausea, vomiting, listlessness, apprehension, muscle weakness, paralytic ileus, hypotension, tachycardia, arrhythmia, and an altered electrocardiogram. The heart may stop in diastole.

Potassium Excess Hyperpotassemia (hyperkalemia) is a frequent complication in renal failure, in severe dehydration, following too rapid parenteral administration of potassium, and in adrenal insufficiency. Hyperkalemia is characterized by paresthesias of the scalp, face, tongue, and extremities; muscle weakness; poor respiration; cardiac arrhythmia; and changes in the electrocardiogram. Cardiac failure may follow with the heart stopping in systole. Hyperkalemia is corrected by using a low-potassium, low-protein, liberal-carbohydrate diet. Carbohydrate intake results in the formation of glycogen and the movement of potassium into the cells.

Chloride

Distribution Chlorine exists in the body almost entirely as the chloride ion. Most of the 100 gm or so of chloride in the body is present in the extracellular fluid but it also occurs to some extent in the red blood cells and to a lesser degree in other cells.

Functions Chloride accounts for two thirds of the total anions of extracellular fluid. It is important in the regulation of osmotic pressure, water balance, and acid-base balance. It is the chief anion of gastric juice and is accompanied by the hydrogen ion rather than the sodium ion, thus providing the acid medium for the activation of the gastric enzymes and the digestion in the stomach. Chloride is one of several activators of amylases.

Metabolism For the secretion of gastric juice chloride is withdrawn from the blood circulation, and changes in dietary intake do not modify its production. The gastric juice mixes with foods and moves along the intestinal tract. The chloride from foods and that from the gastric juice is readily absorbed into the circulation.

The CHLORIDE SHIFT between the red blood cells and the plasma is a mechanism whereby changes in pH are minimized. When the blood reaches the lungs, the blood CO_2 tension is decreased, the bicarbonate ions in the red blood cells decrease, bicarbonate ions move from the plasma into the cells, and chloride and OH ions move from the cells into the plasma. When the blood returns to the tissues, the partial pressure of CO_2 increases and these ionic shifts are reversed.

Chloride, like other ions, is filtered by the glomerulus and selectively reabsorbed from the renal tubules. Excess chloride is readily excreted. The chloride excretion usually parallels the excretion of sodium, but when it is essential to conserve sodium the kidney will substitute the ammonium ion. Sweat and feces contain variable amounts of chloride accompanied by sodium or potassium.

Dietary Intake Most of the chloride intake is from table salt. The amount consumed usually parallels sodium intake and is not deficient under normal circumstances. Estimated safe and adequate intakes for adults have been set at 1,700 to 5,100 mg (48 to 144 mEq) per day. (See also Table 3–2.)

Chloride Imbalance Severe vomiting, drainage, or diarrhea will lead to large losses of chloride and an alkalosis because of the replacement of chloride with bicarbonate.

Role of the Kidney

Structural Unit The NEPHRON, of which there are approximately 1 million in each kidney, is the functioning unit of the kidney. (See Figure 9–2.) Each nephron consists of the GLOMERULUS, which is a tuft of capillaries surrounded by a capsule (Bowman's capsule), and a TUBULE, including (1) the proximal convoluted tubule, (2) the loop of Henle, and (3) the distal convoluted tubule. The nephrons finally empty into collecting tubules.

Blood flows into the glomerulus through an *afferent arteriole* and leaves through an *efferent arteriole* and then flows through a system of *peritubular capillaries* that surround the tubules.

Functions of the Kidney Every meal we eat would seriously upset metabolic balances were it not for the function of the kidneys. The primary function of the kidneys is to maintain the constant composition and volume of the blood. This includes the regulation of (1) the osmotic pressure, (2) the electrolyte and water balance, and (3) the acid-base balance. By regulation of the composition of the blood, homeostasis

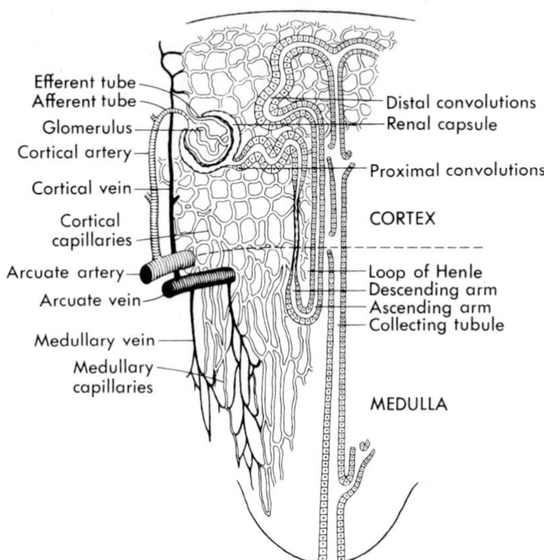

Figure 9–2. The nephron is the functioning unit of the kidney. (Courtesy, Leavell, L. C., and Miller, M. A.: *Anatomy and Physiology,* 15th ed. Macmillan Publishing Co., Inc., New York, 1966.)

in the interstitial and intracellular fluid compartments of the body is achieved.

The production of urine permits the elimination of excess water and solutes such as sodium, chloride, and others, the by-products of metabolism such as urea, and ingested substances that may be toxic.

Glomerular Filtration About 1,200 ml of blood flow through the kidneys each minute, this being about one fourth of the total cardiac output. The total amount of glomerular filtrate produced is about 125 ml per minute for a 24-hour total of 180 liters. The glomerular filtrate has essentially the same composition as the blood plasma except that it contains no protein or other large colloidal particles.

The many branching capillaries in the glomerulus reduce the rate of renal flow, thus promoting filtration. These capillary branches unite to form the efferent arteriole, which has a much smaller diameter. This further resists flow and increases filtration.

Functions of the Tubules There are two broad functions of the tubules: (1) selective reabsorption, and (2) secretion. If it were not for reabsorption from the tubules the body would lose all of its water, sodium, bicarbonate, glucose, and other filtered substances within half an hour and death would ensue.

As the glomerular filtrate moves through the proximal convoluted tubules, all of the glucose, amino acids, acetoacetic acid, and a number of other substances are reabsorbed if blood levels are within normal limits. For example, when glucose loads in the blood are within normal limits, all the glucose will be reabsorbed. Only when glucose levels in the blood exceed normal limits—as in diabetes mellitus—is some glucose not reabsorbed.

About 80 per cent of the water and electrolytes are reabsorbed from the proximal tubule. Since the tubular epithelium is almost impermeable to waste products such as urea, these substances continue to pass along the tubule.

By the time the filtrate has reached Henle's loop, marked changes in composition have occurred. Most of the remaining sodium and some of the remaining water are reabsorbed into the circulation from Henle's loop.

About 3 per cent of the electrolytes and 13 per cent of the water still remain in the filtrate that reaches the distal convoluted tubule. At this point the final adjustments in the concentration of water and solutes are made by mechanisms that are described in more detail on page 173. (See Figure 9–3.)

Energy requirements. Only the liver exceeds the kidney in its metabolic activities. Water and urea move across the membranes by passive diffusion, which does not require energy. However, most substances are reabsorbed by active transport, thus entailing considerable energy expenditure. Fatty acids are the principal source of energy in the aerobic oxidations occurring in the cortex, but glucose, fructose, and other substrates can also be oxidized. In the renal

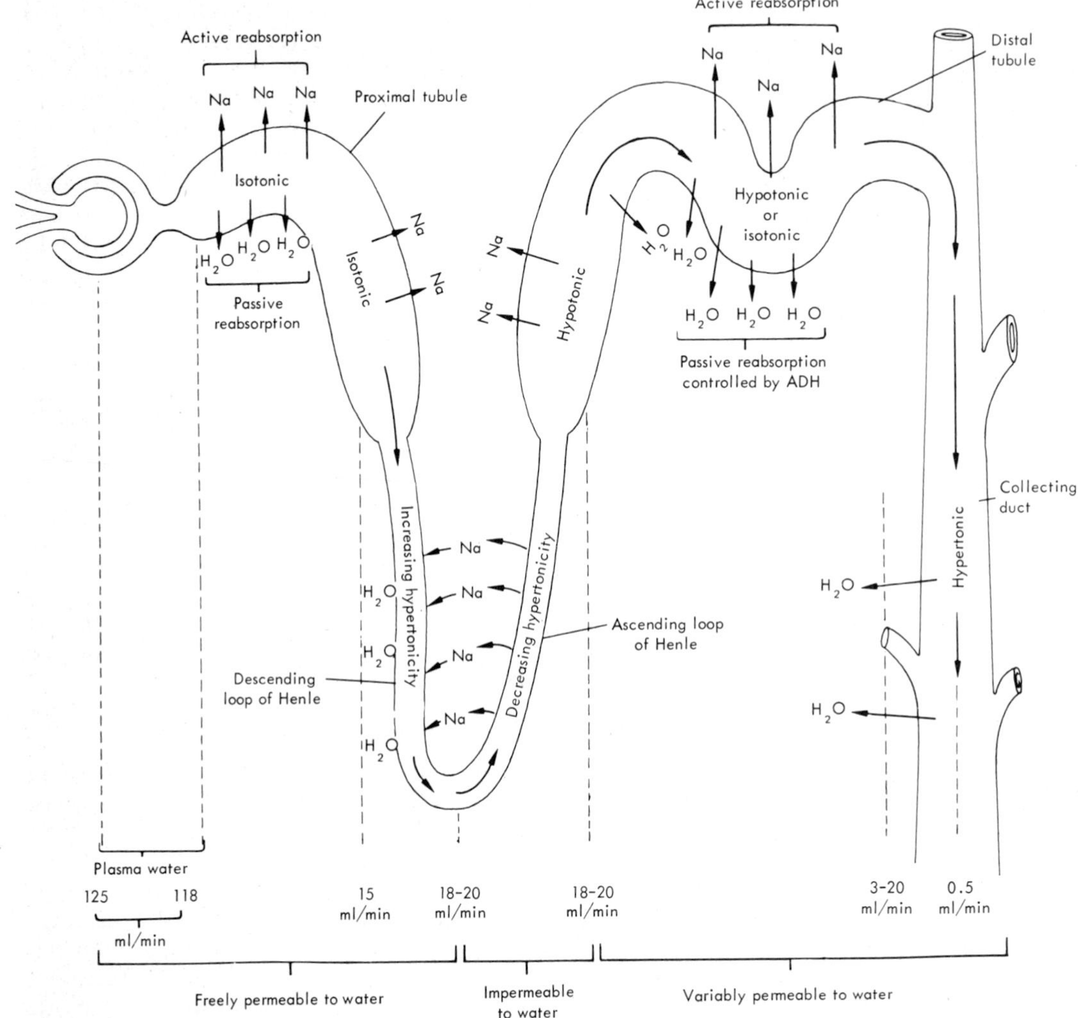

Figure 9–3. Function of the nephron in adjusting the reabsorption of sodium and water, and the formation of urine. (Courtesy, Pansky, B.: *Dynamic Anatomy and Physiology.* Macmillan Publishing Co., Inc., New York, 1975.)

medulla oxidation is principally by anaerobic glycolytic pathway, glucose being the chief substrate. (See page 82.)

Secretory activities. The final control of acid-base balance is brought about by the distal portion of the tubule. Hydrogen ions are continually released from carbonic acid by the action of carbonic anhydrase into the tubules. The tubules synthesize ammonia (NH_3), which then combines with the hydrogen ions to form the ammonium (NH_4^+) ion, thus releasing bicarbonate ions to the blood, thereby replacing the alkaline reserve.

The conversion of absorbed vitamin D to one of its metabolically active forms, 1,25-dihydroxy-vitamin D-3 takes place in the kidney. This form of vitamin D enhances intestinal absorption of calcium. (See page 196.)

Composition of Urine As the glomerular filtrate passes through the tubules, the metabolic wastes—unlike water and electrolytes—are poorly reabsorbed. Their concentration therefore increases as the filtrate moves along the tubules with the resultant formation of urine. Urine consists of about 95 per cent water and 5 per cent solids. The kidney can produce a urine varying in specific gravity from about 1.008 to 1.035 depending upon the proportions of water and solids to be excreted. The average daily excretion of solids is about 50 to 70 gm, with three fifths of this being nitrogenous and two fifths inorganic salts. Urea is the predominating nitrogenous substance in the urine, along with much smaller amounts of uric acid, ammonia, and creatinine. (See Table A–16.)

Inorganic ions in the urine include Na^+, K^+, Ca^{++}, Mg^{++}, Cl^-, SO_4^{--}, and PO_4^{--}. These are not true wastes inasmuch as they are essential to cellular function. They are excreted only when they are in excess of body needs, and the quantity excreted depends upon dietary intake.

With an increase in solid wastes, the fluid required for their excretion would also be increased. Among the situations in which increased solid wastes are produced are the following: (1) protein intake in excess of tissue needs so that large amounts of amino acids are deaminized and the urea production is increased; (2) increased tissue catabolism following any stress such as surgery, injury, burns, or fever; and (3) increased intake of salt. Whenever the kidney is unable to concentrate urine, the fluid requirement for excretion of wastes is greatly increased.

Regulation of Fluid and Electrolyte Balance

Fluid Exchange Although the sources of water to the body and the losses from the body are in balance, the fluid exchanges that take place in a 24-hour period are of tremendous magnitude and impressive in the precision of their regulation. For the digestive process alone the estimated daily volume of fluid that enters and leaves the gastrointestinal tract is estimated to be about 10 liters and is made up of the following:[12]

	ml
Water intake as beverage and in food	2,000
Saliva	1,500
Gastric juice	2,500
Bile	500
Intestinal juice	3,000
Pancreatic juice	700
	10,200

The fluid exchanges between the gastrointestinal tract and the blood circulation are variable from hour to hour; yet they are so balanced that normally the volume of the blood and the fluids within the tract are in equilibrium. Inasmuch as the daily losses from the bowel are no more than 100 to 200 ml, it is evident that the outpouring of digestive juices into the intestinal tract is continuously balanced by the reabsorption of water from the gut. That the kidneys are highly efficient conservators of body water has been pointed out on page 171. The magnitude of water exchange that occurs between the blood circulation, the interstitial fluid, the lymph vessels, and the cells is no doubt very great.

Factors Influencing Fluid and Electrolyte Balance The movements of water and solutes from one compartment to another are influenced by many factors: (1) the permeability of membranes to water and other substances; (2) the hydrostatic pressure within the capillaries; (3) the colloid osmotic pressure exerted by large molecules such as proteins; (4) the osmotic effect of electrolytes in the fluids of extracellular and intracellular fluids; (5) the lymph flow; (6) the mechanisms for active transport; (7) the competition of substances for carriers to transport materials across cell membranes; and (8) the hormonal and nervous controls influencing each of these factors.

The transport of most solutes across cell membranes has been described on page 30. Water can move in and out of cells by OSMOSIS, which is the passage of fluid from the less concentrated to the more concentrated side of the membrane. Osmotic pressure is the difference in the force exerted on each side of the membrane. Thus, the solution that is more concentrated exerts a pull on the water in the more dilute solution.

Sodium has little effect on the osmotic pressure between the capillaries and the interstitial fluid because its concentration in the two fluids is about equal. However, sodium is the principal cation in intercellular fluid and potassium in intracellular fluid so that these electrolytes effect important osmotic controls between these fluid compartments. A reduction of extracellular sodium, for example, results in the entrance of fluid into the cell, whereas an increase in extracellular sodium results in the withdrawal of fluid from the cell.

Proteins are large molecules that form colloidal (gluelike) solutions. They cannot pass through membranes and exert COLLOIDAL OSMOTIC PRESSURE within the blood vessels. Plasma albumin is the principal force that maintains fluid equilibrium between the interstitial fluid and the plasma. The plasma albumin exerts a constant pull of fluid from the interstitial fluid to the plasma. Thus, the colloid osmotic pressure opposes and balances the flow of materials out of the capillaries that is exerted by filtration pressure. When the concentration of plasma albumin is reduced, the osmotic pressure is reduced and the fluid remains in the tissue spaces; this is sometimes referred to as "nutritional edema."

Mechanisms to Regulate Water Balance The sensation of thirst is one means whereby the body meets its water need. When the ionic concentration of the extracellular fluid is increased, the cells in the *drinking center* of the hypothalamus become dehydrated and the desire to drink water is initiated.

Water reabsorption from the renal tubule is modified according to the extracellular fluid concentration. This depends upon the *osmoreceptor system,* which is effective in two ways. One of these is the change in osmotic pressure that occurs in the interstitial fluid of the renal medulla. The loops of Henle of the renal tubules extend into the medulla. Because rapid, active absorption of sodium and chloride occurs, the interstitial fluid of the medulla has a high concentration of sodium and chloride and hence exerts increased osmotic pressure. As the tubular fluid passes into the collecting ducts located in the medulla, water is rapidly absorbed from the ducts.[13]

Water reabsorption by the tubules is also controlled by the secretion of antidiuretic hormone by the posterior pituitary gland. Osmoreceptors especially in the supraoptic nuclei of the hypothalamus are sensitive to increases in the osmolarity of the extracellular fluid. Under conditions of increased concentration, impulses are initiated that stimulate production of ADH. The hormone enters the circulation and passes to the kidney where it increases the permeability of the distal and collecting tubules so that the amount of water that is reabsorbed is greatly increased. If the concentration of electrolytes is low, no stimulation of the osmoreceptors occurs and hence the hormone is not produced. The cell permeability is then decreased so that more water will be excreted, thereby restoring normal electrolyte concentration. (See Figure 9–4.)

Regulation of Ionic Balance The regulation of sodium concentration in the extracellular fluid is better understood than that of other ions, but it is believed that the mechanisms that control the concentra-

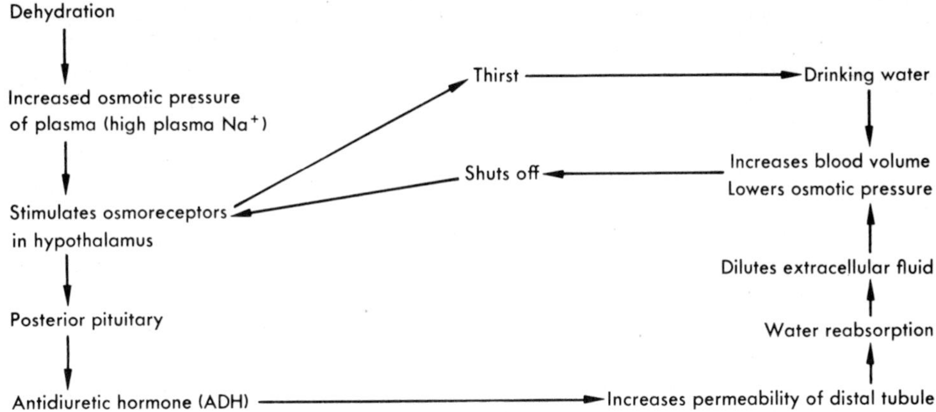

Figure 9–4. The regulation of water balance by thirst and antidiuretic hormone mechanisms.

tions of other electrolytes are similar. These mechanisms are under nervous and hormonal control.

A low concentration of sodium in the extracellular fluid stimulates the secretion of aldosterone and, to a lesser extent, other mineralocorticoids by the adrenal cortex. The sequence for the stimulation of the adrenal is believed to be as follows: with a drop in blood pressure of the juxtaglomerular cells, the kidney is stimulated to produce RENIN, an enzyme, which in turn acts on a globulin substance in blood, ANGIOTENSINOGEN, to convert it to ANGIOTENSIN I, an inactive substance. An enzyme in the plasma converts angiotensin I to angiotensin II; the latter substance in the blood circulation stimulates the production of aldosterone by the adrenal cortex. Upon reaching the renal circulation, aldosterone increases the permeability of the distal and collecting tubules so that more sodium is reabsorbed into the peritubular capillaries. When the extracellular sodium concentration is high, the adrenal cortex stops secreting aldosterone, and thus greater amounts of sodium will be excreted. When sodium is reabsorbed it carries positive electrical charges which draw negative ions, principally chloride, through the tubular membrane. Thus, the reabsorption of chloride closely parallels that of sodium. (See Figure 9–5.)

Potassium ions are passively secreted into the distal and collecting tubules. This secretion is greater when the potassium content of the extracellular fluid is high. The retention of sodium under the influence of aldosterone is accompanied by an increased loss of potassium.

Fluid Imbalance A deficiency of fluid, dehydration, may occur because of inadequate intake, or abnormal loss, or a combination of the two. Abnormal loss of water occurs from prolonged vomiting, hemorrhage, diarrhea, protracted fevers, burns, excessive perspiration, drainage from wounds, and so on. It leads to decrease in peristaltic action, reduced blood volume, poor absorption of nutrients, impairment of renal function, and circulatory failure. Loss of fluid is accompanied by electrolyte losses as well. Thus, the adjustment of fluid balance requires also the consideration of electrolyte concentration.

In some pathologic conditions the body is in *positive* water balance; that is, the intake of fluids is greater than the excretion, and the patient is said to have an edema. The effect of the lowered plasma albumin

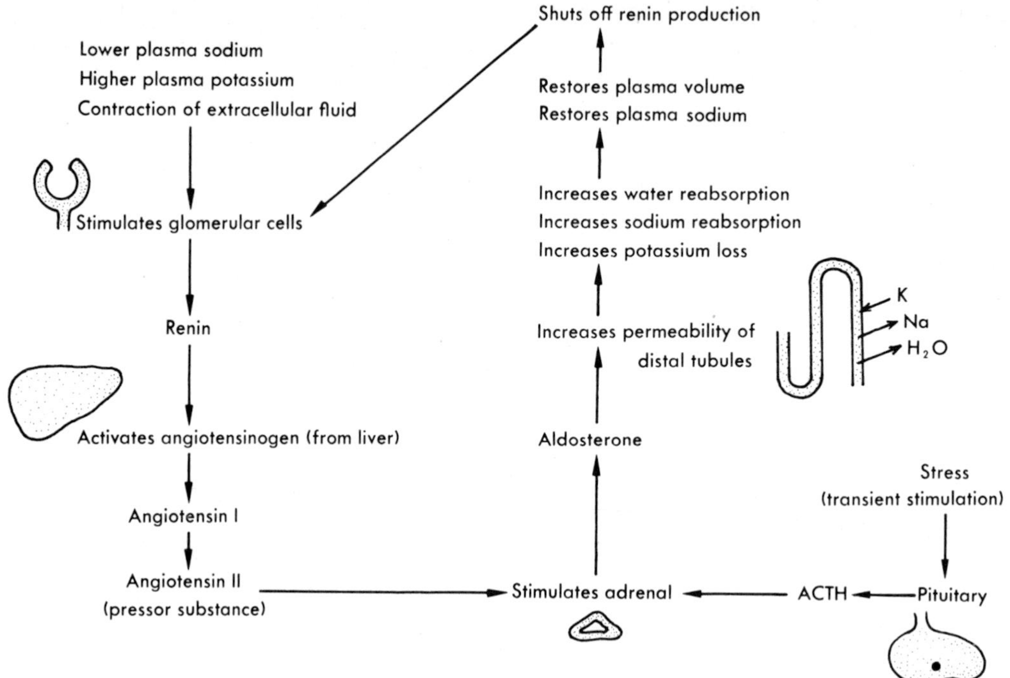

Figure 9–5. The regulation of sodium concentration in extracellular fluid.

has been mentioned. (See page 70.) Congestive heart failure, cirrhosis of the liver, nephritis, and nephrosis are examples of cardiovascular and renal disturbances in which sodium excretion is reduced, thereby contributing to the retention of water.

Acid-Base Balance

Acid-base balance refers to the regulation of the hydrogen ion concentration of body fluids. Normal metabolic processes result in the continuous production of acids that must be eliminated. On a given day, the equivalent of 20 to 40 liters of 1 N acid are eliminated by the lungs and 50 to 150 ml 1 N acid are excreted by the kidney.[14] The mechanisms for maintaining body neutrality are so efficient that the healthy individual does not need to give any thought whatsoever to the nature of his or her diet insofar as acid-producing or alkali-producing elements are concerned.

Many pathologic conditions, however, are characterized by serious disturbances in acid-base balance: for example, acidosis in uncontrolled diabetes mellitus, or fasting for weight reduction, following severe dehydration, and in renal failure. Through the study of physiology and biochemistry the student has gained an understanding of electrolyte and fluid balance, the chemistry of respiration, and the regulation of acid-base balance. Several references at the end of the chapter may be consulted by the student who desires a review or more extensive study than is provided in the following brief summary.

Definitions and Measurements An ACID is a substance that gives off or donates protons (H^+ ions); a BASE is a substance that combines with or accepts protons. The acidity of a fluid is measured by its concentration of hydrogen ions; the greater the concentration of hydrogen ions, the greater the acidity. The pH designation is used to describe the acidity or alkalinity of solutions. The pH is a logarithmic function of the actual hydrogen ion concentration, and a pH difference of one unit represents a tenfold difference in the actual hydrogen ion concentrations. Thus a pH of 4 represents ten times as many hydrogen ions as a pH of 5. Neutrality is an equal concentration of hydrogen and hydroxyl ions and is designated pH 7. Alkaline solutions have pHs between 7 and 14 while acid solutions are designated with pHs below 7. The further the pH is from 7, the more acid or alkaline the solution.

The pH of blood plasma is maintained within very narrow limits of 7.35 to 7.45—a slightly alkaline reaction. The extremes of pH compatible with life are 6.8 and 7.8; obviously, at these extremes individuals are very ill and prompt therapeutic measures must be instituted if the person is to survive.

Acids Formed in Metabolism The principal end products of metabolic activities are acid, chiefly carbonic acid. The oxidation of carbohydrates, fatty acids, and amino acids in the Krebs cycle (see page 84) yields carbon dioxide and water; carbonic acid is the hydrated form of carbon dioxide. Intermediate products in metabolism are also acid, such as lactic and pyruvic acid formed in carbohydrate metabolism, keto acids formed in fatty acid oxidation, and amino acids resulting from the hydrolysis of proteins. Urea synthesis is an acid-producing process, and nucleoproteins give rise to uric acid. Sulfuric acid is formed in the body from the sulfur-containing amino acids and phosphoric acid from the phospholipids and phosphoproteins.

The Reaction of Foods If the cations (Na^+, K^+, Mg^{++}, and Ca^{++}) remaining in the body on the metabolism of a food exceed the anions (PO_4^{--}, SO_4^{--}, and Cl^-), the food is said to produce an ALKALINE ASH and the excess cations will allow the body to retain more bicarbonate ions, thus producing an alkaline reaction. Vegetables, fruits, milk, and some nuts yield excess cations.

Meat, fish, poultry, eggs, cheese, cereals, and some nuts when metabolized yield an excess of anions that are not removed from the body immediately. These foods are said to produce an ACID ASH. The excess anions carrying a negative charge must be balanced approximately with some cations. This yields an acid reaction because less bicarbonate, which also carries a negative charge, can exist in the body. The excess bicarbonate ions form carbonic acid, increasing the acidity.

Fats, sugar, and starches contain no mineral elements and are metabolized quickly to carbon dioxide and water which are rapidly removed from the body. These foods, therefore, do not form excess cations or anions which would disturb the neutrality regulation.

Although lemons, oranges, and certain other fruits contain some free organic acids that give them a taste of acid (sour), they yield an alkaline ash because the body quickly oxidizes the anions of the acid to carbon dioxide and water and leave excess cations that are removed more slowly from the body. Plums, cranberries, and prunes contain aromatic organic acids that are not metabolized in the body, and therefore they increase the acidity of the body fluids.

The Regulation of Body Neutrality The reaction of the body fluids is kept within a narrow range by the following mechanisms:

1. Dilution is an important defense against the effects of the metabolic acids. The total volume of body fluid, representing about two thirds of body weight, is so great that the considerable amounts of carbon dioxide produced result in only a slight increase in the bicarbonate concentration because of the distribution throughout the fluid system.

2. Acid-base buffer systems are an important mechanism for the regulation of acid-

base balance. A BUFFER is a substance that will react chemically with either acids or alkalies so that there is not a marked change in the pH of the solution. The bicarbonate-carbonic acid (HCO_3^-/H_2CO_3) system is one important buffer of the blood in maintaining neutrality. The ease and speed with which the body can get rid of carbon dioxide obtained from this buffer mixture constitute one of the first lines of defense. The plasma bicarbonate is an indicator of the alkaline reserve of the body. Serious disturbances may occur if the alkaline reserve is depleted to a low level. Other buffer systems include

$$\frac{\text{Protein}}{\text{H.protein}} \quad \frac{HPO_4^{=}}{H_2PO_4^-} \quad \frac{Hb^-}{HHb} \quad \frac{HbO_2^-}{HHbO_2}$$

3. Besides its buffer action hemoglobin aids in the transport of carbon dioxide in two ways which prevent great changes in reaction. The acid strength of hemoglobin is decreased when oxyhemoglobin loses oxygen whereby an extra amount of carbon dioxide can be transported without any change of reaction (isohydric transport). Hemoglobin can also transport a limited amount of carbon dioxide by forming a carbamate, which releases most of the carbon dioxide from the hemoglobin complex at the lung as the hemoglobin takes up oxygen.

4. The respiratory rate regulates the losses of carbon dioxide and the intake of oxygen. In one minute the resting individual will have lost about 200 cc carbon dioxide and absorbed about 250cc oxygen. Any increase in activity will raise the exchange of gases taking place by a very large amount. This is accomplished by increasing the respiratory rate. If the hydrogen ion concentration is increased, the respiratory center in the brain causes an increase in the rate of pulmonary ventilation. The increased ventilation increases the loss of carbon dioxide, and the hydrogen ion concentration of the body fluids returns to normal. If the hydrogen ion concentration is lowered, the respiratory center is inhibited and the rate of ventilation is reduced; thus, the carbonic acid concentration of the body fluids rises.

5. The kidney makes the final adjustment that keeps the body pH within normal limits. The glomerular filtrate has a pH of 7.4, but the kidney can excrete a urine that is as acid as pH 4.5 or as alkaline as pH 8; normally, the average urine pH is 6.0. Bicarbonate ions are filtered into the tubular fluid and their loss from plasma represents loss of alkali. Hydrogen ions are secreted into the tubules, and their loss from plasma represents a loss of acid. When the hydrogen ions of the plasma are increased, the secretion of the hydrogen ions into the tubular fluid also increases and exceeds the loss of bicarbonate, thus permitting the return of plasma to its normal pH. The urine excreted is then more acid. Conversely, in alkalosis the hydrogen ion secretion into the tubules is decreased, thus allowing greater loss of bicarbonate. The urine then becomes more alkaline.

The kidney cannot excrete strong acids such as HCl and H_2SO_4. The hydrogen ions secreted into the lumen of the tubule are excreted by combining with disodium phosphate to form monosodium acid phosphate. By excreting practically all of the phosphate as acid phosphate ($H_2PO_4^-$, instead of HPO_4^{--}) only one phosphate is lost instead of two, thus reducing by half the number of milliequivalents of fixed anions that are excreted; this permits the return of more fixed anions to the circulation.

The kidney is also able to synthesize ammonia from glutamine and other amino acids. The ammonia combines with hydrogen ions to form the ammonium ion (NH_4^+), which can then replace cations such as sodium or potassium.

Acidosis and Alkalosis The acid-base balance of the body can be upset by an increase in hydrogen ions, a loss of hydrogen ions, an increase in base, or a loss of base. In each instance the treatment can be instituted only after evaluation of symp-

Death	Acidosis pH 6.8 to 7.3	Normal pH 7.35 to 7.45	Alkalosis pH 7.5 to 8.0	Death

Respiratory: Decreased ventilation
- Pulmonary edema
- Pneumonia
- Asphyxia
- Obstruction in emphysema
- Injury to respiratory center
- Morphine

Metabolic: Uncontrolled diabetes mellitus
- Starvation
- Severe diarrhea
- Chronic renal failure

Respiratory: Increased ventilation
- Hysteria
- Salicylate poisoning
- Infections

Metabolic: Loss of HCl (severe persistent vomiting)
- Excessive intake of bicarbonate
- Loss of H ions in renal dysfunction

Figure 9–6. Normal and abnormal pH ranges in body fluids.

toms that are present, the determination of the pH and the carbon dioxide content of the blood plasma, and the cause of the imbalance. (See Figure 9–6.)

ACIDOSIS is a condition in which the hydrogen ion concentration is increased or there is an excessive loss of base (mineral cations); the ratio of bicarbonate to carbonic acid is less than 20:1 and the pH is below 7.35. ALKALOSIS is a condition in which the hydrogen ion concentration is decreased or the base is increased; the ratio of bicarbonate to carbonic acid is greater than 20:1, and the pH is above 7.45.

With changes in concentrations of hydrogen ions and base, the lungs and kidneys attempt to compensate. Ventilation by the lungs is increased when there is an increase in hydrogen ions, and the kidney attempts to adjust by excreting a more acid urine and conserving base with the synthesis of more ammonia. When there is an increase in base, the respiration is depressed, and the hydrogen ions are retained and more base is excreted by the kidneys. If these adjustments succeed in keeping the bicarbonate-carbonic acid ratio at 20:1, the pH remains at 7.35 to 7.45; the acidosis or alkalosis is said to be "compensated." When the pH is outside these limits, the acidosis or alkalosis is "uncompensated."

Respiratory acidosis or alkalosis results from an abnormality of the control of the normal CO_2 tension. Hypoventilation such as that seen in pneumonia, pulmonary edema, suppression of breathing as with morphine, and asphyxia lead to acidosis. The kidneys partially compensate by increasing the excretion of hydrogen ions and the synthesis of ammonia, thereby increasing the return of bicarbonate to the blood.

Respiratory alkalosis occurs when there is overventilation of the lungs so that excessive amounts of carbonic acid are lost. This may result from hysteria, from salicylate poisoning, in fevers and infections, and at high altitudes. By reducing the excretion of hydrogen ions and the synthesis of ammonia and by increasing the excretion of sodium, the kidneys compensate in part.

Metabolic acidosis or alkalosis refers to changes resulting from faulty intake or output of acids or bases other than carbonic acid. Metabolic acidosis occurs in a variety of circumstances: the rapid production of ketones in uncontrolled diabetes mellitus; the inability of the kidney to excrete acid phosphates in chronic renal failure; the ketosis of starvation; or the loss of bicarbonate and sodium with severe diarrhea. Ventilation of the lungs is greatly increased. The synthesis of ammonia by the kidney may increase tenfold in an effort to conserve base. (Text continues on page 183)

Table 9–3. **Summary of the Minerals**

Minerals	Functions in the Body	Metabolism	Food Sources	Daily Allowances
Calcium	Hardness of bones, teeth Transmission of nerve impulse Muscle contraction Normal heart rhythm Activate enzymes Increase cell permeability Catalyze thrombin formation	*Absorption:* about 15–40 per cent, according to body need; aided by gastric acidity, vitamin D, lactose; excess phosphate, fat, phytate, oxalic acid interfere *Storage:* trabeculae of bones; easily mobilized *Utilization:* needs parathyroid hormone, vitamin D *Excretion:* 60–85 per cent of diet intake in feces; small urinary excretion; high protein intake increases urinary excretion *Deficiency:* retarded bone mineralization; fragile bones; stunted growth; rickets; osteomalacia; osteoporosis	Milk, hard cheese Ice cream, cottage cheese Greens: turnip, collards, kale, mustard, broccoli Oysters, shrimp, salmon, clams	Infants: 360–540 mg Children: 800 mg Teenagers: 1,200 mg Adults: 800 mg Pregnancy: 1,200 mg Lactation: 1,200 mg
Chlorine	Chief anion of extracellular fluid Constituent of gastric juice Acid-base balance; chloride-bicarbonate shift in red cells	*Absorption:* rapid, almost complete *Excretion:* chiefly in urine; parallels intake *Deficiency:* with prolonged vomiting, drainage from fistula, diarrhea	Table salt	Estimated safe and adequate intake: Infants 275–1,200 mg Children 500–2,775 mg Teenagers 1,400–4,200 mg Adults 1,700–5,100 mg Daily diet contains in excess of need
Chromium	Efficient use of insulin in glucose uptake; glucose oxidation, protein synthesis, stimulation of fat, and cholesterol synthesis Activation of enzymes	Usable form in organic compound: glucose tolerance factor	Liver, meat Cheese Whole-grain cereals	Estimated safe and adequate intake: Infants 0.01–0.06 mg Children 0.02–0.20 mg Teenagers 0.05–0.20 mg Adults 0.05–0.20 mg
Copper	Aids absorption and use of iron in synthesis of hemoglobin Electron transport Melanin formation Myelin sheath of nerves Purine metabolism	*Transport:* chiefly as protein, ceruloplasmin *Storage:* liver, central nervous system *Excretion:* bile into intestine *Deficiency:* rare; occurs in severe malnutrition Abnormal storage in Wilson's disease	Liver, shellfish Meats Nuts, legumes Whole-grain cereals Typical diet provides 1 to 5 mg	Estimated safe and adequate intake: Infants 0.5–1.0 mg Children 1.0–2.5 mg Teenagers 2.0–3.0 mg Adults 2.0–3.0 mg
Fluorine	Increases resistance of teeth to decay; most effective in young children Moderate levels in bone may reduce osteoporosis	*Storage:* bones and teeth *Excretion:* urine Excess leads to mottling of teeth	Fluoridated water: 1 ppm	Estimated safe and adequate intake: Infants 0.1–1.0 mg Children 0.5–2.5 mg Teenagers 1.5–2.5 mg Adults 1.5–4.0 mg
Iodine	Constituent of diiodotyrosine, triiodothyronine, thyroxine; regulate rate of energy metabolism	*Absorption:* controlled by blood level of protein-bound iodine *Storage:* thyroid gland; activity regulated by thyroid-stimulating hormone *Excretion:* in urine *Deficiency:* simple goiter; if severe, cretinism —rarely seen in U.S.	Iodized salt is most reliable source Seafood Foods grown in nongoitrous coastal areas	Infants: 40–50 μg Children: 70–120 μg Teen-agers: 150 μg Adults: 150 μg Pregnancy: 175 μg Lactation: 200 μg

Iron	Constituent of hemoglobin, myoglobin, and oxidative enzymes: catalase, cytochrome, xanthine oxidase	*Absorption:* about 3 to 23 per cent, depending on food source and body need; aided by gastric acidity, ascorbic acid *Transport:* bound to protein, transferrin *Storage:* as ferritin in liver, bone marrow, spleen *Utilization:* chiefly in hemoglobin; daily turnover about 27 to 28 mg; iron used over and over again *Excretion:* men, about 1 mg; women, 1 to 2 mg; in urine, perspiration, menstrual flow; fecal excretion is from unabsorbed dietary iron *Deficiency:* anemia; frequent in infants, preschool children, teenage girls, pregnant women	Liver, organ meats Meat, poultry Egg yolk Enriched and whole-grain breads, cereals Dark-green vegetables Legumes Molasses, dark Peaches, apricots, prunes, raisins Diets supply about 6 mg per 1,000 kcal	Infants: 10–15 mg Children: 10–15 mg Teenagers: 18 mg Men: 10 mg Women: 18 mg Pregnancy: 18+ mg Lactation: 18 mg
Magnesium	Constituents of bones, teeth Activates enzymes in carbohydrate metabolism Muscle and nerve irritability	*Absorption:* parallels that of calcium; competes with calcium for carriers *Utilization:* slowly mobilized from bone *Excretion:* chiefly by kidney *Deficiency:* seen in alcoholism, severe renal disease; hypomagnesemia, tremor	Whole-grain cereals Nuts; legumes Meat Milk Green leafy vegetables	Infants: 50–70 mg Children: 150–250 mg Women: 300 mg Men: 350 mg Pregnancy and lactation: 450 mg
Manganese	Activation of many enzymes; oxidation of carbohydrates, urea formation, protein hydrolysis Bone formation	*Absorption:* limited *Excretion:* chiefly in feces *Deficiency:* not known	Legumes, nuts Whole-grain cereals	Estimated safe and adequate intake: Infants 0.5–1.0 mg Children 1.0–3.0 mg Teenagers 2.5–5.0 mg Adults 2.5–5.0 mg
Molybdenum	Cofactor for flavorprotein enzymes; present in xanthine oxidase	Absorbed as molybdate Stored in liver, adrenal, kidney Related to metabolism of copper and sulfur	Organ meats Legumes Whole-grain cereals	Estimated safe and adequate intake: Infants 0.03–0.08 mg Children 0.05–0.31 mg Teenagers 0.15–0.50 mg Adults 0.15–0.50 mg
Phosphorus	Structure of bones, teeth Cell permeability Metabolism of fats and carbohydrates: storage and release of ATP Sugar-phosphate linkage in DNA and RNA Phospholipids in transport of fats Buffer salts in acid-base balance	*Absorption:* about 70 per cent; aided by vitamin D *Utilization:* about 85 per cent in bones; controlled by vitamin D, parathormone *Excretion:* about one third of diet in feces; metabolic products chiefly in urine *Deficiency:* poor bone mineralization; poor growth; rickets	Milk, cheese Eggs, meat, fish, poultry Legumes, nuts Whole-grain cereals	Infants: 200–400 mg Children: 800 mg Adults: 800 mg Pregnancy: 1,200 mg Lactation: 1,200 mg
Potassium	Principal cation of intracellular fluid Osmotic pressure; water balance; acid-base balance Nerve irritability and muscle contraction, regular heart rhythm Synthesis or protein	*Absorption:* readily absorbed *Excretion:* chiefly in urine; increased with aldosterone secretion *Deficiency:* following starvation, correction of diabetic acidosis, adrenal tumors; some diuretics; muscle weakness, nausea, tachycardia, glycogen depletion, heart failure	Widely distributed in foods Meat, fish, fowl Cereals Fruits, vegetables	Estimated safe and adequate intake: Infants 350–1,275 mg Children 550–3,000 mg Teenagers 1,525–4,575 mg Adults 1,875–5,625 mg Diet adequate in calories supplies ample amounts

Table 9–3. **(Continued)**

Minerals	Functions in the Body	Metabolism	Food Sources	Daily Allowances
Selenium	Antioxidant Constituent of glutathione oxidase	Stored especially in liver, kidney Spares vitamin E	Meat and seafoods Cereal foods	Estimated safe and adequate intake: Infants 0.01–0.06 mg Children 0.02–0.20 mg Teenagers 0.05–0.20 mg Adults 0.05–0.20 mg
Sodium	Principal cation of extracellular fluid Osmotic pressure; water balance Acid-base balance Regulate nerve irritability and muscle contraction "Pump" for active transport such as for glucose	*Absorption:* rapid and almost complete *Excretion:* chiefly in urine; some by skin and in feces; parallels intake; controlled by aldosterone *Deficiency:* rare; occurs with excessive perspiration and poor diet intake; nausea, diarrhea, abdominal cramps, muscle cramps	Table salt Processed foods Milk Meat, fish, poultry	Estimated safe and adequate intake: Infants 115–750 mg Children 325–1,800 mg Teenagers 900–2,700 mg Adults 1,100–3,300 mg Diets supply substantial excess
Sulfur	Constituent of proteins, especially cartilage, hair, nails Constituent of melanin, glutathione, thiamin, biotin, coenzyme A, insulin High-energy sulfur bonds Detoxication reactions	Absorbed chiefly as sulfur-containing amino acids Excreted as inorganic sulfate in urine in proportion to nitrogen loss	Protein foods rich in sulfur-amino acids Eggs Meat, fish, poultry Milk, cheese Nuts	Not established Diet adequate in protein meets need
Zinc	Constituent of enzymes: carbonic anhydrase, carboxypeptidase, lactic dehydrogenase	*Absorption:* limited; competes with calcium for absorption sites *Storage:* liver, muscles, bones, organs *Excretion:* chiefly by intestine *Deficiency:* marginal occurs in U.S.	Seafoods Liver and other organ meats Meats, fish Wheat germ Yeast Plant foods are generally low Usual diet supplies 10 to 15 mg	Infants: 3–5 mg Children: 10 mg Teenagers: 15 mg Adults: 15 mg Pregnancy: 20 mg Lactation: 25 mg

Metabolic alkalosis occurs when there is a severe loss of hydrochloric acid as a result of vomiting, or by the ingestion of soluble alkalinizing salts such as sodium bicarbonate.

Some Points for Emphasis in Nutrition Education

1. Mineral elements perform varied and interrelated functions in the body. Among these functions are:
   - **a.** The hardness of bones and teeth especially by calcium and phosphorus.
   - **b.** The association with proteins in numerous ways: potassium with protein within cells; iron with hemoglobin; many minerals with enzymes; and so on.
   - **c.** The regulation of the transmission of the nerve impulses and the contraction of muscles.
   - **d.** The maintenance of the proper environment around and within all cells and tissues of the body–acid-base balance.
2. Mineral elements do not yield energy, as do carbohydrates, fats, and proteins; yet they are essential in the processes whereby the body derives its energy from foods.
3. Only calcium, iron, and iodine require particular attention in the planning of diets for normal individuals. Diets that are adequate in protein, calories, and these minerals and that include a variety of foods can be expected to supply all the other mineral elements in satisfactory amounts.
4. For most persons the calcium allowance can be met only when the diet includes 2 to 4 cups of milk, depending upon age. Cheese may be substituted for part of the milk allowance.
5. A deficiency of calcium may not become apparent for a long time because the bones supply the blood with its needs. Eventually, sufficient calcium is withdrawn from bones so that they may become brittle and break easily, and osteoporosis may occur later in life.
6. Iron deficiency is widely prevalent, especially in infants, preschool children, teenage girls, and pregnant women. The only practical way by which these groups can obtain their iron needs is through the use of foods highly fortified with iron or by oral supplements of iron.
7. Iodine deficiency leads to endemic goiter. It can be prevented by the use of iodized salt.
8. Water is the body's universal solvent and must be supplied in adequate amounts.
9. Variations in the intake of acid-producing or alkali-producing foods do not result in acidosis or alkalosis in healthy individuals.

Problems and Review

1. Give several examples of the ways in which minerals function together in the body structure; in regulatory activities.
2. List four functions of calcium; of phosphorus.
3. What substances may combine with calcium in the intestinal tract and thus interfere with absorption? In which foods do these predominate? Of what practical significance is this in American diets?
4. Many adults believe that their needs for calcium are low because their bones are fully developed. Explain why this reasoning is wrong.
5. Iron is essentially a one-way substance. What does this mean? How does this affect the daily requirement?
6. *Problem.* Calculate your daily intake of calcium and iron for two days. Compare your intake with the recommended allowances. What were the important sources of calcium in your diet? Of iron?

Problem. Using the basic diet calculation on page 262, calculate the amount of iron available for absorption.

8. What is the principal function of iodine? What happens if the intake is inadequate?
9. To which groups of individuals is the prophylactic use of iodine especially important?
10. If you consume 10 gm of iodized salt in a day, how much iodine would you ingest if the level of iodization is 0.005 per cent?
11. What is the significance of fluorine in nutrition? What levels of fluorine are recommended in drinking water?
12. What is meant by dental fluorosis? At what levels of intake does it occur?
13. Name the principal mineral elements that contribute to an alkaline ash. Which foods are classified as alkali producing?
14. Name the principal mineral elements that contribute to an acid ash. Which foods are classified as acid producing?
15. What is the metabolic effect of an excess of acid-producing or of alkali-producing foods?
16. Describe the water compartments of the body in terms of (a) relative size; (b) electrolyte composition.
17. What are the daily sources of water to the body? What are the routes of excretion by the healthy individual?
18. What hormones control the excretion of water? Of sodium and potassium?
19. What is meant by obligatory water loss? If you found yourself in a situation where drinking water was extremely limited in supply, how could you reduce the loss of water from your body?

Cited References

1. Food and Nutrition Board: *Recommended Dietary Allowances,* 8th ed. National Academy of Sciences–National Research Council, Washington, D.C., 1974.
2. Statland, H., cited by Snively, W. D., Jr., and Brown, B. J.: "In the Balance," *Am. J. Nurs.,* **58**:55–57, 1958.
3. West, E. S., et al.: *Textbook of Biochemistry,* 4th ed. Macmillan Publishing Co., Inc., New York, 1966, p. 686.
4. U.S. Senate Select Committee on Nutrition and Human Needs: *Dietary Goals for the United States,* rev. Government Printing Office, Washington, D.C., December 1977.
5. "Addendum to Commentary: Dietary Goals for the United States, Second Edition," *J. Am. Diet. Assoc.,* **74**:533, 1979.
6. *Nutrition and Your Health: Dietary Guidelines for Americans.* U.S. Department of Agriculture and U.S. Department of Health, and Human Resources, Washington, D.C., 1980.
7. Food and Nutrition: *Toward Healthful Diets.* National Research Council–National Academy of Sciences, Washington, D.C., 1980.
8. Prior, I. A. M.: "The Price of Civilization," *Nutr. Today,* **6**:2–11, July 1971.
9. Dahl, L. K.: "Salt and Hypertension," *Am. J. Clin. Nutr.,* **25**:231–44, 1972.
10. American Dietetic Association: "A Statement. Nutrition and Physical Fitness," *J. Am. Diet. Assoc.,* **76**:437–43, 1980.
11. Krehl, W. A.: "The Potassium Depletion Syndrome," *Nutr. Today,* **1**:20, June 1966.
12. Brook, C.E., and Anast, C. S.: "Oral Fluid and Electrolytes," *JAMA.,* **179**:792–97, 1962.
13. Wright, A.: *Rypins' Medical Licensure Examination.* J. B. Lippincott Company, Philadelphia, 1970, p. 98.

14. Frisell, W. R.: *Acid-Base Chemistry in Medicine.* Macmillan Publishing Co., Inc., New York, 1968, p. 51.

Additional References

ABBEY, J. C.: "Nursing Observations of Fluid Imbalance," *Nurs. Clin. North Am.,* **3**:77–86, 1968.
BURGESS, R. E.: "Fluids and Electrolytes," *Am. J. Nurs.,* **65**:90–95, 1965.
CAMIEN, M. N., et al.: "A Critical Reappraisal of 'Acid-Base' Balance," *Am. J. Clin. Nutr.,* **22**:786–93, 1969.
EARLEY, L. E., and DAUGHARTY, T. M.: "Sodium Metabolism," *N. Engl. J. Med.,* **281**:72–86, 1969.
FENTON, M.: "What to Do About Thirst," *Am. J. Nurs.,* **69**:1014–17, 1969.
FRAZIER, H. S.: "Renal Regulation of Sodium Balance," *N. Engl. J. Med.,* **279**:868–75, 1968.
GRANT, M. M., and KUBO, W. M.: "Assessing the Patient's Hydration Status," *Am. J. Nurs.,* **75**:1306–11, 1975.
KLAHR, S., et al.: "Acid-Base Disorders in Health and Disease," *JAMA.,* **222**:567–73, 1972.
KREHL, W. A.: "Sodium: A Most Extraordinary Dietary Essential," *Nutr. Today,* **1**:16, December 1966.
LANE, H. W., et al.: "Effect of Physical Activity on Human Potassium Metabolism in a Hot and Humid Environment," *Am. J. Clin. Nutr.,* **31**:838–43, 1978.
LARAGH, J. H.: "Potassium, Angiotensin and the Dual Control of Aldosterone Secretion," *N. Engl., J. Med.,* **289**:745–47, 1973.
LEE, C. A., et al.: "Extracellular Volume Imbalance," *Am. J. Nurs.,* **74**:888–91, 1974.
Review: "Sodium Intake and Blood Pressure," *Nutr. Rev.,* **27**:280–82, 1969.
ROBINSON, J.: "Water the Indispensable Nutrient," *Nutr. Today,* **5**:16, 1970.
SHARER, J. E.: "Reviewing Acid-Base Balance," *Am. J. Nurs.,* **75**:980–83, 1975.
SIMOPOULOS, A. P., and BARTTER, F. C.: "The Metabolic Consequences of Chloride Deficiency," *Nutr. Rev.,* **38**:201–205, 1980.
TOBIAN, L.: "Dietary Salt (Sodium) and Hypertension," *Am. J. Clin. Nutr.,* **32**:2659–62, 1979.
TOBIAN, L.: "The Relationship of Salt to Hypertension," *Am. J. Clin. Nutr.,* **32**:2739–48, 1979.

10 *The Fat-Soluble Vitamins*

Introduction to the Study of the Vitamins

The story of the vitamins—their discovery, their positive functions in maintaining health, and their usefulness in healing deficiency diseases—is fascinating and deserving of considerable study. Popular interest was early aroused by the discovery of the role of vitamins in preventing such severe deficiency diseases as scurvy, pellagra, beriberi, and others. It is now known that vitamins function primarily in enzyme systems which facilitate the metabolism of amino acids, fats, and carbohydrates. Those who understand the functions of vitamins do not minimize their importance in relation to the utilization of food. However, it is important that no one be misled into believing that vitamins are "cure-alls" for disease. The properties of vitamins, their functions in metabolism, their distribution in foods, and the effects of deficiency will be discussed in the following sections.

Definition and Nomenclature The term *vitamins* was first coined in 1912 by Funk, a Polish chemist, who believed that the water-soluble antiberiberi substance he was describing was a "vital amine"; that is, an amine with life-giving properties. The final "e" was soon dropped because the substance was found, in reality, to be a group of essential compounds not all of which were amines. VITAMINS is the name given to a group of potent organic compounds other than protein, carbohydrate, and fat that are necessary in minute quantities in foods and are essential for specific body functions of maintenance, growth, and reproduction. Vitamins differ from hormones in that they must be supplied by the diet and are not formed by ductless glands in the body. During the last decade important studies have shown that vitamin D is an exception in that its metabolically active form is a hormone. See page 196.

Early classifications listed two groups of vitamins: fat soluble and water soluble. This classification is still used although it is arbitrary. Within each of the classes the vitamins differ widely in their properties, functions, and distribution. Vitamins were first named for their curative properties and were given a convenient letter name according to the order of their discovery; for example, antiscorbutic vitamin or vitamin C. The nomenclature used today includes chemically descriptive terms, but letter designations are also used.

Measurement Before the chemical nature of vitamins was discovered, their potency could be measured only by their ability to promote growth or to cure a deficiency when test doses were fed to experimental animals such as rats, guinea pigs, pigeons, and chicks. Such measurement is known as *bioassay* and has been expressed in units. Vitamins A, D, and E still may be expressed in international units (IU). Other vitamins are measured by their ability to promote the growth of microorganisms; this is known as *microbiologic assay.* Many vitamins formerly measured by bioassay are now measured by *chemical assay* in units of weight. Some vitamins are measured in milligram (mg) amounts; for example, the adult allowance for vitamin C is 60 mg. Other vitamins are measured in microgram (mcg or μg) amounts; the adult allowance for vitamin B-12 is 3 μg. Thus, the weight of ascorbic acid needed is 20,000 times that for vitamin B-12.

Selection of Foods for Vitamin Contents In selecting the foods to furnish vitamins in the diet it is well to keep in mind the following points: (1) under normal circumstances it is better to use common food sources than concentrates, because foods furnish other essential factors as well; (2) it is important to determine how often any given food will be used in the diet; (3) the amount of food which would ordinarily be used must be ascertained; (4) the effects of processing and preparation of foods on the vitamin retention must be clearly understood; and (5) economic factors such as availability and cost must be considered. For example, 100 gm of parsley furnish about 8,500 IU of vitamin A, whereas 100 gm of milk supply only 140 IU of vitamin A. Parsley, as a garnish, will have limited use, whereas 1 pint of milk a day, essential in an adequate diet, furnishes about 670 IU or 15 per cent of the day's allowance for men and women.

Vitamin Supplementation of the Diet Diets which are selected on the basis of the Daily Food Guide and which include a variety of foods usually provide the recommended amounts of vitamins. Although intakes of a few vitamins may not consistently reach the recommended level, the lack of evidence of overt or subclinical deficiency may indicate that the allowances are unrealistically high. Claims for the need and value of vitamin supplements are often exaggerated, and the popularity of megadose supplements is worrisome. Enthusiasm for vitamin pills frequently is based on the erroneous ideas that foods in the United States are depleted of vitamins or that excessive intakes will produce "super" health. In addition to concern about the unnecessary expense associated with purchase of the vitamins, often by those least able to afford them, the possibility of toxicity must be considered. Excessive intakes of vitamins A and D are known to have adverse effects. Traditionally water-soluble vitamins have been assumed to be nontoxic because the excess vitamin is excreted in the urine. This assumption, however, may not be appropriate in view of the number of undesirable side effects of ascorbic acid that have been reported since megadose consumption has become common. Self-medication with vitamins also creates the possibility of delay of proper medical care until a disease state is difficult or impossible to treat.

The value of appropriate use of vitamin supplementation cannot be disputed. Vitamin D supplementation for infants, growing children, and pregnant or lactating women is needed if fortified milk is not available or if exposure to sunlight is inadequate. With diets providing less than 1,400 kcal, the difficulty of selecting foods necessary to supply the recommended intakes of vitamins supports the desirability of supplements for persons on weight reduction regimens or for elderly persons with reduced energy needs.

Vitamin supplements also are needed in some clinical situations, for example, illness characterized by inability to consume a normal diet, following surgery or severe injury such as burns, in diseases of malabsorption, and so on. Sometimes supplements are needed to restore reserves when the diet has been inadequate because of ignorance, poor eating habits, or inability to obtain the necessary foods.

Vitamin A

Discovery In 1913 McCollum and Davis of the University of Wisconsin[1] and Osborne and Mendel of Yale University[2] independently discovered that rats consuming purified diets with lard as the only source of fat failed to grow and developed soreness of the eyes. When butterfat or ether extract of egg yolk was added to the diet, growth resumed and the eye condition was corrected. The term *fat-soluble A* was applied

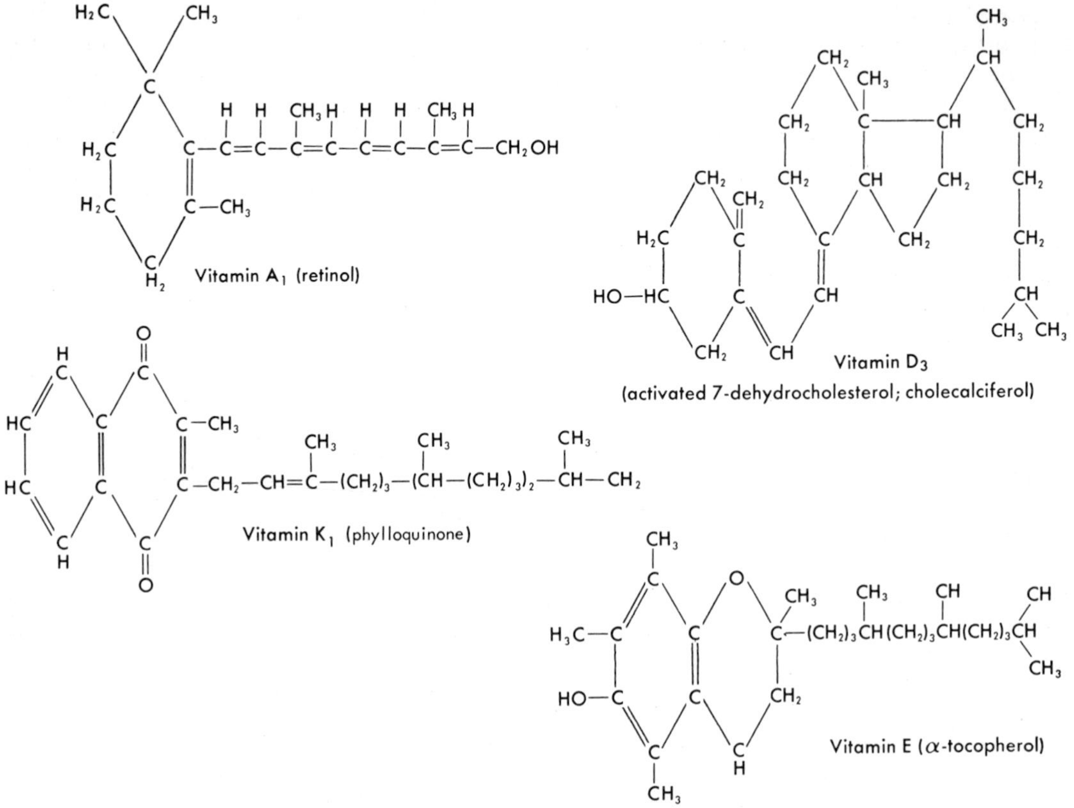

Vitamin A_1 (retinol)

Vitamin D_3 (activated 7-dehydrocholesterol; cholecalciferol)

Vitamin K_1 (phylloquinone)

Vitamin E (α-tocopherol)

Figure 10–1. Each of the fat-soluble vitamins exists in several forms, only one of which is shown here. Note the similarity of structure of vitamin D to that of cholesterol.

by McCollum to the organic complex present in the ether extract that was necessary for normal growth.

A few years later Steenbock at the University of Wisconsin[3] demonstrated that the yellow pigments in plants, the carotenes, had vitamin A activity. Because these carotenes and certain other carotenoid compounds can be converted to vitamin A in the body, they are now often referred to as PRECURSORS of vitamin A or as PROVITAMIN A.

Chemistry and Characteristics Vitamin A is active in many forms, the nomenclature being as follows:[4]

RETINOL—vitamin A, vitamin A alcohol (See Figure 10–1.)

RETINYL ESTERS—vitamin A esters

RETINALDEHYDE—vitamin A aldehyde, retinene, retinal

RETINOIC ACID—vitamin A acid

Collectively, these forms may be referred to as vitamin A.

In its pure form vitamin A is a pale-yellow crystalline compound. It occurs naturally in the animal kingdom and has been synthesized so that it is available commercially. It is soluble in fat and fat solvents. It is insoluble in water, but water-miscible forms are available for use in pharmaceutical products and food fortification. Vitamin A is relatively stable to heat and alkali. It is unstable to light and acid and is easily oxidized. Rapid destruction occurs with exposure to high temperatures in the presence of air, with ultraviolet irradiation, or in rancid fats.

The ultimate source of all vitamin A is the carotenoids which are synthesized by plants. Animals, in turn, and humans as well, convert a considerable proportion of the carotenoids in the foods they eat into vitamin A. The carotenoids are dark red crystalline compounds that give a deep yellow coloration to plants such as carrots and sweet potatoes. In deep green plants, also rich in carotenoids, the color is masked by chlorophyll. The carotenoids having vitamin A activity include alpha-, beta-, and gamma-carotene and cryptoxanthin. Of these precursors, beta-carotene is the most plentiful in human foods and has the highest biologic activity. Upon hydrolysis each molecule of beta-carotene theoretically yields two molecules of vitamin A. Because of physiological inefficiency in this conversion, however, the biologic activity of beta carotene on a weight basis is only half that of vitamin A. The other carotenoid precursors are about half as active as beta carotene.

Measurement Vitamin A is measured in international units. The equivalents are

1 IU = 0.3 μg retinol
1 IU = 0.6 μg beta-carotene
1 IU = 1.2 μg other carotenoids

The Food and Nutrition Board has recommended that RETINOL EQUIVALENTS (RE) replace the international unit.[5] This system of measurement takes into account the amount of absorption of the carotenes as well as the degree of conversion to vitamin A, and thus is a more precise system of measures. The equivalents are

1 RE = 1 μg retinol (3.33 IU)
1 RE = 6 μg beta-carotene (10 IU)
1 RE = 12 μg other carotenoids (10 IU)

Values for vitamin A in this chapter will be expressed in RE with the corresponding values in IU placed in parentheses. Tables of food values at present express the values for vitamin A in international units.

Absorption, Storage, and Transport Preformed vitamin A present in food as retinyl esters is hydrolyzed by pancreatic and intestinal enzymes to form free retinol. After absorption into the mucosal cell, retinol is reesterified to retinyl esters and incorporated into the chylomicrons for transport through the lymphatic system by way of the thoracic duct to the blood stream. Carotenes are split in the intestinal mucosa to form retinaldehyde which is then reduced to retinol. Although the principal conversion of carotenes to vitamin A takes place in the intestine, some carotenes are absorbed intact and converted in other tissues such as liver or kidney. The small amount of retinoic acid that may be present in the intestine is transported directly into the general circulation through the portal vein.

The absorption of vitamin A and the carotenes, like that of fat, is facilitated by bile. When a diet is very low in fat, or when there is an obstruction of the bile duct, the absorption of vitamin A and the carotenes is seriously impaired.

The simultaneous presence of vitamin E in the intestinal tract prevents the excessive oxidation of vitamin A that would otherwise occur. On the other hand, the presence of mineral oil reduces the absorption. Since mineral oil itself is not absorbed, it carries with it vitamin A and other fat-soluble vitamins. When used as a laxative, mineral oil should not be taken at or near mealtime.

Retinol is completely absorbed from the gastrointestinal tract but the absorption of carotenes is about one third. Since about half of the absorbed beta-carotene is converted to retinol, only one sixth of the intake in food is actually utilized. For other carotenoids only one fourth is converted to retinol; thus, only one twelfth of the intake in foods is available[6] (See retinol equivalents, this page.)

Vitamin A transported to the liver by the chylomicrons is removed for storage. About 90 per cent of body stores of vitamin A are found in the liver, with the remainder being present in the kidney, lungs, adrenal glands, and adipose tissue. The healthy adult has reserves that are adequate for several months to a year. Infants and young children have not built up such reserves and therefore are much more susceptible to the effects of deficiency.

When vitamin A is released from the liver stores for use by other tissues, it is transported in the circulation as part of a complex with a specific transport protein called retinol-binding protein (RBP) and prealbumin. Normal concentrations of vitamin A in blood serum range from 25 to 90 μg per 100 ml. The liver maintains the level in the blood as long as there is an adequate reserve. Only when the liver reserves are depleted will the blood concentration be lowered.

Vitamin A and products formed from its breakdown are excreted primarily in the bile. Some reabsorption occurs but most of the vitamin is lost in the feces. Some breakdown products may be excreted in the urine.

Functions Although the existence of vitamin A has been known for over 60 years, its functions have not been fully explained. Retinyl esters, retinol, and retinaldehyde are readily converted from one form to the other, but retinoic acid cannot be converted to other forms. Retinoic acid appears to be the active form of the vitamin in some tissues but it cannot function in the visual cycle or support reproduction in most species. Retinoic acid also cannot be stored in the body.

Vision. The best understood function of vitamin A is related to the maintenance of normal vision in dim light. The retina of the eye contains two kinds of light receptors: the rods for vision in dim light and the cones for vision in bright light and color vision. The rods produce a photosensitive pigment, RHODOPSIN or VISUAL PURPLE, and the cones produce IODOPSIN or VISUAL VIOLET.

In both these pigments vitamin A in the form of retinaldehyde is the prosthetic group, but the proteins to which the aldehyde is attached are different. When light strikes the pigments, changes occur in the chemical configuration of retinaldehydes and the pigments are split into their component parts, retinaldehyde and protein. These changes initiate a nerve impulse that is then transmitted to the brain by way of the optic nerve. Regeneration of rhodopsin occurs in the dark, but some retinaldehyde is lost in each cycle so that a constant supply from the blood must be present. A simplified diagram of the visual cycle is shown in Figure 10–2.

Epithelial tissues. Vitamin A is required for healthy epithelium whether covering the body externally or lining the mucous membranes. It effects the synthesis

Figure 10–2. Metabolism of vitamin A for vision in dim light.

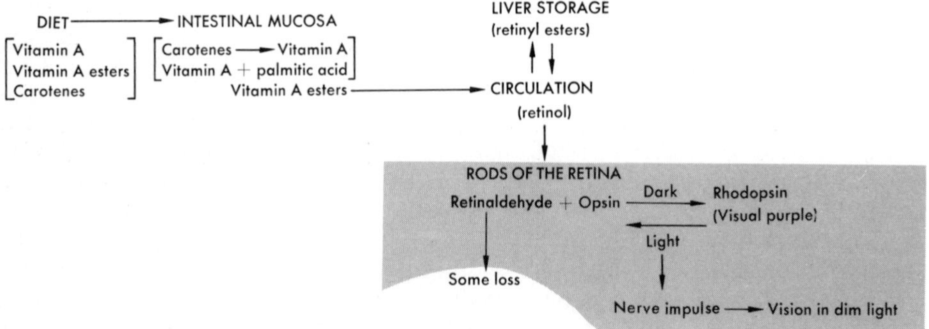

of constituents of mucus such as the mucoproteins and the mucopolysaccharides. The mucous secretions maintain the integrity of the epithelium, especially the membranes that line the eyes, the mouth, and the gastrointestinal, respiratory, and genitourinary tracts. These membranes maintained in their optimum condition offer resistance to bacterial invasion; to that extent vitamin A gives protection against infection. The designation *anti-infective* is unfortunate insofar as it often leads people, mistakenly, to believe that large intakes of vitamin A will confer additional protective benefits.

Growth and Other Functions Vitamin A is essential for normal skeletal and tooth development. With a deficiency of vitamin A bones do not grow in length and the normal remodeling process does not take place. The exact function of vitamin A in these processes is not known but may relate to its role in the synthesis of glycoproteins and maintenance of the stability of cellular membranes. Studies on experimental animals have shown that vitamin A is essential for spermatogenesis in the male and normal estrus cycle in the female. If vitamin A is not available to the animal during fetal development, many malformations result.

The synthesis of hydrocholesterol is facilitated in the adrenal cortex by vitamin A. Vitamin A also influences synthesis of both serum and muscle proteins and its apparent effect on cell differentiation may be related to a role in DNA and RNA metabolism. Development of anemia as a consequence of chronic deprivation of vitamin A suggests that the vitamin may be necessary for normal iron metabolism.

Daily Allowances The recommended allowances for vitamin A are stated in retinol equivalents and international units.[5] When international units are calculated to retinol equivalents, it is assumed that one half of the vitamin A is retinol and one half is beta-carotene. Thus, in the sample calculation 5,000 IU = 1,000 RE:

$$\begin{aligned} 2{,}500 \text{ IU} \div 3.33 &= \phantom{1{,}}750 \text{ RE} \\ 2{,}500 \text{ IU} \div 10 &= \underline{\phantom{1{,}}250 \text{ RE}} \\ & 1{,}000 \text{ RE} \end{aligned}$$

The vitamin A allowance for males over 10 years is 1,000 RE or 5,000 IU and for females over 10 years it is 800 RE or 4,000 IU. The allowances for infants over 6 months and children up to 10 years are 400 to 700 RE, for pregnancy 1,000 RE, and for lactation 1,200 RE.

Food Sources Only animal foods contain vitamin A as such, fish-liver oils being outstanding. These oils are generally not classified with common foods, but milk, butter, fortified margarines, whole-milk cheese, liver, and egg yolk contain vitamin A.

The principal source of vitamin A in the diet is likely to be from the carotenes, which are widespread in those plant foods that have high green or yellow colorings. There is a direct correlation between the greenness of a leaf and its carotene content. Dark-green leaves are rich in carotene, but the pale leaves, in lettuce and cabbage for example, are insignificant sources. Abundant sources of carotene are found in foods such as

- Green leafy vegetables—spinach, turnip tops, chard, beet greens
- Green stem vegetables—asparagus, broccoli
- Yellow vegetables—carrots, sweet potatoes, winter squash, pumpkin
- Yellow fruits—apricots, peaches, cantaloupe

The vitamin A contribution of the Daily Food Guide is indicated in Figure 10–3. The meat group contributes only when liver or an organ meat is served once every week to 10 days. One egg provides about one tenth of the daily allowance.

Retention of Food Values Since vitamin A is stable to the usual cooking temperatures, only slight losses are likely to occur in food preparation. The wilting of

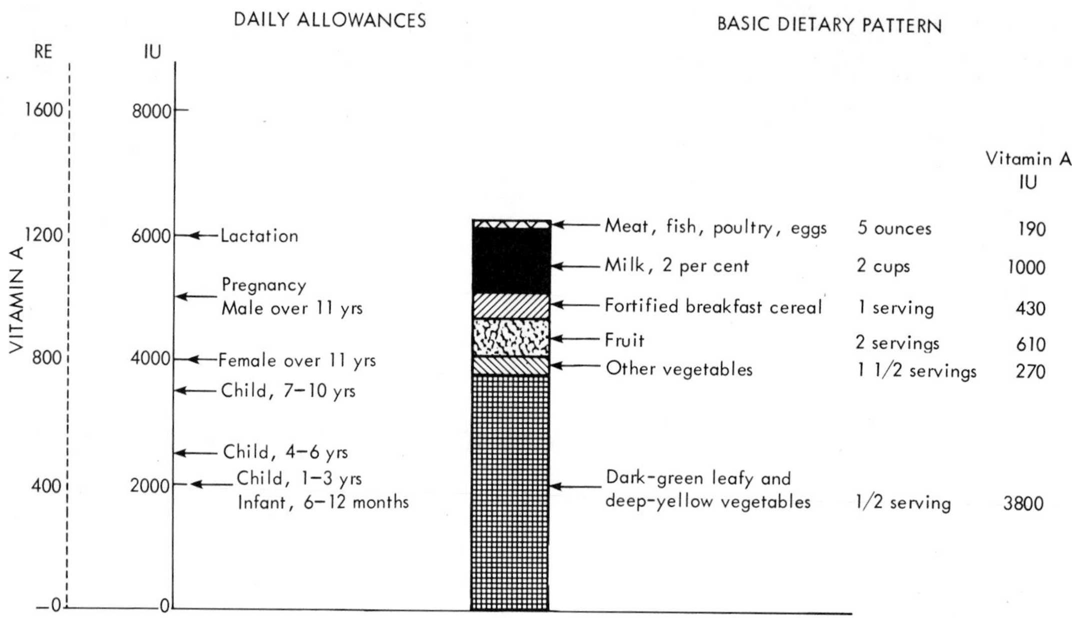

Figure 10–3. The four food groups of the Basic Diet provide a liberal allowance of vitamin A for all age categories. Note the contributions made by dark green leafy and deep yellow vegetables. Some cereals are fortified with vitamin A, but the bread-cereal group is not an important source. See Table 13–2 for complete calculations.

vegetables or dehydration of foods results in considerable losses. Canned and frozen foods retain maximal values for 9 months or longer. Vitamin A activity is rapidly lost in rancid fats.

Effects of Vitamin A Deficiency In the United States vitamin A deficiency should be practically nonexistent inasmuch as there are abundant dietary sources of vitamin A available. Preliminary results of the Nationwide Food Consumption Survey of 1977–78[7] showed that the average intake of vitamin A met the recommended allowance for all sex-age groups. Average intakes reported in the 1971–1974 Health and Nutrition Examination Survey[8] likewise exceeded the recommended allowances except in teenage black males and in most age groups of young females from 15 to 24 years. Although large proportions of individuals reported a 24-hour intake of vitamin A below the standard, preliminary biochemical findings[9] revealed a low incidence of low serum concentrations of vitamin A except in black children 1 to 5 years of age. Low values were found in approximately 10 per cent of these children.

In other parts of the world vitamin A deficiency is the most prevalent vitamin deficiency and ranks second only to protein-calorie malnutrition in its incidence. When the two conditions are present in the same child, the prognosis is very poor. Severe forms of vitamin A deficiency are practically nonexistent in the United States, but throughout the world up to 100,000 persons, chiefly children, become blind each year because of xerophthalmia caused by a lack of vitamin A.[10] The predominant regions of severe deficiency are the Middle East, India, Malaysia, Latin America, and South America.

It is ironic that the most severe forms of vitamin A deficiency occur in areas where there is an abundance of green plant foods. Through ignorance the young child is not given these foods. Vitamin A deficiency has been a major problem in areas where famine has occurred such as Bangladesh and Africa. Vitamin A deficiency also results from faulty absorption in such diseases as sprue, celiac disease, and other malabsorptive disorders.

Night blindness. One of the earliest signs of vitamin A deficiency is night blindness, or NYCTALOPIA. (See Figure 10–4.) This is a condition in which the individual is unable to see well in dim light, especially on coming into darkness from a bright light as in entering a darkened theater. Drivers who are easily blinded (glare blindness) by the headlights of other automobiles and who consequently see road markers, pedestrians, and so on, with difficulty constitute a special traffic hazard.

Nyctalopia occurs when there is insufficient vitamin A to bring about prompt and complete regeneration of visual purple. Blood carotene and vitamin A levels and a substantiating dietary history are useful in establishing a diagnosis of vitamin A deficiency. Other causes of night blindness must be ruled out. If a therapeutic dose of vitamin A does not bring about relief of night blindness after a few weeks' trial, it may be assumed that the condition is not a vitamin A deficiency.

Epithelial changes. An inadequate supply of vitamin A may lead to definite changes in the epithelial tissues throughout the body: KERATINIZATION, or a noticeable shrinking, hardening, and progressive degeneration of the cells, occurs, which increases the susceptibility to severe infections of the eye, the nasal passages, the sinuses, middle ear, lungs, and genitourinary tract.

Skin changes in severe vitamin A deficiency known as FOLLICULAR HYPERKERATOSIS have been described. The skin becomes rough, dry, and scaly. The keratinized epithelium plugs the sebaceous glands so that goose-pimple-like follicles appear first along the upper forearms and thighs, and then spread along the shoulders, back, abdomen, and buttocks.

Xerophthalmia The term XEROPHTHALMIA means dryness of the eye. Development of the condition passes through various stages that may ultimately lead to irreparable damage.[11] The first mild symptoms of epithelial changes in the eye are suggested by night blindness. The young child, most likely to be affected, is unable to describe this condition, but the mother, upon questioning, may be aware that the child does not see well at dusk. Then XEROSIS of the conjunctiva occurs, characterized by dryness and dullness. BITOT'S SPOTS, which are grayish plaques appearing on the conjunctiva, may or may not be seen. This is followed by xerosis of the cornea, which becomes dry and opaque. At this stage the condition is reversible if promptly treated. The corneal xerosis rapidly progresses to involvement of the deeper layers of the cornea, perforation, keratomalacia, scarring, and loss of sight.

Prevention and Treatment Much vitamin A deficiency could be prevented if carotene-rich foods were included in the diet. A very low fat intake, common in many dietaries, reduces the efficiency of absorption. When skim milk is used for the correction of protein-calorie malnutrition, it is essential that it be fortified with vitamin A; such fortification is now prevalent.

When deficiency occurs, treatment is rapidly effective with large doses of vitamin A provided that the eye conditions have not become irreversible. In parts of the world with a high incidence of blindness, strategies to prevent deficiency include intermittent administration of massive oral doses of vitamin A (100,000 to 300,000 IU), fortification of one or more foods that are widely consumed, increased production of vitamin-A-rich foods as well as nutrition education.[12]

Hypervitaminosis A Excessive intakes of vitamin A are toxic to both children and adults and should be avoided. Toxicity in

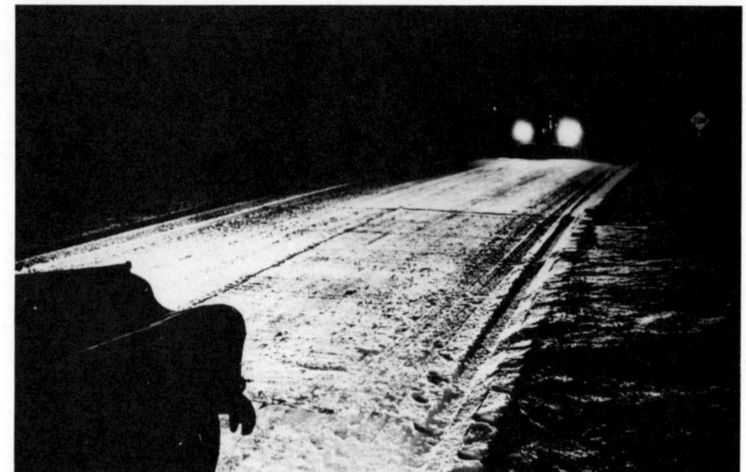

A

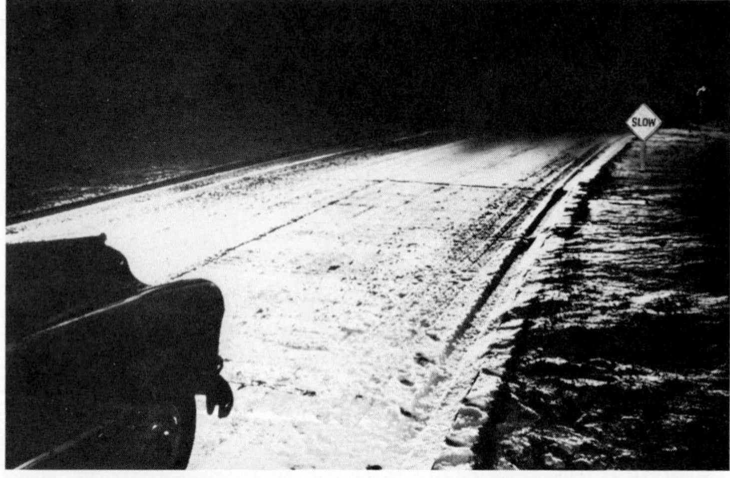

B

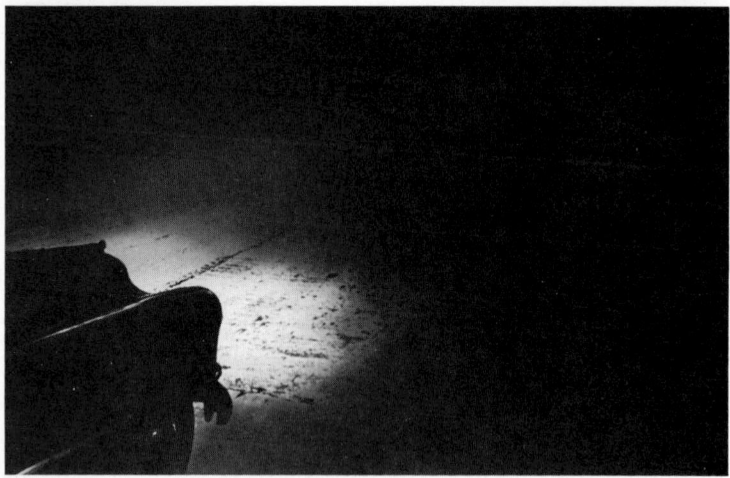

C

Figure 10–4. Night blindness. *(A)* Safe driving at night depends, in part, on the ability of one's eyes to adjust to the glare of headlights. *(B)* Properly focused headlights of an approaching automobile do not impede a good view of the road when the eye has an adequate supply of vitamin A. *(C)* The edge of the road and distances far ahead cannot be seen immediately after meeting an automobile when there is insufficient vitamin A available for the eye. (Courtesy, The Upjohn Company.)

adults is seen with intakes more than 50,000 IU for months or years.[13] In young children administration of doses of 20,000 to 60,000 IU per day for periods of 1 to 3 months has produced vitamin A intoxication.[14] The common symptoms of toxicity are anorexia, hyperirritability, and drying and desquamation of the skin. Loss of hair, bone and joint pain, bone fragility, headaches, and enlargement of the liver and spleen are quite frequent. When vitamin A is discontinued, recovery takes place. Excessive intake of carotenes does not produce toxicity but may produce a yellow discoloration of the skin that disappears when the intake is reduced.

Vitamin D

Cod-liver oil has been recommended as a remedy for rickets ever since the Middle Ages but does not appear to have been used with any consistency until the present century. During World War I, Hess and Unger noted the effect of cod-liver oil in protecting black children in New York City against rickets. Then in 1919 Mellanby found that the skeletal structure of puppies was influenced by some fat-soluble substance in food. McCollum, Steenbock, and Drummond simultaneously reported that cod liver oil in which vitamin A had been destroyed still retained its antirachitic properties, and hence it was shown that vitamin A was not the antirachitic factor. Steenbock and Hess in 1924 independently found that foods that had been exposed to ultraviolet rays possessed antirachitic properties. Pure vitamin D was isolated in crystalline form in 1930 and was called calciferol.

Chemistry and Characteristics Vitamin D is a group of chemically distinct sterol compounds possessing antirachitic properties. The two forms of the vitamin which are of significance nutritionally are vitamin D_2 (ERGOCALCIFEROL, CALCIFEROL, or VIOSTEROL) and vitamin D_3 (CHOLECALCIFEROL). Vitamin D_2 is formed when ergosterol found in plants is exposed to ultraviolet light. Vitamin D_3 is the chief form occurring in animal cells and develops in the skin on exposure of 7-DEHYDROCHOLESTEROL to ultraviolet light from sunshine. (See Figure 10–1.) Pure D vitamins are white, odorless crystals that are stable to heat, alkalies, and oxidation. They are insoluble in water but soluble in fat and fat solvents.

Measurement Traditionally vitamin D has been measured in international units (1 IU = 0.025 μg pure crystalline vitamin D). Based on the recommendations of an international expert committee,[6] the Food and Nutrition Board has decided to express intakes of vitamin D as micrograms of cholecalciferol.

For many years, the LINE TEST has been used to measure the potency of vitamin D in materials. Young rats from mothers having a deficient supply of vitamin D are kept on a rachitogenic diet so that no calcification occurs in the ends of the long bones. When a test material is fed, its value as a source of vitamin D is measured by the amount that must be fed for 7 to 10 days to produce a good calcium line (line test) in the ends of the long bones. Standard codliver oil is fed to a similar group of animals and is used as a basis of comparison. (See Figure 10–5.) Methods have been developed to measure the concentration of vitamin D itself as well as metabolites of the vitamin found in body tissues. However, these methods still are not practical for routine use.

Absorption and Excretion Dietary vitamin D is absorbed along with food fats from the jejunum and ileum and is transported in the chylomicrons through the lymph circulation. Bile is essential for effective absorption, and anything that interferes with fat absorption, such as pancreatitis, sprue, and malabsorption disorders, also affects the completeness of vitamin D absorption. Vitamin D made in the skin enters the blood where it circulates attached to a spe-

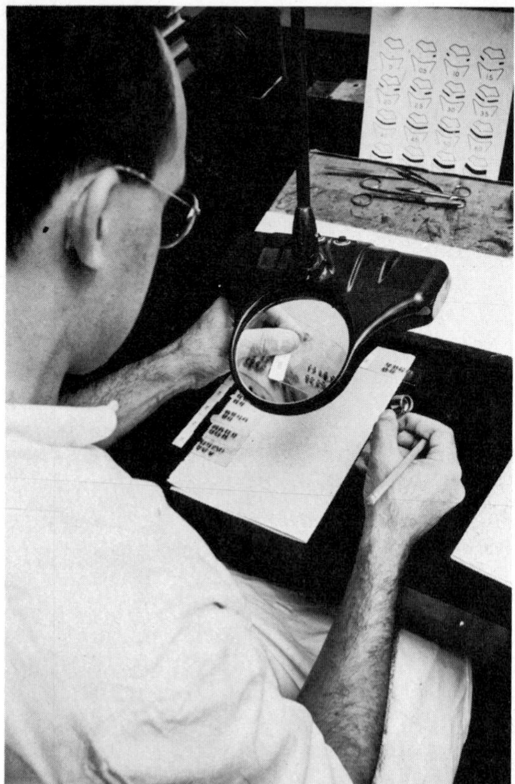

Figure 10–5. The line test is still used for determination of vitamin D. On charts in background, the darker the line, the better the healing. The amount of healing is related to the amount of vitamin D supplied to the test animal by the diet. (Courtesy, Food and Drug Administration.)

cific protein which also transports metabolites of the vitamin formed in other tissues. The major pathway for excretion of vitamin D appears to be through the bile.

Functions Although the importance of vitamin D in calcium and phosphorus metabolism has been recognized for many decades, the mechanisms involved in its actions were poorly understood. Exciting research in the past 10 years by DeLuca and co-workers at the University of Wisconsin[15] and others[16,17] has contributed significantly not only in elucidating the functions of vitamin D but also in making available new forms of the vitamin which have had important applications in the treatment of serious bone diseases.

Vitamin D itself is an inactive, storage form of the vitamin that is concentrated in the liver and to a lesser extent in the skin, spleen, lungs, brain, and kidney. In the liver vitamin D is rapidly hydroxylated to 25-HYDROXYVITAMIN D_3 (25-OH-D_3), also known as 25-HYDROXYCHOLECALCIFEROL. The 25-OH-D_3 released from the liver is the principal form of vitamin D circulating in the blood, but at physiological concentrations it does not appear to act directly on any target tissue. In the kidney 25-OH-D_3 is further hydroxylated to form a number of metabolites, the most important being 1,25-DIHYDROXYCHOLECALCIFEROL [1,25$(OH)_2D_3$]. This compound, considered the active form of vitamin D, circulates to the intestine where it stimulates synthesis of proteins necessary for the transport of calcium across the intestinal mucosa. It also promotes absorption of phosphorus. Formation of 1,25$(OH)_2D_3$ in the kidney occurs in response to the increase in the blood level of parathyroid hormone that is initiated whenever there is a fall in serum calcium. Low serum phosphorus also enhances 1,25$(OH)_2D_3$ formation. In addition to affecting intestinal absorption, 1,25$(OH)_2D_3$ stimulates mobilization of calcium, and consequently phosphorus, from bone and may improve renal reabsorption of calcium. These actions increase the calcium and phosphorus levels of the blood thereby permitting normal mineralization of the bone matrix and cartilage as well as maintaining the correct concentration of calcium in extracellular fluids for muscle contraction and nerve irritability.

Because of its effect on distinct target tissues and the feedback control on its formation mediated by changes in serum calcium and phosphorus, 1,25$(OH)_2D_3$ may be considered a hormone and vitamin D a prohormone. (See Figure 10–6.) Nevertheless,

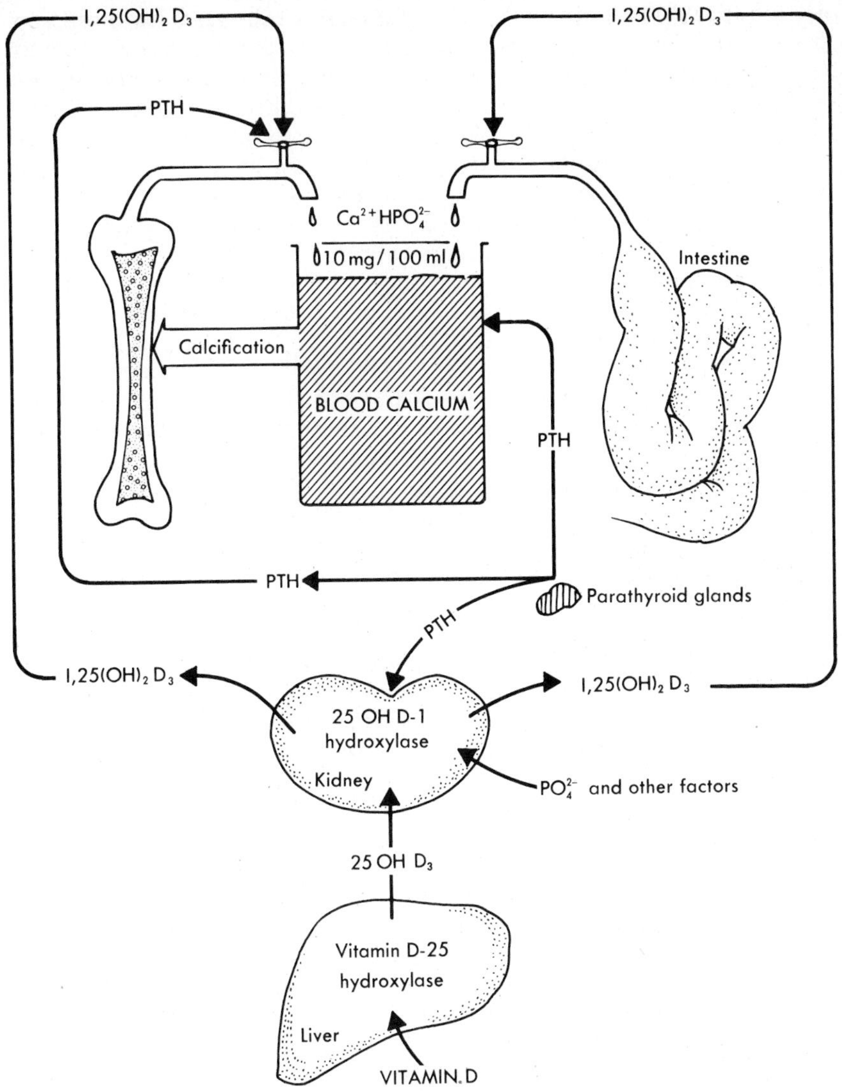

Figure 10–6. Hormonal loop derived from vitamin D. Diagram shows calcium homeostatic system. In the intestine $1,25(OH)_2D_3$ functions without the presence of parathyroid hormone; in bone the presence of parathyroid hormone is essential. (Reprinted from *Federation Proceedings,* 33:2215, 1974. Courtesy, Dr. H. F. DeLuca and *Federation Proceedings.*)

vitamin D still can be considered a vitamin, because many individuals would be unable to meet their requirement for this essential substance if it were not supplied at least in part by the diet.

Daily Allowance As little as 2.5 μg (100 IU) will promote bone development and prevent rickets. The recommended allowance of 10 μg (400 IU) is well documented for full-term and premature infants. Although there is some evidence that the vitamin D content of human milk may be higher than previously estimated, supplements of vitamin D are usually recommended for breast-fed infants.[18] Vitamin D should be supplied to bottle-fed infants either in fortified milk or in supplements.

The allowances for persons of other ages are difficult to establish because of exposure to sunlight, but 10 μg (400 IU) is recommended daily for children and adolescents through 18 years of age. The allowance is reduced to 7.5 μg (300 IU) during the ages of 19 to 22 years and further reduced to 5 μg (200 IU) after the age of 22 years. To meet the increased needs occurring in pregnancy and lactation, an additional intake of 5 μg (200 IU) is recommended.

Sources Exposure to sunlight, fortified foods, fish-liver oils, and commercial vitamin D preparations are the sources of vitamin D. Natural foods are poor sources of vitamin D, although small amounts are present in egg yolk, liver, and fish such as herring, sardines, tuna, and salmon.

About 85 per cent of fresh milk and almost all evaporated milk are fortified with 10 μg (400 IU) vitamin D per quart. Milk is especially suitable for fortification since it contains the calcium and phosphorus whose absorption it facilitates and because it is an important food consumed by children. The fortification of foods other than milk is of dubious value since the ingestion of several foods so treated could lead to excessive intake.

Exposure of the skin to sunlight brings about the synthesis of vitamin D from the precursor 7-dehydrocholesterol. Sunlight cannot always be depended upon to supply the body with adequate ultraviolet rays to manufacture vitamin D, because these rays are so easily strained out by dust, smoke, fog, clothing, and ordinary window glass—all of which act as barriers to prevent the rays from reaching the skin.

Hypervitaminosis D The tolerance for vitamin D varies widely. As little as 45 μg (1,800 IU) over a long period of time may be mildly toxic to children, whereas massive doses of 2500 μg (100,000 IU) may be necessary and are tolerated by those rare individuals who have vitamin-D-resistant rickets. The symptoms of toxicity include nausea, vomiting, diarrhea, excessive thirst, weight loss, polyuria, and nocturia. As the toxicity becomes more severe, renal damage and calcification of the soft tissues such as the heart, blood vessels, bronchi, stomach, and tubules of the kidney occur. Diagnosis is based on history of excess intake and laboratory tests showing hypercalcemia.

Effects of Vitamin D Deficiency A deficiency of vitamin D leads to inadequate absorption of calcium and phosphorus from the intestinal tract and to faulty mineralization of bone and tooth structures. The inability of the soft bones to withstand the stress of weight results in skeletal malformations.

Rickets. Infantile rickets is rarely seen in the United States because of the widespread use of fortified milk or of vitamin D preparations in prophylaxis. When such preventive measures are not taken, rickets is more prevalent in northern regions than in warm, sunny climates. It is more likely to develop in dark, overcrowded sections of large cities where the ultraviolet rays of sunshine, especially in the winter months, cannot penetrate through the fog, smoke, and soot. Poverty and ignorance may account for failure to obtain enough vitamin D from concentrates, fortified milk, or skin exposure. Dark-skinned children are more susceptible to rickets than those of the white race.

Premature infants are more susceptible to rickets than full-term infants since the growth rate and the calcification of the skeleton impose additional demands for vitamin D.

Fully developed cases of rickets present the following characteristics (see Figure 10–7):

1. Delayed closure of the fontanelles, softening of the skull (craniotabes), and bulging or bossing of the forehead, giv-

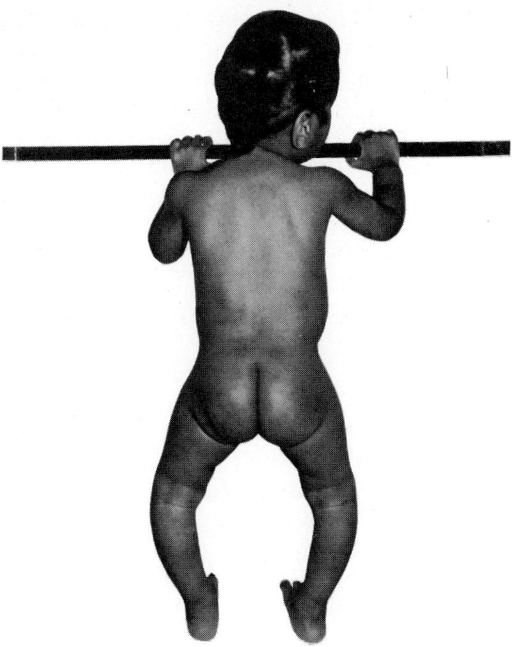

Figure 10–7. Early skeletal deformities of rickets often persist throughout life. Bowlegs that curve laterally, as shown here, indicate that the weakened bones have bent after the second year, as the result of standing. (Courtesy, Dr. Rosa Lee Nemir, Professor of Pediatrics, New York University–Bellevue Medical Center, and The Upjohn Company, *The Vitamin Manual* published by The Upjohn Company.)

ing the head a boxlike appearance.

2. Soft, fragile bones leading to widening of the ends of the long bones; bowing of the legs; enlargement of the costochondral junction with rows of knobs or beads forming the RACHITIC ROSARY; projection of the sternum as in "pigeon breast"; narrowing of the pelvis; spinal curvature.
3. Enlargement of wrist, knee (knock-knees), and ankle joints.
4. Poorly developed muscles; lack of muscle tone—pot belly—being the result of weakness of abdominal muscles; weakness, with delayed walking.
5. Restlessness and nervous irritability.
6. High serum phosphatase; low inorganic blood phosphorus; normal or low serum calcium.

Rickets is treated by giving relatively large amounts of vitamin D concentrates, the dosage being prescribed by the physician.

Tetany. Tetany is characterized by a low serum calcium (7.5 mg per 100 ml or less), muscle twitchings, cramps, and convulsions. It results from insufficient absorption of calcium or vitamin D, or from a disturbance of the parathyroid gland. The physician prescribes calcium salts to control the acute spasms, a diet liberal in calcium, and vitamin D.

Dental health. In rachitic infants and children there may be delayed dentition and malformation of the teeth. Permanent teeth forming in the jaw are more subject to decay.

Osteomalacia. Frequently referred to as "adult rickets," OSTEOMALACIA literally means bone softening. It occurs when there is lack of vitamin D and calcium. In the Orient it is seen in women who have had many pregnancies, who subsist on a meager cereal diet, and who have little exposure to sunshine.

Osteomalacia may occur when there is interference with fat absorption, and hence also vitamin D absorption. The steatorrhea also reduces the absorption of calcium. In chronic renal disease patients often complain of bone pain, and osteodystrophy may be severe. There is little absorption of calcium apparently because the kidney is unable to produce $1{,}25(OH)_2D_3$. Bone abnormalities also are associated with some diseases of the liver because of impaired formation of $25\text{-}(OH)\text{-}D_3$.

The following changes take place in osteomalacia:

1. A softening of the bones, which may be so severe that the bones of the legs, spine, thorax, and pelvis bend into deformities.

2. Pain of the rheumatic type in bones of the legs and lower part of the back.
3. General weakness with difficulty in walking, and especially difficulty in climbing stairs.
4. Spontaneous multiple fractures.

Availability of synthetic forms of 25-(OH)-D_3 and 1,25$(OH)_2D_3$ has led to significant advances in the treatment of these bone disorders. The effective dosages are much smaller than those in vitamin D.

Vitamin E

Discovery Evans and Bishop established the fact that a fat-soluble factor was necessary for reproduction in rats. They showed that absence of vitamin E, or the antisterility factor, as it was designated, led to irreparable damage of the germinal epithelium in male rats, and female rats which had diets deficient in vitamin E were unable to carry their young to term. In severe deficiency the fetus dies and is reabsorbed completely. In the female the damage is not permanent; that is, normal reproduction could again take place if the diet were once more adequate in this factor. The name TOCOPHEROL was suggested for this factor based on the Greek words *tokos* meaning "birth" and *phero* "to carry." The ending *-ol* indicates that the substance is an alcohol.

Chemistry and Characteristics Vitamin E is a generic term for a group of lipid-soluble compounds, the tocopherols and tocotrienols, that possess varying degrees of vitamin activity. Alpha-tocopherol is the most active of these compounds. (See Figure 10–1.) The tocopherols and tocotrienols differ in the chemical structure of their side chains.

High temperatures and acids do not affect the stability of vitamin E, but oxidation takes place readily in the presence of rancid fats or lead and iron salts. Decomposition occurs in ultraviolet light. Vitamin E itself acts as an antioxidant.

Measurement Vitamin E is expressed in international units or in milligrams of α-tocopherol. One international unit of vitamin E is equal to 1 mg synthetic *dl*-α-tocopherol acetate. The activity of the natural form, d-α-tocopherol acetate, is 1.36 IU per milligram; and that of the free alcohol, d-α-tocopherol, is 1.49 IU milligram.[5] Dietary evaluations are concerned primarily with alpha-tocopherol. The other tocopherols and tocotrienols in foods contribute vitamin E activity equal to about 20 per cent of the alpha-tocopherol content of the diet.

Physiology Vitamin E requires the presence of fat and of bile salts for absorption into the intestinal wall. The vitamin is carried with the chylomicrons into the lymph circulation and to the liver. Small amounts of vitamin E are present in all body tissues with the highest concentrations in the pituitary, adrenal gland, and testes. The bulk of the body stores of vitamin E is in the muscle and adipose tissue. There is little transfer of vitamin E across the placenta to the fetus. Hence, newborn infants have low tissue stores.

The total plasma tocopherol ranges from 0.5 to 1.2 mg per 100 ml. A level below 0.5 mg is undesirable. In normal individuals there is a high correlation between plasma total lipids and plasma tocopherol concentration. Thus, conditions that alter blood lipids may lead to changes in plasma tocopherol that may not necessarily reflect changes in tissue concentrations of the vitamin.[19]

Functions The metabolic roles of vitamin E are poorly understood. The principal role appears to be as an antioxidant. By accepting oxygen, vitamin E helps to prevent the oxidation of polyunsaturated fatty acids and phospholipids thereby helping to maintain the integrity of cellular membranes. As a constituent of the enzyme glutathione peroxidase, selenium shares a role with vitamin E in preventing destruction of lipids by oxidation. In animal experiments selenium has been shown to prevent some of the symptoms associated with vitamin E deficiency. Vitamin E has a sparing effect on vitamin A and ascorbic acid by protecting them from oxidation.

Many other functions for vitamin E have been proposed. One of these is the incorporation of pyrimidines into nucleic acids especially in the synthesis of heme in the bone marrow. Vitamin E may also be required for synthesis of coenzyme Q, a factor that is essential in the respiratory chain that releases energy from carbohydrates and fats. Whether these and other proposed functions are secondary to the action of vitamin E as an antioxidant or represent a requirement for the vitamin in specific metabolic reactions remains controversial.[20]

Daily Allowances Intakes of vitamin E recommended by the Food and Nutrition Board are expressed as α-tocopherol equivalents in which 1 mg d-α-tocopherol = 1 αTE.[5] Total vitamin E activity (mg α-TE) in a mixed diet is calculated as follows:

$$\begin{aligned} &\text{mg } \alpha\text{-tocopherol} \\ &+ \text{mg } \beta\text{-tocopherol} \times 0.5 \\ &+ \text{mg } \gamma\text{-tocopherol} \times 0.1 \\ &+ \text{mg } \alpha\text{-tocotrienol} \times 0.3 \end{aligned}$$

These are the only vitamers present in the United States diet that have significant vitamin activity. If only the α-tocopherol content of a mixed diet is known, the value in milligrams should be multiplied by 1.2 to account for the other tocopherols that are present.

Recommended intakes are 3 to 4 mg α-TE during the first year of life, 8 mg α-TE for women, and 10 mg α-TE for men. An additional 2 and 3 mg α-TE are recommended for women during pregnancy and lactation, respectively.

The need for vitamin E is higher when the intake of polyunsaturated fatty acids is increased. Since the principal source of vitamin E is from vegetable oils and margarines, the increased intake of linoleic acid from these fats is accompanied by the satisfactory intake of vitamin E. At the present time evidence indicates that there is no fixed ratio of vitamin E to polyunsaturated fatty acids that can be recommended.[21]

Sources The principal sources of vitamin E in the diet are vegetable oils (corn, soy, cottonseed, safflower), hydrogenated fats from these oils, whole grains, and dark green leafy vegetables, nuts, and legumes. Foods of animal origin are low in vitamin E. Human milk provides adequate vitamin E for the infant, but cow's milk is low. See Table A–2 for alpha-tocopherol content of foods.

The content of tocopherols in foods varies widely. In general, the tocopherol level in oils increases as the linoleic acid content increases. There is considerable loss in fried foods that are frozen and also in the heating of oils. The milling of grains removes about 80 per cent of the vitamin E. Destruction of the remaining vitamin occurs if chlorine dioxide is used in the bleaching process. Typical diets in the United States provide 7 to 9 mg α-tocopherol or a total vitamin E activity of 8 to 11 mg α-TE.[22] In view of the absence of signs of dietary deficiency of vitamin E, the diets in the United States are presumed to meet body needs.

Effects of Deficiency Vitamin E deficiency is extremely rare. In the United States deficiency in adults has been observed only in individuals with chronic fat malabsorption. Changes occurring in severe deficiency included increased hemolysis of red blood cells, creatinuria, deposition of brownish ceroid pigment in smooth muscle and, in some cases, development of a form of muscular dystrophy.[20] When men were fed experimental diets extremely low in vitamin E over a period of several years, there was an increased hemolysis of red blood cells. The length of time to bring about the onset of hemolysis was shortened when the intake of polyunsaturated fats was increased.[23]

Premature and low-birth-weight infants show an extremely low level of tocopherol in the serum and increased hemolysis of red blood cells. When such infants were fed a diet high in polyunsaturated fat and low in vitamin E, they developed a syndrome characterized by edema, skin lesions, and hemolytic anemia. These abnormalities disappeared when vitamin E supplements were given.[24] Evidence of vitamin E deficiency also has been observed in children with cystic fibrosis.

Exaggerated claims for vitamin E. When animals are placed on diets devoid of vitamin E a wide range of symptoms is observed, with considerable variation from one species to another. Among the changes observed have been reproductive failure, macrocytic anemia, shorter life span of the red cells, creatinuria, liver necrosis, encephalomalacia, and muscular dystrophy. The results of these studies have been widely misinterpreted and applied to human nutrition. The fact that human diets generally provide ample amounts of vitamin E is ignored.

Vitamin E has been recommended for such widely varying conditions as heart disease, muscular dystrophy, acne, ulcers, habitual abortion, disorders of the menopause, and sexual impotence. Objective studies, however, have failed to support most of these exaggerated claims, and further research is needed to evaluate new assertions for the possible pharmacologic benefits of vitamin E in certain clinical situations.[25,26]

Toxicity In view of the widespread popularity of megadose supplementation with vitamin E, it is fortunate that the vitamin appears to be relatively nontoxic. Most adults appear to be able to tolerate doses as high as 100 to 1,000 IU per day. However, several reports of adverse effects such as elevation of serum lipids, impaired blood coagulation, and reduction of serum thyroid hormones would suggest that indiscriminate ingestion of excessive amounts of the vitamin over long periods of time should be discouraged.[13,27]

Vitamin K

The existence of vitamin K was first suggested by Dr. Dam of Copenhagen who in 1935 found that a "Koagulations Vitamin" was necessary to prevent fatal hemorrhages in chicks by promoting normal blood clotting.

Chemistry and Characteristics Vitamin K consists of a number of related compounds known as *quinones;* vitamin K_1, also known as *phylloquinone,* was first isolated from alfalfa, and vitamin K_2, also termed *menaquinone,* was produced from putrefied fish meal and is also the form synthesized by intestinal bacteria. (See Figure 10–1.) *Menadione* is a synthetic compound that is two to three times as potent as the natural vitamin. Vitamin K is fat soluble, resistant to heat, but easily destroyed by acids, alkalies, light, and oxidizing agents.

Measurement The activity of test materials is measured in micrograms by its ability to prevent hemorrhage in young chicks. Menadione is used as the standard for measuring vitamin K potency.

Physiology Being fat soluble, dietary vitamin K requires the presence of bile for its absorption, most of which occurs in the upper part of the small intestine. Vitamin K also can be synthesized by bacteria in the lower intestinal tract. It is estimated that approximately 50 percent of the daily requirement is derived from plant sources and the rest from bacterial synthesis.[28] Limited stores of vitamin K are maintained but the concentration is not high in any tissues.

The newborn infant has a very limited supply of vitamin K, and synthesis by the relatively sterile intestinal tract does not take place for several days. Human milk supplies about one fourth as much vitamin K as does cow's milk. Thus, the first few days may be critical for the infant.

Function Vitamin K is essential for the formation of PROTHROMBIN and other clotting proteins by the liver. (See page 133.) It acts as a cofactor for an enzyme in the liver which converts glutamic acid residues in a precursor protein to γ-carboxyglutamic acid, this reaction being necessary before prothrombin can function in blood coagulation. A high prothrombin level indicates good ability to coagulate blood, whereas low blood levels of prothrombin are associated with a slow rate of clotting. Vitamin K also is assumed to be required for the synthesis of other proteins containing γ-carboxyglutamic acid which have been identified in bone and kidney. The functions of these proteins have not been identified.[29]

Daily Allowances Because of variation in intestinal synthesis of vitamin K, no specific allowance is made for this vitamin. The Food and Nutrition Board has established a range of "estimated safe and adequate daily dietary intakes" of vitamin K based on approximately 1 to 2 μg per kilogram body weight. The lower amount is based on the assumption that about one half of the requirement is met by bacterial synthesis; the upper value is calculated assuming that the entire requirement is supplied by diet. The recommended intake for adults, 70 to 140 μg/day, is easily supplied by diet in the United States, and dietary deficiency is not believed to be a problem.

Sources Green leaves of plants such as spinach and kale are excellent sources of vitamin K as are also cabbage, cauliflower, and pork liver. Cereals, fruits, and other vegetables are poor sources.

Effects of Deficiency A low blood level of prothrombin and other clotting factors leads to increased tendency to hemorrhage. Premature infants, anoxic infants, and those whose mothers have been taking anticoagulants are most susceptible to deficiency. The hemorrhagic disease of the newborn can be prevented by a single dose of vitamin K_1 administered to the infant immediately after birth. The practice of giving vitamin K to the mother prior to delivery has been questioned since too much may lead to hemolytic anemia in the infant.

Dietary deficiency of vitamin K is not likely. Deficiency may occur in adults because of a failure in absorption, or interference with the synthesis in the intestine, or inability to form prothrombin by the liver. Oral therapy with sulfa drugs and antibiotics interferes with the synthesis of the vitamin in the intestine. Obstruction of the biliary tract and severe diarrhea as in sprue, celiac disease, and colitis may seriously interfere with absorption. In severe disease of the liver the synthesis of the clotting factors is impaired even though the source of vitamin K is adequate.

If absorption is inadequate, vitamin K may be prescribed orally together with bile salts. Parenteral administration may be required when there is severe intestinal disease. Vitamin K_1 may be used for oral therapy, but menadione taken orally leads to vomiting.

Dicumarol is an anticoagulant often used to treat coronary thrombosis. It is antagonistic to the action of vitamin K and prevents the formation of prothrombin. Anticoagulant therapy carries the risk of hemorrhage. When an excessive amount of anticoagulant is given, vitamin K may be administered to counteract it.

Problems and Review

1. What is the relationship of carotene to vitamin A? What are the important sources of carotene?
2. Why are young children more susceptible than adults to deficiency of vitamin A or D? Describe the signs of deficiency that may be seen in children.
3. *Problem.* Calculate the vitamin A content of your own diet for two days. What percentage of your daily allowance is provided by sources rich in vitamin A? By sources rich in the provitamin?
4. Why is the fortification of milk with vitamin D generally recommended? Why is the fortification of other foods not desirable?
5. Which of the fat-soluble vitamins are toxic? What intakes are likely to lead to toxicity? What are the manifestations of the toxicity?

Table 10-1. **Summary of the Fat-Soluble Vitamins**

Nomenclature	Important Sources	Physiology and Functions	Effect of Deficiency	Daily Allowances*
Vitamin A Retinol Retinal Retinyl ester Retinoic acid Provitamin A Alpha-, beta-, gamma-carotene, cryptoxanthin	*Animal* Fish-liver oils Liver Butter, cream Whole milk Whole-milk cheeses Egg yolk *Plant* Dark-green leafy vegetables Yellow vegetables Yellow fruits Fortified margarines	Bile necessary for absorption Stored in liver Maintains integrity of mucosal epithelium, maintains visual acuity in dim light Large amounts are toxic	Faulty bone and tooth development Night blindness Keratinization of epithelium—mucous membranes and skin *Xerophthalmia*	Children: 400–700 RE (2,000–3,300 IU) Men: 1,000 RE (5,000 IU) Women: 800 RE (4,000 IU) Pregnancy: 1,000 RE (5,000 IU) Lactation: 1,200 RE (6,000 IU)
Vitamin D Vitamin D_2 Ergocalciferol Vitamin D_3 Cholecalciferol Antirachitic factor	Fish-liver oils Fortified milk Activated sterols Exposure to sunlight Very small amounts in butter, liver, egg yolk, salmon, sardines	Synthesized in skin by activity of ultraviolet light Liver synthesizes $25(OH)D_3$ Kidney synthesizes $1{,}25(OH)_2 D_3$ Functions as steroid hormone to regulate calcium and phosphorus absorption, mobilization and mineralization of bone Large amounts are toxic	*Rickets* in children Soft, fragile bones Enlarged joints Bowed legs Chest, spinal, pelvic, bone deformities Delayed dentition *Tetanic* convulsions in infants *Osteomalacia* in adults	Children 0–18 years: 10 μg Adults 19–22 years: 7.5 μg Adults over 22 years: 5 μg Pregnant or lactating women: +5 μg
Vitamin E Alpha-, beta-, gamma-tocopherol Antisterility vitamin	Plant tissues—vegetable oils; wheat germ, rice germ; green leafy vegetables; nuts; legumes Animal foods are poor sources	Not stored in body to any extent Related to action of selenium *Humans:* reduces oxidation of vitamin A, carotenes, and polyunsaturated fatty acids *Animals:* normal reproduction; utilization of sex hormones, cholesterol	*Humans:* hemolysis of red blood cells; mild anemia; deficiency is not likely *Animals:* sterility in male rats; resorption of fetus in female rats; muscular dystrophy; creatinuria; macrocytic anemia	Infants: 3–4 mg α-TE Men: 10 mg α-TE Women: 8 mg α-TE Pregnancy: 10 mg α-TE Lactation: 11 mg α-TE
Vitamin K Phylloquinone (K_1) Menaquinone Menadione	Green leaves such as alfalfa, spinach, cabbage Liver Synthesis in intestine	Bile necessary for absorption Formation of prothrombin and other clotting proteins Sulfa drugs and antibiotics interfere with absorption Large amounts are toxic	Prolonged clotting time Hemorrhagic disease in newborn infants	Estimated safe and adequate intakes Infants: 10–20 μg Adults: 70–140 μg

*See Recommended Dietary allowances for complete listing. Table 3-1.

6. What interrelationship exists between these factors: vitamin A and E; vitamin D and phosphorus; vitamin D and calcium; vitamin E and selenium; vitamin E and polyunsaturated fatty acids?
7. What is the relation of vitamin K to blood clotting? Under what circumstances is a deficiency of vitamin K likely to occur?
8. What is the principal function of vitamin E? What conditions are necessary to produce a deficiency of vitamin E?
9. Which of the fat-soluble vitamins functions as a hormone? How is the hormone formed? What is the role of parathormone?
10. Describe the mechanism by which retinaldehyde participates in night vision.
11. A diet supplies 2,000 IU retinol and 3,000 IU beta-carotene. To how many RE are these equivalent? Does the diet meet the need of the pregnant woman.

Cited References

1. McCollum, E. V., and Davis, M.: "The Necessity of Certain Lipids in the Diet During Growth," *J. Biol. Chem.,* **15**:167–75, 1913. See "Nutrition Classic," *Nutr. Rev.,* **31**:280–81, 1973.
2. Osborne, T. B., and Mendel, L. B.: "The Relation of Growth to the Chemical Constituents of the Diet," *J. Biol. Chem.,* **15**:311–26, 1913.
3. Steenbock, H.: "White Corn Versus Yellow Corn and a Probable Relation Between the Fat Soluble Vitamin and Yellow Plant Pigments," *Science,* **50**:352–53, 1919.
4. "Nomenclature Policy: Generic Descriptions and Trivial Names for Vitamins and Related Compounds," *J. Nutr.,* **110**:8–15, 1980.
5. Food and Nutrition Board: *Recommended Dietary Allowances,* 9th ed. National Academy of Sciences–National Research Council, Washinton, D.C., 1980.
6. FAO/WHO: *Requirements of Vitamin A, Thiamine, Riboflavine, and Niacin.* WHO Tech. Rept. Ser. No. 362, WHO, Geneva, 1967.
7. Pao, E. M.: "Nutrient Consumption Patterns of Individuals, 1977 and 1965," *Family Econ. Rev.,* Spring 1980, pp. 16–20.
8. *Caloric and Selected Nutrient Values for Persons 1–74 Years of Age: First Health and Nutrition Examination Survey, U.S., 1971–1974.* U.S. Department of Health, Education, and Welfare, DHEW Pub. No. (PHS)79–1657, 1979.
9. *Preliminary Findings of the First Health and Nutrition Examination Survey, United States, 1971–1972: Dietary Intake and Biochemical Findings.* U.S. Department of Health, Education, and Welfare, DHEW Pub. No. (HRA)74–1219–1, 1974.
10. Bauernfeind, J. C.: *The Safe Use of Vitamin A.* The Nutrition Foundation, Inc., New York, 1980.
11. Oomen, H. A. P. C.: "Vitamin A Deficiency, Xerophthalmia and Blindness," *Nutr. Rev.,* **32**:161–70, 1974.
12. International Vitamin A Consultative Group: *Guidelines for the Eradication of Vitamin A Deficiency and Xerophthalmia.* The Nutrition Foundation, Inc., New York, 1977.
13. Committee on Safety, Toxicity, and Misuse of Vitamins and Trace Minerals, National Nutrition Consortium, Inc.: *Vitamin-Mineral Safety, Toxicity and Misuse.* American Dietetic Association, Chicago, 1978.
14. Committee on Drugs and on Nutrition, American Academy of Pediatrics: "The Use and Abuse of Vitamin A," *Nutr. Rev.,* **32,** (Suppl. 1):41–43, 1974.
15. DeLuca, H. F.: "The Vitamin D System in the Regulation of Calcium and Phosphorus Metabolism," *Nutr. Rev.,* **37**:161–93, 1979.
16. Fraser, D. R., and Kodicek, E.: "Unique Biosynthesis by Kidney of a Biochemically Active D Metabolite," *Nature,* **228**:764–66, 1970.

17. Haussler, M. R., and McCain, T. A.: "Basic and Clinical Concepts Related to Vitamin D Metabolism and Action," *N. Engl. J. Med.*, **297**:974–83, 1041–50, 1977.
18. Foman, S. J., et al.: "Recommendations for Feeding Normal Infants," *Pediatrics*, **63**:52–59, 1979.
19. Rubenstein, H. M., et al.: "Relation of Vitamin E and Serum Lipids," *Clin. Chim. Acta*, **23**:1–6, 1969.
20. Scott, M. L.: "Vitamin E," in DeLuca, H. F., ed.: *The Fat-Soluble Vitamins.* Plenum Press, New York, 1978, pp. 133–210.
21. Bieri, J. G., and Evarts, R. P.: "Vitamin E Adequacy in Vegetable Oils," *J. Am. Diet. Assoc.*, **66**:134–39, 1975.
22. Bauernfeind, J. C.: "The Tocopherol Content of Food and Influencing Factors," *Crit. Rev. Food Sci. Nutr.*, **8**:337–82, 1977.
23. Horwitt, M. K.: "Vitamin E and Lipid Metabolism in Man," *Am. J. Clin. Nutr.*, **8**:451–61, 1960.
24. Ritchie, J. H., et al.: "Edema and Hemolytic Anemia in Premature Infants: A Vitamin E Deficiency Syndrome," *N. Engl. J. Med.*, **279**:1185–90, 1968.
25. "Vitamin E—Miracle or Myth?" *Nutr. Rev.*, **32** (Suppl. 1):35–36, July 1974.
26. Horwitt, M. K.: "Therapeutic Uses of Vitamin E in Medicine," *Nutr. Rev.*, **38**:105–13, 1980.
27. Tsai, A. C., et al.: "Study on the Effect of Megavitamin E Supplementation in Man," *Am. J. Clin. Nutr.*, **31**:831–37, 1978.
28. Olson, R. E.: "Vitamin K," in Goodhart, R. S., and Shils, M. E., eds.: *Modern Nutrition in Health and Disease,* 6th ed. Lea & Febiger, Philadelphia, 1980, pp. 170–80.
29. Suttie, J. W.: "Vitamin K," in DeLuca, H. F., ed. *"The Fat-Soluble Vitamins.* Plenum Press, 1978, pp. 211–77.

Additional References

Vitamin A

Bernhardt, I. B., and Dorsey, D. J.: "Hypervitaminosis A and Congenital Renal Anomalies in a Human Infant," *Obstet. Gynecol.*, **43**:750–55, 1974.

DeLuca, L. M., et al.: *Recent Advances in the Metabolism and Function of Vitamin A and Their Relationship to Applied Nutrition.* Applied Nutrition. Nutrition Foundation, Inc., New York, 1979.

Hodges, R. E., et al.: "Hematopoietic Studies in Vitamin A Deficiency," *Am. J. Clin. Nutr.*, **31**:876–85, 1978.

Mejia, L. A., et al.: "Vitamin A Deficiency and Anemia in Central American Children," *Am. J. Clin. Nutr.*, **30**:1175–84, 1977.

Muenter, M. D., et al.: "Chronic Vitamin A Intoxication in Adults," *Am. J. Med.*, **50**:129–36, 1971.

Ott, D. B., and Lachance, P. A.: "Retinoic Acid—A Review," *Am. J. Clin. Nutr.*, **32**:2522–31, 1979.

Review: "Vitamin A and the Thyroid," *Nutr. Rev.*, **37**:90–91, 1979.

Rodriguez, M. E., and Irwin, M. I.: "A Conspectus of Research on Vitamin A Requirements of Man," *J. Nutr.*, **102**:909–68, 1972.

Sauberlich, H. E., et al.: "Vitamin A Metabolism and Requirements in the Human Studies with the Use of Labeled Retinol," *Vit. Horm.*, **32**:251–75, 1974.

Shaywitz, B. A., et al.: "Megavitamins for Minimal Brain Dysfunction: A Potentially Dangerous Therapy," *JAMA*, **238**:1749–50, 1977.

Sinha, D. P., and Bang, F. B.: "The Effect of Massive Doses of Vitamin A on the Signs of Vitamin A Deficiency in Preschool Children," *Am. J. Clin. Nutr.*, **29**:110–15, 1976.

SMITH, F. R., and GOODMAN, D. S.: "Vitamin A Transport in Human Vitamin A Toxicity," *N. Engl. J. Med.*, **294**:805–808, 1976.

SOLOMONS, N. W., and RUSSELL, R. M.: "The Interaction of Vitamin A and Zinc: Implications for Human Nutrition," *Am. J. Clin. Nutr.*, **33**:2031–40, 1980.

SPORN, M. B.: "Retinoids and Carcinogenesis," *Nutr. Rev.*, **35**:65–69, 1977.

SWEENEY, J. P., and MARSH, A. C.: "Effect of Processing on Provitamin A in Vegetables," *J. Am. Diet. Assoc.*, **59**:238–43, 1971.

VITAMIN D

BEALE, M. G. et al.: "Vitamin D: The Discovery of Its Metabolites and Their Therapeutic Applications," *Pediatrics*, **57**:729–40, 1976.

COLODRO, I. H., et al.: "Effect of 25-Hydroxy-Vitamin D_3 on Intestinal Absorption of Calcium in Normal Man and Patients with Renal Failure," *Metabolism*, **27**:745–53, 1978.

Committee on Nutrition Misinformation, Food and Nutrition Board: "Hazards of Overuse of Vitamin D," *Nutr. Rev.*, **33**:61–62, 1975.

DELUCA, H. F.: "Some New Concepts Emanating from a Study of the Metabolism and Function of Vitamin D," *Nutr. Rev.*, **38**:169–81, 1980.

GERTNER, J. M., et al.: "Fetomaternal Vitamin D Relationships at Term," *J. Pediatr.*, **97**:637–40, 1980.

KUMAR, R., et al.: "Elevated 1,25 Dihydroxyvitamin D Levels in Normal Pregnancy and Lactation," *J. Clin. Invest.*, **63**:342–44, 1979.

LAKDAWLA, D. R., and WIDDOWSON, E. M.: "Vitamin-D in Human Milk," *Lancet*, **1**:167–68, 1977.

LONG, R. G., et al.: "Serum-25-Hydroxy-Vitamin-D in Untreated Parenchymal and Cholestatic Liver Disease," *Láncet*, **2**:650–52, 1976.

RUDOLF, M., and GREENSTEIN, R. M.: "Unsuspected Nutritional Rickets," *Pediatrics*, **66**:72–76, 1980.

STEICHEN, J. J. et al.: "Vitamin D Homeostasis in the Perinatal Period," *N. Engl. J. Med.*, **302**:315–19, 1980.

WEICK, Sr. M. T.: "A History of Rickets in the United States," *Am. J. Clin. Nutr.*, **20**:1234–41, 1967.

VITAMIN E

BELL, E. F., et al.: "Vitamin E Absorption in Small Premature Infants," *Pediatrics*, **63**:830–32, 1979.

BIERI, J. G., and EVARTS, R. P.: "Tocopherols and Polyunsaturated Fatty Acids in Human Tissues," *Am. J. Clin. Nutr.*, **28**:717–20, 1975.

FARRELL, P. M., and BIERI, J. G.: "Megavitamin E Supplementation in Man," *Am. J. Clin. Nutr.*, **28**:1381–86, 1975.

FARRELL, P. M., et al.: "The Occurrence and Effects of Human Vitamin E Deficiency: A Study in Patients with Cystic Fibrosis," *J. Clin. Invest.*, 60:233–41, 1977.

FARRELL, P. M., et al.: "Plasma Tocopherol Level and Tocopherol-Lipid Relationships in a Normal Population of Children as Compared to Healthy Adults," *Am. J. Clin. Nutr.*, **31**:1720–26, 1978.

GOMES, J. A. C., et al.: "The Effect of Vitamin E on Platelet Aggregation," *Am. Heart J.*, **91**:425–29, 1976.

IFT Expert Panel on Food Safety and Nutrition: "Vitamin E," *Food Technol.*, **31**:77–80, 1977.

Review: "Possible Role of Vitamin E in the Conversion of Cyanocobalamin to Its Coenzyme Form," *Nut. Rev.*, **37**:332–33, 1979.

VATASSERY, G. T., and CHIANG, T.: "Serum α-Tocopherol, Lipids, Potassium, and Creatine Phosphokinase in Normal and Malabsorption Patients," *Am. J. Clin. Nutr.*, **32**:2061–64, 1979.

VITAMIN K

ANSELL, J. E., et al.: "The Spectrum of Vitamin K Deficiency," *JAMA,* **238**:40–42, 1977.

Committee on Nutrition, American Academy of Pediatrics: "Vitamin K Supplementation for Infants Receiving Milk Substitute Infant Formulas and for Those with Fat Malabsorption," *Pediatrics,* **48**:482–87, 1971.

Review: "Evidence for the Occurrence of Gamma-carboxyglutamate in Mineralized Tissue Proteins," *Nutr. Rev.,* **34**:122–24, 1976.

Review: "Osteocaicin: A Vitamin K-Dependent Calcium-Binding Protein in Bone," *Nutr. Rev.,* **37**:54–56, 1979.

STENFLO, J.: "Vitamin K, Prothrombin and γ-Carboxyglutamic Acid," *N. Engl. J. Med.,* **296**:624–25, 1977.

The Water-Soluble Vitamins: Ascorbic Acid 11

Discovery Scurvy has been known as a dread disease since ancient times. It was described as early as 1550 B.C. by the Egyptians in the Papyrus Ebers, a treatise on medicine. It particularly plagued the seagoing adventurers of the sixteenth and seventeenth centuries who lost thousands of men to scurvy. Jacques Cartier in his explorations in Canada was slightly more fortunate for the Indians showed how a brew of pine needles and bark could cure scurvy, and many men were thus saved.

In 1747, Dr. James Lind, a British physician, tested six remedies on twelve sailors who had scurvy. He found that oranges and lemons were curative. But it took another 50 years before the British navy required rations of lemons or limes on the sailing vessels. From that day to the present the British sailor has been known as a "limey." During this same period Captain Cook was able to reduce the incidence of scurvy on his seagoing voyages by stocking up on fresh fruits and vegetables whenever he was in port, and also by including sauerkraut as part of the rations. The sauerkraut kept well and was a good preventive of scurvy.

The scientific era of vitamin C began in 1907 when two Norwegian scientists, Holst and Frölich, produced scurvy in guinea pigs. The isolation and chemical nature of vitamin C, or ascorbic acid, was accomplished by Dr. Charles G. King and his coworkers at the University of Pittsburgh and by Dr. Szent-Györgyi of Hungary in the early 1930s.

Chemistry and Characteristics ASCORBIC ACID is a white crystalline compound of relatively simple structure, and closely related to the monosaccharide sugars. It is synthesized from glucose and other simple sugars by plants and by most animal species. It can be prepared synthetically at low cost from glucose. Vitamin C activity is possessed by two forms: L-ascorbic acid (the reduced form) and L-dehydroascorbic acid (the oxidized form). (See Figure 11–1.) The latter is oxidized further with complete loss of activity. Isoascorbic acid, a compound often used as a preservative in foods, appears to have little or no biological value in humans.

Of all vitamins, ascorbic acid is the most easily destroyed. It is highly soluble in water. The oxidation of ascorbic acid is accelerated by heat, light, alkalies, oxidative enzymes, and traces of copper and iron. Oxidation is inhibited to a marked degree in an acid reaction, and when the temperature is reduced.

Measurement Ascorbic acid is determined by chemical assay, and the concentration in tissues and foods is expressed in milligrams.

Metabolism Only a few species are known to require a dietary source of ascorbic acid: humans, monkeys, guinea pigs, Indian fruit bats, the red-vented bulbul bird, and certain fish such as trout and carp. Ascorbic acid is rapidly absorbed from the gastrointestinal tract and distributed to the various tissues of the body. The adrenal gland and the retina of the eye contain an especially high concentration of vitamin C, but other tissues such as the spleen, intestine, bone marrow, pancreas, thymus, liver, pituitary, and kidney also contain appreciable amounts.

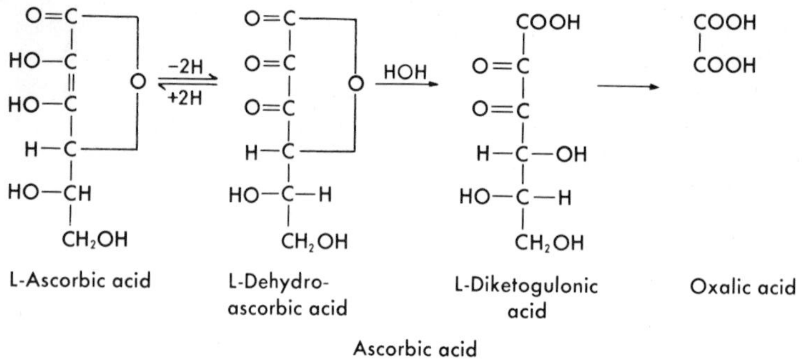

L-Ascorbic acid ⇌ (−2H / +2H) L-Dehydroascorbic acid → (HOH) L-Diketogulonic acid → Oxalic acid

Ascorbic acid

Figure 11–1. Ascorbic acid and dehydroascorbic acid are biologically active. These forms are easily converted to diketogluconic acid which is inactive. Note the similarity of the structure of ascorbic acid to that of glucose.

A plasma concentration of greater than 0.6 mg ascorbic acid per 100 ml indicates tissue saturation and a body pool equivalent to 1,500 mg in the adult. Adequate vitamin C nutrition is indicated when plasma concentrations range between 0.40 and 0.59 mg per 100 ml, representing a body pool of 600 to 1,499 mg.[1] Plasma levels of ascorbic acid tend to be lower in cigarette smokers and women using oral contraceptive agents.[2,3]

The kidney exercises some control over the excretion of ascorbic acid. If tissues are saturated, most of a large dose of vitamin C will be excreted. If tissues are depleted, only a small amount of vitamin C will be excreted. Ascorbic acid is excreted as such, or as metabolites including oxalic acid and ascorbic acid sulfate.

The body efficiently utilizes either synthetic L-ascorbic acid or the vitamin in its natural form as in orange juice.[4]

Functions One of the principal functions of ascorbic acid is the formation of collagen, an abundant protein that forms the intercellular substance in cartilage, bone matrices, dentin, and the vascular epithelium. In the synthesis of collagen ascorbic acid is necessary for the HYDROXYLATION (introduction of −OH groups) of proline and lysine to hydroxyproline and hydroxylysine. These hydroxyamino acids are important constituents of collagen. This function helps to explain the importance of vitamin C in wound healing and the ability to withstand the stress of injury and infection.

Ascorbic acid also plays an important role in other hydroxylation reactions. Conversion of tryptophan to serotonin, an important neurotransmitter and vasoconstrictor, and formation of norepinephrine from tyrosine involve hydroxylation reactions which require ascorbic acid. These reactions may explain some of the abnormalities in vascular and neurologic activity that are observed in persons deficient in the vitamin. Conversion of cholesterol to bile acids is another hydroxylation reaction that may require vitamin C. The effect of ascorbic acid deficiency and excess on serum cholesterol levels in humans remains controversial.[1]

Ascorbic acid is an important antioxidant and thus has a role in the protection of vitamins A and E and the polyunsaturated fatty acids from excessive oxidation. Ascorbic acid enhances iron absorption by reducing ferric iron to ferrous iron, the form which is absorbed most efficiently. It may also bind with iron to form a complex which facilitates transfer of iron across the intestinal mucosa. In the circulation ascorbic acid aids in the release of iron from transferrin so that it can be incorporated into tissue ferritin. Evidence also exists to support a role of vitamin C in biosynthesis of mucopolysaccharides, microsomal drug metabolism, leukocyte function and synthesis of anti-inflammatory steroids by the adrenal gland.[5] It does not appear that vitamin C functions as a coenzyme in these reactions.

Recommended Allowances As little as 10 mg ascorbic acid will prevent scurvy.

This level may be regarded as a minimum requirement but it does not ensure fully satisfactory tissue levels. Each day the adult male removes about 30 mg ascorbic acid from body stores. The recommended allowance has been set at 60 mg for males and females over 14 years, 35 mg for infants, 45 to 50 mg for children, 80 mg for pregnancy and 100 mg for lactation.[5] During infections such as tuberculosis, rheumatic fever, and pneumonia and severe stress such as burn injuries the ascorbic acid requirement is increased.

Food Sources Almost all of the daily intake of ascorbic acid is obtained from the vegetable-fruit group. (See Figure 11–2.) In the American diet the vitamin C in the available food supply is furnished from food groups in these percentages: citrus fruits, 29; other fruits, 12; potatoes and sweet potatoes, 14; dark green and deep yellow vegetables, 9; other vegetables including tomatoes, 28.[6]

Vitamin C has been called the "fresh-food vitamin" since it is found in highest concentrations just as the food is fresh from the plant. In general, the active parts of the plant contain appreciable amounts, and mature or resting seeds are devoid of the vitamin.

Raw, frozen, or canned citrus fruits such as oranges, grapefruit, and lemons are excellent sources of the vitamin. Orange sections including the thin white peel contain

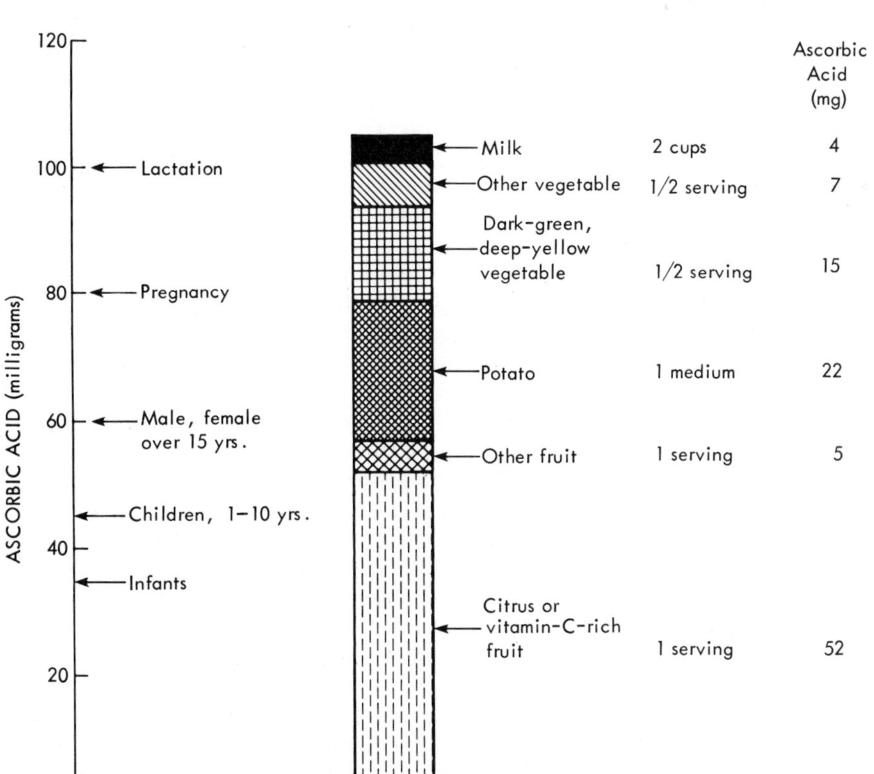

Figure 11–2. The vegetable-fruit group accounts for almost all of the ascorbic acid in the diet. See Table 13–2 for complete calculation of the Basic Diet.

more vitamin C than an equal weight of strained juice.

Fresh strawberries, cantaloupe, pineapple, and guavas are also excellent sources. Other nonacid fresh fruits such as peaches, pears, apples, bananas, and blueberries contribute small amounts of the vitamin; when eaten in large amounts these fruits may be an important dietary source. The concentration of ascorbic acid in the nonacid canned fruits is considerably reduced.

Broccoli, Brussels sprouts, spinach, kale, green peppers, cabbage, and turnips are excellent-to-good sources even when cooked. The use of potatoes and sweet potatoes as staple food items enhances the vitamin C intake considerably provided that preparation methods have been good.

Milk, eggs, meat, fish, and poultry are practically devoid of vitamin C as they are consumed. If the mother's diet has been adequate, human milk contains four to six times as much ascorbic acid as cow's milk and is able to protect the infant from scurvy. Liver contains a small amount of vitamin C, but most of this is lost during cookery.

Retention of Food Values A warm environment, exposure to air, solubility in water, heat, alkali, and dehydration are detrimental to the retention of ascorbic acid in foods. The cutting of vegetables releases oxidative enzymes and increases the surfaces exposed to leaching by water. Since the vitamin is so soluble, losses are considerable when large amounts of water are used. Vegetables should be added to a small quantity of boiling water, covered tightly, and cooked until just tender for high retention of ascorbic acid. Retention is also good when a pressure cooker is used, provided that the cookery time is carefully controlled. The practice of adding baking soda to retain green color of vegetables not only reduces the vitamin C level but may also modify the flavor and texture of the vegetable. Leftover vegetables lose a large proportion of the ascorbic acid, although losses are reduced somewhat when the container is tightly covered in the refrigerator. On the other hand, citrus juices and tomatoes retain practically all the vitamin C value for several days.

Effects of Deficiency Preliminary results of the Nationwide Food Consumption Survey showed that intakes of ascorbic acid in 1977 were considerably higher than average intakes in 1965 and met or exceeded recommended intakes for all sex-age groups. This increased intake was attributed to fortification of beverages and other foods with vitamin C and increased consumption of citrus fruit and juice.[7] Although results of the first Health and Nutrition Examination Survey (1971–1972) likewise showed that the average intake of persons 1 to 74 years of age exceeded the standard, intakes of substantial percentages of persons in the various sex-age categories fell below recommended amounts. The highest prevalence of low intakes was found in low-income white males 45 to 54 years old.[8] Until biochemical or clinical data are available, however, conclusions cannot be made with respect to the prevalence of problems in vitamin C nutriture.

A deficiency of ascorbic acid results in the defective formation of the intercellular cement substance. Fleeting joint pains, irritability, retardation of growth in the infant or child, anemia, shortness of breath, poor wound healing, and increased susceptibility to infection are among the signs of deficiency, but none of these can establish a diagnosis. A dietary history, the concentration of ascorbic acid in the blood plasma and in the white blood cells, and a measure of the excretion of a test dose in the urine help to establish the diagnosis.

Scurvy. The classic picture of scurvy is rarely seen in adults in the United States. The incidence is also uncommon in infants, but a gross deficiency of ascorbic acid results in scurvy during the second 6 months of life. Infections, fevers, and hyperthyroidism may precipitate the symptoms when

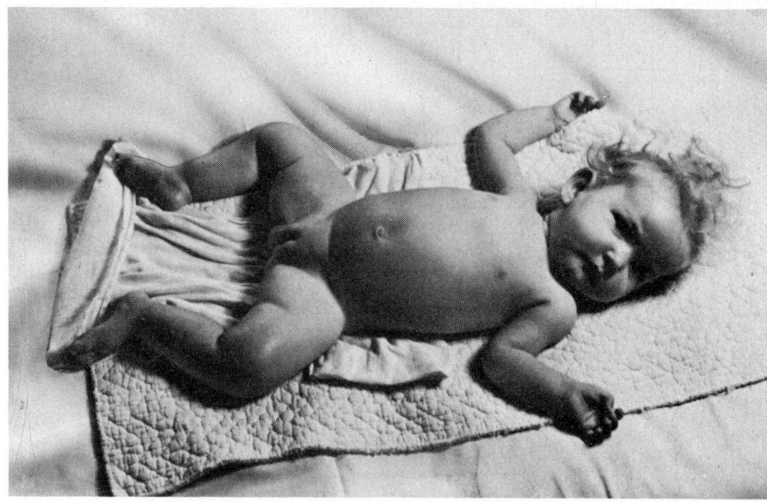

Figure 11–3. Child in scorbutic position (Courtesy, Dr. Bernard S. Epstein, The Long Island Jewish Hospital, New Hyde Park, New York, and *The Vitamin Manual,* published by The Upjohn Company.)

the intake has been inadequate. The symptoms are related to the weakening of the collagenous material.

Pain, tenderness, and swelling of the thighs and legs are frequent symptoms of infantile scurvy. The baby shows a disinclination to move and assumes a position with legs flexed for comfort. (See Figure 11–3.) He is pale and irritable and cries when handled. Loss of weight, fever, diarrhea, and vomiting are frequently present. If the teeth have erupted, the gums are likely to be swollen, tender, and hemorrhagic. Bone calcification is faulty because of degeneration or lack of proper development of the bone matrix. The cartilage supporting the bones is weak, and bone displacement results. The ends of the long bones and of the ribs are enlarged somewhat as in rickets, but tenderness is a distinguishing characteristic in scurvy.

Scurvy in adults results after several months of a diet devoid of ascorbic acid. The symptoms include petechiae or hemorrhagic spots on the skin; swelling, infection, and bleeding of the gums; tenderness of the legs; and anemia. The teeth may become loose and eventually may be lost. As the disease progresses, the slightest injury produces excessive bleeding, and large hemorrhages may be seen underneath the skin. There is degeneration of the muscle structure and of the cartilage generally.

Acute scurvy responds within a few days to the administration of 100 to 200 mg ascorbic acid given in the synthetic form or as orange juice. Chronic changes that have occurred, such as bone deformities and anemia, require much longer periods for their correction.

Megadoses of Ascorbic Acid Since the publication of Dr. Linus Pauling's book,[9] thousands of people have been taking large doses of ascorbic acid to prevent and/or treat colds. The dosages used often are 20 to 100 times the recommended allowances and should be regarded as pharmaceutic agents. Although the results of some controlled studies have suggested that supplements of vitamin C have an effect in reducing the incidence and severity of cold symptoms, other studies have shown little or no effect.[10, 11] In a study of Navajo children in a boarding school in Arizona, administration of 1,000 mg vitamin C resulted in 26 per cent fewer symptomatic days in the younger children receiving the vitamin than in placebo recipients. In older girls receiving 2,000 mg of vitamin C per day a 33 per cent reduction in symptomatic days was observed. Repetition of the study the next year using supplements of 1,000 mg, however, showed only 9 per cent fewer symptomatic days overall in children receiving the vitamin. Average duration of a cold was slightly less in vitamin C recipients in the first study but was about the same in the two groups in the second study.[12]

Claims have also been made for the value of megadose supplements of ascorbic acid in treating cancer patients. In one study administration of ascorbic acid was reported to prolong survival time in patients with terminal cancer.[13] However, other investigators were unable to confirm these results in a controlled study using similar doses of the vitamin.[14]

In view of the widespread use of large amounts of vitamin C, often without medical supervision, the possibility of adverse effects of excessive intakes needs to be considered. Although in the past large doses were generally assumed to be nontoxic, a growing list of complications is now being identified. Formation of kidney stones may be enhanced in certain individuals because of an increase in urine acidity or because of increased oxalate excretion arising from breakdown of the vitamin. An abrupt decrease in intake may precipitate symptoms of scurvy and the possibility of conditioned deficiency occurring in infants of mothers ingesting large amounts of the vitamin is of special concern. Other problems associated with megadoses of vitamin C include gastrointestinal disturbances, interference with anticoagulants, destruction of red blood cells, and excessive absorption of iron.[15] Since many of the claims for megadose use of ascorbic acid have not been documented, and since excessive intakes may have adverse effects, routine use of large supplements of the vitamin C does not appear to be advisable.

A summary of ascorbic acid appears at the end of Chapter 12.

Problems and Review

1. In what way is ascorbic acid related to the functioning of each of these substances: iron, collagen, folacin, cholesterol, vitamin A, tryptophan?
2. What are the clinical manifestations of a deficiency of ascorbic acid?
3. What is the effect of an intake of ascorbic acid in excess of the body's needs?
4. Why is a formula-fed baby more prone to scurvy than a breast-fed baby?
5. List the instructions you would give for the preparation and service of these foods in order that the maximum ascorbic acid would be retained: tossed green salad, buttered cabbage?
6. *Problem.* Calculate the ascorbic acid content of your own diet for two days. Compare your intake with the recommended allowances.
7. *Problem.* Calculate the amounts of each of the following foods necessary to furnish 25 mg of ascorbic acid: orange juice, tomato juice, sweet potato, cabbage, grapefruit, endive, strawberries, cantaloupe, apple, lettuce.
8. Mashed potatoes served in a restaurant probably should not be relied upon as a source of ascorbic acid. Give several reasons why this is true.

Cited References

1. Hodges, R. E.: "Ascorbic Acid," in Goodhart, R. S., and Shils, M. E., ed.: *Modern Nutrition in Health and Disease,* 6th ed. Lea & Febiger, Philadelphia,1980, pp. 259–73, 1980.

2. Pelletier, O.: "Vitamin C and Cigarette Smokers," *Ann. N.Y. Acad. Sci.*, **258**:156–62, 1975.
3. Rivers, J. M.: "Oral Contraceptives and Ascorbic Acid," *Am. J. Clin. Nutr.*, **28**:550–54, 1975.
4. Pelletier, O., and Keith, M. O.: "Bioavailability of Synthetic and Natural Ascorbic Acid," *J. Am. Diet. Assoc.*, **64**:271–75, 1974.
5. Food and Nutrition Board: *Recommended Dietary Allowances,* 9th ed., National Academy of Sciences—National Research Council, Washington, D.C., 1980.
6. Marston, R. M., and Welsh, S. O.: "Nutrient Content of the National Food Supply," *Natl. Food Rev.*, U.S. Dept. of Agriculture, Washington, D.C., Winter 1981, pp. 19–22.
7. Pao, E. M.: "Nutrient Consumption Patterns of Individuals, 1977 and 1965," *Family Econ. Rev.*, Spring 1980, pp. 16–20.
8. *Caloric and Selected Nutrient Values for Persons 1–74 Years of Age: First Health and Nutrition Examination Survey, U.S., 1971–1974.* U.S. Dept. of Health, Education and Welfare, DHEW Publ. No. (PHS) 79-1657, 1979.
9. Pauling, L.: *Vitamin C and the Common Cold.* W. H. Freeman and Company, San Francisco, 1970.
10. Anderson, T. W.: "Large-scale Trials of Vitamin C," *Ann. N.Y. Acad. Sci.*, **258**:498–504, 1975.
11. Chalmers, T. C.: "Effects of Ascorbic Acid on the Common Cold: An Evaluation of the Evidence," *Am. J. Med.*, **58**:532–36, 1975.
12. Coulehan, J. L.: "Ascorbic Acid and the Common Cold: Reviewing the Evidence, *Postgrad. Med.*, **66** (September): 153–60, 1979.
13. Cameron, E., and Pauling, L.: "Supplemental Ascorbate in the Supportive Treatment of Cancer: Prolongation of Survival Times in Terminal Human Cancer," *Proc. Natl. Acad. Sci.*, **73**:3685–89, 1976.
14. Creagan, E. T., et al.: "Failure of High-Dose Vitamin C (Ascorbic Acid) Therapy to Benefit Patients with Advanced Cancer," *N. Engl. J. Med.*, **301**:687–90, 1979.
15. Committee on Safety, Toxicity, and Misuse of Vitamins and Trace Minerals, National Nutrition Consortium, Inc.: *Vitamin-Mineral Safety, Toxicity and Misuse.* American Dietetic Association, Chicago, 1978.

Additional References

ANDREWS, F. E., and DRISCOLL, P. J.: "Stability of Ascorbic Acid in Orange Juice Exposed to Light and Air During Storage," *J. Am. Diet. Assoc.*, **71**:140–42, 1977.

BAIRD, I. MCL., et al.: "The Effects of Ascorbic Acid and Flavonoids on the Occurrence of Symptoms Normally Associated with the Common Cold," *Am. J. Clin. Nutr.*, **32**:1686–90, 1979.

COOK, J. D., and MONSEN, E. R.: "Vitamin C, the Common Cold, and Iron Absorption," *Am. J. Clin. Nutr.*, **30**:235–41, 1977.

DYKES, M. H. M., and MEIER, P.: "Ascorbic Acid and the Common Cold," *JAMA*, **231**:1073–79, 1975.

HOGENKAMP, H. P. C.: "The Interaction Between Vitamin B_{12} and Vitamin C," *Am. J. Clin. Nutr.*, **33**:1–3, 1980.

HOROWITZ, I., et al.: "Bioavailability of Ascorbic Acid in Orange Juice," *JAMA*, **235**:2624–25, 1976.

IRWIN, M. I., and HUTCHINS, B. K.: "A Conspectus of Research on Vitamin C Requirements of Man," *J. Nutr.*, **106**:823–79, 1976.

KALLNER, A., et al.: "Steady-state Turnover and Body Pool of Ascorbic Acid in Man," *Am. J. Clin. Nutr.*, **32**:530–39, 1979.

KALLNER, A., et al.: "On the Absorption of Ascorbic Acid in Man," *Int. J. Vit. Nutr. Res.*, **47**:383–88, 1977.

KARLOWSKI, T. R., et al.: "Ascorbic Acid for the Common Cold: A Prophylactic and Therapeutic Trial," *JAMA.*, **231**:1038–42, 1975.

MACHLIN, L. J., et al.: "Lack of Antiscorbutic Activity of Ascorbate-2-Sulfate in the Rhesus Monkey," *Am. J. Clin. Nutr.*, **29**:825–31, 1976.

MILLER, J. Z., et al.: "Therapeutic Effect of Vitamin C: a Co-Twin Control Study," *JAMA*, **237**:248–51, 1977.

NELSON, E. W., et al.: "Comparative Bioavailability of Folate and Vitamin C from a Synthetic and a Natural Source," *Am. J. Clin. Nutr.*, **28**:1014–19, 1975.

STEIN, H. G., et al.: "Ascorbic Acid-Induced Uricosuria: A Consequence of Megavitamin Therapy," *Ann. Int. Med.*, **84**:385–88, 1976.

12 The Water-Soluble Vitamins: The Vitamin-B Complex

IN areas of the world where polished rice is a staple food, beriberi, a serious disease affecting the nerves, has been known for generations. Takaki, a Japanese medical officer, studied the high incidence of the disease among men of the Japanese navy during the years 1878–1883. Among 276 men serving on one sailing vessel he found 169 cases of beriberi including 25 deaths at the end of 9 months, but only 14 cases with no deaths occurred among a similar number of men on a second vessel who had received more meat, milk, and vegetables in their diet. Takaki believed this difference was related to the protein content of the diet.

About 15 years later (1897) Eijkman, a Dutch physician in the East Indies, noted that illness in fowls that ate scraps of hospital food consisting chiefly of polished rice was similar to beriberi seen in humans. He subsequently showed that the addition of rice polishings to the diet would cure the disease. He theorized that the starch of the polished rice was toxic to the nerves, but that the outer layers of the rice kernel were protective. Another Dutch physician, Grijns, interpreted the findings as a deficiency of an essential substance in the diet.

A number of chemists demonstrated the effects of extracts from rice. Funk in 1912 coined the term *vitamine* for the substance which he found to be effective in preventing beriberi. McCollum and Davis applied the term *water-soluble B* to the concentrates which cured beriberi.

The water-soluble vitamin B described by Funk and others was soon discovered to be not a single substance but a group of compounds which we now designate as the vitamin-B complex. Most of these have been synthesized, and their chemical and physical properties are fairly well understood. Principally these vitamins combine with specific proteins to function as parts of the various enzyme systems which are concerned with the breakdown of carbohydrate, protein, and fat in the body. Thus, they are interrelated and are intimately involved in the mechanisms which release energy, carbon dioxide, and water as the end products of metabolism.

Thiamin

Discovery Crystalline thiamin (vitamin B-1) was isolated from rice bran by Jansen and Donath in Java in 1926. The synthesis and structure were accomplished in 1936 by Dr. R. R. Williams, who had worked for a quarter of a century on studies of beriberi and on the factor in rice polishings which brought about cure of the disease. Because of the presence of sulfur in the molecule, the vitamin was named THIAMIN.

Chemistry and Characteristics Thiamin is available commercially as thiamin hydrochloride in a crystalline white powder. (See Figure 12–1). It has a faint yeastlike odor and a salty nutlike taste, and is readily soluble in water. The vitamin is stable in its dry form, and heating in solutions at 120° C in an acid medium (pH 5.0 or less) has little destructive effect. On the other hand, cooking foods in neutral or alkaline reaction is very destructive.

Measurement Thiamin is now measured in milligrams or micrograms. It is de-

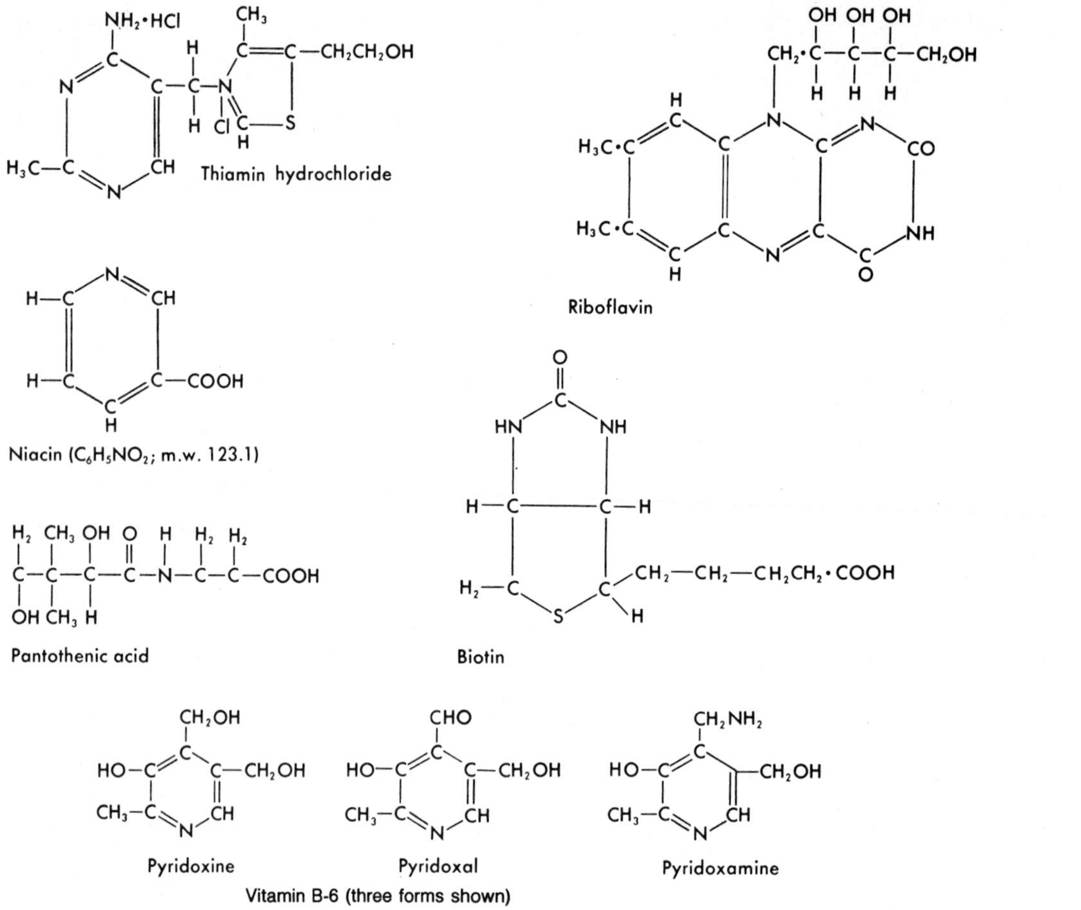

Thiamin hydrochloride

Riboflavin

Niacin ($C_6H_5NO_2$; m.w. 123.1)

Pantothenic acid

Biotin

Pyridoxine

Pyridoxal

Pyridoxamine

Vitamin B-6 (three forms shown)

Figure 12–1. These B-complex vitamins are converted to essential coenzymes in metabolic reactions involving carbohydrates, fats, and proteins. Note the wide variations in structure.

termined by chemical or microbiologic methods.

Physiology The thiamin ingested in food is available in the free form or bound as thiamin pyrophosphate or in a protein-phosphate complex. The bound forms are split in the digestive tract after which absorption takes place principally from the first part of the duodenum. The amount of thiamin stored in the body is not great—probably about 50 mg in all. The liver, kidney, heart, brain, and muscles have somewhat higher concentrations than the blood.

The principal functioning form of thiamin is THIAMIN PYROPHOSPHATE (TPP), also formerly known as cocarboxylase. Conversion of thiamin to this active form requires ATP. Thiamin pyrophosphate acts as a coenzyme for a number of important enzyme systems.

If thiamin is ingested in excess of tissue needs, it is excreted in the urine. With a low dietary intake, the urinary excretion promptly falls.

THIAMINASE is an enzyme present in uncooked clams, some fishes, and shrimp that splits the thiamin molecule, thereby inactivating it. In most situations this presents no problem since cooking inactivates thiaminase. Tea and a few other foods contain compounds that act as thiamin antagonists. Persons on marginal diets consuming large amounts of tea may have an increased risk of developing deficiency.

Functions One of the critical points at which TPP functions in carbohydrate metabolism is in the oxidative decarboxylation of pyruvic acid and the subsequent formation of acetyl coenzyme A, which in turn enters the Krebs cycle. (See Figure 5–5.) This is one of the most complex reactions in carbohydrate metabolism and, in addition to TPP, also requires these cofactors: coenzyme A, which contains pantothenic acid (see page 231); nicotinamide adenine dinucleotide (NAD), which contains niacin (see page 225); magnesium ions; and lipoic acid (see page 240).

Another point in carbohydrate metabolism that involves oxidative decarboxylation is in the Krebs cycle in the conversion of α-ketoglutaric acid to succinic acid. Because breakdown products of fats and proteins as well as carbohydrate can contribute to α-ketoglutaric acid, thiamin, and the other factors listed here are involved in the metabolism of the three energy-producing nutrients.

Thiamin pyrophosphate is also a cofactor for TRANSKETOLASE, an enzyme required to produce active glyceraldehyde through the pentose shunt. (See Figure 5–5.) In addition to its coenzyme function, thiamin may be involved in some aspect of the function of nerve cell membranes or in some way influence the action of neurotransmitters such as acetylcholine or serotonin.[1]

Daily Allowances The thiamin requirement is proportional to the calorie requirement. The minimum requirement is about 0.33 to 0.35 mg of thiamin per 1,000 kcal, and the recommended allowance has been set at 0.5 mg per 1,000 kcal.[2] This provides a margin of safety for individual variation and affords some protection during periods of stress.

The daily allowance for men aged 23 to 50 years is 1.4 mg, and for women of the same age it is 1.0 mg. Elderly persons utilize thiamin somewhat less efficiently, and therefore an allowance of at least 1.0 mg is recommended even though the calorie requirement may be below 2,000. The allowance for pregnant and lactating women is increased by 0.4 and 0.5 mg, respectively. Infants should receive 0.3 to 0.5 mg daily, and children up to 10 years are allowed 0.7 to 1.2 mg daily.

Sources Thiamin is widely distributed in many foods, but most foods do not furnish especially high concentrations. Although brewers' yeast and wheat germ are rich sources, they do not form an important part of most diets. The American food supply provides 2.17 mg per capita.[3] Of this about 40 per cent is furnished by whole-grain or enriched cereals, flours, and breads.

The meat group supplies approximately one fourth of the daily intake of thiamin. Lean pork—fresh and cured—is especially high in its thiamin concentration; its frequent inclusion in the diet thus makes it a highly significant source. Liver, dry beans and peas, soybeans, and peanuts are also excellent sources. The thiamin in egg, a fair source, is concentrated in the yolk.

Although the concentration of thiamin in vegetables and fruits is low, the quantities of these foods eaten may be such that important contributions are made to the daily total. Milk is likewise a fair source because of the amounts taken in the daily diet and because milk is not subjected to treatment other than pasteurization, which does not materially reduce the thiamin level.

The thiamin contribution of the basic diet pattern is shown in Figure 12–2.

Retention of Food Values Little loss of thiamin occurs in the preparation of cooked breakfast cereals inasmuch as the water used in preparation is consumed. On the other hand, losses are considerable when rice is washed before cooking and when it is cooked in a large volume of water that is later drained off. Losses are minimized if rice is cooked in just enough water so

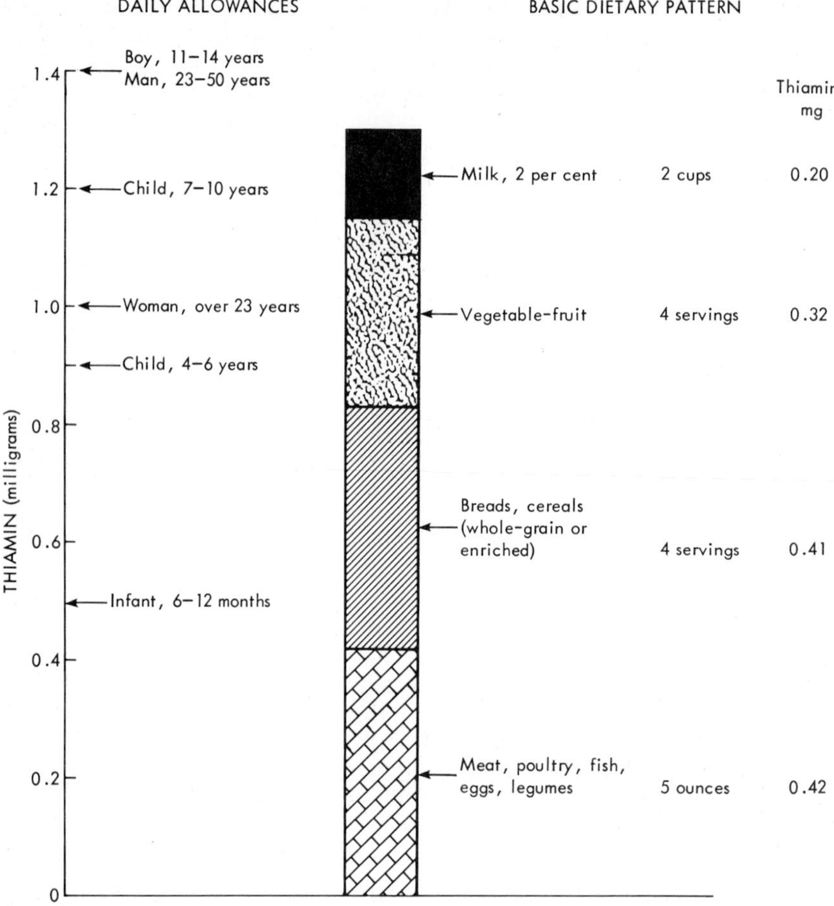

Figure 12–2. Recommended amounts from each of the food groups will provide the thiamin allowances for women and children. The slightly increased allowances for teenagers and men are easily met by increased amounts from one or more of these food groups. See Table 13–2 for complete calculation of the basic dietary pattern.

that all of it is absorbed by the grains. "Converted" rice retains more of the thiamin than does regular rice because in its processing the water-soluble nutrients are distributed throughout the grain. In the baking of bread about 15 to 20 per cent of the thiamin content is lost.

Thiamin losses are 25 per cent or less when meats are broiled or roasted. When meats are cooked in liquid, the losses approach 50 per cent if the liquid is discarded. If the liquid in which meat is cooked is consumed, the loss is about 25 per cent.

Thiamin losses in vegetable cookery are minimal if vegetables are cooked in a small amount of water for a short time without the addition of baking soda. In general, when the principles for retention of ascorbic acid are observed in food preparation, the maximum thiamin content will also be preserved.

Effects of Deficiency Severe thiamin deficiency is rare in the United States. The incidence of mild deficiency is not known. Deficiency may arise following gastrointestinal disturbances accompanied by persistent vomiting or diarrhea or subsequent to febrile diseases or surgery when the dietary intake is poor. One group that is especially susceptible is the alcoholic population. The neurologic disorder, Wernicke-Korsakoff syndrome, which is seen most often in alcoholics is due primarily to a deficiency of thiamin.

Beriberi still occurs in the Orient where high-carbohydrate diets are common and where enrichment of rice and wheat is not practiced. Williams demonstrated the effectiveness of rice enrichment in the Philippines, an area where the incidence of beriberi has been high.[4]

Diagnosis. The symptoms of mild deficiency are so vague that a diagnosis of thiamin lack is difficult. The activity of an enzyme, erythrocyte transketolase, which is found in the red blood cells correlates closely with thiamin nutrition,[5] and is believed to be useful in detecting marginal deficiency before clinical symptoms have become apparent. An elevated level of pyruvic and lactic acids in the blood, especially after exercise and the administration of a standard amount of glucose, together with a low concentration of thiamin in the urine is suggestive of deficiency. If such tests are further substantiated with a dietary history of thiamin lack plus the appearance of peripheral neuritis and disorders of the cardiovascular system, thiamin deficiency is apparent.

Symptoms. The individual who daily receives less than the minimum amount of thiamin builds up an increasing deficiency which affects the gastrointestinal, cardiovascular, and peripheral nervous systems. The early symptoms are nonspecific for thiamin lack and include fatigue, lack of interest in one's affairs, emotional instability, irritability, depression, anger and fear, and loss of appetite, weight, and strength. As the deficiency becomes more marked, the patient may complain of indigestion, constipation, headaches, insomnia, and tachycardia after moderate exercise. There appears a feeling of heaviness and weakness of the legs which may be followed by cramping of the calf muscles and burning and numbness of the feet—an indication of the development of peripheral neuritis.

The neuritic effects are first noted in the foot, then the muscles of the calf, and then the thigh. The muscle degeneration may be so pronounced that coordination is impossible and a characteristic high-stepping gait results. This form of the disease characterized primarily by emaciation and multiple neuritic symptoms often is referred to as "dry" beriberi.

Thiamin deficiency also leads to enlargement of the heart, tachycardia, dyspnea, and palpitations on exertion. In the acute type of beriberi, acute cardiac failure may be fatal before the seriousness of the disease has been fully appreciated. This stage of the disease is known as "wet" beriberi because the chief manifestation is a severe edema which masks the emaciation that is also present.

Infantile beriberi. In the Far East infants are especially susceptible to beriberi because the mother has had a deficient intake of thiamin and the milk she supplies to the infant consequently contains a very low level of thiamin. The onset is often sudden and is characterized by pallor, facial edema, irritability, vomiting, abdominal pain, loss of voice, and convulsion. The infant may die within a few hours. With thiamin therapy, recovery is dramatic.

Treatment. Because beriberi is a complex vitamin deficiency disease, patients make the greatest improvement when B-complex vitamins rather than thiamin alone are prescribed. In addition to the B-complex concentrates, it is customary to prescribe a diet that is high in protein and calories.

Riboflavin

Discovery As early as 1879 a pigment which possessed a yellow-green fluorescence had been discovered in milk. Other workers later obtained it from such widely varying sources as liver, yeast, heart, and egg white. The pigments which possess these fluorescent properties were designated as "flavins."

In the early 1920s the substance in yeast which prevented polyneuritis was shown to be more than one vitamin. The antineuritic fraction which was destroyed by heat was called vitamin B-1. Another fraction not destroyed by heat did not prevent or cure polyneuritis but it was needed for growth. It was designated as vitamin B-2 or vitamin G; it is now known as RIBOFLAVIN.

In 1932 a yellow enzyme necessary for cell respiration was isolated from yeast by Warburg and Christian, who also discovered that a protein and the pigment component were two factors in the enzyme. It then remained for Kuhn and his co-workers in 1935 to report on the synthesis of riboflavin and to note the relation of its activity to the green fluorescence, thereby establishing that lactoflavin and the vitamin are one and the same thing. This was the first example of a vitamin functioning as a coenzyme.

Chemistry and Characteristics Riboflavin was so named because of the similarity of part of its structure to that of the sugar ribose and because of its relation to the general group of flavins. (See Figure 12–1.) In its pure state, this vitamin is a bitter-tasting, orange-yellow, odorless compound in which the crystals are needle shaped. It dissolves sparingly in water to give a characteristic greenish yellow fluorescence. In solution it is quickly decomposed by ultraviolet rays and visible light and is sensitive to strongly alkaline solutions. This vitamin is stable to heat, to oxidizing agents, and to acids.

Measurement Riboflavin is measured in terms of milligrams or micrograms by chemical and microbiologic methods.

Physiology Riboflavin is present in the free state in foods, or in combination with phosphate, or with protein and phosphate. Riboflavin is absorbed from the upper part of the small intestine and is phosphorylated in the intestinal wall. It is present in body tissues as the coenzyme or as flavoproteins.

The body guards carefully its stores of riboflavin so that even in severe deficiency as much as one third of the normal amount has been found to be present in the liver, kidney, and heart of experimental animals. Apparently the flavin content of the body tissues cannot be increased beyond a certain point since the urinary excretion increases markedly if intake exceeds 0.75 mg per 1,000 kcal.[6] On the other hand, a decided reduction in the supply leads to restriction or even curtailment of the urinary excretion.

Functions Riboflavin is a constituent of two coenzymes: riboflavin monophosphate or FLAVIN MONONUCLEOTIDE (FMN) and FLAVIN ADENINE DINUCLEOTIDE (FAD). Both these coenzymes are prosthetic groups for aerobic dehydrogenases that act as hydrogen acceptors. The enzymes are required for the completion of several reactions in the energy cycle by which ATP is generated and in which hydrogen is transferred from one compound to another until eventually it reaches oxygen and forms water. Functionally, these enzymes are closely associated with the niacin-containing enzymes.

Riboflavin is also a component of L- and D-amino acid oxidases that oxidize amino acids and hydroxy acids to α-keto acids, and of xanthine oxidase, an enzyme that catalyzes the oxidation of a number of purines.

Daily Allowances At various times the allowances for riboflavin have been based on the calorie intake, the protein allowance, and the metabolic size. Regardless of the base used, the calculated allowance is about the same. The present recommendation of the Food and Nutrition Board is 0.6 mg per 1,000 kcal for persons of all ages.[2]

The recommended allowance for males 23 to 50 years is 1.6 mg and for females is 1.2 mg. For pregnancy and lactation, the allowances are increased by 0.3 and 0.5 mg, respectively. The infant's allowance is 0.4 to 0.6 mg, and for children to 10 years 0.8 to 1.4 mg are recommended.

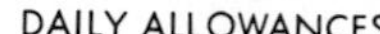

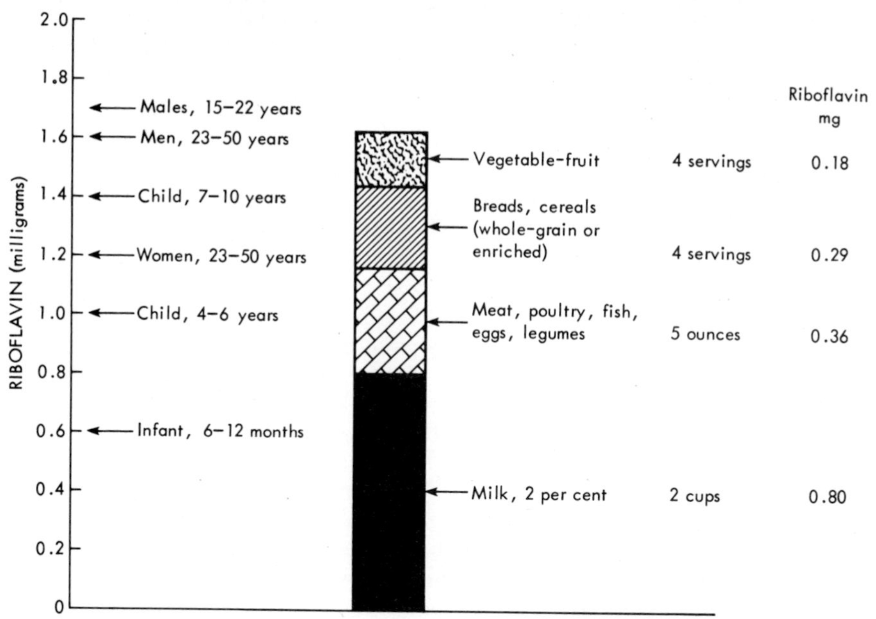

Figure 12–3. Note the important contribution of milk to the total riboflavin content of the diet. See Table 13–2 for complete calculations of the basic dietary pattern.

Hyperthyroidism, fevers, the stress of injury or surgery, and malabsorption are among the factors that increase the requirement. Achlorhydria may precipitate deficiency because the vitamin is so quickly destroyed in an alkaline medium.

Food Sources On a per capita basis the American food supply furnishes 2.44 mg riboflavin daily; 39 per cent of this is supplied by dairy products, 27 per cent by meat, fish, poultry, and eggs; and 22 per cent by cereal and flour products.[3] A diet that supplies 2 cups milk and a serving of meat daily is not likely to be deficient in riboflavin.

Liver, kidney, and heart contain considerable quantities of riboflavin, and other meats, eggs, and green leafy vegetables supply smaller, but nevertheless important, amounts. Cereals and flours are ordinarily low in riboflavin; their enrichment adds significantly to the riboflavin content of the diet.

Fruits, roots, and tubers are poor sources of riboflavin, and fats and oils are practically devoid of the vitamin. The contribution of the basic diet is shown in Figure 12–3.

Retention of Food Values Pasteurization, irradiation for vitamin D, evaporation, or drying of milk accounts for loss of not more than 10 to 20 per cent of the initial riboflavin content of milk. On the other hand, milk that is bottled in clear glass loses up to 75 per cent with 3½ hours exposure in direct sunlight. The distribution of milk in opaque containers prevents this loss.

Meats that have been stewed, roasted, or braised retain more than three fourths of the riboflavin; most of the remainder can be accounted for in the drippings. Because riboflavin is sparingly soluble, the usual cooking procedures for vegetables do not contribute to much loss, but the addition of sodium bicarbonate to preserve green color is destructive.

Effect of Deficiency Riboflavin nutriture is evaluated by determining the activity of the riboflavin-dependent enzyme, glutathione reductase, in red cells. Enzyme activity is measured *in vitro* both in the absence and presence of added FAD. Erythrocytes from persons depleted in riboflavin show a marked stimulation in glutathione reductase activity in response to added FAD. Urinary excretion of riboflavin also has been used to evaluate riboflavin nutriture but is not considered a good test because it reflects primarily recent dietary intake rather than tissue levels of the vitamin.

Little is known about the prevalence of ariboflavinosis. An individual rarely seeks medical advice for this condition alone, but it may accompany other deficiencies especially of the B-complex vitamins. Based on determination of erythrocyte glutathione reductase activity, a deficiency of riboflavin was found in 26 per cent of an adolescent population of low socioeconomic status in New York City. Prevalence of deficiency was highest among those consuming less than 1 cup of milk per week.[7] Depletion of tissue riboflavin may be produced temporarily in babies receiving phototherapy as treatment for hyperbilirubinemia but no long-term effects are believed to occur.

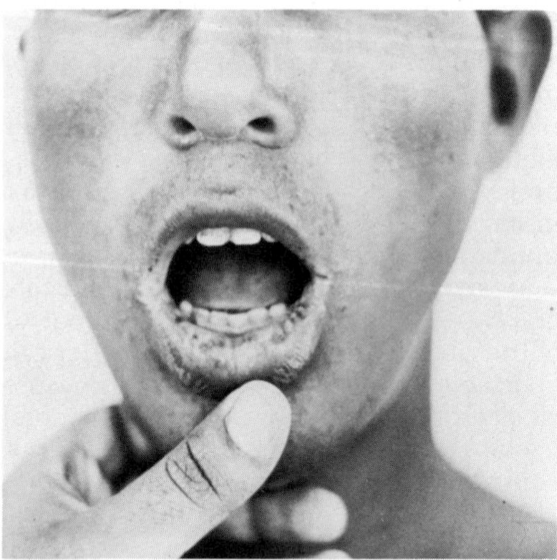

Figure 12–4. Cheilosis—lesions of the lips and fissures at the angles of the mouth. (Courtesy, Nutrition Section, National Institutes of Health.)

Symptoms. In 1939 Sebrell and Butler studied a group of women whom they placed on a diet extremely low in riboflavin. This diet in the course of 94 to 130 days led to such symptoms as a greasy dermatitis around the folds of the nose, a cracking of the lips at the corners (CHEILOSIS), glossitis, and increased vascularization of the cornea.[8] The lips and tongue assumed a purplish red and shiny appearance in contrast to the scarlet color seen in niacin deficiency. (See Figure 12–4.)

Ocular manifestations may be among the earliest signs of riboflavin deficiency. The eyes become sensitive to light and easily fatigued. There is also blurring of the vision, itching, watering, and soreness of the eyes. An increased number of capillaries may develop in the cornea, and the eye becomes bloodshot in appearance. Some of these changes in the eye and appearance of the tongue have not been observed in other controlled studies.[9]

Growth failure is characteristic in young animals, and would also apply if children fail to receive minimum requirements for riboflavin. The appetite, attitude, and activity are not adversely affected with riboflavin lack as they are in thiamin deficiency. No human deaths have been reported because of riboflavin deficiency.

Niacin (Nicotinic Acid and Nicotinamide)

Early Studies In 1735 a Spanish physician, Casals, described a disease, *mal de la rosa,* which came to be known as PELLAGRA, a term of Italian origin meaning "rough skin." In the early part of this century it was one of the leading causes of mental illness and of death in this country. Its causes had been variously ascribed to toxic substances present in corn, infections from microorganisms, of toxicity produced by exposure to the sun, lack of tryptophan in the diet, and amino acid imbalance.

Goldberger, of the U.S. Public Health Service, who was assigned to study the problem of pellagra in the South, early noted that the disease was almost always associated with poverty and ignorance and that hospital attendants who worked with the patients never contracted the disease. In 1915 he performed a classic experiment on twelve prisoners who were promised release in return for their cooperation in eating a diet representative of the poorer classes in the southern states.[10] The diet consisted of sweet potatoes, corn bread, cabbage, rice, collards, fried mush, brown gravy, corn grits, syrup, sugar, biscuits, and black coffee. After a few weeks the prisoners developed headache, abdominal pain, and general weakness, and in about 5 months the typical dermatitis of pellagra appeared. Goldberger then suggested the existence of a pellagra-preventing (P-P) factor and related it to the B vitamins.

Identification of the Vitamin Goldberger in 1922 concluded that blacktongue in dogs was similar to pellagra in humans. Nicotinic acid had been known as a chemical substance since 1867, but it remained for Elvehjem and his co-workers in 1937 to discover its effectiveness as a curative agent for blacktongue in dogs.[11] Following this discovery, Smith, Spies, and others were soon making reports of dramatic clinical improvement in pellagrous patients who had been given nicotinic acid. The term *niacin* was suggested by Cowgill to avoid association with the nicotine of tobacco.

Chemistry and Characteristics NICOTINIC ACID and NIACINAMIDE (see Figure 12–1) are organic compounds of relatively simple structure with equal biologic activity. NIACIN is the generic term that includes both forms. The two forms are white, bitter-tasting compounds, moderately soluble in hot water but only slightly soluble in cold water. Niacin is very stable to alkali, acid, heat, light, and oxidation; even boiling and autoclaving do not decrease its potency.

Measurement Niacin is measured in milligrams by using chemical methods or microbiologic assay.

Physiology Niacin is readily absorbed from the small intestine. Some reserves are found in the body, but, as with other B-complex vitamins, the amount appears to be limited so that a day-to-day supply is desirable. Any excess of niacin is excreted in the urine as N-methylnicotinamide and N-methyl pyridone. In a deficiency such as pellagra the metabolites in the urine diminish markedly or are absent.

Tryptophan, one of the essential amino acids, is a precursor of niacin so that a diet that contains a liberal amount of tryptophan will provide enough niacin even though the diet is low in preformed niacin. Milk and eggs are excellent sources of tryptophan but poor sources of preformed niacin; their pellagra-preventive characteristics have long been known.

Niacin is not toxic in amounts that considerably exceed recommended allowances. In pharmacologic doses nicotinic acid but not nicotinamide brings about some vasodilation and consequent flushing of the skin and tingling sensations. Other adverse effects of long-term use that may occur are elevation of serum uric acid, impairment of glucose tolerance, and liver damage. From 3 to 6 gm of nicotinic acid have been prescribed to reduce the blood levels of cholesterol, beta-lipoproteins, and triglycerides.[12] Although use of nicotinamide would be preferable because of its lack of toxicity, it unfortunately is ineffective in lowering blood lipids.

Functions Like other B-complex vitamins, niacin is a constituent of coenzymes involved in glycolysis, tissue respiration, and fat synthesis. NICOTINAMIDE ADENINE DINUCLEOTIDE (NAD) contains nicotinamide, ribose, two phosphate groups, and adenine; it is also referred to in the literature as diphosphopyridine nucleotide (DPN) or coenzyme I. NICOTINAMIDE ADENINE DINUCLEOTIDE PHOSPHATE (NADP) is similar to NAD except that it contains three phosphate groupings; it was formerly known as triphosphopyridine nucleotide (TPN) or coenzyme II.

NAD and NADP are hydrogen acceptors involved in many reactions. For example, the complex reaction required for the decarboxylation of pyruvic acid and the formation of acetyl coenzyme A requires dehydrogenation by NAD (see also page 84); NAD and NADP are involved in dehydrogenation reactions in the Krebs cycle; hydrogen is transferred from NAD to FAD to cytochrome c in the respiratory chain in which ATP is liberated. (See page 84.)

In the pentose shunt (see page 84) NADP is the hydrogen acceptor for two reactions, thereby forming NADPH. The latter is required for the synthesis of fatty acids and cholesterol, and for the conversion of phenylalanine to tyrosine.

Daily Allowances Recommended intakes of niacin are expressed as niacin equivalents (NE) in which 1 NE is equal to 1 mg niacin or 60 mg of dietary tryptophan. Symptoms of pellagra can be prevented by a daily intake of 4.4 mg niacin per 1,000 kcal. The recommended allowances provide about 50 per cent margin of safety and are based on 6.6 mg NE per 1,000 kcal.[2]

For the reference man, 23 to 50 years, the allowance is 18 mg NE and for the reference woman is 13 mg NE. An addition of 2 and 5 mg NE are recommended during pregnancy and lactation, respectively. From 6 to 8 mg NE are recommended during the first year, and 9 to 16 mg NE for children up to 10 years. For boys and girls 11 to 14 years, allowances are 18 and 15 mg, respectively.

As with the other B-complex vitamins, the niacin requirements are increased whenever metabolism is accelerated as by fever and the stress of injury or surgery.

Sources A diet that furnishes the recommended allowances for protein also provides enough niacin inasmuch as protein will supply tryptophan for conversion to niacin, and the protein-rich foods are generally, except for milk, rich sources of preformed niacin. Animal proteins contain about 1.4 per cent tryptophan, and plant proteins about 1 per cent tryptophan.[2] If one assumes that a mixed diet provides 1 per cent of the protein as tryptophan, then an intake of 65 gm protein is equivalent to 650 mg tryptophan, or 10.8 mg niacin.

Poultry, meats, and fish constitute the most important single food group insofar as preformed niacin is concerned. (See Figure 12–5.) Organ meats, peanuts, peanut butter, and brewers' yeast are rich sources, but are not ordinarily consumed in sufficient amounts to greatly affect the dietary level.

Whole grains are fair sources of niacin but most of this is in a bound form which may not be completely available. The effect of cooking on the bound form is not known.

Potatoes, legumes, and some green leafy vegetables contain fair amounts of preformed niacin, but most fruits and vegetables are poor sources—as are also milk and cheese.

Retention of Food Values The cookery of foods does not result in serious losses of niacin, except insofar as part of the soluble vitamin may be discarded in cooking waters which are not used. The application of principles for the retention of ascorbic acid and thiamin which have been discussed earlier will result in maximum retention of niacin as well.

Effect of Deficiency Pellagra appears after months of dietary deprivation. The phenomenal decrease in the incidence of pellagra in the United States may be attributed to several factors including the enrichment program which is mandatory in some states, the concerted efforts in nutrition education, and the improvement in income. Pellagra is still a public health problem in some countries such as Spain, Yugoslavia, and certain areas of Africa. It tends to occur most often in areas where corn is the major source of protein and calories in the diet.

Symptoms and clinical findings. Pellagra involves the gastrointestinal tract, the

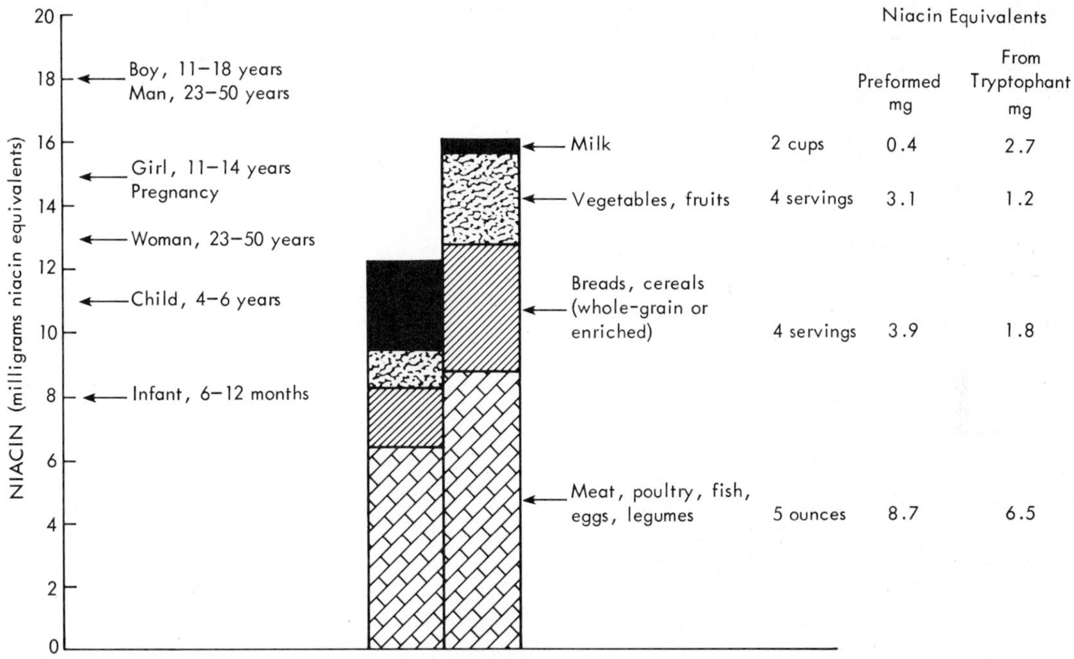

Figure 12–5. Preformed niacin and the niacin equivalents from protein provide the recommended allowances for niacin for all age-sex categories when recommended amounts of the foods in the basic dietary pattern are consumed. Note the important contribution made by the meat group. Note also that milk contributes little preformed niacin but, through its tryptophan content, makes a substantial contribution. See Table 13–2 for calculation of the basic dietary pattern. (Calculations based on tryptophan as 1 per cent of protein. See Table 13–2.)

skin, and the nervous system. Although no two cases of pellagra are exactly alike, the following symptoms are characteristic.

1. Early signs include fatigue, listlessness, headache, backache, loss of weight, loss of appetite, and general poor health.

2. Sore tongue, mouth, and throat, with glossitis extending throughout the gastrointestinal tract, are present. The tongue and lips become abnormally red in color. The mouth becomes so sore that it is difficult to eat and swallow.

3. A deficiency of hydrochloric acid with a resultant anemia similar to pernicious anemia may be found.

4. Nausea and vomiting are followed by severe diarrhea.

5. A characteristic symmetric dermatitis especially on the exposed surfaces of the body—hands, forearms, elbows, feet, legs, knees, and neck—appears. (See Figure 12–6.) The dermatitis is sharply separated from the surrounding normal skin. At first the skin becomes red, somewhat swollen, and tender, resembling a mild sunburn; if the condition is untreated, the skin becomes rough, cracked, and scaly and may become ulcerated. Sunshine and exposure to heat aggravate the dermatitis.

6. Neurologic symptoms which include confusion, dizziness, poor memory, and irritability, and leading to hallucinations, delusions of persecution, and dementia, are noted as severity increases.

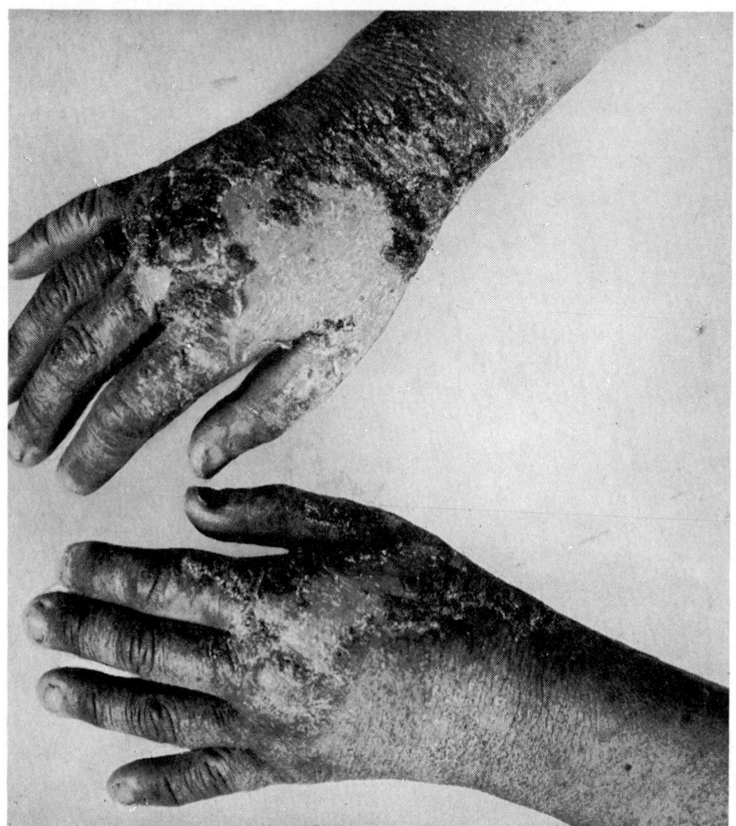

Figure 12–6. Dermatitis of pellagra.

The classic "D's" are the final stages of the disease—dermatitis, diarrhea, dementia, and death.

Treatment and Prophylaxis Treatment includes 300 to 500 mg nicotinamide daily in divided doses as well as supplements of other nutrients which frequently are deficient.[13] Initially the diet should be soft so that it can be easily eaten while the person is acutely ill. Obviously, prophylaxis must include careful and persistent education in dietary improvement, emphasis upon enrichment programs, and efforts to improve the economic status of affected populations.

Vitamin B-6

Discovery Goldberger and Lillie in 1926 provided a description of dermatitis in rats that was recognized several years later to be characteristic of vitamin B-6 deficiency. In 1934 György reported that vitamin B-2 consisted of two factors—riboflavin, and another factor which he named vitamin B-6 prevented skin lesions (acrodynia) in rats. In 1938 the isolation of a crystalline compound with vitamin B-6 activity was reported by several laboratories, followed by identification of the chemical structure by Harris and Folkers and its synthesis by Kuhn and Wendt in 1939.

Chemistry and Characteristics Vitamin B-6 consists of a group of related pyridines: PYRIDOXINE, PYRIDOXAL, and PYRIDOXAMINE. (See Figure 12–1.) These may appear in tissues and foodstuffs in the free form, or combined with phosphate, or with phosphate and protein. The preferred terminology is vitamin B-6; pyridoxine, being only one of the three active forms, is not entirely synonymous.

Vitamin B-6 is soluble in water and relatively stable to heat and to acids. It is destroyed in alkaline solutions and is also sensitive to light. Of the three forms, pyridoxine is more resistant to food processing and storage conditions and probably represents the principal form in food products.

Measurement Vitamin B-6 concentrations are expressed in milligrams or micrograms. The vitamin is determined in tissues and foods by chemical or fluorometric procedures. Because the vitamin occurs in various bound forms, some difficulties have been experienced in providing acceptable tabulations for food values.

Physiology The active form of vitamin B-6 is the coenzyme pyridoxal phosphate, which can be formed from any of the three compounds. Since vitamin B-6 is water soluble, the body stores are small; about half of it is in the form of glycogen phosphorylase. All forms of the vitamin may be excreted in the urine, but the principal metabolite is pyridoxic acid.

Functions Pyridoxal phosphate is the coenzyme for a large number of enzyme systems, most of which are involved in amino acid metabolism. Following are a few examples:

Decarboxylation. The removal of the carboxyl group from amino acids requires enzymes that contain pyridoxal phosphate. Each of the amino acids is decarboxylated by a specific enzyme. For example, the decarboxylation of tryptophan produces tryptamine and carbon dioxide. Serotonin is also produced by decarboxylation of tryptophan and is a potent vasoconstrictor as well as an agent in the regulation of brain and other tissues.

Transamination. Each of the many transaminases involves a distinct protein for which pyridoxal phosphate is the coenzyme. One example of transamination is shown on page 60. In the reaction, the amino group is removed from an amino acid and transferred to a keto acid, thus forming a new amino acid. This reaction is important in the formation of the nonessential amino acids.

Transulfuration. This involves the removal and transfer of sulfur groups from the sulfur-containing amino acids such as cysteine by transulfurases.

Tryptophan conversion to niacin. The importance of tryptophan as a source of niacin has been described on page 225. Several steps are required in this conversion, one of which is catalyzed by vitamin B-6.

Pyridoxal phosphate is also required for glycogen phosphorylase, an enzyme by which glycogen is broken down to glucose; for the formation of antibodies; for the synthesis of a precursor of the porphyrin ring which is part of the hemoglobin molecule; and possibly for the conversion of linoleic acid to arachidonic acid.

Daily Allowances The need for vitamin B-6 is proportional to the amount of protein metabolized. The recommended allowances are 2.2 mg daily for adult men and 2.0 mg for women.[2] These amounts provide a reasonable margin of safety and permit a protein intake of 100 gm or more. Those who ingest a low-protein diet (40 to 50 gm) require only 1.2 to 1.5 mg.

The allowance for infants is 0.3 to 0.6 mg; for children 1 to 10 years, it increases gradually from 0.9 to 1.6 mg; and for adolescents, recommended intakes are 1.8 to 2.0 mg. During pregnancy an additional 0.6 mg is recommended which is decreased to 0.5 mg during lactation.

Food Sources The vitamin B-6 available in the American food supply per capita is 2.05 mg. The principal source is meat, poultry, and fish, with this group accounting for 40 per cent of the total amount available. Potatoes, sweet potatoes and vegetables account for about 22 per cent of the total supply; dairy products, 12 per cent; and flour and cereals, 10 per cent.[3] Whole grains are good sources of pyridoxine, but most of this is lost in the milling of the grains.

Effects of Deficiency The TRYPTOPHAN LOAD TEST has been widely used to measure vitamin B-6 adequacy. In this test a measured dose of tryptophan is given after which the 24-hour urinary excretion of xanthurenic acid is measured. XANTHURENIC ACID is an intermediary metabolite of tryptophan metabolism that is excreted when there is insufficient vitamin B-6 to catalyze the reactions throughout the normal pathway. An excretion of more than 50 mg is indicative of vitamin B-6 deficiency. Reduced levels of serum and red blood cell transaminases and lowered excretion of pyridoxic acid are also found in vitamin B-6 deficiency. With the availability of improved methods of analyses, a reduction in plasma and erythrocyte concentrations of pyridoxal phosphate likewise has been demonstrated.

Deficiency in infants. In the 1950s vitamin B-6 deficiency was reported in infants who had received a commercial formula in which the pyridoxine had been inadvertently destroyed in the processing of the milk. The infants showed nervous irritability and convulsive seizures. Other related symptoms included anemia, vomiting, weakness, ataxia, and abdominal pain. The convulsive seizures responded dramatically to the administration of pyridoxine.[14,15]

Deficiency in adults. A number of studies in college students fed vitamin B-6 deficient diets have shown a rapid fall in urinary excretion of vitamin B-6 and pyridoxic acid as well as decreased blood concentrations of pyridoxal phosphate. Soon after these changes appeared, increased excretion of xanthurenic acid was found with the tryptophan load test.[16] Despite this biochemical evidence of deficiency, no clear-cut symptoms have been observed in adults. However, when an antagonist such as deoxypyridoxine is fed together with a diet deficient in vitamin B-6, seborrheic dermatitis around the eyes, eyebrows, and angles of the mouth has been described.[17] Large doses of vitamin B-6 will counteract the effect of the antagonist.

Isonicotinic acid hydrazide (INH) is widely used in the treatment of tuberculosis. It is chemically related to pyridoxine and acts as an antagonist to vitamin B-6 activity. Patients who have been treated with this drug have experienced neuritic symptoms believed to be caused by the imposed vitamin B-6 deficiency, and the condition was corrected when additional vitamin supplements were prescribed. Penicillamine, a drug used in the treatment of Wilson's disease and cystinuria, is also an antagonist of vitamin B-6. Vitamin B-6 supplements are usually prescribed when this drug is used.

During pregnancy and in women who are using the steroid contraceptive pill there is increased excretion of xanthurenic acid following the tryptophan load test and lower blood transaminase activity. The biochemical changes are readily corrected by increasing the intake of vitamin B-6 but there is little indication that there is any physiologic advantage.[2]

Vitamin B-6 dependency. An inborn error of metabolism has been described in which convulsive seizures are controlled by up to 200 to 600 mg pyridoxine hydrochloride daily.[18]

The effect of megadoses of pyridoxine was tested on normal individuals by giving 200 mg pyridoxine daily for 33 days. When these large doses were withdrawn, the individuals required greater-than-normal intakes of vitamin B-6 to maintain normal biochemical levels.[2] Because such megadoses can induce vitamin B-6 dependency, their use is contraindicated as a routine measure.

Pantothenic Acid

Discovery Pantothenic acid was isolated in 1938 by Dr. R. J. Williams and synthesized in 1940 by workers in the laboratories of Merck and Company. Although tests showed its vitamin nature by its ability to prevent certain deficiencies in animals, little interest was shown in this vitamin until about a decade later. In 1946 Lipmann and his associates showed that coenzyme A was essential for acetylation reactions in the body, and in 1950 reports from this same laboratory showed pantothenic acid to be a constituent of coenzyme A. The name for this vitamin is derived from the Greek word *panthos,* meaning "everywhere." The universal distribution of this vitamin in biologic materials suggests the key role that it plays in metabolism.

Characteristics PANTOTHENIC ACID, as the free acid, is an unstable, viscous yellow oil, soluble in water. (See Figure 12–1.) Commercially, it is available as the sodium or calcium salt, which is slightly sweet, water soluble, and quite stable. There is little loss of the vitamin with ordinary cooking procedures, except in acid and alkaline solutions.

The pantothenic acid content of tissues and foods is determined by microbiological, chemical, or radioimmunoassay methods; values are expressed in milligrams or micrograms.

Functions Coenzyme A is the form in which pantothenic acid functions in the body. Coenzyme A is a complex molecule consisting of a sulfur-containing compound, adenine, ribose, phosphoric acid, and pantothenic acid. The sulfur linkage is highly reactive.

Coenzyme A functions in reactions that accept or remove the acetyl group ($-CH_3CO$). One of these reactions is the formation of acetylcholine, a substance of importance in the transmission of the nerve impulse. Coenzyme A participates in the oxidation of pyruvate, α-ketoglutarate, and fatty acids. (See Figure 5–5 and page 84.) Coenzyme A reacts with pyruvic acid to form acetyl coenzyme A, which, in turn, combines with oxalacetate to form citrate, thus initiating the tricarboxylic acid cycle for the release of energy. Coenzyme A is also involved in the synthesis of fatty acids, cholesterol and other sterols, and porphyrin in the hemoglobin molecule.

Coenzyme A is synthesized in all cells and apparently does not cross cell membranes. Liver, kidney, brain, adrenal, and heart tissues, being metabolically active, contain high concentrations.

Requirement The daily requirement is not known, but the Food and Nutrition Board has estimated the safe and adequate daily intake to be 4 to 7 mg for adults. The customary intake of pantothenic acid from ordinary foods in the United States is approximately 7 mg per day.[3] Intakes of 2 to 3 mg for infants and 3 to 5 mg for children are believed to be satisfactory.

Food Sources Most of the pantothenic acid in animal tissues is in the form of coenzyme A. As its name indicates, pantothenic acid is widely distributed in animal foods and in whole grains and legumes. Liver, yeast, egg yolk, and meat are particularly good sources. Fruits, vegetables, and milk contain smaller amounts. About 50 per cent of the pantothenic acid of grains is lost in their milling, and dry processing of foods also leads to significant losses.

Effects of Deficiency No clear-cut demonstration of pantothenic acid deficiency has been afforded by experimental diets low in pantothenic acid. When an antagonist, omega methyl panthothenic acid, was fed with deficient diets, the following symptoms were observed: loss of appetite, indigestion, abdominal pain; sullenness, mental depression; peripheral neuritis with cramping pains in the arms and legs; burning sensations in the feet; insomnia; and respiratory infections. In these subjects there was an increased sensitivity to insulin, and increased sedimentation rate for erythrocytes, and marked decrease in antibody formation.[19,20]

The neuropathy observed in alcoholics is possibly related to pantothenic acid deficiency. However, when diets are deficient in pantothenic acid, they are also deficient in many other factors, and therefore the separation of symptoms attributable to the lack of various nutrients becomes exceedingly difficult.

Biotin

Discovery In the 1920s a factor essential for the growth of yeast was described and named *bios*. In the 1930s Dr. Helen Parsons and her co-workers and others reported on the symptoms observed in rats that were fed a diet including raw egg white. The animals lost their fur, particularly around the eyes, giving a spectacle-like appearance; there was rapid loss of weight, paralysis of the hind legs, and eventual cyanosis and death. The symptoms did not occur when cooked egg white was used.[21]

Small quantities of the active factor were isolated from egg yolk in 1936 by Kögl and were later established as being identical with the yeast growth factor and the anti-egg-white injury factor.

The substance in raw egg white has been found to be a glycoprotein that binds biotin and thereby prevents its absorption from the intestinal tract. It is called AVIDIN, which means "hungry albumin." Heating of egg white inactivates the binding capacity of avidin.

Characteristics BIOTIN is a relatively simple compound, a cyclic urea derivative, which contains a sulfur grouping. (See Figure 12–1.) In its free form it is a crystalline substance, very stable to heat, light, and acids. It is somewhat labile to alkaline solutions and to oxidizing agents. In tissues and in foods it is usually combined with protein.

Functions and Metabolism Biotin is a coenzyme of a number of enzymes that participate in carboxylation, decarboxylation, and deamination reactions. For example, it is required in the synthesis of fatty acids. Another reaction catalyzed by biotin-containing enzymes is the fixation of CO_2 in the conversion of pyruvate to oxalacetate, an important reaction that generates the tricarboxylic acid cycle (see Figure 5–5). Within the TCA cycle, biotin is also required for the conversion of succinate to fumarate and oxalsuccinate to ketoglutarate.

Biotin is essential for the introduction of CO_2 in the formation of purines, these compounds being essential constituents of DNA and RNA. The deaminases for threonine, serine, and aspartic acid also require biotin as a coenzyme.

Biotin is stored in minute amounts principally in the metabolically active tissues such as the kidney, liver, brain, and adrenal. The biotin content of the feces and likewise of the urinary excretion is considerably greater than the dietary intake. This indicates the intestinal synthesis of biotin and the absorption of the vitamin from this source.

Dietary Needs A recommended dietary allowance for biotin has not been established. The estimated safe and adequate daily intake of 100 to 200 μg recommended by the Food and Nutrition Board for adults is based on reports indicating 100 to 300 μg of biotin in the average American diet.[2] Similar estimates are 35 to 50 μg for infants and 65 to 85 μg for children.

Good dietary sources of biotin include organ meats, egg yolk, legumes, and nuts. Cereal grains, muscle meats, and milk contain only small amounts.

Effects of Deficiency Biotin deficiency has been described in human beings only when large amounts of raw egg whites were fed. Four volunteer subjects were fed an experimental diet containing approximately 3,000 kcal, low in biotin, and including 928 of the total calories from egg white (equivalent to about 60 egg whites!) for a period of 10 weeks. Beginning with the third to fourth weeks symptoms appeared approximately in this order: scaly desquamation, lassitude, muscle pains, hyperesthesia, pallor of skin and mucous membranes, anorexia, and nausea. The hemoglobin levels were lowered, the blood cholesterol levels were increased, and the urinary excretion of biotin dropped to about one tenth of the normal levels. All of these abnormalities were cured within 5 days when 150 μg biotin was given daily.[22]

Recently biotin deficiency was reported in a 62-year-old woman with Laennec's cirrhosis who, on a physician's advice, had ingested six raw eggs daily for 18 months in an effort to regenerate liver tissue. Her symptoms included anorexia, nausea, vomiting, pallor, lassitude, scaly dermatitis, and desquamation of the lips. All these promptly disappeared or significantly improved within a few days following the daily parenteral administration of 200 μg biotin.[23]

Considerable evidence exists indicating that a type of seborrheic dermatitis in young infants is due to biotin deficiency. Blood levels and urinary excretion of the vitamin are depressed. Prompt improvement is achieved by administration of 5 mg biotin daily for 10 days either intravenously or intramuscularly.[24]

Vitamin B-12

Discovery Until the 1920s pernicious anemia was an invariably fatal disease. Then came the dramatic announcement by Minot and Murphy[25] that large amounts of liver—about a pound a day—would control the anemia and prevent the neurologic changes.

Castle set forth the hypothesis that liver contained a substance which he termed the EXTRINSIC FACTOR (now known to be vitamin B-12) and that its absorption required another principle in normal gastric secretion which he called the INTRINSIC FACTOR. Patients with pernicious anemia were lacking the intrinsic factor. Nevertheless, when very large amounts of liver were consumed, some absorption of the extrinsic factor took place by simple diffusion.

The active principle in liver was extracted in the 1930s and provided the basis for the treatment of patients by injection. Then in 1948 came the announcement by Rickes and his associates in the United States[26] and Smith and Parker in England[27] of the isolation of a few micrograms of a red crystalline substance that was shown to be dramatically effective in the remission of pernicious anemia. The structure of this complex molecule was elucidated in 1955, and synthesis was accomplished by Woodward and others just 25 years after its isolation.[28]

Characteristics Vitamin B-12 is the most complex of all vitamin molecules and contains a single atom of cobalt held in a structure similar to that which holds iron in hemoglobin and magnesium in chlorophyll. (See Figure 12–7.) It occurs in several forms designated as COBALAMINS. Cyanocobalamin, the form available commercially, is the most stable form but is present in the body only in small amounts. Forms found in plasma and tissues include methylcobalamin, hydroxycobalamin, and adenosylcobalamin.

Cyanocobalamin forms deep red needlelike crystals which are slightly soluble in water, stable to heat, but inactivated by light and by strong acid or alkaline solutions. Large amounts of ascorbic acid present in a meal or added to serum samples may lead to destruction of vitamin B-12. There is little loss of vitamin B-12 in food by ordinary cooking procedures.

Vitamin B-12 is assayed microbiologically or by radioassay, and is measured in micrograms or picograms (pg, μμg, micromicrograms).

Metabolism Vitamin B-12, being a very large molecule, requires a special mechanism for absorption, including at least five steps: (1) vitamin B-12 is separated from its polypeptide linkages with food by the gastric acid and enzymes; (2) vitamin B-12 is bound to intrinsic factor which is secreted by the parietal cells in the cardia and fundus of the stomach; (3) the vitamin B-12-intrinsic factor complex in the presence of calcium is bound to receptor sites in the ileum; (4) the vitamin is released from the complex and transferred across the mucosal epithelium; (5) vitamin B-12 is bound to a protein, TRANSCOBALAMIN II, for transport in the blood circulation.

Intrinsic factor regulates the amount of absorption to about 2.5 to 3 μg daily.[29] When the dietary intake is only 1 to 2 μg daily, 60 to 80 per cent is absorbed. With good diets young men averaged 10 per cent

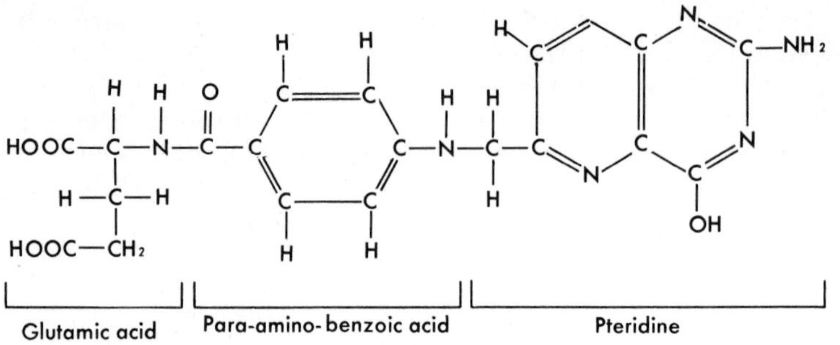

Glutamic acid Para-amino-benzoic acid Pteridine

Folic acid ($C_{19}H_{19}N_7O_6$; m.w. 441.4)

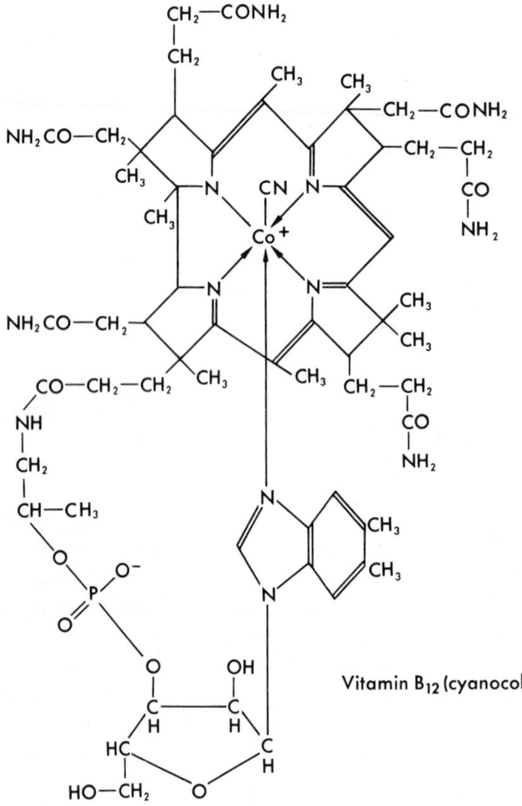

Vitamin B_{12} (cyanocobalamin shown

Figure 12–7. Folic acid and vitamin B-12 are essential for the regeneration of red blood cells. Vitamin B-12 has the most complex structure of any of the vitamins. Note the similarity of the position of cobalt in the structure to the position of iron in hemoglobin and of magnesium in chlorophyll.

absorption and elderly men about 5 per cent. Absorption is greater if the vitamin is present in three meals than if it is all provided in a single meal.

The liver is the principal site of storage for vitamin B-12. Storage in the bone marrow is limited, and amounts to only 1 to 2 per cent of that in the liver. The enterohepatic circulation varies from 0.6 to 6 μg daily of vitamin B-12 with practically complete reabsorption taking place. Thus, the normal liver store of 2,000 to 5,000 μg is sufficient to take care of body needs for 3 to 5 years.

The serum concentration of vitamin B-12 is 200 to 900 pg per milliliter. A level of 80 pg per milliliter represents unequivocal deficiency.

Functions Vitamin B-12 functions in all cells, but especially those of the gastrointestinal tract, the nervous system, and the bone marrow. Within the bone marrow a vitamin B-12 coenzyme participates in the synthesis of DNA. When DNA is not being synthesized, the erythroblasts do not divide but increase in size, becoming megaloblasts which are released into the circulation. Whether the influence of vitamin B-12 is a direct action or a facilitation of the use of folic acid is not understood.

Vitamin B-12 is required for enzymes that accomplish the synthesis and transfer of single-carbon units such as the methyl group, for example, the synthesis of methionine and choline, which are important lipotropic factors. Conversion of methylmalonate, which is formed during degradation of certain amino acids and odd-chain fatty acids, to succinate also requires vitamin B-12 coenzymes. An increase in urinary excretion of methylmalonate occurs in vitamin B-12 deficiency and may be useful in diagnosis.

Dietary Needs A minimum intake of 0.6 to 1.2 μg of vitamin B-12 daily is sufficient for normal hematopoiesis and good health, but will not replenish liver stores. The recommended allowance for persons over 6 years is 3 μg daily, and 4 μg for pregnancy and lactation.[2] For infants from birth to 6 months, 0.5 μg is recommended daily. The allowance is 1.5 μg for older infants, 2.0 μg for children 1 to 3 years, and 2.5 μg for those 4 to 6 years.

The vitamin B-12 available per capita in the American food supply is 9.3 μg of which 68 per cent is supplied by meats, poultry, and fish, 21 per cent by dairy foods excluding butter, and 10 per cent by eggs.[3] Plant foods do not supply vitamin B-12.

Effects of Deficiency Vitamin B-12 deficiency is a defect of absorption and rarely of dietary lack. Pernicious anemia is a disease, probably of genetic origin, in which intrinsic factor is not produced, and consequently vitamin B-12 is not absorbed. The bone marrow is unable to produce mature red blood cells, but releases fewer large cells (macrocytes) into the circulation. Thus, the capacity to carry hemoglobin is reduced. The characteristic symptoms include pallor, anorexia, dyspnea, prolonged bleeding time, abdominal discomfort, loss of weight, glossitis, neurologic disturbances including unsteady gait, and mental depression. Patients respond to as little as 1 μg given parenterally; usually, initial therapy provides 50 to 100 μg until the anemia is corrected, after which maintenance therapy is given monthly and averages 1 μg daily.[30]

Megaloblastic anemia from vitamin B-12 deficiency also occurs following surgical removal of the part of the stomach that produces intrinsic factor, or the part of the ileum where the absorption sites are located. Such deficiency occurs 3 to 5 years following the surgery and can be prevented by injections of vitamin B-12 at periodic intervals. Malabsorption syndromes such as sprue may also be characterized by megaloblastic anemias resulting from deficient absorption of vitamin B-12 as well as folic acid.

Dietary deficiency of vitamin B-12 has been described in vegetarians who consumed no animal foods whatsoever.[31] They showed low serum levels of vitamin B-12, glossitis, paresthesias, and some changes in the spinal cord but did not have the characteristic anemia. For strict vegetarians a supplement of vitamin B-12 is indicated.

A few cases of children with genetic disorders interfering with vitamin B-12 utilization have been described.[32] In one of these the defect was apparently an inability to bind the vitamin B-12-intrinsic factor complex to the ileal receptor sites. In another there was absence of the protein that binds vitamin B-12 in the circulation. A defect in transport across the mucosal membrane was observed in another. Injections of vitamin B-12, sometimes in large doses, were required to maintain normal blood values.

Folacin (Folic Acid)

Discovery During the 1930s and 1940s many investigators had described water-soluble factors required by various animal species and microorganisms and given them names such as factor U (unknown factor required for chick growth); vitamin B_c (antianemia factor for chicks); Wills factor for treatment of tropical macrocytic anemia of pregnancy described by Dr. Lucy Wills; vitamin M, essential for monkeys; L-casei factor, citrovorum factor, and SLR factor for growth of various microorganisms. Folic acid was named in 1941 by Mitchell and his associates. The name was chosen because of the factor's prevalence in green leaves: *folium* is the Latin word for leaf. In 1945 the identification of the structure and the synthesis of folic acid by Angier and his co-workers at Lederle Laboratories established that these variously named factors were one and the same substance. That same year Dr. Tom Spies showed that folic acid was effective in the treatment of megaloblastic anemia of pregnancy and of tropical sprue.

Characteristics FOLACIN is the generic term for folic acid, pteroylglutamic acid, and other compounds having the activity of folic acid. It consists of three linked components: a pteridine grouping, para-aminobenzoic acid, and glutamic acid, an amino acid. (See Figure 12–7).

Polyglutamate forms of folacin having from two to eight glutamic acid groups are common in foods and body tissues.[33] The major form in cabbage, for example, has seven groups and is known as hepta-pteroylglutamic acid.

Pure folic acid occurs as a bright yellow crystalline compound, only slightly soluble in water and quite stable at pH 5 and above even with heating at 100°C. It is easily oxidized in an acid medium and is sensitive to light.

Folic acid is measured in micrograms or nanograms (ng, millimicrograms) and is assayed microbiologically or by colorimetric or fluorometric methods.

Metabolism About 25 per cent of folacin in foods is in the free form and is readily absorbed. Before the polyglutamate forms can be absorbed, the extra glutamate groups must be removed by conjugase, an enzyme present in the mucosal cells of the proximal intestine. Efficiency of absorption of dietary folacin varies considerably depending on the presence of conjugase inhibitors or other unidentified interfering factors in foods.

Folacin is stored principally in the liver. The active form is TETRAHYDROFOLIC ACID. Ascorbic acid prevents the oxidation of this active form and thus maintains an adequate level of the folate for metabolic needs.[34]

Functions After absorption folacin undergoes a series of reactions to form coenzymes known as tetrahydrofolates. These are linked to single carbon groupings: methyl ($—CH_3$); hydroxymethyl ($—CH_2OH$); formyl ($—OCH$); and formimino ($—CH{=}NH$). The ability to link up with and to donate these single carbon units leads to the synthesis of methionine from homocysteine; the formation of choline; and the synthesis of serine, a 3-carbon amino acid, from glycine, a 2-carbon amino acid. Folacin is essential to DNA synthesis, and thus, together with vitamin B-12, regulates the formation of normal red blood cells in the bone marrow.

Because of the importance of folacin in protein synthesis, folacin inhibitors such as methotrexate have been used successfully in the chemotherapy of various types of cancer to inhibit tumor growth and cell proliferation.

Recommended Allowances An allowance of 400 μg is recommended for adults. For pregnancy the allowance is 800 μg and for lactation it is 500 μg; during the first year of life the needs are met with 30 to 45 μg daily.

Food Sources Folic acid is widely distributed in foods in both free and conjugate forms. The availability of the latter to meet body needs is not known. Liver, kidney, yeast, and deep green leafy vegetables are excellent sources; lean beef, veal, eggs, and whole-grain cereals are good sources; and root vegetables, dairy foods, pork, and light green vegetables are relatively low in the vitamin. As much as 50 to 95 per cent of the folacin content of food may be destroyed by extended cooking or other processing.[35]

Effects of Deficiency Folic acid deficiency results from inadequate dietary intake or is secondary to disease. In many instances dietary surveys have shown the intake to be considerably below the recommended allowances, but without accompanying biochemical or subjective signs of deficiency.[36] This suggests that utilization of conjugated forms may be higher than anticipated in setting up the allowances or that the margin of safety is high.

With a deficiency the serum folate level is reduced and changes take place in the production of red blood cells in the bone marrow. The anemia that results from folic acid deficiency is characterized by a reduction in the number of red blood cells, the release into the blood circulation of large nucleated cells (hence the designation macrocytic, or megaloblastic, anemia), low hemoglobin levels but a high color content of each cell, and lowered leukocyte and platelet levels.

The anemia has been observed in elderly patients who have had poor diets and who have various organic diseases, in pregnant women, in some women using contraceptive pills, and in infants whose formulas may be inadequate in folic acid or ascorbic acid. Because of the prevalence of low serum folacin and megaloblastic anemia during pregnancy, supplements frequently are recommended. Folic acid deficiency frequently accompanies disease conditions in which the requirement for the vitamin is greatly increased, as in Hodgkin's disease and leukemia. Malabsorption syndromes, notably tropical sprue, are characterized by the presence of megaloblastic anemias.

The administration of folic acid to patients with megaloblastic anemia brings about dramatic reversal of the changes in the bone marrow. The red blood cells become normal in size, their number increases, the total hemoglobin increases, and the leukocyte levels return to normal. Many of the patients have a glossitis and diarrhea especially associated with malabsorption; these too are improved.

Folacin will bring about remission of the anemia in pernicious anemia but is not effective in preventing or correcting the neurologic disturbances. Therefore, folacin is not a substitute for vitamin B-12 in the treatment of this disorder. In order to avoid masking the existence of vitamin B-12 deficiency and delaying its diagnosis by curing the anemia, the amount of folic acid is regulated in vitamin supplements sold without prescription.

Other Factors

Choline All living cells contain CHOLINE, principally in phospholipids such as phosphotidylcholine (lecithin), which is essential for the structure and function of cell membranes and serum lipoproteins. Another choline-containing phospholipid, sphingomyelin, is found in high concentrations in nervous tissues. As a component of acetylcholine, choline is essential in the transmission of nerve impulses. One of the important functions of choline is the donation of methyl groups that can be utilized in numerous reactions.

Choline has been shown to be essential for various animal species, but the need for it by human beings has not been clearly established. Probably synthesis of choline within the body is sufficient. Large doses of choline have been tried in a number of disorders including fatty liver and cirrhosis and, more recently, memory deficits in the elderly and tardive dyskinesia, a condition characterized by involuntary muscular twitching. Results of such use have been equivocal and any effects probably should be regarded as pharmacologic rather than physiologic.

Egg yolk is especially rich in choline, but legumes, organ meats, milk, muscle meats, and whole-grain cereals are also good sources. A typical diet furnishes from 200 to 600 mg daily. These relatively large amounts indicate that choline is probably not a true vitamin.

Myo-inositol MYO-INOSITOL, also known as inositol or mesoinositol, is a water-soluble, sweet-tasting substance distributed in fruits, vegetables, whole grains, meats, and milk. It possesses lipotropic activity but its significance in human nutrition has not been established.

Lipoic Acid LIPOIC ACID is a sulfur-containing, fat-soluble substance also known as *thioctic acid* and *protogen.* Strictly speaking, it is not a vitamin because it is not necessary in the diet of animals. It functions, however, in the same manner as many of the B-complex vitamins. It is a component of the complexes involved in the decarboxylation of keto acids such as pyruvic acid and α-ketoglutaric acid. (See page 84.)

Bioflavinoids The BIOFLAVINOIDS are a group of chemical substances comprised primarily of flavine and flavinoid compounds found in citrus fruits as well as other fruits and vegetables. In 1936 it was reported that bioflavinoids exerted a synergistic effect on vitamin C in curing scurvy. Because of their effect on capillary permeability they became known as vitamin P. Despite a tremendous amount of work done with these compounds there is no evidence that they are essential for humans or animals and deficiency states have never been produced.

Para-Aminobenzoic Acid PARA-AMINOBENZOIC ACID (PABA) is an integral part of the structure of folic acid. Although some microorganisms may be able to utilize PABA to synthesize folacin, a role for PABA in human nutrition has not been documented in spite of frequent claims for its value.

Non-Nutrients LAETRILE and AMYGDALIN, sometimes referred to as vitamin B-17, are part of a group of cyanide-containing glycoside compounds found in the pits of apricots, peaches, bitter almonds, and apple seeds. Laetrile has been widely promoted for the prevention and cure of cancer but scientific evidence does not exist to support either its effectiveness or lack of adverse effects. Similarly, there is no evidence that physiological or biochemical abnormalities develop when these substances are not included in the diet. Thus, the use of the term "vitamin" is erroneous and misleading.

Another substance erroneously promoted as a vitamin is PANGAMIC ACID or vitamin B-15. Products called vitamin B-15 vary considerably in chemical composition, and the Food and Drug Administration considers pangamic acid an unidentifiable substance. None of the many claims for its value in treating such diverse conditions as allergies, schizophrenia, hepatitis, or autism in children have been documented in controlled studies.

Some Points for Emphasis in Nutrition Education (A General Summary)

1. Vitamins are compounds of known chemical nature occurring in minute amounts in foods. They have exact functions in the body for the use of carbohydrates, fats, and proteins for energy and for the synthesis of tissues, enzymes, and other body regulators. Thus, vitamins help to maintain healthy tissues and normal functions of all organs.
2. Each vitamin has specific functions and cannot substitute for another. Many reactions in the body require several vitamins, and a lack of any one can interfere with the function of another.
3. Synthetic vitamins and the vitamins occurring naturally in foods have the same chemical formulas and, weight for weight, are of equal use in the body.
4. A diet that includes recommended amounts of the Daily Food Guide selected from a variety of foods will furnish sufficient amounts of the vitamins to meet the needs of nearly all healthy persons without the use of supplements.
5. Each food group makes a special vitamin contribution to the diet. All the vitamin needs are not easily met if one or more of these food groups are omitted. For example, fruits and vegetables are the principal sources of ascorbic acid; dark green leafy vegetables and deep yellow vegetables and fruits are a major source of carotene; milk is a principal source of riboflavin; meats, poultry, and fish are outstanding for niacin, vitamin B-6, vitamin B-12, and thiamin; and whole-grain and enriched breads and cereals are especially important for thiamin and niacin.
6. Vitamin D is present in natural foodstuffs in only small amounts. Infants, children, pregnant and lactating women, and people who have little exposure to sunlight should use vitamin D milk or a supplement.
7. All vitamins are susceptible to destruction under certain conditions. However, for practical purposes, if the homemaker observes rules for the preservation of ascorbic acid, thiamin, and riboflavin, all other vitamins are likely to be satisfactorily retained. For riboflavin, the principal destruction comes about when milk in clear-glass bottles is allowed to stand in direct sunlight. The retention of ascorbic acid, thiamin, and other vitamins is assured if (1) some raw foods such as salads are freshly prepared and used daily, (2) cutting and exposure of surfaces are reduced to the shortest possible period of time, (3) cookery takes place in a small volume of liquid, (4) the use of alkali to retain green color is avoided, (5) foods are cooked only to the point of tenderness, and (6) foods are served promptly after preparation.
8. Vitamins A and D are toxic, and high-potency supplements should be used only when prescribed by a physician for specific deficiencies.
9. If taken in greater amounts than the body needs, the water-soluble vitamins are excreted in the urine; hence, supplements in addition to a good diet are probably an economic waste. Long-term intake of excess amounts of certain water-soluble vitamins also may have adverse effects and megadose usage is not advisable without medical supervision.
10. Vitamin deficiencies can be diagnosed only by means of accurate dietary and medical history, physical examination, and laboratory studies. Self-diagnosis and therapy are wasteful and can be dangerous.
11. Vitamin deficiency diseases can occur (1) if the dietary intake is generally poor, (2) if a food group is consistently omitted without making appropriate compensation for such omission, and (3) when there is too little money to buy an adequate diet.
12. A large proportion of vitamin deficiencies in the United States are secondary to disease, including anorexia and vomiting and failure to eat, malabsorption as in

Table 12-1. **Summary of Water-Soluble Vitamins**
(see also Points for Emphasis, pages 239–240)

Nomenclature	Important Sources	Physiology and Function	Effects of Deficiency	Recommended Allowances
Ascorbic acid Vitamin C	Citrus fruits; tomatoes; melons; cabbage; broccoli; strawberries; fresh potatoes; green leafy vegetables	Very little storage in body Formation of intercellular cement substance; synthesis of collagen Absorption and use of iron Prevents oxidation of folacin	Weakened cartilages and capillary walls Cutaneous hemorrhage; sore, bleeding gums, anemia Poor wound healing Poor bone and tooth development *Scurvy*	Men: 60 mg Women: 60 mg Pregnancy: 80 mg Lactation: 100 mg Infants: 35 mg Children under 11: 0.7–1.2 mg Boys and girls: 50 mg
Thiamin Vitamin B-1	Whole-grain and enriched breads, cereals, flours; organ meats, pork; other meats, poultry, fish; legumes, nuts; milk; green vegetables	Limited body storage Thiamin pyrophosphate (TPP) is coenzyme for decarboxylation and transketolation; chiefly involved in carbohydrate metabolism	Poor appetite; atony of gastrointestinal tract, constipation Mental depression, apathy, polyneuritis Cachexia, edema Cardiac failure *Beriberi*	Men: 1.4 mg Women: 1.0 mg Pregnancy: +0.4 mg Lactation: +0.5 mg Infants: 0.3–0.5 mg Children under 11: 0.7–1.2 mg Boys and girls: 1.1–1.5 mg
Riboflavin Vitamin B-2	Milk; organ meats; eggs; green leafy vegetables	Limited body stores, but reserves retained carefully Coenzymes for removal and transfer of hydrogen; flavin mononucleotide (FMN) and flavin adenine dinucleotide (FAD)	Cheilosis (cracks at corners of lips) Scaly desquamation around nose, ears, Sore tongue and mouth Burning and itching of eyes Photophobia	Men: 1.6 mg Women: 1.2 mg Pregnancy: +0.3 mg Lactation: +0.5 mg Infants: 0.4–0.6 mg Children under 11: 0.8–1.4 mg Boys and girls: 1.3–1.7 mg
Niacin Nicotinic acid Nicotinamide	Meat, poultry, fish; whole-grain and enriched breads, flours, cereals; nuts, legumes Tryptophan as a precursor	Coenzyme for glycolysis, fat synthesis, tissue respiration. Coenzymes NAD and NADP accept hydrogen and transfer it	Anorexia, glossitis, diarrhea Dermatitis Neurologic degeneration *Pellagra*	Men: 18 mg NE Women: 13 mg NE Pregnancy: +2 mg NE Lactation: +5 mg NE Infants: 6–8 mg NE Children under 11: 9–16 mg NE Boys and girls: 14–19 mg NE
Vitamin B-6 Three active forms: pyridoxine, pyridoxal, pyridoxamine	Meat, poultry, fish; potatoes, sweet potatoes, vegetables	Pyridoxal phosphate is coenzyme for transamination, decarboxylation, transulfuration of amino acids Conversion of tryptophan to niacin; conversion of glycogen to glucose Requirement related to protein intake	Nervous irritability, convulsions Weakness, ataxia, abdominal pain Dermatitis; anemia	Men: 2.2 mg Women: 2.0 mg Pregnancy: +0.6 mg Lactation: +0.5 mg Infants: 0.3–0.6 mg Children under 11: 0.9–1.6 mg Boys and girls: 1.8–2.2 mg

Pantothenic acid	Meat, poultry, fish; whole-grain cereals; legumes Smaller amounts in fruits, vegetables, milk	Constituent of coenzyme A: oxidation of pyruvic acid, α-ketoglutarate, fatty acids; synthesis of fatty acids, sterols, and porphyrin	Deficiency seen only with severe multiple B-complex deficits; gastrointestinal disturbances, neuritis, burning sensations of feet	Recommended safe and adequate intakes: Adolescents and adults: 4–7 mg Infants: 2–3 mg Children: 3–4 mg
Biotin	Organ meats, egg yolk, nuts, legumes	*Avidin*, a protein in raw egg white, blocks absorption; large amounts of raw eggs must be eaten Coenzyme for deamination, carboxylation, and decarboxylation	Deficiency only when many raw egg whites are consumed for long periods of time Dermatitis, anorexia, hyperesthesia, anemia	Recommended safe and adequate intakes: Adolescents and adults: 100–200 μg Infants: 35–50 μg Children: 65–120 μg
Vitamin B-12 Cyano-cobalamin Hydroxy-cobalamin	In animal foods only: organ meats, muscle meats, fish, poultry; eggs; milk	Requires intrinsic factor for absorption Biosynthesis of methyl groups Synthesis of DNA and RNA Formation of mature red blood cells	Lack of intrinsic factor leads to deficiency: pernicious anemia, following gastrectomy Macrocytic anemia Neurologic degeneration	Adults: 3 μg Pregnancy: 4 μg Lactation: 4 μg Infants: 0.5–1.5 μg Children: 2–3 μg Boys and girls: 3 μg
Folacin Folic acid Tetrahydrofolic acid	Organ meats, deep green leafy vegetables; muscle meats, poultry, fish, eggs; whole-grain cereals	Active form is folinic acid; requires ascorbic acid for conversion Coenzyme for transmethylation; synthesis of nucleoproteins; maturation of red blood cells Interrelated with vitamin B-12	Megaloblastic anemia of infancy, pregnancy, tropical sprue	Adults: 400 μg Pregnancy: 800 μg Lactation: 500 μg Infants: 30–45 μg Children under 11: 100–300 μg Boys and girls: 400 μg
Choline	Egg yolk, meat, poultry, fish, milk, whole grains	Probably not a true vitamin Donor of methyl groups: lipotropic action Component of acetylcholine, lecithin, sphingomyelin	Has not been observed in humans	Not known; typical diet supplies 200–600 mg
Lipoic acid Thioetic acid Protogen		Probably not a true vitamin Coenzyme for decarboxylation of keto acids		Not known
Inositol	Widely distributed in all foods	Lipotropic agent Vitamin nature not established	Has not been observed in humans	Not known

*See also Table 3-1 for complete listing of allowances.

diarrhea, sprue, and other conditions, and increased metabolic requirements because of fever and other stress factors.

13. Specific vitamin deficiencies require therapy with the vitamins that are lacking. Usually, synthetic vitamins are used to correct the deficiency inasmuch as large dosages can bring about rapid improvement.

Problems and Review

1. Explain how the following nutrients are interrelated:

riboflavin and niacin	pyridoxine and protein	cobalt and vitamin B-12
tryptophan and niacin	tryptophan and vitamin B-6	folic acid and ascorbic acid
glucose and thiamin		choline and fat

2. What is the effect on carbohydrate metabolism of a deficiency of thiamin? What are clinical signs of such deficiency?
3. What is the role of niacin in metabolism? What clinical symptoms are observed in a niacin deficiency?
4. How can you explain the fact that milk is a pellagra-preventive food even though it contains very little niacin?
5. The dietary intake of vitamins may appear to be satisfactory when compared with recommended allowances, but a physician may prescribe a vitamin supplement. Under what circumstances would you expect such a supplement to be necessary?
6. What is the possible significance of each of the following in human nutrition: folacin; choline; biotin; panthothenic acid; pyridoxine; inositol; vitamin B-12?
7. *Problem.* Compare the label information on three packages of dry cereal, including whole grain, enriched or restored, and fortified. Which of these would give the highest nutritional value for an expenditure of 10 cents? Show your calculations.
8. *Problem.* Mrs. Smith has asked for your guidance in the selection, storage, and preparation of food so that maximum nutritive value will be retained. On the basis of your information concerning the stability of vitamins, indicate briefly a set of instructions for guiding Mrs. Smith. Show how these rules apply to the preparation of a meal that includes roast beef, potatoes, green beans, cole slaw, milk, and fruit cup. Which vitamin or vitamins are especially concerned in each rule you have laid down?
9. *Problem.* Calculate the thiamin, riboflavin, and niacin content of your own diet for 2 days. Compare your intake with the recommended allowances. If there are any deficits, show how you could correct them.
10. *Problem.* A dietary calculation showed an intake of 80 gm protein and 12 mg niacin. Calculate the total niacin equivalent of this diet.
11. *Problem.* Calculate the percentage of your own daily requirement for thiamin and riboflavin which 2 cups of milk would supply. For each of these nutrients list two foods which would serve as effective supplements to the milk in supplying your daily needs.

Cited References

1. Dreyfus, P. M.: "Thiamin and the Nervous System: An Overview," *J. Nutr. Sci. Vitaminol.*, **22** (Suppl):13–16, 1976.
2. Food and Nutrition Board: *Recommended Dietary Allowances*, 9th ed. National Academy of Sciences–National Research Council, Washington, D.C., 1980.

3. Marston, R. M., and Peterkin, B. B.: "Nutrient Content of the National Food Supply," *Natl. Food Rev.*, U.S. Department of Agriculture, Washington, D.C., Winter 1980, pp. 21–25.
4. Williams, R. R.: "The World Beriberi Problem," *J. Clin. Nutr.*, **1**:513–16, 1953.
5. Wood, B., et al.: "A Study of Partial Thiamin Restriction in Human Volunteers," *Am. J. Clin. Nutr.*, **33**:848–61, 1980.
6. Horwitt, M. K., et al.: "Correlation of Urinary Excretion of Riboflavin with Dietary Intake and Symptoms of Ariboflavinosis," *J. Nutr.*, **41**:247–64, 1950.
7. Lopez, R., et al.: "Riboflavin Deficiency in an Adolescent Population in New York City," *Am. J. Clin. Nutr.*, **33**:1283–86, 1980.
8. Sebrell, W. H., and Butler, R. E.: "Riboflavin Deficiency in Man," *Public Health Rep.*, **54**:2121–31, 1939.
9. Horwitt, M. K., et al.: "Effects of Dietary Depletion of Riboflavin," *J. Nutr.*, **39**:357–73, 1949.
10. Goldberger, J.: "The Prevention of Pellagra. A Test Diet Among Institutional Inmates," *Public Health Rep.*, **30**:3117–31, 1915; nutrition classic reproduced in part in *Nutr. Rev.*, **31**:152–53, 1973.
11. Elvehjem, C. A., et al.: "The Isolation and Identification of the Anti-black Tongue Factor," *J. Biol. Chem.*, **123**:137–49, 1938; nutrition classic reproduced in part in *Nutr. Rev.*, **32**:48–50, 1974.
12. Kudchodkar, B. J., et al.: "Mechanisms of Hypolipidemic Action of Nicotinic Acid," *Clin. Pharmacol. Ther.*, **24**:354–73, 1978.
13. Sandstead, H. H.: "Clinical Manifestations of Certain Classical Deficiency Diseases," in Goodhart, R. S., and Shils, M. E., eds.: *Modern Nutrition in Health and Disease*, 6th ed., Lea & Febiger, Philadelphia, 1980, pp. 685–96.
14. Snyderman, S. E., et al.: "Pyridoxine Deficiency in the Human Infant," *Am. J. Clin. Nutr.*, **1**:200–207, 1953.
15. Coursin, D. B.: "Convulsive Seizures in Infants with Pyridoxine-Deficient Diet," *JAMA*, **154**:406–408, 1954.
16. Linkswiler, H. M.: "Vitamin B_6 Requirements of Men," in Food and Nutrition Board: *Human Vitamin B_6 Requirements*, National Academy of Science–National Research Council, Washington, D.C., 1978, pp. 279–90.
17. Mueller, J. R., and Vilter, R. W.: "Pyridoxine Deficiency in Human Beings Induced with Desoxypyridoxine," *J. Clin. Invest.*, **29**:193–201, 1950.
18. Frimpter, G. W., et al.: "Vitamin B_6-Dependency Syndromes: New Horizons in Nutrition," *Am. J. Clin. Nutr.*, **22**:794–805, 1969.
19. Glusman, N.: "The Syndrome of 'Burning Feet' (Nutritional Melalgia) as a Manifestation of Nutritional Deficiency," *Am. J. Med.*, **3**:211–23, 1947.
20. Hodges, R. E., et al.: "Human Pantothenic Acid Deficiency Produced by Omega-Methyl Pantothenic Acid," *J. Clin. Invest.*, **38**:1421–25, 1959.
21. Parsons, H. T., et al.: "Interrelationship Between Dietary Egg White and Requirements for Protective Factor in Cure of Nutritional Disorder Due to Egg White," *Biochem. J.*, **31**:424–32, 1937.
22. Sydenstricker, V. P., et al.: "Preliminary Observation in 'Egg White Injury' in Man and Its Cure with a Biotin Concentration," *Science*, **95**:176–77, 1942.
23. Baugh, C. M., et al.: "Human Biotin Deficiency: A Case History of Biotin Deficiency Induced by Raw Egg Consumption in a Cirrhotic Patient," *Am. J. Clin. Nutr.*, **21**:173–82, 1968.
24. Bonjour, J. P.: "Biotin in Man's Nutrition and Therapy—A Review," *Internat. J. Vit. Nutr. Res.*, **47**:107–18, 1977.
25. Minot, G. R., and Murphy, W. P.: "Treatment of Pernicious Anemia by a Special Diet," *JAMA*, **84**:470–76, 1926; nutrition classic reproduced in part in *Nutr. Rev.*, **36**:50–52, 1978.
26. Rickes, E. L., et al.: "Crystalline Vitamin B_{12}," *Science*, **107**:396–97, 1948.

27. Smith, E. L., and Parker, L. F. J.: "Purification of Anti-Pernicious Anemia Factors from Liver," *Nature,* **161**:638, 1948.
28. Staff report: "Discovery and Synthesis of Vitamin B_{12} Celebrated," *Nutr. Today,* 8:24–27, January–February 1973.
29. Heyssel, R. M., et al.: "Vitamin B_{12} Turnover in Man," *Am. J. Clin. Nutr.,* **18**:176–84, 1966.
30. McCurdy, P. R.: "B_{12} Shots," *JAMA,* **229**:703–704, 1974.
31. Smith, A. D. M.: "Veganism: A Clinical Survey with Observations on Vitamin B_{12} Metabolism," *Br. Med. J.,* **1**:1655–58, 1962.
32. Review: "Rare Forms of Familial Vitamin B_{12} Malabsorption in Children," *Nutr. Rev.,* **31**:149–51, 1973.
33. Stokstad, E. L. R., et al.: "Distribution of Folate Forms in Food and Folate Availability," in Food and Nutrition Board: *Folic Acid,* National Academy of Science–National Research Council, Washington, D.C., 1977, pp. 56–68.
34. Stokes, P. L., et al.: "Folate Metabolism in Scurvy," *Am. J. Clin. Nutr.,* **28**:126–29, 1975.
35. Herbert, V., et al.: "Folic Acid and Vitamin B_{12}," in Goodhart, R. S., and Shils, M. E., eds.: *Modern Nutrition in Health and Disease,* 6th ed., Lea & Febiger, Philadelphia, 1980, pp. 229–59.
36. Daniel, W. A., Jr., et al.: "Dietary Intakes and Plasma Concentrations of Folate in Healthy Adolescents," *Am. J. Clin. Nutr.,* **28**:363–70, 1975.

Additional References

Thiamin, Riboflavin, and Niacin

Blass, J. P., and Gibson, G. E.: "Abnormality of a Thiamine-Requiring Enzyme in Patients with Wernicke-Korsakoff Syndrome," *N. Engl. J. Med.,* **297**:1367–70, 1977.

Booher, L. E.: "The Concentration and Probable Chemical Nature of Vitamin G," *J. Biol. Chem.,* **102**:39–46, 1933; nutrition classic reproduced in part in *Nutr. Rev.,* 37:257–59, 1979.

Gromisch, D. S., et al.: "Light (Phototherapy)-Induced Riboflavin Deficiency in the Neonate," *J. Pediatr.,* **90**:118–22, 1977.

Katz, S. H., et al.: "Traditional Maize Processing Techniques in the New World. Traditional Alkali Processing Enhances the Nutritional Quality of Maize," *Science,* **184**:765–73, 1974.

Keefer, C. S.: "The Beriberi Heart," *Arch. Int. Med.,* **45**:1–22, 1930; nutrition classic reproduced in part in *Nutr. Rev.,* **32**:304–307, 1974.

Mason, J. B., et al.: "The Chemical Nature of the Bound Nicotinic Acid of Wheat Bran: Studies of Nicotinic Acid-Containing Macromolecules," *Br. J. Nutr.,* **30**:297–311, 1973.

Nail, P. A., et al.: "The Effect of Thiamin and Riboflavin Supplementation on the Level of Those Vitamins in Human Breast Milk and Urine," *Am. J. Clin. Nutr.,* 33:198–204, 1980.

Patterson, J. I., et al.: "Excretion of Tryptophan-Niacin Metabolites by Young Men: Effects of Tryptophan, Leucine, and Vitamin B_6 Intakes," *Am. J. Clin. Nutr.,* **33**:2157–67, 1980.

Rivlin, R. S.: "Hormones, Drugs and Riboflavin," *Nutr. Rev.,* **37**:241–46, 1979.

Shepherd, J., et al.: "Effects of Nicotinic Acid Therapy on Plasma High Density Lipoprotein Subfraction Distribution and Composition and on Apolipoprotein A Metabolism," *J. Clin. Invest.,* **63**:858–67, 1979.

VITAMIN B-6, PANTOTHENIC ACID, AND BIOTIN

BOOSE, T. R., et al.: "The Vitamin B_6 Requirement in Oral Contraceptive Users. I. Assessment by Pyridoxal Level and Transferase Activity in Erythrocytes," *Am. J. Clin. Nutr.*, **32**:1015–23, 1979.

CHARLES, B. M., et al.: "Biotin-Responsive Alopecia and Developmental Regression," *Lancet*, **2**:118–20, 1979.

COHENOUR, S. H., et al.: "Blood, Urine and Dietary Pantothenic Acid Levels of Pregnant Teenagers," *Am. J. Clin. Nutr.*, **25**:512–17, 1972.

FRY, P. C., et al.: "Metabolic Response to a Pantothenic Acid Deficient Diet in Humans," *J. Nutr. Sci. Vitaminol.*, **22**:339–46, 1976.

HEELEY, A., et al.: "Pyridoxal Metabolism in Vitamin B_6-Responsive Convulsions of Early Infancy," *Arch. Dis. Child.*, **53**:794–802, 1978.

KIRKSEY, A., et al.: "Vitamin B_6 Nutritional Status of a Group of Female Adolescents," *Am. J. Clin. Nutr.*, **31**:946–54, 1978.

LEKLEM, J. E., et al.: "Vitamin B–6 Requirements of Women Using Oral Contraceptives," *Am. J. Clin. Nutr.*, **28**:535–41, 1975.

LEWIS, J. S., et al.: "Vitamin B_6 Intakes and 24-Hr 4-Pyridoxic Acid Excretions of Children," *Am. J. Clin. Nutr.*, **30**:2023–27, 1977.

LUMENG, L., et al.: "Adequacy of Vitamin B_6 Supplementation During Pregnancy: A Prospective Study," *Am. J. Clin. Nutr.*, **29**:1376–83, 1976.

MCCORMICK, D. B.: "Biotin," *Nutr. Rev.*, **33**:97–102, 1975.

ROSE, C. S., et al.: "Age Differences in Vitamin B_6 Status of 617 Men," *Am. J. Clin. Nutr.*, **29**:847–53, 1976.

THOMAS, M. R., et al.: "The Effects of Vitamin C, Vitamin B_6 and Vitamin B_{12} Supplementation on the Breast Milk and Maternal Status of Well-Nourished Women," *Am. J. Clin. Nutr.*, **32**:1679–85, 1979.

WEST, K. D., et al.: "Influence of Vitamin B_6 Intake on the Content of the Vitamin in Human Milk," *Am. J. Clin. Nutr.*, **29**:961–69, 1976.

VITAMIN B-12 AND FOLACIN

ASFOUR, R., et al.: "Folacin Requirements of Children. III. Normal Infants," *Am. J. Clin. Nutr.*, **30**:1098–1105, 1977.

BAILEY, L. B., et al.: "Folacin and Iron Status in Low-Income Pregnant Adolescents and Mature Women," *Am. J. Clin. Nutr.*, **33**:1997–2001, 1980.

BAKER, S. J., and DEMAEYER, E. M.: "Nutritional Anemia: Its Understanding and Control with Special Reference to the Work of the World Health Organization," *Am. J. Clin. Nutr.*, **32**:368–417, 1979.

BOTEZ, M. I., et al.: "Polyneuropathy and Folate Deficiency," *Arch. Neurol.*, **35**:581–84, 1978.

CARMEL, R.: "Nutritional Vitamin-B_{12} Deficiency," *Ann. Int. Med.*, **88**:647–49, 1978.

DONALDSON, R. M.: "Serum B_{12} and the Diagnosis of Cobalamin Deficiency," *N. Engl. J. Med.*, **229**:827–28, 1978.

FERNANDES-COSTA, F., and METZ, J.: "Binding of Methylfolate and Pteroylglutamic Acid by the Specific Serum Folate Binder," *J. Lab. Clin. Med.*, **93**:181–88, 1979.

HALSTED, C. H.: "The Small Intestine in Vitamin B_{12} and Folate Deficiency," *Nutr. Rev.*, **33**:33–37, 1975.

HALSTED, C. H., et al.: "Availability of Monoglutamyl and Polyglutamyl Folates in Normal Subjects and in Patients with Coeliac Sprue," *Gut*, **19**:886–91, 1978.

HOGENKAMP, H. P. C.: "The Interaction Between Vitamin B_{12} and Vitamin C," *Am. J. Clin. Nutr.*, **33**:1–3, 1980.

HOPPNER, K., et al.: "Data on Folacin Activity in Foods: Availability, Applications, and Limitations," in Food and Nutrition Board: *"Folic Acid,"* National Academy of Science–National Research Council, Washington, D.C., 1977, pp. 69–81.

MATOTH, Y., et al.: "Folate Nutrition and Growth in Infancy," *Arch. Dis. Child.*, **54**:699–702, 1979.

REISENAUER, A.M., et al.: "Folate Conjugase: Two Separate Activities in Human Jejunum," *Science*, **198**:196–97, 1977.

RODRIGUEZ, M. S.: "A Conspectus of Research on Folacin Requirements of Man," *J. Nutr.*, **108**:1983–2103, 1978.

ROSENBERG, I. H.: "Folate Absorption and Malabsorption," *N. Engl. J. Med.*, **293**:1303–08, 1975.

STRELLING, M. K., et al.: "Diagnosis and Management of Folate Deficiency in Low Birthweight Infants," *Arch. Dis. Child.*, **54**:271–77, 1979.

TOSKES, P. P., AND DEREN, J. J.: "Vitamin B_{12} Absorption and Malabsorption," *Gastroenterology*, **65**:662–83, 1973.

OTHER FACTORS

GROWDON, J. H., et al.: "Oral Choline Administration to Patients with Tardive Dyskinesia," *N. Engl. J. Med.*, **297**:524–27, 1977.

HERBERT, V.: "Laetrile: The Cult of Cyanide. Promoting Poisin for Profit," *Am. J. Clin. Nutr.*, **32**:1121–58, 1979.

KUKSIS, A., AND MOOKERJEA, S.: "Choline," *Nutr. Rev.*, **36**:201–207, 1978.

13 Food Selection and Meal Planning for Nutrition and Economy

FOODS are complex substances that should be evaluated for the variety of nutritive contributions that they make to meeting nutritional needs. The Daily Food Guide and the Dietary Goals are a practical basis for planning meals that are nutritionally balanced and appetizing. Food expenditures are controlled by using the best available purchase information, by menu adjustments, by adequate storage facilities and practices in the home, and by appropriate preparation techniques.

The National Food Supply Are national food supplies adequate for the population needs? What is the relative contribution that may be expected of each of the major food groups to the nutrient supplies? Answers to these questions are provided annually by the U.S. Department of Agriculture. The per capita nutritive value of the available food supply in 1980 was as follows:[1]

Energy, kcal	3,520
Protein, gm	103
Fat, gm	168
Carbohydrate, gm	406
Calcium, mg	891
Phosphorus, mg	1,528
Iron, mg	17.6
Magnesium, mg	343
Zinc, mg	12.5
Vitamin A, IU	8,400
Thiamin, mg	2.2
Riboflavin, mg	2.4
Niacin, mg	26.8
Vitamin B-6, mg	2.0
Vitamin B-12, μg	9.5
Ascorbic acid, mg	123

The percentage of total nutrients contributed by each of the major food groups is shown in Table 13–1. From this table it is easy to see the relative importance of each food group in supplying a given nutrient. This table also demonstrates how some food groups are important suppliers of several nutrients. The following statements represent a summary of the contribution made by each of the major food groups.

1. Milk and dairy products far exceed other food groups for calcium and riboflavin; they are second only to the meat group for the protein contribution.
2. The meat group, including eggs and dry beans, peas, and nuts as well as meat, poultry, and fish, ranks first as a source of protein, phosphorus, magnesium, iron, thiamin, niacin, vitamin B-6 and vitamin B-12. Because of the high level of consumption, this group ranks second for vitamin A and riboflavin.
3. Fruits and vegetables are the only important sources of ascorbic acid and contribute about half of the vitamin A; they supply roughly one fifth of the iron and about one fourth of the magnesium and vitamin B-6.
4. The flour-cereal group takes second place as a source of calories, iron, thiamin, and niacin. This group becomes increasingly important for these nutrients as the income is lowered and the consumption of them is increased.
5. Sugars and sweets and fats and oils each contribute about one sixth of the energy value of the diet but do not add appreciably to the protein, mineral, or vitamin levels.

Table 13-1. **Contribution of Major Food Groups to Nutrient Supplies**[1]

Food Group	Food Energy	Protein	Fat	Carbohydrate	Calcium	Phosphorus	Iron	Magnesium	Vitamin A Value	Thiamin	Riboflavin	Niacin	Vitamin B-6	Vitamin B-12	Ascorbic Acid
1980 Preliminary								Percent							
Meat (Including pork fat cuts), poultry, and fish	21.0	42.9	36.1	.1	4.2	28.6	31.1	14.0	23.9	27.9	23.5	45.4	40.7	71.9	2.1
Eggs	1.8	4.9	2.7	.1	2.4	5.2	5.1	1.2	5.5	1.9	4.9	.1	2.1	8.2	0
Dairy products, excluding butter	9.9	20.2	11.2	5.7	71.6	32.6	2.4	19.8	12.2	7.2	36.3	1.2	10.7	18.4	3.2
Fats and oils, including butter	18.2	.1	43.0	(2)	.4	.2	0	.4	7.8	0	0	0	(2)	0	0
Citrus fruits	1.0	.6	.1	2.1	1.1	.9	.9	2.6	1.7	2.9	.6	.9	1.5	0	29.3
Other fruits	2.3	.7	.3	5.0	1.4	1.3	3.9	4.5	5.9	1.8	1.7	1.7	7.1	0	11.8
Potatoes and sweetpotatoes	2.7	2.3	.1	5.1	1.0	3.6	4.4	7.1	5.0	4.5	1.4	5.9	9.5	0	13.5
Dark green and deep yellow vegetables	.2	.4	(2)	.4	1.5	.6	1.6	2.0	18.5	.7	1.0	.5	1.9	0	9.0
Other vegetables, including tomatoes	2.5	3.3	.4	4.7	5.2	5.1	9.9	10.7	16.7	6.2	4.7	5.7	10.7	0	27.8
Dry beans and peas, nuts, soya flour and grits	3.0	5.5	3.7	2.1	3.1	6.4	6.8	12.3	(2)	5.0	1.9	6.8	5.0	0	(2)
Grain products	19.9	18.8	1.3	36.2	3.8	13.4	31.0	19.1	.4	41.7	23.3	28.4	10.6	1.6	0
Sugar and other sweeteners	17.0	(2)	0	38.1	3.3	.7	.6	.2	0	(2)	(2)	(2)	(2)	0	(2)
Miscellaneous[3]	.6	.3	1.0	.5	.8	1.5	2.1	6.4	2.2	.1	.6	3.3	.1	0	3.3

[1] Marston, R. M., and Welsh, S. O.: "Nutrient Content of the Available Food Supply," U.S. Department of Agriculture, Washington, D.C., Winter, 1981, pp. 19–22.

[2] Less than 0.05 percent.

[3] Coffee, chocolate liquor equivalent of cocoa beans, and fortification of products not assigned to a food group.

Characteristics of Food Groups

Vegetable—Fruit Group

No group of foods lends greater variety to the diet in terms of color, flavor, and texture than the vegetable-fruit group. This group includes practically every part of the plant—leaves, stems, roots, tubers, bulbs, flowers, and seeds. Mature seeds of the grasses are included in the cereal group, and those of leguminous plants such as peas and beans are included in the meat group.

Daily Choices In order to ensure optimum vitamin and mineral contributions, the daily recommendation of four servings from the vegetable-fruit group should be governed as follows:

1 serving daily of a good source of vitamin C such as citrus fruits
1 serving frequently of dark green or deep yellow vegetables for vitamin A
1 serving frequently of unpeeled fruits and vegetables and those with edible seeds such as berries for fiber

A serving is equivalent to ½ cup cooked vegetable, salad, or a whole piece of vegetable or fruit such as a banana, an apple, or medium-sized potato. Teenagers should have larger servings of each, and young children may have smaller-size servings.

Nutritive Characteristics This group is unique for its contribution to the ascorbic acid value of the diet; it is the major source of vitamin A value; it makes an excellent contribution to the iron level of the diet; and it is a fair source of other minerals and B-complex vitamins. The composition of vegetables and fruits covers a wide range depending upon the part of the plant represented. Moreover, the handling of the food from farm to table can be so variable that the amounts of vitamins and minerals retained may be high or low. The vitamin concentration is affected by the season, the degree of maturity, the temperature and length of storage, and the preparation techniques.

Water. As the chief constituent of fruits and vegetables water constitutes 75 to 95 per cent of the weight. Foods relatively high in carbohydrate such as bananas and potatoes are lower in water content than those that are low in carbohydrate such as tomatoes, lettuce, and melons.

Energy. As a group, these foods are not important contributors to the caloric value of the diet, although potatoes and sweet potatoes when eaten in large quantities make an appreciable contribution. Many vegetables such as tomatoes, celery, asparagus, salad greens, and others furnish no more than 25 kcal per serving. Potatoes, Lima beans, fresh corn, and bananas, for example, are slightly below 100 kcal per serving unit. Other vegetables and fruits range from 40 to 80 kcal per average serving.

Protein and fat. The protein concentration of most fresh vegetables ranges from 1 to 2 per cent and is even lower in fruits. Fresh peas and Lima beans are slightly above these levels. All foods of this group are extremely low in fat with the exception of avocados and olives. Vegetables and fruits contain no cholesterol.

Carbohydrate. The carbohydrate composition of this group ranges widely, from as low as 3 to 5 per cent for rhubarb, greens, summer squash, tomatoes, and others, to more than 30 per cent for a few foods such as sweet potatoes. Dried fruits contain about 65 per cent carbohydrate.

The exchange lists (Table A–4) provide a convenient classification of fruits and vegetables according to carbohydrate content. Fruit exchanges (list 3) are stated in amounts required to furnish 10 gm carbohydrate. Most vegetables (list 2) contain about 5 gm carbohydrate per half cup serving. Some vegetables such as chicory, Chinese cabbage, endive, escarole, lettuce, parsley, radishes, and watercress do not contribute significant amounts of carbohydrate. The so-called starchy vegetables including Lima beans, corn, parsnips, peas, potato, pumpkin, winter squash, and sweet potatoes are comparable to a slice of bread in carbohydrate, protein, and energy value (list 4).

Starches, dextrins, sucrose, fructose, glucose, and fiber occur in vegetables and fruits. The starch in immature fruits is converted to sugars during ripening. By contrast, the sweetness of young peas and tender corn is lost as these vegetables become more mature.

Minerals. Turnip greens, dandelion greens, mustard greens, collards, kale, and broccoli are excellent sources of calcium. The calcium of spinach, poke, dock, beet greens, chard, and lamb's quarters is not nutritionally available because the oxalic acid of those plants combines with calcium to form insoluble salts that are not absorbed. Some fruits contribute small amounts of calcium, but the daily contribution cannot be considered important.

The dark green leafy vegetables are fair-to-good sources of iron. Likewise, fresh and dried apricots, raisins, prunes, dates, figs, peaches, and berries are good sources of iron. However, the iron is of lower biologic availability than the iron in meat. The availability is enhanced in the presence of ascorbic acid or in a meal that includes meat.

Fruits and vegetables are rich sources of potassium, but the sodium content is negligible except for a few vegetables such as beets, carrots, spinach, celery, and chard.

Fruits and vegetables contribute to an alkaline ash. The acid or sour taste of some fruits, including citrus fruits, peaches, and others, is accounted for by several organic acids (citric, malic, tartaric) which are fully oxidized in the body. The mineral content of these fruits is such that they also yield an alkaline ash. Plums, prunes, rhubarb, and cranberries, on the other hand, contain benzoic acid, which cannot be utilized by the body; hence, they contribute to an acid reaction.

Vitamins. Among the best contributors to ascorbic acid are the citrus fruits, fresh strawberries, cantaloupe and honeydew melon, broccoli, kale, spinach, turnip greens, sweet green peppers, and cabbage. Potatoes and sweet potatoes contain lesser concentrations of this vitamin, but the amounts eaten daily by some people may appreciably add to the total intake. Dried fruits supply little vitamin C.

Dark-green leafy vegetables and deep yellow vegetables and fruits are outstanding for their carotene content. The concentration of the vitamin is directly proportional to the depth of the color. Lightly colored foods such as lettuce, cabbage, and white peaches are poor sources of the vitamin, although the outer green leaves of lettuce may contain 30 times as much vitamin A as the inner pale leaves.

Vegetables and fruits are fair sources of the B-complex vitamins.

Nutritive Values of Processed Fruits and Vegetables The nutritive values of frozen products are about equal to those of the fresh foods. In fact, fruits and vegetables that have been frozen promptly after harvesting may be superior to fresh foods that have been improperly handled from farm to market to consumer.

Commercially canned fruits and vegetables closely approximate cooked fresh products in their nutritive values since vacuum closure of the cans reduces the rate of oxidation. There is some unavoidable loss of ascorbic acid and thiamin. These losses are accelerated with storage at high temperatures for long periods of time.

The water-soluble nutrients distribute themselves in canned foods so that the concentration is about equal in the liquid and solid phases. Thus, if the contents are two-thirds solid and one-third liquid, two thirds of the vitamin C, for example, would be in the solids and one third in the liquid. Thus, the maximum nutritive value is obtained when liquid as well as solid is consumed.

Selection and Care Fresh fruits and

vegetables are highly perishable so they should be selected with care and used when they are at their peak of quality. Berries, peaches, pears, and tomatoes are highly perishable. Citrus fruits and apples should be refrigerated, but root vegetables can be kept for a short time at cool temperatures.

Crisp, ripe, but not overmature vegetables that are firm in texture and free from blemishes should be selected. As vegetables become too mature, the lignocellulose that is formed gives the characteristic stringy or woody texture which cannot be overcome with cookery. Wilted vegetables are lower in carotene and ascorbic acid content, and recrisping the vegetables will not restore these values.

Fruits improve in flavor and aroma with ripening. Some fruits such as peaches and pears bruise so easily that they are customarily picked before they are fully ripe. They should be allowed to ripen at room temperature before refrigeration.

Bananas are high in starch content when green. During ripening at room temperature, this starch is changed to more digestible sugars. Bananas have the best flavor when the skin shows speckles of brown.

Canned fruits and vegetables are usually sold by grade. Grade A products are uniform in color and size of pieces, practically free of blemishes, and of the proper maturity. Grade B fruits and vegetables are less uniform in color and size of pieces, slightly less tender, and less free of defects. However, they are just as nutritious as grade A vegetables and fruits.

Frozen foods require storage at 0°F, and thus a freezer or a separate freezing compartment in the refrigerator is essential if the foods are to be kept for more than a few days. When frozen foods are to be used within a week, it is satisfactory to keep them in the ice-cube section of the refrigerator. The consumer should select frozen foods only in markets which appear to use care in the display of these foods. If foods are stored above the freezing line indicated in the cabinet, or if frozen foods have thawed, they will lose some of the qualities of texture and may even spoil because of the growth of organisms.

Bread-Cereal Group

Importance in World Diets Today in nearly every country of the world some cereal grain is regarded as the "staff of life." The discovery thousands of years ago that the land could be cultivated to grow grains meant that humans no longer had to lead the nomadic lives of hunters. The word *cereal* is derived from Ceres, the ancient Roman goddess of agriculture and harvest. Numerous references in the Bible attest to the importance of cereals. For example, in Psalm 65:13 we read, "The pastures are clothed with flocks; the valleys also are covered with corn: they shout for joy; they also sing." In the Bible and other early literature *corn* referred to grains such as wheat, millet, and barley.

By reason of its availability, high yield per acre, low production cost, and excellent keeping qualities, grain is used more abundantly than any other food material. Rice is the chief dietary staple for half the world's population and constitutes as much as 80 per cent of the calories for most of Asia's peoples. Wheat ranks second to rice in worldwide use but is the principal cereal grain used in the United States and in some European countries. Corn is widely used in Central and South America. Millet, sorghum, rye, and barley are important in some parts of the world.

Daily Choices The bread-cereal group includes all products made with whole-grain or enriched cereals, flours, and meals: bread, biscuits, muffins, pancakes, waffles; ready-to-eat or cooked breakfast cereals; rice; noodles, spaghetti, macaroni, and other pastas; grits; cornmeal, flours, barley, and bulgur.

Four servings are recommended each

day. Additional servings are desirable to meet caloric requirements and to make adjustments for the Dietary Goals. One serving is one slice of bread, or ½ to ¾ cup cooked cereal, macaroni, rice, and so on, or 1 ounce of ready-to eat cereal.

Nutritional Value of Cereal Foods The seed or kernel of the cereal grain (see Figure 13–1) is divided into three parts, the bran, germ, and endosperm. The aleurone layer just below the bran layer is sometimes identified as a fourth part. Although cereal grains vary somewhat in their composition, the average percentage composition of the whole grain is protein, 12; fat, 2; carbohydrate, 75; water, 10; minerals, especially phosphorus and iron, and the B-complex vitamins, especially thiamin, 1. The mineral and vitamin compositions of market forms of cereal foods vary widely depending upon whether they are whole grain, enriched, or unenriched. Cereal grains contribute importantly to every nutrient need except calcium, ascorbic acid, and vitamin A.

Energy. Cereal foods, it is well known, are the primary source of energy for most of the world's people. Many people infer from this fact that cereals per se are fattening, and so they omit this group of foods from their diets. By such omission they lose the many nutrient benefits provided by whole-grain and enriched products. The average serving of a cereal food furnishes from 65 to 100 kcal.

Protein. The protein of cereal grains is somewhat inferior to that of animal sources because some of the essential amino acids are present in less than needed amounts. Lysine is a limiting amino acid in wheat, rice, and corn, whereas tryptophan and threonine are present in too small amounts in corn and rice, respectively. The aleurone layer of the grain contains protein which is superior to that found in the endosperm, whereas that found in the germ compares favorably in biologic value with animal protein. Unfortunately, these better-quality proteins are removed when cereals are refined. Beans, peas, or soybeans served in

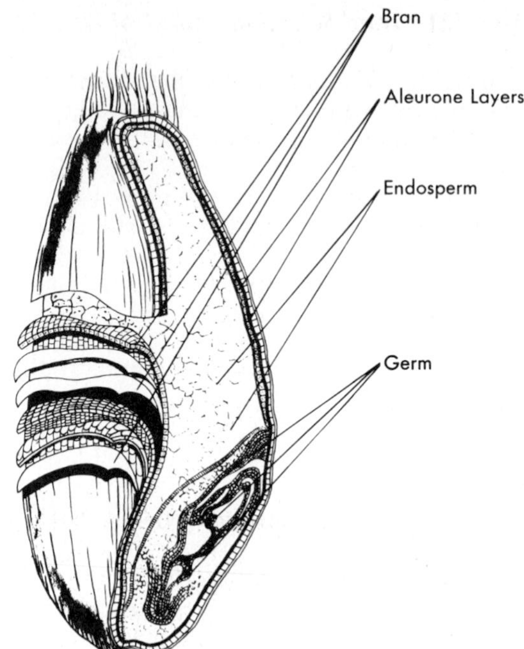

Figure 13–1. Whole wheat—cross section of grain. (Courtesy, the Ralston Purina Company.)

The Bran. The brown outer layers. This part contains:
1. Bulk-forming carbohydrates
2. B vitamins
3. Minerals, especially iron

The Aleurone Layers. The layers located right under the bran. They are rich in:
1. Proteins
2. Phosphorus, a mineral

The Endosperm. The white center. This consists mainly of:
1. Carbohydrates (starches and sugars)
2. Protein

This is the part used in highly refined white flours. Less refined flours and refined cereals are made from this part and varying amounts of the aleurone layer.

The Germ. The heart of wheat (embryo). It is this part that sprouts and makes a new plant when put into the ground. It contains:
1. Thiamin (vitamin B-1). Wheat germ is one of the best food sources of thiamin.
2. Protein. This protein is of value comparable to the proteins of meat, milk, and cheese.
3. Other B vitamins
4. Fat and the fat-soluble vitamin E
5. Minerals, especially iron
6. Carbohydrates

the same meal with foods from the cereal group will supply the limiting amino acids. Thus, rice and kidney beans or brown bread and baked beans are effective combinations. The amino acid deficiency of the cereal group can also be made up by including small amounts of milk, cheese, meat, poultry, or fish in the same meal.

Minerals and vitamins. The greater part of the minerals, iron and phosphorus, and of the B-complex vitamins occurs in the bran and germ of the grain. Consequently, most of these nutrients are lost when cereals are highly milled. Because many people in America and throughout the world prefer white bread and white flour, it is of vast importance that flours, breads, and cereals be enriched.

With increasing emphasis on the inclusion in the diet of foods that are not overly processed, more widespread consumption of whole-grain breads and cereals is taking place. This trend should be encouraged not only for the trace elements that are provided but also for the greater fiber content.

Cereal grains are poor sources of calcium. But breakfast cereals are ordinarily consumed with milk, and many commercial breads contain 2 to 4 per cent nonfat dry milk, thus improving the total calcium content of the diet as well as the quality of the protein intake.

Nutritive Efficiency of Bread The nutritive contribution of bread is illustrated in Figure 13–2. That bread is an important part of the diet was convincingly demonstrated in a study reported by British investigators.[2] The progress of 169 undernourished children, 4 to 15 years of age, was observed in a German orphanage following World War II when food supplies were limited. The calories in the diets consumed by the children were distributed in these percentages: bread, 75; potatoes, 6; soups, vegetables, fruits, butter, margarine, 15; and milk, cheese, meat, and fish, 4. Whole-wheat, enriched, and unenriched white breads were used. The diets were not low in protein, but only 8 to 9 gm were derived from animal sources. Supplements of vitamins A, D, and C were included.

At the end of 1 year the children had

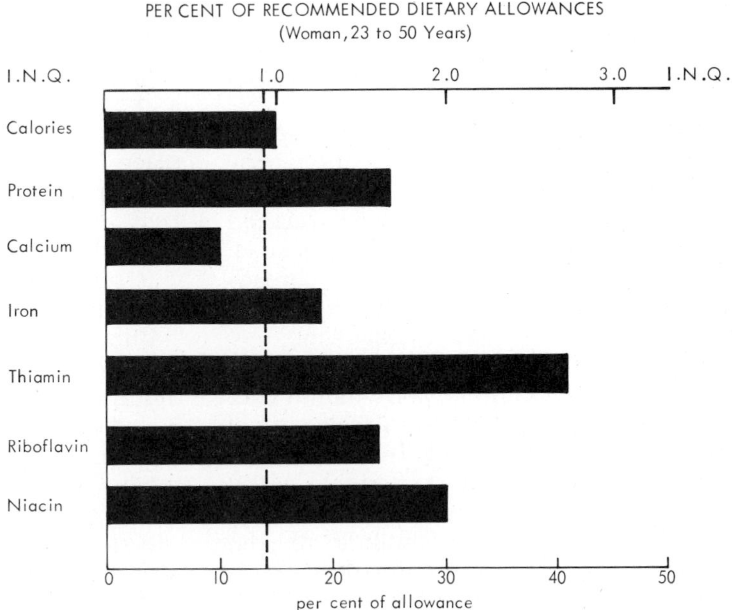

Figure 13–2. Contribution of three slices white enriched or whole-wheat bread plus one serving breakfast cereal to the day's allowance for the woman 23 to 50 years. Note the Index of Nutritional Quality (INQ) over 1.0 for protein, iron, thiamin, riboflavin, and niacin. See Table 13–2 for calculations.

made more rapid gains in height and weight than would be expected of normal children at the same age level; bone development was somewhat more rapid than normal; skin conditions have improved; and muscle tone had increased. The children were judged to be in excellent physical condition. No differences were observed in growth, development, or health with any of the breads tested, but the B-vitamin reserves were somewhat better in those children who had eaten bread enriched to the whole-wheat levels. These results clearly demonstrated the nutritive efficiency of unusually large amounts of bread.

Selection Label reading is important in the selection of foods from the bread-cereal group. The consumer should look for information on enrichment, nutrient fortification, and sugar content.

Bread. About 85 per cent of white bread and rolls sold to the American public are enriched. The B vitamins and iron are included at levels to equal whole-wheat bread.

Whole-wheat flour is the only flour that may be used in bread labeled as "whole-wheat," "graham," or "entire-wheat" bread. Breads labeled as "cracked wheat," "wheaten," "wheat," and "rye" are made with varying proportions of these flours and white flour.

Specialty breads are often advertised as possessing greater nutritional values. Soy flour, wheat germ, molasses, and nonfat milk increase the nutritive value in relation to the amounts used in the bread formula. The greater cost of some of these breads may not justify their selection if the increase in nutritive value is small.

Breakfast cereals. Cereals vary widely in their protein, mineral, and vitamin content. Refined, unenriched cereals supply but a small percentage of the daily allowances for minerals and vitamins. Many breakfast cereals are fortified beyond the usual mineral-vitamin contents of the whole-grain cereal. Indeed, fortification often includes vitamins A, B-12, C, and D, none of which are constituents of the whole grain.

An increasing number of breakfast cereals are presweetened, presumably to appeal especially to children. In some products sugar accounts for as much as 50 per cent. It is preferable to select unsweetened cereals so that the amount of sugar added can be controlled.

Generally, cereals that require cooking are more economical than ready-to-eat cereals. Among the more costly breakfast cereals are those that are sugar coated, with raisins and/or nuts, "natural," and precooked instant cereals as well as those packaged in individual portions.

Other cereal foods. Brown rice is the whole-grain rice with the hull and a little of the bran removed. White rice is milled to removed the hull, bran, and germ. In the milling some of the minerals and vitamins are removed. Since white (polished) rice is a staple for so many of the world's people, enrichment is of major importance. Rice may be enriched by coating the kernels with a premix of vitamins. It should not be washed prior to cooking. The amount of cooking water should be no more than can be absorbed by the rice kernels.

Parboiled rice is steamed by a special process so that the thiamin and other vitamins and minerals are distributed throughout the kernel with only a slight loss taking place in washing and cooking. *Converted rice* is parboiled by a patented process. *Precooked rice* requires the addition of hot water and a short period of standing before it is ready to be served; it is more costly than uncooked rice.

Bulgur is a wheat product of whole or cracked grains with a nutlike flavor and a slightly chewy texture. The wheat is parboiled and dried, and some of the bran is removed. Present methods of processing retain 75 per cent or more of the minerals and vitamins in the wheat.

A special kind of hard wheat flour—durum—is used in the manufacture of some 150 different shapes of pastas, including macaroni, spaghetti, vermicelli, and noodles. The pastas are used in many side dishes for the main meal or as a main dish in combination with cheese, meat, fish, or poultry.

Milk Group

Milk serves as the sole food for the young during the most critical period of life for some 8,000 species. Cow's milk is by far the most commonly used in the United States.

Daily Choices The milk group includes all forms of milk: whole, 1 or 2 per cent fat, nonfat, evaporated—whole or skim, buttermilk or other cultured milks, and chocolate milk. It also includes nonfat dry milk, yogurt, ice cream or ice milk, sour cream, cream, and half-and-half (half whole milk and half light cream), and some 400 varieties of cheese.

One serving of milk is an 8-ounce cup or its equivalent. (See Daily Food Guide, page 41, for equivalents.) The recommended servings of milk are

- 2 cups for adults
- 3 cups for school children and pregnant women
- 4 cups for teenagers and lactating women

The Dietary Goals can be incorporated into dietary planning by making the following adjustments:

1. Substitute skim or 1 or 2 per cent milk for whole milk to reduce the intake of saturated fat.
2. Use low-fat cheeses more frequently and whole-milk cheeses less often.
3. Omit cream and ice cream. Use milk in coffee, and ice milk for desserts. Dairy toppings for desserts are acceptable substitutes for whipped cream.

Nutritive Characteristics Milk is a complex substance in which over 100 separate components have been identified. It is fluid in spite of the fact that it contains more solids than many solid foods. Fresh cow's milk contains 87 per cent water and 13 per cent solids, whereas such foods, as cabbage, strawberries, and summer squash, to name but a few examples, are lower in solids content and higher in water content.

The exact composition of milk varies with the breed of cattle, the feed used, and the period of lactation. Pooled market milk has a uniform composition which may be varied slightly by local or state regulations for butterfat and solids content.

Cultured milks have a nutritive value equal to that of the milk from which they are made. The fermentation of the milk results in the splitting of some of the lactose to lactic acid and in some coagulation of casein. Yogurt is prepared from whole, skim, or partially skimmed milk and is fermented with a mixed culture of microorganisms.

Ice cream supplies the nutrients of cream, milk, and any fruits, nuts, and sugar that are added. Most ice creams contain about 10 per cent fat.

Energy. From Figure 13–3 it may be

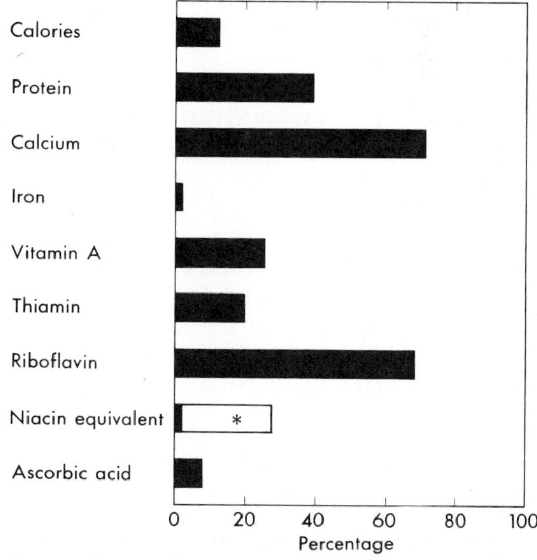

Figure 13–3. Percentage contribution of 2 cups of milk (2 per cent fat) to the recommended dietary allowances for the woman of 23 to 50 years. (Unshaded area represents niacin equivalent from tryptophan.)

seen that 2 cups of 2 per cent milk furnish about 12 per cent of the calories for the woman, but the percentage of contribution for most nutrients is considerably greater. By adjusting the fat level of milk, caloric modifications can be made for low-calorie and high-calorie diets.

1 cut skim milk = 85 kcal
1 cup 2 per cent milk = 120 kcal
1 cup whole milk = 150 kcal
1 cup half-and-half milk and cream = 315 kcal

Protein. One cup of whole, skim, or diluted evaporated milk contains 8 gm protein. Thus, 2 cups daily furnish about one third of the adult protein allowance.

Casein accounts for four fifths of the protein in cow's milk, and various whey proteins, including lactalbumins and lactoglobulins, constitute the remaining protein fractions. The essential amino acids present in milk proteins are supplied in almost ideal proportions for maximum tissue synthesis.

Fat. The fat of milk is highly emulsified and is easily digested. About 60 to 75 per cent of the fatty acids in milk are saturated, 24 to 40 per cent are monounsaturated, and 2 to 10 per cent are polyunsaturated. In modified-fat diets, when saturated fats must be kept to a minimum, skim milk or 1 per cent milk may be substituted for whole milk.

Carbohydrate. Lactose is a carbohydrate occurring only in milk. This sugar is much less sweet, less soluble, and more stable than sucrose and other sugars. It gives to milk a bland flavor. Lactose favors the growth of lactic-acid-producing bacteria which are believed to retard or prevent the growth of putrefying bacteria. Lactose probably favors the absorption of calcium and phosphorus and the synthesis of some B-complex vitamins in the small intestine. Some persons, especially adults, have a lactase deficiency and therefore a poor tolerance for milk. (See Chapter 33.)

Minerals and vitamins. Only the milk group provides a practical basis for meeting the recommended allowance for calcium. Phosphorus occurs in correct proportions with calcium to support optimum skeletal growth. Milk contains appreciable amounts of sodium, potassium, and magnesium, but it furnishes very little iron, so that the infant's diet must be supplemented at an early age to prevent anemia.

Milk is an outstanding dietary source of riboflavin and also supplies fair amounts of vitamin A, thiamin, vitamin B-6, and vitamin B-12. It is low in niacin but is an excellent source of tryptophan, which functions as a precursor of niacin. About 85 per cent of market milk today is fortified with vitamin D to a level of 400 IU per quart. Milk furnishes only small amounts of ascorbic acid.

Cheese The composition of cheese depends upon the kind of milk used—whole or skim—and the amount of water present. A pound of hard cheese contains the casein and fat of 1 gallon of milk. Cheeses, except cream cheese, are excellent sources of protein. The proteins contain all the essential amino acids and are therefore of high biologic value. Only a trace of the lactose in milk remains in the cheese. Some of the water-soluble minerals and vitamins are removed in the whey. Hard cheeses are an important source of calcium, but soft cheeses such as cottage cheese supply much less. See equivalents for 1 cup of milk, page 41. Cheeses also furnish significant amounts of phosphorus, vitamin A (if made with whole milk), riboflavin, and vitamins B-6 and B-12.

Process cheese is a blend of mild cheeses, followed by pasteurization. An emulsifying agent, such as disodium phosphate or sodium citrate, gives a smooth texture and keeps the fat from separating out.

Selection and Care Fresh milk is more economical when purchased in half-gallon or gallon containers at a food or dairy store. Nonfat dry milk costs one half to two thirds as must as fresh milk. When reconstituted it makes an acceptable beverage if well chilled. It may also be mixed with an equal part of whole milk to give a beverage containing about 2 per cent fat. Evaporated milk is less expensive than fresh milk, does not require refrigeration until opened, and lends itself especially to the preparation of cooked dishes. All liquid milks require continuous refrigeration.

For the best buys in cheese select domestic Cheddar, Swiss, process, or cottage cheese, rather than imported cheese. Buy cheese in wedges or sticks, rather than in slices, chunks, or grated. Aged cheeses, imported cheeses, cream, and ice cream are the more expensive items in the milk group. Cheese should be kept refrigerated. When it is to be served as an accompaniment to fruit or crackers, cheese should be brought to room temperature for best flavor.

Meat Group

Daily Choices The meat group includes beef, veal, lamb, pork, poultry, fish, shellfish, dry beans or peas, soybeans, lentils, eggs, seeds, nuts, peanuts, and peanut butter. The daily recommendation from this group is two servings. One serving is 2 to 3 ounces of edible portion of lean cooked beef, veal, pork, lamb, poultry or fish. The equivalents for 1 ounce of meat are

- 1 egg
- ½ to ¾ cup cooked dry beans, dry peas, soybeans, or lentils
- 2 tablespoons peanut butter
- ¼ to ½ cup sesame or sunflower seeds, or nuts

Place of Meat in the Diet The often-heard comment "It doesn't seem like a meal without meat" attests to the popular and psychologic importance of meat. All over the world, as economic positions improve, people are increasing their consumption of meat. In fact, the consumption of meat within a country is probably an indicator of its economic position.

The aromas and flavors provided by meat extractives stimulate the appetite. The protein and fat content increase the satiety value of the meal.

On the basis of available retail food supplies, the per capita consumption of meat is about 147 pounds; of poultry, 62 pounds, and of fish, 13 pounds.[3] About three fifths of the meat consumed is beef, and pork accounts for a little more than a third. Veal, lamb, and mutton together account for about 3 per cent of the meat consumed.

The consumption of chicken and turkey has increased steadily over the years because of the lesser cost. Per capita consumption of eggs, on the other hand, has declined from 42 pounds in 1960 to about 36 pounds at present. This decline has been influenced at least in part by the concern about the cholesterol content in eggs.

Dried peas, beans, and soybeans have not been an important part of diets in the United States, the annual per capita consumption on dry weight basis being about 6 pounds. Per capita consumption of peanuts (shelled), including peanut butter, is about 7 pounds.

Nutritive Characteristics Variations in the composition of meat from one cut to another are due largely to the proportion of lean and fatty tissue. The nutritive value of meat as consumed depends on whether (1) fat was trimmed off before cooking, (2) fat in drippings was used, and (3) surrounding fat on meat was eaten.

Protein. On a cooked basis, 30 gm (1 oz) lean meat, one egg, ½ cup cooked dried beans or peas, and 2 tablespoons peanut butter furnish about 7 gm protein.

Regardless of the species, the amino acid composition of the proteins of flesh foods is relatively constant and of such balance and quality that meats, fish, and poultry rank only slightly below eggs and milk in their ability to effect tissue synthesis. The protein differences between so-called red and white meats are insignificant.

The proteins in beans and nuts are somewhat lower in quality because the amounts of methionine and cystine are below optimum levels. However, when eaten in combination with cereal grains, or with small amounts of milk, eggs, or meat, these deficiencies are corrected.

Fat. In the Exchange Lists (Table A–4, list 5) meat cuts or their equivalents are grouped according to fat content:

1 ounce low-fat meat: 3 gm fat
1 ounce medium-fat meat: 5.5 gm fat
1 ounce high-fat meat: 8 gm fat

The fatty acids in meat are more saturated than those in poultry and fish. Peas, beans, and lentils are very low in fat. Seeds, nuts, and soybeans contain significant amounts of fat, with high proportions of polyunsaturated fatty acids.

Only animal foods contain cholesterol. Egg yolk, liver, and brains are high in cholesterol content. The lean and fat portions of muscle meats contain approximately equal concentrations of cholesterol. Fish and shellfish (except shrimp) are relatively low in cholesterol. (See Table A–5.)

For observance of the Dietary Goals, these adjustments should be made: (1) restrict the total meat intake to 4 to 5 ounces cooked edible portion; (2) select only lean meats, and trim off any visible fat; (3) discard drippings from roasts or broiled meats; (4) use poultry, fish, and legumes frequently in place of meat; and (5) restrict the intake of eggs to 3 or 4 per week—sometimes less than that.

Minerals. The meat group is valuable for its biologically available iron. The inclusion of meat in a meal also enhances the availability of iron from the vegetable-fruit and bread-cereal groups. Red meats and oysters are especially valuable for their zinc content, and dry beans, peas, soybeans and nuts for magnesium. Meats are also rich in phosphorus, sulfur, and potassium and are moderately high in sodium, but they are poor in calcium content. Some shellfish and canned salmon with the bones contain appreciable amounts of calcium. Saltwater fish is a good source of iodine.

Vitamins. All foods of the meat group are good sources of the B-complex vitamins. Pork, liver, and other organ meats and legumes are excellent for their thiamin content; poultry, dry peas, and peanuts are rich in niacin. Vitamin B-12 is supplied by organ meats, muscle meats, poultry, and eggs, but it is not found in the plant foods of this group.

Extractives and purines. Various nonprotein nitrogenous substances give meat its characteristic flavor. They are readily extracted from meat with water, as in the preparation of broth. They have very little nutritive value.

Selection The meat group accounts for a significant part of the food budget. In many families the expenditure for this group is too great, thus reducing the amount of money that can be spent for the other groups.

The standards for various grades of beef, veal, and lamb established by the U.S. Department of Agriculture are based upon the amount of surface fat and marbling (fat interspersed among the muscle fibers), color, firmness of flesh, texture, and maturity.

Prime beef, which is very tender and has a considerable amount of surface fat and generous marbling, is sold chiefly to hotels and restaurants. Many retail markets sell only one grade of meat—either *choice* or *good*, depending upon location. These grades are less generously marbled with fat, but they are juicy and flavorful. Standard-grade beef has very little fat, is less tender and juicy, but quite rich in flavor.

Americans have become accustomed to beef that is well marbled. To bring about marbling, animals must be fed grains for a period of time before marketing. To many concerned people this is extravagant use of grain in a world where severe shortages of food exist for some people.

The costs of protein from various meats or their equivalents are shown in Figure 13–4. Expenditures for the meat group can be reduced if the selection is made according to the market supply. In recent years fish and poultry have been less costly than

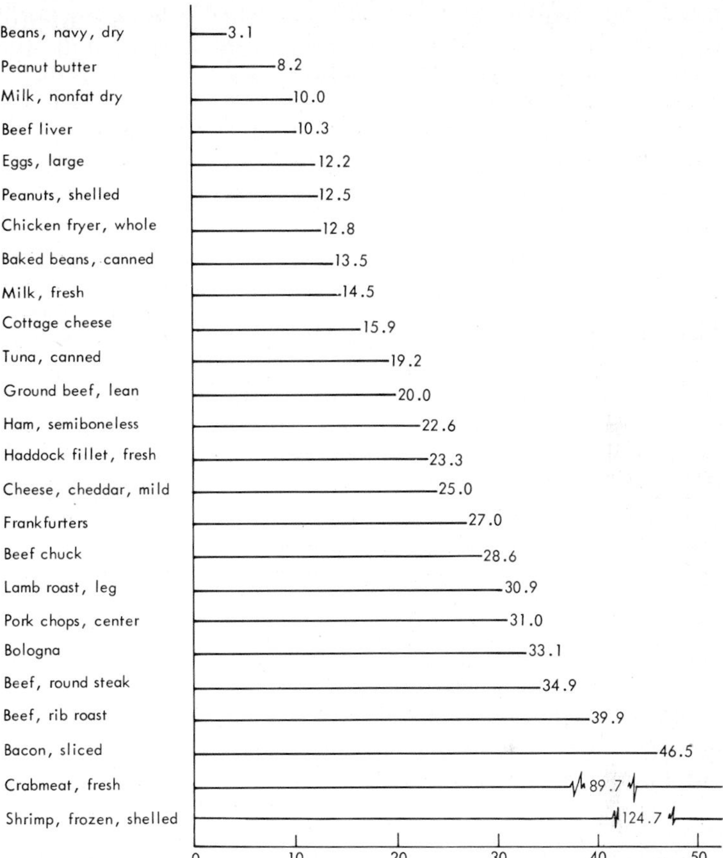

Figure 13–4. Cost of 10 gm protein based on supermarket prices in winter 1981. Although prices vary from week to week, the relative cost positions are not likely to shift greatly.

beef. Larger chickens and turkeys contain a smaller proportion of waste and are a better buy if the family can use the larger sizes. Whole birds are more economical than cut-up pieces.

Tender cuts such as steaks, rib roasts, and chops are more costly than chuck roasts, round steak, and so on. When purchasing meat, one must consider the cost per edible portion. For example, 1 pound of spare ribs will serve only two persons, whereas 1 pound of lean round steak will serve three or four.

Brown or white eggs are equal in nutritive value, and there is no merit in paying additional amounts for one color or the other. Grade A eggs are best for table use, while grade B eggs can be used for cooking and for some table purposes. Small eggs are often a better buy in the fall, whereas large eggs may cost only a few cents more during winter and spring months.

Dried beans and peas, lentils, cowpeas, chickpeas, and peanuts or peanut butter are inexpensive alternatives for meat. Dry beans and peas require a long time for cooking, but are lower in cost than the corresponding canned product.

Fats, Sweets, and Alcohol Group

Choices This group includes butter, margarine, mayonnaise, salad dressings, vegetable oils, and solid shortenings; sugar, syrups, candy, jelly, jams, sweet toppings, honey; soft drinks; and beer, wine, and distilled liquors. It also includes bakery products made with refined, unenriched flours.

There are no recommendations for daily allowances. This group furnishes variety and interest to the meal; for example, dressing on a tossed salad, butter or margarine in a baked potato or on a piece of bread, jelly or preserves with a piece of meat or on a biscuit; or wine with dinner.

This is the group that must be especially restricted to avoid obesity, but it can be used in greater amounts by those who need to gain weight. The Dietary Goals emphasize reduced intake of sugars, and replacement of saturated fats with those that are rich in polyunsaturated fatty acids.

Nutritive Characteristics This group contributes chiefly calories. Ounce for ounce, the fats furnish more than twice as many calories as the sugars. Each gram of pure alcohol yields 7 kcal. The vegetable oils and soft-type margarines are good sources of polyunsaturated fatty acids and vitamin E. Refined, unenriched bakery products and many snack-type foods are low in nutrient density.

Fabricated Foods

Numerous products variously referred to as *fabricated, engineered,* or *simulated* foods are available in today's market. These foods usually simulate a conventional food in color, texture, and flavor. Many of them have been widely accepted by consumers, and their numbers will undoubtedly increase in the next decade.

Imitation milk is a product resembling milk but it contains no milk products such as skim milk or nonfat dry milk. Typical constituents of imitation milk are a protein source such as sodium caseinate or soy protein, corn syrup solids, sugar, and a vegetable fat (usually coconut oil). Additives for color, flavor, and stability are normally present. The nutritive values vary from brand to brand, but they are generally lower in protein, calcium, and vitamins than milk and are not a replacement for whole milk.

Coffee whiteners contain a protein source such as casein, vegetable fat (usually coconut oil), corn syrup solids, emulsifiers, stabilizers, and coloring.

Textured vegetable proteins are the basis for a number of meat analogs. To produce textured vegetable protein, the protein is extracted from grains or legumes, soy protein being widely used. The protein is solubilized and forced through spinnerets to form fibers, which are then coagulated. The fibers are further processed to simulate beef, pork, ham, chicken, or fish by appropriate flavorings, coloring, and texture modification. Minerals and vitamins may be added to correspond to the composition of the product it replaces.

Nutritive Values of Fabricated Foods If fabricated foods comprise only a small part of the diet, there need be no great concern pertaining to nutritive values except in diets that are marginal in quality. However, as the number and variety of these products increase and they become a greater proportion of the total diet, some regulation of nutritive content becomes essential.

One way to measure the nutritive value of simulated foods is to make comparisons with the foods that they would replace in the diet. The information would be available from the labeling of the product. (See regulations for labeling, Chapter 17.) For example, does the breakfast beverage that replaces orange juice contain the same amounts of ascorbic acid and carbohydrate that are present in orange juice? Does the meat analog supply the same amounts and quality of protein as the conventional meat product? Does it also supply the important minerals and vitamins found in meat in the same proportions?

A present area of concern are the numerous nutrients found in conventional foods but lacking in fabricated foods because there is insufficient information on the daily requirements for these nutrients. Thus, when fabricated foods and refined conventional foods comprise an important proportion of the diet, there could well be dietary deficiency of manganese, zinc, copper, chromium, and other trace minerals. Another criticism that may be made of fabricated foods is that many of them have a high content of sodium.

Meal Planning

A Basic Dietary Pattern

Evaluation of the Food Guide The Daily Food Guide and the Dietary Goals are a practical basis for meal planning. Tables 13–2 and 13–3 summarize the nutritive values that may be expected when one selects the recommended amounts of food from each food group.

It becomes evident from the calculations in Table 13–2 and Figure 13–5 that the Basic Diet provides about half of the caloric requirement for adults. The only serious shortcoming of this plan is that the iron level is about half of the recommended 18 mg for women. If a woman were to meet her full caloric needs with emphasis upon iron-rich foods, including liver, dried fruits, molasses, additional meat, and iron-enriched cereals and bread, she might achieve the recommended level. On a day-to-day basis this becomes difficult. Although the recommended allowances furnish a margin of safety for most women, pregnant women and those who are anemic should use an iron supplement. The iron that is supplied by the diet is more biologically available when the meal includes a good source of ascorbic acid or when meat is also present in the meal.

For the man, the basic pattern is below recommended levels for thiamin. When a modest part of the additional calories is selected from the bread-cereal group and/or the meat group, these deficiencies are easily overcome. Although the niacin level appears to be low, it must be taken into account that the tryptophan available from the protein will yield an additional 12 mg niacin.

Other Minerals and Vitamins Table 13–3 is a calculation of the Basic Diet for certain minerals and vitamins for which information at the present time is less complete and reliable. For some of these nutrients the Food and Nutrition Board has pointed out that more research needs to be done upon which to base the allowances and that changes will be made as more information is available. It may be that some of the allowances that have been set are too high.

The tables of food composition for these nutrients are not as reliable as might be desired: (1) only a few analyses have been made for many foods; (2) wide variations exist from one sample to another, depending upon conditions of processing, storage, and cookery; (3) methods for analyses are not always in close agreement, for example, values for folacin will vary widely depending upon the forms of the vitamin that have been determined; and (4) samples are not always fully described in the published reports, and variations could occur because the determinations were made on raw or cooked forms. Although the data presented in Table 13–3 may be less reliable than those in Table 13–2, they do give information on the sources of these nutrients and the relative magnitude.

From Table 13–3 it becomes evident that the Basic Diet does not supply the daily allowances of magnesium, zinc, folacin, vitamin B-6, and vitamin E. If one observes the following guidelines, most of these deficiencies will be corrected.

1. To complete the caloric requirement, select most of the additional foods from the four food groups with minimum choices from the sweets, fats, and alcohol group.
2. From day to day vary the choice of

Table 13-2. Nutritive Value of A Basic Diet Pattern for the Adult in Health*

					Fat				Minerals				Vitamins				
Food	Measure	Weight gm	Energy kcal	Protein gm	Total gm	Saturated gm	Linoleic gm	Carbohydrate gm	Ca mg	P mg	Fe mg	K mg	A IU	Thiamin mg	Riboflavin mg	Niacin mg	Ascorbic Acid mg
Vegetable-fruit group																	
Dark leafy green or deep yellow†	¼–⅓ cup	50	15	1	tr			3	14	16	0.4	112	3,810	0.03	0.04	0.3	15
Other vegetable‡	¼–⅓ cup	50	20	2	tr			4	11	18	0.4	97	270	0.03	0.03	0.4	7
Potato	1 medium	135	90	3	tr			20	8	57	0.7	385	tr	0.12	0.05	1.6	22
Vitamin-C-rich fruit§	½ cup	125	55	1	tr			14	22	22	0.4	226	266	0.11	0.03	0.4	52
Other fruit‖	1 serving	100	60	tr	tr			15	8	15	0.4	180	340	0.03	0.03	0.4	5
Bread-cereal group																	
Cereal, whole-grain or enriched#	¾ cup	30 (dry)	96	3	1	0.1	0.1	21	11	60	1.4	66	433	0.17	0.15	1.6	3
Bread, whole-grain or enriched#	3 slices	75	195	8	3	0.4	0.9	38	70	121	2.1	141	tr	0.24	0.14	2.3	
Milk group																	
Milk (2 per cent fat)	2 cups	488	240	16	10	5.8	0.2	24	594	464	0.2	754	1,000	0.20	0.80	0.4	4
Meat group																	
Meat, fish, poultry, eggs, legumes**	5 ounces (cooked)	140	335	39	18	5.2	2.5	5	41	370	4.3	568	186	0.42	0.36	8.7	
TOTAL			1,106	73	32	11.5	3.7	144	779	1,143	10.3	2,529	6,305	1.35	1.63	16.1††	108
Fats																	
Margarine—soft	1 tablespoon	14	100	tr	12	2.0	4.1		3	3	tr	4	470	tr	tr	tr	0
Oil (corn)	1 tablespoon	14	120	0	14	1.7	7.8	0	0	0	0	0	0	0	0	0	0
			1,306	73	58	15.2	15.6	144	782	1,146	10.3	2,533	6,775	1.35	1.63	16.1	108
Recommended dietary allowances																	
Woman (23–50 years)				44					800	800	18		4,000	1.0	1.2	13	60
Man (23–50 years)				56					800	800	10		5,000	1.4	1.6	18	60

*Values for foods in the vegetable-fruit, bread-cereal, and meat groups are weighted averages based on the approximate consumption in the United States.

†Includes broccoli, carrots, escarole, kale, green peppers, pumpkin, and spinach. Assumes 1 serving (½–⅔ cup) every other day.

‡Includes snap beans, Lima beans, cabbage, cauliflower, celery, corn, cucumbers, lettuce, onions, peas, tomatoes. Assumes ½–⅔ cup every other day.

§Includes oranges, grapefruit, canned and frozen orange, and grapefruit juices.

‖Includes fresh, canned, and frozen fruits: apples, apricots, bananas, cherries, grapes, peaches, pears, pineapple, plums.

#Includes oatmeal, shredded wheat, cornflakes, wheat flakes with added iron, enriched rice, enriched macaroni; whole-wheat and white bread.

**Includes per week: 4 eggs; 2 ounces peanut butter, 1 ounce dry beans; 2 ounces tuna fish; 3 ounces flounder; 7 ounces chicken; 7 ounces pork; 9 ounces beef—based on edible, cooked portion weights for meats.

††The protein in this diet contains about 730 mg tryptophan, equivalent to 12 mg niacin; thus, the niacin equivalent is 28 mg.

Table 13-3. **Additional Mineral and Vitamin Values for the Basic Diet Pattern***

Food	Measure	Weight gm	Minerals: Sodium† mg	Magnesium mg	Copper mg	Zinc mg	Vitamins: Folacin µg	Pantothenic Acid µg	Vitamin B-6 µg	Vitamin B-12 µg	Vitamin E§ mg
Vegetable-fruit group											
Dark green leafy or deep yellow	1/4–1/3 cup	50	18	13	0.06	0.2	23	139	80	0	0.3
Other vegetable	1/4–1/3 cup	50	7	9	0.07	0.2	13	120	56	0	0.2
Potato	1 medium	135	6	24	0.2	0.6	11	540	211	0	0.05
Citrus fruit	1/2 cup	125	1	13	0.03	0.09	47	245	43	0	0.2
Other fruit	1 serving	100	2	13	0.01	0.1	11	139	127	0	0.4
Bread-cereal group‡											
Cereal, whole-grain or enriched	3/4 cup	30 (dry)	1	19	0.05	0.4	11	166	47	0	0.1
Bread, whole-grain or enriched	3 slices	75	15	37	0.2	0.9	37	446	83	tr	0.08
Milk group											
Milk (2 per cent fat)	2 cups	488	244	66	2.0	1.9	24	1,562	210	1.8	0.2
Meat group											
Meat, fish, poultry eggs, legumes	5 ounces (cooked)	140	112	48	0.2	4.0	34	1,386	376	1.6	1.1
Fats											
Margarine—soft (corn)	1 tablespoon	14	1	tr	0.01	0.03	tr	0	0	0	1.8
Oil (corn)	1 tablespoon	14	0	0	0	0	0	0	0	0	2.0
TOTAL			407	242	2.9	8.4	211	4,743	1,233	3.4	6.4
Recommended dietary allowances											
Woman (23–50 years)				300		15	400		2,000	3.0	8
Man (23–50 years)				350		15	400		2,200	3.0	10

*Values calculated on basis of same foods used for Table 13-2. (See footnote descriptions.) Table A-2 used for calculations. Values are to be regarded as approximations because of limited availability of data.

†Sodium values are based upon foods processed and prepared without the addition of salt or other sodium compounds. As consumed in the ordinary diet, the sodium intake would range widely—about 2,500 to 5,000 mg.

‡Average of whole-grain and enriched breads and cereals.

§Values for vitamin E are for alpha-tocopherol only; this slightly underestimates the total vitamin E activity of the diet.

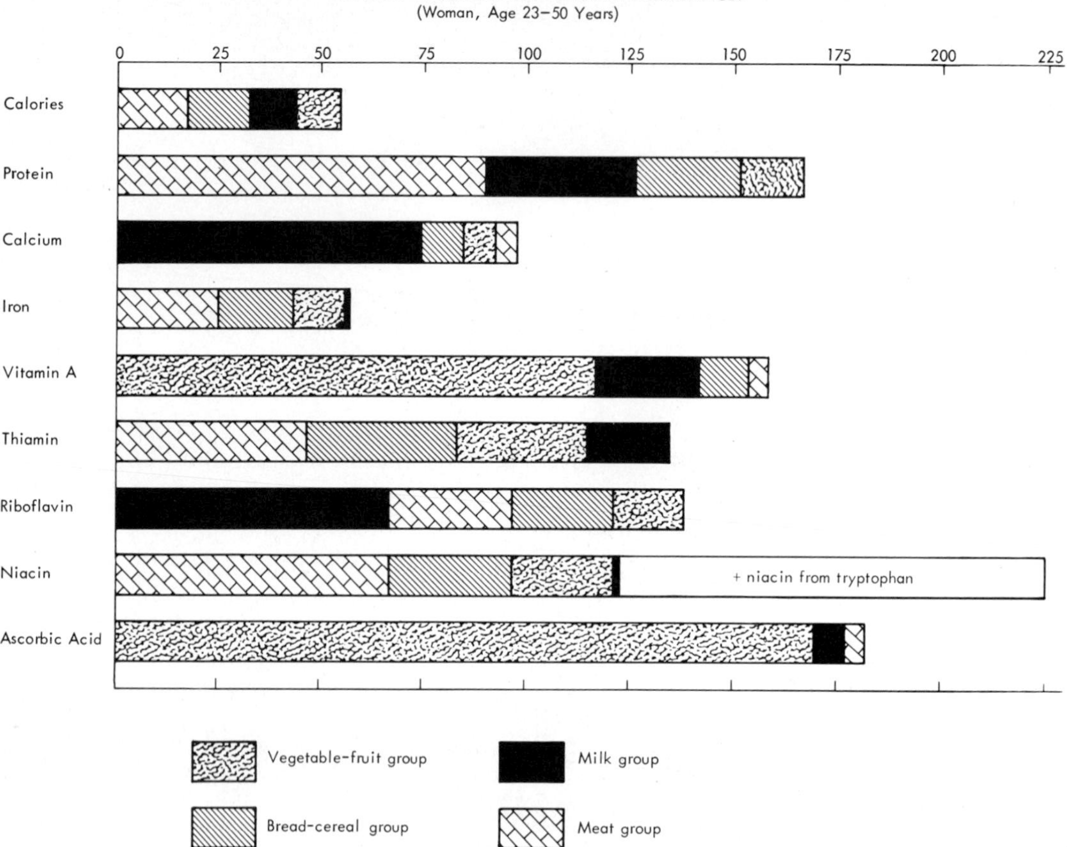

Figure 13–5. The four essential food groups of the Basic Diet meet, or nearly meet, the recommended allowances for nutrients except iron and calories for the woman of 23 to 50 years. See Table 13–2 for calculations.

foods from each group rather than depending upon a few favorite items. A variety of dark green leafy vegetables are excellent sources of magnesium and folacin. Whole-grain breads and cereals are far superior to enriched white breads and refined cereals for magnesium, zinc, folacin, vitamin B-6, and vitamin E.

3. One to two tablespoons of vegetable oils—corn, soybean, cottonseed, safflower—used in cooking, salad dressings, and so on, will furnish sufficient amounts of vitamin E.

Essentials of Meal Planning

In addition to meeting nutritive needs, successful meal planning depends upon many factors that are summarized in Table 13–4.

Begin with a Good Breakfast A great number of adults and children eat an inadequate breakfast or skip it altogether. Studies conducted many years ago at the State University of Iowa[4] showed that (1) efficiency in physiologic performance as measured by bicycle ergometer, treadmill, and maximum grip strength, decreased in late

Table 13-4. **Factors to Consider in Meal Planning**

Essential Factors	Interpretation
Family composition	Adjust amounts for children, teenagers, pregnant and lactating women. For persons with low energy requirements (women and elderly persons) select foods high in nutritive value
Food habits	Consider psychologic and cultural meanings of food. See Chapters 14 and 15 for full discussion
Food costs	Budgeting and food selection for economy are discussed on page 279
Time for food preparation	Budget time for best use, by planning menus for several days; shopping once a week, planning for leftovers; using some convenience foods if homemaker is also employed outside the home
Variety in meals	*Four food groups:* establish menu pattern that includes recommended amounts of each group for each member of the family. Keep selection of sweets, fats, and alcohol to a minimum.
	Variety of choice: vary the choice of foods within each group from day to day; do not use the same meats, vegetables, fruits every day
	Color: be sensitive to color combinations. Avoid meals that are all white, or all one color tone. Use garnishes for a touch of color; for example, paprika, pepper rings, radishes, parsley
	Texture: include some crisp and chewy foods with soft foods
	Flavor: combine bland foods with those that are more strongly flavored; do not use all spicy or all bland foods at one meal
	Preparation: use a variety of preparation methods; for example, boiling, roasting, baking, frying; with or without sauces; various combinations of foods
Season	Hearty foods such as stews and soups are favored in cold weather; lighter foods in hot weather, but including the same nutrients
Satiety	Provide some protein and fat in each meal to allay sense of hunger
Meal spacing	Arrange meal times so that family can be together whenever possible. Plan snacks to include nutrients for the day. Be discriminate in use of high-carbohydrate, high-calorie foods for snacks

morning hours when breakfast was omitted; (2) attitude toward schoolwork and scholastic achievement was poorer when breakfast was omitted; (3) the content of the breakfast did not determine its efficiency so long as it was nutritionally adequate; (4) a breakfast providing one fourth of the daily caloric and protein allowances was superior to smaller or larger breakfasts for maintaining efficiency in the late morning hours; (5) a protein intake of 20 to 25 gm maintained the blood glucose level during the late morning hours; and (6) the omission of breakfast was of no value in weight reduction. In fact, those who omit breakfast while on a weight reduction regimen experience greater hunger in addition to being physiologically inefficient.

A change to better breakfast habits means (1) planning simple, easy-to-prepare, but varied meals; (2) arising sufficiently early so that there is time for eating breakfast; (3) eating breakfast with the family group so that it, like other meals, has pleasant social associations.

Breakfast may include some protein food such as egg or milk, cereal or breadstuff, or both, and a beverage. Children and teenagers should include milk for breakfast. If citrus fruit or another good source of ascorbic acid is included at breakfast, the day's allowance is ensured. Cereal may be hot or cold; breads may vary from plain white enriched or whole grain to muffins, griddle cakes, waffles, or sweet rolls, as the occasion warrants. A breakfast may be light or heavy depending upon the individual's activity and preferences. (See page 266.)

Light Breakfast

Orange juice
Raisin bran with 2 per cent milk
Coffee
Milk for children

Heavy Breakfast

Cantaloupe
Griddle cakes with syrup
Sausages
Coffee
Milk for children

Lunch is Often Neglected Thousands of workers eat lunches that are limited to the choices in a fast-food restaurant or to the sandwich carried from home. The hamburger on a bun, French fries, and a soft drink or coffee is a common pattern. This can be improved by including a salad and a glass of milk or by carrying a piece of fruit from home.

Through school food services lunches that supply about one third of the recommended allowances are available to children and teenagers in most of the nation's schools. Older Americans, too, in many cities and rural communities are able to receive a noon meal at centers for group feeding.

Often the lunch eaten by homemakers and preschool children consists of a day-to-day monotony of leftovers because the homemaker does not take time for adequate planning or preparation. Sometimes this leads to indiscriminate snacking throughout the day. The following menus illustrate good luncheons or suppers that require a minimum of preparation time.

Luncheon or Supper

Tomato soup
Chicken sandwich on whole-wheat bread with celery, lettuce, mayonnaise
Fresh fruit cup
Peanut butter cookies
Milk

Salad bowl with mixed greens, tomato wedges, cauliflower, and cottage cheese
French dressing
Whole-wheat muffin with margarine and jelly
Pumpkin pie (leftover from dinner)
Milk

Dinner Patterns The evening meal is the only meal over which most homemakers have control. For many families it is the only time when all members are together. This meal must make up for any deficiencies that might have occurred earlier in the day.

Meat, fish, fowl, cheese, eggs, or legumes comprise the main dish at dinner. Potatoes or a starchy food and a green or yellow vegetable are generally included. If no salad has been provided in the luncheon it should be served here. Dessert may consist of fruits, simple puddings, cake, or pastries. Milk should be given to children.

Snacks Most people consume snacks and beverages between meals and in the evening. When they are selected as part of the total food pattern for the day, and consist primarily of nutrient-rich foods, they can enhance the nutritive quality of the diet. Far too often, snacks consist of high-calorie foods that are low in nutritive value. This means that some people will exceed their caloric requirements and that others, especially children, may not consume sufficient amounts of essential nutrients.

Some good snack selections for all ages are the following:

Fruit juices without sugar
Fresh fruits
Raw vegetables: celery, cauliflower, broccoli, green pepper, carrots, cabbage wedge, and others
Skim, low-fat, or whole milk
Cereal with milk
Cheese wedge

Meal Patterns The Daily Food Guide and the Dietary Goals are illustrated in the following meal pattern:

Food Groups	Sample Menu Using Food Groups	Completed Menu with Typical Additions
Breakfast		
Fruit, rich in vitamin C	Orange juice	Orange juice
Cereal, whole-grain or enriched	Oatmeal	Oatmeal with milk and sugar
Bread, whole-grain or enriched	Muffin	Muffin with soft-type margarine
Milk	Milk—2 per cent fat	Milk—2 per cent fat
		Coffee or tea for adults; cream and sugar
Luncheon		
Meat—1 to 2 ounces	Sandwich:	Sandwich:
	Tuna fish—2 oz	Tuna fish—2 ounces
Bread—2 slices	Whole-wheat bread—2 slices	Whole-wheat bread—2 slices
		Chopped celery
Fat—2 teaspoons	Mayonnaise—2 teaspoons	Mayonnaise—2 teaspoons
Fruit—1 serving	Fresh plums	Fresh plums
		Spice cupcake
Milk—1 cup	Milk, 2 per cent—1 cup	Milk, 2 per cent—1 cup
Dinner		
Meat—3 to 4 ounces	Meat loaf	Meat loaf with gravy
Potato—1 medium	Mashed potatoes	Mashed potatoes
Leafy green or deep yellow vegetable	Carrots	Parsley carrots with margarine
Raw vegetable or fruit	Lettuce and tomato salad	Lettuce and tomato salad
Fat—3 teaspoons		Italian dressing
		Margarine on vegetables
		Fresh fruit cup
		Milk for children
		Coffee or tea for adults
		Snack
		Apple slices with cheese

Food Budgets

Food Costs in the 1977 Household Survey Preliminary data from this survey indicate, as might be expected, that the expenditures for food both at home and away from home increased as the family income increased.[5] For example, at household incomes between $5,000 and $9,999 the weekly expenditure was $39 for food at home and $8 for food away from home. For households with an income of $20,000 or more the weekly expenditure for food at home was $60 and for food away from home was $25.*

The trend to eat away from home more frequently has been documented. In the 1965 survey about 13 cents of every food dollar was spent for meals away from home and 4 cents for snacks. By 1977 meals away

* Households averaged 3.1 household members.

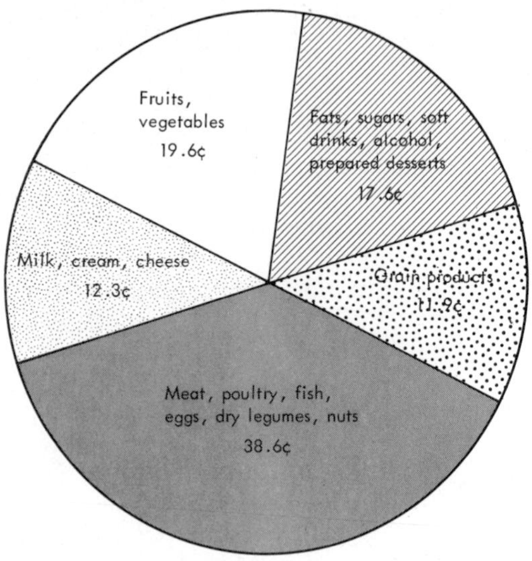

Figure 13–6. Division of food dollar by households in the 1977 Food Consumption Survey. Note that the protein-rich group accounts for almost two fifths of expenditure; also, the sugars, fats, alcoholic and other beverages, prepared desserts, and miscellaneous foods account for more than one sixth, but contribute fewer nutrients than the other groups. (Source: Hama, M.Y.: "Household Food Consumption, 1977 and 1965," *Family Econ. Rev.*, Spring 1980, p. 8.)

from home accounted for 19 cents of every food dollar, and 5 cents for snacks. Each meal away from home cost 2.6 times as much as a meal at home.

The nutrient return per dollar spent was higher for low-income households than for households with higher incomes. This does not mean that people in low-income households chose more nutritious foods consciously. Rather, the foods used in large quantities because they are inexpensive are also significant contributors to nutrient intake: enriched and whole-grain breads, some cereals, dry beans, and potatoes—all of which are eaten in substantial quantities when income is limited. (See Figure 13–6.)

Planning the Food Budget

Factors to Consider in Budgeting Today's homemaker, in most instances in the United States, has more money to spend, spends less time in food preparation, and serves better meals than at any time in history. She has a better education and enjoys more outside activities than did her mother. She lives longer and returns to the work force when her children are in school, if not sooner. During a given year she will purchase about one ton of food for each teenager and adult in her family. All of these circumstances affect the amount of money that will be spent for food and how that money will be spent. Some factors to consider are these:

1. Number of family members, their age distribution, increased needs during pregnancy and lactation and adolescence, or special needs for modified diets.
2. Family income. On a national average about 17 per cent of income is spent for food. But this average can give a false impression. When the income is low the proportion of money spent for food is likely to be 25, 30, or 40 per cent or even more.
3. The availability of supplementary programs when income is limited. Food stamps, free or reduced-cost school lunches and breakfasts, the WIC program for women, infants, and children, and congregate meal programs for the elderly are important ways to increase the available food supply.
4. The location of markets. Although supermarkets generally provide food at less cost than small, neighborhood markets, transportation to these large markets is a problem for some people.
5. Alternative marketing choices. Some community groups have organized cooperatives; that is, they arrange to purchase food in wholesale lots and to sell

them at cost to the members of the group. Usually these cooperatives are restricted to certain foods; for example packaged goods or farm produce. Another alternative is the discount food store that eliminates the frills of merchandising. Foods may be sold directly from the packing carton. In some stores generic rather than trade brands are sold. Although these products may not be graded for quality, the wholesomeness and nutritive values of these foods are good.

6. Home prepared and convenience foods. Some convenience foods compare favorably in cost with home-prepared products: canned soups, fruits, vegetables, and citrus juices; frozen citrus juices and vegetables; muffin, cake, and pudding mixes. Convenience foods that are appreciably more expensive are those that involve much preparation or that have a short shelf life; for example, ready-to-eat salads, packaged salad greens, ready-to-bake rolls, pastries, frozen entrees, and frozen vegetables in sauces. Homemakers who are employed outside the home sometimes balance these additional costs against the time saved in home food preparation.
7. The choice of foods within each major food group. The variations within the food groups have been discussed in the preceding pages.
8. The amount of money that may be spent for snack items and beverages. This category can substantially increase the food expenditure without adding appreciably to the nutrient value of the diet.

Ten Recommendations for Effecting Economy Appreciable savings are possible if the following suggestions are observed.

1. Plan meals several days in advance. Use the Daily Food Guide and the Dietary Goals as a basis for menu planning to ensure good nutrition.
2. Use poultry, fish, peanut butter, and legumes in place of meat for some of the main meals each week. Use smaller portions of meat together with less expensive foods.
3. Eat meals at home or carry meals to work whenever practical.
4. Read newspapers for reports on foods in plentiful supply. Watch advertisements for the items featured as specials for that week. (See Figure 13–7.)
5. Use a market list. Be prepared to make substitutions when other foods of equal value are cheaper. Avoid impulse buying.
6. Purchase foods that the family will eat. Uneaten foods are no bargain, but the wise homemaker introduces new foods attractively prepared from time to time so that the family learns to enjoy a wide variety.
7. Read labels. Look for information on dates and nutritive values. Purchase the grade appropriate for the intended use. Compare unit prices of various brands. (See page 324 for discussion of labeling.)
8. Buy large-size packages only if the price per unit is less, if there is space to properly store the food, and if the food can be used before it spoils.
9. Know the best storage conditions for each food and store food accordingly.
10. Avoid home waste:
    a. Use food when it is at its peak of quality.
    b. Avoid loss of vegetables through excessive peeling.
    c. Cook vegetables in minimum quantities of water until just tender to preserve maximum nutritive value.
    d. Season foods and serve attractively so that they are well accepted.
    e. Use leftovers within 24 hours.

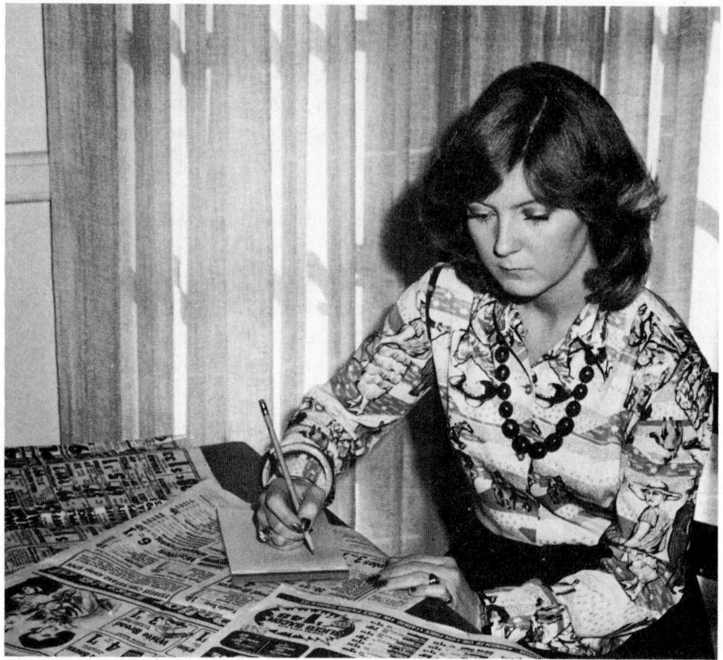

Figure 13–7. Before going to the market this homemaker checks against advertised prices. Menu plans can be adjusted as the market list is prepared. (Courtesy, Ralph E. Pyke and Department of Nutrition and Food Sciences, Texas Woman's University, Denton.)

Master Food Plans

Although the Daily Food Guide is a convenient tool for planning diets that will be nutritionally satisfactory, it does not provide the quantitative basis for estimating the full cost of a diet. Nutritionists, nurses, and other health workers must be able to help families set up food plans that are nutritionally adequate within their incomes. The Consumer and Food Economics Institute of the U.S. Department of Agriculture has set up master food plans at four cost levels: thrifty; low cost; moderate cost; and liberal cost. Each of the plans was designed to furnish the recommended dietary allowances as foods are actually consumed. The plans include recommendations for men, women, and children of differing ages, and for pregnant and nursing women. See Tables 13–5 and 13–6.

The plans take into account the typical patterns of food consumption by most groups of people in the United States. For each category the amounts of food to be brought into the kitchen are listed. Based upon surveys showing practices in typical households at varying levels of income, allowances have been made for waste in preparation, losses of nutrients in cooking, and plate waste. On the low-cost plan 10 per cent waste is allowed and on the moderate-cost plan 20 per cent waste.

Compared with the moderate-cost plan, the low-cost plan calls for more bread, flour, and cereals, but smaller amounts of milk, cheese, ice cream; meat, poultry, and fish; fruits and vegetables other than potatoes; and bakery products. On the low-cost plan it is also necessary to select the less expensive foods within each group. The moderate-cost plan permits more frequent use of expensive cuts of meat and out-of-season foods. The latter also provides greater variety and can make use of more bakery products and other convenience foods.

Twice a year the Consumer and Food Economics Institute determines the cost of food for each age-sex category in each plan. This information provides the basis for set-

Table 13-5. **Low-Cost Food Plan: Amounts of Food for One Week*†**

Family Member	Milk, Cheese, Ice Cream‡ qt	Meat, Poultry, Fish§ lb	Eggs No	Dry Beans and Peas, Nuts‖ lb	Dark Green, Deep Yellow Vegetables lb	Citrus Fruit, Tomatoes lb	Potatoes lb	Other Vegetables, Fruit lb	Cereal lb	Flour lb	Bread lb	Other Bakery Products lb	Fats, Oils lb	Sugar, Sweets lb	Accessories** lb
Child															
7 months to 1 year	5.70	0.56	2.1	0.15	0.35	0.42	0.06	3.43	0.71#	0.02	0.06	0.05	0.05	0.18	0.06
1–2 years	3.57	1.26	3.6	0.16	0.23	1.01	0.60	2.88	0.99#	0.27	0.76	0.33	0.12	0.36	0.68
3–5 years	3.91	1.52	2.7	0.25	0.25	1.20	0.85	2.95	0.90	0.30	0.91	0.57	0.38	0.71	1.02
6–8 years	4.74	2.03	2.9	0.39	0.31	1.58	1.10	3.67	1.11	0.45	1.27	0.84	0.52	0.90	1.43
9–11 years	5.46	2.57	3.9	0.44	0.38	2.13	1.41	4.81	1.24	0.62	1.65	1.20	0.61	1.15	1.89
Male															
12–14 years	5.74	2.98	4.0	0.56	0.40	1.99	1.50	3.90	1.15	0.67	1.88	1.25	0.77	1.15	2.61
15–19 years	5.49	3.74	4.0	0.34	0.39	2.20	1.87	4.50	0.90	0.75	2.10	1.55	1.05	1.04	3.09
20–54 years	2.74	4.56	4.0	0.33	0.48	2.32	1.87	4.81	0.93	0.71	2.10	1.47	0.91	0.81	2.11
55 years and over	2.61	3.63	4.0	0.21	0.61	2.38	1.72	4.92	1.02	0.62	1.73	1.23	0.77	0.90	1.16
Female															
12–19 years	5.63	2.55	4.0	0.24	0.46	2.17	1.17	4.57	0.75	0.63	1.44	1.05	0.53	0.88	2.44
20–54 years	3.02	3.21	4.0	0.19	0.55	2.34	1.40	4.17	0.71	0.55	1.31	0.94	0.59	0.72	2.13
55 years and over	3.01	2.45	4.0	0.15	0.62	2.54	1.22	4.57	0.97	0.58	1.24	0.86	0.38	0.64	1.11
Pregnant	5.25	3.68	4.0	0.29	0.67	2.80	1.65	4.99	0.95	0.66	1.52	1.06	0.55	0.78	2.56
Nursing	5.25	4.16	4.0	0.26	0.66	2.99	1.67	5.33	0.78	0.61	1.55	1.16	0.76	0.91	2.70

*Peterkin, B.: "USDA Family Food Plans, 1974," National Agricultural Outlook Conference, Washington, D.C., December 12, 1974.

†Amounts are for food as purchased or brought into the kitchen from garden or farm. Amounts allow for discard of about one tenth of the *edible* food as plate waste, spoilage, and so on. Amounts of foods are shown to two decimal places to allow for greater accuracy, especially in estimating rations for large groups of people and for long periods of time. For general use, amounts of food groups for a family may be rounded to the nearest tenth or quarter of a pound.

‡Fluid milk and beverages made from dry or evaporated milk. Cheese and ice cream may replace some milk. Count as equivalent to a quart of fluid milk: natural or processed Cheddar-type cheese, 6 ounces; cottage cheese, 2½ pounds; ice cream, 1½ quarts.

§Bacon and salt pork should not exceed ⅓ pound for each 5 pounds of this group.

‖Weight in terms of dry beans and peas, shelled nuts, and peanut butter. Count 1 pound of canned dry beans—pork and beans, kidney beans, and so on—as 0.33 pound.

#Cereal fortified with iron is recommended.

**Includes coffee, tea, cocoa, punches, ades, soft drinks, leavenings, and seasonings. The use of iodized salt is recommended.

Table 13-6. **Moderate-Cost Food Plan: Amounts of Food for One Week*†**

Family Member	Milk, Cheese, Ice Cream‡ qt	Meat, Poultry, Fish§ lb	Eggs No	Dry Beans, and Peas, Nuts‖ lb	Dark Green, Deep Yellow Vegetables lb	Citrus Fruit, Tomatoes lb	Potatoes lb	Other Vegetables, Fruit lb	Cereal lb	Flour lb	Bread lb	Other Bakery Products lb	Fats, Oils lb	Sugar, Sweets lb	Accessories** lb
Child:															
7 months to 1 year	6.46	0.80	2.2	0.13	0.41	0.49	0.06	3.98	0.64#	0.02	0.06	0.05	0.05	0.19	0.08
1–2 years	4.04	1.69	4.0	0.15	0.29	1.24	0.59	3.44	1.03#	0.26	0.81	0.33	0.12	0.28	0.79
3–5 years	4.74	1.88	3.0	0.22	0.30	1.46	0.85	3.51	0.74	0.27	0.82	0.73	0.41	0.81	1.42
6–8 years	5.79	2.60	3.3	0.34	0.37	1.94	1.17	4.39	0.84	0.39	1.14	1.11	0.56	1.03	1.97
9–11 years	6.68	3.31	4.0	0.38	0.45	2.61	1.40	5.76	1.03	0.51	1.47	1.51	0.66	1.31	2.63
Male:															
12–14 years	7.02	3.77	4.0	0.48	0.48	2.44	1.52	4.66	0.94	0.56	1.69	1.54	0.85	1.34	3.65
15–19 years	6.65	4.65	4.0	0.29	0.47	2.73	2.00	5.45	0.80	0.67	1.98	1.82	1.05	1.15	4.41
20–54 years	3.38	5.73	4.0	0.29	0.59	2.92	1.94	5.93	0.76	0.65	1.97	1.65	0.95	0.96	2.95
55 years and over	2.97	4.64	4.0	0.19	0.70	2.91	1.69	5.88	0.89	0.53	1.58	1.45	0.87	1.05	1.50
Female:															
12–19 years	6.22	3.32	4.0	0.24	0.53	2.62	1.21	5.38	0.68	0.56	1.34	1.22	0.56	0.97	3.36
20–54 years	3.35	4.12	4.0	0.19	0.62	2.84	1.35	4.94	0.54	0.49	1.28	1.08	0.65	0.81	2.89
55 years and over	3.35	3.21	4.0	0.14	0.72	3.09	1.17	5.50	0.81	0.52	1.20	0.98	0.45	0.73	1.39
Pregnant	5.44	4.57	4.0	0.25	0.91	3.52	1.60	6.13	0.73	0.83	1.77	1.28	0.46	0.85	3.50
Nursing	5.31	5.01	4.0	0.26	0.91	3.76	1.73	6.52	0.74	0.81	1.84	1.42	0.69	1.00	3.79

*Peterkin, B.: "USDA Family Food Plans, 1974," National Argicultural Outlook Conference, Washington, D.C., December 12, 1974.

†Amounts are for food as purchased or brought into the kitchen from garden or farm. Amounts allow for discard of about one tenth of the *edible* food as plate waste, spoilage, and so on. Amounts of foods are shown to two decimal places to allow for greater accuracy, especially in estimating rations for large groups of people and for long periods of time. For general use, amounts of food groups for a family may be rounded to the nearest tenth or quarter of a pound.

‡Fluid milk and beverages made from dry or evaporated milk. Cheese and ice cream may replace some milk. Count as equivalent to a quart of fluid milk: natural or processed Cheddar-type cheese, 6 ounces; cottage cheese, 2½ pounds; ice cream, 1½ quarts.

§Bacon and salt pork should not exceed ⅓ pound for each 5 pounds of this group.

‖Weight in terms of dry beans and peas, shelled nuts, and peanut butter. Count 1 pound of canned dry beans—pork and beans, kidney beans, and so on—as 0.33 pound.

#Cereal fortified with iron is recommended.

**Includes coffee, tea, cocoa, punches, ades, soft drinks, leavenings, and seasonings. The use of iodized salt is recommended.

ting the amount of money to be included for food in welfare allowances. With the rapid inflation of recent years, these cost adjustments are extremely important. In March 1981 the low-cost plan for a family of four, including two school-age children, for one week cost $73.70; the moderate-cost plan for the same family, $92.00; and the liberal-cost plan, $111.30. Although these costs obviously change from time to time, there is not a great deal of fluctuation in the percentage differences. It may be expected that the moderate-cost plan will cost about 25 per cent more than the low-cost plan, and the liberal-cost plan about 50 per cent more.

Problems and Review

1. *Problem.* Calculate the nutritive values for three foods that you eat regularly. Which of these provides the greatest nutritive value per 100 kcal?
2. *Problem.* Select a series of menus from a popular magazine. Check the menus against the Daily Food Guide for dietary adequacy. Point out examples of good menu planning. What adjustments in these menus would be necessary to incorporate the Dietary Goals?
3. *Problem.* Plan a breakfast for a teenager who does not like cereal. Include some food from each of the groups of the Daily Food Guide.
4. Why are each of the following poor examples of menu planning? How could you change each combination to effect improvement?
   a. Meat loaf, mashed potatoes, mashed winter squash, baked custard
   b. Macaroni and cheese, roast pork, buttered spinach, cheese pie
   c. Broiled flounder, creamed onions, spicy cole slaw, pickles
5. Compare the nutritive values of these snacks: 1 small bag (20 gm) potato chips; one apple; 1 ounce salted peanuts; 4 chocolate chip cookies; 10 thin pretzel twists. How would you rate these for snacks for yourself?
6. *Problem.* Calculate the cost of 25 mg ascorbic acid from each of five fresh fruits available in the market.
7. *Problem.* Compare the unit prices for various size packages of the following cereals: puffed wheat; cornflakes; two brands of sugar-coated cereals; two brands of cereals that are fortified with minerals and vitamins. Tabulate the nutritive value for 1 ounce of each of the cereals, according to information on the label. List the cereals in order of best buys, nutritive values being considered.

Cited References

1. Marston, R. M., and Welsh, S. O.: "Nutrient Content of the National Food Supply," *National Food Rev.*, U.S. Department of Agriculture, Washington, D.C., Winter 1981, pp. 19–22.
2. Widdowson, E. M., and McCance, R. A.: "Studies on the Nutritive Value of Bread and on the Effect of Variations in the Extraction Rate of Flour on the Growth of Undernourished Children," Her Majesty's Stationery Office, Privy Council, Medical Research Council Special Report Series No. 287, London, 1954.
3. "Statistical Highlights: Civilian Consumption of Major Food Commodities (retail weight)," *National Food Rev.*, U.S. Department of Agriculture, Washington, D.C., Winter 1981, pp. 43.
4. *Breakfast Source Book,* Cereal Institute, Chicago, 1959.

5. Rizek, R. L., and Peterkin, B. B.: "Food Costs of U.S. Households, Spring 1977," *Family Econ. Rev.*, Fall 1979, pp. 14–19.

Additional References

BAUMAN, H. E.: "What Does the Consumer Know About Nutrition?" *JAMA,* **225**:61–62, 1973.

CRONIN, F. J.: "Nutrient Levels and Food Used by Households, 1977 and 1965," *Family Econ. Rev.*, Spring 1980, pp. 10–15.

HAMA, M. Y.: "Household Food Consumption, 1977 and 1965," *Family Econ. Rev.*, Spring 1980, pp. 4–9.

KAITZ, E. F.: "Getting the Most from Your Food Dollar," *Nat. Food Rev.*, Winter 1979, pp. 26–29.

PETERKIN, B. B., et al.: "Some Diets That Meet the Dietary Goals for the United States," *J. Am. Diet. Assoc.*, **74**:423–30, 1979.

POPKIN, B. M., and LATHAM, M. C.: "The Limitations and Dangers of Commerciogenic Nutritious Foods," *Am. J. Clin. Nutr.*, **26**:1015–23, 1973.

VERMEERSCH, J. A., and SWENERTON, H.: "Consumer Responses to Nutrition Claims in Food Advertisements," *J. Nutr. Educ.*, **11**:22–26, 1979.

Publications for the Consumer

Publications by the United States Department of Agriculture:

BEEF AND VEAL IN FAMILY MEALS, G 118.
BREADS, CAKES, AND PIES IN FAMILY MEALS, G 186.
CEREALS AND PASTAS IN FAMILY MEALS, G 150.
CHEESE IN FAMILY MEALS, G 112.
EAT A GOOD BREAKFAST, Leaflet 268.
EGGS IN FAMILY MEALS, G 103.
FAMILY FARE: A GUIDE TO GOOD NUTRITION, G 1.
FAMILY FOOD BUDGETING FOR GOOD MEALS AND NUTRITION, HG 94.
FOOD, HG 228.
FOOD GUIDE FOR OLDER FOLKS, G 17.
FOOD FOR FAMILIES WITH SCHOOL CHILDREN, G 13.
FOOD FOR FAMILIES WITH YOUNG CHILDREN, G 5.
FOOD FOR THE YOUNG COUPLE, G 85.
FRUITS IN FAMILY MEALS, G 125.
LAMB IN FAMILY MEALS, G 124.
MILK IN FAMILY MEALS, G 127.
MONEY SAVING MAIN DISHES, G 43.
NUTRITION: FOOD AT WORK FOR YOU, GS-1.
NUTS IN FAMILY MEALS, G 176.
PORK IN FAMILY MEALS, G 160.
POULTRY IN FAMILY MEALS, G 110.
VEGETABLES IN FAMILY MEALS, G105.
YOUR MONEY'S WORTH IN FOODS, HG 183.

14 Factors Influencing Food Intake and Food Habits

FOOD intake is governed by physiologic, environmental, and behavioral factors. Food habits are infinitely complex in their origin, being derived from the earliest experiences in life and influenced by sensory, aesthetic, economic, geographic, social, and cultural factors. Food habits are not necessarily static. They are changed according to the need to adapt to a new environment, to new attitudes, and to new values.

Physiologic Bases for Food Intake

Hunger is a "compelling need or desire for food; the painful sensation or state of weakness caused by need of food."* Contractions of the stomach and a drop in blood sugar accompanied by a feeling of weakness have long been associated with the sensation of hunger.

Mechanisms for Control of Food Intake Mechanical, neural, biochemical, and hormonal interactions regulate the intake of food. The theories for the regulation of food intake are based primarily on animal experiments and are not fully understood.

The hypothalamus is the control center for the regulation of food intake. The ventromedial nucleus is the "satiety" center, and the area lateral to the ventromedial nucleus is the "feeding" center. Thus, the lateral nucleus stimulates the animal to eat until it receives a signal from the ventromedial nucleus to inhibit eating. In experimental animals the bilateral destruction of the ventromedial nucleus leads to overeating and obesity. On the other hand, the destruction of the lateral nucleus leads to cessation of eating and starvation.

Role of the gastrointestinal tract. Walter B. Cannon and Anton Carlson, two famous physiologists early in this century, observed the relationship of the sensations of hunger to increases in the contractions of the stomach and the satiety effect of a filled stomach. There exists a neural link between the gastrointestinal tract and the hypothalamus. This link serves to inform the hypothalamus when the stomach is distended.

Two hormones, gastrin and enterogastrone, exert opposing effects on contractions of the stomach and gastric emptying. Gastrin, a powerful hormone, is produced by the mucous membrane of the pylorus upon vagal stimulation, by distention of the stomach with food, and possibly by the products of protein digestion. It stimulates the secretion of gastric juice and increases contractions. Another hormone, enterogastrone, is produced when fats and fatty acids enter the duodenum. It reduces motility, delays emptying, and suppresses gastric secretion.

Although these mechanisms help to explain feelings of satiety and hunger in normal individuals, these feelings are also experienced by persons who have had a gastrectomy. Thus, other controls must also be operational.

Glucostatic theory. One example of control is the regulation of blood sugar. Insulin is secreted at a controlled rate when the glucose of the blood coursing through the pancreas is high. Conversely, other hor-

* *The Random House Dictionary of the English Language,* unabridged ed., Random House, New York, 1966.

mones such as glucagon, epinephrine, the glucocorticoids of the adrenal cortex, and the adrenocorticotropic and growth hormones of the pituitary can bring the glucose level back to its normal range when the blood concentration is too low. The maintenance of the blood sugar within physiologic limits obviously is a complex interaction involving the liver, pancreas, adrenal, and pituitary.

Mayer and his associates have shown that chemoreceptors in the ventromedial center of the hypothalamus have an affinity for glucose and are activated by it.[1] According to their GLUCOSTATIC THEORY, when glucose utilization is high, these receptors respond by acting as a brake upon the lateral nucleus (the feeding center) and also exercising some control over the hunger contractions of the stomach. When glucose utilization is low, these receptors are not stimulated and the sensation of hunger causes the individual to eat.

Theory of thermostatic control. According to Brobeck, food intake in certain conditions is part of the system of regulation of body temperature.[2] In the cold, food intake is increased and in hot environments intake is reduced. At an environmental temperature of 7°C rats consumed 126 kcal per day, but at 35°C they consumed only 18 kcal per day. If the rats were force-fed at the high temperature, they died of heat stroke. The area in the brain for this control is the preoptic anterior hypothalamus. When this area is destroyed in the rat, there is undereating in a cold environment and overeating in a hot environment.

Adipose tissue and food intake. All factors considered, it is quite remarkable that the body weight for most adults remains fairly constant. Another hypothesis regarding control of food intake asserts that the balance between energy intake and energy loss involves a regulation by body fat.[3] The theory is that some unknown metabolite related to the mass of adipose tissue is sensed by the central nervous system. In turn, the ventromedial hypothalamus in some way acts like a brake to prevent excessive weight gain. In one study rats that were fed excess calories by tube until they became obese consumed little food after tube feeding stopped. Their food intake returned to normal only after they had lost the extra body weight. In other words, the communication from the adipose tissue to the hypothalamus indicated a deviation from the body weight "set point," and correction of the increased body weight was brought about by reducing the food intake.

Sensations Produced by Foods The palatability of food is a composite of taste, smell, texture, and temperature. It is further conditioned by the surroundings in which food is consumed.

Sweet, sour, salty, and bitter are terms used to describe the sensations that result when foods placed in the mouth produce specific stimuli to the taste buds on the tongue. (See Figure 14–1.) The sense of taste is more highly developed in some indi-

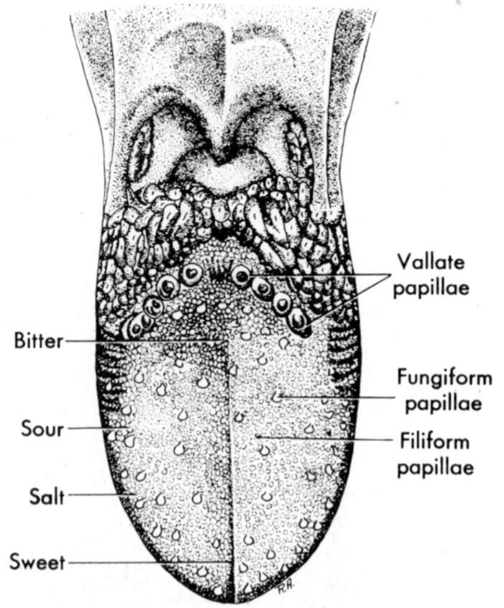

Figure 14–1. The upper surface of the tongue, showing kinds of papilla and areas of taste. (Courtesy, Miller, M. A., and Leavell, L. C.: *Kimber-Gray-Stackpole's Anatomy and Physiology,* 16th ed. Macmillan Publishing Co., Inc., New York, 1972.)

viduals than in others; foods may be too salty for one individual and just right for another; or they may be too sweet for one, but not quite sweet enough for another. Some persons can detect slight differences in taste, others cannot. The number of taste buds varies not only from individual to individual, but also from age to age. Korslund and Eppright found that preschool children who had low taste sensitivities tended to accept more variety of foods than did those with high taste sensitivities.[4] As the taste buds diminish in number later in life, foods that are more highly flavored tend to be preferred, whereas children voluntarily select bland or sweet foods. Taste sensitivity is decreased in those who smoke tobacco.

The taste and smell of foods are directly linked. If one were to hold the nose while eating a piece of fruit, much of the enjoyment would be lost. As a matter of fact, odor is the most important component of flavor, and an individual would derive limited pleasure from food if the tongue were the sole source of the sensations. The stimulation of the olfactory organs is brought about by certain volatile oils. Foods may be accepted because of their aromas, or they may be rejected because of their repulsive odors. No doubt, the odors of certain cheeses, for example, are the determinants in their acceptance by some and their rejection by others.

The sense of touch is highly developed in the tongue. Temperature, pain, and variations in texture or "feel" are experienced. Steaming hot foods are necessary to enjoyment by some, but children usually prefer foods that are lukewarm. A choice of ice cream may be influenced as much by its texture—smooth, creamy, and velvety, or crystalline and grainy—as by its other flavor qualities. Children may reject foods that are slippery such as baked custard or a gelatin dessert only later to learn to enjoy this texture sensation. The stringiness of certain vegetables, the stickiness of some mashed potatoes, the greasiness of fried foods may be important factors in rejection.

Cultural, Social, and Psychologic Factors Influencing Food Acceptance

The theories pertaining to the physiologic and biochemical regulation of food intakes, are based primarily on studies of experimental animals. In humans the regulation of food intake is much more complex. APPETITE is a desire for food and drink. Animals stop eating when satiated, but humans often continue to eat because they derive pleasure from food. Social pressures, habits, prejudices and the communications media are among the many factors that can obscure the mechanisms of the hypothalamus. But in unpleasant situations humans may cease eating even though they are not satiated.

Role of Culture Humans do not choose by instinct that which is best for them. In different environments humans eat what is available and sometimes learn by experience that some foods are better for them than others. The circumstances under which one eats are largely determined by one's culture. Used in this sense, CULTURE is "the sum total of ways of living built up by a group of human beings and transmitted from one generation to another." *

The food culture or foodways may have existed among a given ethnic group for centuries, and such a heritage accounts for great conservatism in accepting change. These patterns reflect the social organization of the people, including their economy, religion, beliefs about the health properties of food, and attitudes toward the various members of the family. The emotional reactions to the consumption of certain foods may be so deeply rooted that effecting acceptance of them is almost impossible.

Food taboos and folklore. In every group of people customs have arisen concerning foods that should and should not be eaten. Although there is little or no sci-

* *Random House Dictionary.*

entific basis for these taboos, they are rigidly held so that change is likely to be resisted. Among people in the developing nations these taboos often accentuate malnutrition. For example, in one ethnic group in Nigeria children are rarely given meat or eggs. These are expensive foods, and it is thought that giving them to children will encourage them to steal. Coconut milk is taboo for children since it is believed to make them unintelligent. Similar taboos prevail for the pregnant woman. She should not eat snails so that her baby will not salivate too much. She should not eat pounded yams because the pounding is likely to have an effect on the child's brain. On the other hand, the pregnant woman is encouraged to eat food left by rats since this will help ensure an easy delivery such as rats are supposed to have![5]

An example of folklore is the belief system held by many Chinese, especially those who are older.[6] These beliefs have their origin in Eastern philosophy, which holds that the universe is regulated by two opposing components, *yin* and *yang*. To maintain health these forces must be in balance. When illness is caused by an excess of yang, "cold" or yin foods should be used, and vice versa. Among the yin or "cold" foods are winter melon, white turnips, and bean sprouts; yang or "hot" foods include scrambled eggs and ginger root. The Zen macrobiotic diet is derived from this earlier folklore. (See page 66.)

The family. The mother has often been referred to as the "gatekeeper" or the one who controls the food that reaches the table. In many families this role is diminishing. Food selection and meal preparation are often shared by parents and older children, and each of these influence the food that is presented to the family. Also, many meals, especially noon meals, are eaten away from home.

Within the home the food choices may reflect the environment in which the parents grew up, including the geographic region from which they came, their level of education, income, and beliefs about food. An atmosphere of security and contentment reinforces the positive values of food. On the other hand, in an environment of hostility, anger, and tension unpleasant images are created for food, often leading to their rejection. In this atmosphere, also, there may be excessive concern about "pure" foods, "pure" morals, and so on.[7]

Meal patterns. Nutritional planning is usually based on a three-meal pattern. Although many people in the United States eat three meals a day, others eat only two, and still others four or five. The coffee break is prevalent in business and industry, and is, for many, a replacement of breakfast. Midafternoon and evening snacks are commonplace.

Breakfasts tend to be light and informal. Family members often eat this meal at different times depending upon the time they must leave for work or school. Such a casual arrangement does not always provide the share of essential nutrients, nor is there the enjoyment that should be experienced at mealtime. In rural areas breakfast is still a substantial meal. Elderly people often enjoy breakfast more than other meals.

A good deal of ritual is part of the mealtime in some homes. Bread becomes the "staff of life" to some people; rice is the basic food for others, and corn to still others. The meal would not be complete if these foods were not included. The art of food preparation is exercised, and food is highly valued for its many properties. Meals are to be enjoyed and relaxation is encouraged. A siesta following meals is customary in some countries. In other homes, mealtime is hurried. It may become the time when members of the family air their problems and when tensions are created.

Communications. The influence of the mass media on food habits can scarcely be overestimated. Those who enjoy an abundant variety of food can no longer be ignorant of the malnutrition and hunger that exist even in the United States as well as in the underdeveloped nations of the world. By these media the poor are also exposed to food products which they are unable to purchase. The affluent and the poor alike know that the distribution of food is decidedly uneven and that the capability exists to feed all people better.

Manufacturers usually create desires for their products by appealing to the emotions. Foods are pictured in forms highly appealing to the eye and in situations that suggest fun, social status, and group acceptance. Foods will consequently be purchased to fulfill these emotional needs rather than for their nutritional content.

Political significance. Large food programs exist in the United States and throughout the world to help the poor meet their nutritional needs. Such programs are important in determining agricultural policies and food prices, on the one hand, and impose regulations for participation by the poor, on the other hand.

During a war food supplies may be rationed and people are forced to substitute one food for another. The scarcity of a given food sometimes creates a tremendous pressure to possess that food. The collapse of a government may indeed be brought about by its failure to provide food for its people.

Throughout history people have gone on "hunger strikes" to achieve some political goal. Gandhi, the great Indian leader, comes to mind for his many fasts. Not many years ago, some people who protested the involvement of the United States in the Vietnam war fasted for brief or long periods of time.

Food movements. Millions of Americans today have adopted eating patterns that differ widely from those of their childhood and that are at variance with so-called typical American diets. Among these groups are (1) those who are vegetarians for ecologic, philosophic, or religious reasons (see also pages 286–88); (2) those who oppose the use of any additives in foods or the use of chemical fertilizers, and who consume only "natural" or "organic" foods (see also page 313); and (3) those who subscribe to the healthful properties of some foods and who proscribe other foods. These groups are often referred to as "faddists" but their adherence to the particular belief is no passing fancy. It is not always possible to change these beliefs, but the counselor for nutrition should recognize what is good in the individual's diet and should attempt to improve the diet within the framework of the beliefs.

Economic Influence on Food Habits Income influences the variety of foods from which people can choose, and also the amount of food that may be purchased from each of the food groups. Generally, people with limited incomes depend on lower cost foods from the bread-cereal group to supply much of the caloric and nutrient needs. They use smaller amounts of the meat and milk groups. Also, the selection from the meat group is restricted to less expensive cuts. From the fruit-vegetable group the selection must be made from a more limited variety of lower cost items.

The meat group, to many people, is essential to meal satisfaction, and the ability to buy it also has a connotation of status. Thus, when the income of poor people improves, the amount of meat purchased is usually increased. Not infrequently, a disproportionate part of the food dollar is spent for meat, leaving too little money for milk and vegetables and fruits.

Preliminary studies of the 1977 Household Consumption Survey have shown that the differences in the selection of foods from various groups by low-income and high-income groups have narrowed.[8] The nutritive values of diets of low-income groups have also improved, when compared with the 1965 consumption survey.

When the income is liberal, people have the freedom to choose from an almost unlimited variety of foods—in or out of season, locally produced or from some distant state or country, fresh or processed. The cost of food is often equated with status. Lobster, prime ribs of beef, fresh asparagus, and champagne are examples of items that one might choose in an expensive restaurant. But beef stew instead of steak, cabbage instead of asparagus, and applesauce instead of fresh strawberries might be more typical choices by people with limited income. Thus, in the hierarchy of food status, these choices may be considered less desirable even though nutritive values might be equal.

People eat more frequently in restaurants. Those who are affluent choose expensive restaurants for the creative menus that sometimes emphasize ethnic gourmet foods, for the excellence of food preparation, for the ambience of the dining room, and even for the association with other persons of affluence. By contrast, persons with low income can afford to eat in restaurants only infrequently or not at all. For them the fast-food restaurant is often the only affordable choice. But people of all income levels have accepted the fast-food place for its convenience and rapid service. The rapid growth of the fast-food industry also characterizes the food habits of many people, especially persons under 35 years.

Social Values of Food "To break bread" together has been from time immemorial an act of friendship. One provides food for friends during a visit in the home; one likewise extends friendship to the stranger by inviting him to share food. The food served to guests is the best that one can afford and the table appointments are as beautiful as one can make them. Important family events are joyously celebrated with meals: the wedding breakfast or reception; birthday parties; Christmas dinner; a Fourth of July picnic. To eat together, whatever the occasion, is to provide friendly relaxation and conversation. The loneliness of eating by oneself, day after day, is not appreciated by those who have never tried it.

Eating together also has connotations of status. Throughout history one's place at the table has been governed by his or her social standing. To be placed "above the salt" at a medieval banquet, to sit at the "head" table at a banquet today, and to be invited to eat at the captain's table while on board ship are marks of social distinction. In some societies women are considered to be inferior to men and must wait to eat until the men and boys have finished the meal. In other authoritarian situations, children may not be permitted to eat until the father has had his meal; in such a society, the father is always served the choicest foods. Many bonds of business or of politics are cemented at businessmen's luncheons or political dinners.

Children too are highly influenced by the foods that are popular with their peer groups. Sometimes they come to scorn certain foods that they have liked because they are different from the prevailing pattern of other children. On the other hand, they are also susceptible to the suggestions of their teachers and classmates and learn to like foods with which they have not been familiar in their homes.

Some people delight in being epicures or gourmets. They derive a certain satisfaction from adventurous eating of food which is unusual to most people—rattlesnake meat, for example. Or they serve food that is difficult to obtain, distinctive in flavor, or exacting and time-consuming in preparation.

Religious and Moral Values Attributed to Foods Almost all religions place some regulations on the use of foods. The association of a food with religion gives some clue to its important in daily living. In the Middle East, bread becomes a symbol in the religious ceremonies of the people; to the Indians of Mexico, corn, the staple food, is invested with religious significance. Christians use bread and wine as symbols of Christ's body and blood in the Eucharist (Lord's Supper or Holy Communion). Religious significance is attached to a number of foods by the Jewish people. (See page 288.)

Certain foods are forbidden by religious regulation. Pork is forbidden to the Orthodox Jews and to the Muslims. Strict Hindus and Buddhists are vegetarians; they will eat no flesh of any animal, and many of them also abstain from eggs and milk. Seventh Day Adventists are lactovegetarians; that is, they will eat milk, cheese, eggs, nuts, and legumes but they eat no flesh foods. (See also Chapter 15.)

Fasting is common to most, if not all, religions. On fast days one food may be substituted for another or foods may be abstained from altogether. A substitute food, such as fish for meat, is likely to be associated with denying oneself, and so when one wishes enjoyment, he doesn't choose to eat fish!

Moral attributes—"good" and "bad"—are often ascribed to foods. A child may be told to eat liver even if he does not like it because it is "good" for him; he may also be told not to eat candy, which he does like, because it is "bad" for him. Or he might be told that he may have candy if he eats some liver!

Food is often used as a reward, punishment, or means of bribery. Thus, a child who has behaved well is rewarded with a prized food—candy, ice cream, cake; but one who has behaved badly may be punished by being deprived of a food such as dessert. Adults, too, may reward themselves after a strenuous day or a trying experience by eating a special food or an expensive meal, saying as they do so, "I certainly earned this today!" The family may feel a sense of reward, as well as the expression of a mother's love, when they sit down to a meal of their favorite foods; they may feel punished and unloved when the meal includes foods they dislike.

Age and Sex Influence Food Choices Some foods are categorized as being suitable for a given age group, or as more suitable for one sex than the other. Peanut butter, jelly, and milk are looked upon as foods for children, but olives and coffee are appropriate for adults! Teenagers adopt current fashions in foods—hot dogs, hamburger, pizza, ice cream with many sauces and toppings. (See Figure 14–2.) Women are said to prefer light foods such as soufflés, salads, fruits, and vegetables, whereas filling meals such as meat, potatoes, and pie represent the more usual choice of men.

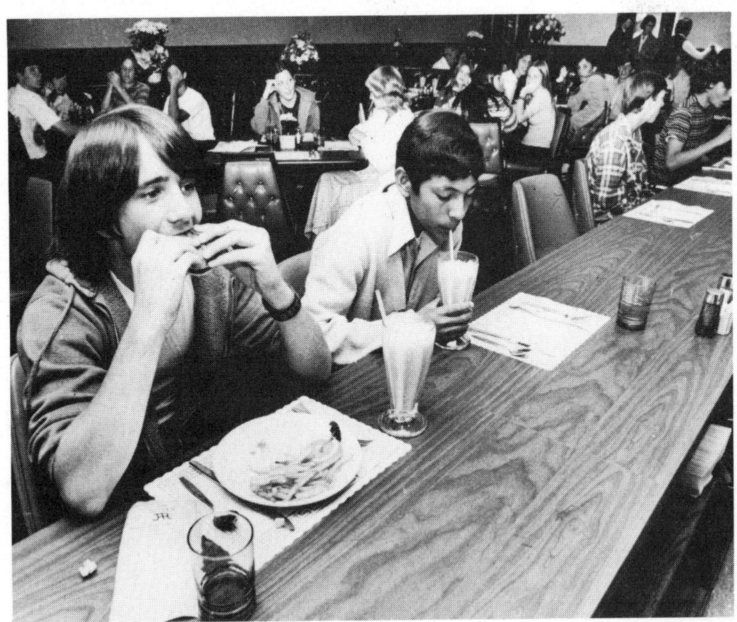

Figure 14–2. Hamburger on bun, French fries, and a milk shake are popular foods for teenagers. They provide substantial amounts of energy and many nutrients. A salad such as coleslaw or a piece of fruit would furnish missing nutrients such as ascorbic acid. (Courtesy, U.S. Department of Agriculture.)

Emotional Outlets Provided by Food Eating provides gratification for life stresses—the difficult examination in school; the homely adolescent who has no date to take her to the movies; the quarrel with a friend; the frustration and loneliness of having no friends; the profound grief at the death of a dear one; and countless others.

Food is a symbol of security to many. Milk, the first food of the infant, is associated with the security of the infant held lovingly in his mother's arms. A person away from home, or ill, looks upon milk as expressing the comfort and security of the home; or, milk might be refused because the individual drinking it experiences a feeling of dependence which he does not want to admit, and so he says he does not "want to be treated like a baby."

Food may be used as a weapon. An insecure child refuses to eat food so that his mother will be concerned about him. The ill and the lonely impose dietary demands upon those caring for them in an effort to gain as much attention as possible.

Illness Modifies Food Acceptance Disease processes and drug therapy often modify the appetite. The anxiety of illness, the loneliness experienced if one eats from a tray alone, the lack of activity, and perhaps a modified diet are likely to interfere with food intake. (See also Chapter 24.)

Problems and Review

1. Key terms: appetite; food culture; food folklore; food taboos; food habits; glucostatic theory; hot-cold theory; hunger; satiety; thermostatic control.
2. How do you feel about food? List insofar as you are able the meanings which you clearly associate with foods. List the foods you especially like; those you especially dislike. Can you give any specific reason for placing the food in one category or another?
3. Note for one day the comments made by people around you about food. Do any of these fall within the physiologic or psychologic categories discussed in this chapter? Do they give you any clue concerning readiness to change food habits?
4. Suppose you were trying to introduce nonfat dry milk to a group of people who were entirely unfamiliar with it. How would you go about gaining their acceptance?
5. Describe the physical factors in food acceptance.

Cited References

1. Mayer, J.: "Why People Get Hungry," *Nutr. Today,* **1**:2–8, June 1966.
2. Brobeck, J. R.: "Food Intake as a Mechanism of Temperature Regulation," *Yale J. Biol. Med.,* **20**:545–52, 1948.
3. Hamilton, C. L.: "Physiologic Control of Food Intake," *J. Am. Diet. Assoc.,* **62**:35–40, 1973.
4. Korslund, M., and Eppright, E. S.: "Taste Sensitivity and Eating Behavior of Preschool Children," *J. Home Econ.,* **59**:168–70, 1967.
5. Ogbeide, O.: "Nutritional Hazards of Food Taboos and Preferences in Mid-west Nigeria," *Am. J. Clin. Nutr.,* **27**:213–16, 1974.
6. Chang, B.: "Some Dietary Beliefs in Chinese Folk Culture," *J. Am. Diet. Assoc.,* **65**:436–38, 1974.
7. Bruch, H.: "The Allure of Food Cults and Nutritional Quackery," *J. Am. Diet. Assoc.,* **57**:316–20, 1970.

8. "Gaps Narrowing Between Diets of Rich and Poor," *Community Nutrition Institute Weekly Reports,* 9(45): 6, November 15, 1979.

Additional References

BROBECK, J. R.: "Nature of Satiety Signals," *Am. J. Clin. Nutr.,* **28**:806–807, 1975.
CHAPPELLE, M. L.: "The Language of Food," *Am. J. Nurs.,* **72**:1294–95, 1972.
FRANKLE, R. T., and HEUSSENSTAMM, F. K.: "Food Zealotry and Youth. New Dilemmas for Professionals," *Am. J. Public Health,* **64**:11–18, 1974.
HODGSON, P. A.: "The Many Faces of Food—As Seen Through the Eyes of the Artist," *J. Am. Diet. Assoc.,* **71**:248–52, 1977.
LEPKOVSKY, S.: "Newer Concepts in the Regulation of Food Intake," *Am. J. Clin. Nutr.,* **26**:271–84, 1973.
LOWENBERG, M. E.: "The Development of Food Patterns," *J. Am. Diet. Assoc.,* **65**:263–68, 1974.
MEAD, M.: "The Changing Significance of Food," *Am. Sci.,* **58**:176–81, 1970.
REABURN, J. A., et al.: "Social Determinants in Food Selection," *J. Am. Diet. Assoc.,* **74**:637–41, 1979.
SHIFFLET, P. A.: "Folklore and Food Habits," *J. Am. Diet. Assoc.,* **68**:347–50, 1976.
WILSON, C. S.: "Food—Custom and Nurture," (an annotated bibliography on sociocultural and biocultural aspects of nutrition), *J. Nutr. Educ.,* **11**(Suppl. 1): 213–61, 1979.
ZIFFERBLATT, S. M., et al.: "Understanding Food Habits. Influence of Ecologic Events on Cafeteria Food Selection," *J. Am. Diet. Assoc.,* **76**:9–14, 1980.

15 *Cultural Food Patterns in the United States*

THE food patterns for a given group of people have their origin in the variety and availability of foods in the country where they live. When people move to another region or country they gradually adapt their traditional diets to the new geographic, economic, and cultural environment. Some of these adaptations are nutritionally advantageous, whereas others have led to imbalance and deficiencies.

Recent Concerns about Food Habits

With individual mobility, rapid communication with all parts of the world, extensive advertising of food through the national media, changes in agricultural and food technology, advances in education, and adoption of new life-styles, it is not surprising that food behaviors also change. Among the important concerns are these:

How do changing values about the environment and life-styles influence food intake and nutrition?

Vegetarian diets have been adopted by several million people in the United States. What are some of the variations within this pattern? What are the health and nutritional implications when these diets are used?

Within the last decade hundreds of thousands of Vietnamese, Mexicans, and Cubans have come to the United States. What are the characteristics of their diets? Given the problems of income and language barriers, what strategies can be used to provide nutritionally adequate diets?

Food Habits Change Rapidly For many groups—for example, the French, German, Italian, Scandinavian, to name but a few—the food habits are those generally prevailing in the United States. Yet, these groups preserve some of their food traditions, especially for holidays and observance of religious customs.

One of the dramatic examples of changing food habits is that of the Japanese in Hawaii as described by Wenkam and Wolff.[1] The Japanese who came to Hawaii at the end of the nineteenth century were mostly agricultural workers who were employed on the plantations. For them, the family was the important social unit. They achieved status through it and were guided by respect for the family, ancestral worship, and so on. Individual desires were subordinated.

The early Japanese immigrants retained the vegetarian food habits of Japan, a diet in which rice, barley, and soybeans were the staple foods. They also used peas and mung beans, cabbage, marine algae, vegetables, roots, and tubers. Those who lived near the seacoast consumed fairly large amounts of fish, but it was not available inland. Scarcely any meat was eaten.

As the immigrants associated with Caucasians and other Orientals they began to include new foods such as Chinese pork, Hawaiian poi, and Portuguese sweet bread. The changing diet was accelerated during World War II when Nisei soldiers were in contact with soldiers of other ethnic groups.

The largest group of Japanese living in Hawaii today have drastically changed their diets. This cosmopolitan group have replaced rice with white flour, bread, and crackers. The consumption of animal foods has increased conspicuously. They have substituted the American breakfast for the traditional rice, soup, and pickled vegetables.

A second, smaller group, mostly older Japanese, are those who have retained the traditions of the Japanese diet, although they eat some American foods. A third group, also small, has become so completely "Americanized" that some of them have even changed their names. To them, the Japanese traditions hold no meaning.

The single most important influence on the food habits has been the American system of education with its emphasis on democracy and the individual.[1] The family controls have also been weakened, and hence the restrictions placed on the use of food, for example, animal foods, are no longer honored. A desire for higher status has been important, and so rice was given up because it no longer was a prestige food. The early immigrants to Hawaii expected to return to Japan as soon as they had earned enough money, and so they retained their Japanese food habits. However, for the present generation of Japanese, Hawaii is the permanent home. Finally, the intermingling of ethnic groups and the availability of foods have contributed to the evolution of the food habits.

Regional Food Patterns of the United States

Perhaps nowhere in the world can one find so great a variety of foods and methods of preparation as in the United States. The dietary patterns are an amalgamation of the foods native to the region and the habits and customs handed down by generations of foreign born. The foods vary from the wheat of the North Central plains to the rice of Louisiana, the potatoes of Maine to the citrus fruits of Florida, the dairy products of Minnesota and Wisconsin to the beef of the western ranges, the fish of the seacoast to the fruits of the Far West. One might associate baked beans with New England, chile con carne with the Southwest, and fried chicken with the South, but today these dishes are served everywhere in the United States.

In addition to the baked beans and brown bread on a Saturday night, in New England one is likely to encounter such favorite dishes as codfish cakes, lobster, clam chowder, and other seafood specialties. Pumpkin pie, squash, Indian pudding, and turkey originated with the Pilgrim fathers, who made adaptations of foods used by the American Indian.

The Pennsylvania Dutch are known for many rich foods including potato pancakes, many kinds of sausage, Philadelphia scrapple, sticky cinnamon buns, pickles and relishes ("seven sweets and seven sours"), and shoofly pie.

Fried chicken, country ham, and hot biscuits are specialties of the South. Green vegetables such as turnip tops, collards, kale, and mustard greens are well liked; they are likely to be cooked for a relatively long time with fat pork as a flavoring agent. Sweet potatoes are preferred to white potatoes, and corn is the cereal of choice, although rice and wheat are also widely used. Corn appears in such forms as corn pone, corn bread, hominy grits, spoon bread, and hush puppies—in Florida and Texas, especially.

Dairy products, meat, and eggs abound in the Middle West. Here one finds dietary patterns similar to those of Scandinavia, Germany, Poland, England, and other northern European countries.

New Orleans is noted for its fine restaurants, which show the influence of French and Creole cookery. Soups and fish dishes are often highly seasoned, and sauces are used for many meats and vegetables.

The Mexican and Spanish influences are felt in the Southwest where pinto beans, tortillas made from flour or lime-treated corn, and chili, a hot pepper, are important constituents of the diet. Usually these staple

for
LACTO-VEGETARIANS
Milk, Cheese
Wheat, Rice, Corn
Nuts, Peanuts
Beans - Navy, Soy,
Kidney, Lima
Dry Peas, ChickPeas
Wheat + Beans
Wheat + Milk
Wheat + Peanuts + Milk
Cheese Pizza
GRADE A
MILK
IDEAL

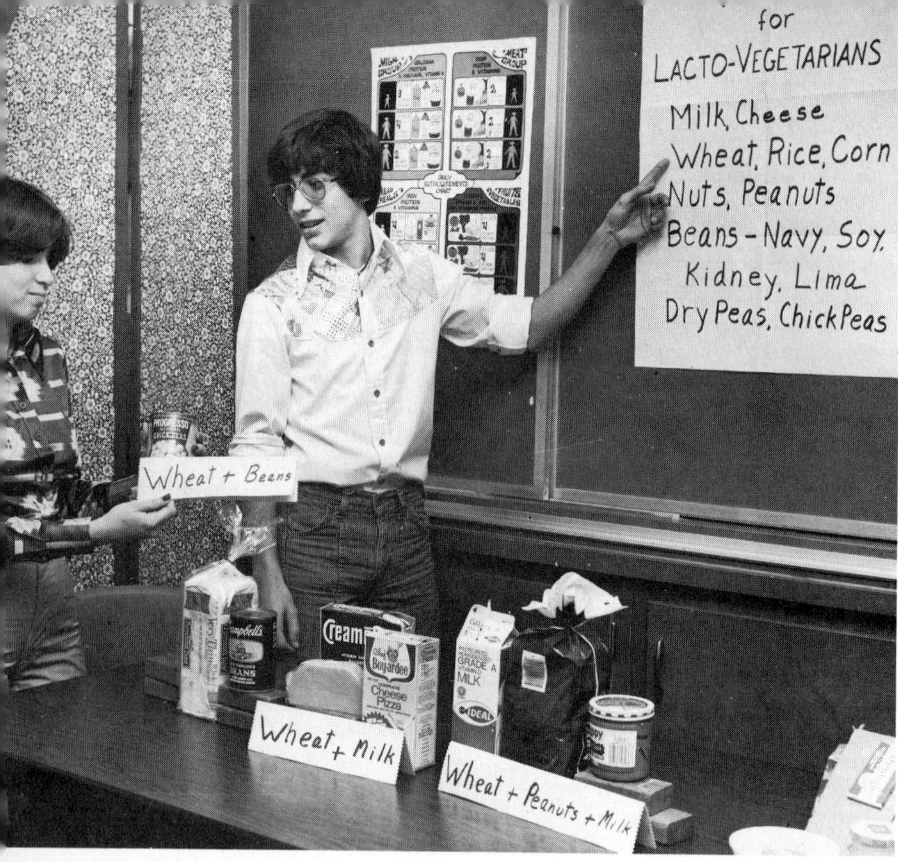

Figure 15–1. High school students study the food combinations that will provide the essential amino acids in a lactovegetarian diet. (Courtesy, Harry Broder and Marple-Newtown School District, Newtown Square, Pennsylvania.)

food items are served with highly seasoned sauces.

The abundance of luscious fruits and vegetables in the Far West leads to a much greater consumption of salads as main dishes as well as accompaniments of the meal. The Oriental influence is especially noted in the delicious vegetables of Japanese and Chinese cookery. Seafoods abound in great variety on the West Coast, as in the East, but the salmon of the Pacific Northwest is especially prized.

Vegetarian Diets

What Is Vegetarianism A VEGETARIAN is a person who uses a diet that includes plant foods but eliminates one or more of these groups of foods: meat; poultry; fish; milk; eggs. (See Figure 15–1.)

LACTOVEGETARIANS include plant foods and milk and other dairy products in their diet. They do not use meat, poultry, fish, or eggs.

LACTO-OVO-VEGETARIANS include plant foods, milk and other dairy products, and eggs. They abstain from meat, poultry, and fish.

PESCO-VEGETARIANS include plant foods and fish but do not use milk, eggs, meat, or poultry.

PURE VEGETARIANS (vegans) include only plant foods in their diets. Some of them use all plant foods, whereas others avoid one or more food groups such as processed foods, cooked foods, legumes, cereals, grains, or fruits. FRUITARIANS limit their food intake to raw and dried fruits, nuts, honey, and oil.

Reasons for Vegetarianism Probably less than 1 per cent of Americans adhere to a vegetarian diet of one kind or another.[2] Unfortunately, vegetarianism has been negatively viewed by some health professionals as an expression of faddism or cultism. Such attitudes fail to recognize that vegetarian diets, like the diets of omnivores, range from those that are nutritionally adequate to those that are bizarre and nutritionally hazardous. Vegetarians, like omnivores, have widely varying beliefs and educational, economic, and cultural backgrounds. Many of them give more than one reason for their adherence to vegetarian diets.

The Seventh Day Adventists and the Trappist monks are lacto-ovo-vegetarians. They also abstain from alcohol, tobacco, and caffeine-containing beverages. Their diet is one of self-discipline but also one that improves health. Studies on males who are Seventh Day Adventists have shown that serum cholesterol levels were lower and that the first heart attack occurred at least a decade later than average. The incidence of heart disease was 60 per cent as high as that of a control group in California. The difference was attributed to the low intake of cholesterol and saturated fat and the higher intake of fiber.[3] Abstinence from tobacco and alcohol might also have contributed to this difference.

The "new" vegetarians[4–6] include mostly young people under 30 years, many of whom have children. Many of them are educated and self-reliant. Some of their diets are nutritionally adequate, but others are dangerously inadequate, especially so for children. The "new" vegetarians often say that they feel better and are "less groggy" when they abstain from animal foods. Those who cite health as a reason for vegetarianism avoid foods that contain additives or hormones or that have been grown on chemically fertilized soils. They also are concerned that animal foods contain toxins, too much uric acid, or are infected with *Salmonella*.[6]

Ecologic reasons are cited by some. In a world where population threatens to exceed the ability to provide food, the rationale is that consuming foods directly is a more efficient use of land resources than feeding plant foods to animals that are subsequently consumed by humans.

Economic reasons are given by some since vegetarian diets can be less expensive than those with animal foods in them. Still others object to the large agribusiness in the United States and choose not to buy their foods from markets that are controlled by the giant corporations.

Nutritional Characteristics Nutritional adequacy is not a problem for lacto- and lacto-ovo-vegetarians. Because meat, poultry, and fish are not used, the diet includes greater amounts of meat analogs, legumes, grains, and milk or milk and eggs.

When planned wisely pure vegetarian diets can be nutritionally adequate. If one or more plant food groups are also omitted, nutritional adequacy is jeopardized. The following are some of the problems that must be considered for pure vegetarian diets.

Calories. The calorie requirement must be met in order to ensure efficient use of protein. Only a minimal amount of fats and sweets can be consumed if all nutrient requirements are to be met. The diets of vegetarians are much more bulky than those that contain animal foods. Vegetarians usually weigh less than nonvegetarians.

Protein. A variety of legumes, nuts, and cereal grains will furnish the essential amino acids. Methionine and lysine are limiting amino acids in plant foods. Cereal grains are deficient in lysine but supply adequate amounts of methionine. Legumes contain inadequate levels of methionine but furnish lysine. Thus, cereals and legumes when eaten together are complementary, and furnish the requirements for the essential amino acids. Fortified soy milk should be used for infants and young children.

Minerals. Calcium, magnesium, iron, zinc, and iodine require particular emphasis in planning the pure vegetarian diet. Calcium is furnished by liberal intakes of dark green leafy vegetables that do not contain oxalate, peanuts, almonds, sesame seeds, and fortified soy milk. Although the amount of iron ingested from a varied vegetarian diet may be equal to that consumed by people who eat meat, the bioavailability of this iron is lower. The availability is improved with the simultaneous ingestion of ascorbic-acid-rich foods. Legumes, peanuts, peanut butter, and whole grains are good sources of zinc but fruits and vegetables are poor sources. Iodized salt should be used.

Vitamins. Vitamin B-12 deficiency is characteristic of all pure vegetarian diets since vitamin B-12 is found only in animal foods. The signs of deficiency are not likely to show up until after several years use of the diet and then correction may be too late. In infants and young children the lack of vitamin B-12 may lead to growth failure. A vitamin B-12 supplement or fortified cereal or soy milk is indicated for pure vegetarian diets.

Except for vitamin B-12 the requirements for B-complex vitamins are met by a diversified selection of whole grains, legumes, nuts, seeds, and vegetables and fruits. Deep yellow and dark green vegetables ensure an ample supply of carotene. Vitamin D should be furnished as a supplement unless there is ample exposure to sunshine.

Typical Food Choices

By selecting a wide variety of foods from the following groups, nutritional adequacy can be achieved.

MILK GROUP All milk and milk products for lactovegetarian diets; 2 cups or more for adults; 3 to 4 cups for children. Milk should be encouraged for infants, children, and pregnant women in pure vegetarian groups, but fortified soy milk can be substituted.

PROTEIN GROUP Choose from dried beans: black, broad, kidney, Lima, mung, navy, pea, soy, white; dried peas: blackeye, chick, split; lentils; nuts: black walnut, Brazil, cashew, peanut, peanut butter, pistachio; seeds: sesame, sunflower; meat analogs, especially those processed to be nutritional replacement for meat. Combine legumes with nuts or cereal foods in the same meal.

VEGETABLE-FRUIT GROUP Generous use of vitamin A- and calcium-rich greens: collards, dandelion, kale, mustard, turnip; also broccoli, okra, rutabaga.

Citrus fruit daily or other good source of ascorbic acid.

BREAD-CEREAL GROUP Preferably whole-grain breads and cereals: barley, buckwheat, bulgur, cornmeal, millet, oatmeal, rice, rye, wheat.

SUPPLEMENTS Vitamin B-12 for pure vegetarian diets; possibly vitamin D, calcium, and iodine, especially for infants, young children, and pregnant women.

Orthodox Jewish Food Habits

Outstanding Characteristics Orthodox Jews observe dietary laws based on biblical and rabbinical regulations (the rules of Kashruth). These laws pertain to the selection, preparation, and service of food. Many Conservative Jews are as observant of dietary laws as are Orthodox Jews. But some conservative Jews nominally observe the laws but make distinctions within and without the home, while Reform Jews minimize the significance of dietary laws. Food habits of the Jewish people are also influenced by the country of origin—for example, Russia, Poland, or Germany.

Religious festivals include certain food restrictions. No food is cooked or heated on the Sabbath. Yom Kippur (Day of Atonement) is a 24-hour period of fasting from food and drink. The Passover, sometimes also referred to as "The Feast of Unleavened Bread," lasts for eight days and commemorates the release of the Israelites from the slavery of Egypt. Only utensils and dishes that have made no contact with leavened foods are used during this time. Thus, the Orthodox Jewish home would have four sets of dishes: one for meat and one for dairy meals during the Passover, and one for meat and one for dairy meals during the rest of the year when leavened breads and cakes may be used.

Typical Foods and Their Uses[7]

MILK GROUP Milk, cottage and cream cheese, sour cream used abundantly. Milk and its products may not be used at same meal as meat (Exod. 23:19; 34:26; Deut. 14:21). Milk may not be taken until 6 hours after eating meat. Separate dishes and utensils must be used for milk and meat dishes.

MEAT GROUP *(Allowed Foods).* All quadruped animals that chew the cud and divide the hoof (Lev. 11:1–3; Deut. 14:3–8); cattle, deer, goats, sheep. Organs of these animals may be used.

Animals must be killed in prescribed manner for minimum pain to animal and for maximum blood drainage. Blood is associated with life and may not be eaten (Gen. 9:4; Lev. 3:17; 17:10–14; Deut. 12:23–27). Meat is made *kosher* (clean) by soaking it in cold water, thoroughly salting it, allowing it to drain for an hour, and then washing it in three waters.

Hindquarters of meat may be used only if the part of the thigh with the sinew of Jacob is removed (Gen. 32:33).

Poultry: chicken, duck, goose, pheasant, turkey. Chicken is common for Sabbath eve meal.

Fish with fins and scales (Lev. 11:9: Deut. 14:9–10): cod, haddock, halibut, salmon, trout, tuna, whitefish, and so on.

Eggs. Fish and eggs may be eaten at both meat and milk meals.

Dried beans, peas, lentils, in many soups.

Corned beef, smoked meats, herring, *lox* (smoked, salted salmon) are well liked.

Cholent: casserole of beef, potatoes, and dried beans. Served on the Sabbath.

Gefillte fish: chopped, highly seasoned fish; a first course for the Sabbath meal.

Kishke: beef casings stuffed with rich filling and roasted.

Knishes: pastry filled with ground meat or potatoes.

Kreplach: noodle dough filled with ground meat or cheese filling.

Prohibited Foods Animals which do not chew the cud or divide the hoof (Lev. 11:4–8): pork.

Diseased animals or animals dying a natural death (Deut. 14:21).

Birds of prey (Lev. 11:13–19; Deut. 14:11–18).

Fish without fins or scales (Lev. 11:10–12): eels, shellfish such as oysters, crab, lobster.

Egg with blood spot.

VEGETABLE-FRUIT GROUP All kinds used without restriction.

Cucumber, lettuce, tomato very frequently used.

Cabbage, potatoes, and root vegetables are often cooked with the meat.

Borsch: soup with meat stock and egg, or without meat stock and with sour cream; includes beets, spinach, cabbage.

Dried fruits are used in many pastries.

BREAD-CEREALS GROUP All kinds used without restriction. Rye bread (pumpernickel), white seed rolls; noodles and other egg and flour mixtures.

Bagel: doughnut-shaped hard yeast roll.

Blintzes: thin rolled pancakes filled with cottage cheese, ground beef, or fruit mixture; served with sour cream.

Bulke: light yeast roll.

Challah: braided loaf or light white bread.

Farfel: noodle dough grated for soup.

Kasha: buckwheat groats served as cooked cereal or as potato substitute.

Kloese: dumplings, usually in chicken soup.

Latkes: pancakes.

Matzoth: flat, unleavened bread.

OTHER FOODS Unsalted butter preferred.

Chicken fat or vegetable oils for cooking.

Rich pastries are common.

Cheese cake.

Kuchen: coffee cake of many varieties.

Leckach: honey cake for Rosh Hashana (New Year).

Strudel: thin pastry with fruit, nut filling.

Teiglach: small pieces of dough cooked in honey, with nuts.

Sponge cake and macaroons at Passover.

Many preserves, pickled cucumbers, pickled green tomatoes, relishes.

Many foods are highly salted.

Black American Food Patterns

Outstanding Characteristics The meals eaten by poor black and white people in southeastern United States were generally similar. For most black Americans in the South poverty was more extreme, and the diet was more restricted. They had small gardens if any at all, and canned less food.

"Soul food" is a term recently used to denote foods of the black culture, especially those foods that prevailed in the South. Many of these foods originated in pre-Civil War days. When black Americans migrate from the South to northern cities, they at first retain most of their favored southern dishes. In time they use more and more foods typical of the area in which they live, but usually retain some of their favorite dishes.

As the income improves, black Americans spend increasing amounts of money for meat. Too little money is spent for vegetables, fruits, and milk. Although lactose tolerance is poor in many adults, most children can drink sufficient milk to meet their calcium needs without untoward symptoms. Meat, poultry, fish, and sweet potatoes are often fried. Greens are usually cooked for a long time and seasoned with salt pork, bacon, or bits of meat. Generally the diet is high in fat and in sweets.

Obesity, hypertension, and anemia are frequent nutritional problems seen in black Americans. Dietary counseling should include emphasis on ways to increase the iron content of the diet and to reduce the salt intake.

Typical Foods and Their Uses

MILK GROUP Little milk is consumed. Most children can tolerate milk well and should be given moderate amounts spaced throughout the meals for the day.

MEAT GROUP Fried chicken and fish are well liked; also catfish stew.

Meat from every part of the pig: bacon, ham hocks, pork chops, salt pork, spareribs (often barbecued); chitterlings (lining of pig stomach boiled and then fried); and pig's feet, tail, and ears.

Wild game when available: beaver, coon, possum, rabbit, squirrel.

Blackeyed peas with molasses and bacon or salt pork: kidney beans; marrow fat beans.

VEGETABLE-FRUIT GROUP Greens: collards, dandelion, kale, mustard, turnip—boiled in salt water with bacon or ham hocks or bits of salt pork; "pot likker" is consumed as well as the greens.

Stewed corn, okra, tomatoes; sweet potatoes.

Fruit sometimes used as snack; needs more emphasis.

BREAD-CEREAL GROUP Baking powder biscuits, served hot.

Corn bread in many ways: crackling bread, hoecakes, hush puppies, spoon bread.

Hominy grits, rice.

Puerto Rican Food Habits

Outstanding Characteristics The quality of the diet of Puerto Ricans living on the mainland of the United States is too often adversely affected by unemployment and poverty. Those who have recently come from the island also find that some foods to which they are accustomed are not always available in local supermarkets. Markets that cater to Puerto Ricans may import these foods, but they are likely to be expensive.

Obesity and iron-deficiency anemia are frequently seen. The intake of calcium, iron, vitamin A, and ascorbic acid is often below recommended allowances.

Rice, legumes, and *viandas* (starchy vegetables) are basic to all diets. Rice and beans offer a combination of high nutritive quality at low cost and their use should be encouraged. When served at the same meal, the rice and beans are complementary in supplying the essential amino acids. The combination also is an important source of calories and B-complex vitamins. Neither milk nor fruits and vegetables are eaten as much as they should be.

Some Puerto Ricans subscribe to the *hot-cold* theory of foods. This refers to inherent properties of heating or cooling that given foods are supposed to possess and is not related to the spiciness or temperature at which food is served. It is believed that some disease conditions are benefited by "hot" foods and others by "cold" foods. Thus, for a given condition there must be the right proportion of "hot" and "cold" foods.

Typical Foods and Their Uses[8]

MILK GROUP Milk is well liked but very little is used. Nonfat dry milk is well accepted; people must be shown how to use it.

Most of the milk is used in strong coffee *(café con leche):* 2–5 ounces milk per cup. Many drink this several times a day.

Cocoa and chocolate used widely.

MEAT GROUP Chicken, pork especially well liked. Seldom used by low-income groups, but liberally by the prosperous.

Chicken often cooked with rice *(arroz con pollo).*

Codfish used frequently; served with viandas.

Legumes *(granos):* chick peas, kidney beans, navy beans, dried peas, pigeon peas, and other varieties. Stewed and dressed with sauce *(sofrito).* About 3–4 ounces legumes eaten daily.

VEGETABLE-FRUIT GROUP *Viandas* (starchy vegetables): sweet potatoes *(batata amarillo)* and white potatoes should be emphasized. Other viandas used on the island may be imported: plantain; white *name;* white *tanier; panapen* (breadfruit); yautia; *yuca* (cassava). Viandas are boiled and served hot with oil, vinegar, and some codfish—often as a one-dish meal.

Beets and eggplant most commonly used vegetables. Some spinach and chard, but insufficient succulent vegetables. Small amounts of carrots, green beans, okra, and tomatoes. Yellow squash *(calabaza)* used in soups or fritters.

Fruits are eaten irregularly, and usually between meals. Preference often shown for canned peaches, pears, apples, and fruit cocktail. Citrus fruits should be emphasized.

BREAD-CEREALS GROUP Rice (arroz) used once or twice daily by all (about 7 ounces per capita). May be boiled and dressed with lard, or combined with legumes, chopped pork sausages, dry codfish, or chicken.

Cornmeal mush made with water or milk is popular.

Oatmeal may be cooked in thin gruel for breakfast.

Cornmeal may substitute for rice and may be eaten with beans and codfish.

Whole-grain or enriched breads should be encouraged.

OTHER FOODS AND SEASONINGS *Sofrito:* sauce made of tomatoes, onion, garlic, thyme, and other herbs, salt pork, green pepper, and fat. This is basis for much of cooking.

Annato: yellow coloring used with rice.

Lard, oil, salt pork, or ham butts used in cooking. Butter and margarine are not used.

Sugar in large amounts in coffee, cocoa, chocolate; molasses.

Coffee (Mocha, never a blend) is very strong; usually served with hot milk. Carbonated beverages are used more frequently.

Pastries and other desserts not widely used.

Mexican-American Food Habits

Characteristics Mexican-Americans are the second largest minority group in the United States. Most of them live in the southwestern states—California, Arizona,

New Mexico, and Texas. Although there is intermingling of Mexican and American cultures, many people still adhere to Mexican traditions.

A number of causes of illness are often cited by Mexican-Americans including those of magical origin, of emotional origin, imbalance of hot and cold foods, and of a scientific nature. Anglo physicians are sometimes mistrusted, and folk medicine is substituted. Treatment for illness at home is preferred since then the patient and family have control of the situation.

According to the hot-cold theory, foods are classified thus:

"Hot" foods: chili pepper, green and red pepper, garlic, onion, potatoes, sweet potatoes; goat milk; fish, turkey, capon; white beans, chick peas, rice, wheat bread, sweet roll, wheat tortillas; honey, sugar, and salt.

"Cold" foods: green beans, beets, cabbage, carrots, cauliflower, cucumber, coriander, parsley, peas, pumpkin, radish, spinach, squash, tomato, turnip; cow's milk, donkey milk, human milk; beef, hen, lamb, mutton, rabbit; red beans, lentils; oatmeal, corn tortillas, vermicelli.[9]

The chief foods of the Mexican-American diet are dried beans, chili peppers, and corn. Many families eat one good meal daily at noon, such as lentil-noodle vegetable soup, and breakfast and supper consist of sweet coffee or sometimes milk and tortillas. When the income is low very little meat is used—usually as flavoring with beans, in soups, or vegetable stews.

The National Nutrition Survey in the Southwest showed that low blood levels of vitamin A, riboflavin, and hemoglobin were prevalent.[10] Deficiencies of thiamin, ascorbic acid, and protein were less frequent but of sufficient magnitude to constitute a problem. Obesity is prevalent.

Typical Foods and Their Uses[10-11]

MILK GROUP Very little milk is used; some evaporated milk for infant feeding.

MEAT GROUP Beef and chicken well liked; meat used only two to three times weekly.

Eggs: two or three times a week.

Fish: infrequently.

Pinto or calico beans: refried *(frijoles refritos);* used daily by some; two or three times weekly by others.

Chile con carne: beef with garlic seasoning, beans, chili peppers.

Enchiladas: tortilla filled with cheese, onion, shredded lettuce, and rolled.

Taco: tortilla filled with seasoned ground meat, lettuce, and served with chili sauce.

Tamales: seasoned ground meat placed on masa, wrapped in corn husks, steamed, and served with chili sauce.

Topopo: corn tortilla filled with refried beans, shredded lettuce, green or ripe olives.

VEGETABLE-FRUIT GROUP Corn: fresh or canned; *chicos,* corn steamed while green and dried on the cob; *posole,* similar to hominy.

Chili peppers: fresh, canned, or frozen are good source of ascorbic acid.

Beets, cabbage, many tropical greens, peas, potatoes, pumpkin, squash, string beans, sweet potatoes, turnips.

Bananas used frequently. *Chayotes* (cactuslike fruit), oranges.

Nopalitos: leaf or stem of prickly pear cactus; diced as vegetable.

BREAD-CEREALS GROUP Corn is staple cereal with wheat gradually replacing it. Rice, macaroni, spaghetti. Some yeast bread; sweet rolls very popular. Increasing use of ready-to-eat cereals.

Atole: cornmeal gruel.

Masa: dried corn which has been heated and soaked in lime water, washed, and ground while wet into puttylike dough; contains appreciable amounts of calcium.

Sopaipillas: puffs of deep-fried dough. Use as bread or dessert, usually with honey.

Tortilla: thin, unleavened cakes baked on hot griddle, using masa; wheat now replacing lime-treated corn.

OTHER FOODS AND SEASONING Ground red chili powder is essential to most dishes; garlic

and onion very common; salt in abundance.
Cinnamon, coriander, lemon juice, mint, nutmeg, oregano, parsley, saffron.
Butter rarely used.
Coffee with much sugar used in large amounts.
Sugar and sweets in large amounts.

Food Habits of Native Americans

Native Americans include diverse ethnic groups such as American Indians who are integrated into the general population, Indians who are relatively isolated on vast reservations, and Eskimos in Alaska. The American Indians live in areas that are vastly different from one another—from Maine to Florida, from Wisconsin to Washington and Oregon and to Arizona, New Mexico, and other states. The Eskimos live on islands, in coastal villages, in mountainous areas, and the Arctic tundra of Alaska and Canada.

American Indians Many foods used throughout the world were probably first used by the Indians of North, Central, and South America: for example, beans, corn, cranberries, peanuts, peppers, potatoes, pumpkin, wild rice, squash, and tomatoes. Because of the diversity of regions in which Indians live there is no single typical diet. Today traditional dishes are prepared infrequently except for ceremonial occasions. Even the Arizona Hopi who still live in old villages that their ancestors inhabited use their native dishes infrequently.[12] The dietary changes have occurred partly because of relocation of the tribes on reservations where the food resources were different. Unemployment and poverty have contributed to a decline in the quality of the diet as has also the excessive use of refined processed foods. Many families live a hand-to-mouth existence with little planning. Nor is there knowledge of the foods that will meet nutritional needs at low cost. Folklore pertaining to the use of foods for health still abounds.

In many Indian diets corn is the staple food. It is eaten fresh roasted or broiled, as hominy, or as cornmeal in a variety of dishes. Meat is eaten when it can be obtained by hunting or fishing, but because of its cost it is used sparingly if it must be purchased in the market. Milk is little used. Lactose intolerance occurs commonly among adult Indians, but children can usually consume enough milk to meet their needs. Berries, wild plants, and roots are used when available, but the intake of fruits and vegetables requires more emphasis. White flour is gradually replacing cornmeal. When corn is soaked in lime and ground it is a good source of calcium. However, the lime treatment is less frequently used, thus bringing about another decline in diet quality. Sugar and sweets, cakes, potato chips, soft drinks, and many snack foods are widely used.

Obesity and diabetes mellitus are prevalent, especially in Indian women. Although the diets are furnishing excess calories for many of them, the intake of calcium, iron, ascorbic acid, and vitamin A are often low.

Eskimos The traditional diet of nomadic Eskimos consisted almost entirely of frozen, dried, or fresh game and fish.[13] Inland Eskimos hunted for caribou while coastal Eskimos caught sea mammals and fish. Fowl, polar bear, musk ox, rabbits, and foxes were eaten depending upon local supply. Berries, leafy greens, roots, and seaweed were seasonally available.

For one meal a day meat might be cooked as soup over a seal-oil lamp, using sea water and seaweed for seasoning. During the remainder of the day the family would nibble on raw *muktuk* (whale skin), caribou, or char (fish). The protein intake was extremely high (average over 300 gm daily) and the carbohydrate intake was insignificant. The meat and fish supplied the minerals and vitamins, including vitamin C from raw liver.

With the transition from a nomadic life to the recent settlements of the white man, the Eskimos were suddenly thrown into a new civilization for which they had no preparation. In the villages the Eskimos still hunt some game and fish. Most of them are unemployed or employed only part time. Profound changes in the composition of the diet have occurred. Store-bought foods were found to be appealing to the taste and also conveyed status.

Sugar, candy, soft drinks, and processed foods are consumed throughout the day and thus contribute to a high intake of simple, rapidly absorbed carbohydrate. The protein intake remains liberal (about 100 gm daily). The adoption of the least desirable aspects of the white culture's diet has led to health problems that did not exist in earlier times. Eskimos had perfect teeth, but dental decay is now rampant. Obesity, gallbladder disease, and acne—hitherto unknown—are now prevalent. Diabetes mellitus occurs more often, and there is a diabetic-type response to the glucose tolerance test. Blood lipid and cholesterol levels are elevated, which suggests that change in physical activity rather than diet may be responsible. Infections and allergic reactions are seen in infants who are bottle fed.[13]

Food Habits of the Vietnamese

Adjustments to Living in the United States More than 130,000 Vietnamese have resettled in the United States since 1975.[14] The nutritional problems of people living in Vietnam and the adjustments of Vietnamese to living in the United States have been described by Kaufman. The largest number have settled in California, but there are also many in eastern, southern, and midwestern states. They find themselves cut off from their own cultural roots. They have had to face problems of finding employment, learning English, managing their money, and becoming accustomed to new life-styles.

Characteristics of Diet In Vietnam three meals a day are preferred with breakfast being the least important meal. Soup *(pho)* made with rice noodles, thin slices of beef or chicken, and greens or bean sprouts is a popular breakfast dish. Another breakfast pattern includes fried eggs, French bread, and café au lait.

Rice with mixtures of vegetables and meat or seafood is used for other meals. The universally used fermented fish sauce *(nuoc mam)* is high in sodium and iodine and also contributes some protein. Poultry, pork, and fish are well liked and used when income permits. Soybeans and peanuts are also important sources of protein. Cabbage, corn, spinach, squash, sweet potato, and watercress are widely used. Bananas, grapefruit, pineapple, mango, lichee, and jackfruit are used for dessert. Tea is drunk daily, but soft drinks and beer are also popular. Lactose intolerance occurs frequently in adults and milk is little used. Children can usually tolerate milk if the amounts given are spaced throughout the day.

The Vietnamese are not familiar with American markets. Although they can purchase the fish sauce, herbs, tea, and rice noodles to which they are accustomed in Oriental food stores in major cities, these imported items are expensive. The Vietnamese are accustomed to buying foods daily since in Vietnam they did not have refrigeration. Steaming, braising, stir-frying, deep-fat frying, and grilling are used. In Vietnam ovens were rare, so baked goods were purchased.

Dietary Patterns of the Near East—Armenia, Greece, Syria, Turkey

Typical Foods and Their Uses[15]

MILK GROUP Cow's, goat's, or sheep's milk; fermented preferred to sweet (yogurt); little used by adults. Often served hot and sweetened to children.

Soft and hard cheeses.

MEAT GROUP Lamb is preferred; also pork, poultry, mutton, goat, beef.

Fish: fresh, salted, or smoked; octopus, squid, shellfish, roe.

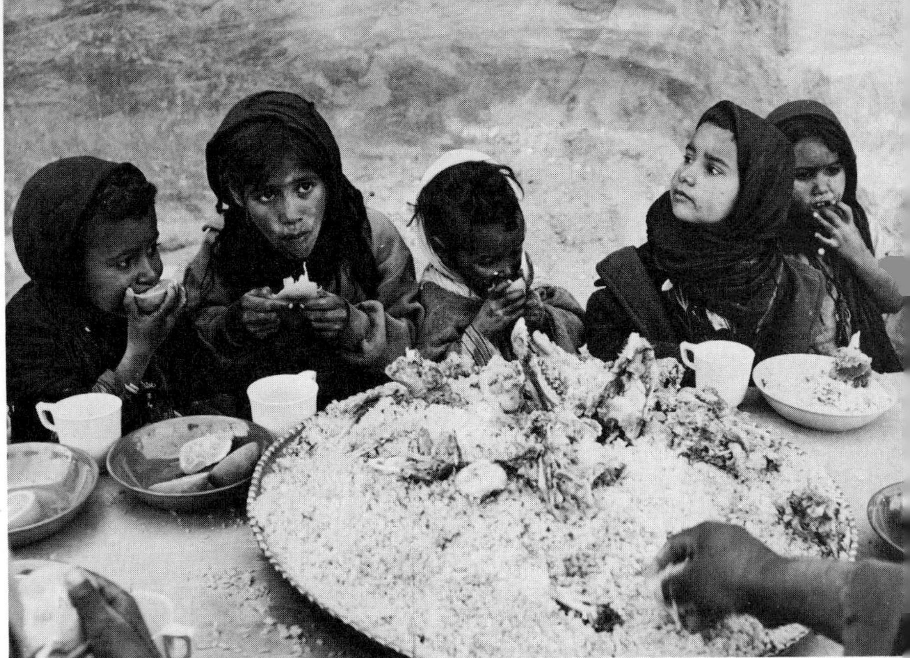

Figure 15–2. This traditional meal of Jordanian children illustrates the use of staple foods supplemented with milk. The common dish of food from which the children help themselves is used by many cultural groups. (Courtesy, UNICEF; photo by George Holton.)

Eggs often used as main dish but not at breakfast.

Beans, peas, and lentils.

Nuts may be used with wheat and rice in place of meat; pignolias, pistachios.

Ground or cut meat often cooked with wheat or rice, or in stews with cereal grains and vegetables. For example:

Breast of lamb stuffed with rice, currants.

Squash stuffed with chopped meat, onions, rice, parsley.

Cabbage rolls with ground meat, rice, and baked in meat stock; served with lemon juice.

Barbecued meats on special occasions: skewered meats are broiled.

Shashlik: mutton or lamb marinated in garlic, oil, vinegar; roasted on skewers with tomato and onion slices.

VEGETABLE-FRUIT GROUP Eggplant, greens, onions, peppers, tomatoes; also cabbage, cauliflower, cucumbers, okra, potatoes, zucchini.

Vegetables cooked with olive oil and served hot or cold; cooked in meat or fish stews; stuffed with wheat, meat, nuts, beans; salads with olive oil, vinegar.

Grapes, lemons, oranges; also apricots, cherries, dates, figs, melons, peaches, pears, plums, quinces, raisins. Fresh fruits widely used in season; fruit compotes.

BREAD-CEREALS GROUP Bread is staff of life; used at every meal. Baked on griddles in round, flat loaves.

Cracked whole wheat *(bourglour)* and rice used as starchy food, or with vegetables, or with meat *(pilavi).* (See Figure 15–2).

Corn in *polenta.*

OTHER FOODS AND SEASONINGS Olive oil and seed oils used in cooking. Butter is not much used.

Nuts (hazel, pignolia, pistachio) used for snacks, in desserts, pastries.

Baklava: pastry with nuts and honey.

Black olives.

Herbs, honey, sugar, lemon juice, seeds of caraway, pumpkin, and sesame.

Apricot candy, Turkish paste.

Wine, coffee.

Dietary Patterns of the Chinese

Typical Foods and Their Uses

MILK GROUP Milk and cheese are well liked but need to be emphasized. Soybean milk for children.

MEAT GROUP Pork, lamb, goat, chicken, duck, fish, and shellfish, eggs, and soybeans.

Organ meats including brain and spinal cord, blood, and bone are used.

Egg rolls: shrimp or meat and vegetable filling rolled in thin dough, and fried in deep fat.

Egg foo yung: combination of eggs, chopped chicken, mushrooms, scallions, celery, bean sprouts cooked similar to an omelet.

Sweet and pungent pork: pork cubes coated with batter and fried in oil; then simmered in a sauce of green pepper, cubed pineapple, molasses, brown sugar, vinegar, and seasonings.

Stir-fried fish with vegetables: diced white meat fish fillets are coated with egg white and fried quickly in deep fat; drained. Sauce of chicken stock, soy sauce, rice wine or sake combined with peas. Scallion, and garlic stir-fried in small amount oil. Bamboo shoots, sauce, and fish added and blended thoroughly. Often served on bed of stir-fried spinach.

Tofu: soybean curd; used in many dishes. An excellent source of protein, iron, and calcium if made with calcium salts.

VEGETABLE-FRUIT GROUPS Cabbage, carrots, onions, peas, cucumbers, many greens, mushrooms, bamboo shoots, soybean sprouts, sweet potatoes.

Stir-fried vegetables are thinly sliced or chopped; cooked in a little oil for a short time before water is added to seal in flavor, preserve crispness, and fresh green color. Any juice remaining is served with the vegetable.

BREAD-CEREALS GROUP Rice is staple food served with every meal.

Wheat and millet are widely used; noodles.

OTHER FOODS AND SEASONINGS Lard, soy, sesame, and peanut oils used in cooking.

Soy sauce present in almost every meal contributes to high salt intake.

Almonds, ginger, sesame seeds, garlic, fresh herbs, for flavoring.

Tea is beverage of choice.

Problem and Review

1. What factors must be kept in mind in teaching normal nutrition to people whose food habits differ widely from our own?
2. What technologic advances of the twentieth century have tended to eliminate regional differences in food patterns of the United States?
3. *Problem.* Select any one ethnic group and plan menus for one day including recipes for special dishes.
4. Make a survey of the ethnic groups represented in the class. List favorite dishes for each of these ethnic groups. Discuss the nutritive values of these dishes. What foods require emphasis in the patterns of these ethnic groups?
5. What problems in dietary adjustment would you expect to encounter for a Puerto Rican child; a student from India who is a strict vegetarian?
6. Compare the principal cereal foods and meats used by the Chinese, the Mexicans, and the Greeks.
7. What problems might arise owing to the bulk of the vegetarian diet?
8. Plan a menu for one day that would be nutritionally adequate for an adult who is a strict vegetarian. What supplements would be indicated?
9. What considerations must be kept in mind in dietary planning for the child whose parents are strict vegetarians?

Cited References

1. Wenkam, N. S., and Wolff, R. J.: "A Half Century of Changing Food Habits Among Japanese in Hawaii," *J. Am. Diet. Assoc.*, **57**:29–32, 1970.

2. Dwyer, J.: "Vegetarianism," *Contemporary Nutrition* **4**(6), June 1979 (General Mills, Minneapolis).
3. Register, U. D., and Sonnenberg, L. M.: "The Vegetarian Diet," *J. Am. Diet. Assoc.*, **62**:253–61, 1973.
4. Erhard, D.: "The New Vegetarians. 1. Vegetarianism and Its Medical Consequences," *Nutr. Today,* **8**:4–12, November 1973.
5. Erhard, D.: "The New Vegetarians. 2. The Zen Macrobiotic Movement and Other Cults Based on Vegetarianism," *Nutr. Today,* **9**:20–27, January 1974.
6. Dwyer, J. T., et al.: "The New Vegetarians: The Natural High?" *J. Am. Diet. Assoc.*, **65**:529–36, 1974.
7. Kaufman, M.: "Adapting Therapeutic Diets to Jewish Food Customs," *Am. J. Clin. Nutr.*, **5**:676–81, 1957.
8. Torres, R. M.: "Dietary Patterns of Puerto Rican People," *Am. J. Clin. Nutr.*, **7**:349–55, 1959.
9. Smith, L. K.: "Mexican-American Views of Anglo Medical and Dietetic Practices," *J. Am. Diet. Assoc.*, **74**:463–64, 1979.
10. Bailey, M. A.: "Nutrition Education and the Spanish-speaking Americans," *J. Nutr. Educ.*, **2**:50–54, Fall 1970.
11. Hacker, D. B., and Miller, E. D.: "Food Patterns of the Southwest," *Am. J. Clin. Nutr.*, **7**:224–29, 1959.
12. Kuhnlein, H. V., *et al.:* "Composition of Traditional Hopi Foods," *J. Am. Diet. Assoc.*, **75**:37–41, 1979.
13. Schaefer, O.: "When the Eskimo Comes to Town," *Nutr. Today,* **6**:8–16, November/December 1971.
14. Kaufman, M.: "Vietnam, 1978: Crisis in Food, Nutrition, and Health," *J. Am. Diet. Assoc.*, **74**:310–16, 1979.
15. Valassi, K. V.: "Food Habits of Greek Americans," *Am. J. Clin. Nutr.*, **11**:240–48, 1962.

Additional References

ALFORD, B. B., and NANCE, E. B.: "Customary Foods in the Navajo Diet," *J. Am. Diet. Assoc.*, **69**:538–39, 1976.

American Dietetic Association: *Cultural Food Patterns in the U.S.A.*, revised, 1976.

American Dietetic Association: "Position Paper on the Vegetarian Approach to Eating," *J. Am. Diet. Assoc.*, **77**:61–69, 1980.

BASS, M. A., and WAKEFIELD, L. M.: "Nutrient Intake and Food Patterns of Indians on Standing Rock Reservation," *J. Am. Diet. Assoc.*, **64**:36–41, 1974.

BERGAN, J. G., and BROWN, P. T.: "Nutritional Status of 'New' Vegetarians," *J. Am. Diet. Assoc.*, **76**:151–55, 1980.

DWYER, J. T., et al.: "Mental Age and I. Q. of Predominantly Vegetarian Children," *J. Am. Diet. Assoc.*, **76**:142–47, 1980.

FITZGERALD, T. K.: "Southern Folks' Eating Habits Aint What They Used to Be—if They Ever Were," *Nutr. Today,* **14**:16–21, July 1979.

HARWOOD, A.: "The Hot-Cold Theory of Disease," *JAMA,* **216**:1153–58, 1971.

KOH, E. T., and CAPLES, V.: "Nutrient Intake of Low-Income Black Families in Southwestern Mississippi," *J. Am. Diet. Assoc.*, **75**:665–70, 1979.

KUHNLEIN, H. V., and CALLOWAY, D. H.: "Contemporary Hopi Food Intake Patterns," *Ecol. Food Nutr.*, **6**:159–73, 1977.

Review: "Growth of Vegetarian Children," *Nutr. Rev.*, **37**:108–109, 1979.

SAKR, A. H.: "Dietary Regulations and Food Habits of Muslims," *J. Am. Diet. Assoc.*, **58**:123–26, 1971.

TABER, L. A. L., and COOK, R. A.: "Dietary and Anthropometric Assessment of Adult Omnivores, Fish-eaters, and Lacto-ovo-vegetarians," *J. Am. Diet. Assoc.*, **76**:21–29, 1980.

YANG, G. I-P., and FOX, H. M.: "Food Habit Changes of Chinese Persons Living in Lincoln, Nebraska," *J. Am. Diet. Assoc.*, **75**:420–24, 1979.

YOHAI, F.: "Dietary Patterns of Spanish-speaking People Living in the Boston Area," *J. Am. Diet. Assoc.*, **71**:273–75, 1977.

Safeguarding the Food Supply 16

EACH year millions of persons experience some foodborne illness caused by microbial infections or intoxications. Most instances of such illness are caused by faulty food handling. Naturally occurring toxicants in foods also cause illness under certain circumstances. A variety of preservation techniques are used to retain nutritive values, esthetic qualities, and safety of the food supply. Many additives serve useful functions in maintaining a high quality food supply and in reducing food waste.

Illness Caused by Food

Following the exodus of the Jews from Egypt, the people had a great craving for meat. When quails were brought in large numbers by winds from the sea, the people gathered them and ate them. This is what happened:*

> While the meat was yet between their teeth, before it was consumed, the anger of the Lord was kindled against the people, and the Lord smote the people with a very great plague. Therefore the name of that place was called Kibrothhattaavah,† because there they buried the people who had the craving.

Recently among some people living on the island of Lesbos (Greece) a syndrome has been observed following the eating of quail.[1] The symptoms include muscular pain, paralysis of used muscles, excretion of myoglobin in the urine, and oliguria. Apparently this illness occurs only in persons who have some enzymatic abnormality and who have become physically fatigued before eating the quail. It is theorized that the eating of quail elicits the abnormality in these persons, thus producing the symptoms. The author of this report believes that this twentieth-century syndrome is the same as that which afflicted the Jews during the exodus.

* *The Holy Bible,* Numbers 11:33–34.
† Graves of craving.

The ancient Egyptians realized that the meat of animals that had died a natural death was unfit for human food. Greek records of many centuries ago note that the wife, daughter, and two sons of the Greek poet Euripides died after having eaten poisonous fungi. For centuries kings were protected against poisoning by employing official food tasters. Thus, history records on numerous occasions the role of food in producing illness.

Illness resulting from the eating of food may be caused (1) by contamination of the food by bacteria, molds, and fungi, (2) by the presence of some natural toxicant in the food, (3) by the contamination of food by a toxic chemical, or (4) by sensitivity of a given individual to one or more foods. Bacterial, parasitic, and chemical contaminations are considered in this chapter.

Foodborne Diseases as a Public Health Problem *Salmonella, Clostridium perfringens,* and *Staphylococci* are considered to be the "big three" responsible for much of the foodborne illness in the United States. For most people in good health an outbreak of food poisoning from these organisms results in an illness of short duration leading to discomfort and absence from work or school. But for the very young, the elderly, and those who are debilitated from other illness, these seemingly mild infections can lead to serious complications or even death. The outbreak of an infection in a child-care institution or in a nursing home is especially life threatening. Therefore, to protect the vulnerable, every precaution must be taken to minimize the occurrence of infection among the more vigorous who in turn become the agents for transmission of organisms.

Other diseases transmitted by foods are typhoid fever, bacillary dysentery, tuberculosis, scarlet fever, streptococcic sore throat, botulism, undulant fever, amebic dysentery, trichinosis, infectious hepatitis, and cholera.

Foodborne diseases result from eating food (1) from an animal or plant that has been infected, (2) that has been contaminated by organisms transmitted by insects, flies, roaches, or rodents, (3) that has had contact with sewage-polluted water (shellfish, for example), or (4) that has been contaminated by a food handler who has not observed good personal hygiene or acceptable food-handling practices.

Some illnesses are enteric in that the symptoms are confined to the gastrointestinal tract with mild to severe nausea, vomiting, abdominal pain, and diarrhea. Other foodborne diseases are systemic; that is, the organisms invade the circulation and produce symptoms in organs and tissues.

Bacterial Food Infections A bacterial *infection* results from the ingestion of food that has been contaminated with large numbers of bacteria. The bacteria continue to grow in the favorable intestinal environment and produce irritation of the mucosa with symptoms occurring in 12 to 36 hours after ingestion of the food.

Salmonellosis. About 1,300 serotypes of the *Salmonella* genus have been identified, each of which is capable of causing infection in humans. The organisms are easily killed by boiling for 5 minutes, but survive in foods that are inadequately heated. Paratyphoid fever (enteric fever) occurs frequently. The symptoms usually last for 2 to 3 days, but the organisms may be present in body wastes for 2 or 3 weeks thereby providing a continuing source of contamination for others.

Typhoid fever, fortunately rare in the United States, is the most serious of the *Salmonella* infections. The symptoms of the gastrointestinal tract may be severe with ulcerations of the mucosa occurring. Unlike most infections by *Salmonella,* typhoid fever is systemic. The organisms particularly affect the liver and gallbladder, but they may also localize in the bone marrow, kidney, spleen, and the lungs where bronchitis and pneumonia may result.

Meat, poultry, fish, eggs, and dairy products that are eaten raw or that have been inadequately heated are most frequently implicated in salmonellosis. Contaminated cake mixes, bakery foods, coloring agents, powdered yeast, and chocolate candy have also caused outbreaks of the infection.

Animals including cattle, swine, poultry, fish, dogs, and birds harbor the organisms. They are usually infected by contact of one animal with another or by animal feeds. A single egg that is infected can contaminate a whole batch of eggs being frozen or dried. A butcher block or kitchen counter with which infected meat has been in contact is a source of contamination for any food placed upon it. Flies and rodents coming in contact with feces of animals or humans are responsible for contamination of food. Food handlers who do not observe good personal hygiene or who do not follow essential directions in the preparation of food are a major source of contamination of the food supplies.

Shigellosis (bacillary dysentery). The *Shigella* genus includes pathogenic organisms widely distributed and capable of producing severe illness. Bacillary dysentery is characterized by fever, abdominal pain, vomiting, and diarrhea. The intestinal mucosa may become ulcerated, and stools often contain blood and mucus. Fatalities from the infections are ordinarily low, but in tropical countries where sanitation is poor and malnutrition is prevalent the disease is fatal to as many as 20 per cent of persons affected.

Infected human feces are the source of the infection, which is transmitted by the direct fecal-oral route or through contamination of food or water.

Clostridium perfringens, the gas gangrene organism, ordinarily inhabits the intestinal tract and in usual numbers does not produce illness. However, when a food is consumed which has been contaminated with large numbers of bacteria, illness results.

Clostridium perfringens appears normally in the soil, in the intestinal tract of humans and animals, and in sewage. The bacteria are destroyed by heat, but the spores they produce will survive boiling for as long as 5 hours. If foods are allowed to remain at temperatures between 10 and 60°C (50 and 140°F) for several hours, the spores germinate and prodigious numbers of bacteria are then present in the food. Food should be refrigerated immediately after heating to prevent rapid germination of spores. Shallow containers are preferred since a large food mass in a deep container cools so slowly that considerable bacterial growth occurs.

Bacterial Food Intoxication Food poisoning frequently results from the ingestion of a food in which a bacterial toxin has been produced. The preformed toxin is responsible for the symptoms, which may be mild to severe. Usually the symptoms are apparent from 1 to 6 hours following a meal.

Staphylococcal poisoning occurs abruptly after the ingestion of food containing the enterotoxin. The gastrointestinal symptoms are often severe but usually the illness lasts for only 1 to 3 days.

Staphylococci are found in the air and occur especially in infected cuts and abrasions of the skin, boils, and pimples. They may be present in the nose and throat of food handlers. Food becomes contaminated through failure to observe rules of hygiene. Rapid growth of the bacteria occurs in contaminated food if it is held at temperatures ranging between 10 and 60°C (50 and 140°F) for 3 to 4 hours. Semisolid foods such as custards, cream fillings in pastries, cream puffs, cream sauces, mayonnaise, chicken and turkey salads, croquettes, potato salad, ice cream, poultry dressing, ham, ground meat, stews, and fish provide the ideal culture media for bacterial growth.

Staphylococci are killed at high temperatures, but the toxin is not inactivated with temperatures ordinarily used in food preparation. The contaminated food usually does not smell, taste, or appear to be spoiled. The best safeguard against staphylococcal poisoning is prompt refrigeration of food so that bacterial growth is retarded and toxin formation does not take place.

Botulism is an extremely rare type of food poisoning but of such serious consequences that it captures the attention of the news media. Each year there are ten to twenty outbreaks of botulism in the United States with two to five deaths. Most instances of botulism are traced to the ingestion of inadequately processed home-canned nonacid vegetables and meats. A few outbreaks in recent years have been reported from commercially processed tuna fish, whitefish, and soup.

Since 1975 over 100 cases of botulism have been diagnosed in infants.[2,3] The disease has resulted from the germination of spores of *Clostridium botulinum* in the lumen of the bowel and the subsequent production of the toxin. One of the sources of these spores has been honey contaminated with the bacterial spores. It is estimated that 10 to 15 per cent of all supplies of honey are contaminated. This poses no problems for older persons, but it is recommended that no honey be given to infants under 1 year of age.

The symptoms of botulism occur 8 to 72 hours after ingestion of the contaminated food and usually begin in the gastrointestinal tract. The principal hazard is the effect on the nervous system. When the toxin enters the circulation, the nerve endings become blocked. Headache, dizziness, double vision, difficulty in swallowing, and paralysis occur. Death is usually the result of respiratory paralysis and cardiac failure. When botulism is suspected early and treatment with antitoxin is initiated, the death rate is about 25 per cent. Failure to initiate early treatment increases the death rate to about 65 per cent.

Clostridium botulinum is present in soils all over the world and in the sediment at the bottom of rivers and lakes. Consequently, vegetables grown on these soils and fish become contaminated. The bacteria do not grow in the presence of oxygen; that is, they are anaerobic. They will grow within a few millimeters below the surface of the foods, however. The bacteria are sporeformers which are resistant to ordinary boiling temperature. As the spores germinate the deadly neurotoxin is produced.

Canned foods that contain little or no acid (pH above 4.6) such as meat, beans, asparagus, corn, and peas are very good media for the growth of the bacillus botulinus, whereas acid-containing foods such as tomatoes and certain fruits are not favorable to growth. Some recently developed varieties of tomatoes, however, do not contain sufficient acid to prevent the growth of the bacteria. The use of sterilization with steam under pressure is absolutely necessary in the home for any nonacid food products, as well as for those processed commercially.

Botulinus-infected foods do not necessarily taste or smell spoiled, so home-canned vegetables should be brought to a vigorous boil and kept boiling for 10 minutes. Any toxin that may be present will thereby be inactivated. Any can of food that shows gas production, change in color or consistency, bulging ends, or leaks should be discarded without even tasting. "When in doubt, throw it out" is a good axiom. The foods must be disposed of so that animals do not have access to them since they too might be poisoned.

Parasitic Infestations of Foods Many protozoa and helminths (worms) gain admission to the body by means of food and parasitize the bowel, thereby causing injury to the intestinal lining. Some of them also invade other tissues of the body.

Among the parasitic protozoa are *Endamoeba histolytica,* which causes amebic dysentery. The source of infection is human feces, and infection is transmitted by a food handler who is a carrier or by contaminated water supplies. The symptoms may be acute, chronic, or intermittent. Erosion of the intestinal mucosa sometimes occurs with profuse bloody diarrhea. The individual with a chronic infection may experience only mild discomfort of diarrhea or constipation. The liver, lung, brain, and other tissues may be infected and abscesses may form. Preventive measures include maintenance of sanitary controls of the water supply and sewage disposal, as well as supervision of public eating places by health agencies.

The helminths that frequently invade the intestinal tract include *nematodes* (roundworms), *cestodes* (tapeworms), and *trematodes* (liver, intestinal, and lung flukes). Trichinosis, one of the more serious infestations, results from the ingestion of raw or partially cooked pork infected with *Trichinella spiralis,* a very minute roundworm barely visible to the naked eye. In the intestinal tract the larvae are set free from their cysts during digestion of the meat and develop into adults within a few days. The females deposit larvae in the mucosa and invade the lymph and blood circulation. The muscles of the diaphragm, the thorax, the abdominal wall, the biceps, and the tongue are frequently involved, there being muscular pain, chills, and weakness.

Trichinella is destroyed by cooking pork until no trace of pink remains. The recommended internal temperature for cooked pork is 77°C (170°F), which allows a margin of about 17°C (30°F) above the lethal point of the organisms. *Trichinella* is also destroyed by freezing at −18°C (0°F) or below for at least 72 hours. Government inspection does not include examination for *Trichinella* at the present time. The cooking of all garbage fed to hogs will go a long way toward reducing *Trichinella* infestation.

Hookworm infestation is a serious problem in children in tropical countries of the world, and in some parts of the United States. The larvae penetrate the exposed skin and reach the lymphatics and blood circulation. They are carried to the lungs and migrate into the alveoli, trachea, epiglottis, and pharynx and are swallowed. They may also be carried from soil to hands to mouth.

It has been estimated that a single hookworm removes almost 1 ml blood per day as it carries on its blood-sucking activity in the intestine. The loss of blood produces an anemia with symptoms of weakness, fatigue, and growth retardation. Usually the infestation is present in children who also are malnourished. A good nutritious diet is always important for these children, but the eradication of hookworm infestation depends upon sanitary measures for disposal of feces so that the cycle of parasite growth in the soil is broken.

Naturally Occurring Toxicants in Foods Foods are exceedingly complex mixtures of chemicals. It has been estimated that the naturally occurring chemicals in the food supply probably number in the hundreds of thousands. For example, potatoes, often considered to be a simple food, contain at least 150 chemical substances including not only the nutritionally important protein, carbohydrate, minerals, and vitamins, but also oxalic acid, tannins, solanine, arsenic, and nitrate.

Two terms must be defined when considering the possible danger from food components. TOXICITY is the capacity of a substance when tested by itself to harm living organisms. HAZARD is the capacity of a substance to produce injury under conditions of use. For example, vitamin A is potentially toxic, but it is a hazard only when ingested over a period of time in amounts that are 10 to 20 times the recommended allowances. Salt is potentially toxic; it is a hazard when ingested in three to five times normal amounts. For hypertensive patients salt may be hazardous at much lower levels of intake.

Foods contain thousands of compounds that are potentially toxic. The hazards are minimal because of several factors: (1) the body has metabolic mechanisms for degrading, detoxifying, and eliminating some substances; (2) some toxic substances are modified by processing—for example, the heating of soybeans to destroy trypsin inhibitor; and (3) some toxic compounds are antagonistic to other toxic compounds, and the net effect is one of neutralization. Molybdenum, an essential nutrient, is toxic in excess; copper, another essential nutrient which is also toxic, is antagonistic to molybdenum. Thus, together they reduce the toxicity of the pair.

Poisoning from natural food toxicants often occurs in times of stress such as famine or war when abnormally large amounts of single foods containing toxic materials are ingested daily for prolonged periods of time.

Alkaloids. The alkaloids such as strychnine, atropine, scopalamine, solanine, and others have long been known as poisonous compounds. Varieties of hemlock have been mistaken for parsley, horseradish, or wild parsnip and eaten in salads and soup only to produce immediate, often fatal, illness. Monkshood, foxglove, and deadly nightshade have from time to time been mistaken for edible plants and have caused violent illness.

Solanine, representing a series of glycosides, occurs in the stems and leaves of the potato plant and in the green part of sprouting potatoes. When potatoes are stored in bright light, significant amounts of solanine are produced in the skin, evidenced by greening. When ingested in sufficient amounts, solanine produces pain, vomiting, jaundice, diarrhea, and prostration. Ordinarily the green parts of the potato are removed with the peel.

Legumes and seeds. Because legumes are important sources of protein and energy in some parts of the world, the presence of toxic factors in them is of nutritional and economic importance. Soybeans are a most valuable source of protein when they are heated. Raw soybeans contain a trypsin inhibitor and probably some other factors that interfere with the metabolism and with growth in animals. In addition, the phytic acid content of soybeans binds zinc so that animals fed a diet in which soybeans are the source of protein develop a severe zinc deficiency. This can be corrected by supplementing the diet with zinc. Soybeans also contain a goitrogen but this is not believed to be a factor in endemic goiter.

Cassava and Lima beans contain *linmarin,* a glycoside that can be split to hydrocyanic acid. People in West Africa, Jamaica, and Malaysia consume up to 750 gm cassava daily. It is thought that the incidence of blindness and tropical ataxic neuropathy, a degenerative disease, may be caused by chronic cyanide poisoning from the cassava.

Lathyrism has been known since the time of Hippocrates. It is observed in India and in Mediterranean countries following the ingestion for 6 months or more of large amounts of the seeds of *Lathyrus sativus,* a legume. These legumes grow under adverse conditions of drought and hence they may be ingested extensively during a famine. Lathyrism is a neurologic disease characterized by weakness of the leg muscles, dragging of the feet, loss of sensation of heat and pain, and spinal cord lesions.

Favism is an inherited sensitivity to fava or broad beans and is fairly common in the Mediterranean area, and in Asia and Formosa. Sensitive individuals have a deficiency of glucose-6-phosphate dehydrogenase and reduced glutathione content of the red blood cells. An unidentified substance in the fava beans leads to hemolysis of the red blood cells and thus hemolytic anemia in the sensitive individuals.

Gossypol is a toxicant in cottonseed that must be removed before the meal can be used in protein mixtures. Some strains of cottonseed are now being developed that are free of this toxic substance.

Mushroom poisoning. A few species of mushrooms are so toxic that eating them may be fatal, others are mildly toxic, and many species are harmless and greatly enjoyed. The *Amanita* is the most poisonous of the mushrooms and produces severe abdominal pain, prostration, jaundice, and death in more than half the people who ingest it. This source of poisoning can be eliminated if people use only the commercially grown mushrooms.

Mycotoxins. In medieval times a poisoning known as "St. Anthony's Fire" was a terrible scourge.[4] It was caused by ergot, a toxic fungus, growing on cereal grains. Ergotism is almost unknown today. Deaths of thousands of people in Russia in times of war and famine have been attributed to the consumption of moldy millet.

Many molds growing on grains and nuts can produce illness in animals and probably in humans. Aflatoxins produced by the mold *Aspergillus flavus* are a class of substances of extreme toxicity to swine, cattle, poultry, and laboratory animals. The aflatoxins are potent hepatocarcinogens. Much attention has been focused on peanuts, Brazil nuts, and grains that are subject to mold growth when they are allowed to remain on damp ground or when they are stored without sufficient drying. The only practical way to prevent the development of the mold is through prompt drying of grains and nuts to a moisture content not over 15 per cent. Allowing crops to remain in fields over winter invites mold growth.

Paralytic shellfish poisoning from oysters, clams, mussels, and scallops has caused many fatal illnesses. The shellfish ingest large quantities of "red tide," the plankton *Gonyaulaux catennela.* Saxitoxin, an extremely toxic metabolite, is produced from the plankton. The toxin resists ordinary cooking procedures.

Interference with nutritive properties. The adverse effect of some chemical substances is an interference with the utilization of a nutrient and thus the imposition of a deficiency. One of the best-known examples of this is the oxalic acid content of certain green leafy vegetables such as spinach, beet tops, and chard that interferes with the absorption of calcium. The occasional use of these vegetables with an adequate calcium intake is of no concern whatsoever. However, if the calcium intake is low and the vegetables are eaten frequently, a problem of calcium deficiency could arise. Rhubarb leaves are so high in oxalic acid content that their ingestion leads to gastrointestinal upsets, and in severe intoxications to hematemesis, hematuria, noncoagulability of the blood, and convulsions.

Goiter is a major public health problem affecting 200 million people throughout the world. Goitrogens, which are antithyroid compounds, are held responsible for about 4 per cent of the goiter incidence, representing a total of 8 million persons. Goitrogens are found in broccoli, Brussels sprouts, cabbage, cauliflower, kale, kohlrabi, rutabagas, and turnips. There is no adverse effect when eating normal amounts of these vegetables, but when they become a major part of the diet for extended periods of time, the antithyroid effect becomes evident. Additional iodine does not counteract this effect.

Thiaminase, an enzyme antagonistic to thiamin, is present in bracken fern, raw fish, and a variety of fruits and vegetables. In an ordinary mixed diet this is of no concern. The enzyme is destroyed by heat.

Excess of nutrients. The toxic effects of vitamins A and D are well known. The ingestion of seal or polar bear liver leads to symptoms of acute vitamin A toxicity, inasmuch as 1 pound of the liver contains about 10 million IU of vitamin A. On a practical basis in the United States the hazards of vitamin A toxicity relate to the indiscriminate use of vitamin supplements and not to excesses in the diet itself. If several foods that are fortified with vitamin D are consumed each day, the intake could be in excess of requirements, and hypercalcemia is a possible outcome. (See Chapter 10.)

Tyramine toxicity. Cheddar cheese and Chianti wine contain appreciable amounts of tyramine, which is produced by the decarboxylation of tyrosine. Tyramine is a potent vasopressor substance but it is normally metabolized in the body by the action of monoamine oxidase. Patients with depressive states are frequently treated with monoamine oxidase inhibitor because of its ability to produce euphoria. Since the inhibitor interferes with the metabolism of tyramine, the ingestion of tyramine-containing foods leads to nausea, vomiting, headache, and severe hypertension, and sometimes death. A glass of Chianti wine or as little as 1 ounce of Cheddar cheese contains enough tyramine to produce some toxic effects, and large amounts may be dangerous for some.

Poisoning by Trace Mineral Elements A number of trace mineral elements are essential nutrients but are also potent toxicants. These include copper, fluorine, manganese, molybdenum, selenium, and zinc. Lead, mercury, and cadmium are serious environmental pollutants. These minerals modify metabolism in several ways: (1) by inactivating enzymes such as ribonuclease, alkaline phosphatase, catalase, and others; (2) by chelating with a nutrient so that the latter is unavailable; (3) by altering cell permeability; and (4) by replacing a structural element—for example, lithium in place of sodium.

Many nutrient-toxicant interactions exist. A few examples follow. Calcium, iron, and protein interact with lead to reduce absorption and thus to lessen the toxic effects. The presence of selenium protects against the toxicity of mercury and cadmium. When a copper deficiency exists, the susceptibility to toxic reactions from cadmium, mercury, and zinc is increased. A zinc deficiency increases the susceptibility to toxicity of cadmium, copper, and mercury.

Lead is a particularly serious contaminant since it accumulates in the body and results in chronic illness characterized by severe anemia and changes in the arteries and kidneys, with death occurring in some instances. A minute quantity of lead occurs naturally in food and is ingested daily, but when the daily intake is 1 mg or more, the eventual accumulations may become toxic. Food becomes contaminated with lead when it is exposed to dust containing lead or when it is kept in containers in which solders, alloys, or enamel containing lead have been used. The canning industry has long since devised containers that are entirely safe for food.

Most lead poisoning occurs in black children who live in ghetto areas where the primary source of lead is the layers of old paint in the interiors of homes. Children from 18 to 30 months chew paint from the woodwork, and a daily ingestion of 3 mg can lead to elevated blood levels in 3 to 4 months. In a number of cities a concerted effort is being made to correct the problem by educating parents, by emphasizing the removal of old paint, and by screening children through blood lead determinations in areas where there is hazard.

A few years ago there was great concern about the mercury content of fish. Strong,[4] an authority on food toxicants, believes the danger was overemphasized and that serious contamination takes place only in areas of pollution by industrial wastes. The mercury in tuna fish appears to be nontoxic because of its interaction with selenium which is also present.

Accidental poisonings occur when chemicals have been mistaken for powdered milk, flour, or baking powder. Some years ago in a state institution 47 deaths resulted when roach powder containing sodium fluoride was mistakenly used as dry milk powder.[5] In another instance boric acid was mistaken for lactic acid for the preparation of infant formulas, again resulting in infant deaths. It goes without saying that insecticides, lye, mothballs, and numerous other poisons should be well labeled, kept away from foodstuffs, and out of the reach of small children.

The metals used in cooking utensils and in food containers have been a source of much controversy. Many studies have shown that glass, stainless steel, aluminum, agate, and tin are suitable containers for food since these materials are practically insoluble or, when dissolved to a slight degree, are not harmful to health. Acid foods may dissolve some of the tin from cans so that a change of flavor results from the iron underneath the tin coating, but the ingestion of these foods is not harmful. It is recommended that acid foods be transferred from the can to a covered glass container if the food is to be refrigerated after opening.

Radioactive Fallout People have always been exposed to the radiation of naturally occurring radioisotopes in the environment. Potassium-40 and carbon-14 are the major contaminants of food from natural sources. The danger from these is slight because carbon-14 is absorbed into the body in very small amounts and potassium-40 remains in the body for only short periods of time.

With the advent of the nuclear bomb and nuclear-powered generator plants the potential for harmful exposure has increased. Following a nuclear detonation there are several pathways by which the radionuclides eventually are ingested by humans. (See Figure 16–1.) For example, contaminated plants may be eaten by cows; much of the element is excreted in the urine of the cow, but some will be secreted in the milk which, in turn, is consumed by humans. Some of the consumed element will be excreted in human feces, but some will enter the metabolism in a manner similar to that of the element with which it is related. Strontium-90 is related to calcium and is deposited chiefly in the bones; cesium-137, like potassium, is distributed throughout the body in the soft tissues; and within 48 hours of ingestion iodine-131 is accounted for in the thyroid gland and in the urine. Excessive deposits of radioactive elements carry the threat of cancer—of the

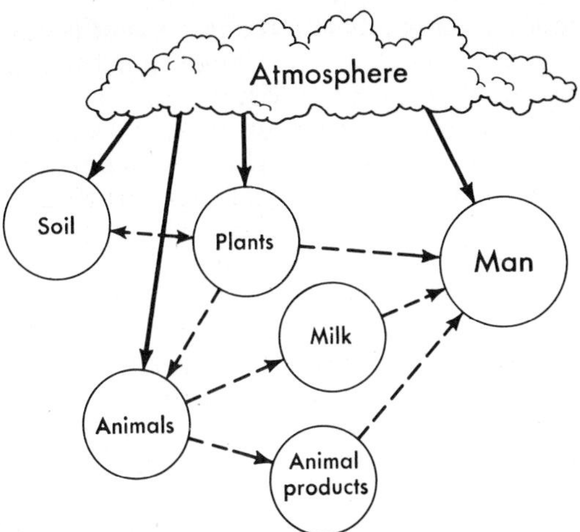

Figure 16–1. Pathways of radioactive fallout. (Courtesy, National Dairy Council, Chicago.)

thyroid with iodine-131, and of the bone with strontium-90.

Each radioisotope has a specific *physical half-life*. This is the amount of time that elapses before half of the element is decayed. The element thus emits radiations to the external environment with consequent exposure of humans, animals, and plants over this period of time. The *biologic half-life* refers to the length of time before half of the element is excreted from the body. Thus, some elements may be rapidly excreted causing little harm, whereas others are retained. Strontium-90 and cesium-137 have a physical half-life of 28 years. Strontium-90 is of much more serious biologic consequence since its rate of turnover is slow in the body, whereas cesium-137 has a biologic half-life of about 140 days.

The Federal Radiation Council has established guidelines which define the potential hazards of radiation. The U.S. Public Health Service, and U.S. Department of Agriculture are among the groups that periodically analyze foods from all over the country to determine levels of radioactivity. About one third to one half of the dietary strontium-90 is present in milk; however, the high calcium intake helps to ensure a preferential use of calcium rather than strontium by the body. The current levels in foods present no risks whatsoever.

Preservation of Foods

Factors Contributing to Food Spoilage Foods are made unsafe to eat or become aesthetically undesirable or both by the actions of bacteria, yeasts, and molds; by enzymatic action; by chemical or physical changes; and by contact with insects and rodents. In food spoilage these factors often coexist. Unsafe foods do not necessarily show any changes in appearance and palatability, and hence the danger from them is great. Foods that are rancid, moldy, or rotting are less likely to be consumed and therefore may not be a direct threat to health, but the economic waste is considerable.

Temperature and growth of organisms. Bacteria, yeasts, and molds grow rapidly at temperatures of 10 to 60°C (50 to 140°F); within this range the rate of growth increases tenfold for each 10°C (18°F) increase in temperature. Thus, the bacteria produced in a food left at room temperature for 3 or 4 hours can reach astronomical numbers.

Growth of microorganisms is retarded at refrigerator temperatures and is stopped at freezing temperatures. Many molds and some bacteria known as *psychrophils* grow even at refrigerator temperatures, leading to spoilage of food. Pathogenic bacteria do not grow at these temperatures. Many bacteria are not killed by freezing—an important fact to remember when frozen foods are thawed and allowed to stand at room temperatures. (See Figure 16–2.)

Some bacteria known as *thermophils* thrive at relatively high temperatures. They are responsible for the "flat sour" which occurs in some home-canned foods.

Many bacteria produce spores that are very resistant to heat. In fact, several hours of boiling do not destroy them. Under fa-

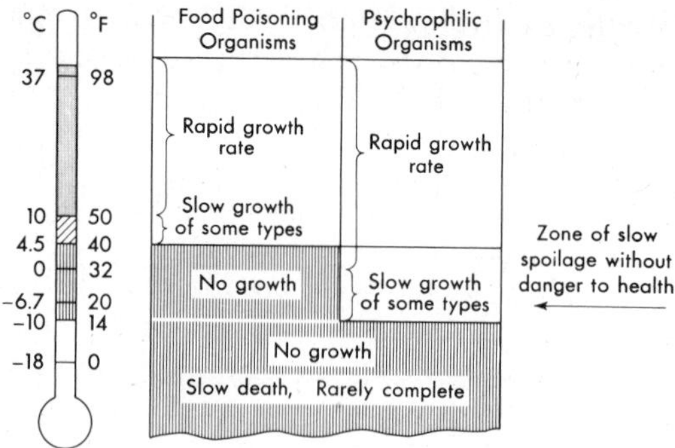

Figure 16–2. Low-temperature limits on growth of food poisoning and psychrophilic organisms. (Courtesy, Dr. Horace K. Burr and the *Journal of the American Medical Association,* **174:**1178–80, 1960.)

vorable conditions such spores will germinate rapidly.

Physical and chemical changes. Appearance, texture, flavor, and the chemical constituents of foods are modified by the influence of air, heat, light, moisture, and time. These changes are accelerated by enzyme action and by the presence of minute traces of mineral catalysts such as copper and iron. All plant and animal tissues contain enzymes that are highly active at room temperatures and above.

The rate of chemical change doubles for each 10°C (18°F) rise in temperature. Rancidity of fats is one example of undesirable oxidation and contributes to the deterioration of flavor even in foods that contain only small amounts of fat. Oxidation also leads to loss of ascorbic acid.

Plant and animal tissue fibers are softened, and the surface of cut nonacid fruits is oxidized and becomes darkened as a result of enzyme action, thereby changing the texture, color, and nutritive value. Some nutrients may be lost by discarding fluids in which they have been dissolved. The exposure of milk to sunlight leads to a tallowy flavor and loss of riboflavin and vitamin B-6. With storage, changes in texture also occur: sugar may crystallize out of jellies; ice cream becomes gummy and granular; and frozen meats and poultry become dry.

Food Preservation The criteria for successful food preservation, whether it be for a day or two or for months, are these: (1) safety from contamination by pathogenic organisms or toxicity through chemicals; and (2) maintenance of optimum qualities of color, flavor, texture, and nutritive value.

Methods of food preservation that destroy bacteria are *bactericidal;* these include the application of heat by cooking, canning, preserving, and irradiation sterilization. Other methods such as dehydration, freezing, treatment with antibiotics, salting, and pickling retard the growth of bacteria, molds, and yeasts; they are *bacteriostatic.*

Pasteurization Of all foods, milk is most susceptible to contamination. The inspection of cows, barns, milk handlers, and dairy-processing plants is essential to the production of milk of high quality. Cattle diseases such as brucellosis, tuberculosis, and mastitis are now rare because of testing and vaccination programs and prompt isolation and treatment of infected animals. Pasteurization, nevertheless, is essential not only for milk but also for the preparation of cheese, butter, and ice cream.

Milk is pasteurized by (1) the *holding* process in which milk is heated to at least 62°C (143°F) and kept at that temperature for at least 30 minutes, or by (2) the *high-temperature short-time* method in which milk is heated to 71°C (160°F) and kept at that temperature for at least 15 seconds.

Milk may be sterilized by boiling it for a specified time as in the preparation of infant formulas or by heat as in the processing of evaporated milk. Pasteurization does not appreciably change the color or flavor of milk, but sterilization deepens the color and gives to milk a slightly carmelized flavor.

Food Preservation by Heat Bacterial destruction by heat depends upon the degree of heat and the length of time it is applied.

Boiling of food (100°C) kills bacteria but

will not destroy the spores of *Clostridium botulinum* or *perfringens.* Toxins formed by staphylococci are not inactivated even with prolonged boiling, but botulin is destroyed with boiling for 10 minutes. Cooking with a pressure cooker will kill bacteria and also destroy the spores of *Clostridium perfringens* and *botulinum.*

Low-heat cookery as for custards and sauces does not destroy *Salmonella* and other bacteria. Likewise the heat produced in the interior of casseroles and stuffed poultry is inadequate for the destruction of bacteria. Thus, such foods should be eaten immediately after cooking, or promptly refrigerated until later use.

Canning. Exact procedures for commercial canning have been developed for each food. Sterilization is brought about by steam under pressure for specified lengths of time.

Home canning. When foods are canned at home, a pressure cooker should always be used for low-acid foods, including most vegetables, poultry, and meat, in order to destroy bacteria and their heat-resistant spores. Fruits and tomatoes, being acid foods, may be safely canned using the boiling-water bath method.

Nutritive values of canned foods. Commercial processes for canning generally result in optimal nutrient retention. Small losses of the heat labile thiamin and ascorbic acid occur. The greater losses occur when canned foods are held for long periods of time at high temperatures. As much as 25 per cent of ascorbic acid and thiamin may be lost from fruits and vegetables stored for a year at 27°C (80°F), but with storage at 18°C (65°F) these losses are reduced to 10 per cent. Meats, likewise, lose 20 to 30 per cent of their thiamin content after 6 months' storage at 21°C (70°F), but the riboflavin content is not adversely affected. Carotene losses in fruits and vegetables are small even after months of storage. Water-soluble nutrients distribute themselves evenly throughout the solids and liquids; thus, if the solids constitute two thirds of the total, one third of these water-soluble nutrients will be lost if the liquid is not used.

Preservation at Cold Temperatures Modern refrigeration has been largely responsible for the tremendous variety of foods available all over the country, in season and out. By means of refrigeration foods can be kept for long periods of time in commercial cold-storage rooms at the proper humidity or transported from coast to coast without danger of loss from spoilage or freezing, and they can be kept in the home refrigerator to reduce the number of trips the homemaker makes to the market.

Cool storage is being gradually extended to canned and dehydrated foods to retain optimum color, flavor, and nutritive values.

Freezing. In the quick freezing of foods, first developed as a practical method of processing some 50 years ago, bacteria are unable to grow and enzymes are inactivated.

Care and use of frozen foods. Because frozen foods contain bacteria and enzymes in a dormant state, it is essential that foods be maintained at −18°C (0°F), or lower, until they are to be used. Bacteria begin to multiply and enzymes begin to bring about oxidative changes as soon as foods begin to thaw. These changes can be rapid if foods are allowed to stand for some time at room temperature. Fully thawed foods should not be frozen again since further deterioration in quality will occur. Fruits retain their best color if they are thawed in the container in which they are packed. Most vegetables are cooked by dropping the frozen product directly into a small quantity of boiling water and rapidly bringing it to the boiling point. Meat and poultry should be thawed in the refrigerator, and not at room temperature. This requires transfer from the freezer to the refrigerator a day or two in advance of cookery.

Nutritive values of frozen foods. The nutritive values of frozen foods compare favorably with those of fresh foods. In fact, the vitamin content of food frozen at the peak of quality may be higher than that of fresh food that is overripe or that has remained for many hours in a warm market.

Slight losses of water-soluble minerals and vitamins occur when vegetables are blanched to inactivate oxidative enzymes. Further small losses of ascorbic acid may occur in frozen nonacid foods kept for a long time. Juice held at 0°C for a year loses not more than 6 per cent of its ascorbic acid content, but nonacid foods lose an appreciable amount at −18°C and much lesser amounts at −23 to −28°C.

Dehydration For centuries people all over the world have dried fruits, vegetables, meats, and fish. The slow drying in the sun resulted in the removal of sufficient moisture to prevent bacterial and mold growth. Salt was usually added to meats and fish to draw out the moisture and hasten drying. Commercial dehydration results in products that have no more than 4 to 5 per cent moisture. Dried foods possess the advantage of light weight and small volume and are easily transported and stored.

Freeze-drying consists of placing the frozen food under vacuum to remove the water and packaging in the presence of an inert gas such as nitrogen. The product retains its original volume and shape and rehydrates readily. Freeze-dried coffee and tea and some soup mixtures are probably the most widely used products prepared by this technique.

Chemical Preservation Sugar is employed in high concentrations for the preparation of jams, jellies, and preserves. The water is made unavailable to the microorganisms and hence spoilage will not occur. However, molds will grow on the surface of these foods if sterility is not maintained. Salt and vinegar are also used for preservation in brining and pickling.

The number of chemicals that may be used for preservation is strictly limited by governmental regulations. For example, sodium benzoate is used in some foods up to a concentration of 0.1 per cent if labels specifically indicate its use. Sulfur dioxide is used in the drying of some fruits to lessen darkening. Meats have been cured by smoking, salting, and treatment with nitrates. (See discussion of nitrates on page 311.) Cured hams are perishable and should be kept under constant refrigeration.

Spices such as cloves and cinnamon have been much overrated for their preservative properties, since concentrations sufficient to inhibit bacterial growth would render food inedible. A number of additives, discussed in the next section, are also used for their preservative qualities.

Food Additives

Chemicals and Our Foods Today's food supply is safer than it has ever been, yet there has never been as much consumer distrust. The mere mention of additives or chemicals often causes highly emotional responses from people. Such persons view with deep distrust any product for which the label lists a chemical. They may say, "We no longer believe that our foods are safe to eat. The chemicals added to our foods are not necessary and can ruin our health—even cause cancer, or produce hereditary defects."

People often forget that they are a fantastically complex organization of chemical substances—the organic compounds such as amino acids, lipids, carbohydrates and vitamins, the inorganic mineral salts, and that marvelous chemical combination of hydrogen and oxygen, water. People forget, too, that their entire living environment—the food they eat, the air they breathe, the clothes they wear, the houses in which they live, the earth on which they walk—all are chemical in nature. Life itself requires a chemical environment. The science of chemistry and the applications by nutrition scientists and food technologists have vastly improved our food supply and extended the quality of our lives. But for all good things there must be limits and safeguards to avoid abuse. Chapter 17 will detail some of the ways in which our food supply is protected.

Additives More than 2,000 additives are used in foods. Yet they make up only a small fraction of 1 per cent of the weight of food.[6] Many of the additives are normal constituents of foods, for example, the nutrients, some natural coloring compounds, flavors, spices, and inorganic and organic salts of sodium, potassium, calcium, and magnesium.

Four points should be made concerning additives: (1) no harm to human health has been clearly demonstrated through the legitimate use of additives in foods,[6] (2) synthetic chemicals and naturally occurring chemicals in foods react identically in the body—e.g., synthetic or naturally occurring ascorbic acid; (3) the food supply would be drastically reduced in the United States if commercial fertilizers and pesticides were not available; and (4) the safety of each new additive—intentional for foods, or incidental through pesticide residues—must be established beyond any doubt by the manufacturer before the Food and Drug Administration or the U.S. Department of Agriculture will permit use.

Intentional Additives An INTENTIONAL ADDITIVE is a substance of known composition that has been added to improve the quality in some way. Some additives perform a single function and others perform several. For example, salt is both a preservative and flavoring agent. Ascorbic acid prevents the discoloration of cut fruit and also adds to the nutritive value. Table 16–1 lists some examples of additives and the functions they perform.

If additives are used, the benefit must outweigh any possible risk. If the risks are high in proportion to the benefit derived, the use of the additive would be contraindicated. For example, the improvement of color, flavor, or consistency would not be justified if a substance had a known risk, even though slight.

The nitrite dilemma. In recent years the use of nitrates and nitrites in the curing of bacon, frankfurters, sausages, ham, and smoked fish has been criticized. Nitrates have been used to impart color and flavor to the product. More important, they protect the product against botulism.

Under certain conditions the nitrites can combine with amines present in meat and in the stomach to form NITROSAMINES. Animal studies have shown that nitrosamines are potent carcinogens, but there is no existing evidence that nitrosamines have caused cancer in humans.[7]

Nitrates occur naturally in many foods: broccoli, beets, celery, collards, radishes, and spinach. Moreover, saliva also contains nitrates. Thus, it remains questionable whether the elimination of nitrates for the curing of meats would be useful. Indeed, the danger of botulism might be greater if nitrates were eliminated. The U.S. Department of Agriculture, the Food and Drug Administration, and an expert panel of the National Research Council continue study of this problem so that appropriate regulations can be developed.

Nitrites do present a problem to some infants under 3 months of age.[8] The low acidity of the gastrointestinal tract of the young infant favors the growth of bacteria that change nitrates to nitrites. Upon absorption, the nitrites change hemoglobin to methemoglobin. The young infant lacks two enzymes that are necessary to convert methemoglobin back to hemoglobin. Thus, there is some reduction in oxygen transport. This is presently not a widespread problem.

Incidental Additives Foods sometimes contain minute traces of a chemical as a result of contact with a substance used in its prodution, processing, or packaging. Since its presence serves no useful purpose in the final food product, such a chemical is considered to be an INCIDENTAL ADDITIVE. For example, food may have picked up a substance from a wrapper or container, either through dissolving it out or by abrasion from the container into the food. Or food may contain a residue of detergents remaining on dishes, or a residue

Table 16-1. Typical Uses of Some Intentional Additives

Function	Chemical Compounds	Examples of Food
Acids, alkalies, buffers		
Enhance flavor	Acetic acid	Cheese, catsup, corn syrup
	Sodium hydroxide	Pretzel glaze
Leavening	Baking powder, baking soda	Cakes, cookies, quick breads, muffins
Antioxidants		
Prevent darkening	Ascorbic acid	Fruit to be frozen
	Sulfur dioxide	Apples, apricots, peaches to be dried
Prevent rancidity	Butylated hydroxyanisole (BHA); butylated hydroxytoluene (BHT)	Lard, potato chips, meat pies, cereals, crackers
	Lecithin	Margarine, candy
	Tocopherol	Candy, oils
Coloring	Annatto; carotene	Butter, margarine
	Certified food colors	Baked goods, soft drinks
Flavoring (over 300 compounds in use)	Aromatic chemicals, essential oils, spices	
Nutritional fortification	Mineral salts, vitamins	Iodized salt; enriched breads and cereals; fortified milk and margarine; see p. 322.
Preservatives	Sodium chloride	Dried pickles, salted meats
	Sodium benzoate	Dried codfish; maraschino cherries
Inhibit mold	Calcium propionate	Bread, rolls
	Sorbic acid	Cheese wrappers
Sweeteners, nonnutritive	Saccharin	Dietetic foods and beverages
Texture	Alum	Firm pickles
Anticaking agents, retain moisture, emulsifiers, give body, jelling, thickening, binding	Disodium orthophosphate	Evaporated milk, cheese
	Mono- and diglycerides	Margarine, chocolate
	Sodium alginate	Cream cheese, ice cream
	Pectin	Jelly, French dressing
Whipping agents	Carbon dioxide	Whipped cream in pressurized can
Yeast foods and dough conditioners	Calcium phosphate; calcium lactate	Bread

of pesticides used in crop control. Dirt, hairs, and insect fragments are also included in this group.

The farmer uses chemicals that destroy insects, control plant diseases, and kill weeds. Without the use of these pesticides it is doubtful that enough food could be produced to feed the population. Nevertheless, these chemicals, if improperly used, pose some hazards.

By their very nature the chemicals used are toxic to some forms of life or they would not be effective in controlling the pests that imperil crops. It is essential that the pesticide residues remaining on foods be at levels that do not constitute any danger to health of the consumer either immediately or through gradual buildup in the body over a long period of time. It is equally important that there be no appreciable increase from year to year in the concentration of pesticides in the environment to endanger animal, fish, or bird life or to increase the levels in soils and water so that future food supplies contain levels that are toxic. Some pesticides meet these criteria but others do not. The kinds and amounts of pesticides that may be used and the residues that may remain in foods are established by regulations formulated by the Food and Drug Administration, the U.S. Department of Agriculture, and the U.S. Department of Interior. (See page 319.)

Polychlorinated biphenyls. A group of compounds known as POLYCHLORINATED BIPHENYLS (PCBs) has recently gained the attention of toxicologists. PCBs are synthetic organic compounds widely used in industry because they are fire resistant and water insoluble. They are used in paints, rubber, plastics, asphalt, adhesives, lubricants, and electrical insulators. They enter the food chain through industrial accidents or improper disposal. A random sample of people in the United States showed that 30 per cent had significant amounts (over 1 ppm) of PCBs in adipose tissue.[9] The cumulative effect is not known.

Monkeys fed diets containing 300 ppm PCBs for 3 months developed hyperplasia of the gastric mucosa together with skin and liver changes.[9] The dosage used was ten times the concentration reported by the Food and Drug Administration present in milk and fish. Environmental control of these compounds is essential, and much study is required to determine the possibility of hazard to humans.

"Organic" and "Natural" Foods Many people use only "organically grown" and "natural" foods, believing them to be more healthful. "Organically grown" foods are those grown on soils enriched with compost and manure and in the absence of chemical fertilizers or pesticides. That foods are organically grown is a misconception. Manures and composts used to enrich the soil must be degraded by bacteria to inorganic phosphates and nitrates since the plant utilizes only the inorganic substances just as it would from the commercial fertilizer. The nutritive values of foods grown on soils enriched in either way are of equal value, and the foods are equally safe and wholesome. Efficient agricultural practices fully utilize the humus resulting from manures and composts together with chemical fertilizers.

"Natural foods" are those that are used in the same form as they were harvested. That is, they have not been processed in any way nor have any additives been used. The term also implies that the foods have been organically grown.

Problems and Review

1. Understanding of the following terms will help you in your review of factors affecting food safety: aflatoxin; alkaloid; amebic dysentery; bactericidal; bacteriostatic; cestode; favism; gossypol; half-life, biologic; hazard; helminth; lathyrism; mycotoxin; nematode; nitrosamine; PCBs; protozoa; psychrophil; solanine; thermophil; toxicity; trematode; tyramine.
2. List several ways by which bacterial diseases are transmitted by foods.
3. Give two examples of bacterial infections transmitted by food; two examples of bacterial intoxication.
4. What organisms are responsible for most cases of summer food poisoning?
5. Explain what is meant by botulism. Which types of foods are most likely to contain botulinus toxin? What measures are necessary to eliminate this hazard?
6. Describe the effects of *Trichinella* infestation. How can it be avoided?
7. Name several plants that are poisonous to humans. What types of chemical compounds produce this poisoning?
8. Lead and mercury are especially toxic to humans. What are some ways by which they contaminate food?
9. What are the causes of food spoilage?

10. Why are commercially canned foods likely to be superior to home-canned foods in their vitamin content?
11. Which method of canning is recommended for home use? Why?
12. Read the labels of a variety of packaged foods and list the additives. What reasons can you give for the use of each? What objections can you see to the use of additives? Would it be advisable to eliminate all additives from foods? Defend your answer fully.
13. What is strontium-90? Why is a liberal intake of milk protective against its effects?
14. Based upon your reading of this chapter, set up some practical rules that you would expect a food handler to observe.

Cited References

1. Ouzounellis, T.: "Some Notes on Quail Poisoning," *JAMA*, **211**:1186–87, 1970.
2. Arnon, S. S., et al.: "Honey and Other Environmental Risk Factors for Infant Botulism," *J. Pediatr.*, **94**:331–36, 1979.
3. Brown, L. W.: "Commentary: Infant Botulism and the Honey Connection," *J. Pediatr.*, **94**:337, 1979.
4. Strong, F. M.: "Toxicants Occurring Naturally in Foods," *Nutr. Rev.*, **32**:225–31, 1974.
5. Lidbeck, W. L., et al.: "Acute Sodium Fluoride Poisoning," *JAMA* **121**:826–27, 1943.
6. Coon, J. M.: "Natural Food Toxicants—A Perspective," *Nutr. Rev.*, **32**:321–32, 1974.
7. IFT Expert Panel on Food Safety and Nutrition: "Nitrites, Nitrates, and Nitrosamines in Foods—A Dilemma," *J. Food Sci.*, **37**:989–92, 1972.
8. Raab, C. A.: "The Nitrite Dilemma: Pink and Preserved?" *J. Nutr. Educ.*, **5**:8–9, 1973.
9. Allen, J. R., and Morback, D. H.: "Polychlorinated Biphenyl- and Triphenyl-induced Gastric Mucosal Hyperplasia in Primates," *Science*, **179**:198–99, 1973.

Additional References

DOULL, J.: "Assessment of Food Safety," *Fed. Proc.*, **37**:2594–97, 1978.

Expert Panel on Food Safety and Nutrition and the Committee on Public Information, Institute of Food Technologists: "The Effects of Food Processing on Nutritional Values," *Nutr. Rev.*, **33**:123–26, 1975.

Food and Nutrition Board: "Symposium: Perspectives on Food Safety," *Activities Report* (Food and Nutrition Board), 1978, pp. 19–58.

FOSTER, E. M.: "Food-borne Hazards of Microbial Origin," *Fed. Proc.*, **37**:2577–81, 1978.

JUKES, T. H.: "Nitrates and Nitrites as Components of the Normal Environment," *Food and Nutrition News* (National Livestock and Meat Board), October/November 1976.

LEVEILLE, G. A., and UEBERSOX, M. A.: "Fundamentals of Food Science for the Dietitian: Thermal Processing," *Dietetic Currents* (Ross Laboratories), May 1979.

RODRICKS, J. V.: "Food Hazards of Natural Origin," *Fed. Proc.*, **37**:2587–93, 1978.

WILSON, B. J.: "Naturally Occurring Toxicants of Foods," *Nutr. Rev.*, **37**:305–12, 1979.

Publications for the Layman

Available from Consumer Information, Manufacturing Chemists Association, 1825 Connecticut Ave., N.W. Washington, D.C.:
Everyday Facts About Food Additives
Food Additives: What They Are. How They Are Used
Why Chemicals?

HAMILTON, L. W., et al.: *Home Canning: The Last Word.* Countryside Press, Philadelphia, 1976.

Keeping Food Safe to Eat, HG 162, Government Printing Office, Washington, D.C.

We Want You to Know about Protecting Your Family from Foodborne Illness, FDA Pub. 74–2003, Government Printing Office, Washington, D.C.

17 Controls for the Safety and Nutritive Value of the Food Supply

You shall not eat anything that dies of itself.
DEUT. 14:21

You shall not have in your bag two kinds of weights, a large and a small. You shall not have in your house two kinds of measures, a large and a small. A full and just weight you shall have, a full and just measure you shall have.
DEUT. 25:13–15

These biblical quotations are but two of the many laws concerning the use of food set down by Moses and others. Throughout history laws have been enacted to protect consumers against fraud and to enhance the safety of the food supply. The most notable advances have occurred in the present century through the passage of food laws by the U.S. Congress and the enforcement of these laws by federal agencies. With continued advances in food and nutrition sciences and applications by the food industry, additional federal legislation and the issuance of new regulations by federal agencies should establish policy for controls of the food supply for the foreseeable future.

Need for Food Laws

Good food laws aid consumers by protecting them against fraudulent manufacturing and labeling practices, and ensuring their right to a safe and nutritious food supply. Good laws aid industry by providing guidelines for good manufacturing practices and protecting against unfair and dishonest competition.

Changing National Environment In the early days of this nation consumers, for the most part, were also the producers. They grew the crops, raised the cattle, preserved the food by methods then available, and cooked the food in their own homes. By and large, those not engaged in agriculture purchased food from sellers who were known on a personal basis. Even in colonial history, however, one can find examples of laws designed to protect consumers against fraud.

With the industrial development and movement to cities people became dependent upon growers, manufacturers, and distributors for the food supply. Not all practices were honest. In fact, the conditions for sanitation in food processing and marketing by the end of the nineteenth century were often described as appalling. Far too common were fraudulent practices whereby the products were diluted with some cheap and unsafe ingredient so that a greater profit could be realized. Over these unsavory practices the consumer had little control.

Advances in science and technology. The twentieth-century developments in microbiology have provided the rationale for good practices in handling food and have served as the basis for setting up controls which might be exercised for a safe food supply. The chemists' laboratory has opened hitherto undreamed-of possibilities for variety in the food supply, preservation, and improvement of nutritional quality, but it has also created vast problems in controls from farm, to factory, to warehouse, and to market. Today's farmer fertilizes the soil with products purchased from a chemical plant; dusts and sprays crops; sometimes uses hormones to accelerate the growth of animals. The manufacturer chooses from hundreds of chemical products to improve the color, flavor, texture, nutritional quality, and keeping properties of the product. Chemicals of some sort enter into the numerous steps in food production—from the sanitation of the plant machinery to the package in which the food is sold. Without these aids from the chemical industry, this country could not produce its abundant supply of high-quality food.

Role of the food industry. Much credit for the remarkable improvements in the food supply must be given to responsible growers, manufacturers, and distributors. A visit to a modern food plant can be an exciting experience. One is impressed with the systems developed for the quality grading of food as it is received, the complex machinery for handling food from raw product to package, the continuous emphasis upon sanitation, and the attractiveness of the finished product. The laboratories in such a plant are at the very center of the successful operation. On the one hand, they are concerned with quality control; on the other, they are developing products for tomorrow's market basket. Many specialists are employed in the maintenance of controls and development of new products—agricultural specialists, food scientists, chefs, microbiologists, chemists, biochemists, nutritionists, and home economists to name but a few.

Consumer interest. Education by various media, advertising, and concern about the environment in which we live have sensitized the public to issues of food and nutrition as never before. People are requesting an accounting from the food industry and from regulatory agencies. The major issue pertains to the right to know what is in the food that is eaten. They want to know what ingredients are present in foods and also the amounts of principal ingredients. In a negative way consumers are concerned about the amounts of sugar, fat, cholesterol, salt, and additives that are present. Many of them also seek information on the nutritive values of the product.

Responses to the Changing Environment Early in 1978 the Food and Drug Administration, the U.S. Department of Agriculture, and the Federal Trade Commission agreed that a thorough review of label regulations was required. Some of the existing regulations were duplicative, while others were inconsistent or in conflict. In 1978 and 1979 public hearings were held with consumer groups, nutrition and health related professional organizations, and representatives from the food industry who presented testimony on labeling problems. Written comments from thousands of individuals and groups were also evaluated. A survey of consumers was conducted to determine how present food labels were being used and what changes should be made.

Based upon the information obtained, the agencies issued in December 1979 the proposed plans for change.[1] Further testimony on these tentative plans was obtained early in 1980, after which regulations and proposals for legislation were revised for eventual implementation. Some of the regulations can be implemented within months, giving manufacturers a period of time in which to comply. Other changes require legislation and the speed with which they can become law depends on the Congress as well as the administration and the priority that can be given to these issues.

Food Legislation

One of the principal crusaders in the movement to secure legislation for a wholesome food supply was Dr. Harvey W. Wiley, who was a chief chemist in the U.S. Department of Agriculture. Through his writings and public appearances he sought the cooperation of women's groups and was instrumental in the enactment in 1906 of the first "pure food" law, the Food and Drug Act. The law, signed by President Theodore Roosevelt, has been represented by some as the most significant peacetime legislation in the history of the country.

Food, Drug, and Cosmetic Act With rapid advances in food technology and industry, the manufacture and distribution of food grew increasingly complex and broader in scale so that the original law became inadequate. Many consumer pressures in the 1930s led to the enactment of the Food, Drug, and Cosmetic Act of 1938. The objectives of the law have been summarized as "safe, effective drugs, and cosmetics; pure, wholesome foods; honest labeling and packaging."* The Food and Drug Administration (FDA) is charged with the responsibility for the enforcement of this act and its amendments.

Additive Amendments The Food, Drug, and Cosmetic Act has been amended a number of times to meet new problems of control as they have arisen. Although additives are essential for high-quality food in sufficient supply for a rapidly expanding population, the introduction of thousands of such products on the market necessitates legal controls for safety and usefulness. For such protection, these amendments to the 1938 law have been enacted:

1954: Pesticides Amendment
1958: Food Additives Amendment, including intentional and incidental additives
1960: Color Additive Amendments

An important regulation in the additives amendment is the Delaney clause. This states that an additive is prohibited if at any level of feeding whatsoever it induces cancer in an experimental animal.

The GRAS list. At the time the Food Additives Amendment was enacted about 600 substances were excluded from testing since they had been used over long periods of time and they were "generally recognized as safe" (GRAS). Among the items on the GRAS list are salt, baking powder, baking soda, spices, and minerals and vitamins for nutritional purposes as well as preservatives, flavorings, and so on.

Cyclamate, a widely used noncaloric sweetening agent in the 1960s, was included in the GRAS list. But a Canadian study had shown that rats developed bladder cancers when given huge doses of cyclamate. Based on the Delaney clause it was necessary to remove cyclamate from the GRAS list and to ban its use. Since that time the National Academy of Sciences has been conducting a thorough study of the items on the GRAS list.[2] They are retained or removed from the list according to the findings. According to the criteria a ban against saccharin was issued. But public outcry against this ban was so great that Congress extended the time that it could be used. At issue here is the benefit that is perceived through the use of saccharin against the small risk of cancer.[3,4] Another sweetener, *aspartame* which is an amino acid derivative, was approved for use by the FDA in 1981.

Introduction of a new additive. Before an additive may be marketed approval must be secured from the Food and Drug Administration, which has spelled out in some detail the requirements that must be met. Essentially, these amendments place the burden of proof for usefulness and safety of a food additive upon the manufacturer, who is required to submit full data which includes name, chemical properties, methods for manufacture, quantities to be used, the conditions for use, the effect of additions on the food, methods for detecting residues in foods, safety, and recommended tolerances. Data pertaining to safety must include toxicity tests on two or more species of animals, usually for a 2-year period; estimates of the maximum amounts which might be consumed in a day; and the cumulative effects upon the body.

The Food and Drug Administration may conduct further tests after examination of the manufacturer's data. Approval will include specific limits for amounts and conditions of use. If a request is denied, the

* Larrick, G. P.: "The Role of the Food and Drug Administration in Nutrition," *Am. J. Clin. Nutr.*, 8:377–82, 1960.

manufacturer may appeal the decision, submit additional data, and request a hearing.

Fair Packaging and Labeling Act In 1966 the Congress authorized the FDA to set up requirements for complete information in labeling and for packaging that is not deceptive in terms of the contents. This act supplements the 1938 law. Included are these label regulations:

1. A statement of identity of a food, under its usual or common name such as *peaches* or *beets,* must appear in bold type on the principal display panel. If a standard of identity (see page 322) has been established for the product, the name shall appear as it is stated in the standard. When a food is packed in various forms such as whole, sliced, or chopped, the form shall be prominently shown with the name of the product except when a see-through container is used.
2. The name and full business address of the manufacturer, packer, or distributor shall be conspicuously shown, indicating "packed for" or "distributed by" if the name is not that of the manufacturer.
3. A statement of the net contents separated from other label information shall appear in legible boldface type within the bottom 30 per cent of the principal display panel.
4. When a label includes a statement of the number of servings, the usual size of that serving shall be stated, for example, in cups or tablespoons.
5. When ingredient listing is required, the information shall appear in a single panel listing by common name in decreasing order of predominance.[5]

Meat and Poultry Inspection Act The "pure food" law of 1906 did not include meat and meat products. The Meat Inspection Act was passed in 1906, the Poultry Inspection Act in 1957, and the Egg Products Inspection Act in 1970. These laws provide for (1) the inspection of animals intended for slaughter; (2) the inspection of carcasses and all meat and poultry products; (3) enforcement of sanitary regulations; and (4) guarding against the use of harmful preservatives.

Federal inspection stamps (see Figure 17–1) are placed upon the surface of an animal carcass if the meat is wholesome. The flesh of an animal that is diseased is stamped "inspected and condemned" and the carcass must be destroyed or may be used for nonfood purposes if warranted.

38
U.S.
INSP'D & P'S'D
U.S.
INSPECTED
AND PASSED BY
DEPARTMENT OF
AGRICULTURE
EST. 38
A
B

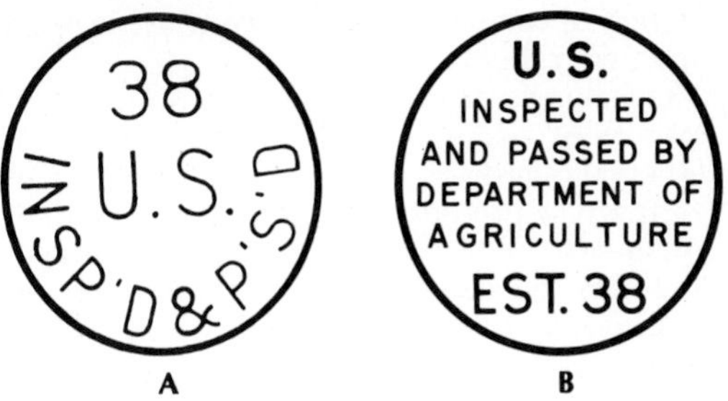

Figure 17–1. *(A)* Seal appearing as purple stamp on cuts of meat passed by the U.S. Department of Agriculture inspector. *(B)* Seal appearing on labels of prepared meat products. (Courtesy, U.S. Department of Agriculture.)

Two amendments to the earlier laws, the 1967 Federal Wholesome Meat Act and the 1968 Federal Wholesome Poultry Products Act, give the U.S. Department of Agriculture the authority to seize meat and poultry products that are moved illegally or that are adulterated or misbranded after leaving official premises. An important part of these laws sets up a cooperative arrangement between state and federal inspection programs. This provides better protection for the consumer for products sold within the state.

Pesticide Regulation Pesticide residues sometimes remain on foods at the time of purchase. What are the tolerable limits for such residues? Industrial pollutants may contaminate soil and water as demonstrated some years ago when some fish contained mercury in excess of tolerances. Therefore, a Commission on Pesticides was set up to study the problem. In the report issued by this commission in November 1969 the following principles were set forth:

1. Chemicals, including pesticides used to increase food production, are of such impor-

tance in modern life that we must learn to live with them;

2. In looking at their relative merits and hazards we must make individual judgments upon the value of each chemical, including the alternatives presented by the nonuse of these chemicals. We must continue to accumulate scientific data about the effects of these chemicals on the total ecology; and
3. The final decision regarding the usage of these chemicals must be made by those governmental agencies with the statutory responsibilities for the public health, and for pesticides regulations.*

The 1954 Miller Pesticide Amendment provided for the establishment of acceptable tolerances for residues on foods. The law provides that the manufacturer must establish to the U.S. Department of Agriculture the usefulness of the product and to the Food and Drug Administration the safety of the product. The World Health Organization and the Food and Agricultural Organization have established acceptable daily intakes of pesticide residues. Because of its persistent retention in the environment, DDT was banned in 1972. The safety of pesticides is under constant scrutiny by the regulatory agencies.

Law Enforcement and Specific Regulations

Responsibility The U.S. Department of Agriculture is responsible for enforcing laws pertaining to meat, poultry, and eggs. The Food and Drug Administration is the regulatory agency for all other foods entering into interstate commerce. The Federal Trade Commission protects the consumer by preventing advertising that is false or deceptive or that is claimed to prevent or treat a disease. To avoid inconsistency in advertising and labeling, close cooperation between the several agencies is essential.

The newest of these regulatory agencies is the Environmental Protection Agency, founded in 1970. It develops and enforces standards for the quality of the air and water and for the levels of noise pollution and toxic substances and pesticides in the environment.

Functions Among the many functions, especially of the USDA and FDA are these:

1. Development of regulations to implement the law.
2. Inspection of factories and warehouses to determine compliance with the law: the raw materials used; the manufacturing process; the packaging and storage practices; and plant sanitation. (See Figure 17–2.)
3. The approval of products for use in manufacture, for example, new additives.
4. Research to determine the physical and chemical characteristics of products; development of methods to detect deviation from standards.
5. Educational programs for the industry and also for consumers.

If inspectors find violations of the law they may remove the food from the market or require that the labeling be revised. Depending on the circumstances, the food may be destroyed or it may be reclaimed and relabeled under the supervision of the inspectors.

Court proceedings become necessary for those who flagrantly violate the laws. Fines or imprisonment or both may be imposed for each violation. Injunctions may be issued by the court to prevent repetition of a violation.

Adulteration and Misbranding Under the law the Food and Drug Administration has defined adulteration and misbranding.

Adulteration of food has occurred if the food contains any substance injurious to health; it contains any filthy, putrid, or decomposed substance; it is prepared, handled, or stored under unsanitary conditions; diseased animals have been used in preparation; the container is made of a poisonous substance which will render the contents harmful; valuable constituents have been omitted; substitutes have been used to con-

* Ramsey, L. L.: "A Twilight for Persistent Pesticides," *FDA Papers*, **4**:14–18, February 1970.

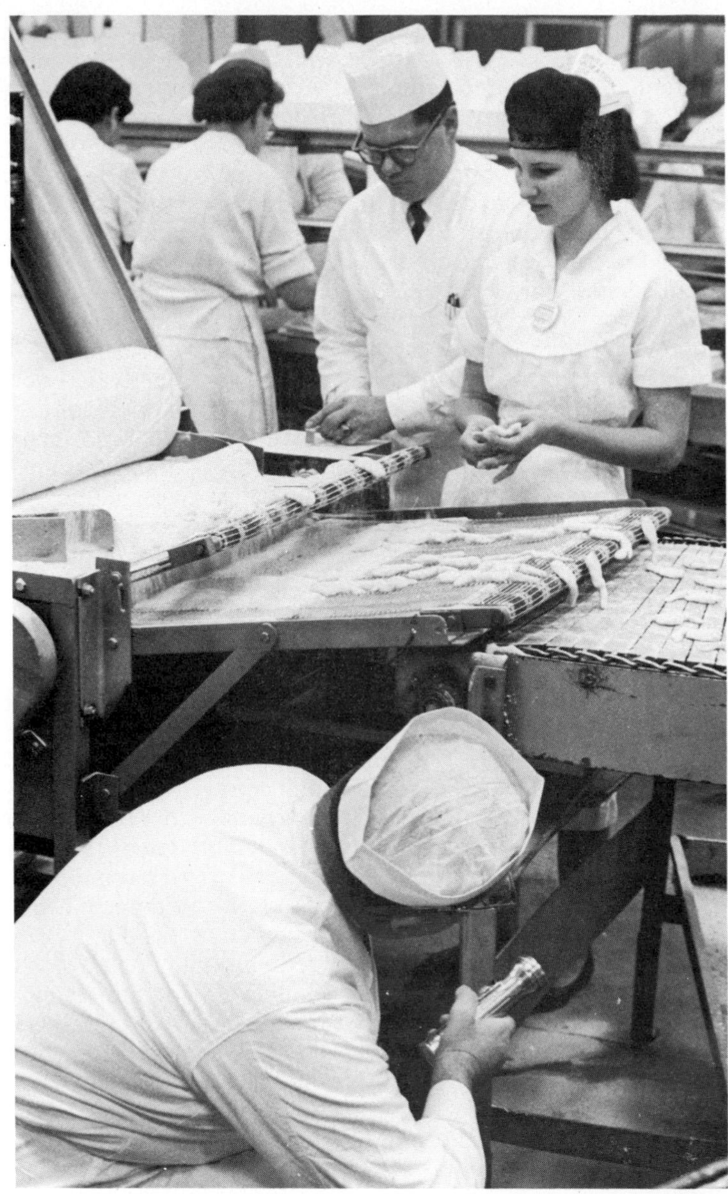

Figure 17–2. Inspectors from the Food and Drug Administration determine that every step of food processing meets standards that ensure the wholesomeness of foods that enter into interstate trade. (Food and Drug Administration photo.)

ceal inferiority; it contains coal-tar colors other than those permitted by law; it contains pesticide residues or additives not recognized as safe.

Misbranding has occurred if the label is false or misleading; the food is sold under another name; imitations are not clearly indicated; the size of the container is misleading; statement of weight, measure, or count is not given or is wrong; manufacturer, packer, or distributor is not listed on the package forms; it is below standard without indication of substandard quality on the label; it fails to list nutrient information when nutrients have been added or when claims are made for nutritional properties; it fails to list artificial colorings, flavorings, and preservatives.

Standards The Food and Drug Administration has established standards of identity, quality, and fill. A *standard of identity* establishes what a product really is. A product which has been so defined must include specified ingredients, often with amounts restricted to designated minimum-maximum ranges. For example, the standard of identity for Cheddar cheese specifies a minimum of 50 per cent milk fat (on a moisture-free basis) and not more than 25 per cent moisture. Fruit jelly and preserves must contain not less than 45 parts by weight of fruit or fruit juice to 55 parts total sweetener. Optional ingredients listed in the standard may be used, but any ingredients that are not mentioned in the standard are forbidden.

The standards are set up after consultation with numerous sources for the customary practices in manufacture and preparation. Proposals for new standards are published in the Federal Register. Opportunity is then given for interested parties, including manufacturers and consumers, to study the proposed regulations and to recommend changes. If there is any controversy, public hearings may be held.

The label for a food for which a standard of identity has been set does not need to include a listing of required ingredients since these are defined within the standard. However, a recently proposed regulation would require the listing of ingredients as for other nonstandardized products. Such listing would be of great assistance to many consumers who have allergies to some food substance or who require some kind of modified diet.

Among the products for which standards of identity have been established are: chocolate and cocoa products; cereal flours and related products; macaroni and noodle products; bakery products; milk and cream; cheese and cheese products; frozen desserts; dressings for foods—mayonnaise, French dressing, salad dressing; canned fruit and canned fruit juices; fruit butters—jellies, preserves; shellfish; canned tuna; eggs and egg products; oleomargarine—margarine; vegetables and vegetable products.

Standards of quality indicate the minimum quality below which foods must not fall. Foods that do not meet the quality specifications must be labeled "Below Standard in Quality" followed by a statement such as "Good Food—Not High Grade" or "Excessively Broken," and so on. Canned foods that do not meet standards of quality are seldom seen on the market.

Standards for fill aim to protect the customer against deception through the use of containers that appear to contain more food than they actually do. Specifications are set up for foods that tend to shake down in the package, or for number of pieces of food within a container.

Food Fortification

Definitions and Purposes ENRICHMENT is a "quantitative increase in content of one or more important nutrients present in lower than desirable amounts."* Generally it has included the addition of thiamin, riboflavin, niacin, and iron to flour and grain products.

FORTIFICATION is the "addition to a food of significant quantities of a nutrient that was initially not present in the food."* Milk fortified with vitamin D, margarine fortified with vitamin A, and salt fortified with iodine are examples.

RESTORATION is the "addition of nutrients to conventional foods in order to restore the level of those nutrients that were present naturally but have been destroyed or lost in processing."*

The central reason for adding nutrients to foods is to enhance the nutritive value

* Darby, W. J., and Hambraeus, L.: "Proposed Nutritional Guidelines for Utilization of Industrially Produced Nutrients," *Nutr. Rev.*, **36**:65–71, 1974.

of a product so that the nutritive intake of the population can promote better health.

General Policies In 1961 the Food and Nutrition Board of the National Research Council and the Council on Foods and Nutrition of the American Medical Association adopted jointly a statement of general policy regarding addition of specific nutrients to foods. This statement was revised and reaffirmed in 1968 and again in 1973. The following continue to be endorsed:

> The enrichment of flour, bread, degerminated cornmeal, corn grits, wholegrain cornmeal, white rice, and certain other cereal grain products with thiamin, riboflavin, niacin, and iron; the addition of vitamin D to milk, fluid skim milk, and nonfat dry milk; the addition of vitamin A to margarine, fluid skim milk, and nonfat dry milk; and the addition of iodine to table salt. The protective action of fluoride against dental caries is recognized and the standardized addition of fluoride to water in areas in which the water supply has a low fluoride content is endorsed.*

The Food and Nutrition Board has developed these guidelines for the improvement of conventional foods by nutrient additions:

1. The potential intake of a nutrient considered for addition to food should be judged to be below a desirable quantity in the diets of a significant number of people.
2. The food that is to carry the nutrient should be consumed by the segment of the population in need, and the added nutrient should make an important contribution to the diet.
3. The addition of the nutrient should not create a dietary imbalance.
4. The nutrient added should be stable under customary conditions of storage and use.
5. The nutrient should be physiologically available from the food.
6. There should be reasonable assurance that an excessive intake to a level of toxicity will not occur.

* "General Policies in Regard to Improvement of Nutritive Quality of Foods," *Nutr. Rev.*, 31:324–26, 1973.

7. The additional cost should be reasonable for the intended consumer.*

Current Practice Enrichment of bread and flour with thiamin, riboflavin, niacin, and iron was introduced in 1940 and was mandated throughout World War II. Federal law does not require enrichment of foods but approximately 85 to 90 per cent of flours and breads are enriched. Some 35 states mandate enrichment of one or more grain products; for example, wheat, corn, or rice products. When foods are enriched they must (1) comply with enrichment standards set by the Food and Drug Administration and (2) must include nutrition information on the label.

Almost all milk is fortified with vitamin D. Many nonfat milks, dry as well as liquid, are also fortified with vitamin A. Most margarines are fortified with 15,000 IU vitamin A per pound. The consumer needs to examine the labeling on salt, since not all salt is iodized.

Fabricated and Formulated Foods A FABRICATED food is a complex mixture of ingredients that may or may not resemble an existing conventional food, for example, a soy protein analog of meat. A FORMULATED food is a mixture of two or more ingredients such as many convenience foods. Nutritional guidelines for such foods have been suggested.[6]

If a food supplies 5 per cent or more of a nutrient or energy need, it is considered to be making a significant contribution to the diet. Thus, it is reasonable to expect such a product to furnish the nutrients based on a calculated nutrient density. For example, if a serving of food furnished 240 kcal or 10 per cent of the caloric requirement, then the nutrient content should also furnish approximately 10 per cent of the recommended allowances.

If a product replaces a meal, for example, a frozen dinner, it should furnish 25 to 50 per cent of the nutrients. Fabricated foods

* Darby: "Proposed Nutritional Guidelines," p. 69.

that are analogs to conventional foods should supply the same variety and quantities of essential nutrients that are present in the foods they replace.

The Food Label

Ingredient Labeling Foods for which there are no standards of identity must include a listing of ingredients in descending order of predominance if they move in interstate commerce. Consumers, however, have been asking for more information regarding ingredients. The FDA and USDA are proposing legislation and developing regulations to supply information such as the following:

Complete ingredient listing for products that have a standard of identity.
Quantitative information on ingredients that characterize a product, for example, the percentage of beef in a beef stew.
Specific names for spices and colors.
Specific names for some designated flavorings; because many flavorings might be used in a single product it is not practical to list all of them on label space available.
Specific source of fat or oil (for example, corn, cottonseed, and so on) if a food contains 10 per cent or more of fat.
The total sugar content of specified foods. The total would include sugar naturally present in a product as well as all added sugars—white, brown, natural, honey, and so on. Some cereal manufacturers now voluntarily state carbohydrate information on the label, including total carbohydrate, starch, and sugar.
The total sodium content.

Open Date Labeling This is a system that is intended to assure the consumer that the product is fresh. Food processors are gradually replacing private codes with one of these methods of date labeling: date when product was packed; last date at which a product should be sold; last date at which quality can be ensured. A consistent approach is needed to the kind of dating that should be used and to the classes of foods for which dating should be mandated.

Universal Product Code Labels on many packaged foods now include a symbol unique for each product that consists of a linear bar system and a 10-digit number. These codes are being used in some supermarkets at the checkout counter. The code is placed over a scanner that reads the line pattern and feeds it into a computer coupled with a cash register. As each food is checked out, the description of the item and the price is printed on the customer's receipt. The system also maintains a constant inventory for each product.

Nutrition Labeling

Labeling for nutrition information has been mandatory for (1) any food to which a nutrient has been added—enrichment, fortification, or restoration—and (2) any food for which a claim is made for nutritional properties either on the label or in advertising. All foods for special dietary use require labeling.

At present most nutrition labeling is voluntary, but many manufacturers have adopted it for their products. Studies are now in progress by FDA and USDA to determine for which foods nutrition labeling should be required.

Purposes Served The principal reason for nutrition labeling is that the consumer has a right to know what is in the foods being purchased in order to be able to make better decisions for personal well-being and that of his or her children. A consumer can compare one product with another to determine which product offers the best nutritive values for the money. One important result of such comparisons is that the consumer gradually becomes aware of the good and poor sources of nutrients. Labeling also leads food processors to be constantly aware of the nutritive values of the foods that they produce. Nutrition labeling is a useful teaching tool in the classroom and in education of the public. Labeling will help persons who require modified diets to select those foods appropriate for their needs. One urgent reason for labeling is the identification of the nutritive values of the numerous fabricated foods that food technology has made possible. With such information the consumer can decide whether the fabricated food is an appropriate replacement for an ordinary food. (See Figure 17–3.)

The Labeling Standard For labeling purposes the Food and Drug Administration has developed the U.S. Recommended Dietary Allowances (USRDA). (See Table 17–1.) It was not practical to adopt the recommended dietary allowances set up by the Food and Nutrition Board because of the seventeen age-sex categories, and because the RDAs are revised at approximately 5-year intervals. The USRDA for adults and children over 4 years of age is based on the highest level for a given nutrient (usually the adult male) in the 1968 RDAs. For example, the vitamin A level of 5,000 IU for the adult male was adopted; the iron level of 18 mg for the female was chosen.

Two standards are given for protein. When the quality of protein is equivalent to that found in casein, the standard has been set at 45 gm; this would include milk, eggs, poultry, meat, and fish, and also combinations of vegetable protein that equal casein in value. Single-plant protein foods or combinations of plant foods that have a quality less than that of casein are evaluated at a higher standard—65 gm.

For healthy adults the standards afford a margin of 30 to 50 per cent to allow for individual variations. Many adults need only two thirds to three fourths of the

NUTRITION INFORMATION
(PER SERVING)
SERVING SIZE = 1 OZ.
SERVINGS PER CONTAINER = 12

CALORIES	110
PROTEIN	2 GRAMS
CARBOHYDRATE	24 GRAMS
FAT	0 GRAM

PERCENTAGE OF U.S. RECOMMENDED DAILY ALLOWANCES (U.S. RDA)*

PROTEIN	2
THIAMIN	8
NIACIN	2

*Contains less than 2 percent of U.S. RDA for vitamin A, vitamin C, riboflavin, calcium and iron.

This is the minimum information that must appear on a nutrition label.

NUTRITION INFORMATION
(PER SERVING)
SERVING SIZE = 8 OZ.
SERVINGS PER CONTAINER = 1

CALORIES	560	FAT (PERCENT OF CALORIES 53%)	33 GM
PROTEIN	23 GM	POLYUNSATURATED*	2 GM
CARBOHYDRATE	43 GM	SATURATED	9 GM
		CHOLESTEROL* (20 MG/100 GM)	40 MG
		SODIUM (365 MG/100 GM)	830 MG

PERCENTAGE OF U.S. RECOMMENDED DAILY ALLOWANCES (U.S. RDA)

PROTEIN	35	RIBOFLAVIN	15
VITAMIN A	35	NIACIN	25
VITAMIN C (ASCORBIC ACID)	10	CALCIUM	2
THIAMIN (VITAMIN B_1)	15	IRON	25

*Information on fat and cholesterol content is provided for individuals who, on the advice of a physician, are modifying their total dietary intake of fat and cholesterol.

A label may include optional listings for cholesterol, fats, and sodium.

Figure 17–3. Regulations for nutrition labeling have been established by the Food and Drug Administration. (Courtesy, Food and Drug Administration.)

Table 17-1. United States Recommended Daily Allowances (USRDA) for Labeling Purposes (for adults and children over 4 years)

Mandatory Nutrients		Optional Nutrients	
Protein		Vitamin D	400 IU
Protein quality equal to or greater than casein	45 gm	Vitamin E	30 IU
Protein quality less than casein	65 gm	Vitamin B-6	2.0 mg
Vitamin A	5,000 IU	Folic acid (folacin)	0.4 mg
Vitamin C (ascorbic acid)	60 mg	Vitamin B-12	6 μg
Thiamin (vitamin B-1)	1.5 mg	Phosphorus	1.0 gm
Riboflavin (vitamin B-2)	1.7 mg	Iodine	150 μg
Niacin	20 mg	Magnesium	400 mg
Calcium	1.0 gm	Zinc	15 mg
Iron	18 mg	Copper	2 mg
		Biotin	0.3 mg
		Pantothenic acid	10 mg

USRDA and many children about half. The standards include some nutrients not listed in the recommended dietary allowances but for which requirements have been estimated. The nutrient information listed by the manufacturer on a label must be based upon laboratory analyses of the product; calculations of nutritive values are not adequate.

Labeling standards have also been set up for infants under 12 months and for children under 4 years for the labeling of baby foods and vitamin-mineral supplements. Another standard has been set up for pregnant and lactating women pertaining especially to the mineral and vitamin supplements often recommended for use.

Mandatory and Optional Labeling A standard format for listing nutrition information was adopted by the Food and Drug Administration. The kinds of information required and the sequence on the label are as follows:

1. Serving size and number of servings in container
2. Calories in one serving
3. Protein, carbohydrate, and fat in grams per serving
4. Percentages of the USRDA provided by one serving for protein, vitamins A and C, thiamin, riboflavin, niacin, calcium, and iron

Optional minerals and vitamins may also be declared on the label. They include phosphorus, iodine, magnesium, zinc, copper, vitamins B-6, B-12, D, and E, biotin, folacin, and pantothenic acid. When these minerals are declared they shall be stated in the percentages of the USRDA for these nutrients.

Except where claims are made for specific nutritional properties, the declaration of cholesterol and fatty acids has been optional. When the information is included, it shall include:

1. Per cent of calories from fat
2. Amounts of saturated and polyunsaturated fatty acids in grams per serving
3. Amount of cholesterol in milligrams per serving and per 100 gm of food

The Food and Drug Administration is seeking legislation that would require fatty acid and cholesterol labeling on specified foods. Because there has been much criticism of the format for displaying nutrition information, several alternatives such as graphs and charts are being studied.

Special Dietary Foods In addition to the standard and format for labeling just described, five prohibitions have been set up for the labeling of these foods:

1. With certain exceptions, it prohibits any claim or promotional suggestion

that products intended to supplement diets are sufficient in themselves to prevent, treat, or cure disease.

2. It prohibits any implication that a diet or ordinary foods cannot supply adequate nutrients.
3. It prohibits all claims that inadequate or insufficient diet is due to the soil in which a food is grown.
4. It prohibits all claims that transportation, storage, or cooking of foods may result in inadequate or deficient diet.
5. It prohibits nutritional claims for non-nutritive ingredients such as rutin, other bioflavonoids, paraaminobenzoic acid, inositol, and similar ingredients, and prohibits their combination with essential nutrients.*

So that claims for special dietary foods can be standardized, the FDA and USDA are developing definitions for such terms as "low calorie," "reduced calorie," "low sodium," "reduced sodium," "low cholesterol," and "cholesterol free."

What Labeling Does Not Do People could add up the percentages for each nutrient from various foods and thus conclude that their diets were fully adequate if the total were 100 per cent or more for each listed nutrient. Such a conclusion might, in fact, be justified if the totals resulted from a wide variety of ordinary foods. However, if the choice is restricted to a few food items or if an important part of the intake consists of fabricated foods, it is quite likely that the combinations will not furnish all of the 45 to 50 nutrients required by humans even though the percentages for the listed nutrients all add up to 100 or more. As fabricated foods become more prominent in the diet, the danger of nutritive inadequacy increases. Although the manufactuers of such products may indeed be producing a food that is high in the listed nutrients, some trace elements about which realtively little is known could be omitted, for example, chromium, selenium, molybdenum, and manganese. The best advice for dietary planning still is the selection of a wide variety of foods from each of the important food groups. The selection should include fresh as well as processed foods.

* "The New Look in Food Labels," DHEW Pub. (FDA)73–2036, Washington, D.C., 1973.

Other Agency Activities

U.S. Public Health Service One of the concerns of the Public Health Service is the effect of diet on nutritional status and health, and it has sponsored research to make these determinations. The safety of the food supply is another concern that leads to the promulgation of sanitary codes and ordinances. During outbreaks of food poisoning the Public Health Service conducts tests to determine the source and nature of the poisoning.

The Public Health Service has defined standards for milk production and quality that provide the basis for the codes used in most states and communities. It also certifies interstate milk shippers.

Food Protection Committee To study the legitimate uses of chemical additives, the Food Protection Committee was established in 1950 as a permanent committee of the Food and Nutrition Board. The membership of the committee includes specialists who are qualified to establish criteria for the evaluation of additives on the basis of their chemical and physical properties, their toxicologic aspects when tested in several species, and their metabolic and nutritional aspects.

The Food Protection Committee acts as a clearing house for information on pesticides and intentional additives; it reviews the information and makes it available; it assists in the integration and promotion of research on foods; it aids regulatory agencies such as the Food and Drug Administration in the formulation of principles and standardized procedures; it aids in the dissemination of accurate information to the public.

State and Local Regulations Food that is produced and sold within state boundaries does not come under control of federal agencies. Therefore, states and communities must establish their own regulations for the safety and quality of foods. The identity of foods, the labeling, and the inspection of plants, markets, and public eating places are subject to controls set up by the state departments of agriculture and health. Some cities and states require periodic, medical examination of food handlers. Most of the regulations are patterned after those of federal laws, but considerable variations exist, nevertheless, from state to state.

Problems and Review

1. Key terms: adulteration; enrichment; fabricated food; formulated food; fortification; GRAS list; misbranding; restoration.
2. What is the aim of the Food, Drug, and Cosmetic Act? Under its provisions what is meant by misbranding? Adulteration?
3. What provisions are included in the Meat Inspection Act?
4. Where does the primary responsibility for proving the safety of an additive rest? What information is essential for establishing this safety?
5. What purposes are served by nutrition labeling?
6. Compare the nutrition labeling for three brands of ready-to-eat cereals. Which is the best buy? Why?
7. Compare two margarines that carry nutritional labeling for fat and cholesterol. Which supplies the greater amount of polyunsaturated fatty acids? On the basis of cost is such a difference justified?
8. *Problem.* Watch television advertising for three food products. Note especially the words used to describe products and the claims for the products. Look for labels on the packages of these products in a market. What conclusions can you make regarding this advertising?
9. Determine the governmental agency in your community that is responsible for controlling the sale of milk; the sale of meat within your state; the inspection of public eating places.
10. *Problem.* Prepare a short paper (about 300 words) that describes the activities of any one of the following organizations in promoting a safe food supply: Food Protection Committee; your state department of health; your state department of agriculture; the U.S. Public Health Service; the Federal Trade Commission.

Cited References

1. "Food Labeling; Tentative Positions of Agencies," *Federal Register,* **44**:75990–76020, December 21, 1979.
2. Irving, G. W.: "Safety Evaluations of the Food Ingredients Called GRAS," *Nutr. Rev.,* **36**:351–56, 1978.
3. American Diabetes Association: "Saccharin. A Policy Statement," *Diabetes Care,* **2**:380, 1979.
4. American Dietetic Association: "The Saccharin Question Re-examined: An ADA Statement," *J. Am. Diet. Assoc.,* **74**:574–81, 1979.
5. Friedelson, L.: "Fair Packaging," *FDA Papers,* **1**:21–24, October 1967.
6. Darby, W. J., and Hambraeus, L.: "Proposed Nutritional Guidelines for Utilization of Industrially Produced Nutrients," *Nutr. Rev.,* **36**:65–71, 1978.

Additional References

Board of the National Nutrition Consortium: "Nutritional Labeling Statement," *Am. J. Clin. Nutr.*, **32**:1753–55, 1979.

Food and Nutrition Board: "General Policies in Regard to the Improvement of Nutritive Quality of Foods," *Nutr. Rev.*, **31**:324–26, 1973.

HAGER, C. J.: "Consumers and Food Labels," *National Food Rev.*, Summer 1979, pp. 37–38.

JUKES, T. H.: "Carcinogens in Food and the Delaney Clause," *JAMA*, **241**:617–19, 1979.

Review: "Standards of Identity," *Nutr. Rev.*, **32**:29–30, 1974.

Symposium: "Risk Versus Benefits: The Future of Food Safety," *Nutr. Rev.*, **38**:35–64, 1980.

Publications for the Consumer

DEUTSCH, R.: *Nutrition Labeling—How It Can Work for You,* The Nutrition Consortium, The American Dietetic Association, Chicago, 1976.

Food and Drug Administration, U.S. Department of Health, Education, and Welfare:
Additives in Our Foods, Pub. 43.
Metric Measures in Nutrition Labels, Pub. 74–2022.
FDA—What It Is and Does, Pub. 1.
How Safe Is Our Food? Pub. 41.
Nutrition Labeling—Terms You Should Know, Pub. 74–2010.
Nutrition Labels and U.S. RDA, Pub. 73–2042.
We Want You to Know About the Laws Enforced by FDA, Pub. 73–1031.
We Want You to Know About Nutrition Labels on Food, Pub. 74–2039.

PETERKIN, B., et al.: *Nutrition Labeling—Tools for Its Use,* Information Bull. 382, U.S. Department of Agriculture, Washington, D.C., 1975.

18 Nutrition During Pregnancy and Lactation

The object of maternity care is to ensure that every expectant and nursing mother maintains good health, learns the art of child care, has a normal delivery, and bears healthy children. Maternity care in the narrower sense consists in the care of the pregnant woman, her safe delivery, her postnatal care and examination, the care of her newly born infant, and the maintenance of lactation. In the wider sense, it begins much earlier in measures aimed to promote the health and well-being of the young people who are potential parents and to help them to develop the right approach to family life and to the place of the family in the community. It should also include guidance in parentcraft and in problems associated with infertility and family planning.*

Important Concerns

The position of the World Health Organization just cited is a comprehensive statement of the objective of maternity care. In the United States there has been steady improvement in achieving a successful outcome of pregnancy. Yet, these improvements are not evenly distributed throughout the population.

About 1 million pregnancies (one in ten teenage girls) occur each year in adolescents; of these, 600,000 babies are born. A quarter of a million births are to girls 17 years and under; 13,000 are to girls under 15 years. The mortality rate is higher in pregnant adolescents; the younger the girl, the greater the risk.

For nonwhite women the mortality rate is higher and appears to be associated with low income. Nonwhite and white women of similar income show no such difference.

The infant with a birth weight of less than 2,500 gm has less chance of survival than does the infant who is larger. Even when the low-birth-weight infant survives, there remains a long period of costly care and a continuing concern about establishing normal growth and development patterns.

About two thirds of infant deaths occur within the first month of life. Again, the mortality rate is higher in infants born to mothers of low income and to teenage mothers. These differences reflect the adverse effects of low income, limited education, faulty nutrition, and other environmental factors.

Oral contraceptives are widely used. They bring about biochemical changes, and their effects on nutritional status are not fully understood.

Nutritional Studies

Folklore and Diet in Pregnancy Since earliest times the diets of pregnant women have been considered to be of importance. The foods eaten by the pregnant women were believed to convey to the unborn child not only certain physical characteristics but also desirable or undesirable attributes of behavior. Consequently, various societies set up rigid rules for the pregnant

* World Health Organization: *The Organization and Administration of Maternal and Child Health Services.* Fifth Report of the World Health Organization Expert Committee on Maternal and Child Care, WHO Tech. Rep. Ser. No. 428, Geneva, 1969.

woman, including the foods she could eat, the foods she must not eat, and even the foods she must not touch lest she contaminate them for the rest of the community. Even today superstitions about foods and their desirability for the pregnant woman prevail among some people.

Some of the theories relating to nutrition that have been practiced by physicians are now known to be incorrect: the semistarvation of the mother with the view of a smaller baby and easier delivery; the restriction of salt and fluids to reduce the incidence of toxemia; and the theory the maternal organism will produce a healthy baby regardless of the mother's own state of nutrition.[1]

Factors Influencing the Outcome of Pregnancy On a probability basis, a mother who is well nourished prior to and during pregnancy is likely to have an uncomplicated pregnancy and to deliver a healthy infant. A poorly nourished woman is more likely to have complications during pregnancy and to bear a small infant in poor physical condition. There are, of course, exceptions. Some well-nourished mothers have problems during pregnancy and may not bear a healthy infant. Also, some poorly nourished mothers may have a successful pregnancy. Such exceptions are understandable when one considers the numerous factors influencing the outcome of pregnancy. (See Figure 18–1).

When one or more of the following factors are present in the mother, the risk of low-birth-weight infant and the related neonatal mortality is increased:[2]

Biological immaturity (under 17 years of age)
High parity
Small stature
Low prepregnancy weight for height
Low gain in weight during pregnancy
Poor nutritional status
Smoking; certain medications; drugs
Certain infectious agents
Complications of pregnancy
History of unsuccessful pregnancies
Poverty
Unfavorable social environment

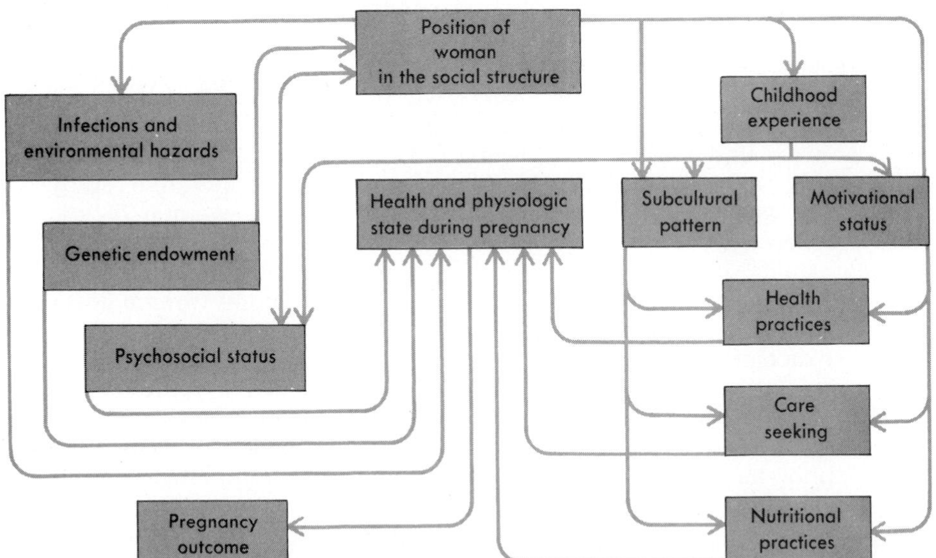

Figure 18–1. Factors influencing pregnancy outcome: a theoretical model. (Reprinted with permission of *Nutrition Today.* Copyright Summer 1970 by Nutrition Today, Inc.; chart adapted by permission of the Food and Nutrition Board.)

Prematernal Nutrition The PERINATAL CONCEPT[3] assumes that the mother is in a good nutritional state prior to conception, and that this status will be maintained throughout pregnancy, labor, and the period after birth. Fewer complications in pregnancy, fewer premature births, and healthier babies result when the mother is well nourished prior to conception.

The influence of the quality of prematernal nutrition was strikingly demonstrated in World War II.[4] In Holland food rations were severely restricted from October 1944 to May 1945 so that pregnant women early in 1945 had less than 1,000 kcal and 30 to 40 gm protein available. Prior to this period women had ingested diets that were reasonably adequate. The babies conceived before the hunger period and born during the hunger period were shorter and had lower birth weights than those born before this time, this being a direct result of the mother's diet during the latter half of pregnancy. However, there was no increase in the rate of still births, prematurity, and malformations but the rate of conception fell off markedly during the hunger period.

During the siege of Leningrad acute food shortages occurred between August 1941 and February 1942. Prior to this time the food supplies had been inadequate so that women were chronically undernourished. During 1942 the birth rate fell off markedly, the stillbirth rate was twice as high, and prematurity had increased 41 per cent. The infants had low vitality, had poor resistance to infection, and did not suckle well. The better outcome in Holland was directly related to the better diets of women prior to conception.

Studies by Tompkins in Philadelphia showed that women who are underweight at the time of conception have the greatest probability of premature labor and toxemia. He found a strikingly high incidence of prematurity in infants born of mothers who were both underweight and anemic.[5]

Difficult deliveries are more frequent in short than in tall women, according to studies reported from Scotland.[6] The more frequent occurrence of "flat pelvis" in short women was believed to be related to inadequate diet in childhood. Thus, a short stature may mean that a woman has not achieved the full genetic possibilities of body structure because of dietary inadequacies.

Prenatal Nutrition Burke and her coworkers in Boston[7] studied 216 pregnant women over an extended period during which the women were examined and their diets were rated as excellent, good, fair, poor, and very poor.

These studies indicated that a woman who has a poor or a very poor diet during pregnancy will in all probability have a poor infant; that is, prematurity, congenital defects, and stillborn infants occurred almost entirely in this group. On the other hand, the women who had good-to-excellent diets almost invariably bore infants in good physical condition. The mother's protein intake correlated well with the infant's physical condition, weight, and length. Inadequate nutrition resulted in relatively greater harm to the fetus than to the mother. No cases of eclampsia were noted in those women having excellent or good diets, whereas 50 per cent of those receiving poor or very poor diets developed toxemia of varying degrees of severity.

The Vanderbilt cooperative study of 2,338 pregnant white women of low income showed the effects of weight status and hemoglobin levels of the mother on the infant.[8] Underweight women (less than 85 per cent of standard) produced smaller babies, prematurity occurred more frequently, and artificial feeding was more common. The overweight group (120 per cent of standard) had more stillborn children and a threefold increase in preeclampsia. Women who gained too much, especially during the second trimester, had more toxemia.

Low intakes of iron and ascorbic acid were correlated with lower hemoglobin levels and blood levels of vitamin C. However, during the first year of life the infants of these mothers maintained hemoglobin levels equal to those whose mothers had higher hemoglobin levels, showing that appropriate infant feeding practices can make up for the deficient infant stores of iron.

The Vanderbilt study did not fully establish nutritional deficiency as a primary causative factor in metabolic diseases of pregnancy. The investigators point out that the patient cannot be assured of freedom from complications simply through a satisfactory intake of nutrients. They did observe that diets which contained less than 50 gm protein and less than 1,500 kcal resulted in a greater frequency of complications of pregnancy and of the newborn, but they felt that the low levels of intake were a result of the complications rather than the cause.

Nutrition and Brain Development The first stage of cellular growth is characterized by a rapid increase in cell numbers (HYPERPLASIA) but without increase in cell size. During the second stage there is HYPERTROPHY or increase in cell size, and also a continuation of the increase in cell numbers, though at a slower rate. In the third stage, hyperplasia ceases but hypertrophy continues at a rapid rate.

For each organ there is a critical time table for each stage of cellular growth and development. The brain develops rapidly in the fetus and in the early postnatal period. Research on animals has shown that severe malnutrition during pregnancy and in the first weeks of life leads to reduced cell numbers and reduced brain weight. If the increase in cell numbers is impaired, there is no reversal if an adequate diet is provided after stage two of cell development has been completed. If malnutrition occurs during the third stage of growth, the cells do not achieve their full size. However, with later improvement in nutrition this can be reversed and the cells achieve their normal size. In research on malnourished animals the dietary restriction is usually much greater than that encountered in human beings, and the results should not be extrapolated fully to human beings.

Some postmortem studies on tissues of severely malnourished fetuses and infants have shown reduced brain weight, cell number, and cell size. Whether such changes could be interpreted in terms of impaired mental performance is not known. The development of the brain and resulting behavior are dependent upon the interaction of genetic and environmental factors including nutrition, illness, psychologic factors, and cultural variables. Interference with learning and behavior could occur in three ways: (1) abnormalities of the biochemical and physiologic characteristics of the brain; (2) reduced exposure and stimulation because of the unfortunate social-familial environment; and (3) interruptions in learning because of emotional, personality, and behavioral changes in the child.[9] Intrauterine malnutrition can result from a poor maternal diet before and during pregnancy or from insufficiency of the placenta.

The mental performance of men born during the severe famine in Holland (see page 332) was studied when they enrolled for military service.[10] There was no difference in the mental performance of men from western Holland where the famine was severe and men from other parts of Holland not subjected to the severe food privations. This study does not support the view that severe undernutrition during pregnancy will affect the intellectual development. It must be remembered that the mothers were generally well nourished prior to the famine and thus their bodies were a reasonable reserve for the fetus. On the other hand, in the developing countries where prematernal as well as prenatal nutrition is extremely poor, the effect on intellectual ability might be adversely affected.

Pregnancy during Adolescence Pregnant adolescents are "medically, nutritionally, and socially at risk."[11] If they have two or more babies during their teens the risk is extremely high. Among the frequent undesirable outcomes for the mother are these: anemia, preeclampsia and toxemia, premature labor, prolonged labor, and an increased rate of maternal deaths. For the infant the risks are greatly increased for premature birth, low birth weight, and neonatal death. The younger the girl, the greater her vulnerability is.

In addition to the physical risks, the pregnant adolescent often has serious psychologic, social, and economic problems. She often encounters the disapproval of her family and her friends, thus becoming isolated from the support she needs. She may be unable to complete her education. When the family income is low and the family is large it may be impossible for her to get the amount of food she needs for a successful pregnancy. Often the pregnant adolescent does not receive the medical care and the counseling she needs at an early stage of her pregnancy.

Many adolescent girls, especially in the lower socioeconomic classes, are poorly nourished. They know little about the nutritive values of foods and have often pursued unwise weight-reducing programs. Their intake of calories, calcium, iron, and vitamin A, and sometimes even protein has frequently been inadequate to meet the growth requirements of their own bodies. If the pregnant girl is under severe emotional stress, the nutrient balances such as calcium and nitrogen are often negative even though an adequate diet may be consumed. Thus, during pregnancy she must provide the additional demands for the fetal and maternal tissues as well maintain her own satisfactory growth pattern.

Physiologic and Biochemical Changes in Pregnancy

Three Stages of Pregnancy Pregnancy may be considered in three stages.

1. The first 2 weeks following conception: the fertilized ovum becomes implanted in the endometrium of the uterus and rapid cell proliferation occurs. Initially the uterine glands and the outer layers of the germ plasm nourish the embryo, and the placenta begins to develop.

2. About 2 to 8 weeks: all the major organs are formed during this period—heart, kidneys, lungs, liver, and skeleton. Studies on experimental animals have shown that congenital malformations occur during this stage when the pregnant animal has had a diet grossly deficient in vitamin A, riboflavin, vitamin B-6, vitamin B-12, or folacin. However, it is difficult to correlate poor nutrition with malformations sometimes seen in humans.

3. Eighth week to term: rapid growth of the fetus and the establishment of the maternal reserves in preparation for labor, the puerperium, and the production of milk are taking place. During each of these stages, both cell hyperplasia and hypertrophy are occurring with the rate of each varying from one organ to another.

The Placenta There is no direct connection between the mother's circulation and that of the fetus. The placenta is the organ to which the fetus is attached by means of the umbilical cord and by which the transfers between the two circulatory systems occur. The placenta achieves its maximum size early in gestation. Its large surface area is estimated to be between 10 and 13 m^2.

Some nutrients such as water, oxygen, and electrolytes diffuse through the placental membrane to the fetal circulation. Others such as glucose and amino acids require active transport from the maternal to the fetal circulation. Just as nutrients are transported to the fetus, so metabolic wastes from the fetus are returned to the maternal circulation.

The placenta also has synthetic functions and regulates selectively the transfer of nutrients and hormones according to the changing needs of the fetus. Many drugs such as tranquilizers, sedatives, and some antibiotics are not filtered out by the placenta and thus have access to the fetal circulation. The pregnant woman should consult her physician about the possible effects of any prescribed or proprietary drug that she might use.

Undernourishment leads to smaller placental size. There are fewer cells available for the transfer of nutrients and oxygen to the fetus, thus leading to lower birth weight. Also the placenta is less able to dispose of any toxic substances including catabolites, the effects of smoking, and so on.

Hormones Progesterones, the estrogens, and the gonadotropins are the hormones primarily involved in reproduction. PROGESTERONE is secreted by the corpus luteum and brings about increased secretion by the endometrium, as well as developing glycogen and lipid stores. It also inhibits contraction of the uterine smooth muscle layers thereby preventing expulsion of the embryo. In these ways progesterone has prepared for the implantation of the fertilized ovum and its early growth. Between the second and third months of gestation the formation of progesterone is taken over by the placenta.

GONADOTROPINS are especially concerned with organ formation up to about the fourth month of pregnancy and with fetal growth. Chorionic gonadotropin is produced by the *trophoblastic* cells (outer layer of cells of the dividing ovum) and has the same effects on the corpus luteum as the luteinizing hormone and the luteotropic hormone from the pituitary gland. It keeps the corpus luteum from degenerating and keeps it secreting large quantities of estrogen and progesterone. The endometrium remains in the uterus and is gradually phagocytized by the growing fetal tissues, thereby furnishing a major portion of the nutrition to the fetus during the first weeks of pregnancy.

ESTROGEN production increases appreciably after about the one-hundredth day of gestation. Estrogen and progesterone stimulate the growth of the mammary glands and also inhibit the lactogenic function of the pituitary gland until birth of the infant.

Steroid hormones are produced in greater amounts with the result that water and sodium are more readily retained in the body. The thyroid gland is less active during the first four months of pregnancy, and thereafter is somewhat more active than normal.

Body Fluids During pregnancy a gradual increase in the volume of intracellular and extracellular fluids accounts for several pounds of the total increase in body weight. Late in pregnancy some fluid retention is fairly common.

The total blood volume is increased by as much as one third by the end of pregnancy. With the increase in blood volume, the concentration of serum albumin, hemoglobin, and other blood constituents is reduced. The average hemoglobin level of 13.7 gm per 100 ml (range, 12.0 to 15.4 gm) for healthy nonpregnant women drops to about 12.0 gm per 100 ml despite the ingestion of supplemental iron.[2] Although the concentration of hemoglobin is lower, with the increase in blood volume the total circulating hemoglobin is much greater. A level of 11.0 gm hemoglobin per 100 ml blood is considered to be the border below which true anemia exists.

Gastrointestinal Changes Pregnant women sometimes have cravings for some foods and aversions to others. Whether there is an alteration in taste sensitivity is not known. Especially during the first half of pregnancy some women experience distaste for meat, poultry, sauces flavored with oregano, coffee, soda, beer, wine, and alcoholic spirits.[12] Coffee provokes nausea in some, while the elimination of sodas and alcoholic beverages may be linked more closely with concern for the developing fetus. Women often express cravings for foods such as milk, ice cream, sweets, chocolate candy, and fruits.

PICA or the appetite for abnormal nonfood substances such as clay, starch, ice, and dirt occurs in some women, especially in lower socioeconomic classes.

Less acid and pepsin are produced by

the stomach, and regurgitation of stomach contents into the esophagus (heartburn) sometimes occurs. This may become more pronounced with the increasing pressure of the growing fetus. The motility of the intestinal tract is reduced, thus contributing to constipation. The absorption of important nutrients, however, is enhanced.

Weight Gain The gain in weight for the healthy woman who enters pregnancy at her desirable weight level should average 11 kg (24 pounds).[13] Gains in weight vary widely, being somewhat greater in young women than in those who are older, and greater in those who are having their first babies.

The weight gain is accounted for by the weight of the full-term infant, the increase in size of the uterus, the placenta, amniotic fluid, breast tissue, expanding blood circulation, and the reserves of nitrogen and lipids that help to meet the needs during parturition and lactation. (See Table 18–1.)

The pattern of weight gain is as important as the total weight gain. During the first trimester there is little or no increase in weight; from 0.7 to 1.4 kg (1.5 to 3.0 pounds) is appropriate. Thereafter, a steady gain of 0.35 to 0.40 kg (0.8 to 0.9 pounds) per week is desirable. In addition to the expected gains for pregnancy, the adolescent girl should also increase her weight by an amount that is appropriate for the nonpregnant girl of her age. (See Figure 18–2.)

Faulty patterns of weight gain cannot be fully corrected. For example, a woman who has gained 8 to 10 kg during the first trimester should not be held down to the recommended 11 kg. Such restriction could seriously interfere with the supply of nutrients to the fetus. On the other hand, a woman who has gained little during most of her pregnancy cannot expect to make up entirely for this deficiency by considerable increase in weight during the last trimester.

For obese women, restriction of caloric intake to maintain weight or even to lose weight, is no longer advocated. Although obesity increases the risk of pregnancy, the correction of it during pregnancy imposes even greater risks on the fetus. If a woman is fasting or is restricting her caloric intake, her blood glucose will be lower, glycogenesis will be reduced, and ketosis will be increased. With a reduced supply of glucose, the fetus is unable to synthesize glycogen

Table 18-1. **Average Components of Weight Gain in Pregnancy***

	Cumulative Gain (kg) at End of Each Trimester		
	First	Second	Third
Fetus	Negligible	1.0	3.4
Placenta	Negligible	0.3	0.6
Amniotic fluid	Negligible	0.4	1.0
(Fetal subtotal)		(1.7)	(5.0)
Increased uterine size	0.3	0.8	1.0
Increased breast size	0.1	0.3	0.5
Increased blood volume	0.3	1.3	1.5
Increased extracellular fluid	0	0	1.5
(Maternal subtotal)	(0.7)	(2.4)	(4.5)
Total gain accounted for	0.7	4.1	9.5

*Pitkin, R. M., et al.: "Maternal Nutrition. A Selective Review of Clinical Topics," *Obstet. Gynecol.*, **40**:777, 1972.

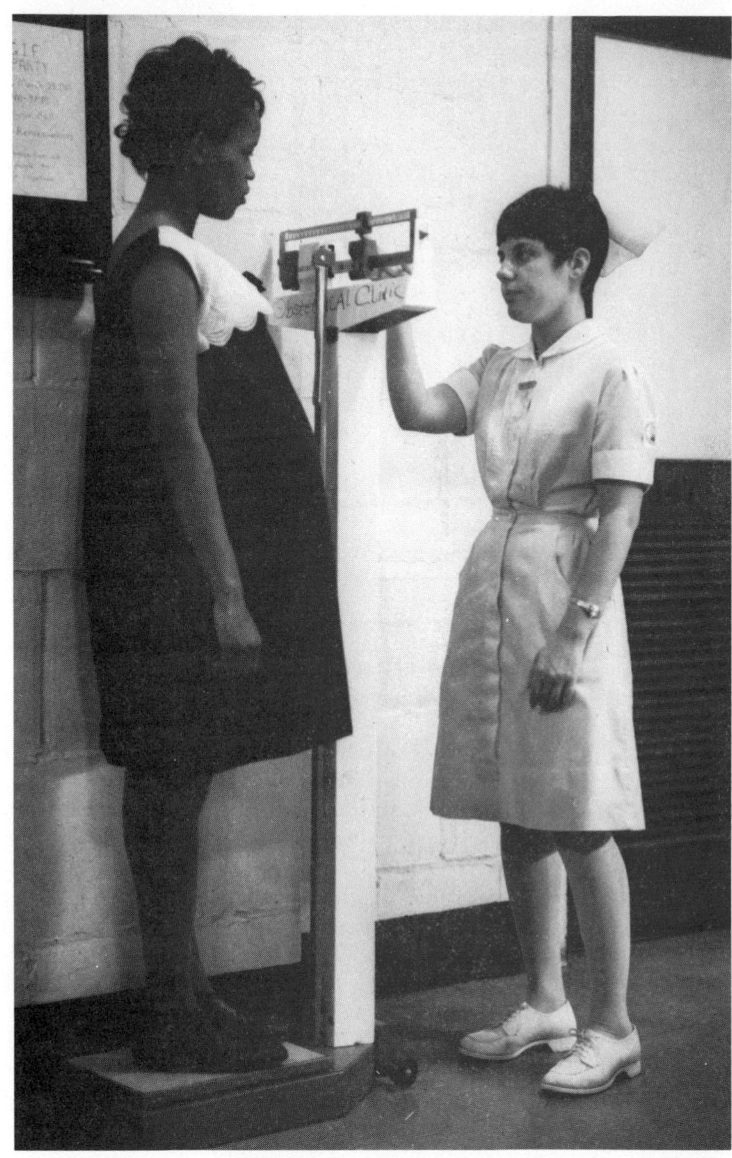

Figure 18–2. Weight is checked at each clinic visit. After the first trimester the weekly gain should be about 0.4 kg. (Courtesy, School of Nursing, Thomas Jefferson University.)

and fat. Ketosis may impair neurologic development.[14]

Nutritional Considerations

The recommended allowances for nutrients are listed in Table 18–2. The recommended intakes for protein, calcium, phosphorus, magnesium, folacin, and vitamin D are increased by 50 per cent or more.

Energy The total caloric cost of producing the fetus, the placenta, and other maternal tissues and of establishing reserves is about 80,000 kcal. For most women an

Table 18-2. **Recommended Dietary Allowances Before and During Pregnancy and Lactation***

Nutrient	11–14 Years	15–18 Years	19–22 Years	23–50 Years	Pregnancy	Lactation
Energy, kcal	2,200	2,100	2,100	2,000	+300	+500
Protein, gm	46	46	44	44	+30	+20
Vitamin A, RE	800	800	800	800	+200	+400
IU	4,000	4,000	4,000	4,000	+1,000	+2,000
Vitamin D, μg	10	10	7.5	5	+5	+5
Vitamin E, mgα TE	8	8	8	8	+2	+3
Ascorbic acid, mg	50	60	60	60	+20	+40
Thiamin, mg	1.1	1.1	1.1	1.0	+0.4	+0.5
Riboflavin, mg	1.3	1.3	1.3	1.2	+0.3	+0.5
Niacin, mg equiv.	15	14	14	13	+2	+5
Vitamin B-6, mg	1.8	2.0	2.0	2.0	+0.6	+0.5
Folacin, μg	400	400	400	400	+400	+100
Vitamin B-12, μg	3.0	3.0	3.0	3.0	+1.0	+1.0
Calcium, mg	1,200	1,200	800	800	+400	+400
Phosphorus, mg	1,200	1,200	800	800	+400	+400
Magnesium, mg	300	300	300	300	+150	+150
Iron, mg	18	18	18	18	†	†
Zinc, mg	15	15	15	15	+5	+10
Iodine, μg	150	150	150	150	+25	+50

**Recommended Dietary Allowances*, 9th ed., Food and Nutrition Board, National Academy of Sciences, National Research Council, Washington, D.C., 1980.

†Supplemental iron, 30–60 mg daily, is recommended.

extra allowance of 300 kcal daily will permit satisfactory weight gain. An allowance of at least 36 kcal per kg pregnant weight is needed for satisfactory utilization of protein.[13]

The caloric requirement may vary as much as 800 to 900 kcal, depending upon the activity of the woman. Some adolescent pregnant girls are so sedentary that their caloric need is increased by only 150 kcal. But women who have several children and the associated household duties or women whose employment involves body movement require more than the 300 kcal daily increase. The adequacy of the caloric requirement can be evaluated by maintaining a desirable rate of weight gain.

Protein About 925 gm protein is deposited in the fetus and maternal tissues during pregnancy. The rate of deposit in these tissues averages 0.6, 1.8, 4.8, and 6.1 gm daily during the four quarters of pregnancy.[13] Protein may be stored in the body at a uniform rate during the entire pregnancy and is made available to the specialized tissues as needed.

The recommended allowance during pregnancy is increased by 30 gm. Nonpregnant girls 15 to 18 years should have an intake of 0.9 gm protein per kg, and girls 11 to 14 years an intake of 1.0 gm per kg. To this allowance, an additional 30 gm protein per day should be included during pregnancy.

Minerals The efficiency of absorption of minerals such as calcium and iron improves during pregnancy, but the demands of the fetus and other developing tissues necessitate increases in the diet during the second and third trimesters. The full-term fetus contains about 28 gm calcium. Some calcium and phosphorus deposition takes place early in pregnancy, but most of the calcification of bones occurs during the last 2 months of pregnancy. The first set of teeth begins to form about the eighth week of prenatal life, and they are well formed by the end of the prenatal period. The 6-year molars, which are the first permanent teeth to erupt, begin to calcify just before birth.

If the mobile reserve of calcium is lacking in the mother, the demands of the fetus can be met, perhaps inadequately, only at severe expense to the mother. For many women it is advisable to increase the calcium intake early in pregnancy even though fetal calcification does not occur until later. The phosphorus allowance should be about equal to that for calcium and will be readily supplied through the calcium-rich and protein-rich foods.

Iron. The amount of iron in the full-term fetus is about 300 mg. For the maternal tissues and the increase in blood volume, an additional 500 mg is required. To these must be added the losses of about 300 mg through normal excretion from the skin, hair, urine, and stools. The prematernal stores are about 300 mg iron or less.

To cover the needs during pregnancy about 3.5 mg iron must be absorbed daily (range 2 to 4 mg).[13] Many factors determine the availability of dietary iron. (See Chapter 8.) Assuming an average absorption of 10 to 15 per cent, between 23 and 35 mg iron would need to be ingested daily. Such an intake, even with a carefully planned diet, is unlikely, and a supplement of 30 to 60 mg iron is recommended.

Iodine. The daily allowance of 175 μg iodine is easily met by using iodized salt. If sodium restriction is required for any reason, the physician may prescribe a supplement.

Sodium. During pregnancy the sodium requirement increases to take care of fetal needs, the enlarging maternal tissues, and the expanding blood volume. The homeostatic mechanisms spare sodium loss that might otherwise occur because of the increased glomerular filtration rate. There is no convincing evidence that sodium restriction has any effect on the incidence of preeclampsia. The woman should be permitted to salt food to her taste.

Vitamins The thiamin, riboflavin, and niacin allowances are slightly increased to correspond to the increase in calories. There is also an increased allowance for vitamins A and D.

Folacin deficiency manifested as megaloblastic anemia occurs occasionally in women whose dietary intakes have been low. The recommended allowance is 800 μg, a level that is not easily achieved by food selection alone. An oral supplement is considered to be advisable.[13]

Blood levels of vitamin B-6 are often low in pregnant women. Although supplementation with vitamin B-6 will restore blood levels to the normal range, there is no evidence that such supplementation confers any physiologic advantage.

Dietary Counseling

ATTITUDES TOWARD COUNSELING Although most women believe strongly that diet is important for a successful outcome of pregnancy, many of them do not feel the need for dietary counseling.[15] Negative attitudes are expressed in this way: "it makes you feel bad"; "difficult to follow"; "like being sent to the principal"; "feel guilty." Women especially view the dietary advice given by physicians as being restrictive inasmuch as recommendations are still being made for caloric and sodium restriction. Women who have the least education and the least income often do not attend classes concerning prenatal care for a variety of reasons. Obviously, the dietary counselor must give advice that emphasizes the positive aspects of diet, realistic suggestions for food choices according to available income, and adaptations to individual needs.

Dietary counseling of the pregnant adolescent is especially important but not always well accepted. An interdisciplinary approach through an educational component within the school curriculum, together with prenatal care and counseling, delivery, family planning, and child care can be effective.[11]

THE BASIC DIET The basic diet plan (Table 13–2) furnishes about half of the calories needed by the pregnant woman and provides ample amounts of protein, vitamin A, and ascorbic acid. The addition of 1 to 2 cups milk ensures satisfactory intakes of calcium, thiamin, and riboflavin as well as additional protein. (See Table 18–3 and Figure 18–3.)

Good sources of vitamin B-6, folacin, magnesium, iron, and zinc should be emphasized since diets of many pregnant women do not supply the recommended allowances.

SUPPLEMENTS TO DIET Many physicians routinely prescribe multivitamin-mineral supplements to pregnant women. For women who are well nourished, vitamin-mineral supplementation does not change the blood levels of various nutrients.[16] When the nutritional status is poor, the primary emphasis should be placed on dietary improvement. In addition, a supplement may be prescribed to hasten the improvement of nutritional status.

Iron supplementation—30 to 60 mg daily —is recommended since even a carefully planned diet cannot meet both the maternal and fetal needs for iron. (See page 339.) Unfortunately, many women do not take the iron because of nausea, constipation, or, in some cases, diarrhea.[15] Thus, the dietary counselor should monitor and promote compliance by explaining the need for iron and by suggesting the correction of constipation through fiber and fluid intake. (See page 341.)

When there is biochemical and clinical evidence of deficiency, a supplement of folacin (200 to 400 μg) may be recommended. A calcium supplement is required only when there is intolerance to milk or for strict vegetarians.

NUTRITION PROGRAMS The Supplementary Food Program for Women, Infants, and Children (WIC) administered by the Food and Nutrition Services of the U.S. Department of Agriculture and available in designated health centers and clinics throughout the country is intended for pregnant women who are at risk and who qualify on the basis of low income. Nutritional anemia, a history of miscarriage or premature births, underweight, obesity, or poor food habits place women in the at-risk category. The supplemental foods are available throughout pregnancy and for 6 months postpartum; for the lactating woman they are available for 1 year. The foods provided are milk and cheese, iron-fortified cereals, eggs, and vitamin-C-rich fruit or vegetable juices.

Table 18-3. Food Allowances for Pregnancy and Lactation

	Pregnant Woman	Pregnant Teenage Girl	Lactating Woman
Milk, whole or low-fat	3–4 cups	4–5 cups	4–5 cups
Meat, fish, poultry (liver once a week), cooked weight	4 ounces	4 ounces	4 ounces
Eggs	3 to 4 per week	3 to 4 per week	3 to 4 per week
Vegetables, including			
Dark green leafy or deep yellow	½ cup	½ cup	½ cup
Potato	1 medium	1 medium	1 medium
Other vegetables	½–1 cup	½–1 cup	½–1 cup
One vegetable to be raw each day			
Fruits, including			
Citrus	1 serving	1 serving	1 serving
Other fruit	1 serving	1 serving	1 serving
Cereal, whole grain or enriched	1 serving	1 serving	1 serving
Bread, whole grain or enriched	4 slices	4 slices	4 slices
Butter or fortified margarine Desserts, cooking fats, sugar, sweets	To meet caloric needs	To meet caloric needs	To meet caloric needs
An iron supplement is usually prescribed.			
Iodized salt			

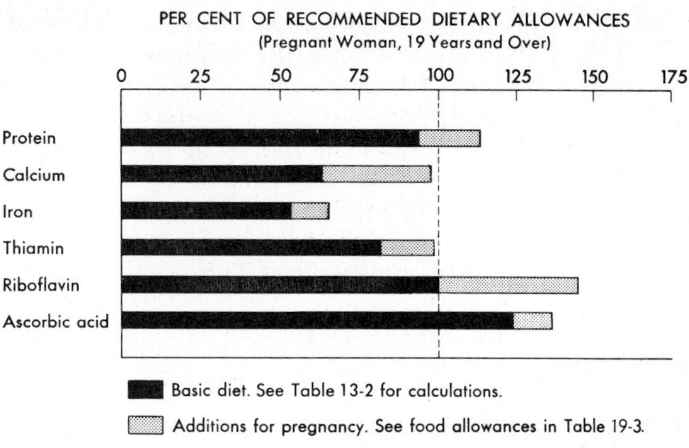

Figure 18–3. The Basic Diet (page 262) furnishes sufficient protein, riboflavin, and ascorbic acid for the pregnant woman. It also provides ample amounts of vitamin A and niacin (not shown in the chart). The addition of 1 to 2 cups of milk supplies the needed calcium as well as additional protein and riboflavin. The iron intake can be increased by including liver weekly and by eating more meat, dark green leafy vegetables, and enriched bread. An iron supplement prescribed by the physician will be less costly and also helps the woman to keep her caloric intake at the desired level.

The Maternal and Infant Care Projects (MIC) provide a comprehensive range of prenatal services, including screening for nutritional problems and dietary counseling. Eligible clients may be referred to the WIC program for supplemental foods or to the Food Stamp Program.

Complications of Pregnancy

Mild Nausea and Vomiting During the first trimester, the physiologic and biochemical balances are often disturbed, possibly because of excessive hormone production. Gastrointestinal upsets, including loss of appetite, nausea, and vomiting, are relatively frequent; loss of weight occasionally takes place because of inability to eat sufficient food.

Mild early morning nausea may usually be overcome by the use of high-carbohydrate foods such as crackers, jelly, hard candies, and dry toast before arising. Frequent small meals rather than three large ones are preferable. Fluids should be taken between meals rather than at mealtime. Fatty, rich foods such as pastries, desserts, fried foods, excessive seasoning, coffee in large amounts, and strongly flavored vegetables may be restricted or eliminated if the nausea persists or if the patient complains of heartburn or gastric distress.

Constipation The occurrence of constipation especially during the latter half of pregnancy is common. The amount of pressure exerted by the developing fetus on the digestive tract, the limitation of exercise, and insufficient bulk may be contributing factors. The normal diet outlined in Table 18–3 provides a liberal allowance of whole-grain cereals, fruits, and vegetables, and consequently of fiber. It is also necessary to stress the importance of adequate fluid intake and of regular habits of exercise, elimination, sleep, and recreation.

Toxemia By toxemia is meant that combination of symptoms including hypertension, edema, and albuminuria. Preeclampsia is the appearance of hypertension, edema of the face and hands, and/or albuminuria about the twentieth week of pregnancy. It should be suspected when there is a sudden gain in weight, indicating fluid retention rather than tissue building. Eclampsia is the end result of preeclampsia; it includes the earlier symptoms but may culminate in convulsions.

The treatment of toxemias is highly controversial. In fact, toxemia has been called the "disease of theories."[2] Protein and calorie restriction are no longer recommended, and sodium restriction should be used with caution.

Chronic Conditions Preexisting conditions such as diabetes mellitus, heart disease, hypertension, inborn errors of metabolism, and others increase the risks of pregnancy just as pregnancy adds to the stress of these conditions. With good prenatal care and adjustment of the diet to meet the dual requirements of the pregnancy and the disease condition, a successful outcome is likely. See chapters pertaining to specific disease conditions in Part Two.

Lactation

With a resurgence of interest in breast feeding, three of every four women in middle and upper socioeconomic groups breast feed their babies, at least for a short time. But in lower socioeconomic groups the rate of breast feeding is more nearly one of every four women. The advantages as well as disadvantages are discussed fully in Chapter 19.

Nutritive Requirements When one considers the nutritive value of human milk, and that the nursing mother will produce 20 to 30 ounces each day, it becomes apparent that the requirements for protein, minerals, vitamins, and energy are even greater than they were during pregnancy. See Tables 18–2 and 18–3 for recommended dietary allowances and suggested food intake.

Energy. Each 100 ml breast milk supplies 67 to 77 kcal. The conversion of food energy to milk energy is 80 to 90 per cent efficient, thus necessitating 80 to 95 kcal to produce 100 ml milk. The average daily production of 850 ml milk, representing 600 kcal, necessitates an expenditure of 750 kcal.[13]

If weight gain followed recommended levels during pregnancy, the fat deposits will furnish 200 to 300 kcal for the first 100 days of lactation. Thus, an added allowance of 500 kcal to the diet is recommended.

Protein. Each 100 ml of human milk contains 1.2 gm protein. Thus, 850 ml milk daily would yield 10 gm protein. Since the efficiency of conversion of dietary protein to milk protein is about 70 per cent, and individual variations also occur, the recommended allowance for lactation is an additional 20 gm protein.[13]

The need for protein is greatest when lactation has reached its maximum, but it is a need that should be anticipated and planned for during pregnancy.

Minerals. Even liberal intakes of calcium may not be successful in completely counteracting a negative calcium balance. Consequently, a high level of calcium intake and the building of reserves during pregnancy cannot be overemphasized. Four to five cups of milk daily is recommended during lactation.

The infant is born with a relatively large reserve of iron since milk is not a good source of iron. A good allowance of iron in the mother's diet during lactation does not convey additional iron to the infant. Nevertheless, iron-rich foods are essential for the mother's own health, and supplements are included early in the infant's diet.

Vitamins. The adequacy of the mother's intake of vitamins is reflected to some extent in the vitamin levels of the milk she produces. For example, low levels of intake of thiamin and vitamin B-6 have been shown to result in low levels of these vitamins in the milk. Ascorbic acid is transferred to the milk, and the needs of the infant are fully met if the mother's diet is adequate.

Dietary Counseling

Successful lactation is dependent not only upon an adequate diet but also upon a desire to nurse the baby, freedom from anxiety, and sufficient rest. The decision to nurse the baby should be made early in pregnancy, and the woman needs the support and counseling of her physician, nurses, nutritionists, and family.

The choice of foods during lactation should be wide. No specific foods need to be omitted unless there is evidence of distress caused by them. Occasionally strongly flavored vegetables or highly seasoned or spicy foods may be implicated.

Alcohol, tobacco, marijuana and other street drugs, and some proprietary and prescribed medications are transmitted to the milk and infants may be adversely affected. The lactating woman is well advised to omit these except upon the specific recommendation of her physician.

Oral Contraceptives

With the widespread use of oral contraceptives there is much interest in the possible effects of these compounds on nutritional status. The preparations in common use contain varying proportions of estrogens and progestogens. In some respects the metabolic effects are similar to those observed in pregnancy.

Reports of numerous studies on the metabolic changes resulting from the use of oral contraceptives are often contradictory. Although biochemical changes occur, clinical manifestations of nutritional deficiency are rare. The significance of the observed biochemical changes is by no means clear.

The biochemical changes are more likely to be observed in women whose nutritional status is poor than in those who are well nourished. Among these changes are the following:[13, 17–20]

Impaired glucose tolerance
Increased concentrations in the blood of
- phospholipids, cholesterol, triglycerides
- plasma vitamin A; plasma retinol-binding protein
- plasma copper; plasma ceruloplasmin
- serum iron; total iron-binding component

Decreased concentration in the blood of
- ascorbic acid content of leukocytes, platelets
- riboflavin in red blood cells
- serum folacin (megaloblastic anemia is rarely seen)
- red blood cell folacin
- serum vitamin B-12
- plasma pyridoxal phosphate
- plasma zinc

Changes in urinary excretion:
- decrease in riboflavin
- increase in xanthurenic acid and kynurenine

Particular emphasis has been placed on vitamin B-6 deficiency and its relationship to changes in tryptophan metabolism and also to the occasional incidence of mental depression. If the vitamin B-6 intake is deficient, the excretion of xanthurenic acid and kynurenine is increased, indicating interference with the normal pathways of tryptophan metabolism. For example, conversion of tryptophan to niacin does not occur.

The changes observed for vitamin B-6 and other nutrients can be reversed by improvement of the diet alone so that it meets the RDA. Routine supplements of vitamin B-6 and other nutrients are not justified.[13]

Problems and Review

1. Key words: amniotic fluid; corpus luteum; endometrium; estrogen; gonadotropin; hyperplasia; hypertrophy; implantation; low-birthweight; organogenesis; perinatal concept; pica; placenta; prematernal nutrition; prematurity; progesterone.
2. What evidence exists that diet is of importance in the development of the fetus and the health of the mother?
3. What physiologic changes occur during the course of pregnancy?
4. Name the hormones which are especially important in controlling the changes occurring during pregnancy? What is the effect of an excess production?
5. In what way do the nutritional practices of teenage girls affect the outcome of pregnancy?
6. What weight increases are recommended for each trimester? What are the dangers of underweight or insufficient weight gain?

7. What foods are especially important for their protein content in the diet during pregnancy and lactation?
8. What mineral elements require especial attention during pregnancy? What changes occur in the rate of absorption of calcium and iron?
9. Discuss the need for an increased vitamin intake. What foods would you recommend for this?
10. Mrs. A. does not like milk and is taking calcium gluconate to correct calcium deficiency. Why is this less desirable than taking milk? List ways by which she could incorporate milk into her diet.
11. What recommendations can you make to a woman with complaints of nausea, vomiting, and gastric distress?
12. What instructions are in order for the woman who complains of constipation?
13. What is meant by the "physiologic anemia of pregnancy"? What are the hazards of iron-deficiency anemia? What measures are essential for its prevention and treatment?
14. A woman secretes 800 ml milk daily. What amount of protein is here represented? What allowances must be made in the diet for protein?
15. *Problem.* Plan a low-cost diet for a woman of moderate activity during the second half of pregnancy. Calculate the nutrients in this diet and compare them with the recommended allowances.
16. *Problem.* Modify the diet in problem 14 for a woman who is lactating.

Cited References

1. Shank, R. E.: "A Chink in Our Armour," *Nutr. Today,* **5**:3–11, Summer 1970.
2. Committee on Maternal Nutrition, Food and Nutrition Board: *Maternal Nutrition and the Course of Pregnancy, Summary Report,* National Research Council–National Academy of Sciences, Washington, D.C., 1970.
3. Macy, I. G.: "Metabolic and Biochemical Changes in Normal Pregnancy," *JAMA,* **168**:2265–71, 1958.
4. Stearns, G.: "Nutritional State of the Mother Prior to Conception," *JAMA,* **168**:1655–59, 1958.
5. Tompkins, W. T., and Wiehl, D. G.: "Nutritional Deficiencies as a Causal Factor in Toxemia and Premature Labor," *Am. J. Obstet. Gynecol.,* **62**:898–919, 1951.
6. Thomson, A. M., and Hytten, F. E.: "Nutrition in Pregnancy and Lactation," in *Nutrition, a Comprehensive Treatise, Vol III.* G. H. Beaton and E. W. McHenry, eds. Academic Press, New York, 1966, pp. 103–45.
7. Burke, B. S., et al.: "Nutrition Studies During Pregnancy," *Am. J. Obstet. Gynecol.,* **46**:38–52, 1943.
8. McGanity, W. J., et al.: "Vanderbilt Cooperative Study of Maternal and Infant Nutrition. XII. Effect of Reproductive Cycle on Nutritional Status and Requirements," *JAMA,* **168**:2138–45, 1958.
9. Subcommittee on Nutrition, Brain Development and Behavior, Food and Nutrition Board: "The Relationship of Nutrition to Brain Development and Behavior," *Nutr. Today,* **9**:12–17, July 1974.
10. Review: "Effect of Famine on Later Mental Performance," *Nutr. Rev.,* **31**:140–42, 1973.
11. Alton, I. R.: "Nutrition Services for Pregnant Adolescents within a Public High School," *J. Am. Diet. Assoc.,* **74**:667–69, 1979.
12. Hook, E. B.: "Dietary Cravings and Aversions During Pregnancy," *Am. J. Clin. Nutr.,* **31**:1355–62, 1978.
13. Food and Nutrition Board: *Recommended Dietary Allowances,* 9th ed. National Research Council–National Academy of Sciences, Washington, D.C., 1980.

14. Review: "Maternal Weight Gain and the Outcome of Pregnancy," *Nutr. Rev.*, **37**:318–21, 1979.
15. Orr, R. D., and Simmons, J. J.: "Nutritional Care in Pregnancy: The Patient's View," *J. Am. Diet. Assoc.*, **75**:126–31, 131–36, 1979.
16. Thomas, M. R., and Kawamoto, J.: "Dietary Evaluation of Lactating Women with or Without Vitamin and Mineral Supplementation," *J. Am. Diet. Assoc.*, **74**:669–72, 1979.
17. Roe, D.: "Nutrition and the Contraceptive Pill," in *Nutritional Disorders of American Women*, M. Winick, ed. John Wiley and Sons, New York, 1977.
18. Hudiburgh, N. K., and Milner, A. N.: "Influence of Oral Contraceptives on Ascorbic Acid and Triglyceride Status," *J. Am. Diet. Assoc.*, **75**:19–22, 1979.
19. Review: "The Effect of Oral Contraceptives on Blood Vitamin A Level and the Role of Sex Hormones," *Nutr. Rev.*, **37**:346–48, 1979.
20. Review: "The Vitamin B_6 Requirement in Oral Contraceptive Users," *Nutr. Rev.*, **37**:344–45, 1979.

Additional References

ASHE, J. R., et al.: "The Retention of Calcium, Iron, Phosphorus, and Magnesium During Pregnancy. The Adequacy of Prenatal Diets with and Without Supplementation," *Am. J. Clin. Nutr.*, **32**:286–91, 1979.

BEAL, V. A.: "Nutritional Studies During Pregnancy," *J. Am. Diet. Assoc.*, **58**:312–20, 321–26, 1971.

BLACKBURN, M. W., and CALLOWAY, D. H.: "Energy Expenditure and Consumption of Mature Pregnant and Lactating Women," *J. Am. Diet. Assoc.*, **69**:29–36, 1976.

COURSIN, D. B.: "Maternal Nutrition and the Offspring's Development," *Nutr. Today*, **8**:12–18, March/April 1973.

EDOZIEN, J. C., et al.: "Medical Evaluation of the Special Supplemental Food Program for Women, Infants, and Children," *Am. J. Clin. Nutr.*, **32**:677–92, 1979.

HANSEN, C. M., et al.: "Effects on Pregnant Adolescents of Attending a Special School. Nutritional Status and Outcome of Pregnancy," *J. Am. Diet. Assoc.*, **68**:538–41, 1976.

JACOBSON, H. N.: "Maternal Nutrition," *Mod. Med.*, **39**:102–105, October 18, 1971.

LINDHEIMER, M. D., and KATZ, A. I.: "Sodium and Diuretics During Pregnancy," *N. Engl. J. Med.*, **288**:891–94, 1973.

OAKES, G. K., et al.: "Diet in Pregnancy. Meddling with the Normal or Preventing Toxemia?" *Am. J. Nurs.*, **75**:1134–36, 1975.

PIKE, R. L., and GURSKY, D. S.: "Further Evidence of Deleterious Effects Produced by Sodium Restriction During Pregnancy," *Am. J. Clin. Nutr.*, **23**:883–88, 1970.

WEIGLEY, E. S.: "The Pregnant Adolescent," *J. Am. Diet. Assoc.*, **66**:588–92, 1975.

19 Nutrition During Infancy

EACH infant's physical growth and development are determined by genetically acquired characteristics, the prenatal quality of nutrition, and the nutritional adequacy of the postnatal diet. Satisfying relationships developed between mother and infant from the earliest days influence not only the establishment of desirable food behavior, but are important also for their social and psychologic value. In addition to achieving one's potential in growth and development, many clinicians and nutrition scientists maintain that the initiation in early life of preventive measures including diet and life-style can reduce the risks of chronic disease in the middle and later years of life.

Changing Feeding Patterns and Current Issues

Infant feeding practices change as research identifies new and better ways. But they also change for environmental, cultural, and socioeconomic reasons. Sometimes the issues are emotionally charged–among pediatricians and nutritionists as well as parents!

In the United States and other developed countries there has been a resurgence of interest in breast feeding, especially among educated women of middle and higher socioeconomic classes. For those who use artificial feeding, commercial formulas now account for about 90 per cent of all bottle feedings. In the developing countries, by contrast, breast feeding has been declining; yet, for a number of reasons, bottle feeding becomes a hazardous substitute.

With understanding of the adequacy of human milk for the infant and in consideration of the development of feeding behavior, the introduction of solid foods before the infant is 4 to 6 months old is now believed to be undesirable. There are, likewise, proponents of home-prepared rather than commercially produced baby foods. Parents often express concern about modified starches and additives in commercial foods.

The emphasis in recent years on the prevention of diseases has raised the question: Will modification of the infant's diet help to reduce the risks or to prevent chronic disease? Thus there are concerns, and indeed controversies, about the intake of energy, sugar, fat, cholesterol, and salt.

Each of these issues will be considered in this chapter. Although some controversies persist, the health professional can help parents to make prudent choices for the well-being of their children.

Growth and Development

GROWTH is an increase in the size of the body or any parts of the body. It includes an increase in cell numbers and cell size. DEVELOPMENT entails the maturation of body tissues, organs, and metabolic systems so that the intended functions can be performed.

Body Size Next to the fetal period, the infant's first year is the time of most rapid growth. Each week during the first 4 or 5 months the infant will gain 140 to 225 gm (5 to 8 ounces), thereby doubling the birth weight. For the remainder of the year he or she will gain 110 to 140 gm (4 to 5 ounces) each week, so that the weight is tripled by the time the infant is 10 to 12 months old. On his or her first birthday the infant will have achieved one sixth to one seventh of the adult weight.

The normal birth length of 50 to 55 cm (20 to 22 inches) increases by another 23 to 25 cm (9 to 10 inches) during the first year. With the increase in length the body proportions are also changing. The trunk becomes longer as do also the short arms and legs. The baby's head grows rapidly during fetal life and during the first year. By the end of the second year the head circumference is about two thirds of its final size.

Body Composition Weight gains consist of water, muscle and organ tissues, adipose tissue, and skeletal structures. At birth the infant's body consists of as much as 75 per cent water, about 12 to 15 per cent fat, and poorly developed muscles. By the end of the first year the water content has decreased to about 60 per cent, the fat has increased to about 24 per cent, and lean body mass has correspondingly increased. From birth onward girls have more adipose tissue than boys.

The skeleton contains a high percentage of water and cartilage at birth and is gradually mineralized throughout childhood and adolescence. The calcium content of the skeleton at birth of about 25 to 28 gm is tripled by the end of the first year.

Cardiovascular-Respiratory Systems Infants have rapid heart (120 to 140 per minute) and respiratory (20 per minute) rates. At birth the hemoglobin level of the well-nourished infant is 17 to 20 gm per 100 ml. This provides a reserve for expansion of the blood circulation and adequate oxygen-carrying capacity to the growing tissues during the first 4 to 6 months. By 6 months of age the hemoglobin level has dropped to 11 to 12 gm per 100 ml or lower. The failure to anticipate this decline and to supply iron can lead rapidly to anemia.

Gastrointestinal System The full-term infant is able to digest protein, emulsified fats, and simple carbohydrates such as lactose. There is little secretion by the salivary glands until 2 to 3 months at which time the increased salivation becomes evident with drooling. Also, during the first few months the starch-splitting enzymes are not produced at levels of satisfactory digestion of complex carbohydrates. Gastric acidity is low in infants under 3 months. One of the effects of this is the growth of bacteria that bring about the conversion of nitrates to nitrites. Nitrites, when absorbed, change some of the hemoglobin to methemoglobin so that the oxygen-carrying capacity of the blood is reduced.[1] Home-prepared baby foods such as beets, spinach, carrots, and broccoli contain appreciable amounts of nitrates. Although methemoglobinemia is not a widespread problem, it provides an additional reason for delaying the introduction of solid foods.

Renal System The kidneys reach their full functional capacity by the end of the first year. During the first few months the glomerular filtration rate is somewhat lower, and therefore the excretion of a high concentration of solutes is more difficult. Young infants also excrete greater amounts of some amino acids, but the reabsorption of other amino acids such as phenlyalanine is high. Thus, 97 to 98 per cent of phenylalanine may be reabsorbed even though blood levels are high, as in phenylketonuria, one of many genetic diseases.

Brain Development The brain develops rapidly in fetal life and during infancy and early childhood. By the age of 4 years the brain has reached 80 to 90 per cent of its adult size. The increase in the number of brain cells is most rapid during fetal life and in the first 5 to 6 months after birth. Thereafter, the rate of cell division declines but continues into the second year. If malnutrition is unusually severe during pregnancy and during the first few months of life, as in the marasmic infant, the number of brain cells is greatly reduced. Once the critical period of cell division has passed, an adequate diet given subsequently cannot bring about an increase in cell numbers.

Feeding Behavior The development of feeding behavior depends on maturation of the nervous system which controls muscular coordination. At birth the baby is able to coordinate sucking, swallowing, and breathing. The eyes cannot yet be focused, but by the ROOTING REFLEX the baby can find nourishment; that is, when the cheek and lips nearest the nipple are stroked the infant will turn toward the stimulus and seek the nipple and suckle.

For about 3 months the baby suckles rhythmically with an up and down movement of the tongue. If solid food is placed on the tongue at this age, the same tongue movements result in food being pushed out of the mouth (EXTRUSION REFLEX).

At 12 to 16 weeks the sucking pattern changes and the tongue moves back and forth instead of up and down. When food is placed on the tongue the baby is able to draw in the lower lip when the spoon is withdrawn, transfer the food to the back of the tongue and swallow it.

By 6 months of age the infant has better coordination of eyes and hands, grasps objects within reach, and puts them into the mouth. The baby also develops chewing movements and it is appropriate to give him or her zwieback or crackers.

Nutritional Assessment

Measurements Each infant is individual and serves as his or her own best control in the measurement of progress. Although it is useful to make comparisons with stated norms such as length and weight, it is also dangerous to expect every infant to conform exactly to such norms. No single criterion of physical status by itself is indicative of the quality of nutrition, but a series of measurements over a period of time are likely to be reliable indicators. (See also Chapter 22.)

Weight, length, head circumference, and skinfold thickness can be compared with standards for infants of a given age. (See Length and Weight Charts, Tables A-6 and A-8.) An infant that falls within the 25th and 75th percentile is within the range of most infants. If the baby falls within the 90th to the 95th percentile for weight and/or length, he or she exceeds all but 5 to 10 infants in each 100. Thus, weight at the 90th percentile should be monitored for the onset of obesity. Conversely, an infant that falls at the 5th to 10th percentile may be experiencing growth failure, and its causes should be sought.

Other criteria of satisfactory quality of nutrition are these:

Normal levels of hemoglobin and hematocrit for age
Steady rate of weight gain, but some weekly fluctuations to be expected
Healthy, smooth skin
Firm muscles with moderate amount of subcutaneous fat
Tooth eruption beginning at about 5 to 6 months; 6 to 12 teeth by end of first year
Normal elimination for type of feeding
Vigorous and happy; sleeps well

Nutritional Status Many studies have shown that most infants in the United States receive an adequate intake of all nutrients except iron and are well nourished. A deficient intake of iron leads to iron-deficiency anemia, especially during the second half of the first year. The prevalence is relatively high in infants from low socioeconomic groups and among multiple births or premature infants.[2]

Overnutrition of infants, with particular reference to excessive weight gain, is deemed to be undesirable because it is associated with a great increase in the number of adipocytes, thus possibly paving the way for obesity in later life.[3]

Even in the United States there are occasional instances of failure to thrive, vitamin deficiencies such as scurvy or rickets, deficiencies in trace minerals such as zinc, and protein-calorie malnutrition. When such conditions are encountered, the underlying causes must be sought for they may range from poverty to ignorance of the infant's needs to infant neglect to metabolic errors that have not been diagnosed.

Nutritional Requirements

The amount of human milk ingested by the healthy infant from a well-nourished mother has been used as the primary basis for the recommended allowances during the first 6 months.[4] In some instances the nutrient levels have been set higher for babies who are receiving formulas. For the second 6 months the allowances are based on the consumption of a formula and a mixture of solid foods. The recommended allowances are listed in Table 19–1.

Energy The energy needs of the infant for the first 6 months range from 95 to 145 kcal per kilogram and for the second 6 months from 80 to 135 kcal per kilogram.[4] About half of the energy expenditure is ac-

Table 19-1. **Comparison of Recommended Dietary Allowances for Normal Infants with Composition of Human Milk, Cow's Milk, and Milk-based Formula***

Nutrient	Dietary Allowances 0-6 Months	Dietary Allowances 6-12 Months	Human Milk per 1,000 ml†	Cow's Milk (Whole) per 1,000 ml	Milk-based Formula per 1,000 ml
Weight, kg	6	9			
lb	13	20			
Height, cm	60	71			
in	24	28			
Water, ml			897	894	875
Energy, kcal	kg × 115	kg × 105	718	620	670
Protein, gm	kg × 2.2	kg × 2.0	10.6	33.4	15-16
Fat, gm			44.9	33.9	36-37
Carbohydrate, gm			70.6	47.3	70-72
Vitamin A, RE	420	400	656	315	340-500
IU	1,400	2,000	2,470	1,279	1,700-2,500
Vitamin D, μg	10	10		10‡	10
Vitamin E, mg TE	3	4	1.3-3.3	5.7	5.7-8.5
Ascorbic acid, mg	35	35	51	10	55
Thiamin, mg	0.3	0.5	0.14	0.39	0,4-0.7
Riboflavin, mg	0.4	0.6	0.37	1.65	0.6-1.0
Niacin, mg NE	6	8	2.0	0.85	7-9
Vitamin B-6, mg	0.3	0.6	0.11	0.43	0.3-0.4
Vitamin B-12, μg	0.5	1.5	0.46	3.63	1.5-2.0
Folacin, μg	30	45	51	51	50-100
Calcium, mg	360	540	328	1,208	550-600
Phosphorus, mg	240	360	144	945	440-460
Sodium, mg	115-350§	250-750§	141	498	250-390
Potassium, mg	350-925§	425-1,275§	523	1,544	620-1,000
Magnesium, mg	50	70	31	132	40-50
Iodine, μg	40	50	30-100		40-70
Iron, mg	10	15	0.3	0.5	1.4-12.5**
Zinc, mg	3	5	1.8	3.9	2.0-4.0

*Food and Nutrition Board: *Recommended Dietary Allowances,* 9th ed. National Research Council–National Academy of Sciences, Washington, D.C., 1980.

†One liter of human milk = 1.025 gm; 1 liter of cow's milk = 1.017 gm.

‡Assumes fortification of cow's milk with 10 μg vitamin D.

§Allowances for sodium and potassium are ranges considered to be safe and adequate.

**Values for formula not fortified and fortified with iron.

counted for by the basal metabolism alone in order to regulate the temperature of the body with its high skin surface, and to maintain the high level of metabolic activities. The caloric requirement for growth is higher during the first half of the year when growth is most rapid. Babies who are active and who cry a lot have much higher energy requirements than those who are placid. The general well-being, rate of weight gain, and appetite give clues to the adequacy of the energy intake.

Protein The infant adds about 3.5 gm protein daily to his or her body during the first 4 months and thereafter about 3.1 gm per day for the rest of the year. This results not only in a net increase in body size but also in an increase of the percentage of body protein from 11 to 14.6.[4]

Human milk furnishes about 2 to 2.4 gm protein per kilogram per day during the first month of life, but by the sixth month this has fallen to 1.5 gm per kilogram per day. In the recommended allowances this lower level has been adjusted to 2.0 gm per kilogram for the second 6 months in order to allow for the lesser efficiency of the protein in a mixed diet.

Carbohydrate There is no recommended allowance for carbohydrate for infants. Lactose accounts for about 38 to 40 per cent of the calories in human milk. Since the lactose content in cow's milk is lower, lactose or another simple carbohydrate is added to commercial formulas. Sucrose, cane syrup, or dextrimaltose are commonly added to home-prepared formulas.

Fat About 45 to 50 per cent of calories in human milk and in most formulas are provided by fat. Such a proportion helps to meet the high energy requirements of the infant in an efficient way.

Human milk supplies from 6 to 9 per cent of its calories as linoleate. A formula that furnishes 3 per cent of calories as linoleic acid will meet the infant's needs.[4]

Low-fat formulas are contraindicated since it is difficult to achieve sufficient caloric intake for satisfactory weight gain. Low-fat formulas will not furnish enough linoleic acid unless it is added to the formula. If the concentration of the formula is increased, there will be greater deamination of amino acids and thus a considerable increase in the renal solute load.

The desirable level of cholesterol intake is not known. Human milk contains significantly more cholesterol than commercial formulas made with vegetable oils. Cholesterol is required for the synthesis of bile salts, the development of the central nervous system, and the elaboration of enzymes that control the body's synthesis of cholesterol.[5] Two questions remain unanswered: Does restriction of cholesterol in the formula impair the synthetic processes? Does restriction of cholesterol in infancy and early life help to reduce the incidence of atherosclerosis?

Water The normal daily turnover of water by the infant is about 15 per cent of body weight. The water loss from the skin is large because of the greater surface area in relation to body weight. The ability of the kidneys of the young infant to concentrate urine is much less than that of older children or adults. Hence, to excrete a given amount of solute, chiefly urea and sodium chloride, a larger volume of fluid is required. The osmolar load of breast milk is well within the excretion capacity of the kidney, but more concentrated formulas could present an excessive osmolar load.

Infants require about 150 ml water per 100 kcal. This requirement is met by breast milk, and by formulas containing 5 to 10 per cent sugar and enough water to give a concentration of 65 to 70 kcal per 100 ml.

Minerals Iron is probably the mineral that requires most emphasis in infant feeding, especially for infants of lower socioeconomic groups. An intake of 1 mg iron per kilogram per day beginning about the third month will maintain hemoglobin levels in normal infants. The recommended allowance of 10 and 15 mg, respectively, for the first and second half of the year is based on an average need of 1.5 mg per kilogram.[4]

The American Academy of Pediatrics recommends that iron supplementation (not more than 15 mg per day) should begin at 4 to 6 months for normal infants and at 2 months for preterm infants.[6]

The recommended allowance for calcium is based on about 60 mg calcium per kilogram body weight, the amount supplied to breast-fed infants.[4] Breast-fed infants retain about 50 to 60 per cent of the total calcium intake, whereas bottle-fed infants retain 25 to 30 per cent of a cow's milk formula. Since formulas contain a much higher proportion of calcium, the net retention is approximately the same. The calcium to phosphorus ratio during the first year should be 1.5 to 1 in order to offset the tendency toward hypercalcemia that sometimes occurs with a high phosphorus intake.

Allowances for zinc, magnesium, and iodine, listed in Table 19–1, are adequately met by human milk or formulas. The ranges for safe and adequate intakes of electrolytes and some trace minerals are listed in Table 3–2 (page 36).

The infant requires about 1.0 to 1.5 mEq sodium for daily growth, and losses from the skin and excretions are about 1 to 2 mEq daily. The total sodium needs are estimated to be 2 to 5 mEq (46 to 115 mg) daily.[7] The average daily intake of sodium ranges from 13 mEq (300 mg) at 2 months to 60 mEq (1,400 mg) at 12 months.[4]

Vitamins Human milk from a healthy, well-nourished mother supplies sufficient levels of vitamins for the infant with the possible exception of vitamin D. Although some studies have indicated that a water-miscible form of vitamin D is present in human milk and will meet the infant's needs, a supplement is usually recommended. Formulas generally contain the 10 μg vitamin D recommended for the first year.[4]

The plasma vitamin E content of newborn infants is low but rises rapidly to normal levels by the end of the first month. The need for vitamin E is normally met by human and cow's milk. A vitamin E supplement may be required if formulas have an increased level of polyunsaturated fatty acids and are also fortified with iron. The presence of iron increases lipid peroxidation, reduces the available level of vitamin E, and leads to anemia, reticulocytosis, and thrombocytosis.[8]

Because human milk supplies low levels of vitamin B-6, the infant is born with a store of the vitamin. Vitamin B-6 gained some attention years ago when infants displayed symptoms of deficiency following ingestion of a formula in which vitamin B-6 had been inadvertently destroyed by overheating. There have been no further instances of such formula deficiencies.

Human milk will meet the ascorbic acid needs of normal infants. Formula-fed infants require supplementation if the formula itself is not fortified. When increased amounts of protein are given, infants require additional amounts of ascorbic acid for the metabolism of tyrosine.

Breast Feeding

Human milk is the natural food for the infant. If breast feeding is to be successful, the advantages must be sold to the mother early in pregnancy. An adequate diet, exercise, rest, and freedom from anxiety are important during the prenatal period as well as during lactation.

For the first few days after delivery the breasts yield 10 to 40 ml of a clear yellowish secretion known as COLOSTRUM. By the tenth day the composition and amount of this secretion has changed until it has the properties of mature milk.

Breast feeding for as little as 2 or 3 months confers advantages to the infant. Some women breast feed their babies for 5 to 6 months, gradually weaning to a formula and then to the cup. Others continue breast feeding up to a year and occasionally longer.

Advantages Human milk is the most nutritionally balanced food for the infant. The solute content of human milk is lower than that of cow's milk and entails less excretory load for the immature kidneys. However, most commercial formulas now compare favorably with human milk in their solute load.

With breast milk there are fewer and less serious illnesses and allergies. The colostrum and mature milk confer immune properties that are low or missing in cow's milk.[9] Human milk contains about as many leukocytes as are found in blood. They bring about phagocytosis, and also secrete complement, lysozyme, and lactoferrin. Most classes of immunoglobulins (IgA, IgG, and IgM) are present. Lysozymes split bacterial walls, while lactoferrin retards growth of bacteria such as *E. coli* and *Shigella*. The BIFIDUS factor in human milk increases the growth of lactobacilli and helps to convert lactose to lactic and acetic acids. With the consequent lowering of the pH of the intestinal tract, the growth of enteropathogenic organisms is reduced. Lipid factors (lipase and monoglyceride) have also been identified as antimicrobial agents.

In lower socioeconomic groups breast-fed infants have a lower mortality rate, probably because there is no problem of sanitation. On a practical basis breast feeding eliminates preparation of a formula; the feeding is immediately available at the proper temperature; and errors in formula dilution or home preparation of a formula are avoided.

Claims are often made for psychologic advantages of breast feeding. A bonding between mother and child is established; that is, the baby feels safe, warm, and protected and the mother has a sense of satisfaction and closeness to the baby. Yet it is difficult to prove that the formula-fed baby is in any way disadvantaged in this respect. Health care professionals must exercise discretion so that they do not make the mother feel guilty if she chooses not to breast feed her baby.

The cost of the additional foods needed to produce milk by the mother varies widely depending upon choices made. Generally, the cost of the added foods is about comparable to that of a home-prepared formula using evaporated milk, and considerably less than some commercial formulas.[10]

In the developing countries breast feeding can be lifesaving. Yet in many countries breast feeding is declining. This has come about because some mothers are working and are unable to feed their babies, while others have come to regard bottle feeding as a status symbol. Many people in these countries do not have sufficient income to purchase the amounts of formula that the infant requires. They resort to excessive dilution and the infant becomes malnourished. Water supplies are often contaminated and refrigeration is lacking. With the contamination of the formulas, the subsequent diarrhea leads to loss of nutrients, dehydration, acidosis, and a high mortality rate. (See Figure 19–1.)

Contraindications Breast feeding must be discontinued when (1) chronic illnesses are present in the mother, such as cardiac disease, tuberculosis, severe anemia, nephritis, and chronic fevers; (2) another pregnancy ensues; (3) it is necessary for the mother to return to employment outside the home; or (4) the infant is weak or unable to nurse because of cleft palate or harelip. Some places of employment are now providing day-care nurseries and in some of them it is possible for the woman to breast feed her baby.

If the mother has an acute infection it may be necessary to temporarily halt breast feeding. In such a situation the mother's breasts should be completely pumped at regular intervals so that the breast supply will not diminish.

A number of drugs are transmitted to the mother's milk and the baby may have adverse reactions to them. These include anticoagulants, some antibiotics, anticancer drugs, nicotine from heavy cigarette smoking, tranquilizers and sedatives, and

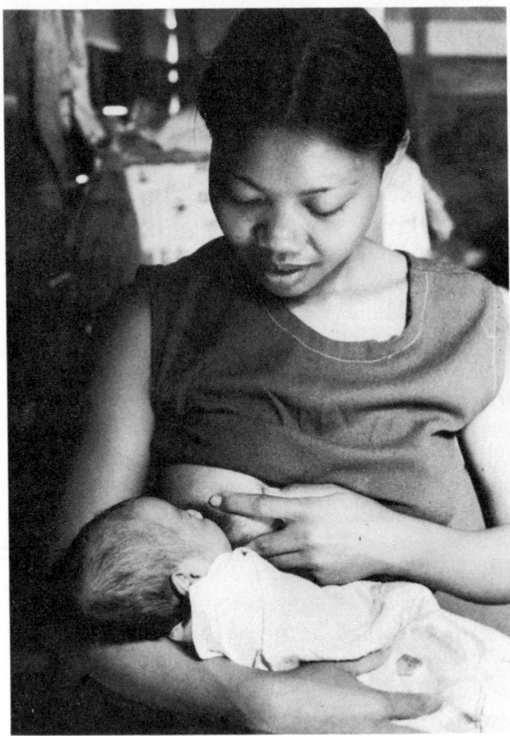

Figure 19–1. Breast feeding provides the best nourishment for the baby. It also confers immunity against some infections during the early months of life. (WHO photo by J. Abcede.)

"street" drugs. Occasionally breast milk can be contaminated by environmental pollutants such as DDT and PCBs. (See page 313.)

Initiation of Feeding In order to foster breast feeding the mother and infant should not be separated during the first 24 hours after delivery. The sucking of the hungry infant stimulates the flow of milk. At first the infant will ingest only small amounts of colostrum. The weight drops for a few days, but will be regained by the tenth day.

The baby may get enough food by emptying one breast, but if the baby is still hungry he or she should be offered the other breast. At the next feeding the breast that was not emptied should be offered first.

When the baby stops sucking he or she should be held over the shoulder and patted on the back to release any air that may have been swallowed. Some babies burp best if they are laid across the knee, abdomen down, and patted. Some babies suckle so vigorously and swallow so much air that they require two or three burpings for each feeding.

Self-Demand Feeding Healthy infants will establish, after a few weeks, schedules of their own that are reasonably regular from day to day if they are fed when they indicate they are hungry.

The success of self-demand feeding depends upon the mother's ability to determine when the child is hungry. The infant who cries at intervals much shorter than 3 hours may be underfed, may have swallowed too much air at the previous feeding, or may be crying because of other discomforts.

The very young infant may require as many as 10 or 12 feedings at first but soon establishes a rhythm of feeding which falls into approximately 3- to 4-hour intervals. After the second month, the night feeding usually may be discontinued. By the end of the fourth or fifth month, the infant sleeps through the night and will no longer require a feeding around 10 P.M.

Adequacy of Feeding About 150 to 165 ml human milk per kilogram body weight (2.5 ounces per pound) result in satisfactory weight gain. The baby is getting enough milk if he or she is satisfied at the end of a 15-to-20-minute feeding, falls asleep promptly and sleeps quietly for several hours thereafter, and makes satisfactory gains from week to week. The infant should be weighed once a week in the same amount of clothing each time. If the milk intake is inadequate one or more breast feedings may be replaced with a formula. At 4 to 6 months supplementary foods may be added.

During the first 5 or 6 months the breast-fed baby who is gaining at a normal rate receives all the nutrients needed with a few exceptions. These supplements are generally recommended:

Vitamin K is usually given parenterally shortly after birth

10 μg (400 IU) vitamin D as a water-miscible preparation, beginning a week to 10 days after birth[11]

Iron (not more than 15 mg) at 4 to 6 months; may be given as iron-fortified cereal or as iron drops[6]

Vitamin B-12 if the mother is a strict vegetarian

At 4 to 6 months baby foods are introduced and will gradually contribute increasing amounts of nutrients. (See page 357.)

Weaning When the supply of milk declines or breast feeding must be terminated for any reason, the baby is gradually weaned by offering a formula for a single feeding. After 4 to 5 days the baby is offered the bottle for the second feeding, and so on. When breast feeding has been successful for most of the year the baby can be weaned directly to cup feedings of formula.

Bottle Feeding

Comparison of Human and Cow's Milk Human and cow's milk are similar in their energy value and in the amount of fat. Cow's milk contains substantially higher levels of most nutrients, but supplies less lactose, ascorbic acid, niacin, and vitamin A than does human milk. (See Table 19–1.)

Lactalbumin accounts for 60 per cent of the protein in human milk, while in cow's milk only 15 per cent of the protein is lactalbumin. The remaining protein in both milks is primarily casein. For the infant lactalbumin provides an amino acid pattern that most nearly approaches that of the body tissues. However, the protein of cow's milk is also well utilized by the infant.

Newborn babies absorb about 95 to 98 per cent of the fat from human milk but only about 80 per cent of fat from a milk-based formula.[9] Human milk has a high lipase activity, and also a higher level of linoleic acid.

Cow's milk contains about three times as much ash as does human milk. Most of this is accounted for by higher contents of calcium, phosphorus, sodium, and potassium. The calcium to phosphorus ratio in cow's milk is about 1 to 1 and in human milk 2 to 1.

Human and cow's milk differ considerably in their vitamin contents. Human milk can furnish the ascorbic acid needs of the infant, but cow's milk cannot. Both milks provide satisfactory levels of other vitamins except vitamin D.

Human milk forms fine flocculent curds in the stomach, and the emptying time is more rapid than for cow's milk. The curd of cow's milk is larger, tougher, and more slowly digested; it is modified by homogenization, heating, or acidification.

Proprietary Premodified Formulas About 90 per cent of formula-fed infants are now being given commercially prepared formulas. Some of these are available in dry form; some are concentrated, requiring dilution with water; some are ready-to-use to be measured into the bottle; and some are available in disposable nursing bottles. Their cost is moderate to expensive; packaging in disposable bottles for each feeding increases the cost considerably.

Proprietary formulas are available not only for healthy babies but for a variety of conditions such as lactose intolerance, allergies, and inborn errors of metabolism. (See also pages 551, 696, and 707.) The formulas for healthy infants are patterned on human milk and are adjusted to meet the nutrient requirements set by the Food and Drug Administration.[12] They are homogenized and have a low curd tension. Nonfat dry milk is used for milk-based formulas. Typical modifications in the formulas include the following:

Protein content is lowered; the protein is treated to produce a fine, flocculent, easily digested curd.

Butterfat is removed, and vegetable oils, such as corn oil are substituted to increase the linoleic acid content.

The cholesterol content is usually low.

Lactose or other carbohydrate is added.
Calcium, phosphorus, and other mineral levels are lowered by dilution.
Vitamins A, D, E, and ascorbic acid are added to meet the infant's needs.
Iron may be added; iron-fortified formulas should be encouraged throughout the first year.

Home-Prepared Formulas A formula prepared in the home using evaporated milk, cane sugar, and ascorbic acid tablets is relatively inexpensive. Although some savings can be effected by preparing the formula in the home and most babies thrive on them, the families that can most benefit from these savings are sometimes least able to understand the importance of proper measurements and sanitary preparation.

The following guidelines may be used for a satisfactory formula using evaporated milk.

Amount of milk. About 50 to 65 ml of evaporated milk per kilogram of body weight (¾ to 1 oz per pound).

Sugar. Sucrose and corn syrup are inexpensive, easily digested, and lend themselves to formula preparation. Lactose dissolves poorly and is expensive. Dextrimaltose is less sweet than sugar and is sometimes used. Honey is not recommended inasmuch as its use has occasionally led to infant botulism.[13]

During the first 2 weeks about 15 gm (½ oz) sugar is added to the day's formula. Thereafter, 30 gm (1 oz) is sufficient. Sugar is discontinued at the time the baby is taking appreciable amounts of other foods.

Liquid. At 2 months the infant will take about 120 ml (4 oz) of formula. This is increased about 30 ml each month until the infant is taking a maximum of 240 ml at approximately 6 months of age.

Intervals of feeding. As with breast feeding, the number of feedings and the amount taken at each feeding should be flexible. Formula-fed babies should not, as a rule, be fed at less than 3-hour intervals since the cow's milk remains for a longer time in the stomach.

Calculation of the formula. The calculation of a formula using evaporated milk is as follows:

Infant, 5 months old, weighs 7 kg
Number of feedings. . . . 5 (assuming approximately 4-hour intervals)
Volume of feeding: 210 ml (7 oz)
Total volume of formula: 5×210 ml = 1050 ml (35 oz)
Evaporated milk: 7×55 ml = 385 ml (13 oz)
Water: $1050 - 385 = 665$ ml (22 oz)
Sugar: 30 gm (2 tablespoons)

This formula provides 527 kcal from milk and 120 kcal from sugar, or a daily intake of 92 kcal per kilogram of body weight. Food supplements given at this age will increase the caloric intake to the desired level. (See page 357.) The formula contains 27 gm protein, or about 3.8 gm per kilogram of body weight.

Sterilization of formula. Terminal sterilization of the formula is preferred. The steps are as follows: (1) Pour measured amount of formula into thoroughly washed bottles. (2) Put nipples on bottles and test the flow of milk. (3) Cover loosely with nipple covers. (4) Place bottles on rack in sterilizer and add water to halfway level of bottles. (5) Cover sterilizer, bring water to boiling, and maintain boiling for 25 minutes. (6) Remove bottles as soon as they can be handled, and cool slightly. (7) Store in refrigerator.

Technique of Feeding The feeding is usually warmed to body temperature, but no adverse effects have been noted when it is given cold. As with breast feeding the baby should be held in a semireclining position. The baby should never be propped up and allowed to feed alone. (See Figure 19–2.)

An overly large hole in the nipple leads to rapid taking of the formula and excessive swallowing of air, discomfort, and perhaps regurgitation. On the other hand, a very small hole in the nipple will necessitate too long a period of feeding. During the feed-

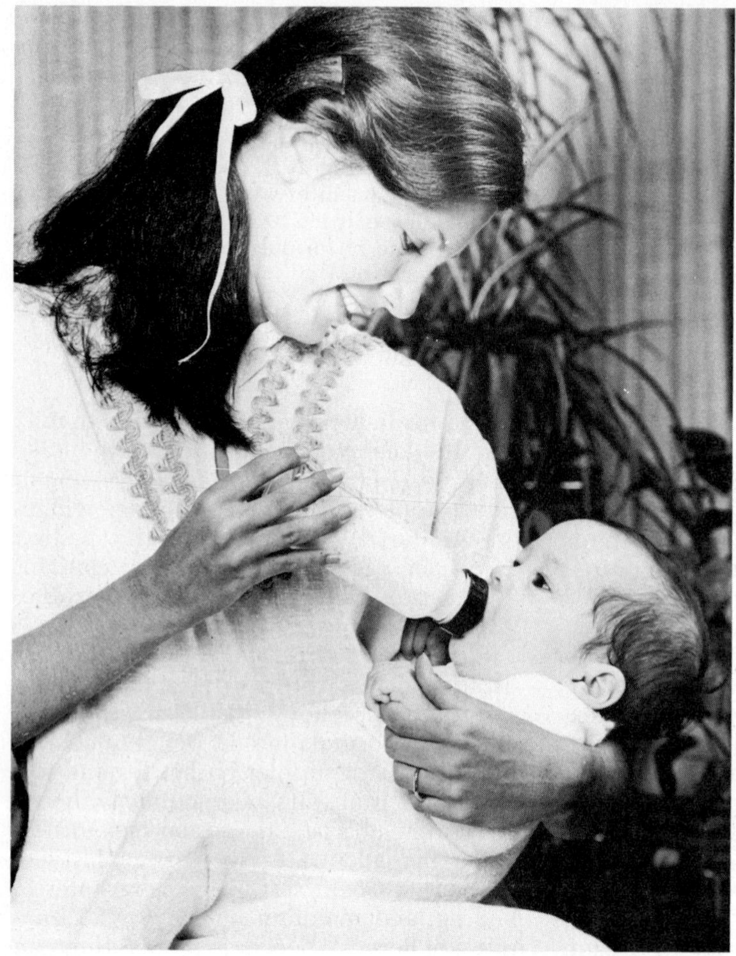

Figure 19–2. Infants are successfully fed by formulas when breast feeding is not possible. The baby should be held comfortably during the feeding. (Courtesy, Ross Laboratories, Columbus, Ohio.)

ing the nipple should be filled with fluid, and not air, so that less air is swallowed. Even so, the infant will need to be "burped" one or more times as experience shows to be necessary.

The baby should not be expected to finish the entire amount of formula in the bottle at each feeding. The mother soon learns how much the baby will usually take at each feeding and can adjust the amounts of formula in the bottle. Any formula remaining at the end of each feeding must be discarded.

Supplements for Formula Feeding Proprietary formulas fortified with iron require no supplementation except for fluoride if the water supply is not fluoridated. Home-prepared formulas should be supplemented with 35 mg ascorbic acid within 2 weeks after birth. Synthetic ascorbic acid is preferable since young babies are sometimes allergic to citrus juices. This may be added to the formula or given with water. At 4 to 6 months iron-fortified cereal is given to meet the iron need. If the water is not fluoridated a fluoride supplement is indicated. When soy-milk formulas are used it is essential that a vitamin B-12 supplement be provided if the formula itself is not fortified.

Solid Foods

Rationale for Timing In the last quarter century most babies have been introduced to solid foods at an early age—sometimes within a few weeks after birth. It was believed that such foods would help the baby to sleep through the night although there is no evidence for this. Many also believed that the early introduction of solid foods would improve acceptance of a variety of foods. However, the sense of taste is not well developed until 3 to 4 months. Mothers were often prodded to early feeding by relatives and friends. Indeed, it was considered to be an accomplishment for the baby to be accepting solid foods!

Pediatricians and nutritionists now recommend that solids be introduced at about 6 months for breast-fed babies and at 4 to 6 months for formula-fed babies. This is more in accord with the time at which lessening of the extrusion reflex occurs and the increased ability to transfer food to the back of the mouth and to voluntarily swallow it. Moreover, fewer allergic reactions are likely when the mucosa of the intestinal tract is less permeable to foreign proteins. Each baby should be allowed to develop a feeding behavior according to his or her neuromuscular coordination.

Proprietary and Home-Prepared Baby Foods Commercially prepared baby foods are convenient, bacteriologically safe, moderate in cost, and available in considerable variety. Baby meats contain more protein than do soups and meat dinners. Desserts that contain sugar contribute to a liking for sweets. Manufacturers have eliminated sugar in some fruits and have reduced the amounts in desserts and fruits that are more acidic. Likewise, the salt content has been reduced or eliminated.

Modified food starches have been added to dinners, high-meat dinners, fruits, and desserts in order to retain proper texture, consistency, and uniformity of ingredient distribution. In a study of 430 infants modified starches provided an average of only 2 per cent of caloric intake and appeared to be well utilized. Only four of the infants in this study had a modified starch intake accounting for as much as 10 per cent of total caloric intake.[14]

With a little expenditure of time and careful attention to sanitary handling of food, the mother can prepare satisfactory foods for the infant, usually at lower cost. Many of the foods prepared for the family can be used, but they should not be salted or sweetened. The mineral and vitamin content is more variable than that of commercial foods. If foods are cooked in a minimum amount of water, puréed or chopped as soon as cooked, and fed to the baby promptly, the nutrient retention should be good. Individual portions may be frozen in ice-cube trays, and stored in plastic bags kept in a freezer for several weeks.

Choices for Solid Foods By the end of the year the baby will be consuming 300 to 450 gm (10 to 15 oz) of solid foods. Correspondingly, the amount of breast milk or formula ingested will decline to about three fourths of a liter. Iron-fortified formula, rather than fresh whole cow's milk, should be continued throughout the first year. Fresh whole cow's milk is low in iron and unless heated at a high temperature (as in evaporated milk) occasionally causes gastrointestinal bleeding. A typical sequence for adding solid foods is shown in Table 19–2.

Cereals. Iron-fortified rice cereal is preferred initially since it is less likely to produce allergic reactions than are wheat and oats. The dry cereal is mixed with some of the formula, initially using a semiliquid and, later, a more solid consistency.

Crisp toast, zwieback, and graham crackers may be given when teeth appear.

Fruits. Mashed ripe banana or mild-flavored cooked or canned puréed and later chopped fruits without added sugar—applesauce, pears, peaches, prunes—are accepted well. Orange, grapefruit, grape, and apple juices—all unsweetened—are initially diluted with water, given in very

Table 19–2. **Typical Sequence for Adding Solid Foods***

The amounts stated below for each age grouping are approximate, and will vary from one infant to another.

5 to 6 months if breast-fed; 4 to 6 months if formula-fed
- Dry, iron-fortified infant cereal—2 to 3 tablespoons
- Strained, unsweetened fruit—2 tablespoons
- Strained vegetable—2 tablespoons

6 to 7 months
- Dry infant cereal—¼ cup
- Fruits and vegetables—3 tablespoons each
- Start strained meat—2 tablespoons

7 to 8 months
- Fortified infant cereal—½ cup
- Mashed or chopped fruits and vegetables—¼ cup each
- Meat—3 tablespoons
- Add zwieback, toast, potatoes

8 to 12 months
- Cereal—½ cup
- Chopped fruits and vegetables—⅓ cup of each
- Meat—¼ cup; may be chopped or ground
- Add mashed cooked egg yolk, cottage cheese or other soft cheese, or mashed dried cooked beans or peas

*See page 357 for guidelines for introduction of new foods.

small amounts, and then given full strength.

Vegetables. Puréed carrots, peas, green beans, and squash are better accepted initially than are spinach, beets, asparagus, or broccoli.

Protein-rich foods. Hard-cooked egg yolk should be mashed and mixed with a little formula, cereal, or vegetable. Only ½ teaspoon should be given initially lest there be an allergy to egg protein. Egg white is not given until the infant is a year old, and then it must be well cooked.

Strained, and later ground or chopped, beef, chicken, turkey, tuna fish, and other fish (with careful removal of all bones) are added by the seventh or eighth month. Cottage cheese or other soft cheese, peanut butter, or mashed dried cooked beans may be substituted occasionally for the meat or egg.

Feeding Problems and Nutritional Issues

Regurgitation and Colic The small amounts of food regurgitated by many babies is no cause for concern. Vomiting is more serious and should receive the prompt attention of the pediatrician.

Some babies cry loudly and for long intervals following feeding. Usually they have swallowed excessive amounts of air and have been inadequately burped. However, some babies continue to cry even with burping and the parents become quite distraught. These colicky babies usually grow well, and the parents need reassurance that they are progressing satisfactorily and will usually outgrow the colic within a few months. Colic sometimes occurs because the baby is overfed, is tired, or is cold.

Constipation Formula-fed infants usually have but one bowel movement daily, whereas breast-fed infants have two or three. Only when the stools are hard and dry and eliminated with difficulty does constipation exist. Prune juice or strained prunes given daily usually suffice to correct the constipation.

Diarrhea Infantile diarrhea is sometimes caused by improper preparation or storage of the formula. The incidence is several times higher in bottle-fed than in breast-fed infants and is greatly increased in the summer months, especially in infants from lower socioeconomic groups. Serious consequences including dehydration and acidosis follow diarrhea in infants under 1 year if treatment is not given promptly.

Hazards of Overconcentrated Formulas Formulas are sometimes insufficiently diluted with water because of error, or because the mother mistakenly believes that the baby will be better nourished if the formula is more concentrated. Also, if skim milk is boiled, as is sometimes recommended for infants with diarrhea, the solute concentration increases unless the water lost by evaporation is replaced. With the higher solute concentration the kidney requires additional water for the excretion of metabolic wastes. Dehydration becomes increasingly severe, and, if not corrected, could lead to renal failure and coma.

Bottle Mouth Syndrome This is a condition of rampant dental caries affecting especially the maxillary incisors (four upper anterior teeth). Infants who are allowed to use the bottle with milk in it as a pacifier at bedtime, or who breast feed at night after 1 year, or who suck on a pacifier dipped in a sweetener are especially prone to the condition. The teeth are bathed with the liquid containing the fermentable carbohydrate, and in severe cases may be destroyed.

Salt Intake Salt taste is a learned behavior. Babies will accept unsalted and salted foods equally well, and much of the salt added to infant foods seems to be a response to the mother's, and not the infant's, taste. Normal salt intakes exceed requirements by a wide margin. (See page 351.) The healthy baby readily excretes the excess and seems to be able to adapt to a wide margin of intake. Based on animal research and also epidemiologic studies, many clinicians are concerned that excessive salt intake could lead to hypertension in later life.[15] Manufacturers of baby foods have eliminated or reduced the salt content of their products. Mothers, likewise, need to take the same steps in the preparation of foods for their infants and young children.

Sugar Intake Breast-fed babies as well as most babies given commercial formulas ingest lactose, a sugar that is not very sweet. When home-prepared formulas are used, the sugar or corn syrup added to meet the caloric requirement should be used only until solid foods are added.

Infants do not need to be taught to like sweet foods. Three objections can be raised to the use of sugar in the infant diet: (1) the role in dental caries; (2) the contribution of energy without a corresponding contribution of other nutrients; (3) the initiation of a lifetime habit of overuse of sweet foods. (See also Bottle Mouth Syndrome.)

Obesity Infants who remain in the 90th percentile of weight during the first year are more likely to become obese in later life than are infants whose weight remains within the 25th to 75th percentile. Excessive weight gains during infancy are accompanied by an enormous increase in the number of adipocytes. If overfeeding persists throughout childhood, the number of adipocytes increases at an abnormal rate until adolescence. Thereafter, the number of cells remains fixed throughout life, but the size of each cell can increase enormously. When weight is lost the size of the cells decreases but the cells themselves remain intact. In a recent study a close correlation was found between excessive weight gains at 6 weeks, 3 months, and 6 months, and overweight and obesity at 6 to 8 years.[3]

Infantile obesity must be approached individually.[16] It is not necessarily caused by bottle feeding instead of breast feeding, or the early introduction of solid foods. Nor is it caused by a mother's inability to heed the baby's satiety signals. Some mothers, however, may prod the baby to finish the bottle, thinking that the baby will be undernourished if the amounts recommended by the nutritionist or pediatrician are not consumed. Babies that are inactive will have lower than average energy requirements, and their caloric intake needs to be monitored. Nonfat milk formulas should not be used for the baby's first year, and formulas with 2 per cent fat should not be used for the first half year. (See page 350.)

Growth Failure Infants sometimes fail to thrive because they are deprived of the normal emotional environment. This occurs occasionally when infants are placed in an institution and also in the home when parents reject their children, neglect them, or provide an otherwise hostile environment. Given adequate emotional support and appropriate diet these babies again begin to thrive.

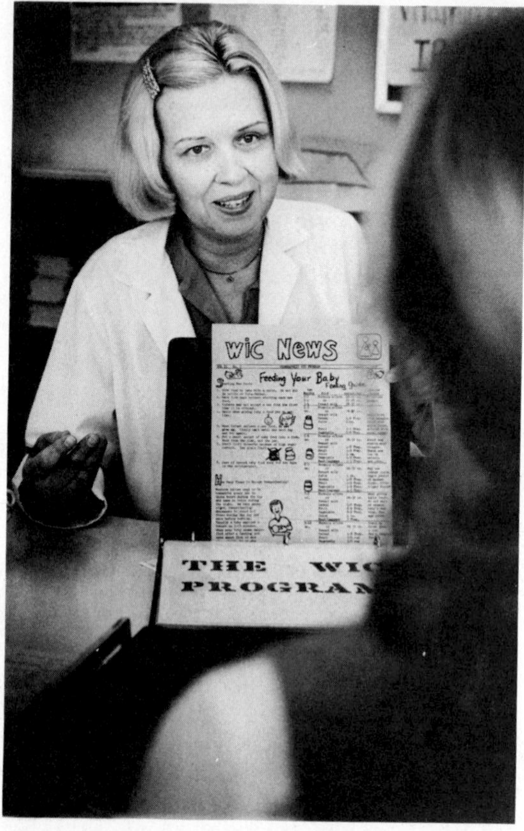

Figure 19–3. The mother who receives food supplements for her baby through the WIC program is also counseled concerning the steps to take to ensure safe and adequate food intake by her baby. (Courtesy, Jeffrey Grosscup and Hennepin County Medical Center, Minneapolis.)

Counseling the Mother

COMMUNITY RESOURCES The La Leche League International is a lay group that supports breast feeding.* It issues practical guidelines for the pregnant woman in preparation for breast feeding, and also for initiation of the new infant to the breast. Through local chapters new mothers can talk with other mothers to air their concerns and to receive advice.

To families who qualify on the basis of low income, the WIC program (see page 340) provides food supplements for infants who are at high nutritional risk, for example, low-birth-weight infants, those who fail to gain or who gain excessively, and those who are anemic. A typical food allowance for the infant includes iron-fortified formula, cereal high in iron, and fruit juice. (See Figure 19–3.)

INFANT FEEDING The nutritionist or nurse who counsels the pregnant woman should present the advantages of breast and formula feedings, but the choice should be freely made by the woman without any pressures whatsoever. If she chooses to breast feed, she needs guidance prior to delivery on diet and care of the breasts. The new mother nursing a baby for the first time sometimes needs guidance and encouragement from the nurse and directions for support of the breast and care of the nipples.

If commercial formulas are selected, these points must be emphasized: reading of labels for proper dilution of formulas; sanitation of bottles into which formulas are placed; refrigeration of formula once it is mixed.

If formulas and baby foods are to be home prepared, detailed written and illustrated instructions should be provided. In addition the dietary counselor should demonstrate measurements, sanitation of utensils, and terminal sterilization of the formula.

* La Leche League International, 9616 Minneapolis Avenue, Franklin Park, IL 60131.

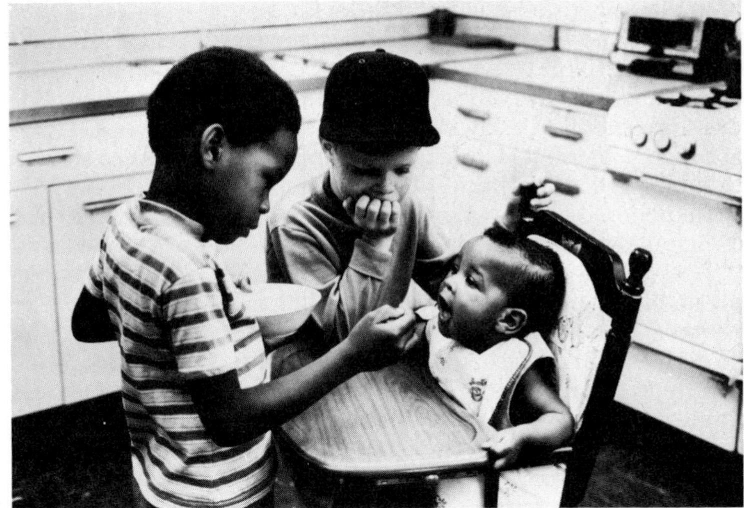

Figure 19–4. Meal time is also a means whereby happy relationships are established with others. (Courtesy, The Equitable Life Assurance Society of the United States.)

INTRODUCTION OF NEW FOODS These practical suggestions are intended to help the mother give the baby a smooth adjustment to new foods. (See Figure 19–4.)

1. Hold the baby upright while feeding to facilitate swallowing and to enhance the baby's feeling of security.
2. Give very small amounts of any new food—teaspoonfuls or even less—at the beginning.
3. Introduce only one new food at a time. Allow the infant to become familiar with that food before trying another. Watch for any allergic symptoms.
4. Use foods of smooth rather thin consistency at first. Gradually the consistency is made more solid as the infant learns how to use the tongue in propelling food to the back of the mouth. With a small spoon food is placed on the middle of the tongue, thereby facilitating swallowing.
5. Never force an infant to eat more of a food than he or she takes willingly.
6. If, after several trials, it is apparent that a baby has an acute dislike for a food, omit that item for a week or two and try it again. If the dislike persists it is better to forget about that food for a while and substitute another.
7. Gradually introduce variety from each group of foods. Babies, like older persons, tire of repetition of certain foods.
8. When the baby is able to chew, gradually substitute finely chopped foods for strained foods. Include some zwieback or dry toast.
9. Avoid showing in any way a dislike for a food that is being given.

Nutrition for Low-Birth-Weight Infants

Definitions A low-birth-weight infant (LBW) is one whose weight at birth is 2,500 gm (5½ pounds) or less. A very-low-birth-weight infant (VLBW) infant weighs 1,500 gm or less. Infants that are born prior to term (less than 38 weeks) are premature. Infants may be small for gestational age (SGA) or "light-for-date" because of severe maternal undernutrition, genetic abnormalities, or insufficient transfer of placental transfer of nutrients. The SGA infant may be full-term or premature.

Developmental Problems The LBW infant is born with poorly developed muscle tissues, very little body fat, low stores of iron, and an inadequately mineralized skeleton. Because there is very little fat and practically no glycogen, the energy stores are minimal and hypoglycemia, hyperbilirubinemia, and starvation result unless calories are supplied early. The energy needs are high because the surface area is proportionately great and because the extremely small deposits of subcutaneous fat result in a higher rate of heat loss.

The capacity of the stomach is about 5 ml at birth and increases to about 20 ml per kilogram by the end of the first week. The activity of sucrase, maltase, and lactase is reduced or may be nonexistent. Lactose intolerance is not uncommon during the first weeks of life. The digestion of fats is reduced, but some fat excretion is not harmful. The digestion of protein is adequate.

Because the kidneys are immature there is a reduced capacity to excrete wastes and consideration must be given to the concentration of nitrogenous constituents and electrolytes. When there is evidence of growth, the renal solute load is reduced because of the storage of nitrogen and minerals in the body.

The infant of less than 34 weeks has poor sucking and swallowing reflexes, and regurgitation of feedings is common. Aspiration and pneumonia are ever-present dangers.

Nutritional Requirements Premature infants are especially vulnerable to the effects of inadequate nutrition. Weight loss during the first few days should not exceed 5 to 10 per cent of body weight, and the birth weight should be regained in 1 to 2 weeks.[17] Infants that weigh 1 to 2 kg should then gain about 20 gm a day. The estimated requirements are as follows:

Water: up to 200 ml per kilogram
Energy: 110 to 125 kcal per kilogram
Protein: 3 to 4 gm per kilogram

Supplements. In addition to the formula, supplements of iron and of the fat-soluble and water-soluble vitamins are indicated.[17] Anemia is common in premature infants and a daily supplement of 2 mg iron per kilogram is advisable. Larger iron supplements can lead to vitamin E deficiency and increased hemolytic effects. Not only are the vitamin E stores in the infant low, but the absorption of the vitamin is also likely to be reduced.[8] The multivitamin supplement includes 5 IU (3.3 mg α-tocopherol) vitamin E and 50 μg folacin. The infant has reduced ability to metabolize the aromatic amino acids, phenylalanine and tyrosine, and to correct this defect 60 mg ascorbic acid is recommended. Because of the increased tendency to rickets, 10μg vitamin D is also included.

Selection of Formula The formula must be appropriate for the nutritional requirements, the gastrointestinal osmotic load, and the renal osmotic load. For premature infants the protein content of the formula can be 16 per cent of the calories. Protein levels at 5 to 6 gm per kilogram may present an excessive renal solute load. Concentrated formulas increase the gastrointestinal osmotic load and can lead to loose stools and diuresis. Rickard and Gresham[17] suggest that human milk and several commercial formulas* avoid excessive osmotic load when fed at a concentration of 85 kcal per 100 ml (24 kcal per ounce) or less. When the concentration of the formula is increased, the specific gravity of the urine should be watched closely.

Methods of Feeding The oral route, as often as every hour or two, is the preferred method if the baby is able to suck or swallow. Since the initial amounts taken are very small, parenteral feeding by peripheral vein may be used as a supplement, including synthetic amino acids, multivitamins, and minerals.

If the baby is unable to suck or swallow, gavage feedings can be given every 2 or 3 hours. The capacity of the stomach is easily exceeded, and careful monitoring is necessary to avoid overdistention, regurgitation, and aspiration. An indwelling na-

* Enfamil, Mead Johnson Laboratories, Evansville, Indiana. Similac, Isomil (soy-based formula), Ross Laboratories, Columbus, Ohio.

sogastric or nasojejunal tube with constant drip has been used with some success.[17]

Total parenteral alimentation through an indwelling catheter in the superior vena cava permits adequate caloric and nutrient intake. It is not a routine procedure for LBW infants, but is an alternative when oral or tube feeding is not feasible or when these feedings remain inadequate for prolonged periods.

Schedule of Feeding The schedule suggested by Rickard and Gresham is as follows:[17]

First day. Give 65 to 150 ml per kilogram of 10 percent glucose intravenously with multivitamin supplement and iron.

Second day. By gavage or nipple give 3 ml per kilogram of a formula providing 70 kcal per 100 ml (20 kcal per ounce). Give feedings every 2 hours for the smallest babies. At every other feeding increase the amount of formula by 1 to 2 ml, provided there are no adverse effects. Include oral multivitamins and iron. Continue the intravenous glucose, allowing a total volume, including the formula, of 80 to 150 ml per kilogram.

Third day. Increase the strength of the formula to 85 kcal per 100 ml (24 kcal per ounce). Gradually increase the size of the feedings as on day 2. Continue the multivitamins and iron. Continue the intravenous glucose allowing a total volume of intake, including the formula, that ranges between 100 to 200 ml per kilogram.

By the fourth day the caloric intake should reach 90 kcal per kilogram, and by the seventh day 100 kcal per kilogram. If the caloric intake is less, it becomes necessary to consider intragastric infusions or transpyloric feeding.

Problems and Review

1. Key words: bifidus factor; colostrum; development; extrusion reflex; growth; LBW infant; rooting reflex; SGA infant; terminal sterilization of formula.
2. Select an article from the list of references pertaining to breast feeding and on the basis of your reading prepare a 200-word summary of viewpoints on breast feeding.
3. What advantages can be claimed for a commercially prepared formula compared with one prepared in the home? What disadvantages could be cited?
4. What adjustments must be made in cow's milk to make it suitable for infant feeding?
5. *Problem.* Examine the labeling of four popular brands of premodified formulas. How much of each would be required for a 4-month infant weighing 5.5 kg? Are any supplements required? Calculate the cost of each formula for one day.
6. What important nutrients are provided by each of the following additions to the infant's diet: cereal; fruits; vegetables; meat; citrus juices?
7. *Problem.* Develop a lesson plan that you could use for counseling a group of mothers on the home preparation of vegetables that could be used for 6-month-old babies.
8. What are the possible consequences of each of the following: an overconcentrated formula; overweight; addition of salt to baby's foods; ice cream, gelatin, or pudding for dessert; raw egg added to formula at 4 months; certified raw milk at 6 months?
9. How do the nutritional requirements of low-birth-weight infants differ from those of normal full-term infants?

Cited References

1. Raab, C. A.: "The Nitrite Dilemma: Pink and Preserved?" *J. Nutr. Educ.*, 5:8–9, 1973.

2. Owen, G., and Lippman, G.: "Nutritional Status of Infants and Young Children: U.S.A." *Pediatr. Clin. North Am.*, **24**:211–27, 1977.
3. Eid, E. E.: "Follow-up Study of Physical Growth of Children Who Had Excessive Weight Gain in First Six Months of Life," *Brit. Med. J.*, **2**:74–77, 1970.
4. Food and Nutrition Board: *Recommended Dietary Allowances*, 9th ed. National Research Council–National Academy of Sciences, Washington, D.C., 1980.
5. Jackson, R. L.: "Maternal and Infant Nutrition and Health in Later Life," *Nutr. Rev.*, **37**:33–37, 1979.
6. Committee on Nutrition, American Academy of Pediatrics: "Iron Supplementation for Infants," *Pediatrics*, **58**:765–67, 1976.
7. Filer, L. J.: "Salt in Infant Foods," *Nutr. Rev.*, **29**:27–30, 1971.
8. Williams, M. L., et al.: "Role of Dietary Iron and Fat on Vitamin E Deficiency Anemia of Infancy," *N. Engl. J. Med.*, **292**:887–90, 1975.
9. Kabara, J. J.: "Lipids as Host-Resistance Factors in Human Milk," *Nutr. Rev.*, **38**:65–73, 1980.
10. Peterkin, B., and Walker, S.: "Food for the Baby—Cost and Nutritive Value Considerations," *Family Econ. Rev.*, U.S. Department of Agriculture, Fall 1976.
11. Fomon, S. J., et al.: "Recommendations for Feeding Normal Infants," *Pediatrics*, **63**:52–59, 1979.
12. Committee on Nutrition, American Academy of Pediatrics: "Commentary on Breast-feeding and Infant Formulas, Including Proposed Standards for Formulas," *Nutr. Rev.*, **34**:248–56, 1976.
13. Arnon, S. S., et al.: "Honey and Other Risk Factors for Infant Botulism," *J. Pediatr.*, **94**:331–36, 1979.
14. Filer, L. J., Jr.: "Modified Food Starches for Use in Infant Foods," *Nutr. Rev.*, **29**:55–59, 1971.
15. Committee on Nutrition, American Academy of Pediatrics: "Salt Intake and Eating Patterns of Infants and Children in Relation to Blood Pressure," *Pediatrics*, **53**:115–21, 1974.
16. Dubois, S., et al.: "An Examination of Factors Believed to Be Associated with Infantile Obesity," *Am. J. Clin. Nutr.*, **32**:1997–2004, 1979.
17. Rickard, K., and Gresham, E.: "Nutritional Considerations for the Newborn Requiring Intensive Care," *J. Am. Diet. Assoc.*, **66**:592–600, 1975.

Additional References

ABRAMS, C. A. L., et al.: "Hazards of Overconcentrated Milk Formulas," *JAMA*, **232**:1136–40, 1975.

BEAL, V. A.: "Breast- and Formula-feeding of Infants," *J. Am. Diet. Assoc.*, **55**:31–37, 1969.

Committee on Nutrition, American Academy of Pediatrics: "Breast-feeding. A Commentary in Celebration of the International Year of the Child," *Pediatrics*, **62**:591–601, 1978.

HIMES, J. H.: "Infant Feeding Practices and Obesity," *J. Am. Diet. Assoc.*, **75**:122–25, 1979.

LACKEY, C. J.: "International Symposium on Infant and Child Feeding," *Nutr. Today*, **13**:11–16, 31–32, November/December 1978.

MARLIN, D. W., et al.: "Infant Feeding Practices," *J. Am. Diet. Assoc.*, **77**:668–76, 1980.

PAO, E. M., et al.: "Milk Intakes and Feeding Patterns of Breast-fed Infants," *J. Am. Diet. Assoc.*, **77**:540–45, 1980.

Review: "Vitamin B_{12} Deficiency in the Breast-fed Infant of a Strict Vegetarian. Clinical Nutrition Case," *Nutr. Rev.*, **37**:142–144, 1979.

Nutrition for Children and Teenagers 20

EACH person inherits a unique genetic pattern upon which the environment throughout life brings about modifications in physical, biochemical, mental, and emotional characteristics. The rate of growth and maturation and the activity of the child and teenager, rather than chronological age, are the more accurate predictors of nutritional needs. Desirable food behaviors for a lifetime have their beginnings in childhood and adolescence.

Current Issues

Parents, as well as health workers, continue to seek answers to questions concerning the nutritional care of children. Among the recent concerns are these:

What dietary measures can be taken during childhood to reduce the risks of chronic diseases later in life?

Can nontraditional diet patterns, for example, vegetarian diets, meet the nutritional needs of children?

The consumption of fast foods has increased greatly during the past decade. How well do these foods provide nutritional needs? What restraints, if any, are advisable concerning their use by teenagers?

What dietary regimen can be recommended for athletes?

Nutritional Requirements

Changes in Growth and Development Neither growth nor development occurs at a uniform rate. The rapid growth in overall size that occurred in fetal life and during infancy is followed by a long period of very gradual growth that accelerates again in the adolescent years. The three phases of cellular growth continue: rapid cell division; slowing of cell division but increase in cell size; and cessation of cell division with continuing protein synthesis and increase in cell size. These phases follow a chronological schedule with the timing differing for the various organs and tissues of the body. For example, brain development is rapid during fetal life and infancy whereas sexual maturation takes place during the teen years.

During the second year the toddler increases in height by 7 to 8 cm and gains 3 to 4 kg, approximately quadrupling the birth rate. Thereafter, until the preadolescent period the annual gains in height are 6 to 7 cm and in weight 1½ to 3 kg. Boys are taller and heavier at each age than girls, except about 11 to 12 years when girls are usually heavier.

As growth proceeds there are changes in the proportions of water, muscle tissue, fat deposits, and skeletal structures. The body water decreases gradually with the addition of adipose tissue and of minerals to the bones. The body protein content has increased from 14.6 per cent at the end of the first year to the adult level of 18 to 19 per cent of body weight by 4 years of age.[1] At a given age girls have a higher percentage of body fat than boys but less muscle tissue.

The number, size, and composition of the bones change from birth to maturity. The skeleton has reached its full size in girls by the age of 17 years, and in boys at 20 years. The water content of the bones gradually diminishes as the mineralization increases. Provided that the diet remains good, bone mineralization continues for several years after the attainment of full size.

Adolescent Growth and Development The adolescent period covers almost a decade. It is characterized by rapid increase in height and weight, by hormonal changes, by sexual maturation, and by wide swings in emotions. The patterns of body water, lean body mass, bone, and fat show increasing differences between boys and girls.

For a year or two before and during adolescence the growth rate accelerates and is second only to that of infancy. The growth spurt in girls occurs at approximately 11 to 14 years and in boys between 13 and 16 years. The annual peak rate for height and weight in girls averages about 9 cm and 8 to 9 kg, respectively. For boys the annual peak rate, reached about 2 years later, is 10 cm and 10 kg.

Along with the spurt in height of girls, development of the breasts and axillary and pubic hair takes place. Menarche occurs after the peak velocity in growth. With these changes in growth the fat content of the girl's body has increased from about 10 per cent at 9 to 10 years to 20 to 24 per cent at the beginning of menarche. The fat content of the girl's body at age 20 is about 1½ times that of boys.

By 18 to 20 years boys have achieved their full height, but small increases in stature are often observed during the next decade. At the end of the growth period boys will have 1½ times as much lean body mass as girls. At the beginning of the growth spurt sexual changes in boys appear: deepening of the voice; broadening of the shoulders; development of axillary, body, and pubic hair; and growth of the penis and testicles.

Dietary Allowances Because the anabolic activities are considerable during the entire period of childhood, the nutritional requirements in proportion to body size are much higher than they will be in the adult years. Moreover, childhood and adolescence are times of considerable physical activity and hence the energy requirement is greater. The recommended dietary allowances are designed to support optimum growth and development. When using these allowances it is important to interpret them in terms of the child's size as well as with reference to chronologic age. (See Table 3–1.)

Energy. At any given age the energy requirements will vary widely depending upon the level of growth and activity. A deficit of as little as 10 kcal per kilogram body weight can lead to growth failure and reduced nitrogen retention even though the protein intake is adequate.[2] Average energy requirements for each age category are listed in Table 20–1. Although the total energy requirements increase with age, the per kilogram allowances gradually decline.

Protein. The protein allowances range from 1.8 gm per kilogram at 1 to 3 years to the adult level of 0.8 gm per kilogram by 18 years of age. (See Table 20–1.) From 10 to 15 per cent of calories are normally derived from protein—a level that exceeds the recommended allowances.

Minerals. The recommended calcium and phosphorus allowances are 800 mg for

Table 20-1. Recommended Energy and Protein Allowances for Children and Teenagers*

Age	Energy		Protein	
Years	Per Day kcal	Per Kg kcal	Per Day gm	Per Kg gm
Children				
1–3	1,300	100	23	1.8
4–6	1,700	85	30	1.5
7–10	2,400	85	34	1.2
Boys				
11–14	2,700	60	45	1.0
15–18	2,800	42	56	0.85
Girls				
11–14	2,200	48	46	1.0
15–18	2,100	38	46	0.84

*Calculations per kilogram body weight are based on mean weights for each age category. See Table 3-1.

children from 1 to 10 years, and 1,200 mg for adolescents. The greatest retention of calcium and phosphorus precedes the period of rapid growth by 2 years or more, and liberal intakes of these minerals before the age of 10 are a distinct advantage. Children whose diets have been poor require a diet adequate in nutrients for as long as 6 months before they can equal the calcium and phosphorus retention of children on a good diet.[3] Such a lag in retention can be a special hazard for the poorly nourished girl who becomes pregnant.

Adequacy of calcium intake is directly correlated with the intake of milk or milk foods. All nonmilk foods in the diet can be expected to yield only 0.2 gm calcium to young children, and 0.3 gm calcium to older children.

The data on magnesium requirements for children are limited. The allowances range from 150 mg for children at 1 to 3 years to 250 mg at 7 to 10 years. Boys from 11 to 18 years should receive daily allowances of 350 to 400 mg and girls should receive 300 mg. One quart of milk furnishes about 120 mg magnesium, and dark green leafy vegetables are also good sources. Although many diets reasonably adequate in other nutrients fail to provide the recommended allowances for magnesium, symptoms of magnesium deficiency have not been demonstrated.

The recommended allowances for iron are 15 mg at 1 to 3 years, 10 mg at 4 to 10 years, and 18 mg at 11 to 18 years. The iron needs are met only when emphasis is given to factors that favor iron absorption (see Chapter 8) and to inclusion of a wide variety of meats, legumes, whole-grain or enriched breads and cereals, and green leafy vegetables and fruits. Some children consume milk in excessive amounts thus crowding out other essential iron-rich foods.

Iodized salt should be used throughout childhood and adolescence because of the high rate of energy metabolism and the increased activity of the thyroid gland.

The allowance for zinc is 10 mg for preadolescent children and 15 mg for boys and girls. Animal foods furnish higher levels of available zinc than do vegetable foods.

Vitamins. The vitamin requirements of children have not been extensively studied. Throughout childhood and adolescence 10 μg (400 IU) vitamin D should be provided—an allowance met by 1 quart of fortified milk. The vitamin A needs are related to body weight with the allowance increasing from 400 RE (2,000 IU) at 1 to 3 years to 1,000 RE (5,000 IU) for boys and 800 RE (4,000 IU) for girls. These allowances are easily met by including milk, margarine or butter, dark green or deep yellow vegetables and fruits, egg yolk, and liver. The vitamin E allowances ranging from 5 to 10 mg α-tocopherol equivalents are provided by vegetable oils, margarines, whole grains, legumes, nuts, and dark green leafy vegetables.

Ascorbic acid allowances range from 45 mg for 1-to-6-year-olds to 60 mg for 15-to-18-year-olds. Thiamin and niacin allowances are 0.5 and 6.6 mg, respectively, for each 1,000 kcal. The range of riboflavin allowance is from 0.8 to 1.4 mg for children, up to 1.7 mg for boys, and up to 1.3 mg for girls.

Vitamin B-6 allowances are based upon 0.02 mg per gram of expected protein intake as estimated from surveys of food consumption.[1] Thus, toddlers should receive 0.9 mg daily whereas teenage girls and boys need 1.8 and 2.0 mg.

Folacin allowances supply 8 to 10 μg per kilogram body weight. Green leafy vegetables, fruits, legumes, and liver supply generous amounts. Vitamin B-12 needs ranging from 1.5 to 3.0 μg are readily met when the diet includes foods from animal origin.

Nutritional Status of Children

Assessment of Nutritional Status The determination of nutritional status can be made only by specialists qualified to give comprehensive physical and dental examinations, to make biochemical studies of the blood and urine, and to evaluate patterns of growth and measurements of body size. (See Chapter 22.) However, every mother, teacher, or nurse should be aware of these characteristics of the well-nourished child:

SENSE OF WELL-BEING: alert, interested in activities usual for the age; vigorous; happy
VITALITY: endurance during activity, quick recovery from fatigue; looks rested; does not fall asleep in school, sleeps well at night
WEIGHT: normal for height, age, and body build
POSTURE: erect; arms and legs straight; abdomen pulled in; chest out
TEETH: straight, without crowding in well-shaped jaw
GUMS: firm, pink; no signs of bleeding
SKIN: smooth, slightly moist; healthy glow; reddish-pink mucous membranes
EYES: clear, bright; no circles of fatigue around them
HAIR: lustrous; healthy scalp
MUSCLES: well developed; firm
NERVOUS CONTROL: good attention span for age; gets along well with others; does not cry easily; not irritable and restless
GASTROINTESTINAL FACTORS: good appetite; normal, regular elimination

Dietary Adequacy Numerous surveys of the diets of children have shown that the intakes of calcium, iron, ascorbic acid, and vitamin A are often below recommended allowances. The National Food Consumption Survey of 1977 identified the age groups that had average intakes of nutrients below the RDA.[4] It must be remembered, however, that average intakes conceal those persons who might have had intakes much lower or higher than the RDA. In this survey the averages that were significantly low were these:

Toddlers, 1 to 2 years: iron
Females, over 12 years: calcium, iron
Females, over 15 years: vitamin B-6

Surveys on the diets of children have shown that a direct correlation exists between the adequacy of the diet and the socioeconomic status. Based on the caloric level, the quality of the diet of children in poor families is generally good. The principal problem lies in an insufficient quantity of food to meet the child's need. The diets of Hispanic and black children were often low in iron, ascorbic acid, and vitamin A.[5]

Nutritional Status Because the RDAs provide a margin of safety for most persons, a diet that fails to meet these standards cannot be interpreted as a decline in nutritional status. Indeed, national studies[5-7] have shown that children and teenagers, for the most part, have satisfactory nutritional status. Better economic conditions and access to assistance in nutrition programs have contributed substantially to improvement in recent years. Nonetheless, several nutritional problems persist to a varying degree and these should be addressed so that they can be prevented or corrected. These problems occur more frequently in the lower socioeconomic groups.

Dental caries is widespread and occurs in all economic groups. Among preventive measures are these: prenatal and postnatal nutrition with special emphasis on calcium, phosphorus, vitamins A and D, and ascorbic acid; use of fluoridated water throughout childhood; reduced frequency of contact of sticky carbohydrates with tooth surfaces; and good dental hygiene.

Anemia caused by iron deficiency is present in 5 to 10 per cent of children in some groups and as high as 25 to 30 per cent in other groups. Preschool children are especially vulnerable. Intestinal parasites contribute to the incidence of anemia in some geographic areas. Many children have normal hemoglobin and hematocrit values but have a low transferrin saturation. Thus, in times of stress such as infections there could be limited iron stores upon which to draw.

Obesity. About 10 to 20 per cent of children and teenagers are overweight and the likelihood is great that they will be obese as adults. Some but not all obese infants are obese at 8 to 10 years, during adolescence, and into adult life. However, environmental factors are likely to be more important contributors to obesity such as a sedentary life-style with too many hours spent watching television; too little activity even though participating in outdoor sports; ready access to calorie-rich foods; and substitution of food for social relationships and to counteract emotional problems.

Growth failure. A significant number of children are underweight and undersized. (See Figure 20-1.) Such children usually tire easily, are irritable and restless, and are more susceptible to infections. Underweight especially in teenagers increases the risk of tuberculosis. Adolescent girls sometimes make exaggerated efforts to lose weight and may succumb to *anorexia nervosa,* a serious nutritional and psychologic problem. (See also Chapter 42).

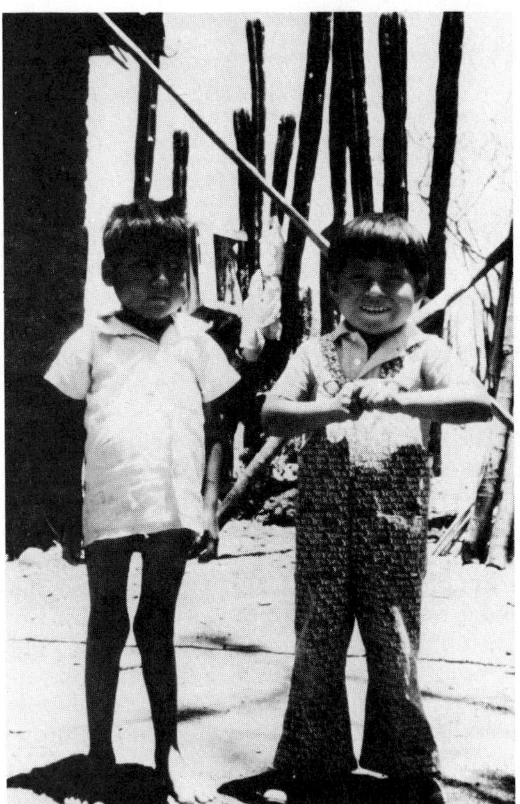

Figure 20–1. Growth retardation. The child on the right is 3 years younger than the child on the left. Not only is he better nourished and healthier than the other child, but his parents who are equally poor keep their child cleaner and better dressed. (UNICEF photo by Chavez.)

"Catch-up" growth can take place within predetermined limits. The undernourished child, if given an adequate diet, will gain weight rapidly until he or she approaches the norm for height. Then weight and height increase together toward the expected norm. The degree to which such "catch-up" growth occurs seems to be related to the length of the period of undernutrition, the stage of development, and the interaction of other factors such as illness.

Pregnancy in adolescent girls is a nutritional problem of considerable importance. (See Chapter 18.)

Food Behavior

Food Habits and Development Food continues to be a major factor in the development of the whole person throughout the growing years. Food becomes a means of communication; it has cultural and social meanings; it is intimately associated with the emotions; and its acceptance or rejection is highly personal.

The environment in which the child lives determines the food behavior and the quality of nutrition. Sims and Morris[8] have studied environmental factors by considering the family as one ecosystem and the child as a second ecosystem. The family has responsibility for the child's food, controls the child's access to the foods, and establishes the emotional climate. Interacting factors within the family include the family composition, income, general education, the stability of the family, the quality of housing, the attitudes toward food, parental knowledge of nutrition, attitudes toward child rearing—authoritarian or nonauthoritarian—and others.

The child is the second ecosystem. From the family ecosystem he or she uses information, materials, and energy, and nutrient intake is the output of the family ecosystem. The nutrient supply is processed by the child to the output of his or her own ecosystem, namely an individual development and nutritional status.

Good food habits have several characteristics. First, the pattern of diet permits the individual to achieve the maximum genetic potential for his or her physical and mental development. Second, the food habits are conducive to delaying or preventing the onset of degenerative diseases that are so prevalent in American society today. Third, the food habits are part of satisfying human relationships and contribute to social and personal enjoyment. The development of food habits is a continuous process in which each year builds upon what has gone before. The responsibility of parents and all who work with children goes far beyond ensuring the ingestion of specified levels of nutrients. It requires the application of knowledge from the fields of human behavior and development, psychology, sociology, and anthropology.

Common Dietary Errors Studies of food habits of children have shown repeatedly that the foods requiring particular emphasis for the improvement of diets are milk, dark green leafy and deep yellow vegetables, and whole-grain or enriched breads and cereals. Among the food habits that contribute to these deficiencies are these:

POOR BREAKFAST OR NONE AT ALL: lack of appetite; getting up too late; no one to prepare breakfast; monotony of breakfast foods; no protein at breakfast, meaning that the distribution of good quality protein is poor even though the day's total may be satisfactory; too little fruit, meaning that ascorbic acid often is not obtained.

POOR LUNCHES: failure to participate in school lunch program; poor box lunches; spending lunch money for snacks or other items; unsatisfactory management of school lunch program with resultant poor menus, poor food preparation, excessive plate waste.

SNACKS: account for as much as one fourth of calories without providing significant amounts of protein, minerals, and vitamins; often eaten too near to mealtime thus spoiling the appetite. (See also page 372.)

OVERUSE OF MILK, ESPECIALLY BY YOUNGER CHILDREN: other foods are not eaten so that the intake of iron and certain vitamins may be low.

SELF-IMPOSED DIETING, ESPECIALLY BY TEENAGE GIRLS: caloric restriction but no consideration given to protein, minerals, and vitamins.

IRREGULAR EATING HABITS: few meals with the family group; no adult supervision in eating; children often prepare own meals without guidance.

FOOD DISLIKES: little exposure to new foods; limited variety from day to day.

Diet for the Preschool Child

Food Selection Correlated with Behavioral Changes The nutritional requirements of the child cannot be satisfied apart from an understanding of behavioral changes that occur. Toddlers have a short attention span and are easily distracted from eating. Their response to food is often inconsistent. They have limited muscle coordination at this age, and their eating behavior can best be described as messy. Also, by handling food they learn about its textures. If given the opportunity the toddler quickly learns to take advantage of parents through his or her food behavior. As the child enters the 3-to-5-year-old group the attention span is somewhat longer, and muscle coordination is much better although the child still has some problems from time to time in the handling of utensils. (See Figure 20–2.)

During the second year the appetite tapers off corresponding to the slower rate of growth. Beal[9] found that healthy, well-nourished girls reduced their milk intake as early as 6 months and returned to higher intakes at 2 to 3 years of age. Boys also reduced their milk intake at about 9 months,

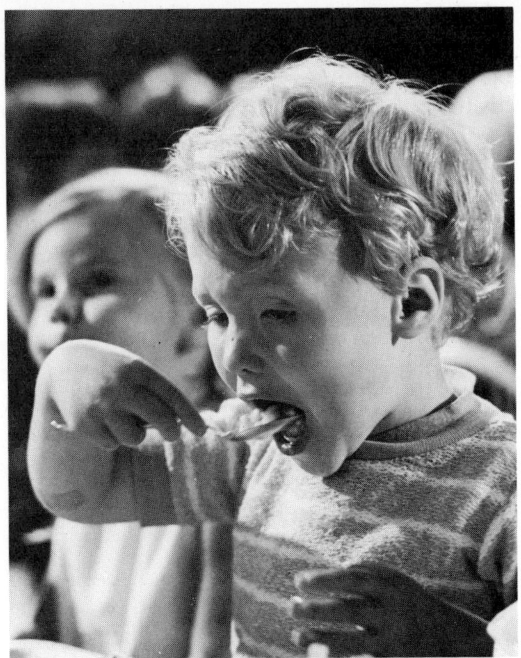

Figure 20–2. The young child gradually develops muscle coordination as he tries to feed himself. A word of encouragement now and then is helpful. (Courtesy, U.S. Department of Agriculture.)

but started to increase their consumption between 1 and 2 years. An intake of 2 cups or less is not uncommon for a period of time. Some children's appetities improve by 5 years or earlier, but other children have poor appetities well into the school years.

Many mothers must be reassured that the child will remain well nourished provided that foods of high nutrient density are offered, and that feeding does not become an issue between mother and child. Some compensation for the reduced consumption of milk may be made by incorporating milk into foods such as simple puddings. The occasional use of flavorings such as molasses or cocoa may increase milk acceptance. Children are sometimes encouraged to drink milk if they are permitted to pour it for themselves from a small pitcher. Cottage cheese, yogurt, and mild American cheese are often well liked and help to increase the calcium intake as well as the protein.

Because young children have a high taste sensitivity they prefer mildly flavored foods. Generally they like meat, chicken, and milk. Fruits are well liked but vegetables are frequently disliked. Plain foods are preferred to mixtures such as casserole dishes, creamed dishes, and stews. Preschool children do not like extremes of food temperatures, and may seem to dawdle until the mashed potatoes are lukewarm or the ice cream is beginning to melt.

The feel of food is important to young children, and they enjoy foods that can be picked up with the fingers such as pieces of raw vegetables, small sandwiches, strips of cheese or meat, and narrow wedges of fruit. The ability to chew food should determine the textures that are given. Toddlers may be given chopped vegetables and ground meat, whereas the 3- to 5-year-old can manage diced vegetables and minced or bite-size pieces of tender meat. Foods that are stringy such as celery, sticky such as some mashed potatoes, or slippery such as custard are often disliked because the child is not familiar with the texture.

Food jags are not uncommon, especially between the ages of 2 and 4 years. The child may shun all but a few foods, such as milk or peanut-butter-and-jelly sandwiches. Such occurrences do not last too long, if the parent does not show concern, and if the foods which constitute the child's preference at the moment are nutritious in general.

Preschool children are almost constantly active. Their interest is readily diverted from food. If they become overtired or excessively hungry, their appetites may lag a great deal.

Daily food allowances. A selection of a variety of foods from the milk, meat, vegetable-fruit, and bread-cereal groups provides a sound basis for the child's diet. Although intakes vary widely, the following amounts provide a guide:

2 cups milk, fortified with vitamin D
3–4 eggs per week
1–3 ounces chopped meat, fish, or poultry; or equivalent of cheese, legumes, or peanut butter
4 ounces orange juice or other source of ascorbic acid
2–4 tablespoons other fruit such as banana, peaches, pears, apple, apricot, prunes
2–4 tablespoons vegetables, including deep yellow and dark green leafy
1 potato
1 raw vegetable such as carrot sticks, cabbage slices, lettuce, tomato
⅓ to ⅔ cup enriched dry or cooked cereal
1–3 slices enriched or whole-grain bread

The three-meal pattern used for adult members of the family is appropriate for the child, but some snacks in midmorning and midafternoon are also necessary. Very active children become excessively fatigued and hungry if they are not fed between meals. Snacks should make a liberal contribution to the nutrient requirements. Some that are suitable for preschool children are

Fruit juices without sugar
Milk and milk beverages; yogurt, plain or with fruit
Cheese cubes
Fruit of any kind
Raw vegetables: carrot sticks, celery sticks, cauliflower buds, green beans, rutabaga sticks, broccoli buds, zucchini slices, cherry tomatoes, green pepper slices
Molasses, oatmeal, or peanut butter cookies
Dry cereal from the box or with milk
NOTE: Very young children should not be given nuts, popcorn, seeds, or vegetable sticks since they may choke on them and aspirate the food items.

Establishing Good Food Habits Suggestions have been made in the preceding chapter for the establishment of good food habits in the infant. In addition, the following considerations are conducive to the development of good food habits in the preschool child.

Meals should be served at regular hours in a pleasant environment. The child should be comfortably seated at a table. Deep dishes permit the child to get the food onto the fork or spoon with greater ease. A fork, such as a salad fork with blunt tines, and a small spoon can be handled comfortably. A small cup or glass should be only partially filled with liquid to minimize spilling; however, the coordination of eye, hand, and mouth is difficult and some spilling is to be expected.

Children enjoy colorful meals just as adults do. Their appetites also vary from day to day, and like adults they react strongly to portions that are too large. It is much better to serve less than the child is likely to eat and to let him or her ask for more.

Even favorite foods should not be served too often. Breakfasts do not need to be stereotyped. A hamburger or sandwich and an orange cut in sections to be picked up with the fingers is just as satisfactory as a juice, cereal, and egg breakfast.

Fewer difficulties are likely to be encountered if new foods are given at the beginning of the meal when the child is hungry. A food is more likely to be accepted if it is given in a form which can be easily handled, which can be chewed, and if some favorite food is also included in the same meal. A taste or two is enough for any new food that is offered. Encouragement and praise are helpful, but favorite foods should not be used as a bribe or reward for taking the new food. Any new food should be offered at regular intervals until the child learns to accept it.

Whether or not the preschool child should eat with other members of the family or alone is a matter that individual parents must determine for the child's greatest good and the family's convenience. In most situations the young child should eat with the rest of the family because the interactions between family members are a part of normal development. If, however, the evening meal must be late, if the child becomes overexcited about the family doings, or if the child is expected to live up to a code of behavior beyond his or her young years, it is better that the child be allowed to eat before the rest of the family in a pleasant, quiet atmosphere with the parent nearby. Even so, an occasional meal with the family is a treat for the child and parent if tension can be avoided. Since children are great imitators, they enjoy doing just as the parents or the other children are doing.

The child may well learn early in life that he or she is expected to eat foods that are prepared, but this does not mean that nagging or bribery will accomplish anything. Children, like adults, enjoy attention, and they are quick to realize that food can be a powerful weapon for gaining such attention. A display of concern or the use of force in getting a child to drink milk or to take any other food can have nothing but unfavorable effects. When a child refuses to take a food, the unwanted item should be calmly removed without comment after a reasonable period of time. If the child is refusing to eat because this behavior attracts attention, the parent should make certain that the child receives a full share of affection and companionship at other than mealtimes. If this is done the child will lose interest in using food as a weapon.

Diet for the Schoolchild

Characteristics of Food Acceptance Elementary-school children are usually better fed than preschool children or adolescents. Group acceptance is extremely important at this time, and the child needs to be able to keep up with classmates and to have a sense of accomplishment. When the child goes to school for the first time he or she makes acquaintance with food patterns that may be different from those at home. The child learns that certain foods are acceptable to the peer group, whereas other foods from a different cultural pattern may be looked upon with disdain; as a result he or she may be unwilling to accept these foods at home—good though they may be. On the other hand, within a group the child is willing to try foods with which he or she is unacquainted and would not try alone.

Schoolchildren have relatively few dislikes for food except possibly for vegetables, which are usually not eaten in satisfactory amounts. By the time children reach 8 to 10 years of age the appetite is usually very good. Feeding problems are more likely to result because parents are unduly concerned with behavior at mealtime which does not come up to adult standards. Most children of this age are in a hurry, and do not like to take time for meals. Breakfast, especially, is likely to be skipped.

Schoolchildren are subject to many stresses which affect the appetite. Communicable diseases occur often in this age group. They reduce the appetite on the one hand, but they increase body needs on the other. Schoolwork, class competition, and emotional stresses in getting along with many children may have adverse effects on appetite, as may also an unbalanced program of activity and rest.

Choice of Foods Table 20–2 lists the kinds and amounts of foods which may be taken in a day by healthy schoolchildren. A number of other equally satisfactory patterns could be devised for different cultural groups. A diet for adults which places emphasis first on the inclusion of protein, minerals, and vitamins is also a good one for schoolchildren. The amount of milk given to children should be greater than that for the adult. Although no foods need to be forbidden to this age group, it is extremely important that high-carbohydrate and high-fat foods not be allowed to replace essential items of the diet.

Food Habits The suggestions concerning good food habits for preschool children also apply to schoolchildren. A good school lunch program (see page 378) may introduce new foods in a setting where the child is anxious to conform to the group. The ele-

Table 20-2. **Foods to Meet Nutritional Needs of Elementary-School Children and Teenagers**

Food	6 to 10 Years	10 to 12 Years	12 to 16 Years
Milk, vitamin-D fortified	2–3 cups	3–4 cups	4 cups or more
Eggs	3–4 per week	3–4 per week	3–4 per week
Meat, poultry, fish	2–3 ounces (small serving)	3–4 ounces (average serving)	4 ounces
Dried beans, peas, or peanut butter	2 servings each week. If used as an alternative for meat, allow ½ cup cooked beans or peas or 2 tablespoons peanut butter for 1 ounce meat		
Potatoes, white or sweet (occasionally spaghetti, macaroni, rice, noodles, etc.)	1 small or ⅓ cup	1 medium or ½ cup	1 large or ¾ cup
Other cooked vegetable (green leafy or deep yellow 3 to 4 times a week)	¼ cup	⅓ cup	½ cup or more
Raw vegetable (salad greens, cabbage, celery, carrots, etc.)	¼ cup	⅓ cup	½ cup
Vitamin C food (citrus fruit, tomato, cantaloupe, etc.)	1 medium orange or equivalent	1 medium orange or equivalent	1 large orange or equivalent
Other fruit	1 portion or more as: 1 apple, 1 banana, 1 peach, 1 pear, ½ cup cooked fruit		
Bread, enriched or whole grain	3 slices or more	3 slices or more	4–6 slices or more
Cereal, enriched or whole grain	½ cup	¾ cup	1 cup or more
Additional foods	Butter or margarine, desserts, etc., to satisfy energy needs		

mentary teacher should integrate nutrition education with the total classroom experience so that good food habits are strengthened.

Since children are likely to be in a hurry, it is often wise to require that a certain time be spent at the table—say 15 or 20 minutes—so that the child will take time to eat. Children learn good manners by imitation of adults, and not by continuous correction at the table. During the elementary-school years, little can be gained by overemphasis of manners. In fact, the food intake may be adversely affected.

Diet for the Teenager

Adolescent Dietary Problems Even boys and girls who have had an excellent pattern of food intake are likely to succumb to bizarre, unbalanced diets during the adolescent years. Teenagers have many concerns about their development such as the size and shape of the body, sexual development, skin conditions, vitality, attractiveness, and approval by their peers. They feel independent and seek freedom to make their own decisions. It is a period when family conflict is likely to increase. The advice of teachers and coaches is often taken more seriously than that of parents.

Failure to maintain normal weight is a frequently recurring problem. Obesity occurs more frequently in girls, whereas underweight is more prevalent in boys. The caloric intake by overweight girls is often no greater than that of girls of normal weight, but the caloric expenditure is less because of limited activity.

The teenager is concerned about his or her weight. Most girls want to weigh less; they want smaller hips, smaller thighs, and smaller waists but larger busts. Most boys want to weigh more and they equate overweight with muscle development which is desirable. They want a larger upper torso and arms, an indication of strength.[10]

Stresses of various kinds have an adverse effect on nutrition. The incidence of tuberculosis is higher than it should be in adolescent years and in early adulthood and is believed to occur more frequently in those who have inadequate diets, especially with respect to protein and calcium. Teenage pregnancy can have serious effects on the girl who has a poor intake of essential nutrients. (See page 333.)

Emotional difficulties often stem from the feeling of social inadequacy or the pressures of schoolwork. Where there is conflict within the home because of the teenager's food choices, failure to accept responsibilities, the use of money, dating hours, and so on, the emotions not only determine the food intake but also modify nutrient utilization. For example, negative nitrogen and mineral balances have been observed when students were taking examinations or when young women were upset about a pregnancy.

Selection of Foods Because of their high energy requirements boys are more likely to meet their nutrient needs than are girls. Emphasis upon green leafy and deep yellow vegetables is necessary for both boys and girls. In addition girls need to increase their intake of milk and whole-grain or enriched breads and cereals. The list in Table 20–2 serves as a starting point for the planning of meals.

Snacks furnish about one fourth of the energy requirement of most adolescents. They should also furnish an equivalent amount of the day's allowance for protein, minerals, and vitamins. Thus, sandwiches, hamburgers, pizza, fruit, and milk are types of snacks to be encouraged. A recent study has shown that typical teenage snacks are better nutritionally than many people have believed them to be. For each 100 kcal supplied by the snacks there are substantial contributions of protein, calcium, iron, vitamin A, thiamin, riboflavin, and ascorbic acid.[11] (See Figure 20–3.)

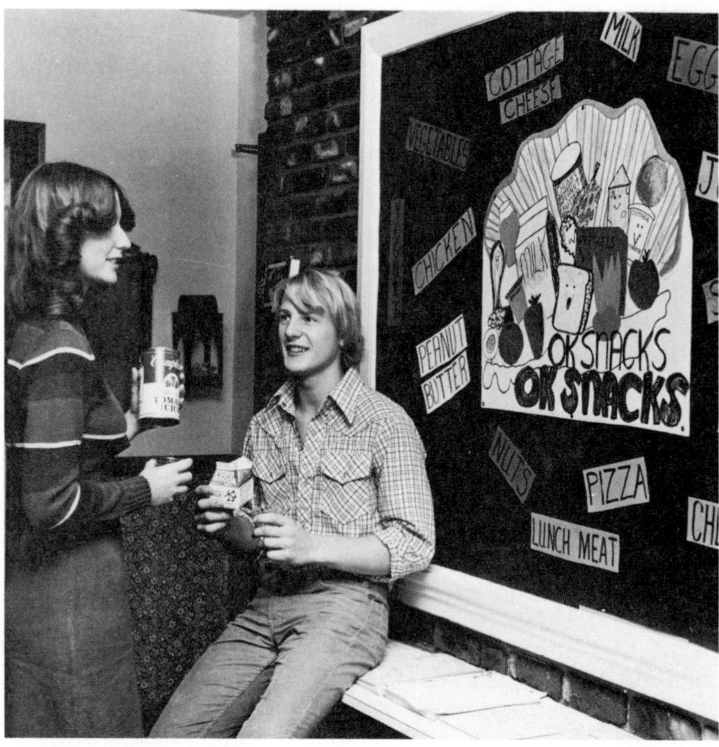

Figure 20–3. Well chosen snacks contribute an important share of nutrients toward the day's allowance. (Courtesy, Harry Broder and Marple-Newtown School District, Newtown Square, Pennsylvania.)

Diet for Athletes

High-school and college-age youth often participate in competitive sports. Many of them are poorly informed about appropriate diets and resort to faddish and even dangerous practices regarding food and fluid intake.

Nutritional Requirements The nutrient levels set forth in the Recommended Dietary Allowances are satisfactory for planning the diet for athletes. The athlete's primary increased need is in the caloric intake which ranges from 3,000 to 6,000 kcal, and occasionally more. In proportion to the caloric intake, the need for thiamin, riboflavin, and niacin is increased. (See pages 219, 222, and 226.) These needs are more than met by the increased amounts of foods consumed from nutrient-rich food groups.

Protein. The recommended allowances for protein will meet the needs for growth of adolescents, for tissue turnover, and for development of muscles during athletic conditioning. A high protein intake does not increase the efficiency of muscle performance. However, in a hot, humid environment during vigorous activity the nitrogen losses from the skin are considerable, and total daily body losses may necessitate a protein intake up to 100 gm.[12] Such intakes are actually commonplace since food selections for a palatable diet are likely to include more protein-rich foods as the caloric requirement increases.

Fluid needs. Fluid losses during prolonged, vigorous activity may account for up to 4 liters per hour. Dehydration reduces performance, and, if extreme, can be life-threatening. About 2 hours before the event the athlete should consume about 500 ml water, and 10 to 15 minutes prior to the competition another 500 ml water. During the competition it is better to ingest small amounts (100 to 200 ml) every 10 to 15 minutes rather than a large amount at one time. Fluid consumed prior to and during the competition will not fully restore fluid balance, and the athlete should continue to drink water for the next 24 to 36 hours until his or her initial weight is restored.[13]

Electrolytes. Profuse sweating increases the losses of sodium, potassium, and chloride. Ordinary mixed diets furnish generous amounts of these electrolytes and replacement is not necessary during a competition. Following the competition any deficits can be corrected by consuming foods whose content is high in sodium chloride and potassium.[13] When fluid losses in excess of 4 liters per hour are anticipated, the team physician may recommend some electrolyte replacement during the competition.

Weight Control During the period when muscles are being developed some weight gain is experienced. A shift from fatty tissue to lean tissue also occurs. Following seasonal activity in sports athletes need to reduce their caloric intake or substitute other activities of equal energy output so that weight remains at desirable levels.

Athletes who must meet specific weight requirements, as for wrestling, should achieve the necessary weight loss by losing fat, not water. A nutritionally adequate low-calorie diet and the maintenance of physical activity over a period of time will accomplish such weight loss. Starvation and dehydration reduce effective performance and are dangerous.

Carbohydrate Loading The ability to sustain peak performance over an extended period of time (as in a marathon race) is influenced by the availability of muscle glycogen. To build up glycogen stores, two phases of preparation are recommended: (1) About a week before the competition the athlete exercises vigorously to deplete glycogen stores and consumes a diet high in protein and fat and restricted to about 100 gm carbohydrate. (2) After 2 to 3 days of the glycogen-depleting phase, a diet low in fat, moderate in protein, and high in carbohydrate (250 to 500 gm) is consumed for 3 to 4 days. Complex carbohydrates that also furnish minerals and vitamins are preferred to simple sugars.[14]

Carbohydrate loading is not recommended for short-time competition since it can lead to a feeling of heaviness that is a disadvantage in high-intensity competition. Occasional adverse effects of carbohydrate loading including myoglobinuria, chest pains, and change in the electrocardiogram have been observed when glycogen loading has been used persistently. Carbohydrate loading is not advised for athletes in early adolescence and should be used no more than two or three times a year by high-school- and college-age athletes.[13]

PreGame Meal Exercise immediately after a meal could lead to nausea, vomiting, distention, and cramping. In addition the blood flow is diverted to the gastrointestinal tract and not to the working muscles. A rapidly digested meal low in fat, moderately low in protein, and high in complex carbohydrate should be eaten 3 to 5 hours prior to the competition. It may include some lean meat, fish, or poultry, vegetables, fruits, bread, and 250 to 500 ml beverage. Contrary to popular opinion, there is no evidence that milk needs to be omitted. Because of their diuretic effects, coffee, tea, and caffeine-containing soft drinks should be avoided. Athletes sometimes have strong opinions about specific foods that will help them to win, and such preferences should be respected within the general bounds of good nutrition and fluid balance.

Ergogenic Properties Substances that increase the ability to work are ERGOGENIC AIDS. There is no evidence that wheat germ, honey, bee pollen, lecithin, protein supplements, gelatin, brewer's yeast, sunflower seeds, vitamin E, ascorbic acid, or vitamin-mineral supplements have any special value in promoting endurance or skills.[13]

Some Current Nutrition Issues

"Junk Food" The term *"junk food"* has been applied indiscriminately to menu items in a fast-food restaurant, numerous snack-type crackers, pretzels, chips, cakes, cookies, pies, sweets, and soft drinks. The nutrient content of some of these items is good and that of others is insignificant. But even foods such as sweets, fats, and some snack-type items that are lacking in essential nutrients furnish energy and can be used in moderation in an otherwise well-balanced and varied diet. The nutrient-poor foods are harmful when they replace foods that supply the needed nutrients, and when they are superimposed on an adequate diet so that the caloric intake exceeds the caloric requirement. The designation "junk food" is misleading at best.

Fast Foods The phenomenal growth of the fast food industry continues. Fast-food restaurants appeal especially to persons under 35 years. For those who eat a meal or a snack in a fast-food restaurant once a week or so, the effect on the nutritive adequacy of the diet is not great. But for workers and teenagers who might eat a meal daily at these places the nutritive contributions must be carefully considered.

A typical meal in a fast-food restaurant (hamburger, french fries, milk shake) furnishes about half of the caloric requirement of a teenage boy, 40 per cent or more of his protein allowance, and up to one third of his thiamin, riboflavin, and niacin allowances. The meal also provides significant amounts of calcium and iron. But if coffee or a soft drink is substituted for the milk shake the calcium content of the meal is very low.

Most fast-food meals are low in fiber, vitamins A and C, folacin, and some trace minerals. Many are also low in calcium and iron. Gradually fast-food restaurants are introducing breakfast items, orange juice, frozen yogurt, and salad bars to provide wider choice and more opportunity to meet nutrient requirements.

Vegetarian Diets Children can be nourished satisfactorily on a lacto-ovo-vegetarian diet. Strict vegetarian diets must be planned with great care, and are not generally recommended. A recent study of preschool children living in a commune using a strict vegetarian diet showed that the mean intakes of most nutrients met or exceeded the recommended allowances, although variations were wide. The diets were extremely high in vitamins A and C, the vitamin B-12 intake was satisfactory because of supplementation with soy milk, but the mean intake of calcium was less than half of the recommended allowance.[15]

If strict vegetarian diets are used these points require emphasis: (1) sufficient calories to meet growth as well as activity requirements; (2) inclusion of foods that complement each other for amino acids; and (3) supplementation with calcium, zinc, and vitamin B-12. (See also page 286.)

Preventive Aspects of Children's Diets Controversy continues about the value of restricting the intake of fat and cholesterol in children's diets on the prevention of atherosclerosis and other pathologic changes later in life. But there is general agreement that a nutritionally adequate diet, weight control, and physical activity are sound measures for health maintenance. In order to keep caloric intake within desirable bounds some reduction in the intake of fats and sugars is usually indicated. But it must also be remembered that even nutrient-rich foods consumed in excess of caloric needs will contribute to overweight.

Children, like adults, consume far more salt than they need. A substantial reduction in salt intake may be useful in reducing the incidence of hypertension later in life. Teenagers should also recognize the increased health risks that pertain when they smoke or consume alcohol.

Some children are at increased risk because their blood lipid levels are elevated or because of a family history of cardiovascular diseases. Nutritionists and clinicians agree that they should follow modified diets planned according to the specific lipid profiles. (See Chapter 39.)

Community Resources

WIC Program The Special Supplemental Feeding Program for Women, Infants, and Children (WIC) provides food vouchers for children up to 5 years who are at risk from economically deprived families. Children at risk include those known to have inadequate diets, who are anemic, or who have deficient growth patterns. Food supplements that meet standards set by the U.S. Department of Agriculture include milk, eggs, fruit juices, and iron-fortified cereals.

School Food Services Of approximately 41 million elementary and secondary students in attendance on a given day, about 27 million participate in the school lunch program. Over 3 million students are given school breakfasts each day. In addition, day-care and summer feeding programs qualify for assistance through federal regulations. (See Figure 20–4.)

The National School Lunch Act was passed in 1946 "to safeguard the health and well being of the nation's children." It provides participating schools with cash assistance; donation of surplus food commodities; and technical assistance in the purchase and use of foods and in the management and equipment of the school lunchroom. The school lunch program has always been regarded as a laboratory for nutrition education.

To participate in the program a school must agree to operate the program on a nonprofit basis; provide free or reduced-price lunches for needy children; serve all children regardless of race, color, or national origin; and serve lunches that meet the requirements established by the Secretary of Agriculture. Children who are eligible for free or reduced-price meals must not be identified by placing them in separate lines, requiring them to sit in places set apart, or requiring them to provide service as a reimbursement for the meal.

New regulations for the school lunch were not available at this writing (October 1981). The most recent Type A pattern for preschool and school children includes the following:

MILK: ½ cup, 1 to 2 years; ¾ cup, 3 to 8 years; and 1 cup, 9 years and over. In addition to

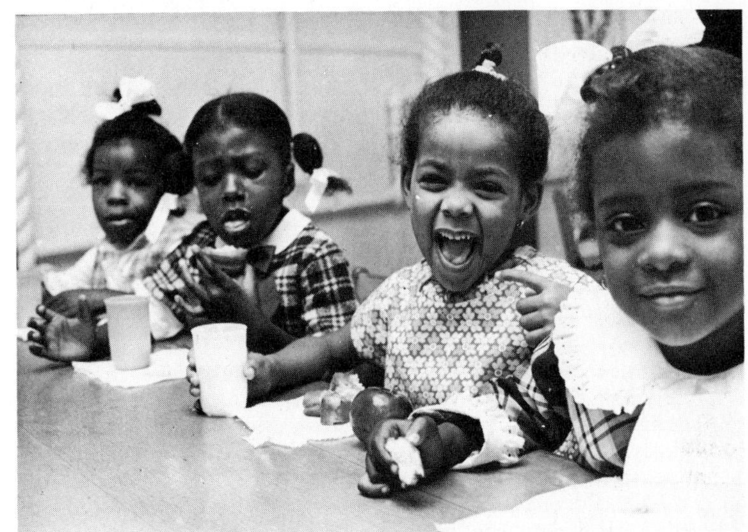

Figure 20–4. Preschool children in a day-care center are provided nutritious meals and snacks. The food service program is similar to that in the elementary and secondary schools. The Child Nutrition Program provides cash and USDA donated foods. (Courtesy, USDA)

whole milk schools may offer unflavored lowfat milk, skim milk, or buttermilk.

PROTEIN-RICH FOOD: equivalent of 1 oz, 1 to 2 years; 1½ oz, 3 to 8 years; 2 oz, 9 to 11 years; and 3 oz, over 12 years. Equivalents for 1 oz meat: 1 oz cheese, 1 egg, 2 tablespoons peanut butter, or ½ cup cooked dry beans or peas.

VEGETABLES AND FRUITS: 2 servings equal to ½ cup at 1 to 8 years and ¾ cup at 9 years and over. A vitamin-C-rich food should be served daily and a vitamin-A-rich food at least twice a week.

WHOLE-GRAIN OR ENRICHED BREAD OR ALTERNATE: 5 slices per week, 1 to 2 years; 8 slices per week, 3 to 11 years; 10 slices per week, 12 years and over. Alternative for 1 slice bread: biscuit, muffin, roll, or ½ cup whole-grain or enriched rice, macaroni, noodles, bulgur, corn grits.

Junior and senior high school students are eligible for the "offer vs. serve" pattern; that is, the five items of the type A pattern (milk, meat, vegetables, fruits, breads-cereals) are offered and the student may select three of these items. This option is intended to reduce plate waste by omitting foods that the student doesn't like. A study of free-choice lunches actually consumed by high school students showed that the nutritional values were as high as type A lunches actually eaten.[16] Intakes by girls of vitamins A and C and iron were marginal. Free-choice programs should be combined with an ongoing program of nutrition education.

A controversial issue for nutritionists and parents has been the introduction of fast foods into some school lunch programs. Proponents of such a program maintain that participation is much better than with the traditional type A lunch. When salads and citrus juices are provided with the usual fast-food items, the nutrient requirements of the type A lunch can be met. Opponents point out that the limited variety of foods can result in deficient intakes of some nutrients such as trace minerals, and that few choices will not help children to develop acceptance of a wide range of foods.

School Breakfast Program Breakfasts are planned to provide one fourth to one third of the recommended allowances. A breakfast includes:

1. One-half pint milk.
2. One-half cup fruit, or fruit or vegetable juice.
3. One serving bread or cereal; may be 1 slice of whole-grain or enriched bread, or an equivalent amount of corn bread, biscuits, or muffins; or ¾

cup of whole-grain or enriched or fortified cereal.

4. As often as practicable, a serving of protein-rich food such as 1 egg, or 1 oz meat, fish, or poultry, or 1 oz cheese, or 2 tablespoons peanut butter.

Additional foods to round out the breakfast and to satisfy the appetite may include foods of popular appeal such as doughnuts, potatoes, or bacon; sweeteners; butter or margarine.

Problems and Review

1. Key terms: catch-up growth; carbohydrate loading; ergogenic aids; fast foods; type A lunch.
2. In terms of food habits, what can be expected at each of these ages: 18 months to 2 years; 5 years; 10 years; 14 years?
3. Discuss the role of cultural pressures on food habits and attitudes to food.
4. Why is skipping breakfast a serious problem? What factors interfere with the child's appetite for breakfast?
5. *Problem.* Record the food intake of a child for one day, and calculate the nutritive values. How does the intake compare with the recommended allowances? What suggestions can you make for improvement of the diet?
6. *Problem.* Plan two menus for packed lunches for an 8-year-old boy that furnishes one third of the day's allowances.
7. *Problem.* List several ways in which a school nurse could assist in bringing about the improvement of food habits of schoolchildren.
8. A friend asks you about the changes he should make in his diet now that he is jogging 4 miles a day. What suggestions can you offer?
9. Comment on each of the following practices:
   a. Candy, pretzels, snack-type crackers, and soft drinks are available in a vending machine in the school with profits being used for band uniforms.
   b. A couple are raising their preschool child on a strict vegetarian diet.
   c. An athlete takes salt tablets with a little water during an athletic competition.
   d. A high-school junior eats a fast-food lunch each day: cheeseburger, french fries, cola beverage, and pie.
   e. A couple have adopted a low-fat, low-cholesterol diet for themselves and their children, believing that they can reduce the risk of chronic disease later in life.

Cited References

1. Food and Nutrition Board: *Recommended Dietary Allowances,* 9th ed. National Academy of Sciences–National Research Council, Washington, D.C., 1980.
2. Macy, I. G., and Hunscher, H. A.: "Calories—A Limiting Factor in the Growth of Children," *J. Nutr.,* **45**:189–99, 1951.
3. Ohlson, M. A., and Stearns, G.: "Calcium Intake of Children and Adults," *Fed. Proc.,* **18**:1076–85, 1959.
4. Pao, E. M.: "Nutrient Consumption Patterns of Individuals, 1977 and 1965," *Family Econ. Rev.,* Spring 1980, pp. 16–20.
5. Owen, G. M. et al.: "A Study of Nutritional Status of Preschool Children in the United States, 1968–70." *Pediatrics,* **53**(Suppl.):597–646, 1974.
6. *Ten-State Nutrition Survey 1968–1970.* Pub. No. (HSM) 72–8132, U.S. Department of Health, Education, and Welfare, 1972.

7. Abraham, S. et al.: *Preliminary Findings of the First Health and Nutrition Examination Survey, United States, 1971–72. Anthropometric and Clinical Findings.* Pub. No. HRA 75–1229, U.S. Department of Health, Education, and Welfare. 1975.
8. Sims, L. S., and Morris, P. M.: "Nutritional Status of Preschoolers. An Ecologic Perspective," *J. Am. Diet. Assoc.,* **64**:492–99, 1974.
9. Beal, V. A.: "Dietary Intake of Individuals Followed Through Infancy and Childhood," *Am. J. Public Health,* **51**:1107–17, 1961.
10. Huenemann, R. L. et al.: "A Longitudinal Study of Gross Body Composition and Body Conformation and Their Association with Food and Activity in a Teen-age Population. View of Teen-age Subjects on Body Conformation, Food and Activity," *Am. J. Clin. Nutr.,* **18**:325–38, 1966.
11. Thomas, J. A., and Call, D. L.: "Eating Between Meals—A Nutrition Problem Among Teen-agers?" *Nutr. Rev.,* **31**:137–39, 1973.
12. Consolazio, C. F. et al.: "Protein Metabolism During Intensive Physical Training in the Young Adult," *Am. J. Clin. Nutr.,* **28**:29–35, 1975.
13. American Dietetic Association: "Statement on Nutrition and Physical Fitness," *J. Am. Diet. Assoc.,* **76**:437–43, 1980.
14. Forgac, N. T.: "Carbohydrate Loading. A Review," *J. Am. Diet. Assoc.,* **75**:42–45, 1979.
15. Fulton, J. B. et al.: "Preschool Vegetarian Children. Dietary and Anthropometric Data," *J. Am. Diet. Assoc.,* **76**:360–65, 1980.
16. Jansen, G. R., and Harper, J. M.: "Nutrition vs. Waste in School Menus," *National Food Rev.,* Winter 1980, pp. 32–34.

Additional References

American Dietetic Association: "Position Paper on Child Nutrition Programs," *J. Am. Diet. Assoc.,* **64**:520–21, 1974.

Committee on Nutrition, American Academy of Pediatrics: "Should Milk Drinking by Children Be Discouraged?" *Nutr. Rev.,* **32**:363–69, 1974.

FISK, D.: "A Successful Program for Changing Children's Eating Habits," *Nutr. Today,* **14**:6–10, 28–33, May/June 1979.

HANLEY, D. F.: "Athletic Training—And How Diet Affects It," *Nutr. Today,* **14**:5–9, November/December 1979.

HURSH, L. M.: "Practical Hints About Feeding Athletes," *Nutr. Today,* **14**:18–20, November/December 1979.

LARKIN, F. A. et al.: "Etiology of Growth Failure in a Clinic Population," *J. Am. Diet. Assoc.,* **69**:506–10, 1976.

MARTIN, E. A., and BEAL, V.A.: *Roberts' Nutrition Work with Children.* University of Chicago Press, Chicago, 1978.

MARTIN, H. P.: "Nutrition: Its Relationship to Children's Physical, Mental and Emotional Development," *Am. J. Clin. Nutr.,* **26**:766–75, 1973.

Review: "Protein Energy Intake and Weight Gain," *Nutr. Rev.,* **38**:13–15, 1980.

SHANNON, B. M., and PARKS, S. C.: "Fast Foods: A Perspective on Their Nutritional Impact," *J. Am. Diet. Assoc.,* **76**:242–47, 1980.

YOUNG, E. A. et al: "Perspectives on Fast Foods," *Dietetic Currents* (Ross Laboratories), **5**, September/October 1978.

21 *Nutrition for Older Adults*

THE goal of nutritional care for the vast majority of persons in the later years of life is to help achieve healthful, purposeful, and independent living. A much smaller segment of the population requires coordinated health and social services including nutritional rehabilitation because they have suffered illness, physical disability, socioeconomic deprivation, or other handicap.

Concerns Related to Nutritional Care

Although older adults have essentially the same human needs as do younger adults, many circumstances in their lives lead to a number of concerns.

Negative stereotypes exist not only in the general population, but are also held by health workers whose services are provided largely to a small percentage of the aging population.

With advancing years, especially after age 75, more people are frail, physically disabled, lonely, and poor, and need many kinds of services including comprehensive arrangements for nutritional care.

Some older people are especially susceptible to the exaggerated claims that certain foods or supplements will sustain health and vigor, prevent disease, or lengthen life.

By a physician's prescription or by self-medication many elderly are taking a variety of drugs. These can compromise good nutrition, but food intake can also interfere with the effectiveness of certain medications.

Who Are the Elderly

Demographic Profile About one person in nine in the United States is 65 years or older, which accounts for approximately 24 million individuals. Today at birth the white male has a life expectancy of almost 69 years and the white female of 77 years. The life expectancy for blacks is about 5 years less. Most of the increase in life expectancy since the early years of this century has resulted from greatly reduced infant mortality and not from the lengthening of the life span in the later years.

Upon reaching age 65, men can expect to live about 14 years longer and women 18 years. For every 100 men over 65 years there are 146 women. There are five times as many widows as there are widowers. One third of older women live alone, but most men over 65 years are living with their wives. Thus the problems of aging are much more acute for women since they live longer, more frequently live alone and are isolated, and have lower incomes.

Low income and lack of education are more characteristic of blacks and Spanish-Americans. Although most older persons are healthy, the average per capita expenditure for health care for the over-65-year group is about three times as high as that for the 19-to-64-year group. Although persons over 65 years account for about 11 per cent of the population, they utilize about one third of the nation's hospital beds.

Stereotypes and Realities Some unfortunate stereotypes about older persons exist in all segments of our society: that they are set in their ways, lonely, sick, poor, handicapped, no longer able to contribute to society, senile, living in nursing homes, and so on. Although some of these characteristics apply to millions of older persons, they are not descriptive of most older persons. The elderly who have lived 60, 70, or 80 years have been molded by their heredity, health, family, education, occupation, and numerous social, economic, and cultural factors. With the passage of time they have become increasingly complex individuals, and they comprise a highly heterogeneous population.

Older adults fall into three subgroupings: those in middle age are likely to be at the peak of their careers and the fulfillment of their hopes, but are beginning to think about retirement; those for whom retirement has become a fact rightfully should be able to live up to high expectations; those in old age experience a decline with increasing dependency based upon state of health, economics, and social change.

Most older Americans have had a good marriage and family life, have financial security, and live comfortably. They live independently in their own homes, some live with their children, relatives, or friends, and only about 5 per cent are confined to nursing homes. These older adults have learned to cope with many changes that occur in the later years: retirement, reduced income, death of loved ones, physiologic and pathologic changes, and so on. They lead productive lives by engaging in volunteer activities in the community, by working part time and sometimes full time, and by contributing to family welfare. They are physically active and enjoy life. They manage their own resources for healthful living, for pursuit of hobbies, and for travel. They have a strong sense of personal worth and spiritual values. In every sense they are a part of the community in which they live and not apart from it. They are a valuable source of experience, skills, and talents.

Physiologic and Biochemical Changes

AGING is a continuous process that begins with conception and ends with death. The Greek word for *old man* is *geron* and that for *treatise* is *logos;* therefore, the term GERONTOLOGY refers to the science that deals with the physiologic, psychologic, and socioeconomic aspects of aging. The suffix *-iatrics* means *the treatment of;* thus, GERIATRICS is the specialty in medicine concerned with the prevention and treatment of disease in older persons.

Body Composition With aging a progressive decline in the water content and the lean body mass is accompanied by an increasing proportion of body fat. By 80 years it is estimated that half of the muscle cells remain.[1] Specific functioning cells are replaced in part by nonspecific fat and connective tissue.

The changes in connective tissue, which is so abundant in the human body, are of especial significance. Collagen is one of the fibrous materials found in tendons, ligaments, skin, and blood vessels. With aging the amount of collagen increases and it becomes more rigid; the skin loses its flexibility, the joints creak, and the back becomes bent.

Cellular Changes For each species there appears to be a built-in limitation of the life span. Moreover, within the organism each cell type has a given life span. Some cells, such as those of the gastrointestinal mucosa have a very short life span, whereas others such as those of the brain have a long life span. In addition some cells continue to divide and reproduce throughout life—for example, cells of the gastrointestinal mucosa, skin, and hair, while others appear to be programmed to divide a specific number of times and then cease reproducing—such as muscle and nerve cells.

With time there is a decline in the number of functioning cells of various organs so that performance is reduced. Two quite different examples illustrate the problem:

a reduction in the number of taste buds reduces taste acuity and may modify the acceptance of food; a reduction in the number of functioning nephrons reduces glomerular filtration and renal blood flow so that wastes are less efficiently removed.

Theories of Aging The causes of cell aging are not known. On a molecular basis aging is the result of changes in cell metabolism or of cell death. Both genetic and environmental factors determine the rate of aging. No single theory of aging is generally accepted. Among the theories that have been set forth are the following:[2, 3, 4]

1. Modification of biologic information. The nuclear DNA may be damaged faster than it can be repaired, or there might be a defect in the repair mechanism. Alteration in the DNA can lead to transcription of faulty information to mRNA. Errors in the RNA assembly of amino acids lead to faulty protein synthesis so that enzymes required for normal cellular function are not produced.
2. Programmed life span or biologic time clock. Cells may be programmed to divide and replicate a given number of times, after which they lose their capacity to replicate. By genetic coding in the brain according to a precise timetable, signals are sent by neural and hormonal stimulation or inhibition to organs and peripheral tissues. Thus, the "self-destruct" mechanism of the cells is ordered.
3. Wear and tear. Cells are subjected to insults and injuries by mechanical and thermal alterations, ionizing radiations, and uncontrolled chemical reactions. Highly reactive free radicals can react with polyunsaturated fatty acids to form peroxidation products that disrupt the cell membrane; that produce disintegration of the mitochondria (the cell's energy powerhouse) so that the ability to bring about electron transport and phosphorylation is reduced; or that release lysosomes (the "suicide bags" within the cells) so that cell death occurs. Some research indicates that vitamin E, selenium, and ascorbic acid may play a role in reducing the peroxidation reactions.
4. Cross linkage. Because collagen accounts for about 40 per cent of all protein in the body, there is a great interest in studying the changes that occur in it with advancing years. With aging there appears to be an increased number of hydrogen and ester bonds forming cross links between molecules of the collagen fiber. As the number of cross links increases, the collagen is immobilized. With the increasing rigidity of collagen, the skin, blood vessels, and respiratory system lose their elasticity, and the joints become stiff.
5. Immunologic changes. Immunologic function declines with age. On the one hand, the antibody synthesis may be defective so that the body's ability to counteract damaging substances is reduced. On the other hand, an increased response to endogenous antigens (autoimmune reactions) leads to increased destruction of normal body cells.

Function of the Gastrointestinal Tract The senses of taste and smell are less acute in later years so that some of the pleasure derived from food is lost. Less saliva is secreted so that swallowing becomes more difficult. Because of tooth decay and periodontal disease a high percentage of persons over 70 years have lost some or all of their teeth. Many have ill-fitting dentures or none at all so that chewing is difficult. Consequently, these persons eat more soft, carbohydrate-rich foods that fail to provide adequate intakes of protein, minerals, and vitamins.

Digestion in later years is affected in a number of ways. Annoying delay of esophageal emptying occurs in many older persons.[1] Hiatus hernia leads to increased complaints of heartburn and intolerance to foods. A reduction of the tonus of the musculature of the stomach, small intestine, and colon leads to less motility so that the likelihood of abdominal distention from certain foods is greater, as is also the prevalence of constipation. The volume, acidity, and pepsin content of the gastric juice is sometimes reduced. In turn there is interference with the absorption of calcium, iron, zinc, and vitamin B-12.

Fats are often poorly tolerated because they further retard gastric emptying, because the pancreatic production of lipase is inadequate for satisfactory hydrolysis and because chronic biliary impairment may reduce the production of bile or interfere with the flow of bile to the small intestine.

Cardiovascular and Renal Function The progressive accumulation of atheromatous plaques leads to narrowing of the lumen of the blood vessels and loss of elasticity. There is a decline in cardiac output, an increased resistance to the flow of blood, and a lessened capacity to respond to extra work. As the rate of blood flow is reduced the digestion, absorption, and distribution of nutrients is retarded. A reduced blood flow together with a smaller number of functioning nephrons lessens the glomerular filtration and the tubular reabsorption so that the excretion of wastes and sometimes the return of nutrients to the circulation is less efficient.

Metabolism From age 25 years the basal metabolism decreases about 2 per cent for each decade owing to the increasing proportion of body fat and the lesser muscle tension. The decline in basal metabolism is less in persons who remain healthy and pursue vigorous activity in their later years. The ability to maintain normal body temperature is also lessened and hypothermia in the elderly can be especially dangerous.

Carbohydrate metabolism. Usually the fasting blood sugar is normal. Likewise, the absorption of carbohydrate is not imparied. However, when a carbohydrate load is presented, as in the glucose tolerance test, the blood sugar remains elevated for a longer period of time than it does in younger persons. Following exercise, the levels of blood lactic acid and pyruvic acid are often above normal limits.

Fat metabolism. With increasing age the blood cholesterol and blood triglyceride levels gradually increase. The kind and amount of fat and carbohydrate in the diet, the degree of overweight, the stresses of life, and many other factors are believed to be responsible for these changes.

Nutritional Status and Health

Nutritional Status Data on the nutritional status of the elderly population is limited. Many studies have been carried out on selected population groups such as the elderly in nursing homes, or on those with low incomes. Such studies are useful for identifying the nutritional problems of these particular groups, but they are hardly representative of the needs of all older Americans. In general, surveys have shown that blacks and Spanish Americans are most likely to have deficient diets and to show evidence of biochemical deficiency. Low income and lack of education are important contributing factors.

Based on nutrient intakes per 1,000 kcal, most studies show that the quality of the diets of the elderly is generally good. However, significant numbers fail to eat enough food so that the total nutrient intake does not meet recommended allowances. According to the 1977 Household Food Consumption Survey[5] calcium and vitamin B-6 intakes were found to be most significantly below recommended allowances for women.

Important nutrition-related problems occurring in large numbers of the elderly population include decayed or missing teeth accompanied by lack of dentures, obesity, and anemia. Hypochromic, microcytic anemia characteristic of iron deficiency is surprisingly common in older persons. It could reflect a lifelong inadequacy of iron intake, or, not frequently, it is caused by a small, undetected loss of blood from the gastrointestinal tract. Folacin deficiency is fairly common and leads to macrocytic anemia. Pernicious anemia results from a lack of intrinsic factor in the gastric juice and failure to absorb vitamin B-12.

Health Problems About one person in five over 65 years identifies some serious health problems. Some of these problems are the consequence of poor nutrition throughout life. Others are not caused by faulty nutrition but may have profound effects on nutritional status because they affect appetite, ability to digest, absorb, and metabolize nutrients, or because of limited physical powers that affect the ability to obtain an adequate diet. Arthritis afflicts many to the extent that shopping, food preparation, or even feeding oneself may be difficult. Fine neuromuscular coordination may be reduced so that it is difficult to hold and use utensils or to manage food preparation safely.

Osteoporosis (bone loss) is highly prevalent after age 50 in women and age 60 in men. There is a high rate of spontaneous fractures. Although hormonal imbalances are frequently seen, the causes of osteoporosis are not fully understood. Some protection against the bone loss seems to be afforded by a lifetime adequate intake of calcium, vitamin D, and fluorine. (See Chapter 38.)

Disorders of the gastrointestinal tract ranging from functional disorders such as heartburn, hiatus hernia, and irritable colon to pathologic changes such as diverticulitis and colon cancer account for a large proportion of health problems.

The highest incidence of coronary heart disease and hypertension leading to stroke occurs in those who are over 45 years. An excessive intake of salt, calories, saturated fat, and cholesterol over a lifetime are among the many factors that increase risk in susceptible individuals. Adult-onset diabetes is seen especially in obese women after age 50, and its presence increases susceptibility to atherosclerosis and its complications.

Medications With increasing health problems in later years there is also an increasing use of medications either according to a physician's prescription or through use of over-the-counter preparations. Some drugs can have a profound effect on nutritional status, and their properties must be considered in nutritional planning. Many medications reduce the appetite or cause nausea, vomiting, abdominal distress, and diarrhea. Others interfere with the absorption of nutrients; for example, chronic use of laxatives. Antibiotics such as tetracyclines interfere with the absorption of carotene, calcium, iron, vitamin B-6, and vitamin B-12. Another antibiotic, neomycin, reduces the synthesis of folacin and vitamin K in the intestinal tract. Other medications affect fluid and electrolyte balance. Many elderly who must take antihypertensive drugs should be aware of the potential loss of potassium. (See Chapter 24 for further discussion of the effects of medications on nutrition.)

Factors Influencing Food Habits

The food habits of the elderly are the result of the lifetime influences of cultural, social, economic, and psychological factors. The individual who has had poor food habits throughout life is not likely to be in as good health as the one who has enjoyed the benefits of a good diet. Good diet in later years cannot completely make up for the years of inadequacy or correct irreversible changes. Furthermore, an older individual cannot completely change his or her whole pattern of eating. Nevertheless, even the individual with poor food habits who is in a poor state of nutrition can benefit greatly from the application of the principles of good nutrition.

Socioeconomic Factors Insufficient income is probably the chief factor that limits dietary adequacy. About one fourth of all persons over 65 years are poor or near the poverty level. Many persons must rely solely on Social Security income. Others have pensions and some savings, but fixed incomes make it increasingly difficult to meet ever-increasing costs for the essentials of life. Although Medicare and Medicaid provide substantial benefits for health care, the costs of medications and catastrophic illness can use up life savings and reduce the available income.

Housing is a major problem for many older persons. Most older people continue to live in their own homes but find it increasingly difficult to pay the exorbitant charges for fuel and other utilities and the ever-increasing taxes. Those who live in apartments are often unable to afford higher rents so they are forced to move to less desirable places. Many live in neighborhoods where they are afraid to walk on the streets because they might be robbed or physically assaulted. Living in a single room with no facilities for food preparation is the lot of many elderly.

Transportation to shopping facilities, physician, dentist, and churches is a serious problem for many older people. Some cannot afford to drive an automobile and others have lost the ability to drive safely. Even those who live near public transportation find it difficult to manage bags of groceries while boarding or getting off vehicles. Nearby independent food stores offer convenience but the food costs are likely to be higher.

Shopping itself can be a problem. With thousands of items in supermarkets, the shopper finds it more difficult to make economical, nutritious choices. Failing vision means that one cannot read the fine print on labels or compare costs of various brands.

Psychological Factors Loneliness and social isolation powerfully affect food intake. Upon retirement some elderly persons lose their sense of worth since they are no longer consulted for advice or see their former co-workers. Some older adults have lost their loved ones, live far away from their children, or are neglected by their relatives. They often have little desire to prepare meals and may eat only those foods that are conveniently available. Others eat compulsively to assuage their feelings of loneliness, depression, and despair. Erratic eating habits in turn perpetuate the mental depression.

Food Misinformation and Faddism Older adults are justified in their hopes that a nutritionally balanced diet throughout life will improve health and prolong life. However, many of them are susceptible to exaggerated claims for health foods and supplements. Advertising for these products usually extols the values they have in correcting deficiencies and removing symptoms. The individual makes a self-diagnosis based on the graphic description of symptoms to which he or she is subjected and buys the product to alleviate these symptoms, real or imagined. Although the product is likely to be safe, it is often not needed and the money spent could better be used for a good diet. More important, by self-diagnosis one may wait too long before seeking medical advice. Among the exaggerated claims being made for special products are these:

Typical diets do not furnish sufficient amounts of trace minerals and a supplement should be taken daily. (NOTE: a diet consisting mostly of *highly processed* foods could indeed be lacking some trace minerals.)

Vitamin E will prolong life and prevent heart attacks.

Garlic parsley reduces blood pressure.

Lecithin supplements will prevent or treat heart disease.

The elderly also hold a variety of erroneous beliefs about foods that are normal constituents of the diet. Among these are:

Older people do not need milk. It is expensive, and also causes flatulence and constipation.

Fruits are too "acid."
Raw vegetables and whole-grain breads and cereals irritate the lining of the stomach and intestines and cause diarrhea.
Pork causes high blood pressure. (NOTE: persons using antihypertensive drugs are sometimes advised by their physicians not to eat pork. They should avoid salted meats such as bacon, salt pork, and ham, but there is no reason to restrict fresh pork.)
Honey and vinegar reduce the symptoms of arthritis.

Dietary Management

Dietary Allowances Although only limited data are available on the nutritional needs of older persons, it is generally believed that the nutrient requirements for the healthy older individual do not differ appreciably from those of younger persons. Thus, the Food and Nutrition Board has set nutrient allowances for adults over 51 years at the same level as for the earlier adult years. (See Table 3–1.) These allowances should be adjusted for individual needs. Infections, interference with digestion or absorption, deficiencies in cardiovascular and renal function, and medications are among the factors that require dietary adjustment. These are discussed more fully in Part Two of this text.

Energy. The mean energy requirement for men 51 to 75 years is 2,400 kcal and, for those 76 years and above, 2,050 kcal. For women of 51 to 75 years the mean energy requirement is 1,800 kcal, and for those 76 years and above, 1,600 kcal. It is expected that for any individual the actual need may vary as much as 400 kcal below or above these means.

Meal Plans Since the caloric requirement for older persons is lower than that for younger adults, the diet must be one of higher nutrient density. Especially for women, there is little margin remaining for foods high in sugar and fat that are nutrient-poor but that also can lead to weight gain and obesity. The basic diet outlined for adults on page 262 serves as a foundation for the diet after 50 years. It furnishes about 1,200 kcal and most of the nutrients at recommended levels. The levels of folacin, vitamin B-6, magnesium, and zinc do not meet the recommended levels. Thus, in the selection of foods to add to the basic diet, particular emphasis should be given to good sources of these nutrients.

Daily meal patterns followed in earlier years are satisfactory for older persons. Breakfast is often the best meal of the day and it should be planned to contribute a significant proportion of the day's nutrients. Some prefer to have the heavier meal at noon rather than at night. Others enjoy a midafternoon snack.

Community Resources The intention of the revised Older Americans Act (1978) is to provide essential services to older Americans so that they can remain in their homes rather than being forced into more expensive institutional facilities. This act provides funding for meals and supporting social services that are provided in senior centers or to persons who are homebound. Although all persons over 60 years are eligible for the programs, priority is given to those who have low income, physical limitations, live alone, and are over 75 years.

A noon meal that furnishes at least one third of the recommended dietary allowances is served at community centers at least 5 days a week. (See Figure 21–1.) Modified diets are furnished according to need. Some centers also serve breakfasts or afternoon snacks. The supporting services may include information and referral, outreach activities, health screening, health and nutrition education, diet counseling, transportation to centers, shopping, and physician's offices, legal aid, crafts and recreational activities, and so on.

For individuals who are homebound, one and sometimes two meals a day are furnished 5 to 7 days weekly. Other services to the homebound include home health aide or homemaker assistance, dietary counseling, chore services, case management, and protective services.

Food Stamps Many older Americans are unaware that they may be eligible to receive food stamps, while others refuse to accept stamps because they feel they do not want to accept charity. Dietary counselors should encourage eligible individuals to use the stamps, thereby increasing the likelihood of an adequate diet.

Meals-on-Wheels Voluntary civic and religious organizations throughout the nation sponsor programs that deliver meals to ill and disabled persons of any age who have no one to prepare food for them. In some communities that do not have access to the federally funded programs for the elderly the Meals-on-Wheels program is another resource for the older person. Also, the availability of Meals-on-Wheels extends the services that are available in communities that have federally funded programs.

Usually the program provides a hot noon meal and a sack lunch for the evening meal 5 days a week. Each recipient pays for the cost of the food, but the meals are packed and delivered by volunteers. For those who cannot pay the full food cost, a sliding scale of payment can usually be arranged.

Dietary Counseling

With increasing age the problems of meal management become greater. The dietary counselor must consider the individual's income, the facilities for food preparation, the physical ability to shop for food and prepare it, the social and cultural background, and the individual attitudes toward food together with the motivation for obtaining an adequate diet. The counselor must be especially alert

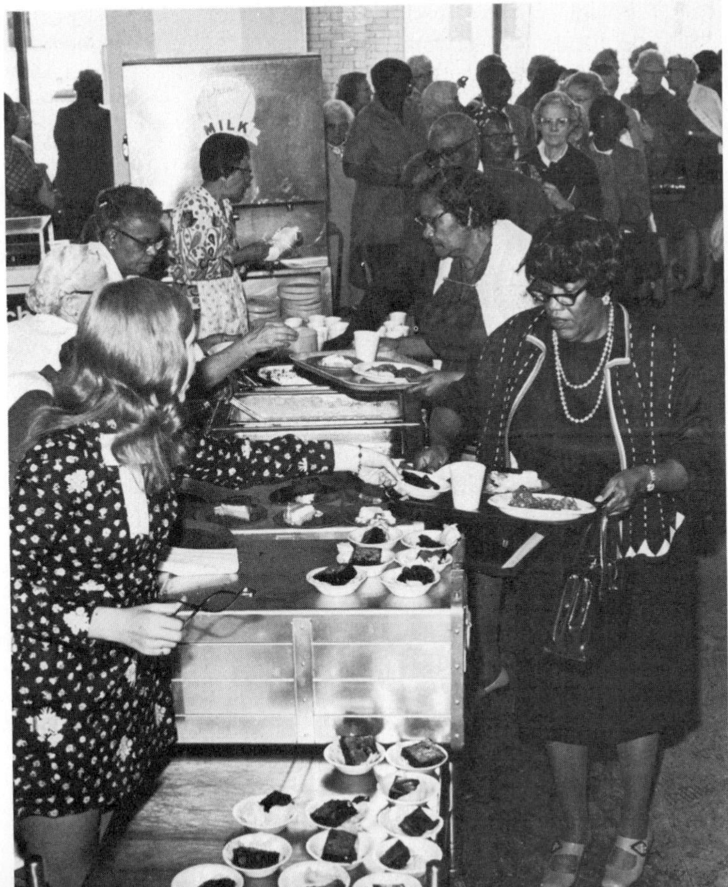

Figure 21–1. Through the Older Americans Act and by state and community support a noon meal and a spectrum of social services are available in senior centers 5 days a week. (Courtesy, *Aging Magazine,* October 1975, Administration on Aging, Department of Health, Education, and Welfare, Washington, D.C.)

to the food beliefs held by the client and to the possibility that medications might interfere with food utilization.

Most older adults are anxious to improve their diets, but they also need assurance that some of their present practices have merit. They need assistance in planning simple meals that not only meet their nutritional requirements but are satisfying; advice concerning the best food buys for the money; information on the interpretation of labels; recipes suitable for one or two people; and suggestions for simple food preparation. (See Figure 21–2.)

The Daily Food Guide can be adapted to various cultural patterns. Special emphasis should be given to the inclusion of milk daily, except for those occasional persons who have lactose intolerance; of good sources of fiber including some fresh fruits and raw vegetables as well as whole-grain breads and cereals; and at least 1,200 to 1,800 ml water daily. Some salt restriction is desirable for most older persons. They need information not only on foods that contain much salt, but also on ways to reduce the use of salt in food preparation.

The elderly who live alone need encouragement to take time to prepare attractive meals and to make mealtime enjoyable. The following suggestions may help.

1. Serve colorful foods attractively on a tray if eating alone. Invite relatives or friends to share a meal from time to time.
2. Eat leisurely in pleasant surroundings; for example, by a window with a good view.
3. Include essential foods first. Sweets and fats should be moderately restricted. Use fresh fruits for dessert, with a calorie-rich dessert included occasionally as a special treat.
4. Adjust food selection to individual tolerance. For some this might indicate that one or more strongly flavored vegetables are not included, whereas others find fatty foods, fried foods, gravies, pastries, and rich cakes give discomfort. No foods need arbitrarily be omitted for all elderly just because a few have a poor tolerance.
5. Avoid coffee, tea, and cola beverages late in the day if insomnia is a problem.

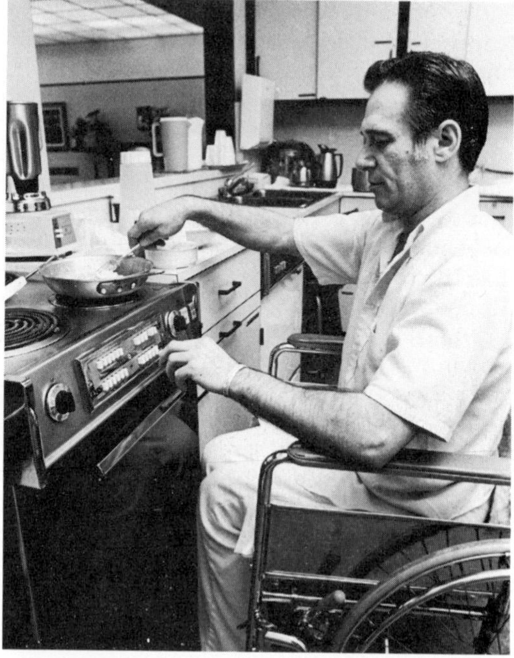

Figure 21–2. Older man who wants to be independent learns how to prepare his meals before discharge from the hospital. (Courtesy, Metropolitan Medical Center, Minneapolis, and Jeffrey Grosscup, photographer.)

Many older people are unable to chew food well. Yet, ground meats and purées are very unpopular. Soft foods such as those in the following list offer many possibilities for attractive meals.

Milk as a beverage
  Cottage cheese; American cheese in sauces or casserole dishes
Eggs, soft cooked, scrambled, poached
Tender meat, or poultry, finely minced or ground; flaked fish; finely diced meat in sauces often taken more readily
Soft raw fruits as banana, berries; canned or cooked fruits; fruit juices
Soft-cooked vegetables, diced, chopped, or

mashed. Raw vegetables such as tomatoes can often be eaten if finely chopped—skin and seeds removed
Cooked and dry cereals with milk
Bread, crackers, and toast with hot or cold milk
Desserts: diced cake with fruit sauce; fruit whips; gelatin; ice cream and ices; puddings; pie, if crust is tender and cut up

Problems and Review

1. Key terms: aging; cross-linkage theory; geriatrics; gerontology; immune response; lipid peroxidation; programmed life span.
2. List five factors that could be responsible for loss of appetite in older persons.
3. What changes occur with aging that may modify the digestion of foods?
4. What reasons can you give for the difficulty some older women experience in the healing of a bone?
5. What are the dangers of overweight in the middle aged?
6. A widow has no cooking facilities in her room and eats her noon meal at a senior center. She cannot afford to eat breakfast and supper in a restaurant. How would you go about helping her to get a nutritionally adequate breakfast and supper?
7. *Problem.* Plan a menu for one day that could be prepared with only a single hot plate available for cooking.
8. *Problem.* Using the low-cost plan on page 271 plan a week's menu for a couple, both of whom are over 65 years.
9. Determine what nutrition programs are available for older persons in your community. If possible, visit such a program or interview a participant in the program. Describe the characteristics of the program, including the priorities for participation.

Cited References

1. Busse, E. W.: "Eating in Late Life: Physiologic and Psychologic Factors," *Contemporary Nutrition* (General Mills Nutrition Department) November 1979.
2. Marx, J. L.: "Aging Research. I. Cellular Theories of Senescence," *Science,* **186:**1105–07, 1974.
3. Timiras, P. S.: "Biological Perspectives on Aging," *Am. Scientist,* **66:**605–13, 1978.
4. Hayflick, L.: "Current Theories of Biological Aging," *Fed. Proc.,* **34:**9–13, 1975.
5. Pao, E. M.: "Nutrient Consumption Patterns of Individuals, 1977 and 1965," *Family Econ. Rev.,* Spring 1980, pp. 16–20.

Additional References

American Dietetic Association: "Position Paper on Nutrition and Aging," *J. Am. Diet. Assoc.,* **61:**623, 1972.

KLINGER, J. L.: *Mealtime Manual for People with Disabilities and the Aging.* Campbell Soup Company, Camden, N.J., 1978.

KOHRS, M. B.: "The Nutrition Program for Older Americans. Evaluation and Recommendations," *J. Am. Diet. Assoc.,* **75:**543–46, 1979.

KRITCHEVSKY, D.: "Diet, Lipid Metabolism, and Aging," *Fed. Proc.,* **38:**2001–06, 1979.

LUTWAK, L.: "Continuing Need for Dietary Calcium Throughout Life," *Geriatrics,* **29:**171–78, 1974.

LYTLE, L. D., and ALTAR, A.: "Diet, Central Nervous System, and Aging," *Fed. Proc.,* **38:**2017–22, 1979.

MARRS, D. C.: "Milk Drinking by the Elderly of Three Races," *J. Am. Diet. Assoc.*, **72**:495–98, 1978.

O'HANLON, P., and KOHRS, M. B.: "Dietary Studies of Older Americans," *Am. J. Clin. Nutr.*, **31**:1257–69, 1978.

ROWE, D.: "Aging—A Jewel in the Mosaic of Life," *J. Am. Diet. Assoc.*, **72**:478–86, 1978.

SCHLENKER, E. D., et al.: "Nutrition and Health of Older People," *Am. J. Clin. Nutr.*, **26**:1111–19, 1973.

SHANNON, B., and SMICIKLAS-WRIGHT, H.: "Nutrition Education in Relation to the Needs of the Elderly," *J. Nutr. Educ.*, **11**:85–89, 1979.

SHERWOOD, S.: "Sociology of Food and Eating: Implications for Action for the Elderly," *Am. J. Clin. Nutr.*, **26**:1108–10, 1973.

SHOCK, N. W.: "Physiologic Aspects of Aging," *J. Am. Diet. Assoc.*, **56**:491–96, 1970.

WEG, R. B.: *Nutrition and the Later Years.* University of Southern California Press, Los Angeles, 1978.

WEINBERG, J.: "Psychologic Implications of the Nutritional Needs of the Elderly," *J. Am. Diet. Assoc.*, **60**:293–96, 1972.

YOUNG, V. R.: "Diet as a Modulator of Aging and Longevity," *Fed. Proc.*, **38**:1994–2000, 1979.

22 Nutritional Assessment and Dietary Counseling

NUTRITIONAL ASSESSMENT is the process whereby the state of nutritional health of an individual, or group of individuals, is determined. It includes anthropometric, clinical, biochemical, and dietary data. The conclusions reached through nutritional assessment become the basis for the development of intervention programs in the community, and for the planning and implementation of nutritional care for individuals. Dietary counseling is based upon the information obtained by nutritional assessment, and entails planning, implementation, and evaluation.

NUTRITIONAL STATUS refers to the health of an individual as it is affected by the intake and utilization of nutrients. Nutritional health can be described at several levels. Normal nutrition implies a sufficiency of nutrients and energy intake—neither deficiency or excess—that affords the highest level of wellness. At one extreme are the manifestations of severe nutritional deficiency in which the sequence has consisted of tissue depletion, followed by biochemical alterations, and finally by clinical signs. At the other extreme are the signs related to excessive intake of one or more nutrients. A given individual, however, may show signs of deficiency and excess at the same time; for example, an obese person sometimes has an inadequate intake of some nutrients despite an excessive caloric intake.

Procedures commonly used in nutritional assessment are described in the sections that follow. Readers who desire detailed descriptions of these procedures are encouraged to consult some of the sources listed at the end of this chapter. In each community setting or clinical situation, a plan for nutritional assessment is first developed that identifies those items that will lead to the most useful information for the given circumstances. For persons who are ill, for example, a preliminary screening helps to identify those that should be studied further and what studies should be initiated. See Chapter 24.

Assessment of Nutritional Status

Anthropometric Measurements

ANTHROPOMETRY deals with comparative measurements of the body. These are the most frequently used for screening children since various body measurements made under controlled conditions can give important clues to nutritional status.

Measurements must be made by trained personnel who use instruments that are accurate and that are frequently checked for their reliability. For example, lever balances with weights that cannot be removed are required; tapes that do not stretch are used for linear measurements. Finally, measurements must be compared with standards that are appropriate for the population. Unfortunately, standards are not yet available that are appropriate for people in some geographic areas and of some ethnic groups.

Weight Serial measurements of weight help to establish the pattern of growth during childhood. For healthy adults, increase in body weight usually, but not always, indicates an increase in body fatness. In some pathologic conditions such as diseases of the heart, kidney, or liver, a rather sudden increase in body weight is an indication of fluid retention. A decrease in body weight of an adult or a child often accompanies a disease process in which there is a reduction of appetite, a defect in absorption or utilization, or an increase in metabolism. In each of these instances, the cause must be determined.

The individual should be weighed on a beam-type scale without shoes and with the same light garments each time. The interpretation of any weight change is important. Although weight can provide some valuable clues, it also has limitations. Body weight is a composite of body water, lean mass, and adipose tissue. The average percentage of fat in healthy, nonobese women is 24, and that for men is 17. Correspondingly, the percentage of body water and lean mass differ in men and women. The proportions of water, lean mass, and fat also change with age and are modified by diet and exercise. One individual may have a high proportion of fat while another individual of the same height and weight has a highly developed musculature and much less body fat. Or, for a given individual with a change in activity, a shift in the proportion of fat and lean mass can occur without change in body weight.

Height and Length Although height is genetically determined, it can be modified according to dietary adequacy. Socioeconomic deprivation is a leading cause of failure to reach genetic potential.

Under 2 years of age recumbent length (crown to heel) is measured by means of a specially designed board or table. The measurement is recorded to the nearest centimeter or fourth of an inch. For young children the recumbent length is 1 to 2 cm greater than that for standing height. For children over 3 years sitting height is sometimes determined.

Height-Weight Standards for Adults The body weight most conducive to health for a given age, height, and sex is not known. For adults a widely adopted standard gives "desirable" or "ideal" weight for men and women of varying heights and body frames. (See Table A-10.) Desirable weight is that weight that is normal for an individual of a given height and body frame at age 25 years. This weight is 7 to 11 kg (15 to 25 pounds) lower than the average weights that are found throughout life. Desirable weight assumes that the gradual weight increase that occurs so commonly after age 25 is not conducive to optimum health.

The determination of body frame is subjective and requires a good deal of judgment. Three types of body build have been identified. (See Figure 22–1.) The ECTOMORPH ("small" or "low" frame) is a tall, slender person with long limbs, narrow head, narrow chest, small hip measurement, and a low percentage of body fat. The ENDOMORPH has short limbs, a round head, a short, thick neck, large bone structure, wide chest and hip measurements, and a higher percentage of body fat.

Height-Weight Standards for Children The height-weight standards of 20 to 30 years ago are no longer applicable for determining patterns of growth. They are based on data from a relatively small number of children from selected geographic areas and ethnic origin. The National Center for Health Statistics has published data for boys and girls from birth to 36 months, and from 2 to 18 years. See Tables A 6–9. These include curves for length or stature and for weight at these percentiles: 5, 10, 25, 50, 75, 90, and 95. Thus, a single value plotted on such a chart indicates where a child ranks in relation to other children of the same age and sex in the United States. The child that falls within the 25th and 75th percentiles is within normal limits. A single weight above or below these limits is not significant, but if values fall consistently below or above these limits the child should be monitored more closely to determine the pattern of growth. Children who fall above the 95th or below the 5th percentile

of the long bones, bones of the chest, spine, and pelvis
Neuromuscular: poor coordination; flabby muscles; sore, painful muscles; muscle weakness
Thyroid: enlarged
Infections: frequent colds and other infections
Gastrointestinal: poor appetite; diarrhea; fear of eating many foods

Many of the signs that suggest nutritional lack are also the result of other factors. For example, a student who obtains only 5 or 6 hours of sleep may complain of being unable to concentrate well, being irritable, and always feeling tired. These symptoms are also characteristic of a continuing dietary lack of B-complex vitamins. A differential diagnosis and correct treatment can be arrived at only when there is correlation of a complete dietary and medical history, a thorough physical examination, and laboratory studies. Table 22–1 summarizes signs that physicians may use in the clinical examination.

Biochemical Studies

Scope and Purposes With some biochemical tests deficiencies or excesses can be detected before symptoms are apparent, thus, making it possible to institute nutritional corrections early. Some biochemical determinations also help to confirm clinical and dietary data so that a diagnosis can be made and nutritional care can be planned and implemented. Other biochemical studies do not necessarily give a clue to nutritional status, but the findings may be significant for the initiation of appropriate therapeutic diets.

Whole blood, blood serum, blood plasma, urine, feces, hair, and biopsy of liver and bone are among the materials used for biochemical studies. Analyses may be made for *nutrient levels* such as glucose, lipids, amino acids, vitamins, and minerals, for concentrations of *metabolic products* such as serum proteins, hemoglobin, and en-

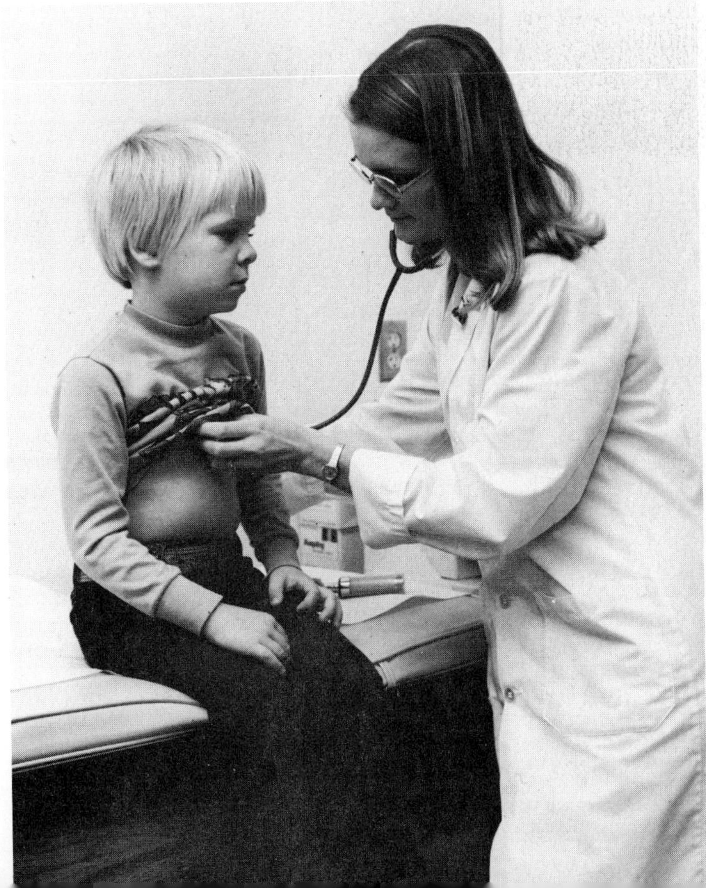

Figure 22–3. The physical examination is an important part of the assessment for nutritional status. (Courtesy, Diabetes Education Center, Minneapolis.)

Table 22-1. **Classified List of Signs Used in Nutrition Surveys***

Area of Examination	Group 1: Signs Known to Be of Value in Nutrition Surveys	Group 2: Signs that Need Further Investigation	Group 3: Some Signs Not Related to Nutrition
(1) Hair	Lack of luster Thinness and sparseness Dyspigmentation of proximal part of hair Flag sign Easy pluckability		Alopecia Artificial discoloration
(2) Face	Diffuse depigmentation Nasolabial dyssebacea Moon face	Malar and supraorbital pigmentation	Acne vulgaris Acne rosacea Chloasma
(3) Eyes	Xerosis conjunctivae Xerophthalmia (including keratomalacia) Bitot's spots Angular palpebritis	Conjunctival injection Circumcorneal injection Circumcorneal and scleral pigmentation Corneal vascularization Corneal opacities and scars	Follicular conjunctivitis Blepharitis Pingueculae Pterygium Pannus
(4) Lips	Angular stomatitis Angular scars Cheilosis	Chronic depigmentation of lower lip	Chapping from exposure to harsh climates
(5) Tongue	Edema Scarlet and raw tongue Magenta tongue Atrophic papillae	Hyperaemic and hypertrophic papillae Fissures Geographic tongue Pigmented tongue	Aphthous ulcer Leukoplakia
(6) Teeth	Mottled enamel	Carles Attrition Enamel hypoplasia Enamel erosion	Malocclusion
(7) Gums	Spongy, bleeding gums	Recession of gum	Pyorrhea
(8) Glands	Thyroid enlargement Parotid enlargement	Gynecomastia	Allergic or inflammatory enlargement of thyroid or parotid
(9) Skin	Xerosis Follicular hyperkeratosis, types 1 and 2 Petechiae Ecchymoses Pellagrous dermatosis Flaky paint dermatosis Scrotal and vulval dermatosis	Mosaic dermatosis Intertriginous lesions Thickening and pigmentation of pressure points	Folliculosis Ichthyosis Acneiform eruptions Miliaria Epidermophytoses Sunburn Onchocercal dermatosis
(10) Nails	Koilonychia	Brittle, ridged nails	
(11) Subcutaneous tissue	Edema Amount of fat		

Table 22-1. **(Continued)**

Area of Examination	Group 1: Signs Known to Be of Value in Nutrition Surveys	Group 2: Signs that Need Further Investigation	Group 3: Some Signs Not Related to Nutrition
(12) Muscular and skeletal systems	Intramuscular or subperiosteal hematomas Craniotabes Frontal and parietal bossing Ephiphyseal enlargement (tender or painless) Beading of ribs Knock knees or bow legs Diffuse or local skeletal deformities	Winged scapula Deformities of thorax	Funnel chest Kyphoscoliosis
(13) Internal systems:			
(*a*) Gastro-intestinal	Hepatomegaly Ascites		Splenomegaly
(*b*) Nervous	Psychomotor change Mental confusion Sensory loss Motor weakness Loss of position sense Loss of vibratory sense Loss of ankle and knee jerks Calf tenderness	Condition of ocular fundus	
(*c*) Cardio-vascular	Cardiac and peripheral vascular dysfunction Pulse rate	Blood pressure	

**Expert Committee on Medical Assessment of Nutritional Status.* Tech. Rep. Series, No. 258, World Health Organization, Geneva, 1963, pp. 57–58.

zymes, or for *excretory substances* such as urea, creatinine, ketones, vitamins, and intermediary metabolites. The selection of the tests to be made is determined by the data from clinical, anthropometric, and sometimes dietary studies. (See Figure 22–4.)

Table 22–2 lists some of the common biochemical studies useful in nutrition surveys. Those listed in the first category are relatively simple and adaptable to population surveys. Those in the second category are more complex and would be selectively used depending upon results in the first category or on other information relative to nutritional inadequacies in the individual or population group.

Interpretation Normal values for various blood and urine constituents are listed in Tables A-15 and A-16. The interpretation of biochemical data requires an understanding of the metabolic pathways of the constituent being tested and of the factors that influence the levels of this constituent in the body. For some constituents, the normal range of values differs for men, women, and children—for example, hemoglobin and hematocrit values for various age groups of children may differ from each other and from those for adults.

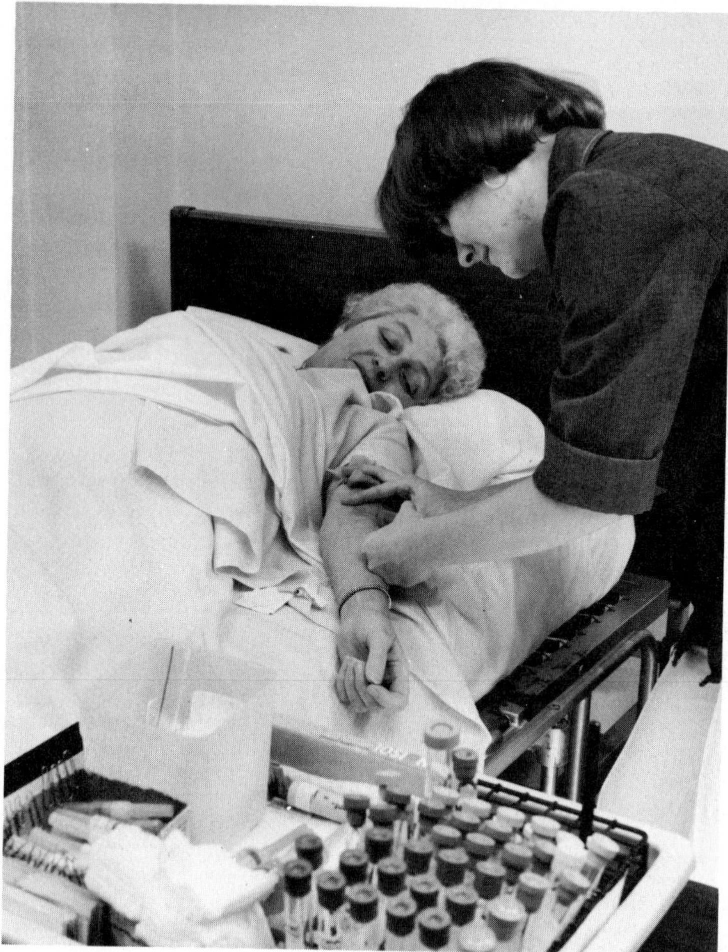

Figure 22–4. Blood studies are useful for assessment of nutritional status as well as for the purposes of diagnosis and therapy. (Courtesy, University of Minnesota Health Sciences Center, Minneapolis.)

The measured constituents may deviate from normal values because of inappropriate nutrient intake, faulty absorption, alterations in intermediary metabolism, increased destruction of specific components, defective waste elimination, or a combination of two or more of these. Some findings may reflect current nutrient intake whereas others are the result of long-term effects.

The interpretation of biochemical data is sometimes controversial. For example, some clinicians make a diagnosis of anemia if the hemoglobin level is less than 12 gm per 100 ml, while others set 10 gm per 100 ml as the lower limit for normal value.

Various homeostatic mechanisms maintain normal levels in the blood at the expense of tissue and storage forms, or by reducing the excretion of a given substance. Only when dietary and tissue sources no longer suffice to replenish the blood constituents, or when there is interference with release from the stores, will the blood levels fall.

Several examples illustrate some problems of interpretation. A normal value for total serum protein does not always rule

Table 22-2. **Biochemical Studies Applicable to Nutrition Surveys***

Nutritional Deficiency	First Category†	Second Category
(1) Protein	Total serum protein Serum albumin Urinary urea (F)‡	Serum protein fractions by electrophoresis Urinary creatinine per unit of time (T)
(2) Vitamin A	Serum vitamin A Serum carotene	
(3) Vitamin D	Serum alkaline phosphatase in young children	Serum inorganic phosphorus
(4) Ascorbic acid	Serum ascorbic acid	White blood cell ascorbic acid Urinary ascorbic acid Load test
(5) Thiamin	Urinary thiamin (F)‡	Load test Blood pyruvate Blood lactate Red blood cell hemolysate transketolase
(6) Riboflavin	Urinary riboflavin (F)‡	Red blood cell riboflavin Load test
(7) Niacin	Urinary *N*-methylnicotinamide (F)‡	Urinary pyridone (*N*-methyl-2-pyridone-5-carbonamide)
(8) Iron	Hemoglobin } Thin blood Hematocrit } smear	Serum iron % saturation of transferrin
(9) Iodine		Urinary iodine (F) Tests for thyroid function

**Expert Committee on Medical Assessment of Nutritional Status.* Tech. Rep. Series, No. 258, World Health Organization, Geneva, 1963, p. 29.

†Urinary creatinine used as reference for expressing other urine measurements in first category.

‡Expressed per gram of creatinine.

(F) In a single urine specimen, preferably fasting.

(T) In timed urine specimens.

Serum cholesterol levels vary widely in population groups with different dietary habits. The determination may often be included in nutrition surveys because of the reported association of serum cholesterol levels with atherosclerosis.

out protein deficiency. A fractionation of the serum proteins might indicate hypoalbuminemia together with elevated globulin fractions. The serum albumin concentration is not a sensitive indicator of early protein deficiency, since it is reduced only when the tissues have been severely depleted. When the serum albumin is reduced, there remains the question of etiology: Was there extreme dietary lack of protein over a prolonged period? Is there a defect in the formation of albumin by the liver? Are there large daily losses in the urine?

Biochemical findings do not always correlate with dietary findings. For example, suppose the hemoglobin and hematocrit levels were found to be normal, but the diet study indicated that the iron intake did not meet the recommended allowances. How shall this be interpreted? On one hand, the iron allowances include a margin of safety for most people and it may be that in the given instance the need for iron was less than the allowances so that the hemoglobin level was normal. But there is another consideration: because of homeostatic mechanisms, the hemoglobin level might be normal but tissue reserves are depleted. Thus, values for serum iron and for transferrin saturation might be sought to define the body's iron reserves.

Immune Response System

A study of the various components of the immune systems also gives some clues to nutritional status. The synergism between malnutrition and infection is widely recognized. Immunity refers to the ability of the host to resist the damaging effects of foreign materials that can result in disease. Immunity involves three major responses: (1) cell-mediated immune response, the thymus-dependent system; (2) humoral-antibody response, the bone-marrow-dependent system; and (3) nonspecific immunity response which includes phagocytosis and macrophage-mediated cytotoxicity.[3] Among the changes that might occur with undernutrition are these:

Cell-mediated immunity—lymphocyte T cells: depressed

Specific antibody production: often impaired. Skin tests to many antigens are frequently negative. Immunization of children who are severely malnourished may not be effective.

Humoral immunity—B cells: immunoglobulins IgG, IgM, and IgA are usually normal in malnutrition alone; in the presence of infection these immunoglobulins are usually elevated. Secretory IgA (S-IgA) secreted in the tears, nasal secretions, and saliva: depressed with malnutrition

Polymorphonuclear leukocytes and macrophages: normal levels in malnutrition, but bacterial killing may be impaired because of enzyme deficiency.

Complement system, consisting of nine protein fractions, activated when antibody is formed: except for C4, concentrations are depressed.

Dietary Assessment

Dietary assessment, of itself, cannot be used for diagnosis of nutritional status, but it may correlate with biochemical and clinical findings, thereby pointing to the appropriate therapy. A study of the diet provides the foundation for individualized dietary counseling.

The dietary study may be brief or detailed depending upon the purposes for which it is intended. Some of the information can be assembled by a nurse or dietetic technician. Or information may be obtained by means of a questionnaire that the client completes before an interview. Only a dietitian is qualified to make a comprehensive assessment and to evaluate it.

Twenty-four-hour Recall This is probably the most widely used method on which subsequent dietary counseling is based. The client recalls food intake for the preceding 24 hours by interview or by completing a questionnaire. He or she recalls what was eaten, how much food was eaten, how the food was prepared, and when it was eaten. By itself, the 24-hour recall is not a reliable indicator of food intake. If it is used together with a food frequency study or cross-check, or if it is used randomly when the client has a follow-up counseling session, the 24-hour intake is a more useful tool.

Among the disadvantages of the 24-hour recall are these: some people find it difficult to remember everything they ate on the preceding day, especially if their eating pattern is irregular; the recalled day may not be typical of the usual intake; or the person may not be entirely truthful, citing what he or she wants the interviewer to think he or she ate.

Food Frequency This consists of asking the client (by interview or by a check-off list) how often (daily, weekly, monthly) specific foods are eaten. The food frequency list might be inclusive of a wide variety of foods in order to get a clue to nutritive adequacy or for diagnosis of food allergies; or it might be selective as for the frequency with which certain categories of foods are eaten, for example, cholesterol-containing foods, or certain salty foods.

Food Diary Persons are sometimes asked to keep a food diary for 3 to 7 days. Such records are more reliable than the 24-

hour recall. Midweek days, rather than weekends, should be selected if the record is to be kept for only 3 days.

When the record is carefully kept, as by a mother for her child or by an adult who is motivated to effect improvement in his or her diet, much useful information on food habits is made available. But this method too has its disadvantages. People who are illiterate obviously cannot keep the record. Other persons modify their diets during the record-keeping period to simplify the recording; still others are unable to estimate food portions accurately; and for many it is burdensome to keep the record.

Weighed Intake This method consists of weighing, on a gram scale, the amount of food served, and the amount of food not eaten. The procedure is used primarily for research on food consumption and for controlled diets used for the study of nutritional requirements.

Diet History As the term implies, the diet history is a record of dietary practices of the individual over a period of time. The food intake by recall, frequency, or diary is a part of the diet history. Information is also obtained on the environment in which the individual lives, for example, socioeconomic history; clinical findings; home-family environment; dietary practices. The following items are among those commonly included in forms that have been developed for recording data conveniently and uniformly. Much of this information is available from medical or health records and the client should not be subjected to a second questioning on these items.

Socioeconomic History

Occupation: hours for work; travel time to work
Education: ability to read
Language spoken
Ethnic background: influence on eating habits
Residence: house, apartment, room
Income: employment, pension, Social Security, welfare, and so on
Family relationships: living with whom
Leisure activities: type, how often, how much time spent on these
Religious beliefs regarding food

Medical History

Present illness: chief complaints, especially those relating to nutrition; diagnosis
Weight: any recent changes; comparison with desirable weight
Appetite: good, fair, poor; any recent changes; taste and smell of food
Dental and oral health: ability to chew, salivation; ability to swallow
Digestion: anorexia, vomiting, distention, cramps
Elimination: regular, constipation, diarrhea
Handicaps related to feeding: need for self-help devices for preparing food or eating it
Medications

Dietary History

Meals: where eaten, when, with whom
Meals away from home: which, how often, type of facility (lunch counter, cafeteria, school lunch, restaurant, vending machine)
Meals skipped: which, how often
Food preparation: by whom, facilities
Typical day's meals—24-hour recall
Frequency check of day's meals
Snacks: how often, types, amounts
Food supplements: protein, minerals, vitamins; how often, reasons for use
Food likes and dislikes: food intolerance, food allergies
Attitudes toward food: food and nutrition beliefs
Previous dietary restrictions: reasons for, type, how long, response to modified diet
Sources of nutrition information

Dietary Evaluation Once the data have been assembled, what methods can be used for dietary evaluation?

Food groups and dietary inspection. Typical diet patterns according to 24-hour recall or food diary can be checked against the food groups to determine whether the amounts eaten from each group are equal to the amounts recommended. This is a rapid but rather crude evaluation technique. It is most useful when the client eats a wide variety of food from each group rather than a limited choice. It is also more useful when it is used randomly for follow-up counseling sessions.

Dietitians who are conversant with the nutritive values of various foods can often make important evaluations by review of the food intake. For example, a diet that supplies little or no milk suggests that the intake of calcium and riboflavin, and possibly protein, are likely to be inadequate. A diet that includes no animal foods is one that lacks vitamin B-12, and so on.

Calculation of nutritive values. For some patients a daily record of the intake of calories and sometimes energy-yielding nutrients is ordered. The exchange lists for meal planning (see Table A-4) provide a rapid method for estimating such intakes. For foods not included in the exchange lists, information on nutritive values is obtained from a table of food composition. (See Table A-1.)

Detailed calculations for many nutrients are used for surveys of nutritional status and for research pertaining to nutritional requirements. They are also used for setting up appropriate rations for normal nutrition for feeding programs as in school food service, for the elderly, in prisons, hospitals, and extended care facilities. They are applicable to setting standards for therapeutic diets as described in diet manuals of various health-care facilities.

Because calculations are time consuming they are rarely used for the assessment of diets as a basis for dietary counseling. With the development of nutrient data banks and the wider availability of computers, the evaluation of diets according to food composition data can be accomplished more rapidly.

The limitations of calculations must also be recognized. Portion sizes must be carefully determined if the calculations are to be meaningful. Also, food composition varies widely, depending upon variety, environmental conditions in production, and methods of food preparation. There is also considerable variability in the availability of nutrients to the body, depending upon food source, the mixture of foods that is ingested, and the environment within the gastrointestinal tract.

After calculations have been completed, comparisons are often made with the recommended dietary allowances for the age and sex category of the individual. When such comparisons reveal intakes below the RDA, they cannot be interpreted as indicating nutritional deficiency. It must be remembered that the RDA furnish a substantial margin of safety for most individuals. Nonetheless, nutrient intakes substantially below the recommended levels can provide further documentation of abnormal clinical or biochemical findings.

Food Analysis is used for some metabolic studies. All food to be eaten is weighed. Duplicate samples of each food are weighed for analysis in a laboratory for energy and nutrient content.

Dietary Counseling

Dietary counseling is the process whereby people are helped to deal with their dietary and nutritional problems. The goal of the counseling is to bring about a desirable change in food behavior. In the process the principles of food and nutritional sciences are translated into practices that are appropriate and acceptable to the client.

Clients and Counselors

Clients Nurses and dietitians often think of counseling in terms of patients who require modified diets. To be sure, such counseling is essential to nutritional care of the patient, but it is a limited view. Many healthy people will have an enhanced sense of well-being if their diets are improved. With today's emphasis on prevention of disease, most people can be helped to reduce the risk of some illness by appropriate dietary counseling. Thus, the client might be a child in school who is becoming obese; a mother enrolled in a WIC program; an elderly person participating in a congregate feeding program; a homemaker receiving food stamps, and so on. It could be someone who receives such counseling as part of the program of a health maintenance organization, or an executive in a corporation that provides surveillance of the health of its employees. Some clients are counseled toward better behavior patterns, whereas others can receive assurance that their present diets are indeed satisfactory.

Client Responsibility Each person is responsible for his or her own health. Thus, the individual must be an active participant throughout the counseling process. In many instances members of the family must be involved. For a very young child the parent, of course, is the principal participant in the counseling process. For the child old enough to take some responsibility for his or her nutritional health, the counseling involves the child, with the parent as an observing supporter whose actions will help the child to implement the needed changes. The spouse of a client provides support and willingness to help in the change process. But only the client can effect the modification of behavior, so it is essential that he or she be directly involved.

Counselors The dietitian is the professional person who by education and experience is best qualified to provide dietary counseling. But in the absence of a dietitian, a nurse often provides dietary counseling to clients, for example, in a school, or in the home, or in an extended care facility. Other members of the health team are often involved. In some situations the client may be referred to a social worker to help solve some financial problem that requires welfare assistance, or to arrange for supportive services such as home-delivered meals, homemaker services, and transportation. Modified diets are usually prescribed by a physician who should also assume responsibility for discussing the reasons for such a prescription with the patient.

Attributes of a Successful Counselor Needless to say, thorough knowledge of the sciences of food and nutrition and of their practical applications are prerequisite to satisfactory counseling. One can scarcely advise on low-cost diets if one is not familiar with food costs and budgeting. Nor can one advise on food substitutions without being able to make comparisons of nutritive values. If one does not have an understanding of the basic principles of food preparation, there is little likelihood that sound directions can be given to the client. Equally important is an understanding of factors that influence food behavior and of techniques that can be used to help the client arrive at decisions to make the necessary change.

The counselor makes every effort to make the client feel comfortable and at ease. She or he shows genuine interest in the client, makes "eye-to-eye" contact, and inspires confidence and trust. The counselor avoids facial expressions or conversation that conveys ideas of impatience, intolerance, pity, or superior intelligence. The counselor is one who helps but does not threaten or dictate.

Steps in the Counseling Process

Each step leads to the next:

Assessment → Planning →
Implementation → Evaluation

Assessment This is a process of gathering data and evaluating data as a means of improving the client's nutritional practices. It describes the client with respect to nutritional status, food behavior, and environment. It includes the social, medical, and dietary history. (See page 403.) Each assessment must arrive at a conclusion upon which the plan is developed.

Planning Based upon the assessment (1) reasonable objectives are set toward which the client is willing to work; (2) ways are described to achieve the stated objectives; and (3) a plan is devised for evaluation of the results. A satisfactory plan applies the principles of food and nutrition sciences within the context of the client's social, economic, psychological, and physical environment. The plan is the blueprint for action.

The objectives must be within the client's ability to implement them. They must include short-range and long-range goals. People often feel overwhelmed by many problems and are unable to make progress in solving them. A small problem that seems important to the individual and toward which some success can be anticipated should be singled out for attention. Then, with time, other problems can be attacked. For example, learning to cook an inexpensive one-dish meal may be a genuine accomplishment for an unskilled homemaker. Or increasing the caloric intake by 200 each day for a period of time might be a good beginning for one who needs to gain weight, whereas a larger goal—500 to 1,000 kcal a day—would be too difficult.

Each client should receive an individualized written plan that includes not only a list of the objectives to which he or she is committed but also a detailed description of the changes that are required to achieve these objectives. The plan itself is developed with the client and not imposed by the counselor. The plan may be supplemented with printed materials such as the exchange lists or other food lists, guidelines for food preparation, pamphlets, books, programmed instruction, or teaching machines. Food models, household measuring equipment, and rulers are useful for estimating portion sizes. Any printed materials, of course, should be explained fully to the client.

Implementation Understanding and attitude are basic to putting a plan into action. Implementation means that the client is able, independently, to plan his or her own menus, to prepare foods appropriate to the needed changes (or to supervise such preparation), and to consume the needed amounts of food. It includes the client's selection of food in the marketplace with respect to cost, information on labels, and so on. It means that the client applies each day those modifications of food behavior to which he or she is committed.

Evaluation The progress of a client toward achieving personal goals should be evaluated from time to time by the client and the counselor. The evaluation confirms the degree of success by the client. Did the client understand the plan that was set? Was he or she motivated to make the needed changes? What support systems were available to the client? How consistently was the plan followed? Were the counselor's techniques appropriate for the client?

Each evaluation becomes, in effect, a reassessment or addition to the initial assessment. This may lead to revision of the plan, if needed, and then to changes in implementation. Sometimes the evaluation may show that an individual cannot be helped or does not want to be helped; this too should be recognized.

Some Counseling Guidelines

Timing is Important At certain stages of the life cycle people are particularly receptive to making changes in their food behavior. The teenager is intent upon improving his physique or her figure; the young couple planning for their first baby want the best environment for the developing fetus; the new mother desires a long, healthy life for her baby; and the older person often looks to nutrition as valuable in maintaining or improving health.

For patients in a hospital, the timing of counseling is of great importance. Indeed, counseling can become a part of daily nutritional care. For example, each meal for the patient with diabetes illustrates the use of the exchange lists. A complaint about unsalted food gives opportunity to tell about the use of flavoring aids, and so on. Formal counseling sessions with the patient should be planned well in advance of the time of discharge. For persons who are ill and fatigued, several brief sessions are likely to be more helpful than long sessions. Neither hunger just before a meal nor satiety after a meal are conducive to learning about diet.

Be an Effective Listener Allow ample time for the client to voice problems and frustrations. What does the client say first? How intense are the feelings expressed? Do the client's words mask his or her true feelings?

When the client is describing problems, the counselor should avoid frequent interruptions except those that might be essential to clarify a point or that may be needed if the client strays to some irrelevant topic. But sometimes a seemingly unrelated subject may have an important bearing on the nutritional problem.

Ask Questions in a Nondirective Way The question: "What kind of cereal do you eat for breakfast?" suggests to the client that he or she should have eaten breakfast and that it should have included cereal. It is better to say: "Tell me when you first ate yesterday." Then, "What did you eat?" and "How much did you eat?" and "How was it prepared?"

Begin Where the Client Finds Himself Something good can be found in every dietary pattern, and efforts should be made to make as few changes in the pattern as necessary. Any change in diet represents a threat to the patient's way of life. Negative, critical attitudes toward current practices are rarely helpful.

Use Appropriate Communication Skills Counseling means talking together with the client, not lecturing. It means conversation at the level of the client's understanding. Any scientific terms should be used with full explanation of their meaning. Counseling means answering questions as well as asking them; it also means showing and doing. Learning has been described in this way:

> One remembers *best* what one does
> Next best, what one *sees,*
> Least well what one hears.

Group Counseling

In a food clinic or health center, classes may be held for groups with similar diet problems: pregnant women, mothers with preschool children, diabetic patients, those requiring sodium restriction, weight-control groups, and so on. Economy of time for the professional worker is an apparent advantage of using group instruction. Many patients are helped by this approach inasmuch as they learn to appreciate that others have similar problems and that they can share experiences with one another. The person who is given to much self-pity may receive encouragement toward a more positive outlook on his or her problems if proper guidance is provided in the group setting. Group instruction may be supplemented by individual teaching, particularly with respect to problems of finance and emotional reactions to the diet.

Group instruction must be a democratic process in which everyone feels free to participate. The nurse or dietitian cannot be authoritarian, the talkative patient should not monopolize all of the time, and the self-conscious, shy patient should not be made uncomfortable by having to respond when not ready. Verbal instruction should be coordinated with visual aids, including dietary lists, leaflets, posters, food models, and films as the occasion may warrant. The leader of the group cannot change the individual or the group; she or he can only help them to recognize their own goals and to make their own decisions for change.

Problems and Review

1. Key words: anthropometry; assessment; cross-sectional study; densitometry; dietary counseling; dietary history; dietary survey; evaluation; food behavior; food frequency; longitudinal study; monitoring; multiple isotope dilution; skinfold measurement; total body potassium.
2. List some physical and behavioral signs that might suggest to a teacher that a child should be further assessed for nutritional status.
3. *Problem.* Develop a list of five foods commonly used from each of the food groups. Then interview a classmate to determine the frequency with which he or she consumes these foods. Determine the amounts of food consumed. What are the advantages of this approach? What limitations did you encounter?
4. Based on a dietary history, including a 3-day food record, it was determined that the diet furnished the recommended allowances for protein, calories, and ascorbic acid. All of the B-complex vitamins and iron fell within 70 to 90 per cent of the allowances. What evaluation would you make of such information? Explain fully.
5. *Problem.* Using the height-weight chart (Tables A–7,9), evaluate the growth status of a 10-year-old boy who weighs 25 kg and is 130 cm tall; a 12-year-old girl who weighs 55 kg and is 160 cm tall.

Cited References

1. Rathbun, E. N., and Pace, N.: "Studies on Body Composition. I. The Determination of Total Body Fat by Means of the Body Specific Gravity," *J. Biol. Chem.*, **158**:667–76, 1945.
2. *Obesity and Health.* PHS Pub. 1485. National Center for Chronic Disease Control, U.S. Department of Health, Education, and Welfare, Arlington, Va., 1966, p. 13.
3. Vitale, J. J.: *Impact of Nutrition in Immune Function.* Ross Laboratories, Columbus, Ohio, 1979.

Additional References

AUSTIN, J. E.: "The Perilous Journey of Nutrition Evaluation," *Am. J. Clin. Nutr.*, **32**:2324–38, 1978.

BAIRD, P. C., and SCHUTZ, H. G.: "Life Style Correlates of Dietary and Biochemical Measures of Nutrition," *J. Am. Diet. Assoc.*, **76**:228–35, 1980.

CHRISTAKIS, G., ed.: "Nutritional Assessment in Health Programs," *Am. J. Public Health*, **63** (Suppl.):1–82, November 1973.

DANSKY, K. H.: "Assessing Children's Nutrition," *Am. J. Nurs.*, **77**:1610–11, 1977.

Expert Committee on Medical Assessment of Nutritional Status. Tech. Rep. Series No. 258, World Health Organization, Geneva, 1963.

FRANKLE, R. T., and Owen, A. Y.: *Nutrition in the Community.* The C. V. Mosby Company, St. Louis, 1978, chaps. 7 and 8.

GARN, S. M., and Clark, D. C.: "Problems in the Nutritional Assessment of Black Individuals," *Am. J. Public Health*, **66**:262–67, 1976.

GERSOVITZ, M. et al.: "Validity of the 24-hour Dietary Recall and Seven-day Record for Group Comparisons," *J. Am. Diet. Assoc.*, **73**:48–55, 1978.

HAMILL, P. V. V., et al.: "Physical Growth: National Center for Health Statistics Percentiles," *Am. J. Clin. Nutr.*, **32**:607–29, 1979.

MASON, M., et al.: *The Dynamics of Clinical Dietetics.* John Wiley & Sons, New York, 1977, pp. 99–173.

SHAPIRO, L. R.: "Streamlining and Implementing Nutritional Assessment: The Dietary Approach," *J. Am. Diet. Assoc.*, **75**:230–37, 1979.

TROWBRIDGE, F. L.: "Clinical and Biochemical Characteristics Associated with Anthropometric Nutritional Categories," *Am. J. Clin. Nutr.*, **32**:758–66, April 1979.

ZERFAS, A. J.: "The Insertion Tape. A New Circumference Tape for Use in Nutritional Assessment," *Am. J. Clin. Nutr.*, **28**:782–87, 1975.

23 Nutritional Problems and Programs in the Community

THE nutritional problems of a community, state, or nation are identified by many interrelated studies including data on food production and consumption, morbidity and mortality statistics, levels of income, and surveys of nutritional status. Strategies for the prevention and correction of nutritional problems of individuals or groups are developed by a network of agencies within the community.

Focus on Community Nutrition The term PUBLIC HEALTH NUTRITION is generally understood to be concerned with those problems of nutrition that affect large numbers and that can be solved most effectively through group action. The term COMMUNITY may be used to refer to any group of people; it might be, for example, a small, closely knit group such as the student community, or the low-income area of a city, or an entire city.

Physicians, nurses, dietitians, nutritionists, social workers, home economists, and teachers must be informed citizens regarding nutrition concerns of the local community, the state, the nation, and even the world. They have a responsibility to assume leadership in identifying nutritional problems and in finding solutions to these problems. The solutions might result in direct services to clients, in expanded programs of nutrition education, in committee activities to develop new programs, and in taking a position on proposed legislation that affects the nutritional well-being of the population.

The purposes of this chapter are to give the reader an appreciation of the scope of nutrition problems in the nation and throughout the world; to describe the broad range of nutritional services that are needed in varying circumstances; to create an awareness of the many resources that exist for solving these problems; and to develop a sense of individual responsibility toward the improvement of nutrition and health.

Identifying Problems Related to Nutrition

Scope of Studies

Per Capita Food Consumption Each year the U.S. Department of Agriculture accumulates data pertaining to the per capita consumption of food and calculates the per capita nutritive value of that food (see p. 247). Such data include inventories of food on hand, food imports, and agricultural production from which are subtracted food exports, nonfood use of agricultural products (industrial use, feed use), and losses in distribution. These data provide information on the adequacy of the food supply and national trends in food consumption over a period of time. These data give no information on the variability of individuals nor of the nutritional status of the population.

Vital Statistics Morbidity and mortality rates for various age groups provide clues to the level of nutritional health. Such data may be especially significant in the developing countries. The possibility of malnutrition as an etiologic agent should be investigated when (1) maternal and infant deaths are high; (2) death rates for children 1 to 4 years are high; (3) when the incidence of diseases such as measles, tuberculosis, parasite infestation, dysentery, and malaria is high. The lack of sanitation and failure to immunize children against a number of diseases as well as malnutrition contribute to rising morbidity and mortality rates. (See *synergism*, page 421.)

Economic Data The distribution of wealth in a community is an important indicator of nutritional adequacy. Where there are areas of poverty, the quality of the diet is compromised and the incidence of malnutrition is thus increased.

Congressional Action Physicians testified in 1967 that hunger and some deficiency diseases had been diagnosed especially among poor people in the South. This led Congress to mandate an investigation of malnutrition in the United States and to authorize the formation of the U.S. Senate Select Committee on Nutrition and Human Needs. This committee held hearings on many nutrition-related topics during the 9 years of its existence (1968–1977). The Ten-State Nutrition Survey (p. 413) was authorized by Congress, as was also the White House Conference on Food, Nutrition, and Health in 1969.

White House Conference on Food, Nutrition, and Health. The almost 4,000 participants in the 1969 conference included nutrition scientists, dietitians, nutrition educators, physicians, public health workers, representatives from agriculture and the food industry, clergymen, consumer organizations, civil rights organizations, ethnic minorities, welfare administrators, and the poor. Among the many recommendations set forth were that food assistance programs be expanded; that the coordination of nutrition programs in various governmental agencies be improved; that nutrition education be expanded in the elementary and secondary schools, and also incorporated into the medical curricula; that research be conducted on food safety and quality, including additives, environmental contaminants, and foodborne diseases; and that labeling regulations be developed by the Food and Drug Administration. Although not all recommendations have been adopted, the decade of the 1970s brought about significant improvements in food assistance, education, research, and labeling.

The Dietary Goals. One of the final acts of the Senate Select Committee on Nutrition and Human Needs was the publication of the Dietary Goals. (See Chapter 3.) Adherence to these goals could improve the nutritional status of many persons. Research to date indicates that adherence to the goals may reduce the risk of some chronic diseases. As with any guideline, these goals are subject to modification as additional data become available.

World Food Conference The participants in this conference held in Rome in 1974 declared that hunger and malnutrition should be eliminated. They identified the needs of the developing countries as capital, technology, fertilizers, insecticides, and energy.[1] They called for (1) increased food production by all countries; (2) commodities and financial assistance to provide food (grain) aid; (3) development of a world network of grain reserves; (4) a global information system; (5) the elimination of trade barriers, and (6) the establishment of a world food council. Recommendations for programs to improve nutrition included nutrition education, fortification of foods to improve the nutritive content, an inventory of vegetable food sources other than cereals, modernization of consumer education and food legislation programs, a global nutrition surveillance system, and applied nutrition research. (See Figure 23–1.)

Surveys of Food Consumption and Nutritional Status

The Nature of Dietary and Nutrition Surveys A SURVEY is an "examination of the

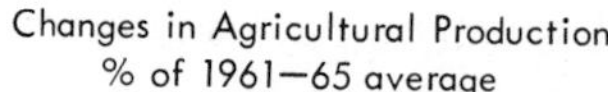

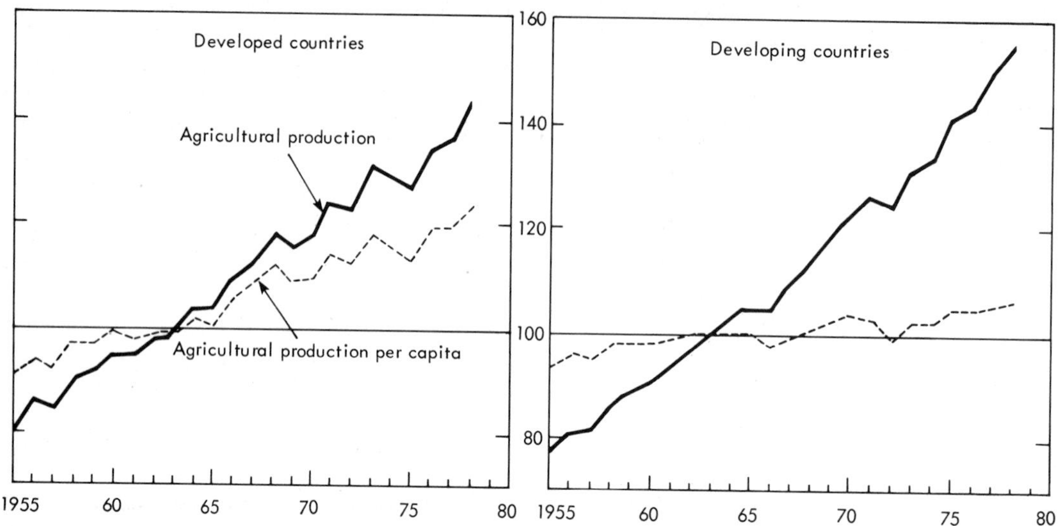

Developed countries include United States, Canada, Europe, USSR, Japan, Republic of South Africa, Australia and New Zealand.
Developing countries include South and Central America, Africa (except Republic of South Africa), Asia (except Japan, Communist Asia).

Figure 23–1. Agricultural production has increased substantially in the developing and the developed countries. But the population continues to increase faster in the developing countries. Thus, there is little improvement in the amount of food available per capita. (Courtesy, U.S. Department of Agriculture.)

particulars of something, in order to ascertain condition, character, etc."* CROSS-SECTIONAL STUDIES are made once on many people. They establish the number of people that fall within or outside the criteria that have been established. They help to identify the problems that exist so that intervention programs can be initiated. The Ten-State National Nutrition Survey is an example of cross-sectional studies.

LONGITUDINAL STUDIES are those in which individuals are observed at specified time intervals over a period of time. They help to identify physiologic and pathologic changes that occur. The Harvard growth study including observations on children over an 18-year period is an example of a longitudinal study. Another example is the Multiple Risk Factor Intervention Trial (MRFIT) conducted in twenty research centers throughout the country over a 6-year period on approximately 12,000 men to determine the effects that modification of life-style might have on the incidence of cardiovascular diseases.

A DIETARY SURVEY is concerned with the food intake of persons included in the sample. The food inventory, food diary, 24-hour recall, and dietary history are methods that may be employed in making a dietary survey. These have been discussed more fully in Chapter 22. The data collected might reveal the adequacy of diet consumed by various age groups as measured against a standard such as the recommended dietary allowances; the food preferences of ethnic groups or in varying geographic areas; the

* *The Random House Dictionary of the English Language,* Unabridged Edition, 1966.

expenditures for food; the practices in food buying, food storage, and food preparation. The dietary survey may help to identify groups that might be vulnerable, but it does not establish the nutritional status of the group.

A nutritional status survey identifies the nutritional health of a selected population at a given time. It includes anthropometric measurements, physical and clinical findings, biochemical data, and dietary studies as described in Chapter 22. Surveys of nutritional status help to identify persons who are at risk or are malnourished and to set the bases for intervention programs. They also help to motivate a population to better nutritional patterns and to wider acceptance of programs for education in nutrition. A follow-up survey can establish the effectiveness of intervention programs.

Dietary and nutritional status surveys may be based on a sampling that is representative of the entire national population (see HANES); on a selected age group (Preschool Nutrition Survey, 1968–70); on a given economic group (see Ten-State, low-income). Or surveys might be restricted to pregnant women, the elderly, adolescent girls, and so on.

National Surveys The U.S. Department of Agriculture and the U.S. Department of Health, Education, and Welfare have conducted surveys that yielded important information on food consumption and nutritional status. Three of these are described briefly in the following paragraphs.

National Food Consumption Survey. At approximately 10-year intervals the U.S. Department of Agriculture has conducted six national food consumption surveys. The most recent of these, 1977–78, included data on food consumption and dietary levels of households and also studies of food and nutrition intake of individuals. Data were collected from 15,000 households in the 48 conterminous states and the District of Columbia, with one fourth of these occurring in each quarter of the year. In addition, 1,200 households in Alaska and 1,200 households in Hawaii were surveyed for the first quarter of 1978. Thus, the data are representative of the population of the United States. The data when processed can be used for economic and marketing information; to assess the adequacy of the food and nutrition programs of the department; to update the USDA food plans (see p. 270); and to evaluate the effects of fortification, additives, pesticides, and residues in foods so that proper regulations can be developed. Special attention has been given in this survey to the nutritional well-being of the elderly.[2] (See also p. 385.)

Ten-State Nutrition Survey. This survey conducted in 1968–70 focused on the nutritional status of people living in low-income areas of ten states: California, Kentucky, Louisiana, Massachusetts, Michigan, New York, South Carolina, Texas, Washington, and West Virginia. Some middle- and upper-income families who were living in the low-income areas were also included in the survey.

Health and Nutrition Examination Survey (HANES). The HANES I survey examined over 20,000 persons, ages 1 to 74, between April 1971 and October 1975. Data were collected on disease conditions by region, race, sex, age, and level of income, and of any association of these conditions with nutritional status. Of about 100 anticipated reports from this survey, many are not yet completed.

HANES II was begun in February 1976 and ended in March 1980. This sample again includes about 21,000 persons aged 6 months to 74 years. In addition to data collected for HANES I, this survey includes studies on the levels of copper, zinc, and lead in the diet and in the body.

Results of Surveys Nutritional failure was observed at all income levels but was most acute at the low income level. Obesity, especially in women, dental caries, growth failure in children, and iron-deficiency anemia were the major nutritional problems encountered.

The most vulnerable groups in the population were found to be Indians, migrant workers and their families, Spanish Americans, Eskimos, the poor, and the elderly. Irregular income, large families, and lack of knowledge of food values contributed to the problems. In the Ten-State study there was an important correlation between the level of education of the mother and the nutritional status of the child.

Malnutrition—A Worldwide Concern

Scope of Malnutrition

Incidence and Nature of Malnutrition Malnutrition is an inclusive term that involves the lack, imbalance, or excess of one or more of some 50 or so nutrients that are required by the body. The classic nutritional deficiencies are rarely encountered in the United States and Western Europe. Occasionally beriberi is seen in severe alcoholics. Marasmus, a severe form of protein-calorie malnutrition, is not unknown in the United States but is almost always traceable to child neglect. Iatrogenic malnutrition in hospital patients has also been described (see p. 451).

A report to the World Food Council in October 1979 indicated that about 1 billion people suffer from chronic undernutrition. Over three fourths of the world's undernourished live on the Indian subcontinent, in Southeast Asia, and in Africa below the Sahara desert. Children are most severely affected. Protein-calorie malnutrition is the chief problem, but usually there are also deficiencies of minerals and vitamins. (See Figure 23–2.)

Nutritional excesses or imbalances are important problems in the United States. Obesity and dental caries assume epidemic proportions in the population. Dietary excesses are also implicated as risk factors in cardiovascular diseases, cancer, diabetes, and other chronic conditions.

Nutritional Deficiencies The nutritional deficiencies arising from lack of specific nutrients, the nutritional problems encountered at various stages of the life cycle, and the effects of disease upon nutrition are discussed in detail in appropriate chapters of this text. Table 23–1 summarizes the principal nutritional deficiencies on the world scene today and includes a cross-reference to the chapters within this text where a fuller description is available.

In the initial stages of development a deficiency is so mild that physical signs are absent and biochemical methods generally cannot detect the slight changes. As tissue depletion continues the biochemical changes can be measured in body fluids and tissues. With further depletion the physical signs become apparent until finally the full-blown signs of the predominating classic deficiency can be recognized.

Nutritional deficiencies rarely occur singly inasmuch as an inadequacy of food almost always reduces the intake of more than one nutrient. Moreover, the metabolic interdependence of nutrients means that a lack of one will interfere with the proper utilization of another, many examples of which have been cited in Chapters 4 through 12.

Primary nutritional deficiencies are those that are caused by inadequate or imbalanced intake of food. These conditions are the result of many environmental factors, some of which are discussed more fully on page 418.

Secondary deficiencies are those that result from some fault in digestion, absorption, and metabolism so that tissue needs are not met even though the ingested diet would be adequate in normal circumstances. Thus, the restoration and maintenance of good nutrition are important concerns in clinical nutrition.

Classic deficiency diseases are diagnosed relatively easily because the physical and biochemical findings are prominent and specific. Nevertheless, the diagnosis of even these may be missed when the disease is seldom seen by clinicians, as is the case in the United States.

Economic Cost of Malnutrition The maintenance of health and the treatment of disease are important not only for humanitarian reasons but also in economic terms. What is good nutrition really worth? Can a preventive program in nutrition be economically justified? The answers are not easy to obtain. According to testimony given by Dr. George Briggs at 1972 hearings before the Senate Select Committee on Nutrition and Human Needs, poor dietary habits may account for as much as one third of the total health care bill.[3]

Programs to prevent nutritional deficiencies, excesses, or imbalances must emphasize lifelong attention to diet. Effective preventive programs can be expected to reduce the costs of medical services including hospital care, extended-care services,

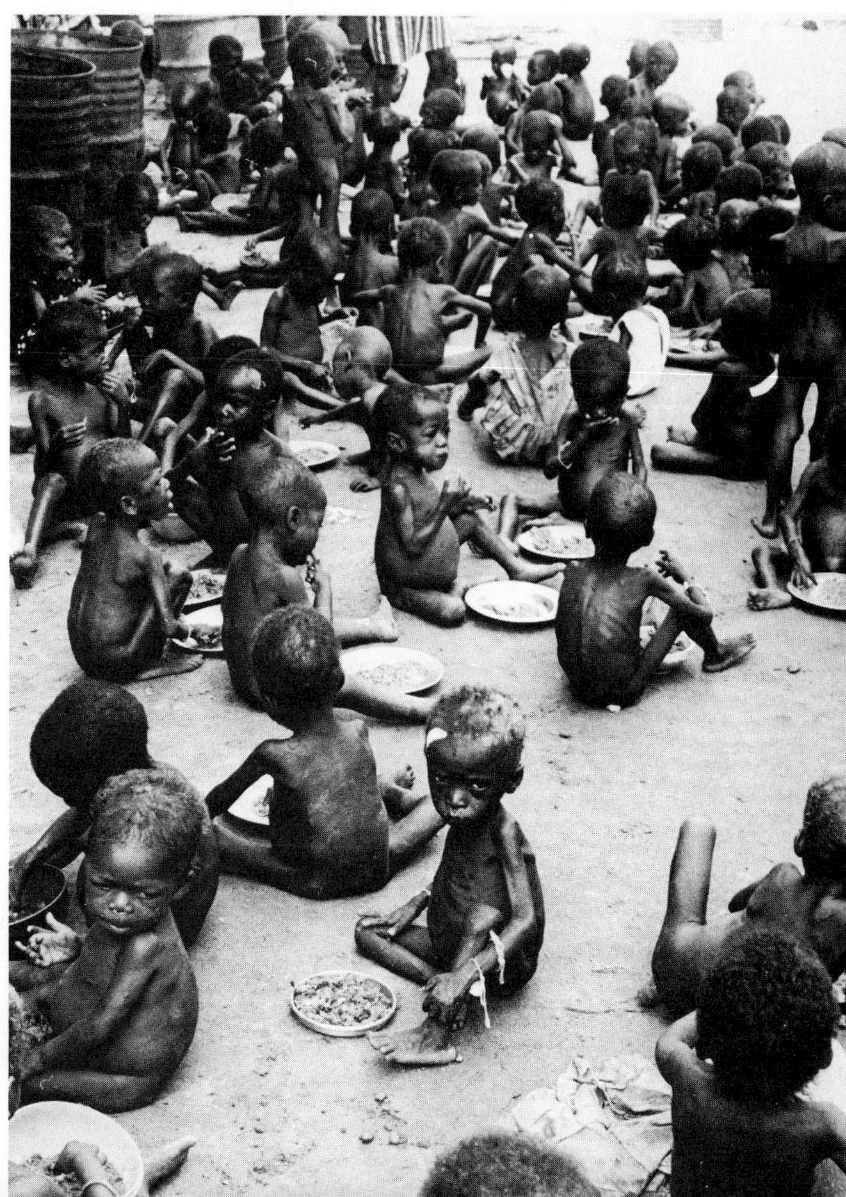

Figure 23–2. Children are among the first victims of food scarcity. Here some children are being fed a mixture of stockfish and beans from an improvised kitchen in a Niger clinic. Note the emaciation and pot bellies in some of the children. (UNICEF photo by Poul Larsen.)

Table 23-1. **Summary of Diseases of Malnutrition**

Principal Disease Conditions	Nutrient Imbalances
Deficiencies	
Underweight	Calorie deficit (Chapter 28)
Protein-calorie malnutrition	
Kwashiorkor	Principally protein lack (page 421)
Marasmus	Calorie-protein lack (page 422)
Dental caries	Calcium, phosphorus, fluorine, vitamins A and D (Chapters 8, 10)
Anemia, microcytic, hypochromic	Iron (Chapters 8 and 30)
Macrocytic in infancy, pregnancy, malabsorption	Folacin (Chapters 12 and 30)
Pernicious (absorptive defect)	Vitamin B-12 (Chapters 12 and 30)
Goiter, endemic	Iodine (Chapter 8)
Osteoporosis	Possibly calcium, vitamin D; endocrine factors (Chapter 38)
Osteomalacia	Vitamin D, calcium, phosphorus (Chapter 10)
Scurvy; hemorrhagic tendency; inflamed gums; loose teeth	Ascorbic acid (Chapter 11)
Beriberi; polyneuritis, circulatory failure; emaciation; edema	Thiamin (Chapter 12)
Pellagra; glossitis; dermatitis; diarrhea; nervous degeneration; dementia	Niacin (Chapter 12)
Cheilosis; scaling of skin; cracking of lips; light sensitivity; increased vascularization of eyes	Riboflavin (Chapter 12)
Growth failure, anemia, convulsions in infants	Vitamin B-6 (Chapter 12)
Night blindness; keratomalacia; xerophthalmia blindness	Vitamin A (Chapter 10)
Rickets; bone deformities	Vitamin D (Chapter 10)
Hemorrhagic tendency in infants	Vitamin K (Chapter 10)
Excesses	
Obesity	Calorie excess (Chapter 27)
Toxicity; changes in skin, hair, bones, liver	Vitamin A excess (Chapter 10)
Hypercalcemia, calcification of soft tissues	Vitamin D excess (Chapter 10)
Dental caries	Sticky sugars (Chapter 5)
Atherosclerosis; cardiovascular and cerebrovascular disease*	Too much saturated fat, cholesterol; ?simple sugars (Chapter 39)
Hypertension*	Calorie excess; ?too much salt (Chapter 40)
Diverticulosis; irritable colon*	Excessively refined diets (Chapter 32)
Cancer of the colon*	?Excessively refined diets; ?excess of fat leading to excess metabolites of sterols and bile acids (Chapter 35)

*In these diseases diet is only one of a number of risk factors that must be considered; more research is needed to fully establish the role of diet.

physician's fees, laboratory studies, medications, and other expenses. Illness also means loss of income through absence from work and loss of time in school. In the marginally ill and the physically and mentally handicapped it means reduced efficiency at work, reduced ability to learn, and the ability to perform only a limited range of tasks.

Child wastage because of malnutrition has been singled out as being especially restrictive in an economic sense. Children comprise up to half of the population in many developing countries, but most of them will never reach maturity. The costs involved in their short lives include extra food consumed by the mother during pregnancy, the costs of childbirth, the food, clothing, and shelter consumed by the child while living, and even the costs of burial. These malnourished children are consumers without ever reaching the status of producers and their own brief existence has usually been miserable.

When malnourished children survive to adulthood their stunted growth, retarded mental development, lessened ability to learn, reduced work efficiency, and physical defects including blindness are among the handicaps that beset them.

The costs of preventive action must also be considered; these include feeding programs for the vulnerable, subsidies to promote better nutrition through food stamps, food supplements to women, infants, and children, and others, and educational programs. One can expect, however, that the benefits of a preventive program far outweigh the costs of such action.

Factors Contributing to Malnutrition

The causes of malnutrition are complex. They include conditions that preexist within the individual—the *host*, the quality of the *environment*, and the specific *agents* that provoke the problem. Each element of this triad interacts with others. For example, many people in the United States suffer from some degree of malnutrition but the food supply, water, and waste disposal meet high standards of sanitation and safety so that health remains relatively good. On the other hand, people in some developing countries suffer the same degree of undernutrition but are exposed to grossly contaminated food and water so that life-threatening illness results. (See Figure 23–3.)

Susceptibility of the Individuals Within a given environment some individuals are more susceptible than others to malnutrition. Normal adults can usually survive moderate nutritional deficits rather well. Among the vulnerable groups are these:

1. Infants and preschool children: their nutritional requirements are high during rapid growth. When nutrients are not available for a given stage of development, the physical or mental retardation may be irreversible.

2. Pregnant women: inadequate diets

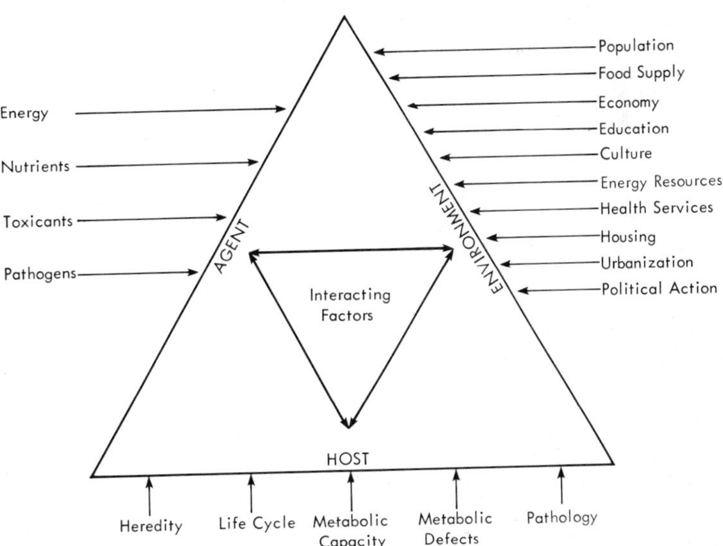

Figure 23–3. Many factors of the host-agent-environment triad interact to determine the quality of nutrition.

compromise the development of the fetus and also the mother's own nutritional status and her freedom from the complications of pregnancy.

3. The elderly: malnutrition results from chronic ill health and long-standing nutritional deficiency; endocrine imbalances; inability to chew; physical handicaps that prevent adequate shopping or food preparation; loneliness and lack of interest in eating; and misconceptions concerning diet.

4. The sick: poor appetites; psychiatric disorders that prevent eating; infections; fevers and metabolic disorders that increase nutritional requirements; allergy; blood losses; injuries; gastrointestinal disorders that lead to fear of eating; diarrhea; malabsorption; and so on.

The vulnerability of these groups to malnutrition is considered when priorities are assigned to food assistance and to educational programs.

Environmental Factors that Favor Malnutrition In the United States and throughout the world poverty and ignorance are leading causes of malnutrition. Lack of available food is a principal cause of malnutrition in the underdeveloped and the developing countries of the world, but not in North America, Europe, and Oceania.

Poverty. Two billion people live in about 100 poor underdeveloped nations of the world. Two thirds of these people live in Asia. In most African and Latin American countries the per capita income ranges from moderate to extreme poverty.

Even in the United States approximately 30 million people are living at or below the poverty level. They are to be found in the slums of the cities and in rural areas as well. Minority groups including blacks, Puerto Ricans, Spanish Americans, American Indians, and many people living in Appalachian regions constitute important segments of the poor population. The plight of no group in the United States is less favorable than that of the migrant farm workers who have few if any roots in a community and who often do not have the services of agencies that can provide assistance.

Inflationary food costs in recent years have worsened the plight of the poor. Poverty means too few dollars to spend for food; competition between food and other necessities of life as well as things that give personal satisfaction for the available income; lack of food storage and preparation facilities; inability to purchase foods under the most favorable price conditions; and crowded, often unsanitary housing. Poverty results in a vicious cycle: poverty→inadequate diet→undernutrition→illness→inability to work→poverty.

Population growth. At present the food supply in the developing countries is just about keeping pace with the growth in population. (See Figure 23–1.) Half of the world's population live in the Far East but only one fourth of the world's food supply is produced there. If the entire world food supply could be evenly distributed, it would just about meet the energy needs of the people.

By the year 2000 a population of 6.5 to 7 billion persons is predicted. Thus, it will be necessary within less than 20 years to almost double the food supply even at the present inadequate standards. There is, however, a finite limit to the acreage available for agriculture, for water resources, and for fertilizers to increase crop yields. Control of population growth is especially difficult to achieve in countries where infant and child mortality is high and each couple wants survivors who can care for them in their old age.

Lack of education. People of all income classes and at all educational levels lack knowledge regarding the essentials of an adequate diet. Those who are ignorant concerning nutrition are particularly susceptible to food faddism, superstition, and nutritional quackery.

A limited education exacts a particularly severe toll from those who are also poor. It is, for many of them, the cause of their poverty inasmuch as people with minimal education and technical skills are unable to secure employment to earn a satisfactory living wage. Somehow, the poor must use each dollar more carefully but they have too little consumer information to help them. Moreover, inasmuch as the amount and quality of food available to them are limited, they need to employ the best techniques in food preparation to preserve nutritive values—but they lack the facilities and skills to do so.

Cultural factors. Malnutrition sometimes results because people refuse to eat foods prohibited by religious beliefs or taboos and superstitions, those that lack prestige value, and those that are unfamiliar.

The taking of life is prohibited by some religions and no flesh foods may be eaten. This restriction excludes even eggs and milk for some. The prohibition against the taking of life may also mean that pesticides will not be used against rodents, thus resulting in high food losses in some countries. In India the sacred cows still compete seriously for the food supply of humans.

Social customs, taboos, and superstitions interfere with adequate food intake, especially by vulnerable groups. In some of the developing countries the father and other men in the family eat first and are given the choicest share of food. When food is scarce, women and children may get less than they need. Many primitive people believe that foods are endowed with specific qualities that can influence the personality of the unborn child or that can mark him or her physically. Thus, animal foods in particular may be taboo for pregnant and lactating women.

To be accepted food must be familiar. People to whom rice is the staple do not quickly change to a diet consisting principally of wheat. Even a change in a familiar food will reduce its acceptability. The new high-yielding varieties of rice and corn are less well liked by the people who use them because they are slightly different in color and texture and have somewhat different cooking qualities.

Plentiful foods may be ignored because they lack status value even though they are of excellent nutritive quality, whereas other foods of more marginal value may be selected because of their prestige value. Poor people often resent gifts of food that are classified as surplus. In the developing countries spices, fats, oils, sweets, tea, coffee, and cola beverages are often purchased because they are equated with a higher standard of living.

Misinformation and Faddism A fad is a fashion of the moment—here today, gone tomorrow. Fads sometimes disappear, only to reappear some years later in a new form. Persons of all ages fall prey to exaggerated claims: the teenage girl looking for a quick way to lose some weight; the teenage boy seeking athletic prowess; the elderly person hoping for some panacea for impaired health. In each instance lack of education in nutrition, the influence of peers, and the pressures of advertising may have been influential.

During the past decade the words *natural, organic,* and *health* have been used to characterize certain foods, these attributes being "good." The words *synthetic, chemical, additive,* and *processed* have often been used to denote "bad" characteristics. Herein lies much misinformation about the quality of the food supply.

At the least, such characterizations are misleading. Probably $1 billion is spent annually for "natural," "organic," and "health foods." Such foods are neither more nor less nutritious than their counterparts available in supermarkets, but they are usually much more expensive. For persons with limited income the additional expenditure for such foods could mean the elimination of other needed foods.

Urbanization. Jelliffe[4] has described the flood of rural dwellers to the cities that is now occurring throughout the entire world as "disurbanization" because the influx is too rapid to accommodate people in terms of employment, housing, food, and services. The shanty towns and ghettos provide surroundings that are often worse than the rural areas left behind. Because they need cash to purchase food, people find themselves with diets that are more meager than their rural fare.

Infants and children suffer most from this trend. Infants are often weaned early, partly because the mother seeks employment and partly because she is trying to emulate the women of the Western world who do not breast feed their babies. Unfortunately, the substitute feedings for the baby are insufficient in quantity, often poor in quality, and likely to be grossly contaminated with bacteria. Jelliffe deplores the use of highly advertised expensive proprietary infant formulas because few people in the developing countries can afford them and mothers use too little of the formula to meet the baby's needs.

Inadequate supply of food. Since 1972–1973 there has been a deepening food crisis throughout the world. Natural disasters such as the floods in Bangladesh and India, the severe droughts for several years in the Sahel, Africa, and political upheaval as in Campuchia have severely curtailed food production thus leading to starvation for millions of people. People in affluent countries are demanding more and more animal foods, especially meat, and thereby excessive amounts of grain are fed to animals rather than being used directly as human food.

Tremendous increases in oil prices have made it impossible for farmers in developing countries to adopt modern methods of agriculture that depend upon energy resources, or to purchase fertilizers that are dependent upon oil for their production. Food spoilage is excessively high because of lack of processing, storage, and distribution facilities. Where agriculture is most primitive the diets are almost always at the subsistence level. Thus, there is no food left over for an emergency. In the developing countries governments are usually unable to finance the irrigation programs needed for crops, the industrial plants for food processing and storage, and the roads for food distribution.

Protein-Calorie Malnutrition

Protein-calorie malnutrition (PCM), the world's most serious nutritional problem, to some degree affects up to 70 per cent of infants and preschool children in the developing countries of Africa, the Middle East, southeastern Asia, and Central and South America. Millions die annually and millions more will go through life stunted in their physical growth and unable to achieve their potential mental development. PCM is an inclusive term that embraces mild deficiency, kwashiorkor, and marasmus. (See Figure 23–2.)

Etiology Dr. Cicely Williams, a pediatrician, in the 1930s observed a syndrome in infants and children in Ghana which was called kwashiorkor. This is "the disease the deposed baby gets when the next one is born."[5] In the developing countries babies are usually breast fed for 18 to 24 months, and sometimes longer. Upon the birth of another child, the older child is deposed from the breast and subsists largely on a high-carbohydrate low-protein diet provided by the staple foods of the country. The symptoms become apparent about 3 to 4 months after the child has been weaned and have their highest incidence between 2 and 5 years of age.

In Africa the staples to which the child is weaned are manioc, cassava, plantain, and millet; in Central America and South America they are corn and beans; and in Asia, rice and some legumes. These foods do not provide sufficient amino acids for the rapid growth needs of the infant. The ignorance of the mother concerning food needs of the baby may further reduce the intake of protein. In Iran, for example, many babies are given tea sweetened with as much as 40 gm sugar daily.[6] Formulas are often diluted excessively so that they provide neither the calories nor the protein the infant needs. When diarrhea is present, the concerned mother often resorts to feeding of dilute gruels for extended periods of time.

Marasmus results from a deficiency of calories as well as protein. It occurs at an earlier age than does kwashiorkor and is usually evident by the second half of the first year. The incidence of marasmus is increasing with urbanization in the developing countries because infants are being weaned at a very early age. The low-protein formulas and other staple foods, poverty, poor sanitation, and cultural patterns all contribute to the high incidence. The occurrence of PCM in mild to severe stages accelerates rapidly in countries afflicted by drought, floods, and war.

Synergism between Malnutrition and Infection When a diet is nutritionally inadequate but the sanitation is good and infections are minimal, the onset of deficiency symptoms is gradual. Likewise, when a well-nourished child succumbs to an infection, the period of illness is usually short, the residual effects are few, and the mortality rate is low. Conversely, the coexistence of malnutrition and infection vastly increases the severity of both; that is, a synergism exists between the two. (See Figure 23–4.) The child with prekwashiokor rapidly advances to kwashiorkor if gastroenteritis, measles, or some other infection is also present. Infections that are ordinarily mild become so severe in the malnourished that the resulting death rate is high. In some countries the mortality from measles is 400 times greater than in the United States—not because of increase in virulence but because of coexisting malnutrition.

Mild Deficiency The symptoms of mild deficiency of calories and protein are nonspecific. Most infants and preschool children in the developing countries suffer from mild deficiency of calories or protein or both. The outstanding characteristic is growth retardation or growth failure. The deficiency is not always detected unless one determines the age of the child, since the height and the weight may be proportionate. There is delayed maturation of the bones and other biologic systems. Anorexia, mental apathy, infections, and diarrhea are common findings.

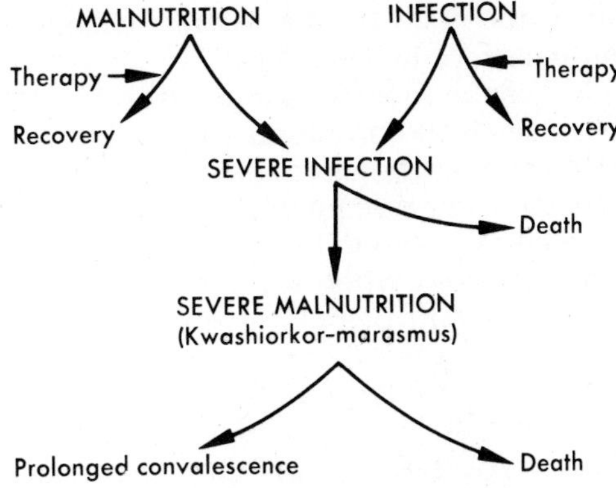

Figure 23–4. The prognosis in malnutrition or infection occurring independently is good if appropriate therapy is instituted promptly. When malnutrition and infection interact, the severity of both is greatly increased and the prognosis is guarded.

Kwashiorkor Moderate to severe failure of growth is present in kwashiorkor. For the first few months of life the breast-fed infant in the developing countries grows at a rate that is comparable to that of well-fed infants in the Western world. Thereafter, the increase in stature and in tissue development is increasingly retarded. The muscles are poorly developed and lack tone.

Edema is the cardinal symptom in kwashiorkor. It is usually severe, resulting in a large pot belly and swollen legs and face and masking the muscle wasting that has occurred. (See Figure 23–2.)

The skin, especially in the pelvic region and the thighs often becomes dry and flaky, peeling, and sometimes ulcerated. The hair is easily plucked out, thin, and takes on a reddish color.

Anorexia and diarrhea are common. In fact, poor sanitation is likely to be the cause of the diarrhea, which, in turn, rapidly advances the child from moderate malnutrition to severe kwashiorkor.

One of the more striking features of the deficiency is the profound apathy and general misery of the child. He whimpers but does not cry or scream. He is not interested in or curious about his surroundings, but remains seated wherever he is put down. When he again begins to smile he is said to be on the road to recovery.

Pathologic and biochemical changes. Fatty infiltration of the liver is usually extensive. The serum levels of triglycerides, phospholipids, and cholesterol are reduced indicating an inability of the liver to manufacture and release these substances to the circulation. Atrophy of the pancreas results in a lessened production of amylase, lipase, and trypsin.

The total serum protein and albumin fractions are markedly reduced thus accounting for the severe edema that is present. Hemoglobin levels are low, especially if parasitism is also present. The serum vitamin A levels are usually reduced; profound vitamin A deficiency is a serious complication leading to blindness and death in some children.

Marasmus Severe growth failure and emaciation are the most striking characteristics of the marasmic infant. The wasting of the muscles and the lack of subcutaneous fat are extreme. As in kwashiorkor, the incidence of diarrhea is high. (See Figure 23–5.)

Marasmus differs from kwashiorkor in several important respects: the onset is earlier, usually within the first year of life; growth failure is more pronounced; there is no edema and the blood protein con-

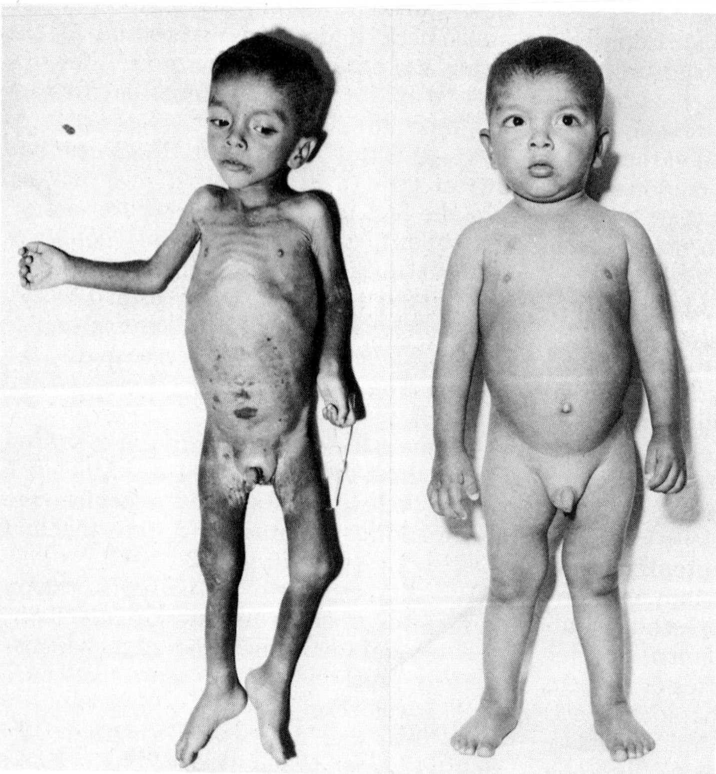

Figure 23–5. Severe protein-calorie malnutrition. Two-year-old child 2 weeks after admission and 10 weeks after treatment with INCAPARINA. (Courtesy, Institute of Central America and Panama, and the *Journal of The American Dietetic Association.*)

centration is reduced less markedly; skin changes are seen less frequently; the liver is not infiltrated with fat; and the period of recovery is much longer.

Mental Development Possibly the most serious problem of PCM is in the mental retardation that may occur. It must be emphasized that the effects of malnutrition on mental development and learning are exceedingly difficult to measure. As a rule, the malnourished child is also exposed to environmental influences that interfere with rapid learning. Moreover, the methods for testing children in one cultural environment are not applicable in an entirely different cultural setting. If brain development is irreversibly retarded, this could mean that nations with large numbers of malnourished children might be unable to achieve their economic and social equality with the rest of the world.

The marasmic infant is in great danger of retarded mental development. Retardation is less frequent and less severe in kwashiorkor. Malnutrition can have two effects on the child's potential mental development. First, if the nutrients required for multiplication and growth of the brain cells are lacking during the period of most rapid development, it appears highly unlikely that the deficiency can be corrected by improved nutrition once the time cycle for brain development has gone by. It would be expected that the effects would be most profound in severe malnutrition during the first year of life. If nutrition is satisfactory during infancy and subsequently deteriorates, the effects are less devastating.

The second effect of malnutrition in the preschool years may be on the interference of learning that normally occurs in healthy preschool children at a truly fantastic rate. The apathy, lack of curiosity, and reduced activity of the malnourished child over a protracted period of time will greatly reduce the amount of learning. Thus, the development of behavioral characteristics expected of the normal child at any given age may be delayed for months or years and may sometimes never be fully corrected.

Prevention and Treatment of PCM The growth chart is the best tool for the early detection of growth failure. In the developing countries breast feeding should be urged since it helps to ensure more nearly adequate protein and caloric intake. The most practical approach to the prevention of PCM is to improve the food supply of the entire family because this is the best way to ensure that the preschool child will receive his or her needed share. Such a goal involves the improvement of locally available food supplies, income, and education. These measures of course are not of much help to the child in immediate need.

Food mixtures that contain sufficient quantities of essential amino acids to meet the growth needs of the child have been developed in a number of countries.

Another approach of considerable importance is the improvement of sanitation and programs of immunization so that the incidence of infections is greatly reduced.

When properly planned, a milk formula is curative of mild malnutrition. For some children a lactose-free formula is required. At later stages a milk formula or food mixtures bring about weight gain, a return of the appetite, and increased interest in surroundings. The liver and pancreas rapidly return to normal and the blood proteins are increased to normal levels. The effects on brain development are not as likely to be reversed if therapy has been delayed.

The prognosis for children with alterations in fluid and electrolyte balance is not good. A deficit of potassium is usually present in severe malnutrition and this may lead to cardiac failure if food therapy is too vigorous in the beginning. Also, an excess of sodium in the feedings can precipitate cardiac failure.

When electrolyte imbalance is present, the initial therapy should be directed to restoration of electrolyte and fluid balance.

Thereafter, a half-strength formula of skim milk is fed, with gradual increases to a whole-milk formula that furnishes 125 to 150 kcal and 3 to 4 gm protein per kilogram.

Anemia and vitamin A deficiency become more apparent as growth resumes and blood volume increases. These complications can be prevented by using formulas that are fortified with vitamins A and D, and with iron and folacin. A single injection of 100,000 IU water miscible vitamin A may be given instead of the daily supplementation of the formula.

Community Nutrition Services for Prevention and Intervention

National Food and Nutrition Policy Unemployment, poverty, worldwide inflation, dwindling food stockpiles, rapid developments in food technology, regulation of food quality and safety, concerns about diet and health—all of these factors and others point to the need for a food and nutrition policy at the highest levels of government. A national food and nutrition policy is a constantly evolving concept. The directions that a policy should take are recommended by consumer and industry groups, by professional organizations, and by concerned citizens. Policies are adopted in part by educational programs that bring about change in practices and in part by legislative action.

The Nutrition Consortium (The American Dietetic Association, the American Institute of Nutrition, the American Society for Clinical Nutrition, the Institute of Food Technologists, and the Society for Nutrition Education) has developed guidelines for a national nutrition policy.[7] The aim of such a policy is "to provide an adequate diet at a reasonable cost to every person within the United States." This aim has never been realized even in the United States, let alone in other nations of the world.

The food and nutrition policy stated by the U.S. Department of Agriculture is "to ensure that there will continue to be an adequate, safe, palatable, nutritionally balanced, and reasonably priced food supply, equitably available to all Americans."* The very low incidence of deficiency disease is evidence that such a policy has been successful. But it has become increasingly apparent that a nutritionally adequate diet is not enough and that overconsumption, widely prevalent in the United States, becomes a risk factor for a number of diseases. Thus, the dietary guidelines described in Chapter 3 represent another component of food and nutrition policy.

Prior to the 1970s the government programs in the agricultural sector dealt primarily with the needs of farmers. But the nation's economy and inflation, the world's inability to meet the expanding needs for food, the interdependence of nations, and even the changing perceptions of dietary needs required a reorientation of policy. Thus, the Food and Agriculture Act of 1977 was a response to the needs of consumers as well as farmers. The 1977 act provides for expansion of human nutrition research. It provides for the first federally mandated program of nutrition education for children. Another consideration is that "nutritional goals may require changes in the types of commodities at the farm level and thus change the emphasis of government programs for producers, marketing promotion, regulation, and research."† Other important provisions of this act are the food assistance programs. (See Table 23-2.)

* *Food and Nutrition for the 1980's: Moving Ahead.* U.S. Department of Agriculture, Washington, D.C., April 1979, p. iii.

† *Agricultural-Food Policy Review,* Economics, Statistics, and Cooperative Services, U.S. Department of Agriculture, Washington, D.C., February 1980, p. 81.

Nutrition Education

Scope of Educational Programs Education means change in behavior. It moves the individual from lack of interest and ignorance to increasing appreciation and knowledge and finally to action. Nutrition education offers a great opportunity to individuals to learn about the essentials of nutrition for health and to take steps to improve the quality of their diets and thus their well-being.

In 1977 an amendment to the Child Nutrition Act mandated that 50 cents per child be allocated to each state for education in nutrition. If this education is to succeed, it must become an essential component of the curriculum for each of the elementary and secondary school years. The content must be sequential and coordinated from year to year. Classroom instruction is effectively enhanced by experiences through the school food services. To succeed, the teachers in the nation's schools must have opportunity for nutrition study while in college or through in-service courses. (See Figure 23–6.)

Dietary counseling, described in Chapter 22, is an example of education in nutrition on a one-to-one basis and is designed to bring about desired changes in food behavior as identified by nutritional assessment. Educational activities at the community level are available at health centers, maternal and child-care centers, day-care centers, programs for the elderly, youth organizations, women's clubs, and special purpose programs such as those for alcoholism, drug abuse, and the handicapped.

Nutrition education must continue throughout the individual's life in order to accommodate for developments in nutrition science and for changing economic circumstances, health requirements, and the new food products appearing in the nation's markets. This requires a greatly expanded use of the mass media, and the involvement of governmental and private agencies, universities, as well as the food industries.

What Knowledge Is Essential The Interagency Committee on Nutrition Education developed basic concepts on the nutrition information needed to make wise choices of food for individuals and families. The concepts are not facts to be memorized as such, but they serve as guidelines for the selection of content, learning experiences,

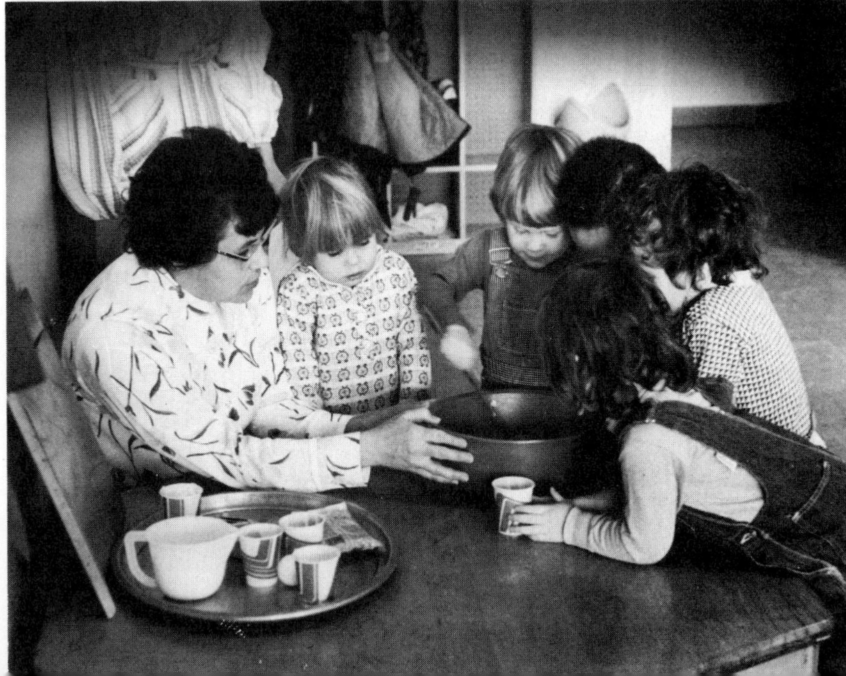

Figure 23–6. Nursery school children enjoy food preparation. They learn about food and develop muscle coordination. (Courtesy, University of Delaware.)

and teaching materials in a program of education.

Basic Concepts in Nutrition

1. Nutrition is the food you eat and how the body uses it.
   We eat food to live, to grow, to keep healthy and well, and to get energy for work and play.
2. Food is made up of different nutrients needed for health and growth.
   All nutrients needed by the body are available through food. Many kinds and combinations of food can lead to a well-balanced diet. No food, by itself, has all the nutrients needed for full growth and health. Each nutrient has specific uses in the body. Most of the nutrients do their best work in the body when teamed with other nutrients.
3. All persons, throughout life, have need for the same nutrients, but in varying amounts.
   The amounts of nutrients needed are influenced by age, sex, size, activity, and state of health. Suggestions for the kinds and amounts of food needed are made by trained scientists.
4. The way food is handled influences the amount of nutrients in food, its safety, appearance, and taste.
   Handling means everything that happens to food while it is being grown, processed, stored, and prepared for eating.*

Dietary excesses. In addition to stressing a sufficiency of all nutrients to meet the metabolic needs of the individual throughout the life cycle, nutrition educators must emphasize the importance of avoiding excesses of calories, saturated fats, simple sugars, refined foods, and salt. These excesses over the course of a lifetime lead to obesity and dental caries and are considered to be risk factors in heart disease, hypertension, diabetes mellitus, and various gastrointestinal disorders. (See pages 522, 631, and 656.)

Nutritional Services

Nature of Services In the hospital or clinic the nurse and dietitian give direct service to the individual. Nutrition services of the community are also provided on an individual basis, especially at the city-county level. For example, such direct services are given by a public health nurse, a nutritionist, a homemaker from a welfare agency, or a volunteer who delivers a hot meal to an aged person.

Community programs in nutrition seek to improve nutrition through research, education, improvement of the food supply, and feeding. The individual reaps the rewards of activities such as these: legislation which makes funds available for feeding vulnerable groups and which protects the food supply; research concerning the preventive and therapeutic aspects of diet with respect to disease; methods for preserving the food supply; the development of new and better foods through food technology; a more abundant food supply because of research on plant varieties, soil conservation, pest control; education for an adequate diet—and so on.

Typical Community Services A complex network of agencies exists at the local, state, and national level for providing nutrition services to the people at all stages of the life cycle. Health workers must know what public and private resources exist in the community so that they are able to make appropriate referrals for assistance.

Nutritionists in local and state programs work closely with physicians, nurses, dentists, dental hygienists, social workers, administrators of institutions, food service managers, dietitians, and others. The following activities are representative of those included in nutrition programs.

1. Define the place of nutrition in program areas.
   a. Conduct surveys of the community needs.
2. Provide materials on nutrition information.
   a. Analyze and interpret findings of science.
   b. Prepare leaflets on topics such as: weight control; meal planning; in-

* Hill, M. M.: "I.C.N.E. Formulates Some Basic Concepts in Nutrition," *Nutrition Program News,* September–October 1964, U.S. Department of Agriculture, Washington, D.C.

fant feeding; food misinformation; diet patterns for various cultural groups; teenagers; senior citizens.
   c. Prepare diet manuals, food value charts, exhibits, newspaper, magazine, radio, and television releases.
3. Consultant service to agencies and institutions: child care, nursing homes, small hospitals, mental hospitals, homes for the elderly.
   a. Planning food service facilities.
   b. Personnel training; budgeting; menu planning; purchasing; sanitation; preparation and service of food; therapeutic diets.
4. Work with schools: elementary, secondary, college, medical, nursing, allied health.
   a. Plan and conduct dietary surveys as part of research program.
   b. Assist in developing programs in nutrition education.
   c. Conduct workshops for school faculty.
   d. Assist in training programs for school food service personnel; help to interpret educational value of school meals.
5. Cooperate with other health groups in rehabilitation and in chronic disease programs: cardiovascular disease, cancer, diabetes, tuberculosis, arthritis, cerebral palsy, orthopedic disabilities, mental retardation, and so on.
   a. Preparation of materials for professional and lay instruction.
   b. Conduct of institutes for staff education of nurses, nutritionists, physicians.
6. Work with patients individually or in groups.
   a. Clinics: child health, crippled children, cardiovascular, diabetes, prenatal, tuberculosis.
   b. Food budgets.
   c. Home visits.
7. Work with other groups:
   a. Social and welfare agencies on dietary standards and budgets.
   b. Public instruction.
8. Assist in programs of research with schools of home economics, medical schools, departments of health, federal and private agencies.

Federal Nutrition Programs The *Inventory of Federal Food, Nutrition and Agriculture Programs* describes 359 programs administered by 28 agencies. Some of the major programs are listed in Table 23-2 and are described at appropriate points throughout the text.

Helping People with Low Incomes

Characteristics of the Poor The poor are often thought of as a single group that can be described in terms of a "culture of poverty." Although certain characteristics of behavior are enforced upon them by reason of poverty, it is a serious error to regard the poor as a homogeneous group.[8]

Variations in environment and culture. Poor people living in Appalachia, the Mexican-Americans of the Southwest, the Puerto Ricans, the American Indians, the black people in city ghettos, and many people in cities and in rural areas have one thing in common—lack of sufficient income to meet their basic needs. Their cultures, however, have little in common. Moreover, within each of these groups, individuals and families differ from one another in their values, aspirations, and style of living just as people of the more affluent society differ from one another. Some poor people come from families that have been poor for generations and have never known any other way of life; other people are poor because of changed circumstances brought about by unemployment, inflation, and health costs. Some of the poor have a fair level of education, whereas others are illiterate. Some homemakers are good managers and do a remarkable job in keeping the family together, whereas others lack even the simplest skills in homemaking and in child care. Some constantly strive for a better way of life, whereas others regard their

Table 23-2. **Some Examples of Federally Sponsored Nutrition Programs**

Program	Description
Administered by the Food and Nutrition Service, U.S. Department of Agriculture	
National School Lunch Program	Cash and food subsidies to school programs; reduced and free meals for the poor. See page 378.
School Breakfast Program	Especially for low-income areas. See page 379.
Special Milk Program	Reimbursement for milk served to children.
Summer Food Service Program	Assistance to public and nonprofit institutions operating recreational programs in low-income areas.
Food Stamp Program	See page 429.
Supplemental Food Program for Women, Infants, and Children (WIC)	Food supplements to supply nutrients low in diets of high-risk persons. See page 378.
Education in schools	Allocates 50 cents per child in each state for education in nutrition.
Administered by Cooperative Extension Service, U.S. Department of Agriculture	
Expanded Food and Nutrition Education Program (EFNEP)	See page 429.
Administered by the U.S. Department of Health and Human Resources	
Nutrition programs for the elderly Congregate meals Home-delivered meals Nutrition education	See page 388.
Early and Periodic Screening, Diagnosis, and Treatment	Preventive medical care for persons under 21 who are Medicaid beneficiaries.
Maternity and Infant Care Projects (MIC, M&I)	Multidisciplinary prenatal care to high-risk women, and to high-risk infants. See page 341.
Children and Youth Projects (C&Y)	Comprehensive health care to preschool and school children in low-income areas.
Head Start	Multiple health services to children 3 years to school age in low-income areas.

present status as permanent and they can do little about it.

The limitations of poverty. A limited income restricts people to living in declining neighborhoods with deteriorating houses, inadequate sanitation, crowding, and lack of privacy. There is a constant fear of eviction because of loss of income and failure to pay the rent.

The poor are isolated from society. They move about from place to place—usually not by choice but by necessity—and therefore establish no roots in the community. Their participation in community activities is minimal and their contact with the outside world through newspapers and magazines is small. This isolation encourages suspicion of the motives of those who may try to help them; it also means that they are poorly equipped to cope with emergencies because they do not know what resources are available to them.

The poor must live from day to day and are unable to plan ahead. The future is uncertain, they are fatalistic about what is to come, and setting goals for the future seems pointless.

Lacking education, the poor may not be able to make the best use of the little money they have. They are often at the mercy of credit schemes that, over a period of time, exact large interest payments.

Poor people have known little success. They feel that people look down on them and have little concern for them. They will often place more confidence in the advice of a neighbor, a faith healer, or a practitioner of folk medicine—all of whom are attuned to their way of living.

Social problems are not unique to the poor but they are likely to be more frequent. Many of the families have only one parent, usually the mother. Men in many households are unable to fulfill their roles as providers, and they leave their homes so that their families can qualify for public assistance.

Better Nutrition for the Poor Adequate income is basic to an adequate diet. Before you can tell people what foods they require and how to prepare them, there must be food in the home to prepare or money with which to purchase it. Many people who receive welfare allowances or whose sole source of income is Social Security are unable to provide the amounts of foods recommended for the low-cost plan (see page 271). The problem has become increasingly acute with the rapid increase in fuel and other utility services; for some it could mean choosing between staving off hunger or keeping warm.

Food Stamp Program. Some 16 to 21 million persons from year to year have been eligible for the Food Stamp Program first authorized in 1964. The stamps are issued to families and single persons who meet income eligibility standards. They may be used instead of money to purchase food and to buy seeds or plants for producing food. The elderly may use the stamps for their contribution to congregate meal programs.

It is the intention of the program to increase food purchasing power. Although the stamps may be used only for the purchase of food, there is no guarantee that some of the income ordinarily spent for food might be released for nonfood purchases. It should be obvious that consumer education along with the distribution of the food stamps is needed so that maximum nutritional benefits are realized.

Expanded Food and Nutrition Education for the Poor (EFNEP). Home economists and nutritionists in the Cooperative Extension Service of the U.S. Department of Agriculture give intensive training to nutrition aides. The aides are mature, nonprofessional women selected from the community in which they will serve. These women are usually aware of the problems of families with whom they will work. They know from their own experience what it means to have little money to spend for food. Their assistance is less likely to be viewed with suspicion than is that of a helper who comes from a middle-class environment with different standards and values, and with little understanding of what it means to be poor.

Program aides work with homemakers on an individual basis in their homes and give assistance on the problems associated with foods, child care, housekeeping and management, clothing repair, and so on. The assistance for better nutrition is on such practical points as how to prepare simple dishes, how to make the best use of the food money, how to use food stamps, what to look for on a label or on unit pricing, how to use a food guide, and easily prepared breakfasts. Very easy to read booklets are often made available. (See Figure 23–7.)

International Agencies for Nutrition

Food and Agriculture Organization The Food and Agriculture Organization of the United Nations (FAO) was founded in Quebec, Canada, in October 1945 the aims being:

To help the nations raise the standard of living;
To improve the nutrition of the people of all countries;
To increase the efficiency of farming, forestry, and fisheries;
To better the condition of rural people;

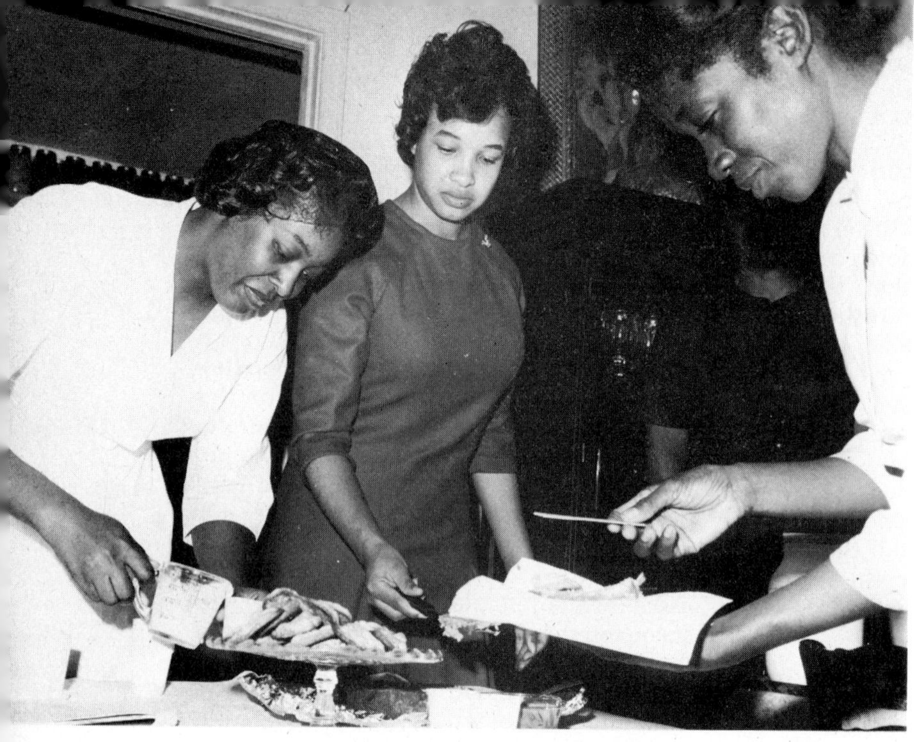

Figure 23–7. Nutrition aides prepare foods to be used in a demonstration in a home. (Courtesy, Kevin Shields and U.S. Department of Agriculture.)

And, through these means, to widen the opportunity of all people for productive work.*

The headquarters office of FAO is in Rome where the work of the organization is supervised by a director-general. FAO maintains an intelligence service which gathers, analyzes, and distributes information on which action can be based, and advises governments on actions to take.

Technical assistance is provided in agriculture, economics, fisheries, forestry, and nutrition to member countries. The diversified projects have included development of food storage, processing, and marketing facilities; land reclamation through irrigation and drainage; control of animal diseases; development of grains of higher nutritive value; increased yields of crops and greater resistance to disease; inland fish culture in ponds and rice fields; establishment of home economics programs in colleges; school feeding; and many others.

World Health Organization The World Health Organization (WHO) was created in 1948 and is administered by a director-general with headquarters in Geneva, Switzerland, and with six regional offices, one of which is in Washington, D.C.

WHO is "the directing and coordinating authority for international health work." It is governed by two principles defined in its constitution:

UNIVERSALITY: The health of all peoples is fundamental to the achievement of peace and security. The enjoyment of the highest attainable standard of health is one of the fundamental rights of every human being without distinction of race, religion, political belief, economic or social condition.

CONCEPT OF HEALTH: Health is a state of complete physical, mental and social well-being and not merely the absence of disease or infirmity.†

The assistance which WHO renders to government includes

. . . strengthening national health services; establishing and maintaining epidemiological and

* *Food and Agriculture Organization—What It Is—What It Does—How It Works.* Leaflet, Food and Agriculture Organization, Rome, 1956.

† *World Health Organization—What Is It—What It Does—How It Works.* Leaflet, World Health Organization, Geneva, 1956.

statistical services; controlling epidemic and endemic diseases; maternal and child health; promotion of mental health to foster harmonious human relations; improvement of sanitation and of preventive and curative medical services.*

United Nations Children's Fund To children in different countries UNICEF means different things. It may mean an injection to cure them of yaws, a crippling disease, or vaccination to protect against tuberculosis; or protection against blindness caused by lack of vitamin A; or food to stave of starvation.

Organized in 1947, UNICEF continued the emergency feeding in war-devastated countries of Europe, with emphasis upon protein-rich foods, especially milk. Now, in developing countries all over the world, programs are directed to infants, children, and pregnant and lactating women. Although UNICEF continues to provide emergency relief, most of its funds are now diverted to long-range programs, for it is realized that countries must be able to solve their own nutritional problems.

United States Responsibility in World Nutrition Each nation justifies its participation in programs to solve world nutrition problems on the basis of economic and political considerations as well as humanitarian concerns. The needs were identified at the World Food Conference held in Rome in 1974. "The penalty of failure is a spectre of want, of need and starvation of inconceivably disastrous proportions."†

Food must be a vehicle for promoting peace and not a political tool used only at high levels of government. Public Law 480, the Food for Peace Program, was adopted by the Congress in 1954 as a means of using agricultural surpluses for feeding the world's needy people. The program has been administered by the Agency for International Development (AID) in the Department of State.

Throughout the years the program has provided food through UNICEF, CARE, and other relief agencies working in maternal and child health centers. (See Figure 23–8.) Food has been available for refugees and to feed people in disasters such as floods, hurricanes, and crop failures. Food has also been used as part payment for laborers working on development programs: irrigation projects, dams, roads, drainage, and so on. Assistance has been given to business investors by providing guarantees against losses of investments in developing countries through war, revolution, and expropriation. Loans have been made to the development of food industry in various countries including dairy plants, bakeries, fertilizer plants, and tractor manufacture.

The people of the United States can set an example by modest changes in their own food habits so that there is less demand for meat from grain-fed animals. (See pages 68 and 432.) Much food is wasted each day in the United States, and in the homes as well as institutions this can be greatly reduced.

Increasing the World Food Supply

Priorities At least 20 per cent of the people in less developed countries receive far too few calories and 60 per cent receive diets of poor quality. People who are poor and for whom the food supply is scarce are in need of (1) sufficient calories to sustain life and (2) protein of adequate quality and amount. The food must be culturally acceptable and must have taste, odor, and texture properties that provide palatability. The foods must be locally available, easily transported, stable for long periods without spoilage in the absence of refrigeration, and low in cost.

Important enterprises of AID and foundations such as the Ford and Rockefeller Foundations have included the development of better agricultural practices, im-

* *World Health Organization—What Is It—What It Does—How It Works.* Leaflet, World Health Organization, Geneva, 1956.

† Darby, W. J.: "Nutrition, Food Needs and Technologic Priorities: The World Food Conference," *Nutr. Rev.*, 33:233, 1975.

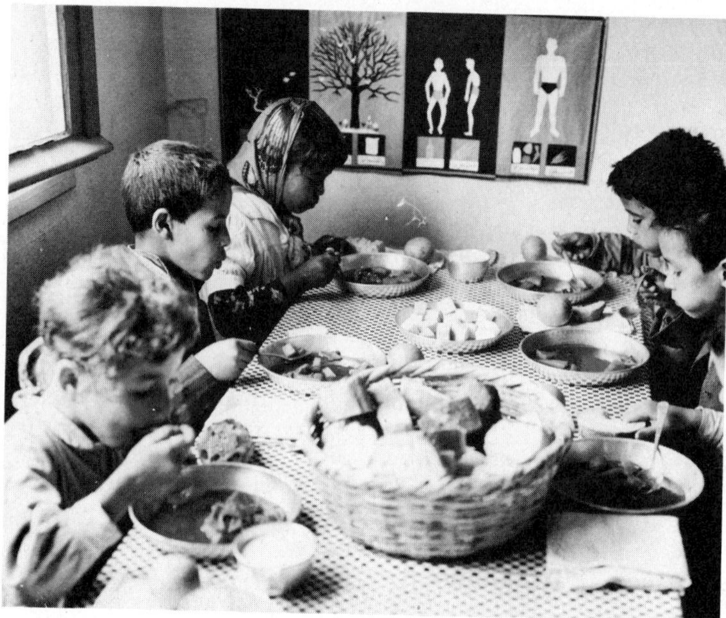

Figure 23–8. A nourishing meal of soup, bread, cheese, and fruit helps to teach children the basic principles of nutrition as well as to provide the nourishment they need. (UNICEF Photo/Almasy)

proved strains of plants, and protein mixtures of high nutritive value. In turn the skills of the agriculturist, food technologist, nutrition scientist, marketing expert, anthropologist, and many others have been involved in the governmental research programs, in universities, and in the food industries.

Potential Sources of Food Cereal grains today comprise the principal source of food for the world's people and will, undoubtedly, continue to rank first throughout the world. In recent years agricultural scientists have brought about the so-called "green revolution." In many less developed countries high yields of cereals are being achieved by using improved strains of rice, wheat, and corn, and by emphasizing modern agricultural practices including fertilizers and equipment. The green revolution buys time, but eventually food production will not be able to keep up with the present rapid growth in population.

Improved cereal quality. Cereal grains are deficient in one or more of the essential amino acids and thus do not meet the needs for rapid synthesis of proteins required for growth. (See page 66.) An outstanding example of an improved cereal grain is opaque-2 corn, a hybrid variety that has been developed in which the lysine and tryptophan content of the endosperm is 50 per cent higher than in regular varieties.[9] Also, the leucine content is lower so that the balance with isoleucine is improved. This development is of considerable significance to Central American, Latin American, and some African nations where corn is a staple food. In 1973 two varieties of high-lysine sorghum were developed. Eventually, this will be of benefit in arid regions of Asia and Africa where sorghum is a staple food.

Triticale is a man-made grain, combining the properties of wheat and rye. It contains a higher quality of protein than other grains, and it is more resistant to drought and cold than is wheat.

Amino acid supplementation. To improve the protein quality of wheat requires additional lysine; rice needs lysine and threonine; legumes require methionine;

and corn requires tryptophan and lysine. Although supplementation with lysine and methionine is now economically feasible, the cost of tryptophan is still too high for practical application. Moreover, amino acid supplementation is not readily accomplished except in large-scale flour mills.

Nutrition scientists have been cautious about amino acid supplementation because an excess of certain amino acids can create an increased need for the next most limiting amino acid. Amino acid imbalances in low-protein diets can result in growth failure and other metabolic problems.

Other plant sources. Legumes, including chick peas, peanuts, and many varieties of beans, are important sources of protein and calories in Central America, Africa, and India. Soybeans contain protein of superior quality and probably have not been utilized for human food as much as they might be. Cottonseed is a useful source of protein when the toxic pigment, gossypol, is removed.

Soybean, wheat, cottonseed, and peanuts can be processed to provide protein-rich foods that simulate chunks of beef, chicken, ham, or bacon bits. These products find wide use in restaurants and institutions. Meat dishes used in school food services may contain up to 30 per cent of such products.

Fish. Japan leads the world with an annual per capita consumption of 32 kg fish. In the Soviet Union the per capita intake is 10 kg and in the United States 6 kg. In recent years fishing has exceeded the capacity to regenerate the seas, and since 1970 there has been a steady decline in the catch of fish. Much competition exists today between nations concerning fishing rights. Another serious problem is the pollution of the seas by oil, and agricultural, industrial, and municipal wastes. Polluted waters may kill fish, interfere with their reproduction, or render fish unfit to eat, for example, the mercury poisoning that has been traced to fish in isolated instances in Japan.

Fish protein concentrate is a low-fat, bland powder produced from whole fish. It contains in excess of 80 per cent protein, but problems of production and palatability have prevented wide use of this product.

Food mixtures. Many food mixtures that apply the principle of the supplementary value of the proteins of various foods have been developed, particularly for the relief of protein-calorie malnutrition in children. These mixtures do not yet account for a sizable proportion of the world's protein needs. Among the mixtures that have been shown to be nutritionally satisfactory, economically feasible, and acceptable to the consumers are these:

C.S.M.: corn, soy, milk blend; developed for use in U.S. AID programs

INCAPARINA: the first mixture to be developed; cottonseed and corn flours, vitamins, minerals, and torula yeast; protein efficiency equal to milk; 26 per cent protein; Central America.

BAL AHAR: a farina-like blend of bulgur wheat, peanut flour, nonfat dry milk, vitamins, minerals; 22 per cent protein; India.

GOLDEN ELBOW MACARONI *(General Foods):* corn, soy, and wheat flours; calcium carbonate, calcium phosphate, iron, B vitamins; 20 per cent protein; Brazil.

LECHE ALIM: A cereal food of toasted wheat flour, fish protein concentrate, sunflower meal, skim milk powder; 27 per cent protein; Chile.

PUMA *(Monsanto):* SACI *(Coca-Cola);* and VITASOY *(Lo):* beverages containing vegetable protein, sugar, vitamins; compete with soft drinks in price and are well accepted; 2.5 to 3 per cent protein; Brazil, Guiana, Hong Kong.

Food for the future. Leaves of plants such as alfalfa and single-celled plants, including yeasts, fungi, and algae, may become important sources of food in the more distant future. The techniques for producing them at low cost are not yet known, and major problems remain in developing products that are aesthetically acceptable. The high nucleic acid content leads to increased uric acid production and subsequent problems of excretion.

Problems and Review

1. Key terms: etiology; kwashiorkor; malnutrition; marasmus; nutritional status survey; protein-calorie malnutrition; synergism.
2. What problems of malnutrition are you aware of in your community? What factors may be contributing to these problems?
3. Explain why the rapid urbanization of the world's population is especially devastating to infants and preschool children.
4. Describe the differences between kwashiorkor and marasmus.
5. List the public and private agencies in your own community that work for better nutrition in one way or another. If possible, arrange for an interview to learn more about the activities of one of these.
6. *Problem.* Plan a lesson on one of these topics to help a homemaker who has a low income:
   a. How to obtain and use food stamps.
   b. How to use nonfat dry milk in some cooked foods.
   c. What to look for on labels of packages.
   d. Buying protein-rich foods for economy.
7. *Problem.* Determine the current regulations for assistance through food stamps in your community.
8. *Problem.* Determine the current public assistance allowance in your community for:
   a. A husband and wife over 65 years.
   b. A mother with four children: girls, 6 and 10 years; and boys, 4 and 14 years.
   Based on the current cost of foods for a low-cost diet, what per cent of this assistance allowance must be spent for food?

Cited References

1. Darby, W. J.: "Nutrition, Food Needs and Technologic Priorities: The World Food Conference," *Nutr. Rev.*, **33**:225–34, 1975.
2. Rizek, R. L.: "The 1977–78 Nationwide Food Consumption Survey," *Family Econ. Rev.*, Fall 1978, pp. 3–7.
3. Briggs, G. M., cited by Frankle, R. T., and Owen, A. Y.: *Nutrition in the Community.* The C. V. Mosby Company, St. Louis, 1976, p. 12.
4. Jelliffe, D. B., and Jelliffe, E. F. P.: "The Urban Avalanche and Child Nutrition," *J. Am. Diet. Assoc.*, **57**:111–18, 1970.
5. Williams, C. D.: "Kwashiorkor. A Nutritional Disease Associated with a Maize Diet," *Lancet*, November 16, 1935, p. 1151; reprinted in *Nutr. Rev.*, **31**:350–51, 1973.
6. Review: "Childhood Malnutrition in Iran," *Nutr. Rev.*, **27**:69–71, 1969.
7. National Nutrition Consortium: "Guidelines for a National Nutrition Policy," *Nutr. Rev.*, **32**:153–59, 1974.
8. Shoemaker, L.: *Parent and Family Life Education for Low-Income Families.* Children's Bureau Pub. 434–1965. U.S. Department of Health, Education, and Welfare, Washington, D.C. 1965.
9. Clark, H. E.: "Meeting Protein Requirements of Man," *J. Am. Diet Assoc.*, **52**:475–79, 1968.

Additional References

NUTRITION EDUCATION

American Dietetic Association: "Position Paper on the Scope and Thrust of Nutrition Education," *J. Am. Diet. Assoc.*, **72**:302–5, 1978.

BOSLEY, B.: "Nutrition, Human Welfare, and Economics," *J. Am. Diet. Assoc.*, **67**:104–6, 1975.

CELENDER, I. M. et al.: "What Are the Needs of Nutrition Educators?" *J. Nutr. Educ.*, **10**:82, 1978.

DARBY, W. J.: "The Renaissance of Nutrition Education," *Nutr. Rev.*, **35**:33–38, 1977.

DWYER, J. T.: "Point of View: Challenges in Nutrition Education of the Public," *J. Am. Diet. Assoc.*, **72**:53–55, 1978.

JOHNSON, M. J., and BUTLER, J. L.: "Where is Nutrition Education in the Public Schools?" *J. Nutr. Educ.*, **7**:20–21, 1975.

LEVINE, R. R. et al.: "An Assessment of High School Nutrition Education," *J. Nutr. Educ.*, **11**:124–26, 1979.

ROBINSON, C. H.: "Nutrition Education—What Comes Next?" *J. Am. Diet. Assoc.*, **69**:126–32, 1976.

NUTRITION POLICY

American Dietetic Association, Commentary: "Dietary Goals for the United States (Second Edition)," *J. Am. Diet. Assoc.*, **74**:529–33, 1979.

DWYER, J. T., and MAYER, J.: "Beyond Economics and Nutrition: The Complex Basis of Food Policy," *Science*, **188**:566–70, 1975.

HEGSTED, D. M.: "Food and Nutrition Policy: Probability and Practicality," *J. Am. Diet. Assoc.*, **74**:534–38, 1979.

HILLEBOE, H. E.: "Modern Concepts of Prevention in Community Health," *Am. J. Publ. Health*, **61**:1000–06, 1971.

QUELCH, J. A.: "The Role of Nutrition Information in National Nutrition Policy," *Nutr. Rev.*, **35**:289–93, 1977.

NUTRITIONAL STATUS AND NUTRITIONAL SERVICES

AUSTIN, J. E.: "What Comes First in Feeding the Hungry?" *Nutr. Today*, **13**:21–26, November/December 1978.

BIRO, L. "Home Health Agencies: Federal and State Requirements for Nutrition Intervention," *J. Am. Diet. Assoc.*, **73**:536–40, 1978.

HEGSTED, D. M.: "Protein-Calorie Malnutrition," *Am. Scientist*, **66**:61–65, 1978.

LANGHAM, R. A..: "A State Health Department Assesses Undernutrition," *J. Am. Diet. Assoc.*, **65**:18–23, 1974.

LATHAM, M. C.: "Strategies to Control Infections in Malnourished Populations—Holistic Approach or Narrowly Targeted Interventions?" *Am. J. Clin. Nutr.*, **32**:2292–2300, 1978.

NICHAMAN, M. Z.: "Developing a Nutritional Surveillance System," *J. Am. Diet. Assoc.*, **65**:15–17, 1974.

Review: "Adaptation in Protein Calorie Malnutrition," *Nutr. Rev.*, **37**:250–52, 1979.

SABRY, Z. et al.: "Nutrition Canada," *Nutr. Today*, **9**:5–13, January/February 1974.

SHAW, S. H., and MILLER, D.: "Preventive Medicine Through Nutrition: A Model Health Care Delivery System in San Diego County," *J. Am. Diet. Assoc.*, **75**:49–51, 1979.

WORLD NUTRITION

BERG, A.: "Fear of Trying," *J. Am. Diet. Assoc.*, **68**:311–16, 1976.

BROWN, L. R., and ECKHOLM, E. P.: *By Bread Alone.* Praeger Publishers, New York, 1974.

HARLAN, J. R.: "The Plants and Animals That Nourish Man," *Sci. Am.*, **235**:88–97, September 1976.

HOPPER, W. D.: "The Development of Agriculture in Developing Countries," *Sci. Am.*, **235**:197–205, September 1976.

JELLIFFE, E. F. P.: "When the Answer Is Not a Bottle," *UNICEF News*, Issue 107, 1981, pp. 3–7.

MAYER, J.: "The Dimensions of Human Hunger," *Sci. Am.*, **235**:40–49, September 1976.

WORTMAN, S.: "Food and Agriculture," *Sci. Am.*, **235**:31–39, September 1976.

part two

Therapeutic Nutrition

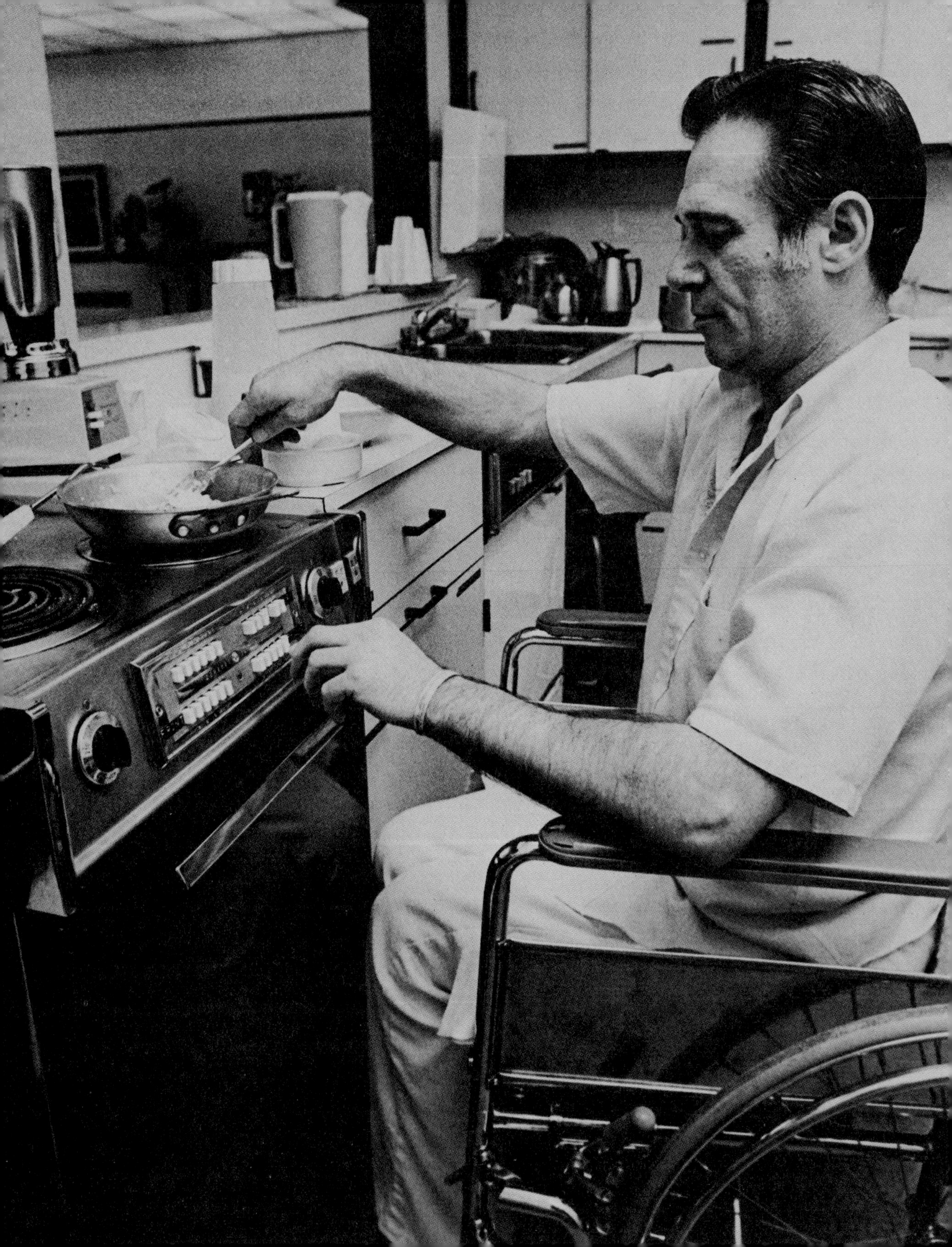

24 Comprehensive Nutritional Services for Patients

SOONER or later most individuals will experience an acute or chronic condition that requires hospitalization. To the uninitiated, hospitals can be very frightening places. Food often is the only aspect of the daily routine that is familiar to hospitalized patients; if the usual food intake is not permitted because of the need for a therapeutic diet, food may become a source of apprehension. Regardless of the diagnosis or the type of diet prescribed, the satisfactory intake of food by the patient is essential for maintenance of tissue structures and body functions so that recovery from illness is not impeded. Inadequate intake of the proper nutrients, or impaired ability to digest, absorb, or metabolize foods leads to nutritional deficiency. This lowers the body's resistance and may initiate or aggravate diseases of nonnutritional origin. Illnesses such as infections, injuries, and metabolic disturbances lead to deficiencies even in previously well-nourished persons because of failure to ingest sufficient food or because the disease process greatly increases nutritional needs. Thus, a vicious cycle of disease, malnutrition, and prolonged convalescence ensues.

The attributes of good nutrition and the principles and practices for achieving them have been discussed for all age categories in Part One of this text. The adaptation of the normal diet to the needs of individuals with some pathologic conditions is the objective of Part Two. This introductory chapter in therapeutic nutrition presents an overview of some of the factors that may have a bearing on the nutritional status of hospitalized persons and the role of the health care team in meeting their nutritional needs. Much concern has been expressed about the prevalence of malnutrition in hospitalized patients and on the role of the health care team in assessing, preventing, and treating hospital malnutrition. Nutritional assessment has been described in Chapter 22. Further techniques for assessing nutritional status of hospitalized patients are described in detail in this chapter. Also described are the importance of nutrition in comprehensive health care and some ways in which nutritional services are provided for persons with health problems of a temporary or chronic nature that do not require hospitalization.

Purposes of Modified Diets Most patients do not require dietary modification. Good nutritional care for them consists of supplying a normal diet that furnishes their nutritional, psychologic, and aesthetic needs and taking measures to enable them to consume it. On the other hand, modified diets are the principal therapeutic agents in some metabolic diseases such as Type II (noninsulin-dependent) diabetes mellitus. In other instances diet therapy supports the overall therapeutic program; for example, a sodium-restricted diet may be prescribed in addition to diuretics for some patients with hypertension. Modified diets are also used as preventive measures. One example of this is the fat-controlled diet prescribed for individuals with elevated blood lipids who are at increased risk for ischemic (coronary) heart disease. For some conditions in which diet therapy formerly played a major role, drug therapy is now a more effective means of controlling symptoms. Use of cimetidine in peptic ulcer or allopurinol in gout has largely superseded the need for bland and purine-restricted diets in patients receiving these medications. Nevertheless, these diets are still used in some circumstances.

Team Approach to Nutritional Care Meeting the patient's nutritional needs involves the coordination of several hospital departments. The core team is composed of the physician, nurse, and dietitian. With the advent of enteral and parenteral feeding formulas and greater awareness of drug-diet interactions, the role of the clinical pharmacist is becoming increasingly recognized. At times, other health professionals, such as the social worker or physical therapist become directly involved. The relationships of each of these team members to one another and to the patient might be depicted as shown in Figure 24–1. The focus, of course, is on the patient who must actively participate, insofar as possible, in his or her health care. The physician prescribes the diet and should also give the patient some information concerning the reasons that a modified diet has been ordered. The dietitian is the specialist who translates the physician's written order into practicality in terms of foods or nutritional products or formulas. The dietitian assesses and evaluates the patient's nutritional status; formulates nutritional care plans; designs meal patterns individualized according to the patient's food habits and modified according to the therapeutic need; and recommends appropriate proprietary formulas for enteral feeding. The dietary staff is also responsible for the preparation and service of food to the patient, the evaluation of the patient's response to the diet, and the subsequent counseling of the patient and family if a home diet is required. The clinical pharmacist formulates solutions for parenteral feedings and advises on nutritional effects of drug therapy.

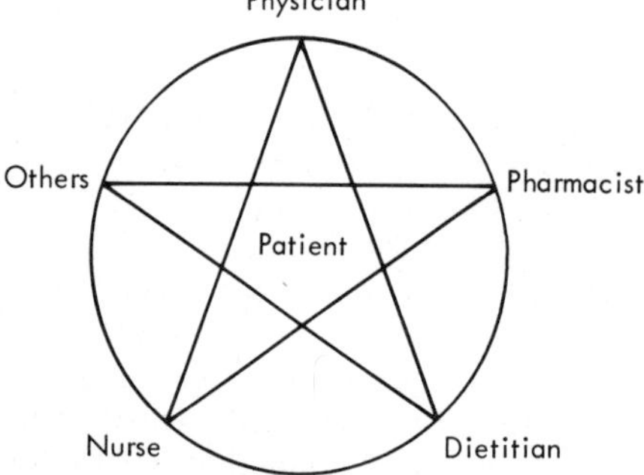

Figure 24–1. The central or "star" member of the health care team is the patient. The lines connecting the points of the star illustrate the lines of communication among all members of the team.

The nurse is the member of the health team who has the most constant and intimate association with the patient, and the direct services she or he gives to the patient differ from those of the physician and the dietitian. Some specific means by which nursing personnel assist in nutritional care include the following:

1. Maintaining lines of communication with the physician and dietitian regarding the patient's dietary needs:
   a. Obtaining a diet prescription if there is none, and arranging for food service to the patient.
   b. Providing the dietitian and physician with information regarding the patient's response to the diet.
   c. Serving as liaison between the patient and the physician and dietitian.
2. Assisting the patient at mealtimes:
   a. Providing a pleasant environment conducive to eating.
   b. Preparing the patient for the meal.
   c. Giving assistance to the patient as needed, including feeding.
   d. Helping the handicapped to adjust to self-feeding.
   e. Giving encouragement and support to the patient.
3. Interpreting the diet to the patient:
   a. Explaining the reasons for a modified diet and what may be expected of the diet.

   b. Answering questions about the diet.
4. Observing, recording, and reporting the patient's response to diet:
   a. Eliciting information regarding food habits, likes and dislikes, and attitudes toward diet.
   b. Noting adequacy of food intake.
   c. Reporting patient's response to dietitian and physician.
5. Planning for home care:
   a. Identifying needs for outside assistance.
   b. Arranging for counseling regarding home diet with member of family as well as patient.

Factors to Consider in the Study of Diet Therapy In order to function effectively in the provision of nutritional care students of nursing and dietetics must have an understanding of (1) acute and chronic conditions which require a change in diet; (2) the rationale for dietary changes, characteristics of the diet, its beneficial and possible adverse effects, nutritional limitations of the various modified diets, and indications and contraindications for use; (3) ways in which drug therapy may influence food intake or utilization; and (4) the patient's tolerance for food.

A correctly planned diet is successful only if it is eaten. The dietitian and nurse must be able to apply the principles pertaining to the preparation and service of appealing, palatable, and nutritious food. They must have the necessary understanding of the psychologic and emotional factors influencing food acceptance.

Patient care includes planning for full rehabilitation. For some patients a modified diet may be required for weeks, months, or even a lifetime; for others, guidance may be desirable in the improvement of a normal diet. Such planning necessitates consideration of social, religious, and cultural patterns, availability of foods, cost of food, suitable methods of food preparation, and so on.

The hospital or regional diet manual is used as the basis for planning modified diets. The American Dietetic Association has compiled a handbook in which the scientific basis for dietary modification in treatment of disease, dietetic terminology, and contents of various diets are listed.[1]

Effect of Illness on Food Acceptance and Utilization

The physiologic, psychologic, and emotional factors governing food acceptance have been discussed in Chapter 14. Likewise, a number of cultural food patterns have been presented in Chapter 15. Illness may modify or accentuate the influence of any of these factors.

The Stress of Illness The sick person has many fears: those relating to the outcome of the illness itself; economic concerns for self and family; emotional adjustments to having to depend on others during the illness; anxiety about loss of love and self-esteem. The sick person may express fears in a number of ways: by being angry, self-conscious, talkative or reticent, uneasy, depressed, indifferent, impatient, hostile, apologetic for failure, or resentful.

When hospitalization becomes necessary, the sick person experiences additional stress. Some patients adjust easily to a hospital routine, but for others it is difficult. The patient is subjected to seemingly endless questions, physical examinations, laboratory tests, and ministrations of therapy by a parade of specialists and auxiliary workers who, too often, do not explain what is happening, thus causing much needless anxiety. On the other hand, the patient often experiences long delays when he or she requires attention to personal needs. Especially if primary care nursing is not provided, patients may feel that there is no specific person who has the primary concern and responsibility for his or her care. The loss of privacy is an especial embarrassment and even shock to an elderly individual who has never before been in a hospital. Likewise the loss of independence to eat when and what one wishes, to get out of bed or not, to come and go as one wishes, and so on, can be frustrating. Each member of the health care team should be concerned that the patient is treated with dignity and that his or her rights are observed. The American Hospital Association has prepared a bill of rights for patients in the interest of better patient care.[2]

Illness Modifies Food Acceptance Hospitalization itself may influence food acceptance. When the patient most needs the comfort and companionship of family and friends, he or she is relegated to eating alone. Perhaps the meal hours are different from those to which the patient is accustomed; the foods appearing on the tray may be unlike those usually eaten with respect to choice, or flavoring, or portion size; a single food to which the patient has a strong aversion may be so upsetting that he or she is unable to eat anything served with it; managing a tray and the utensils for eating may be awkward when one is in bed; the patient may perceive expressed needs as being minimized or brushed aside. Some patients, under stress, use diet as a means of gaining attention from hospital personnel and later from family members. They may insist upon meticulous attention to the minutest of details, in order to be noticed.

The disease process itself may have a profound effect on food acceptance. Some foods may produce marked anorexia, others may be distending, and still others may be irritants to the gastrointestinal tract. Food preferences may revert to those of earlier years. These may be bland foods of childhood, but they might be the special dishes associated with one's ethnic origin.

Modified Diets Impose Additional Problems When a patient is confronted with the need for a therapeutic diet, he or she may respond with comments such as these: "I just can't get it down." "This food is tasteless." "I can't afford such food when I go home." "Who is going to prepare my food at home?" "I can't buy these foods at work." Remarks such as these may indicate unwillingness to accept change; anger at those associated with the diet—nurse, dietitian, physician, or even mother or spouse who has nagged about the food habits at home; or fears—of having to eat disliked foods; of having to forego favorite foods; of loss of social status and self-esteem; or the feeling that diet is, in some way, a punishment.

The nurse and dietitian must try to allay the patient's fears by empathetic understanding and by providing help in budgeting, arrangements for food preparation, suggestions for making the diet more palatable, and other useful advice.

Nutritional Stress Emotional stress such as the taking of examinations leads to increased losses of nitrogen and calcium. In fact, persons under such stress may achieve balances only with considerable difficulty. One may reasonably assume that the anxiety concerning illness may also accentuate such losses.

Immobilization is also a stressful situation in which nitrogen and calcium excretions are elevated. In long-term illness, immobilization may be responsible for serious demineralization of bones.

Any trauma to the body such as bone fracture, wound injury, or infection increases the losses of nitrogen and various electrolytes. The secretion of several hormones is often increased, thereby elevating the needs for vitamins required to carry on metabolic processes.

Effect of Drugs Drug therapy may have profound effects on nutritional status by interfering with food intake, decreasing nutrient absorption, or altering metabolic responses. (See Figure 24–2.) Frequent gastrointestinal manifestations of drug intolerance are anorexia, nausea, and diarrhea. A listing of some commonly used drugs and some of the often reported nutritional effects is shown in Table 24–1. The listing of drugs is not all-inclusive. Many of the gastrointestinal side effects listed are also

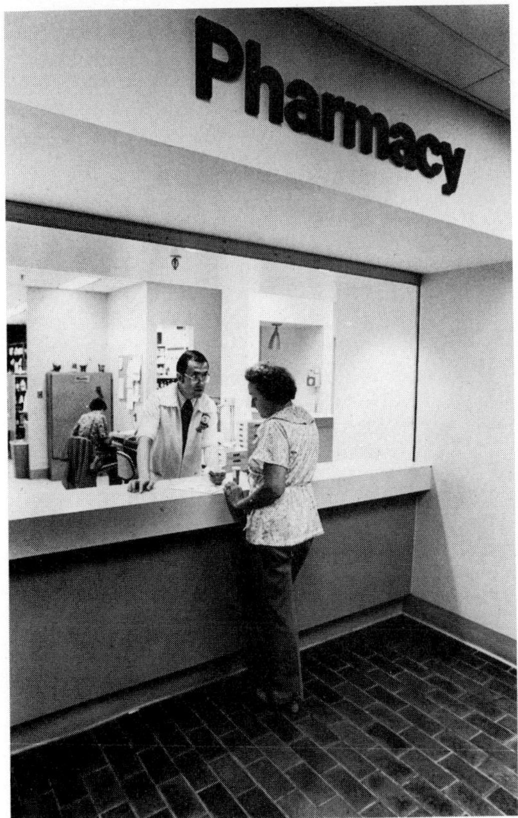

Figure 24–2. Because food and drug interactions are common, the pharmacist advises a patient regarding not only dosages, but also the time for taking the medication with reference to food intake. (Courtesy, Metropolitan Medical Center, Minneapolis.)

characteristic of other drugs in the same class which are not listed for the sake of brevity.

Interpersonal Relationship with the Patient

The Needs of the Patient Each patient has physical, psychologic, social, and spiritual needs. The pathophysiologic aspects of illness are the immediate reasons for care by the health team, but other needs must not be overlooked. Each member of the health team has a unique contribution to make in providing for these needs. Some examples relating to nutritional care follow.

1. Each person wants to be treated as an individual. He or she has specific needs and values that are unique for him or her, and care should be personalized rather than making the patient fit into a general mold.

Listening. Those who care for the patient must learn to listen carefully—not only to the words themselves but also to their tone and inflection. By taking time to listen, one may be made aware of a legitimate complaint about something wrong with the meals a patient receives—for example, cold coffee, an egg not cooked to his or her liking, or a vegetable the patient thoroughly dislikes. Such details are relatively easy to correct, and the patient is thereby made quite comfortable and satisfied. The seemingly casual conversation with the patient may bring to light that the past diet has been inadequate for a long period of time because of lack of teeth, poor health, inadequate income, or the inability to prepare food. Permitting the patient to talk about other things as well as the diet will often reveal that the problems encountered in food acceptance are actually a by-product of the deep anxieties caused by other problems; through understanding, the patient can often be helped. (See Figure 24–3.)

2. Each person has a right to know what should be expected from the health team and what is expected of the patient. If a modified diet is prescribed, the patient should be given some understanding of the reasons for it and what he or she may expect by way of needed change in food habits. Reassurance with respect to the diet is essential, but it must be realistic in terms of the difficulties of adjustment to it and its legitimate role in the total therapeutic program. To illustrate, appropriate diets for obesity and diabetes are basic to treatment, but some patients may find the adjustment to the restrictions extremely difficult; to

Table 24-1. **Some Effects of Drug Therapy of Nutritional Significance**

Drug Group	Effects of Nutritional Significance	Proposed Mechanism
Adrenocortical Steroids		
ACTH	Gastric inflammation, ulcer	Breaks gastric mucosal barrier
Glucocorticoids	Gastric inflammation, erosion, ulcer with bleeding; pancreatitis; ↓ calcium, iron	↓ Active transport; stimulates pancreatic secretion in partially obstructed gland; breaks gastric mucosal barrier
Prednisone	Gastrointestinal hemorrhage; ↑ liver fat; ↓ muscle protein; peptic ulcer; ↓ glucose tolerance; iron-deficiency anemia	
Alcohol	Inflammation of gastric mucosa; interferes with activities of liver and pancreas; ↑ magnesium excretion; ↓ absorption: folic acid, B-12, thiamin hydrochloride, vitamin A, nitrogen	Mucosal blockade; direct toxic effect on pancreas
Antacids		
Nonsystemic		
Aluminum hydroxide	Constipation; nausea, vomiting; ↓ absorption vitamin A; phosphate depletion (with anorexia, weakness, progressive debility) in persons on low-phosphate diets; hypomagnesemia; if severe: urinary calculi, osteomalacia, osteoporosis, muscle weakness	
Calcium carbonate	Constipation; nausea; hypercalcemia with alkalosis, calcinosis, and azotemia in chronic use, especially with milk-alkali syndrome; acid rebound; electrolyte imbalance	
Magnesium hydroxide	Cathartic effect; flatulence	
Systemic		
Sodium bicarbonate	Belching; sodium retention; alkalosis; milk-alkali syndrome if taken with milk	
Antibiotics and Other Antiinfective Agents		
Ampicillin	Oral lesions; diarrhea	
Chloramphenicol	↓ Lactose absorption; ↑ protein synthesis; aplastic anemia	Inhibits disaccharidases
Lincomycin	Glossitis; stomatitis; nausea, vomiting, diarrhea	Irritant; stimulates myenteric nerve reflexes
Neomycin	Steatorrhea; binds bile acids; ↓ absorption: glucose, sucrose *d*-xylose, nitrogen, iron, electrolytes, carotene, fat-soluble vitamins; ↓ synthesis of folic acid and vitamin K; ↓ serum cholesterol	Binds bile acids; precipitates fatty acids; produces histologic changes in mucosa (clubbing of villi, etc.), toxic effect on mucosa
Penicillins	↑ Malabsorption syndrome; nausea, diarrhea	
Tetracyclines	Stomatitis; esophagitis; nausea, vomiting; colitis; diarrhea; gastric ulcer; ↓ absorption fat, protein, glucose, *d*-xylose, lactose, carotene, ferrous sulfate, sodium; binds calcium → hypoplasia; ↓ absorption B-6, B-12	Reduces protein synthesis in body cells; may block normal carrier function of proteins; direct toxic effect on liver
Sulfonamides	Hepatitis; pancreatitis; ↓ bacterial synthesis of folate and B vitamins	
Anticoagulants		
Coumarin	↑ Prothrombin activity with green leafy vegetables	
Heparin	Intestinal bleeding	

Table 24-1. **(Continued)**

Drug Group	Effects of Nutritional Significance	Proposed Mechanism
Anticonvulsants		
Phenytoin	Anorexia, nausea, vomiting; gingival hyperplasia; osteomalacia; ↓ absorption: B-12, folic acid, *d*-xylose	Inhibits folic acid conjugase
Phenobarbital	Osteomalacia; ↓ activity of folic acid and B-12	
Antidepressants		
MAO inhibitors	React with tyramines in foods → headache, hypertensive crises; diarrhea	
Tricyclic	Substantial weight gain	
Antihypertensives		
Diuretics	Gastrointestinal irritation; many types → hypokalemia	
Chlorothiazide	Sodium and water losses; large doses → pancreatitis	Unknown
Ethacrynic acid	Fluid and electrolyte imbalance; ↓ carbohydrate tolerance; interference with amino acid transport; ↓ serum sodium	Unknown
Furosemide	Fluid and electrolyte imbalance; hyperglycemia; hyperuricemia; ↓ serum potassium	
Guanethidine	Diarrhea	Augments parasympathetic activity
Hydralazine	Nausea and vomiting	
Methyldopa	Gastrointestinal upset	
Reserpine	Gastric inflammation, ulcer with bleeding	Breaks gastric mucosal protective barrier
Antimetabolites		
Aminopterin	↓ Absorption: B-12, folic acid, *d*-xylose	Mucosal damage
Fluorouracil	Sore mouth; oral ulcers; esophagitis; gastrointestinal bleeding; diarrhea; altered taste acuity	
Methotrexate	↑ Prothrombin; ↓ absorption: B-12, folic acid, *d*-xylose; weight loss; nausea; vomiting; anorexia; diarrhea; gastrointestinal ulceration; mucosal damage	Inhibits dihydrofolate reductase; mucosal damage
Antipyretics		
Acetylsalicylic acid	Nausea, vomiting; gastric ulcer; pancreatitis; ↓ absorption: glucose, amino acids	Unknown
Indomethacin	Anorexia, nausea; mucosal ulceration	
Phenylbutazone	Nausea, vomiting; epigastric distress; peptic ulcer; stomatitis; anticoagulant effect; edema; diarrhea	
Antituberculars		
Aminosalicylic acid	Anorexia, nausea, vomiting; abdominal distress; peptic ulcer; steatorrhea; ↓ absorption: *d*-xylose, cholesterol, iron, B-12	Unknown
Isoniazid	Dry mouth; epigastric distress; hepatitis; antipyridoxine effect	
Ganglionic Blockers		
Atropine	Bitter taste; dry mouth; nausea; vomiting; heartburn; constipation; occasional diarrhea; ↓ gastric secretion, motor activity of gastrointestinal tract	
Ganglionic Stimulators		
Nicotine	↑ Tone and motor activity of bowel; occasional diarrhea	
Hypocholesterolemic Agents		
Cholestyramine	Nausea; constipation; steatorrhea; osteomalacia; ↓ absorption of fat-soluble vitamins	Binds bile acids

Table 24-1. (Continued)

Drug Group	Effects of Nutritional Significance	Proposed Mechanism
Clofibrate	Unpleasant or altered taste sensation; occasional nausea, diarrhea; ↓ absorption: sugar, iron, electrolytes, B-12	↑ Fecal neutral sterol excretion; ↓ carbohydrate enzyme activity
Nicotinic acid	Dyspepsia; vomiting; diarrhea; peptic ulcer	
Laxatives		
Bisacodyl Cascara Phenolphthalein	Chronic use: mild steatorrhea, protein-losing enteropathy, osteomalacia; ↓ absorption: glucose, *d*-xylose, calcium, electrolytes	"Intestinal hurry"
Mineral oil	↓ Aborption: fat-soluble vitamins	Unknown
Oral Contraceptives		
Estrogen and progesterone compounds	↓ Serum folate levels	Inhibits folic acid conjugase enzyme secondary to underlying malabsorption
Oral Hypoglycemic Agents		
Sulfonylureas Tolbutamide	Nausea; vomiting; cholestasis; peptic ulceration or perforation	
Others		
Colchicine	Nausea; vomiting; abdominal pain; diarrhea; ↓ serum cholesterol; high doses ↓ absorption: amino acids, fats, sterols, bile acids, lactose, glucose, *d*-xylose, iron, electrolytes, carotene, B-12	Damages mucosal enzymes; inhibits mitosis
Digitalis	Nausea; vomiting	Stimulates central or peripheral nerve receptors
Ferrous sulfate	Nausea; vomiting	Gastric irritation
Griseofulvin	Unpleasant or altered taste sensation; absorbed better with fatty meal; nausea; vomiting; diarrhea; epigastric distress	
Potassium chloride	Nausea; vomiting; ↓ absorption: B-12	Gastric irritation; ileal acidification
Levodopa	Anorexia; nausea; vomiting	Stimulates central or peripheral nerve receptors
Probenecid	Gastrointestinal irritation	Unknown
Triparenol	↓ Absorption: fat, glucose	Mucosal damage

minimize the problems involved is to invite failure. A fat-restricted diet may be helpful to the patient with gallstones, but it should never be held as a guarantee that surgery would not be required at a later time. Likewise, benefit may accrue to a patient with cardiovascular disease who is placed on a diet with modification of the amount and nature of the fat, but success is so variable that promises of marked improvement would be ill-advised and rash.

3. Each patient should be helped to participate in his or her own care. A selective menu can be a useful tool to help in making good choices for a normal as well as a modified diet. If dietary counseling is begun early, each meal helps the patient to learn what changes will be needed in the diet when the patient goes home. A patient who has a physical handicap should be helped to feed himself or herself as much as is possible, thereby increasing independence.

4. Each person expects that his or her behavior during illness will be accepted as part of the illness. The modification of food acceptance during illness as described on page 442 is an important expression of the change in behavior.

5. Each person expects to be treated with kindness, thoughtfulness, and firm-

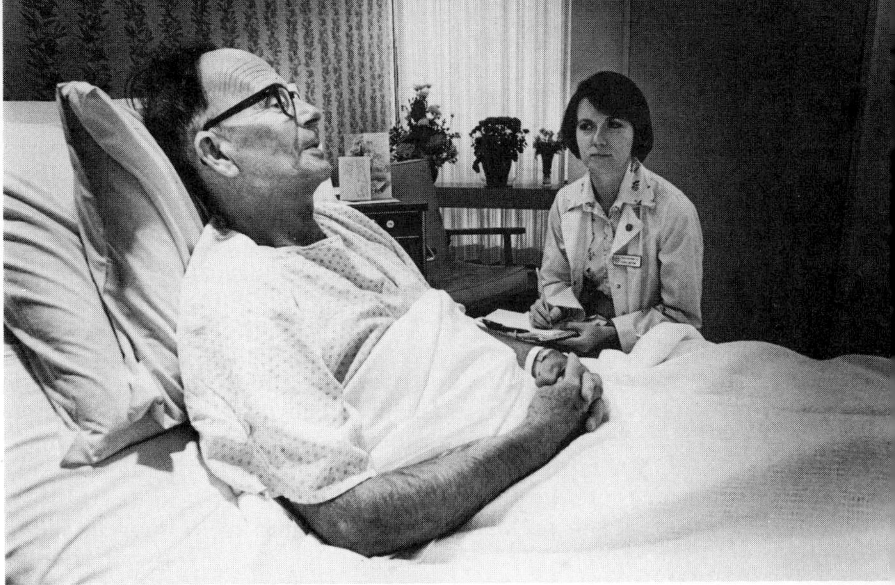

Figure 24–3. The dietitian interviews the patient in a relaxed environment. She is nonjudgmental as she listens to him, and she skillfully elicits information by interjecting a question now and then. (Courtesy, Metropolitan Medical Center, Minneapolis.)

ness. The work of the dietitians, nurses, or homemakers is often more successful if they can place themselves in the patient's role, although they must guard against overidentification; if they become too close to the patient, they may accept his or her reactions as being always so reasonable that they are unable to do anything about changing them.

Recognition of attitudes. How does the nurse or dietitian feel about the patient who does not eat the food, who eats too much, or who complains about the food a great deal? When the patient expresses resentment or hostility toward nurses or dietitians, do they realize that this may be against the restrictions the diet puts upon the patient and not against them as individuals? It is important that they recognize their own attitudes toward the patient, lest they give the impression that they are pitying, superior, intolerant, resentful, or critical of him or her. Moreover, they must avoid an expression of any negative attitudes they may have toward food.

Documentation of Nutritional Care

The Medical Record The medical record is the primary instrument for communication among those directly concerned with the care of the patient; therefore, it should contain ongoing documentation of all aspects of health care provided to the patient, including nutrition. Many institutions use the "problem-oriented" approach. The record is organized according to the patient's key problems. This approach permits ready access to the problem of interest and knowledge of its current status by each member of the health care team. Entries into the record by team members are identified according to the problem and are organized so as to distinguish subjective and objective information, assessment data, and plans for resolution of the problem.

Nutritional Care Plans The dietitian is responsible for the nutritional care plan for each patient. Many hospital dietary departments have developed forms for this purpose. Information from the medical record, such as the diagnosis, pertinent laboratory values and medications, height, and weight are entered as well as information obtained directly from the patient regarding the dietary history, food preferences, food allergies, and so on.

The care plan includes (1) an estimate of the adequacy of the patient's usual dietary intake; (2) any nutritional problems and (3) plans for resolving these; (4) objectives for patient education, stated in terms of patient outcomes; (5) progress notes; and (6) evaluation of nutritional care. Individualized meal patterns are often included. Patients at risk for malnutrition require more extensive nutritional evaluation using the techniques described on page 444.

Nutritional Assessment of the Hospitalized Patient

For many patients the nutrition assessment techniques described in Chapter 22 are adequate. However, additional measurements are needed for those at increased risk for protein-calorie malnutrition. Those considered to be at high risk are listed in Table 24–2.

All patients have the right to expect assessment of their nutritional status as a routine part of their care while they are hospitalized. Obviously, not all are malnourished, thus, the extent of the evaluation will vary from one individual to another. Preliminary screening will identify those who are at increased risk for malnutrition; for these individuals more detailed assessment is required in order to define the extent of the nutritional problem and to plan and implement appropriate nutritional support. The particular techniques used in screening and in further assessment will depend upon the patient population and the resources and personnel available.

Determinations of energy stores, lean body mass, visceral protein status, and immune competency are of particular interest to clinicians. It should be noted that few patients will have a completely normal profile of anthropometric, biochemical, and immune factors; however, the patient who is moderately or severely depleted in several of these parameters is likely to benefit from nutritional support. The validity of these measurements has been questioned by some on the grounds that they do not reflect changes in body composition[3] and do not accurately predict nutritional risk for individuals,[4] as opposed to groups of patients. Nevertheless, the techniques will continue to be important because of ease

Table 24–2. **Some Factors that Increase Risk for Hospital Malnutrition**

1. Abnormal weight patterns
   a. Children—weight for height outside the normal range
   b. Adults— ≥ 20 per cent above or > 10 per cent below desirable weight
   c. Significant recent weight loss though the individual has not been on a weight reduction diet
2. Any condition characterized by insufficient intake of energy and nutrients
   a. Impaired ability to chew, swallow, taste, or smell food
   b. Diets with multiple restrictions in types of food and/or levels of nutrients; for example, clear liquid; extremely low protein diets
   c. "Nothing by mouth" or use of intravenous feedings for more than a few days
   d. Chronic disease such as cancer or ulcerative colitis that influences appetite or ability to digest or absorb food
3. Increased nutritional needs
   a. Pregnancy, malabsorption, diarrhea, postoperative states, fever, sepsis, burns
   b. Continued external losses of bodily constituents; open, draining wounds; chronic hemorrhage; chronic dialysis
4. Drug therapy that interferes with nutrient utilization
5. Conditions characterized by abnormal levels of hemoglobin, hematocrit, lymphocytes, albumin, transferrin, cholesterol, blood urea nitrogen, etc.

of use, convenience, and low cost. It must also be remembered that deficiencies of vitamins and minerals, especially trace minerals, are likely in patients whose protein or energy stores are depleted using these parameters. Some indexes of nutritional status are listed inside the back cover of this text.[5] Values 60 to 80 per cent of the accepted standards are usually interpreted as moderate depletion and those less than 60 per cent of standard as severe depletion. For triceps skinfold, midarm circumference, and midarm muscle circumference values below the 5th percentile indicate depletion; those between the 5th and 15th percentiles indicate increased risk for nutritional depletion.[6]

Initial Screening Preliminary information obtained from the medical record and dietary history is useful in determining those patients likely to have nutritional problems that require intervention. (See Table 24–2.) Some rely on these two sources; others add anthropometric determinations—triceps and subscapular skinfolds, midarm muscle circumference, height, and weight.[7] One group has reported that serum albumin and total lymphocyte determinations are as useful as more detailed methods in identifying those at risk for nutritional complications.[8] If the initial evaluation suggests malnutrition, more extensive evaluation is needed.

Assessment of Energy Stores Determination of height and weight provides an indirect estimate of fat stores, assuming the patient is not edematous. The actual weight is compared with the patient's desirable weight. Height-weight standards for children and adults are shown in Tables A–6 through A–10. A weight loss of 10 per cent or more over a period of 3 months or less indicates losses of both adipose tissue and muscle mass and is suggestive of protein-calorie malnutrition.

Measurement of the triceps skinfold using calipers is also used to estimate fat stores. The technique has been described in Chapter 22. Based on data from the Ten-State Nutrition Survey, acceptable values in adult males range from 10 to 12 mm and from 17 to 22 mm in adult females. (See Table A–11.)

Lean Body Mass This represents the body weight devoid of fat. Lean body mass is estimated by the upper midarm muscle circumference and the creatinine height index. Midarm muscle circumference is derived from midarm circumference and triceps skinfold. Ranges for circumferences of arm and arm muscle are shown in Tables A–11 and A–12. A nomogram for obtaining arm muscle circumference is shown in Tables A–13 and A–14.

A more sensitive indicator of lean body mass is the creatinine height index. Creatinine, a normal product of muscle metabolism, is excreted in urine at a relatively constant rate for a given amount of muscle. As muscle mass is lost in wasting diseases creatinine excretion falls. The creatinine height index (CHI) compares the patient's 24-hour urinary creatinine excretion to that excreted by a reference individual of "ideal" body weight (according to Metropolitan Life Insurance standards), who is of the same sex and height as the patient. The normal creatinine excretion is 23 mg per kilogram body weight for males and 18 mg per kilogram for women. Normal renal function and accurate 24-hour urine collection are essential for this method to yield reliable data.

Visceral Protein Status The serum albumin level is correlated with arm muscle circumference. As lean body mass becomes depleted, the serum albumin level falls. Values less than 3.5 gm per deciliter indicate depletion. Transferrin is a more sensitive indicator of visceral protein status because it has a shorter half-life than albumin and will, therefore, indicate protein deficiency more rapidly. Transferrin is measured directly or is calculated from knowledge of the total iron-binding capacity.

Immune Competency Cell-mediated immunity is an important host defense mechanism for resistance to infection. Morbidity and mortality from infections are increased when cellular immunity is depressed. One indicator of immune status is the total lymphocyte count. A value of less than 1,000 per mm is associated with impaired cellular immunity.

Delayed hypersensitivity skin tests using intradermal injections of recall antigens such as candida, streptokinase-streptodornase (SK-SD), and mumps are another means of evaluating immune competency. An induration of 5 mm or more in diameter at the site of the injection at 24 and 48 hours indicates a positive response. Normally positive responses to two or more antigens occur. Failure to respond to any of the antigens is termed *anergy* and indicates increased risk for sepsis. Relative anergy refers to a positive response to only one antigen. The delayed hypersensitivity response is often depressed in stress, chemotherapy, radiation therapy, after major surgery, in sepsis, and with certain drug therapy.

Apparent Nitrogen Balance A rough estimate of nitrogen balance can be made from nitrogen intake and urinary urea nitrogen excretion. The latter accounts for about 80 per cent of the nitrogen excreted from the body. Nitrogen losses are subtracted from nitrogen intake. Total nitrogen loss is estimated by adding a constant factor of 4 to urinary urea nitrogen to account for nonurea nitrogen losses. Nitrogen balance is dependent on protein and energy intake. The balance data are of limited value in the initial assessment of protein depletion because such patients tend to conserve nitrogen more efficiently than better nourished individuals. Nitrogen excretion tends to increase as the severity of nitrogen depletion increases, however.

Vitamins and Minerals It is important to recognize that malnutrition in hospitalized patients is not limited to depletion of energy and protein reserves. Vitamin and mineral deficiencies may also occur. In one large study about 30 per cent of hospitalized patients were found to have biochemical evidence of marginal or deficient status of thiamin, riboflavin, and vitamin C.[9] Individuals whose vitamin nutriture is marginal are at increased risk for deficiencies of these vitamins in infectious and catabolic diseases. Requirements for water-soluble vitamins, in particular, are increased in disease. Vitamin status is assayed by clinical observations, determination of blood levels, or by enzyme assays. Plasma levels reflect recent dietary intake whereas intracellular levels are a better index of whole body status.

Recent mineral intake is evaluated by measurement of both blood and urine levels. A fall in blood levels and a low urinary excretion are generally suggestive of an inadequate intake. Blood levels of trace minerals may shift in acute infections. For example, plasma zinc falls while plasma copper increases. Urinary excretion of zinc is increased in a number of catabolic conditions.[10]

Follow-up Assessment If the initial assessment has indicated that nutritional support is needed, periodic follow-up is done to evaluate the effectiveness of nutritional therapy. One group recommends the following schedule: body weight, three times weekly; total lymphocyte count, weekly; albumin and transferrin, every 10 to 14 days; cell-mediated immunity, anthropometrics, and creatinine height index, every 21 to 30 days.[7]

Limitations of Nutritional Assessment The following points should be kept in mind concerning the various parameters used to assess nutritional status:

1. No one test is an accurate predictor of increased risk for nutritional complications. The best combination of tests is not known. Conflicting reports in the literature seem to suggest that the particular patient population, the number of patients studied, and the severity of stress may all influence the usefulness of certain tests as predictors.

2. Few patients have a completely normal profile when a number of parameters are assessed. In one study of surgical patients, only 3 per cent had no abnormal measures. About one third of patients had three or more abnormal measurements of nutritional and immunologic status.[11]

3. Although some tests are useful in predicting increased risk of nutritional complications in groups of patients, the applicability of the data to individuals is meaningful only when associated with functional consequences. The measurements associated with functional consequences are recent weight loss of more than 10 per cent, serum albumin less than 3.0 gm per deciliter, weight and height less than 85 per cent of standard, and anergy.[12]

4. In general, anthropometric data are not useful predictors of increased risk. Nevertheless, many malnourished patients have abnormal anthropometric measurements. Depressed levels of serum albumin and transferrin and the presence of anergy are all associated with increased morbidity and mortality.

Classification of Hospital Malnutrition Based on the information obtained from anthropometric, biochemical, and immune status determinations, three types of malnutrition have been described:

1. Marasmus, or protein-calorie malnutrition, is associated with depletion of energy reserves and lean body mass. Cellular immunity is impaired when weight is less than 85 per cent of desirable weight. Significant depletion of triceps skinfold, arm circumference, arm muscle circumference, and creatinine height index is seen, while visceral protein status is maintained. The patient has a wasted appearance.

2. Hypoalbuminemic malnutrition (kwashiorkor or protein malnutrition) is characterized by depressed serum albumin and transferrin levels and impaired cellular immunity. Patients often appear to have adequate energy stores.

3. A combination state is characterized by acute visceral protein depletion superimposed on protein-calorie malnutrition.

Nutritional Intervention Determination of protein and energy requirements is discussed in Chapter 28.

Feeding the Patient

Environment for Meals Time and effort directed toward creating an atmosphere conducive to the enjoyment of food are well spent. Such an environment implies that the surrounding areas are orderly and clean; that ventilation is good; and that distracting activities such as treatment of patients and doctors' rounds are not occurring at mealtime except as emergencies may arise.

Patients who are ambulatory enjoy eating with others. In some hospitals a dining room is provided for patients, and in others food service may be easily arranged at small tables set up in the patients' lounge.

Readiness of the Patient The patient should be ready for the meal whether in bed or ambulatory. This may entail mouth care, the washing of the hands, and the positioning of the patient so that eating can take place in comfort. If tests or treatment unavoidably delay a meal, arrangements must be made to hold trays so that the food can be fresh and appetizing when the patient is ready to eat.

The Patient's Tray The appearance of the tray is of the utmost importance since the patient's consumption of the food presented is the goal to be achieved. Some of the items listed following, which describe standards for tray service, are the primary responsibility of the dietary department, but others require the maximum cooperation of nursing and medical staffs with the dietary department.

1. Variations in color, flavor, and texture for appeal to the senses are essential in menu planning and food preparation. (See Chapter 13.)

2. The tray should be of a size suitable for the food to be served—small trays for liquid nourishment and large trays for full meals.
3. The tray cover and napkins should be of suitable size for the tray, immaculately clean, and unwrinkled.
4. Everything on the tray must reflect cleanliness—sparkling glassware, shining flatware, attractive china.
5. The tray should be symmetrically arranged for the greatest convenience. All necessary flatware and accessories should be included.
6. Foods should be attractively served, with the size of portions not being overlarge. Spilled liquid or sloppy serving of food is inexcusable. Garnishes help to make foods more appealing.
7. Meals should be served on time. This requires careful planning so that foods will be prepared in the proper sequence.

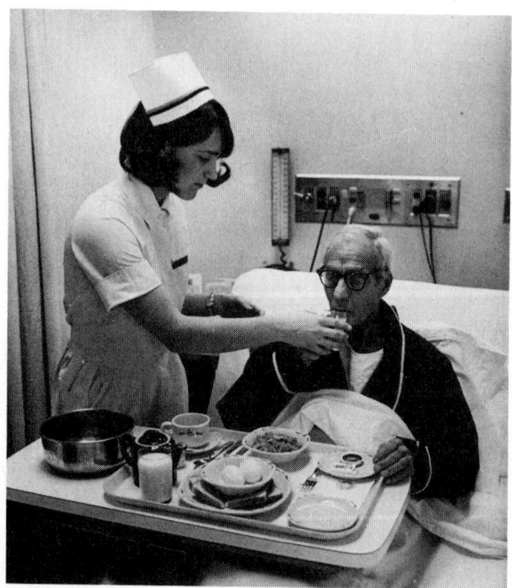

Figure 24–4. Some patients require assistance at meals because they are too weak to feed themselves, while others need the encouragement to eat. (Courtesy, Yale–New Haven Medical Center.)

8. Foods should be served at the proper temperature. Hot foods should be served on hot plates, protected with a cover, and cold foods should be served on chilled dishes.
9. A final check of the tray should establish that it fully meets the requirements of the diet order and that the patient's preferences have been implemented.

Assistance in Feeding Some patients may require assistance in the cutting of meat or other dense foods, the pouring of a beverage, or the buttering of a piece of toast. Very ill or infirm patients must be fed. Ideally, the nurse should sit while feeding the patient so as to be at ease and avoid undue haste. Food will be enjoyed more if it can be eaten with reasonable leisure and if there is some conversation. Obviously, the nurse responsible for feeding several patients will make arrangements to delay tray service or to keep foods hot for those who must await their turn. (See Figure 24–4.)

Comprehensive Care Services

Concepts of Comprehensive Care The provision of all necessary health services so that the patient can maintain or be restored to independent living is implied in the term *comprehensive care.* The components of comprehensive health care include screening, assessment, intervention, and follow-up. Careful evaluation and reevaluation of the client's physical, psychologic, economic, and social needs are required so that referral is made to the appropriate personnel in essential services. (See Figure 24–5.) The services may be provided on an in-patient basis, including hospital care for the acutely ill, a minimum-care facility within a hospital, or convalescent care in a nursing home. Care may be furnished through an out-patient clinic, utilizing a single service in a physician's office or multiple services

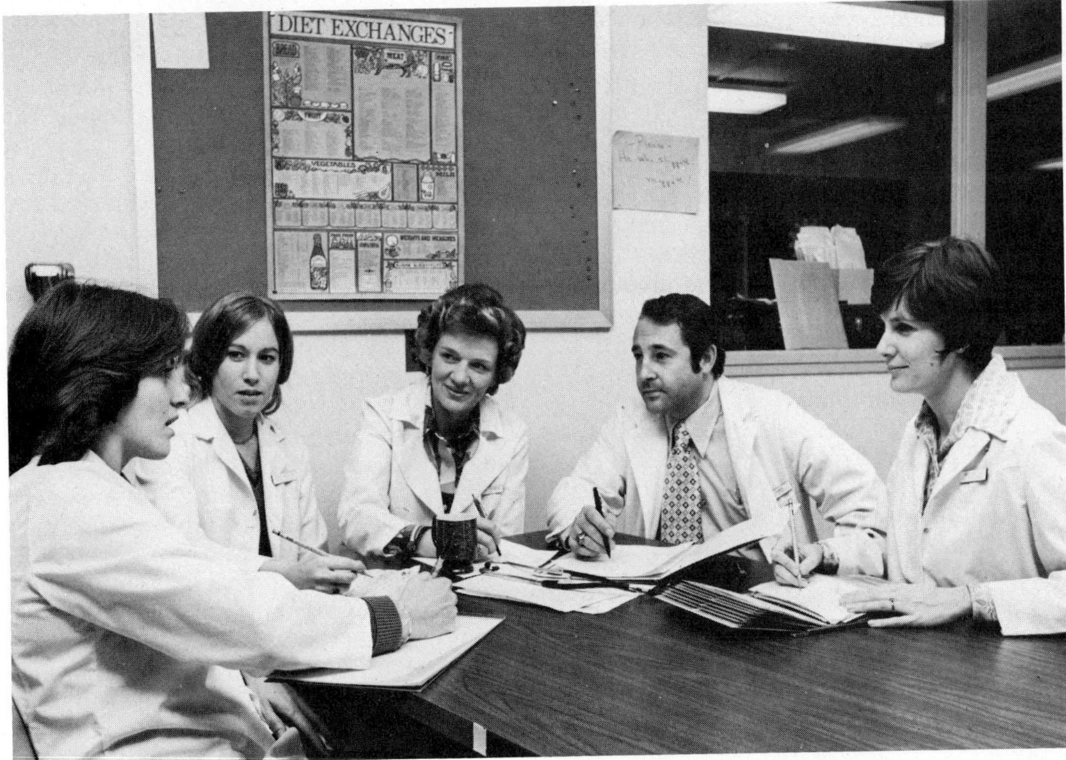

Figure 24–5. An important part of patient care involves adequate planning for the patient's discharge. Here the social worker shares information with the occupational therapist, nurse, physician, and dietitian. (Courtesy, University of Minnesota Health Sciences Center, Minneapolis.)

provided by a clinic or health center. Home care, of course, implies services provided in the home, and can range from a single service such as nursing to coordinated services by many disciplines that could include medical, nursing, dental, dietetic, social, occupational therapy, physical therapy, and others.

Many home-care programs are now available, some of which are sponsored by the hospital whereas others are directed by a public or voluntary health agency. Such services require the assistance of a variety of technicians so that the services of the professional nurse, nutritionist, and others may be most effectively used.

Home parenteral nutrition is an example of one of the newer programs which require periodic monitoring by health team members. Family members are increasingly assuming responsibility for care of relatives who are terminally ill from cancer. The programs permit the patient to spend his or her last weeks or months among loved ones in a more comfortable environment.

Federal legislation has greatly expanded the opportunities for better health care of the population. Especially significant are Medicare, children and youth programs, and regional medical programs. The impact these programs have is exemplified by Medicare coverage for patients with end-stage renal disease. In 1979, just 7 years after coverage became available, approximately 50,000 patients were participating in the program at a cost over $1 billion.[13] Undoubtedly further legislation will be enacted for programs designed to promote the maintenance of health of the entire population as well as care during illness.

Nutritional care is an essential and dynamic component of comprehensive health care. In fact, the ability to deliver the needed nutritional services and the quality of nutrition that the patient can maintain are often the decisive factors in restoring health or in maintaining it. A brief discussion of some elements of home care follows.

Home-delivered meals Many individuals or couples with physical limitations can remain in their own homes rather than be institutionalized if some provision can be made for their meals. Others who are temporarily disabled by illness but who are ambulatory and can feed themselves may find it possible to return to their homes at an earlier time if they can procure their meals. Two programs are available in many communities for providing home-delivered meals. Under Title III-C of the Older Americans Act one or two meals may be delivered daily to homebound persons over 60 years of age. For these meals the elderly person makes a voluntary confidential contribution. The "Meals-on-Wheels" program is a voluntary nonprofit service available to persons of all ages. It is usually operated by church groups, family service organizations, women's clubs, and so on. Generally, in this program a hot noon meal and a packaged evening meal are delivered by a volunteer on a 5-day basis. The recipient pays a fee for these meals, with gradations according to ability to pay.

In both programs each meal is planned to provide about one third of the recommended allowances. When the services of a dietitian are available, it is often possible to provide modified as well as normal diets.

Homemaker Services The purpose of this service is to maintain the family in a healthful setting when no one in the family can fulfill the homemaking function. For example, the mother may be ill or convalescing from physical or mental illness; an aging person or couple is unable to perform the necessary tasks in the home, but could remain at home at less expense with homemaker assistance; death of the mother in a home with young children presents a major problem to the working father unless relatives help out or homemaker service is available.

The sponsoring organization may be a public or voluntary agency such as the welfare division, the family service organization, or the community nursing service. The organizations recruit, define duties, provide formalized training and in-service programs of education, and provide supervision on the job.

The terms *homemaker, home health aide, housekeeper,* and *visiting homemaker* are used interchangeably by many agencies. The duties of the homemaker may include light housekeeping, meal preparation, marketing, laundry, and escort services to medical facilities. In some instances the homemaker also provides personal care such as bathing and grooming as supportive assistance.

A home health aide provides personal care to the client as supportive assistance and also as part of a medical care plan. She also assumes the general duties of homemaking listed previously. Generally she is employed by a nursing agency that is responsible for the supervision of the medical care plan. These services may be reimbursable through present regulations of Medicare when the medical care plan follows a period of hospitalization.

Physical Handicaps, Rehabilitation, and Nutrition

Physical Handicaps Millions of Americans have physical handicaps that restrict their ability to care for themselves and to work. Physical disabilities cover a wide range: the individual who has lost a hand or an arm, or who is hemiplegic and has the use of only one arm; arthritics with stiff, swollen, painful joints and who have a limited range of motion; those with cerebral palsy, Parkinson's disease, or multiple sclerosis and for whom uncoordinated movements are a constant trial; those bound to a wheelchair; the blind; those who have limited cardiac and respiratory reserves such as patients with cardiac disease or emphysema; and many others.

Nutrition of the Physically Handicapped Adequate nutrition is essential in restoring a patient to his or her potential capacity for independence, yet the handicap itself may be the principal factor that favors malnutrition even though the supply of food is plentiful. The use of only one arm, or stiff, painful joints, or incoordinated movements present tremendous difficulties in feeding oneself and may limit the performance of simple kitchen tasks such as opening packages, cutting foods, peeling vegetables, and using appliances.

The energy balance is an important consideration. Some handicapped individuals have an increased energy requirement because they must exert a tremendous effort to complete tasks. The increased requirement, on the one hand, and the difficulties experienced in eating, on the other hand, lead to excessive weight loss and to tissue depletion. Other individuals confined to wheelchairs and who exert little effort may become obese and require a diet restricted in calories. (See Chapter 27.)

Good protein nutrition is essential for restoration of body tissues, to reduce the incidence of infection, and to maintain the integrity of the skin. For immobilized individuals decubitus ulcers are a frequent problem. During the early stages of immobilization the nitrogen losses from the body greatly exceed the intake. The accelerated catabolism of protein tissues appears to run a time sequence that is not wholly reversed in the early stages even though a high-protein diet may be used. Nevertheless, the replacement of these losses requires a high-protein diet over an extended period of time. (See Chapter 28.)

Excessive losses of calcium from the bones may lead to urinary calculi. A liberal fluid intake is essential to facilitate the excretion of calcium, and some restriction of the calcium intake is often prescribed. (See Chapter 41.)

Constipation is a frequent complication of those who are immobilized. Its prevention or correction requires a liberal intake of fluids, a diet containing sufficient bulk, and regular habits of elimination. (See Chapter 32 for further details.)

The Nature of Rehabilitation Rehabilitation is the return of a handicapped individual to his or her maximum potential—to what the person will be able to do in the future. It is an individualized process in which therapy is designed specifically in terms of the patient's handicap, psychologic problems, family situation, and economic circumstances. It is individualized in that each patient's progress is measured against that person's own possibilities, not against some normal standard.

Rehabilitation may occur in a rehabilitation center, in a school for handicapped children, or in the home. The economic consideration is important inasmuch as rehabilitation is costly in terms of weeks or months in a rehabilitation center and the involvement of many specialists in the process. In addition, when the homemaker is handicapped, additional costs for a substitute in the home are likely to be appreciable.

The handicapped individual experiences helplessness, defeat, frustration, and even neglect. To surmount these difficulties becomes a constant uphill battle. Rehabilitation itself is usually slow, sometimes painful, and fatiguing both physically and emotionally. The patient needs the support of every member of the rehabilitation team.

The rehabilitation team. The skills and techniques in physical medicine, physical therapy, occupational therapy, nursing,

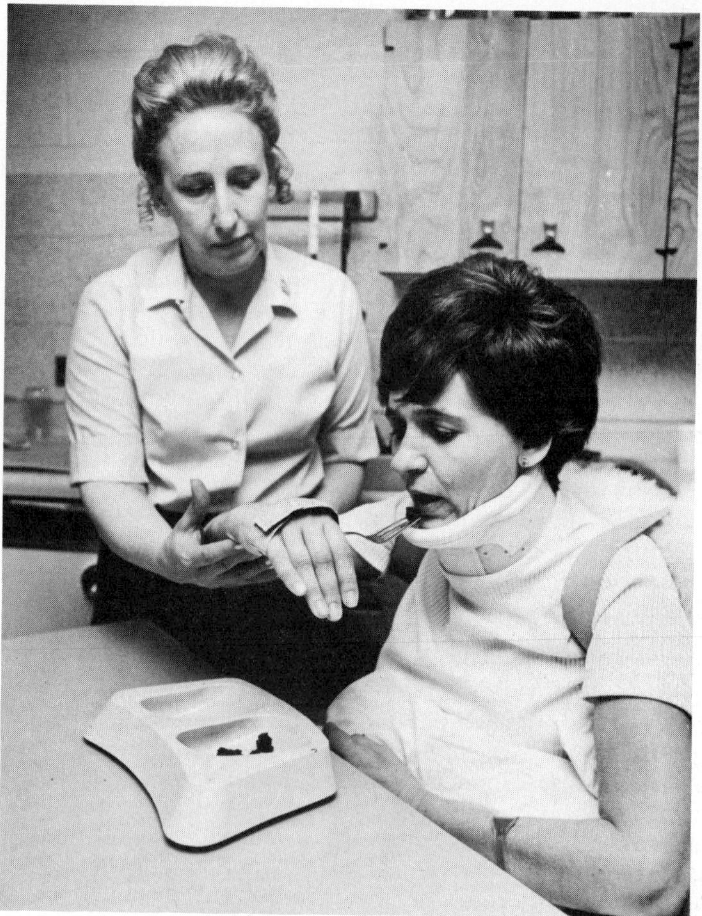

Figure 24–6. This patient is learning to use a universal cuff to become independent in self-feeding activities. A bowl with suction cups adheres to the table and prevents slipping. This will be used to make learning less difficult and will be replaced with regular utensils when the skill is perfected. (Courtesy, Allied Services for the Handicapped, Inc., Scranton, Pennsylvania.)

home economics, nutrition, social work, and psychology are utilized in rehabilitation. The patient is not only the focus of these specialized skills but part of the team and a participant in the plans for his or her restoration—as are members of the family. Each member of the team contributes skills in a way that complements but does not overlap or duplicate the efforts of another. The nurse is usually the coordinator of these services in the rehabilitation center.

Self-help Devices for Eating Numerous devices for daily activities have been designed at the Institute of Rehabilitation Medicine of the New York University Medical Center. In addition, publications such as the *Mealtime Manual for People with Disabilities and the Aging* are valuable.[14] Many of the devices can be made in the home, and others are available at moderate costs. A few of the devices that are helpful to those who have only one arm or who have difficulty in holding articles or bringing food to the mouth are described in the following. (See Figure 24–6.)

Jointed handles for spoons and forks. When the motions of the arm and wrist are restricted, the joints of the utensil permit an angle that can approach the mouth.

Knife for cutting. A knife needs a firm support, and cutting is difficult for persons with the use of only one arm. A cuff fitted over the hand permits the knife to be held firmly. A serrated edge is better than one with a smooth edge.

Plate guards. These are placed at the edge of the plate; they keep food from spilling and provide a surface against which food can be pushed. A deep dish with straight sides is also helpful. The plate can be kept from sliding by placing it in a support constructed to hold it, or by setting it on a sponge.

Buttering bread. A right-angle ledge affixed to the corner of the breadboard will hold a piece of bread in place while it is being buttered.

Drinking glass and tube. A drinking glass can be fitted with a holder that has a wide handle easily grasped by the hand. If it is difficult to bring the glass to the mouth, a wooden block into which a hole has been cut to hold a standard-size glass will hold the glass firmly on the table. A piece of plastic tubing bent at an angle for approach to the mouth can be used. To keep the plastic tube from slipping, a bulldog clip can be fastened to the edge of the glass and the tubing can be placed through the hole of the handle of the clip.

Aids in food preparation Homemaking is the single most frequent occupation of the physically handicapped. The rehabilitation of the homemaker in terms of food preparation skills and in overall homemaking activities benefits the entire family. Home economists, occupational therapists, and dietitians have specialized skills by which they are able to help the homemaker in simplification of procedures in food preparation and in more convenient kitchen arrangements.

The handicapped homemaker will find that each task requires a longer time to complete. As much food preparation should be completed in advance as possible so that there are few last-minute tasks. Arthritics fatigue easily and they should not attempt tasks that cannot be interrupted for a rest period. For many homemakers a list of things to be done is helpful.

Electric mixers, blenders, wedge-shape jar openers, electric can openers, long-handled tongs to reach packages and equipment out of reach, turntables in cupboards to hold supplies, sliding racks, magnetized equipment holders, and carts on wheels are among the pieces of equipment that facilitate work for the handicapped homemaker.

The person who has the use of only one arm needs firm support for devices. For example, a board with two stainless steel nails serves as a holder for vegetables to be peeled. A sponge underneath a bowl helps to keep it from sliding. Boxes can be held firmly between the knees and a scissors can be used with one hand to cut off tops.

For those who will be confined to a wheelchair indefinitely or who must sit while working, a redesign of the kitchen is essential. Counter surfaces need to be lowered so that work can be done while sitting. Kneehole spaces are needed so that the chair or wheelchair can be partially underneath the work surface. Equipment and storage shelves must be within reach.

Problems and Review

1. Define the following terms: hospital malnutrition, visceral protein status, creatinine height index, comprehensive health care.
2. *Problem.* Obtain a diet history from one of your patients who is receiving a normal diet. Use a form available in your hospital or develop one of your own. Evaluate the adequacy of the patient's diet according to the Daily Food Guide. What recommendations can be made to the patient? How would you plan for this counseling?
3. Make a list of drugs received by several of your patients. What are the nutritional side effects of these drugs?

4. How is nutritional status evaluated at your hospital? Which tests are used? What are the advantages and limitations of these particular tests?
5. Study the charts of three patients who have been hospitalized for two weeks or more. Indicate the type of diet each is receiving. Are there any indications in the record that nutritional status is compromised? How was this determined? What steps are to be taken to improve nutritional status in these individuals?
6. Identify some home health services available in your community. How is nutritional care provided?

Cited References

1. American Dietetic Association: *Handbook of Clinical Dietetics,* Yale University Press, New Haven, Conn., 1981.
2. American Hospital Association: "Statement on a Patient's Bill of Rights," *Hospitals,* **47**:41, February 16, 1973.
3. Forse, R. A., and Shizgal, H. M.: "The Assessment of Malnutrition," *Surgery,* **88**:17–24, 1980.
4. Buzby, G. P. et al.: "Prognostic Nutritional Index in Gastrointestinal Surgery," *Am. J. Surg.,* **139**:160–67, 1980.
5. Blackburn, G. L. et al.: "Nutritional and Metabolic Assessment of the Hospitalized Patient," *J.P.E.N.,* **1**:11–22, 1977.
6. Gray, G. E., and Gray, L. K.: "Anthropometric Measurements and Their Interpretation: Principles, Practices, and Problems," *J. Am. Diet. Assoc.,* **77**:534–39, 1980.
7. Blackburn, G. L., and Thornton, P. A.: "Nutritional Assessment of the Hospitalized Patient," *Med. Clin. North Am.,* **63**:1103–15, 1979.
8. Seltzer, M. H. et al.: "Instant Nutritional Assessment," *J.P.E.N.,* **3**:157–59, 1979.
9. Lemoine, A. et al.: "Vitamin B_1, B_2, and C Status in Hospital Inpatients," *Am. J. Clin. Nutr.,* **33**:2595–2600, 1980.
10. Shenkin, A.: "Assessment of Nutritional Status: The Biochemical Approach and Its Problems in Liver Disease," *J. Human Nutr.,* **33**:341–49, 1979.
11. Mullen, J. L. et al.: "Implications of Malnutrition in the Surgical Patient," *Arch. Surg.,* **114**:121–25, 1979.
12. Bistrian, B.: "Anthropometric Norms Used in Assessment of Hospitalized Patients," *Am. J. Clin. Nutr.,* **33**:2211–14, 1980.
13. Kolata, G. B.: "Dialysis After Nearly a Decade," *Science,* **208**:473–76, 1980.
14. Klinger, J. L. et al.: *Mealtime Manual for People with Disabilities and the Aging,* Campbell Soup Company, Camden, N.J., 1978.

Additional References

American Dietetic Association: *Handbook: Interactions of Selected Drugs with Nutritional Status in Man,* 2nd ed., American Dietetic Association, Chicago, 1978.

ANNAS, G. J.: *The Rights of Hospital Patients,* Avon Books, New York, 1975.

BRODY, D. S.: "The Patient's Role in Decision Making," *Ann. Intern. Med.,* **93**:718–22, 1980.

HOOLEY, R. A.: "Clinical Nutritional Assessment: A Perspective," *J. Am. Diet. Assoc.,* **77**:682–86, 1980.

PREVOST, E. A., and BUTTERWORTH, C. E.: "Nutritional Care of Hospitalized Patients," *Am. J. Clin. Nutr.,* **27**:432, 1974.

SALMOND, S. W.: "How to Assess the Nutritional Status of Acutely Ill Patients," *Am. J. Nurs.,* **80**:922–24, 1980.

SHAVER, H. J. et al.: "Nutritional Status of Nursing Home Patients," *J.P.E.N.*, **4**:367–70, 1980.

WARNOLD, I. et al.: "Energy Intake and Expenditure in Selected Groups of Hospitalized Patients," *Am. J. Clin. Nutr.*, **31**:742–49, 1978.

WATESKA, L. P. et al.: "Cost of a Home Parenteral Nutrition Program," *JAMA*, **244**:2303–04, 1980.

WEINSIER, R. L. et al.: "Hospital Malnutrition. A Prospective Evaluation of General Medical Patients During the Course of Hospitalization," *Am. J. Clin. Nutr.*, **32**:418–26, 1979.

25 Adaptations of the Normal Diet for Texture:

NORMAL, SOFT, AND FLUID DIETS

Therapeutic Nutrition Begins with the Normal Diet Normal and therapeutic diets are planned to maintain, or restore, good nutrition in the patient. In diet manuals the normal diet may be designated as *regular, house, normal,* or *full diet.* It consists of any and all foods eaten by the person in health. Fried foods, pastries, strongly flavored vegetables, spices, and relishes are not taboo, but good menu planning means that these foods are used judiciously. The normal diet satisfies the nutritional needs for most patients and also serves as the basis for planning modified diets.

The nutritive contributions of a basic diet composed of recommended levels from the Daily Food Guide were discussed in Chapter 13 and are summarized in Table 13–2. One of the many ways by which such a foundation diet may be amplified to provide meal patterns that are typical in many hospitals is shown in Table 25–1. In the suggested additions to the basic list of foods an additional cup of milk is included because it provides important amounts of several nutrients that are likely to be needed in increased amounts by many patients. Contrary to the opinion held by some, milk is one of the best-accepted foods in the hospital dietary.

To use the normal diet as the basis for therapeutic diets is sound in that it emphasizes the similarity of psychologic and social needs of those who are ill with those who are well, even though there may be differences in quantitative or qualitative requirements. Insofar as possible the patient is provided a food allowance that avoids the connotation of a "special" diet that sets him or her apart from family and friends. Moreover, in the home, food preparation is simplified when the modified diet is based upon the family pattern, and the number of items requiring special preparation is reduced to a minimum.

Although it is desirable that the normal diet provide the basis for planning modified diets, it must be remembered that the nutritional requirements of patients are likely to vary widely. The recommended dietary allowances are designed to meet the nutritional needs for almost all healthy persons in the United States, and they should not be interpreted as being appropriate allowances during illness. For any given patient the nutritional requirements depend upon nutritional status, modifications in activity, increased or decreased metabolic demands made by the illness, and the efficiency of digestive, absorptive, and excretory mechanisms.

Many adaptations to the plan presented in Table 25–1 could be devised for varying cultural and socioeconomic circumstances. The calculated values for the basic plan are useful in determining the effects of the omission or addition of foods to such a plan. For example, if a patient is allergic to milk, the plan shows that adjustment would need to be made especially for calcium, riboflavin, and protein. Or, if the intake of vegetables and fruits were to be curtailed, it is obvious that there would be a deficiency of vitamin A and ascorbic acid and that a supplement of vitamins should be prescribed.

Therapeutic Modifications of the Normal Diet The normal diet may be modified (1) to provide change in consistency as in fluid

Table 25-1. **Nutritive Value of the Normal Diet Pattern as a Basis for Therapeutic Diets***

Food	Measure	Weight gm	Energy kcal	Protein gm	Fat gm	Carbohydrate gm	Minerals: Ca mg	Minerals: Fe mg	Vitamins: A I.U.	Vitamins: Thiamin mg	Vitamins: Riboflavin mg	Vitamins: Niacin mg	Vitamins: Ascorbic Acid mg
Milk	2 cups	488	320	18	18	24	576	0.2	700	0.14	0.82	0.4	4
Meat Group													
Egg	1	50	80	6	6	tr	27	1.1	590	0.05	0.15	tr.	0
Meat, fish, poultry (lean, cooked)	4 ounces	120	240	33	10	0	17	3.6	35	0.32	0.26	7.4	0
Vegetable-Fruit Group													
Leafy green or deep yellow	1/2–2/3 cup	100	30	2	tr	6	28	1.0	7,400	0.06	0.08	0.6	28
Other vegetable	1/2–2/3 cup	100	30	2	tr	6	20	0.8	480	0.06	0.06	0.6	14
Potato	1 serving	122	80	2	tr	18	7	0.6	tr	0.11	0.04	1.4	20
Citrus fruit†	1 serving	100	40	1	tr	10	10	0.2	160	0.07	0.02	0.3	40
Other fruit	2 servings	200	120	2	tr	32	24	1.0	1,200	0.08	0.08	0.8	18
Bread-Cereal Group													
Cereal, enriched or whole grain	3/4 cup	30 (dry)	105	3	tr	22	10	0.8	0	0.12	0.04	0.8	0
Bread, enriched or whole grain	3 slices	75	210	6	3	39	63	1.8	tr	0.18	.0.15	1.8	tr
Fats-Sweets Group													
Butter or margarine	4 pats	28	200	tr	24	tr	6	0	940	—	—	—	—
Sugars, sweets	3 tablespoons	33	120	0	0	33	0	0	0	0	0	0	0
Desserts‡	1 serving	varies	190	4	6	30	70	0.3	190	0.03	0.10	0.1	tr
			1,765	79	67	220	858	11.4	11,695	1.22	1.80	14.2	124
Additional Foods													
Milk	1 cup	244	160	9	9	12	288	0.1	350	0.07	0.41	0.2	2
Bread	3 slices	75	210	6	3	39	63	1.8	tr	0.18	0.15	1.8	0
Total nutritive value			2,135	94	79	271	1,209	13.3	12,045	1.47	2.36	16.2§	126

*The nutritive values of the foods listed for the normal diet, page 462, have been calculated using Table A-1 in the Appendix. The additional foods listed at the bottom of the table suggest one of many ways to complete the diet.

†Other ascorbic-acid-rich foods such at cantaloupe and strawberries are also included.

‡Desserts include plain gelatin, cake with icing, custard, ice cream, cookies, and plain pudding.

§The tryptophan content of this diet is about 940 mg, equivalent to 15.7 mg niacin, thus providing a niacin equivalent of 31.9 mg.

Regular or Normal Diet

Include These Foods, or Their Nutritive Equivalents, Daily:

2–3 cups milk

4 ounces (cooked weight) meat, fish, or poultry; cheese, additional egg or milk, or legumes may substitute in part

1 egg (3 to 4 per week)

4 servings vegetables and fruits including:
- 1 serving of citrus fruit, or other good source of vitamin C
- 1 serving dark green leafy or deep yellow vegetable
- 2 or more servings of other vegetables and fruits, including potatoes

4 or more servings whole-grain cereals or bread

Additional foods such as butter or margarine, soups, desserts, sweets, salad dressings, or increased amounts of foods listed above will provide adequate calories. See calculation in Table 25–1.

Meal Pattern	Sample Menu
BREAKFAST	
Fruit	Sliced banana in orange juice
Cereal, enriched or whole-grain	Oatmeal
Milk and sugar for cereal	Milk and sugar
Egg	Soft-cooked egg
Whole-grain or enriched roll or toast	Whole-wheat toast with margarine
Butter or margarine	
Hot beverage with cream and sugar	Coffee with cream and sugar
LUNCHEON OR SUPPER	
Soup, if desired	
Cheese, meat, fish, or legumes	Cheese soufflé
Potato, rice, noodles, macaroni, spaghetti, or vegetable	Peas with margarine
Salad	Lettuce and tomato salad
	Russian dressing
Enriched or whole-grain bread	Hard roll with margarine
Butter or margarine	
Fruit	Royal Anne cherries
Milk	Milk
DINNER	
Meat, fish, or poultry	Meat loaf with gravy
Potato	Mashed potato
Vegetable	Carrots with margarine
Enriched or whole-grain bread	Enriched white, rye, or whole-wheat bread with margarine
Butter or margarine	
Dessert	Apple Betty
Milk	Milk
Coffee or tea, if desired	

and soft diets to be described later; (2) to increase or decrease the energy values; (3) to include greater or lesser amounts of one or more nutrients, for example, high-protein and sodium-restricted diets; (4) to increase or decrease bulk—high- and low-fiber diets; (5) to provide foods bland in flavor; (6) to include or exclude specific foods, as in allergic conditions; and (7) to modify the intervals of feeding.

Rationale for Modified Diets The principles for diet therapy in many pathologic conditions are well established, and dietary regimens are based upon a sound rationale. In such regimens the food allowances may vary according to ethnic and socioeconomic factors. It is to be expected that differences in interpretation will be found in the detailed descriptions of diet that are presented in the diet manuals of hospitals. Some of these differences are caused by the fact that some modified diets have only an empirical basis. Research to establish the merits of a particular regimen as opposed to another is difficult to control because of the numerous physiologic and psychological variables in human beings. Fortunately, a number of widely varying dietary programs may be equally effective because of the remarkable response of the human body.

Probably no diets are more subject to criticism than those modified for fiber and flavor. In order to reduce the fiber content of a diet, meats may be ground and vegetables and fruits strained. Yet, experience has shown that few patients consume such foods in satisfactory amounts, and the harm to nutritional status is likely to be greater than the possible insult to the mucosa of the gastrointestinal tract.

Some patients experience heartburn, abdominal distension, and flatulence following the ingestion of strongly flavored vegetables, dry beans or peas, and melons. Other patients refuse to eat these foods simply because they have been told that they are poorly digested. There is no evidence that justifies the omission of these foods for all patients. Although dietitians and nurses have a responsibility to correct food misinformation whenever it is encountered, little is gained by coercing someone who is ill into eating a food that he or she dislikes intensely or has a prejudice against.

Diet Manuals and Dietary Patterns The American Dietetic Association has prepared a *Handbook of Clinical Dietetics* which documents the scientific basis for dietary modification in treatment of specific disorders and includes food lists and sample menus for the various modified diets.[1] Numerous local or regional manuals are available as guides in the standardization of dietary procedures for a given hospital. The best of these manuals have been prepared by committees including representatives of the various medical specialties, nursing, and dietary departments. The manual generally includes statements concerning principles of diet, food allowances with detailed lists of foods to use and to avoid, typical meal patterns, and nutritive evaluations. They serve as a guide for the physician in prescribing a diet, a reference for the nurse, a procedural manual for the dietary department, and a teaching tool for professional personnel.

Although a manual achieves standardization in procedures, it does *not* mean that every patient on a given diet must have exactly the same food allowances as every other patient. In fact, within the guide ample opportunity is provided for individualization of a given patient's regimen. The diet manual is *not* an instructional guide for the patient for whom individualized and more detailed aids are necessary. It may, however, serve as the basis for the development of such teaching aids.

Throughout this text dietary regimens which are representative of those used in many hospitals are presented. Each description includes a statement of characteristics, lists of foods to include, detailed lists of foods permitted and contraindicated, a typical meal pattern, and a sample menu. The student will learn much by comparing one regimen with another and will begin to understand the rationale for diet therapy and how the goals may be achieved in a number of ways.

Nomenclature of Diets Insofar as possible, the nomenclature used in this text will describe the modification in consistency, in nutrients, or in flavor; thus *bland* diet *1,200-kcal* diet, and so on. When the quantity of one or more nutrients is important to the success of the diet, it is essential that these quantities be specified in the diet prescription. Thus, the term *diabetic diet* has little meaning, but a prescription for 245 gm carbohydrate, 70 gm protein, and 60 gm fat can be accurately interpreted. Likewise, a *sodium-restricted* diet gives no indication of the exact level of restriction required, but the designation *500-mg sodium diet* leaves no room for misinterpretation.

Several undesirable practices have been, and still are, common in the naming of diets. The literature is replete with illustrations of diets named for their originators. The Sippy diet is a classic example, but there have been others from time to time. Unfortunately, such nomenclature tells nothing about the diet, and the practice should be discouraged.

Others have used the name of a disease condition to specify a given diet, such as ulcer, ambulatory ulcer, ulcer discharge, cardiac, and gallbladder diets. Psychologically, this is not good practice, for patients should not need to be reminded of their condition every time they look at a diet on a tray card. Moreover, the diets used for many of these conditions have multiple uses, and the uninitiated may overlook the full usefulness of a given regimen with such disease-oriented terminology.

Frequency of Feeding Research on experimental animals and on humans has shown that more than three meals daily may be desirable for some patients. When the patient eats five, six, or more meals a day which are approximately balanced for protein, fat, and carbohydrate, the metabolic load at a given time is less, and the nutrients can be more effectively utilized. It is well known that protein is inefficiently used if the day's allowance is more or less concentrated in one meal. Large amounts of carbohydrate at a given meal require the use of alternate metabolic pathways which favor the deposition of fat.

Irwin has described guidelines for health care facilities using menu patterns with four or five meals daily. Each meal provides at least three menu items and 10 per cent or more of calories as protein. Between-meal snacks are not considered as meals. In compliance with federal guidelines the time lapse between the last meal of one day and the first meal of the next is not more than 14 hours. From 20 to 50 per cent of total calories are given in consecutive five-hour periods between 7 A.M. and 10 P.M.[2]

Sometimes it is desirable to adapt home diets of patients to a six- or seven-meal program. Some protein, fat, and carbohydrate should be given at each meal. Thus, milk or a protein sandwich may be useful for interval feedings, but juices or sweets alone do not satisfy the requirements. The interval between meals should be 1½ to 3 hours, with meals spread throughout the waking hours. Any of the modified diets might be presented in more than three meals. A judicious choice of bedtime snacks apparently does not modify sleep. (See Figure 25–1.)

Mechanical Soft Diet Many persons require a soft diet simply because they have no teeth. It is neither desirable nor essential to restrict the patient to the selection allowed on the customary soft diet (page 466 employed for a postoperative patient or for a patient with a gastrointestinal disturbance. For example, stewed onions, baked beans, and apple pie are foods considered to be quite unsuitable for the latter patients but which may be enjoyed by those who simply require foods that are soft in texture. The terms *mechanical soft* and *dental soft* are used in some diet manuals to describe such a dietary modification. The following changes in the normal diet will usually suffice for individuals without teeth:

Meats should be finely minced or ground.
Soft breads are substituted for crusty breads.
Cooked vegetables are used without restriction, but dicing or chopping may be desirable for

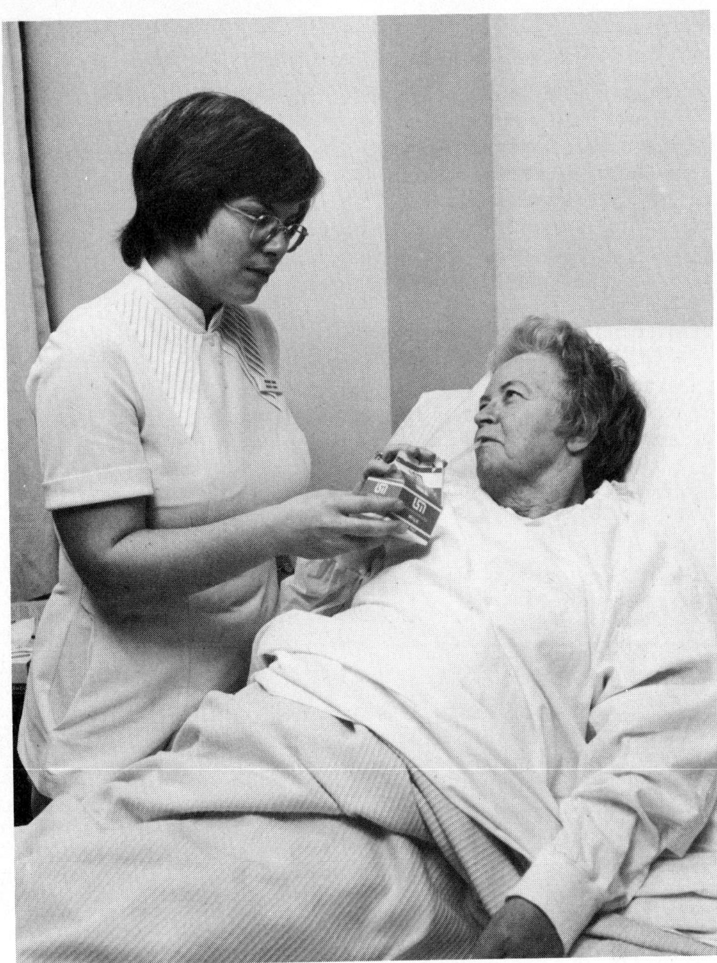

Figure 25–1. Milk is well accepted by most patients and provides important nutrients for liquid diets or between-meal feedings. (Courtesy, University of Minnesota Health Sciences Center, Minneapolis.)

some; for example, diced beets, chopped spinach, corn cut from cob.

Most raw vegetables are omitted; raw tomatoes, cut finely, may usually be used. Sometimes finely chopped lettuce in a sandwich may be accepted.

Many raw fruits may be used: banana, orange, grapefruit, soft berries, soft pear, apricots, peaches, grapes with tender skins.

Hard raw fruits such as pineapple and apple are usually avoided; but finely diced apple in fruit cup may be used.

Tough skins should be removed from fruits: raw, soft pear, or baked apple, etc.

Nuts and dried fruits, when used in desserts or other foods, are acceptable if finely chopped.

Soft Diet This diet represents the usual dietary step between the full fluid and normal diet. It may be used in acute infections, some gastrointestinal disturbances, and following surgery. The diet is soft in consistency, easy to chew, made up of simple, easily digestible food, and contains no harsh fiber, no rich or highly flavored food. It is nutritionally adequate when planned on the basis of the normal diet.

Soft Diet

Include These Foods, or Their Nutritive Equivalents, Daily:

2–3 cups milk
4 ounces (cooked weight) very tender or ground meat, fish, or poultry; soft cheese, legumes, or additional milk may substitute in part
1 egg (3 to 4 per week)
4 servings vegetables and fruits including:
- 2 servings of citrus fruit or juice
- 1 serving dark green leafy or deep yellow vegetable—tender chopped or strained
- 1 medium potato
- 1 or more servings of other tender chopped or strained vegetables, or cooked fruits without skin or seeds, or strained cooked fruit

4 or more servings strained whole-grain cereals or fine whole-grain bread
Additional foods such as butter or margarine, soups, desserts, sweets, or increased amounts of the above will provide adequate calories.

Nutritive value. See calculation for the normal diet in Table 25–1.

Foods Allowed

All beverages
Bread—white, fine whole-wheat, rye without seeds; white crackers
Cereal foods—dry, such as cornflakes, Puffed Rice, rice flakes; fine cooked, such as cornmeal, farina, hominy grits, macaroni, noodles, rice, spaghetti; strained coarse, such as oatmeal, Pettijohn's, whole-wheat
Cheese—mild, soft, such as cottage and cream; Cheddar; Swiss
Desserts—plain cake, cookies; custards; plain gelatin or with allowed fruit; Junket; plain ice cream, ices, sherbets; plain puddings, such as bread, cornstarch, rice, tapioca
Eggs—all except fried
Fats—butter, cream, margarine, vegetable oils and fats in cooking
Fruits—raw: ripe avocado, banana, grapefruit or orange sections without membrane; canned or cooked: apples, apricots, fruit cocktail, peaches, pears, plums—all without skins; Royal Anne cherries; strained prunes and other fruits with skins; all juices
Meat—very tender, minced, or ground; baked, broiled, creamed, roast, or stewed: beef, lamb, veal, poultry, fish, bacon, liver, sweetbreads
Milk—in any form
Soups—broth, strained cream or vegetable
Sweets—all sugars, syrup, jelly, honey, plain sugar candy without fruit or nuts, molasses Use in moderation.

Foods to Avoid

Bread—coarse dark; whole-grain crackers; hot breads; pancakes, waffles
Cereals—bran; coarse unless strained
Cheese—sharp, such as Roquefort, Camembert, Limburger
Desserts—any made with dried fruit or nuts; pastries; rich puddings or cake
Eggs—fried
Fats—fried foods
Fruits—raw except as listed; stewed or canned berries; with tough skins
Meat—tough with gristle or fat; salted and smoked meat or fish, such as corned beef, smoked herring; cold cuts; frankfurter; pork
Soups—fatty or highly seasoned
Sweets—jam, marmalade, rich candies with chocolate

Foods Allowed

Vegetables—white or sweet potato without skin, any way except fried; young and tender asparagus, beets, carrots, peas, pumpkin, squash without seeds; tender chopped greens; strained cooked vegetables if not tender; tomato juice

Miscellaneous—salt, seasonings and spices in moderation, gravy, cream sauces

Foods to Avoid

Vegetables—raw; strongly flavored, such as broccoli, Brussels sprouts, cabbage, cauliflower, cucumber, onion, radish, sauerkraut, turnip; corn; dried beans and peas; potato chips

Miscellaneous—pepper and other hot spices; fried foods; nuts; olives; pickles; relishes

Meal Pattern	Sample Menu
BREAKFAST	
Fruit or fruit juice	Orange sections and banana slices
Cereal—strained, if coarse	Oatmeal
Milk and sugar for cereal	Milk and sugar for cereal
Egg	Soft-cooked egg
Soft roll or toast	Toast with margarine
Butter or margarine	
Hot beverage with cream and sugar	Coffee
LUNCHEON OR SUPPER	
Strained soup, if desired	Cream of tomato soup
Mild cheese, tender or ground meat, fish, or poultry	Cheese soufflé
Potato without skin, rice, noodles, macaroni, or spaghetti; or	
Cooked vegetable	Tender peas
Enriched bread	Soft roll
Butter or margarine	Butter or margarine
Fruit	Royal Anne cherries
Milk	Milk
Coffee or tea, if desired	Coffee or tea, if desired
DINNER	
Orange, grapefruit, or tomato juice	Grapefruit juice
Tender or ground meat, fish, or poultry	Meat loaf (no onion or pepper) with gravy
Potato, any way except fried	Mashed potato
Cooked vegetable	Carrots with margarine
Enriched bread	Rye bread without seeds
Butter or margarine	Butter or margarine
Dessert	Baked apple without skin; cream
Milk	Milk
Hot beverage with cream and sugar, if desired	Tea with sugar and lemon

Liquid Diets Fluid diets are used in febrile states, postoperatively, or whenever the patient is unable to tolerate solid foods. The degree to which these diets are adequate will depend upon the type of liquids permitted.

Clear-fluid diet. Whenever an acute illness or surgery produces a marked intolerance for food as may be evident by nausea, vomiting, anorexia, distension, and diarrhea, it is advisable to restrict the intake of nutrients. A clear-fluid diet is usually

Full-Fluid Diet

General Rules

Give six or more feedings daily.

The protein content of the diet can be increased by incorporating nonfat dry milk in beverages and soups. Strained canned meats (used for infant feeding) may be added to broths.

The caloric value of the diet may be increased by: (1) substituting 10 percent cream for part of the usual milk allowance; (2) adding butter or margarine to cereal gruels and soups; (3) including glucose in beverages; (4) using ice cream as dessert or in beverages.

If a decreased volume of fluid is desired, nonfat dry milk may be substituted for part of the fluid milk.

Include These Foods, or Their Nutritive Equivalents Daily:

6 cups milk
2 eggs (in custards or pasteurized eggnog)
1–2 ounces strained meat
½ cup fine or strained whole-grain cooked cereal for gruel
¼ cup vegetable purée for cream soup
1 cup citrus fruit juices; plus other strained juices
½ cup tomato or vegetable juice
1 tablespoon cocoa
3 tablespoons sugar
1 tablespoon butter or margarine
2 servings plain gelatin dessert, Junket, soft or baked custard, ices, sherbets, plain ice cream, or plain cornstarch pudding
Broth, bouillon, or clear soups
Tea, coffee, carbonated beverages as desired
Flavoring extracts, salt

Nutritive values of foods listed in specified amounts: kcal, 1,950; protein, 85 gm; calcium, 2.1 gm; iron, 7.7 mg; vitamin A, 7,150 I.U.; thiamin, 1.1 mg; riboflavin, 3.2 mg; niacin equivalents, 19.1 mg; ascorbic acid, 160 mg.

Meal Pattern	**Sample Menu**
BREAKFAST	
Citrus juice	Orange juice
Cereal gruel with butter, sugar Milk	Cream of wheat with milk, butter, and sugar
Beverage with cream, sugar	Coffee with cream and sugar
MIDMORNING	
Milk, plain, malted, chocolate, or eggnog (pasteurized)	Eggnog, pasteurized
LUNCHEON OR SUPPER	
Strained soup	Beef broth with strained meat
Tomato juice	Tomato juice
Custard, Junket, ice cream, sherbet, ice, gelatin dessert, or plain pudding	Maple Junket
Eggnog, milk, or cocoa	Milk
Tea with sugar, if desired	Tea with sugar and cream

Meal Pattern	Sample Menu
MIDAFTERNOON	
Milk, ice cream, custard, or gelatin dessert	Vanilla milkshake
DINNER	
Strained cream soup	Strained cream of mushroom soup
Citrus juice	Grapefruit juice
Custard, Junket, ice cream, ice, sherbet, or gelatin dessert	Gelatin dessert
Milk or cocoa	Cocoa
Tea, if desired	Tea with sugar and lemon
EVENING NOURISHMENT	
Milk, custard, or juice	Custard

used for 1 to 2 days, at the end of which time the patient is usually able to utilize a more liberal liquid diet.

Tea with lemon and sugar, coffee, fat-free broth, and carbonated beverages are the usual liquids permitted. In addition, strained fruit juices, fruit ices, and plain gelatin are often included.

The amount of fluid in a given feeding on the clear-fluid diet is usually restricted to 30 to 60 ml per hour at first, with gradually increasing amounts being given as the patient's tolerance improves. Obviously, such a diet can accomplish little beyond the replacement of fluids.

Full-fluid diet. This diet is indicated whenever a patient is acutely ill or is unable to chew or swallow solid food. It includes all foods liquid at room temperature and at body temperature. It is free from cellulose and irritating condiments. When properly planned, this diet can be used for relatively long periods of time. However, iron is provided at inadequate levels.

Other Methods of Feeding Food by mouth is the method of choice when the patient can eat, digest, and absorb sufficient food to meet nutritive requirements. In illness, however, it is occasionally necessary to augment the oral intake by giving parenteral feedings of one type or another.

When the patient is unable to chew or swallow because of deformity or inflammation of the mouth or throat, corrosive poisoning, unconsciousness, paralysis of the throat muscles, and so on, tube feeding is used (see page 590).

Semisynthetic fiber-free diets are used in situations in which it is desirable to have a minimum of residue in the intestine. These preparations are administered orally or by tube and may be used for extended periods.

Intravenous feeding is used when it is necessary to rest the patient's gastrointestinal tract. Fluids given by such means include solutions of glucose, amino acids, salts, and vitamins. Transfusions of whole blood or of plasma are commonly used. For selected patients who are seriously depleted nutritionally, total parenteral nutrition is used.

Problems and Review

1. What is meant by routine house diets?
2. Why is the normal diet used as a basis for planning therapeutic diets?
3. What are the advantages of using a diet manual for planning diets? What are the limitations?

4. What objections can you see to the following examples of dietary nomenclature: nephritic diet; Kempner diet; low-protein diet; ulcer discharge diet? Examine the nomenclature used for diets in your hospital, and suggest ways for improvement.
5. *Problem.* Write a menu for one day for a patient to receive a regular diet. Modify this pattern for a patient who is unable to chew foods well.
6. *Problem.* Prepare a table that shows the food intake for one day by a patient receiving a full-fluid diet. Calculate the protein, energy, and ascorbic acid intake.
7. *Problem.* Prepare a chart that shows the dietary orders for five patients. On this chart include a statement concerning the reasons for the diet order and the patient's acceptance of the diet.

Cited References

1. American Dietetic Association: *Handbook of Clinical Dietetics.* Yale University Press, New Haven, Conn., 1981.
2. Irwin, E. R.: "Alternate Menu Patterns—Survey and Nutritional Guidelines," *J. Am. Diet. Assoc.,* **65**:291–93, 1974.

26 Dietary Calculation Using the Exchange Lists for Meal Planning

NURSES and dietitians are frequently expected to make quick, yet reasonably accurate estimations of the nutritive value of diets or to calculate diets that must be controlled for one or more nutrients. The Exchange Lists for Meal Planning provide the basis for the rapid calculation of diets that require control of energy, carbohydrate, fat, and protein. These lists are also used for counseling patients on the kinds and amounts of foods that are included in their diets. (See Figure 26–1.)

Food Exchange Lists

Six Exchange Lists The exchange lists were first published by a joint committee of the American Dietetic Association, the American Diabetes Association, and the U.S. Public Health Service.[1] They were revised in 1976.[2] (See Table A–4.)

An exchange list is a grouping of foods in which specified amounts of all the foods listed are of approximately equal carbohydrate, protein, and fat value. Specific foods within the lists may differ slightly in their nutritive value from the averages stated for the group. (See Table 26–1.) These differences in composition tend to cancel out because of the variety of foods selected from day to day. Thus, any food within a given list can be substituted or exchanged for any other food in that list. In the fruit list, for example, 1 small apple, or ½ banana, or

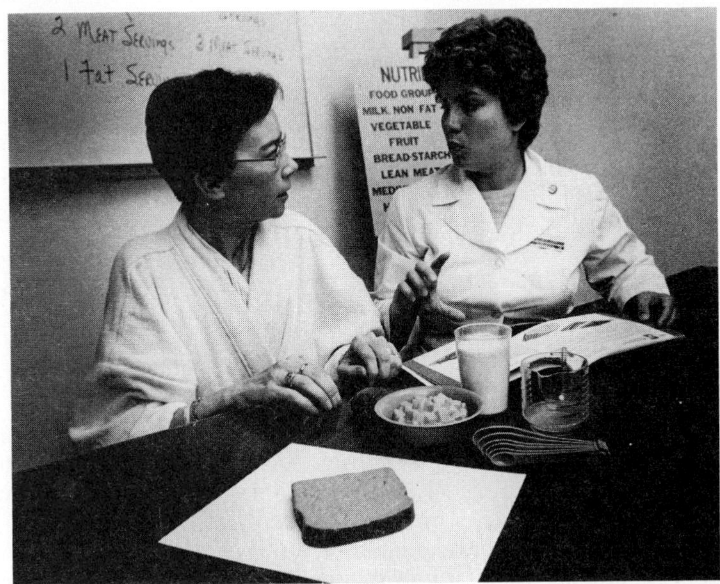

Figure 26–1. The diet counselor teaches the patient how to use the Exchange Lists for planning menus within her daily food allowance and in accordance with cultural food patterns. (Courtesy, Hennepin County Medical Center, Minneapolis.)

Table 26-1. **Composition of Food Exchange Lists***

Food Exchange	Measure	Weight gm	Carbohydrate gm	Protein gm	Fat gm	Energy kcal
Milk, nonfat	1 cup	240	12	8	—	80
Milk, whole	1 cup	240	12	8	10	170
Vegetables	½ cup	100	5	2	—	25
Fruit	Varies		10	—	—	40
Bread	Varies		15	2	—	70
Meat, low fat	1 ounce	30	—	7	3	55
medium fat	1 ounce	30	—	7	5	75
high fat	1 ounce	30	—	7	8	100
Fat	1 teaspoon	5	—	—	5	45

*Consult Table A-4 for food selections for each of the exchange lists.

2 prunes, or ½ cup orange juice would contain 10 gm carbohydrate.

Milk list. One cup of skim milk is the basis for this list. If 2 per cent fortified skim milk is used in place of skim milk, an adjustment must be made. For each cup of 2 per cent milk one fat exchange should be omitted from the diet. If whole milk is used regularly, the milk allowance is calculated to provide 12 gm carbohydrate, 8 gm protein, and 10 gm fat per cup.

Note that cheeses are listed with meat exchanges; cream, cream cheese, and butter are listed as fat exchanges.

Vegetable lists. An exchange of most vegetables in this list is ½ cup and provides 5 gm carbohydrate and 2 gm protein. Vegetables high in carbohydrate are included in the bread list. A few salad greens and radishes may be used as desired.

Fruit list. Each fruit in the amount stated supplies 10 gm carbohydrate. Many of the fruits are in average-size servings, but some are not. For example, 2 prunes, 1 fig, and ¼ cup grape juice would be smaller-than-average servings. It is important, therefore, not to use the terms *exchange* and *serving* interchangeably.

Bread list. One slice of bread is the basis for the exchanges in this list. Included are biscuits, muffins, and rolls; dry and cooked breakfast cereals; grits, macaroni, noodles, spaghetti, and rice; crackers; and a number of vegetables—corn, Lima beans, baked beans, cooked dry beans, peas, white potato, and lentils, winter squash, sweet potato, and others.

Meat list. Meats are listed in three groups: low, medium, and high fat. Protein sources in the low-fat group are used for planning diets low in saturated fat and cholesterol. (See Chapter 39.) One ounce of cooked meat, poultry, or fish is used as the basis for each list. On a raw-weight basis this is equivalent to about 1⅓ ounces of edible portion; thus, one would need to purchase 4 ounces of raw meat, edible portion to equal a 3-ounce serving of cooked meat. It is assumed that the visible fat is trimmed off, but a wide selection of choices is permissible from each list.

Luncheon meats, canned fish, shellfish, Cheddar, American, Swiss, and cottage cheese, eggs, and peanut butter in the amounts listed are exchanges for meat.

Fat list. This list is based upon 1 teaspoon of margarine. It includes butter, solid fats and oils used in cooking, bacon, light and heavy cream, cream cheese, salad dressings, nuts, avocado, and olives.

Miscellaneous list. Coffee, tea, broth, spices, herbs, and some other items are insignificant for their nutritive values but they lend interest to the diet. They may be included in dietary plans without calculation.

Supplementary lists. Some hospital dietary departments have calculated the carbohydrate, protein, and fat content of various commercial products and have determined the amount of the food that can be substituted for items in the traditional exchange lists. In using these supplementary lists, it is well to remember that it is not possible to have an up-to-date, accurate list of products because of the rapidity with which new products are introduced and because formulations may change from time to time.

Assuring Mineral and Vitamin Adequacy Since the exchange lists do not provide information on mineral and vitamin values it becomes evident that some degree of discretion must be used in establishing the daily food allowances and in selecting specific menus. For example, 2 cups of milk daily will supply sufficient calcium and riboflavin for the adult; 3 to 4 cups of milk would be included in the diet plan of children and pregnant or lactating women. At least two fruit exchanges are included daily, one of these being selected from those fruits rich in ascorbic acid. Fruits that are good sources of this vitamin are marked with an asterisk in the listing. Vegetables are often neglected in dietary planning or are restricted to a few choices. Those that are dark green or deep yellow are excellent sources of vitamin A, and one of these should be included frequently. Note that vitamin-A-rich vegetables have been indicated in the vegetable lists.

Procedure for Calculation The calculation of a diet requires only the nutritive values of Table 26–1. Let us suppose that the following diet prescription is to be cal-

Table 26–2. **Calculation of Diet Using Food Exchange Lists**
(*Carbohydrate, 245 gm; Protein, 70 gm; Fat, 60 gm*)

List	Food	Measure	Weight gm	Carbohydrate gm	Protein gm	Fat gm
1	Milk, skim	2 cups	480	24	16	—
2	Vegetables	3 exchanges	300	15	6	—
3	Fruit	7 exchanges	Varies	70	—	—
				109		
4	Bread	9 exchanges	Varies	135	18	—
					40	
5	Meat, low fat	2 exchanges	Varies	—	14	6
	medium fat	2 exchanges	Varies	—	14	10
						16
6	Fat	9 exchanges	Varies	—	—	45
				244	68	61

245 gm carbohydrate prescribed total
109 gm carbohydrate from milk, vegetables, and fruit

136 gm carbohydrate to be supplied from bread exchanges
136 ÷ 15 = 9 bread exchanges

70 gm protein prescribed total
40 gm protein from milk, vegetable, and bread exchanges

30 gm protein to be supplied from meat exchanges
30 ÷ 7 = 4 meat exchanges

60 gm fat prescribed total
16 gm fat from meat exchanges

44 gm fat to be supplied from fat exchanges
44 ÷ 5 = 9 fat exchanges

culated: carbohydrate, 245 gm; protein, 70 gm; and fat, 60 gm. A daily food allowance for this prescription is shown in Table 26–2 using the following procedures.

1. Estimate the amounts of milk, vegetables, and fruits to be included. The allowances are dictated somewhat by the preferences of the patient, but the following amounts are minimum levels that should ordinarily be included:

Milk—2 cups for adults; 3 to 4 cups for children and for pregnant or lactating women
Vegetables—2 exchanges
Fruit—2 exchanges

2. Fill in the carbohydrate, protein, and fat values for the tentative amounts of milk, vegetables, and fruits.

3. To determine the number of bread exchanges: Total the carbohydrate value of the milk, vegetables, and fruit. Subtract this total from the total amount of carbohydrate prescribed. Divide the remainder by 15 (the carbohydrate value of one bread exchange). Use the nearest whole number of bread exchanges. Fill in the carbohydrate and protein values.

4. Total the carbohydrate column. If the total deviates more than 3 or 4 gm from the prescribed amount, adjust the amounts of vegetables, fruits, and bread. No diet should be planned with fractions of an exchange since awkward measures of food would sometimes be encountered.

5. To determine the number of meat exchanges: Total the protein value of the milk, vegetable, and bread. Subtract this total from the amount of protein prescribed. Divide the remainder by 7 (the protein value of one meat exchange). Use the nearest whole number of meat exchanges. Fill in the protein and fat values.

6. To determine the number of fat exchanges: Total the fat values for milk and meat. Subtract this total from the amount of fat prescribed. Divide the remainder by 5 (the fat content of one fat exchange). Fill in the fat value.

7. Check the entire diet for the accuracy of the computations. Divide the daily food allowance into a meal pattern suitable for the individual. For some diets the distribution of food may be specified in the prescription.

The following menu illustrates one way that the day's food allowance for the diet shown in Table 26–2 could be used. Another menu is shown on page 608 in the adaptation for a patient with diabetes.

BREAKFAST
Stewed prunes—4
Dry cereal—¾ cup
Skim milk—1 cup
Toast, whole-wheat—2 slices
Butter or margarine—2 teaspoons

LUNCHEON
Tomato juice—½ cup
Saltines—6
Sandwich
  Rye bread—2 slices
  Sliced ham—1 thin slice (1 ounce)
  Swiss cheese—1 slice
  Lettuce
  Mayonnaise—2 teaspoons
Celery and radishes
Olives—5 small
Honeydew melon—¼ medium

DINNER
Skewered lamb and vegetables
  Lamb—2 ounces (3 ounces raw)
  Onions—4 small
  Tomato wedges
  Mushroom caps
  Green-pepper strips
  Oil—2 teaspoons for basting meat and vegetables while cooking
Rice—½ cup
Dinner roll—1
Butter or margarine—2 teaspoons
Fruit cup (2 exchanges fruit)
  Banana, small—½
  Blueberries—⅓ cup
  Grapes—6

EVENING SNACK
Skim milk—1 cup
Graham crackers—2
Apple, small—1

Problems and Review

1. How do you explain the fact that Cheddar and cottage cheese are listed as meat exchanges but they are included in the milk group of the Daily Food Guide (page 40)?
2. Which vegetables are especially rich in vitamin A? In iron? In ascorbic acid?
3. Explain the placement of potatoes, corn, Lima beans, and baked beans in the bread exchange list.
4. *Problem.* Plan a menu for a lunch that permits the following exchanges: one milk; two vegetables; one fruit; three bread; two meat; three fat.
5. *Problem.* Write three breakfast menus based upon the following exchange requirements: one milk; one fruit; two bread; two meats; and three fat.
6. *Problem.* Keep a record of your food intake for one day and calculate the carbohydrate, protein, fat, and caloric value using the exchange lists.

Cited References

1. Caso, E.: "Calculation of Diabetic Diets," *J. Am. Diet. Assoc.*, **26**:575–83, 1950.
2. American Diabetes Association, Inc., and The American Dietetic Association: *Exchange Lists for Meal Planning.* The American Dietetic Association, Chicago, 1976.

Additional Reference

WYSE, B. W., and HANSEN, R. G.: "Nutrient Analysis of *Exchange Lists for Meal Planning.* II. Nutrient Density Food Profiles," *J. Am. Diet. Assoc.*, **75**:242–49, 1979.

Patient Education Materials

American Diabetes Association, Inc., and The American Dietetic Association: *Exchange Lists for Meal Planning.* The American Dietetic Association, Chicago, 1976.

Exchange Lists for the Blind. Volunteer Braille Services, P. O. Box 1592, Houma, La. 70361.

HELSEL, J., and LANSING, E.: *The ABC's of Diabetic Cooking and Dining.* Dell Publishing Co., Inc., New York, 1979.

Meredith Corporation: *Eat and Stay Slim,* Meredith Publishing Co., Des Moines, Iowa, 1979.

27 Overweight: Low-Calorie Diets

THE problem of overweight is one of great frustration for many North Americans. Relative affluence, abundance of a wide variety of foods, and lack of physical activity are a few of the factors that contribute to excessive calorie intake for many. Numerous weight reduction regimens have been described; yet the long-term success rate with all of these is limited. Because of the difficulty in achieving and maintaining desirable weight once obesity is established, emphasis must be on prevention of overweight beginning early in life. Several approaches to weight control are described in this chapter. None of these is appropriate for all patients; nevertheless, each has advantages for certain patients.

Importance of Weight Control

Hazards of Obesity The health consequences of obesity have been studied both retrospectively and prospectively. Life insurance statistics provide retrospective data suggesting that life expectancy is shorter in overweight individuals. For example, if one's weight is 20 per cent more than the average, life expectancy is decreased by 20 per cent in males and 10 per cent in females. (See Table 27–1.) The principal causes of death in these individuals are diabetes mellitus, gallbladder disease, and cardiovascular-renal disease.[1] Data from the Framingham study also show increased mortality for persons weighing more or less than average.[2]

In morbidly obese men, the mortality is markedly higher than that of the U.S. male population as a whole. A longitudinal study of 200 morbidly obese men revealed a twelve-fold excess mortality rate in 25 to 34-year-olds, and a sixfold increase in 35 to 44-year-olds. The most common cause of death in these men was cardiovascular disease; the incidence was 30 per cent higher than that of U.S. males in general. Obesity appeared to favor the development of degenerative diseases at an earlier age, with more rapid progression to clinical events.[3]

Prospective studies have shown that obesity correlates with increased incidence of hypertension, impaired glucose tolerance, increased plasma insulin levels, gallbladder disease, elevated serum lipid levels, with the exception of HDL-cholesterol, and hyperuricemia. Correction of the obesity is associated with improvement in these parameters.[1] The obese are at increased risk for cardiovascular disease although

Table 27-1. Mortality According to Per Cent Deviation from Average Weight*

Per Cent of Average Weight	Per Cent Mortality	
	Males	Females
80	105	110
90	94	97
100	100	100
110	111	107
120	120	110
130	135	125
140	153	136
150	177	149
160	210	169

*Adapted from Van Itallie, T. B.: "Obesity: Adverse Effects on Health and Longevity," *Am. J. Clin. Nutr.*, 32: 2723–33, 1979.

obesity per se is not a risk factor. It can, however, indirectly increase risk by causing or exacerbating known risk factors such as hypertension, hyperlipidemia, and diabetes mellitus. Obesity is considered to be a risk factor for endometrial cancer.[1]

Obesity entails a respiratory cost in normal persons by increased work of breathing, a decrease in lung volume, and pulmonary hypertension. In any person with chronic pulmonary disorders such as emphysema and asthma obesity greatly increases the respiratory stress. The hazards of surgery and of pregnancy and childbirth are multiplied in the presence of excessive adipose tissue.

Overweight is a physical handicap as well as a primary health hazard. Obese people are more uncomfortable during warm weather because the thick layers of fat serve as an insulator. More effort must be expended to do a given amount of work because of the increase in body mass. Because of their lessened agility, obese people are more susceptible to accidents. Fatigue, backache, and foot troubles are common complaints of the obese.

Obesity and Faddism For a significant portion of the American population, weight control is a perplexing problem. For many, constant vigilance is necessary to prevent gain of unwanted pounds and for maintenance of the slim physique so highly valued in the American culture. This cultural attitude toward slimness is evident everywhere—television and magazine ads for reducing aids such as low-calorie formula diets, appetite suppressants, and special clothing designed to promote quick weight loss; use of slim models in advertising everything from clothing to work tools; book clubs and bookstores with their abundance of books on reducing diets—such books are frequently best sellers; women's magazines—practically every month one of these has a new weight-loss diet; drugstores and supermarkets which feature a wide variety of reducing candies, "dietetic" and "low-calorie" items. Especially among American women emphasis on slimness contrasts sharply with that of other cultures, southern Europe, for example, where women generally weigh more than their American counterparts.

Evaluation of Weight Status and Body Composition

Desirable Weight The best weight for a given individual's height, age, bone structure, and muscular development is not known. For adults over age 25, height-weight tables compiled by the life insurance industry provide a rough guide for estimating desirable weight according to height and frame. The tables are based on the weight ranges associated with the lowest mortality rates, and on the philosophy that the ideal weight for one's height and build at age 25 should be maintained throughout adult life. See Table A–10. Limitations of the tables should be kept in mind: (1) They are based on data obtained from a large group of insured persons over a quarter of a century ago and are not necessarily representative of the population as a whole. (2) Although the tables allow for differences in body frame, criteria for determining frame size are not defined. (3) The level of weight that is considered abnormal is not defined. (4) The tables do not provide information on body composition, that is, the degree of fatness.

A deviation of not more than 10 per cent above or below the desirable weight for a given individual is not considered to be significant. The term *overweight* is applied to persons who are 10 to 20 per cent above desirable weight. It usually represents excessive fat stores but may also reflect increased muscle mass or abnormal fluid retention. *Obesity,* on the other hand, is characterized by an excessive amount of adipose tissue, and the term is applied to persons 20 per cent or more above desirable weight. The term *severe* or *morbid* obesity is applied to persons who are 100 per cent or more overweight.

Body Composition Gross obesity is easily identified by visual observation alone, but errors in making a diagnosis of moderate obesity are frequent by reference to height-weight tables. The concern in obesity, from a clinical point of view, is the excessive amount of adipose tissue and not overweight per se. A football player may be overweight by the usual height-weight standards but he has a well-developed musculature and does not have excessive fat deposits, and therefore is not classified as obese.

Body fatness can be measured by determining the thickness of subcutaneous tissues at designated body locations by means of calipers. (See Chapter 22 for a description of tests used to determine body composition.) The subscapular skinfold provides a better indication of fatness than does the triceps skinfold; nevertheless, the triceps skinfold is frequently used since it is conveniently measured. In adults, values greater than 18 mm in males and 25 mm in females indicate obesity.[4]

Estimation of Weight Loss Adipose tissue in adults consists of about 75 per cent fat, 23 per cent water, and small amounts of protein and mineral salts.[5] Each kilogram of adipose tissue represents 7,700 kcal (1 pound = 3,500 kcal). An individual who consumes 100 kcal in excess daily ingests an excess of 3,000 kcal by the end of 1 month. Theoretically, this would result in a weight gain of 0.4 kg monthly, or 4.8 kg (about 10 lb) in a year. The weight gain from consistently overeating by this amount over a 5- to 10-year period would be considerable. It requires about 2 teaspoons of butter, or two 1-inch squares of fudge, or an oatmeal cookie to supply the additional 100 kcal each day.

Conversely, the loss of 1 kilogram of adipose tissue means that the diet would be deficient by 7,700 kcal for the total time period of the weight loss. A young woman requiring 2,000 kcal a day to meet her energy needs who consumes a diet that supplies only 1,200 kcal has a weekly deficit of 5,600 kcal, and the predicted adipose tissue loss would be 5600 ÷ 7,700, or 0.7 kg (1.6 pounds).

Weight loss does not always follow the predicted straight line for several reasons: (1) The type of diet may influence losses—on very low carbohydrate diets rapid weight loss occurs initially, due principally to losses of sodium, potassium, and water; on more conventional diets, such losses are less conspicuous. (2) As weight loss continues, the basal metabolic rate per unit of active tissue mass declines, resulting in a slower rate of weight loss. (3) The energy cost of activity decreases as a function of lower body weight. Furthermore, subjects tend to decrease overall activity in response to reduced caloric intakes. (4) Adherence to the diet may change over time.[6]

The composition of the tissue losses is influenced by the dietary regimen. Losses of protein, fat, and water are greatest during total fasting; protein and fat losses are similar on isocaloric ketogenic (high fat) diets and mixed diets. Greater water losses on a ketogenic compared to a mixed diet give the appearance of a more rapid weight loss.[7] Introduction of carbohydrate following use of total fast or a ketogenic diet is associated with a temporary weight gain due to fluid retention.

Obesity

Incidence Obesity, according to some, is the most prevalent nutritional disorder in the United States. The exact incidence is not known, but the HANES data, based on triceps skinfold thickness, indicate that 14 per cent of men and 24 per cent of women are 20 per cent or more overweight.[8] (See Table 27–2.) Estimates of the prevalence in children vary from 3 to 20 per cent depending on the criteria used.[9] Based on skinfold thickness, about 5 per cent of adult men and 7 per cent

Table 27-2. **Prevalence of Overweight. Percent of Population Deviating by 10 to 19 Per Cent and by 20 Per Cent or More from Desirable Weight:* United States, Health and Nutrition Examination Survey, 1971–1974†**

	Men		Women	
Age	10–19%	20% or More	10–19%	20% or More
20–74	18.1	14.0	12.6	23.8
20–24	11.1	7.4	9.8	9.6
25–34	16.7	13.6	8.1	17.1
35–44	22.1	17.0	12.3	24.3
45–54	19.9	15.8	15.1	27.8
55–64	18.9	15.1	15.5	34.7
65–74	19.1	13.4	17.5	31.5

*Estimated from regression equations of weight on height for men and women ages 20 to 29 years, obtained from HANES I.

†Bray, G. A., ed.: *Obesity in America*, U.S. Department of Health, Education, and Welfare, Public Health Service, 1979.

of women can be considered severely obese.[10]

Causes Obesity is invariably caused by an intake of calories beyond the body's need for energy. Theoretically, it can easily be corrected by bringing the energy intake and expenditure into balance; practically speaking, however, this is not easily accomplished. The reasons for an existing imbalance are many and complex, and some understanding of the problems of the individual must be gained before therapy can be effectively instituted. A thorough physical examination, a dietary history, and an investigation of habits relating to activity, rest, and family and social relationships are indicated.

Food habits. Eating too much becomes a habit for many people. Sometimes this is the result of ignorance of the calorie value of food. The amounts of food are not necessarily excessive, but it is the extra foods, beyond the calorie need, that account for the gradual increase in weight, for example, the extra pats of butter, the spoonful of jelly, the second roll, the preference for a rich dessert, or the TV snack. Eating too much may result from having to maintain social relationships including rich party foods in addition to usual mealtime eating. Excessive amounts of carbohydrate-rich foods are sometimes eaten because they are cheaper than lower-calorie fruits and vegetables.

Activity patterns. Many persons continue to gain weight throughout life because they fail to adjust their appetites to reduced energy needs. The many laborsaving devices in homes and in industry reduce the energy requirement. Most people enjoy sports as spectators rather than as participants. Riding rather than walking to school or work is common practice even for short distances. Other circumstances may further reduce the energy needs: (1) basal metabolism is gradually decreased from year to year (see Chapter 7); (2) changes in occupation may result in reduced activity; (3) the middle years of life sometimes bring about a repose and consequent reduction of muscle tension; (4) periods of quiet relaxation and sleep may be increased; and (5) disabling illness such as arthritis or cardiac disease may reduce markedly the need for calories.

Psychological factors. For the individual who is bored, lonely, discontented, or depressed, eating can be a solace. Food often becomes the focal point of the day for those with little else to do or who are not motivated to seek another outlet for their problems.

Genetic· influences. Several investigators have shown that there is a high correlation between obesity in parents and their children. Data from the Ten-State Nutrition Survey indicate that triceps skinfold is greater in children whose parents are obese than in children of lean parents. By age 17, children of two obese parents are three times as fat as children of two lean parents.[11] Mayer noted that if both parents are of normal weight, only 7 per cent of children will be obese; if one parent is obese, the incidence in children is 40 per cent, and it climbs to 80 per cent if both parents are obese.[12] His observations led him to conclude that food habits alone do not explain these differences; further, he found a correlation between obesity and body build.

The *endomorphic* or round, soft individual gains weight readily, whereas the *ectomorphic* or slender, wiry person rarely becomes overweight.[13] This does not mean that obesity is inevitable for the endomorph, but it does mean that constant vigilance is required to avoid it. (See Figure 22–1.)

Metabolic abnormalities. Only a small percentage of obese cases can be attributed to endocrine disorders. A deficiency of the thyroid gland can reduce the basal metabolism, but overweight from this cause can be prevented if the diet is sufficiently restricted in calories.

A number of biochemical parameters are altered in obesity. These include abnormal glucose tolerance and elevations in fasting levels of plasma glucose, insulin, glucagon, free fatty acids, triglycerides, cholesterol, and uric acid. These tend to revert to normal as the individual loses weight.

Types of Obesity Based on anatomical characteristics of adipose tissue two types of obesity have been described.[4] *Hypercellular* obesity is characterized by an increase in the *number* of fat cells, as much as three to five times above normal. Onset of this type generally occurs early in life, and the fat is distributed over the entire body. Fat cells may or may not be enlarged. In *normocellular* obesity the number of adipocytes is normal but the cells are greatly enlarged, or *hypertrophied.* Onset of this type occurs during the adult years or pregnancy, and is likely to be associated with Type 2 (noninsulin-dependent) diabetes mellitus, hyperlipidemia, or hypertension. Fat distribution is more centralized.

Classification of obesity on the basis of fat cell characteristics is not yet feasible in the clinical setting because the techniques for fat cell biopsy are not generally available. However, valuable clues can be obtained from the history of onset, biochemical alterations, and type of fat distribution. Weight reduction can bring about a decrease in the fat content of adipose cells, but probably not in the number of fat cells; thus, the adult-onset type may have a better prognosis for achieving normal weight than does the individual with an increased number of fat cells.

Prevention of Obesity

Identifying Those Who Are Likely to Become Obese The most vigorous efforts to prevent obesity should be directed to those individuals who are most susceptible, namely, children of obese parents and children who have stocky frames. Certain periods of life are also likely to bring about obesity. Men of normal weight often begin to gain weight in the 20s and early 30s and women are more likely to gain in the mid-30s and 40s.[14] Following pregnancy weight gain is common. If these trends are recognized, the individual can elect to reduce caloric intake, or increase exercise, or both.

Education for Prevention The best hope for the prevention of obesity is through greatly expanded programs of nutrition education directed particularly to schoolchildren, teenagers, and mothers. The pattern for obesity is often set in infancy when the mother overfeeds the baby in the erroneous belief that a "fat baby is a healthy baby." Sometimes overeating becomes a habit with a child following an illness because the mother keeps urging food upon the child through her concern for his or her state of nutrition. During adolescent years food is often used to submerge the many problems that face the boy and girl. By recognizing these trends, the mother can do much to redirect the food habits. The education of the mother in terms of weight control for her family and the education of the child in the elementary and secondary school can be effective.

Increased activity. In these times of affluence, mechanization, and automation many individuals become overweight because of lack of exercise. A pattern of activity is best taught during childhood and must also be emphasized during the school years. Too often competitive sports exclude the child who most needs the exercise. Physical education should be directed to those activities that are likely to carry over into adult life.

Treatment of Obesity

Two criteria must be satisfied if the treatment is to be considered successful: (1) weight loss must be such that desirable weight according to body frame and state of health is achieved; and (2) the desired weight must be maintained. The essential components of treatment are calorie restriction, nutrition education, exercise, and psychologic support.

Assessment of the Patient The treatment of obesity is a frustrating problem to the physician, nutritionist, and nurse because failures are so frequent. To a patient a failure can be demoralizing. Therefore, it is important that each patient be evaluated in terms of his or her medical and dietary history and emotional stability. Weight reduction should be guided by a physician since the physiologic and psychological stresses of weight loss are not well tolerated by all.

Some persons lose weight satisfactorily when shown how to keep the calorie intake within prescribed limits; others benefit from group methods or behavior modification; for others, a program designed to promote rapid weight loss initially is an important motivating factor.

Behavior Modification This is based on the premise that excessive food intake is a learned response that can be changed. By means of this technique the individual learns to focus attention on the environmental factors that influence his or her food intake and gradually to modify these so that a change in eating habits and subsequent weight loss occurs.

Initially the client is asked to keep a detailed record of food intake and activity patterns. From this, the client and counselor identify problem areas and outline strategies to overcome them. Emphasis is on changing eating patterns rather than on caloric intake or pounds lost. For example, if the problem is too much unstructured eating, such as frequent snacking while watching television, knitting or other activities might be recommended as a diversion. Some techniques that have been used successfully to control food intake include (1) eating only at specified times and places; (2) learning to eat more slowly; (3) omitting other activities, such as reading or watching television while eating; (4) using smaller plates and placing portions directly on the plate rather than serving family style; (5) use of a reward system; and so on. Individualized stepwise behavioral changes are sought.

The behavioral approach to weight control involves detailed record keeping by the client; thus, it is not suitable for all. Not all such programs include nutrition education in the essentials of a well-balanced diet. Subjects may thus lose weight initially by eliminating excessive eating, yet fail to improve their nutritional habits.

The long-term efficacy of behavior modification for weight control is not known. Limited data suggest that initial weight loss is greater than with conventional methods; however, for most subjects, weight loss by the end of the program is modest, 5 to 15 pounds, and only a small percentage of subjects achieve substantial weight loss after termination of the program. One year follow-up results indicate that regaining the weight lost is common unless an exercise or contingency component is built into the program.[15, 16] In one study of patients treated by behavior modification with or without appetite suppressants, weight loss was greater in those receiving the appetite suppressants than in those receiving only behavior modification. At 1 year follow-up, however, the weight gain among subjects in the group receiving only behavior modification was only 20 to 25 per cent of that regained by subjects receiving appetite suppressants alone or in combination with behavior therapy.[17]

Self-help Groups Some persons find that group support, such as that provided by TOPS or Weight Watchers, is a valuable aid in helping them to continue a weight reduction program. Most of these groups require the individual to weigh in at a weekly meeting; some charge a small fee. These groups are most effective for persons who need to lose only a modest amount of weight, and the attrition rate is relatively high after a few months.

In general, results of dietary treatment of obesity have been disappointing in the majority of patients. In a review of the literature, Stunkard noted that only 25 per cent of patients were able to lose as much as 20 pounds and only 5 per cent lost as much as 40 pounds.[18]

Calorie-restricted Diets Many widely accepted nutritionally sound diets are available and are designed to bring about steady weight loss, to establish good food habits, and to promote a sense of well-being. Such diets must be palatable, must fit into the framework of family food habits, and must not require additional expense or long preparation time. Basic considerations in planning weight reduction diets include the following:

Energy. A diet that provides 800 to 1,000 kcal below the daily requirement leads to a loss of 3 to 4 kg (6 to 8 pounds) monthly. This gradual loss does not result in severe hunger, nervous exhaustion, and weakness that often accompany drastic reduction regimens. For most men 1,400 to 1,600 kcal is a satisfactory level, and for women 1,200 to 1,400 kcal are indicated. Diets that supply 1,000 kcal or less are rarely necessary except for individuals who are bedfast. In many elderly persons satisfactory weight loss is achieved only when energy intake is limited to 1,000 to 1,200 kcal; this is because of their reduced basal metabolism and reduced physical activity.

Protein. Although 0.8 gm protein per kilogram desirable body weight is sufficient,

Table 27-3. **Food Allowances for Calorie-Restricted Diets**

	Normal Protein, Moderate Carbohydrate, Low to Moderate Fat			High Protein, Low Carbohydrate, Moderate Fat
Food for the Day	1,000 kcal	1,200 kcal	1,500 kcal	1,500 kcal
Milk, 2%, cups	3 (skim)	3	3	3
Vegetable, raw, cups	1	1	1	1
cooked, cups	½	½	½	½
Fruit, unsweetened, exchanges	4	4	4	3
Bread, exchanges	2	3	5	2
Meat, medium-fat, exchanges	5	5	6	5
low-fat, exchanges	—	—	—	4
Fat, exchanges	1	1	3	5
Nutritive Value				
Protein, gm	67	69	80	95
Fat, gm	30	45	60	77
Carbohydrate, gm	116	131	161	106
Energy, kcal	1,002	1,205	1,504	1,497

an allowance of 1½ gm per kilogram improves the satiety value of the diet. Most dietary plans can include 70 to 100 gm protein daily.

Fat and carbohydrate. Many diets drastically restrict the fat intake and allow a moderate carbohydrate intake. (See the 1,000-kcal diet in Table 27–3.) Some patients prefer a more liberal fat intake and a reduced carbohydrate level as in the high-protein moderate-fat 1,500-kcal diet, Table 27–3.

Minerals and vitamins. A multivitamin preparation, iron salts, and possibly calcium are indicated for diets containing 1,000 kcal or less. Calorie-restricted diets for obese children and for pregnant women must be planned with the increased mineral and vitamin requirements in mind. For these reasons the diets used for them are usually less restricted.

Daily Meal Patterns The diets in Table 27–3 have been calculated with the food exchange lists (Table A–4). The vitamin and mineral values in most instances equal or exceed the RDA; the levels of some trace minerals such as zinc, copper, and others may be marginal.

These diets include 3 cups of milk, thus enhancing the calcium intake, and also providing a convenient bedtime snack, if desired. Some adults will prefer 2 cups of milk and more meat. This can be arranged by substituting one medium-fat meat exchange for 1 cup of skim milk. The caloric exchange for 1 cup of 2 per cent milk would

Sample Meal Patterns

	Normal Protein, Moderate Carbohydrate, Moderate Fat (1,500 kcal)	High Protein, Low Carbohydrate, Moderate Fat (1,500 kcal)
BREAKFAST		
Unsweetened citrus fruit	1 exchange	1 exchange
Eggs	1	2
Bread	2 slices	1 slice
Butter or margarine	1 teaspoon	1 teaspoon
Milk, 2 per cent fat	1 cup	1 cup
Coffee or tea		
LUNCH		
Meat, poultry, or fish	2 oz, medium-fat	4 oz, lean
Vegetable, raw or cooked	1 exchange	1 exchange
Bread	1 slice	None
Butter or margarine	1 teaspoon	2 teaspoons
Unsweetened fruit	1 exchange	1 exchange
Milk, 2 per cent fat	1 cup	1 cup
DINNER		
Meat, poultry, or fish	3 oz, medium-fat	3 oz, medium fat
Potato	1 small	1 small
Vegetable, cooked	½ cup	½ cup
raw	1 serving	1 serving
Bread	1 slice	None
Butter or margarine	1 teaspoon	2 teaspoons
Unsweetened fruit	2 exchanges	1 exchange
Milk, 2 per cent fat	1 cup	1 cup
Coffee or tea, if desired		

be one medium-fat and one low-fat meat exchange, thus giving a higher protein intake.

A great deal of flexibility in food choices is possible with the exchange lists. One important consideration is the satiety value of the diet. Inasmuch as proteins and fats remain in the stomach longer, the protein and fat allowance should be divided approximately equally between the three meals.

Some plans permit six meals a day instead of three; in these, some protein should be provided at each feeding. Part of the success of a reducing diet depends upon learning to be content with smaller portions of food and less concentrated foods.

Foods to restrict or avoid. The individual who learns to select foods in appropriate amounts from the exchange lists does not require specific lists of foods to avoid. For some persons, however, it may help to create calorie consciousness if listings of concentrated foods are provided. Some of the foods in the following list are permitted in specified amounts in the exchange lists, but others are best avoided altogether.

HIGH-FAT FOODS: butter, margarine, cheese, chocolate, cream, ice cream, fat meat, fatty fish, or fish canned in oil, fried foods of any kind such as doughnuts and potato chips, gravies, nuts, oil, pastries, and salad dressing

HIGH-CARBOHYDRATE FOODS: breads of any kind, candy, cake, cookies, corn, cereal products such as macaroni, noodles, spaghetti, pancakes, waffles, sweetened or dried fruits, legumes such as Lima beans, navy beans, dried peas, potatoes, sweet potatoes, honey, molasses, sugar, syrup, rich puddings, sweets

BEVERAGES: all fountain drinks, including malted milks and chocolate, carbonated beverages of all kinds, rich sundaes, alcoholic drinks, sweetened drink mixes

Other Dietary Regimens Commercial low-calorie meal substitutes, as *formulas* in liquid or powder form, cookies, and combination dishes are popular. Generally, they are nutritionally adequate and possess the advantages of convenience and strict calorie control. Some persons find them useful initially while they are learning the essentials of dietary planning. Others substitute these preparations for one meal a day.

The principal disadvantages of the formula diets are these: (1) they do not retrain the individual to a new pattern of food habits that must be followed once the weight is lost; (2) they are monotonous if used for a long period of time; and (3) they may be constipating for some patients, whereas others occasionally experience diarrhea.

Starvation. Total starvation for weeks or months has been used in treatment of persons who fail to achieve weight loss by conventional methods. Prolonged fasting requires hospitalization to monitor for side effects that include postural hypotension, acidosis, transient liver and kidney impairment, and hyperuricemia. Rapid weight loss is accompanied by substantial loss of lean body mass in addition to adipose tissue loss. Subjects who are overweight, but not obese, tend to have greater losses of body weight and nitrogen during fasting than do the obese. The large losses of lean body mass that occur in these subjects concern many workers, and some have suggested that total fasting for weight reduction be used only for very obese persons.

One group has shown that during caloric restriction cumulative nitrogen balance is highly correlated with the serum insulin concentration. This, in turn, is related to total body fat mass. Thus, the hyperinsulinism of obese subjects with greater fat stores helps to preserve protein homeostasis. In overweight subjects without massive fat stores, the lower serum insulin concentration may not be sufficient to prevent protein catabolism nor to stimulate protein synthesis enough to offset losses of lean tissue.[19] Theoretically, protein supplementation would replace some of the nitrogen losses in these subjects. Unfortunately, most subjects who fast tend to rapidly regain the lost weight when the fast is discontinued because they have not been educated to adopt a new pattern of eating habits.

Protein-sparing modified fast. Decreased losses of body protein have been reported with use of the protein-sparing modified fast which provides approximately 400 kcal per day and consists of 1.5 gm of high quality protein per kilogram of desirable body weight. No other calorie sources are permitted. Vitamin and mineral supplements are needed. About 2 gm potassium and 5 gm sodium chloride are required to prevent orthostatic hypotension.[20] Modifications of this regimen permit a small amount of carbohydrate in the diet. Nitrogen metabolism is not significantly different on the latter diet compared to the hypocaloric protein diet, but sodium depletion is less, thus lessening the possibility of orthostatic hypotension.[21] These programs require careful medical supervision, but not hospitalization. The long-term results in maintaining weight loss do not appear to be any more promising than with other approaches for the majority of persons; nevertheless, some individuals will find this approach to be highly effective.

Liquid protein diet. This modification of the protein-sparing modified fast has had some unfortunate outcomes. The plan involves consumption of a 300 to 600 kcal diet composed of low quality protein, collagen hydrolysate, supplemented with tryptophan, as the sole source of calories. Rapid weight loss occurs and subjects report absence of hunger sensations; this may be due to ketosis. Electrocardiographic changes indicative of cardiac arrhythmias have been associated with use of the diet.[22] A number of these have been fatal following prolonged use of the diet.[23] Protein malnutrition and excessive mineral loss have been proposed as possible causes.

Ketogenic diets. Periodically, low-carbohydrate ketogenic diets are publicized as an aid to rapid weight reduction. Advocates of these diets claim that one need not be concerned about calorie intake as long as carbohydrate is sharply restricted or even eliminated from the diet; and that the diet will produce more rapid weight loss than more conventional calorie-restricted diets. The American Medical Association has pointed out some of the facts and fallacies concerning ketogenic weight reduction diets.[24] There is no scientific evidence that this type of diet is any more effective than better balanced diets in promoting weight reduction. Weight loss is attributed to a decrease in calorie intake as a result of the high satiety value of the diet, and to increased urinary excretion of water and sodium. Potential adverse effects include elevations in serum lipids, increased blood uric acid levels, postural hypotension, and fatigue. The effects of long-term ketosis are not known. The practicality of such diets for long-term weight reduction is questionable inasmuch as most subjects are unable to persevere in the regimen for long periods.

Exercise and Weight Loss Moderate exercise on a consistent daily basis is an important aid in weight loss and should be a required component of any weight reduction program. The exercise program should be determined by the physician on the basis of the client's age, state of health and physical condition, and activity preferences. (See Figure 27–1.) Contrary to popular opinion, moderate exercise does not lead to increased appetite; conversely, a diminution of activity does not lead to a corresponding decrease in appetite. The exercise program should involve continuous use of large muscle groups and should be rhythmic and aerobic in nature, such as running, walking, or swimming. A duration of at least 20 to 30 minutes for a minimum of 3 days per week is needed for weight reduction and loss of fat stores.[25] On the other hand, passive exercise devices, such as mechanical vibrators and spot reducers, are ineffective methods of achieving loss of body fat. Some beneficial effects of regular sustained exercise include increased work capacity and cardiovascular efficiency, reduction in total fat stores, increased HDL-cholesterol, and

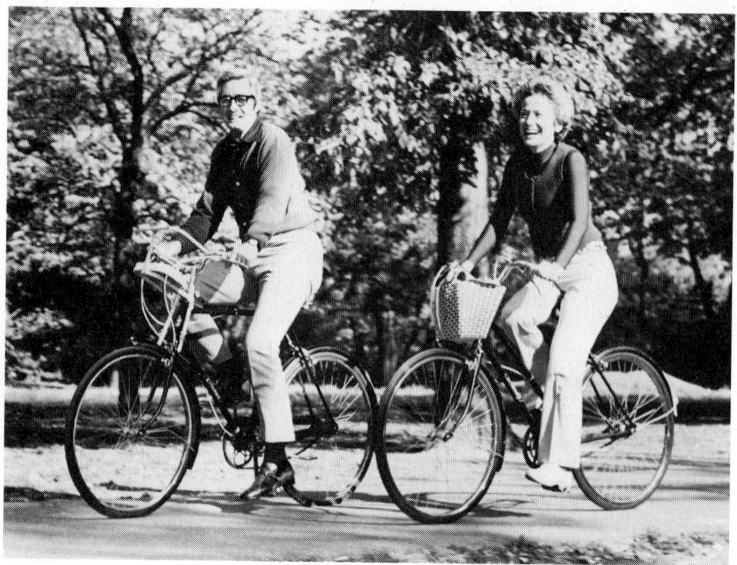

Figure 27–1. Exercise such as bicycling is not only enjoyable but it also increases energy expenditure, thereby helping to maintain normal weight. (Courtesy, National Association Plans, Inc., Philadelphia.)

improved muscle tone. Strenuous activity is accompanied by an increase in the metabolic rate for up to 24 hours; thus, expenditure of calories continues after the exercise is stopped. The energy costs of some popular forms of exercise are shown in Table 27–4. Several studies have shown that vigorous walking, alone or in combination with moderate calorie restriction promotes weight loss.[26, 27] The importance of exercise can be illustrated by calculating the energy equivalents of foods in terms of various kinds of activity. Six foods shown in Figure 27–2 illustrate the wide ranges of time required to utilize the energy provided by various foods at sedentary to moderate activities.

Role of Hormones and Drugs Most overweight persons have no deficiency of endocrine secretions and should not be led to believe that they have glandular disturbances, nor should they be exposed to the increased nervousness and irritability that result from such medication. Thyroid hormone is sometimes prescribed; however, it promotes loss of lean body mass rather than adipose tissue.

Anorexigenic drugs, such as amphet-

Table 27–4. **Energy Cost of Exercise***

Activity	Energy Cost†‡ kcal/kg/1.6 km	Kcal Expended	
		(70 kg Man)	(55 kg Woman)
Walking	1.15	80.5	63.3
Running	1.70	120.0	93.5
Bicycling	0.60	42.0	33.0

*Adapted from Franklin, B. A., and Rubenfire, M.: "Losing Weight Through Exercise," *J. Am. Med. Assoc.*, **244**: 377–79, 1980.

†Caloric cost is relatively independent of speed.

‡1.6 km is approximately 1 mile.

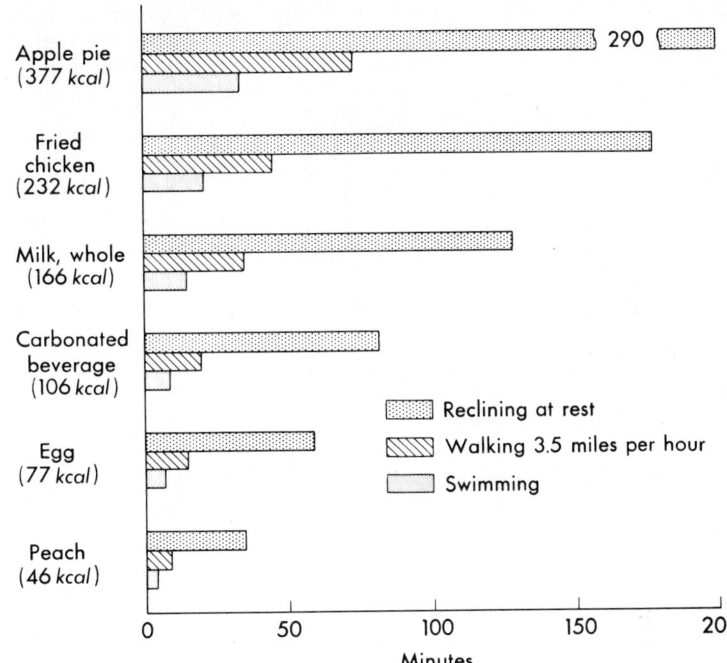

Figure 27–2. The energy value of foods expressed as number of minutes of activity for three levels of energy expenditure. (Data from Konishi, F.: *J. Am. Diet. Assoc.,* **46**:187, 1965.)

amines, are often used to suppress the appetite. These drugs are only temporarily effective, however, and require an ever-increasing dosage for sustained weight loss. They may produce insomnia, excitability, dryness of the mouth, gastrointestinal disturbances, and other toxic manifestations. For some patients they are a crutch and for others they have no effect on decreasing the appetite. Human growth hormone offers theoretical advantages over other drugs since it mobilizes fatty acids and decreases fat stores without enhancing nitrogen loss; however, inadequate supply and cost factors limit its potential use. The Food and Drug Administration has cautioned that most drugs are of limited value in the treatment of obesity and should be used with great care because of the possibility of dependence and abuse. The label must state that they are for short-term use and only when a calorie-restricted diet is also used.[28]

Surgical Treatment

Surgical treatment of obesity is used for selected patients who are more than 100 pounds over their ideal body weight and who meet certain other criteria. Both jejunoileal bypass and gastric bypass are used. These procedures exclude 90 percent of the small bowel and gastric reservoir, respectively.

Jejunoileal bypass This procedure involves anastomosis of a short section of the proximal jejunum, about 14 inches in length, to a 12- to 18-inch section of terminal ileum in end-to-end or end-to-side fashion. (See Figure 27–3.) The closed end of the bypassed jejunum is sutured to the mesentery to prevent displacement and the end of the bypassed ileum is anastomosed to the transverse or sigmoid colon for drainage. The procedure decreases the absorptive surface and reduces transit time, thereby resulting in malabsorption. For

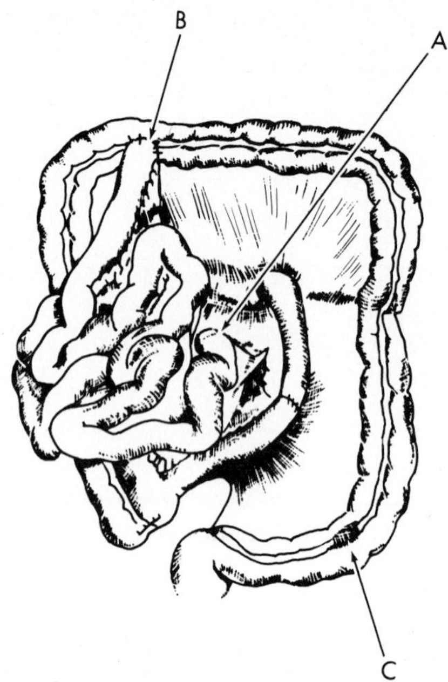

Figure 27–3. End-to-end jejunoileostomy. The closed end of the bypassed jejunum is sutured to the mesentery to prevent displacement *(A)*. The end of the bypassed ileum is drained by end-to-side anastomosis with the transverse *(B)* or sigmoid *(C)* colon. (From: Scott, H. W.: "Surgical Experience with Jejunoileal Bypass for Morbid Obesity," *Surg. Clin. North Am.*, **59**:1033–41, 1979. Used with permission.)

most patients, steady weight loss occurs for 1 to 2 years following the surgery, after which weight stabilizes. Average weight loss at 2 years is about 35 per cent of the preoperative weight; most do not reach their ideal weight. Besides weight loss, there are reductions of serum lipids and blood pressure, and improvement in Type II (noninsulin-dependent) diabetes mellitus. Complications of the surgery include diarrhea, steatorrhea, electrolyte imbalance, liver disease, cholelithiasis, renal calculi, polyarthritis, trace mineral deficiencies, and loss of lean body mass, among others. These tend to improve with time; however, some deaths have occurred as a consequence of liver failure.

Gastric Bypass In this procedure, the stomach is divided by means of several rows of staples into a small proximal pouch of 50- to 60-ml capacity, and a nonfunctioning distal compartment. The small proximal pouch is then anastomosed to the jejunum. (See Figure 27–4.) A modification of this procedure, *gastroplasty,* retains normal anatomical structure by incomplete staple division of the stomach. A small opening, approximately 12 mm or ½ inch in diameter, permits passage of food between the small upper pouch and the distal stomach. Both procedures result in rapid filling and slow emptying of the stomach, giving a feeling of satiety and forcing the individual to eat small meals. Nausea and vomiting follow over-indulgence. Ingestion of hypertonic sweets can provoke symptoms of the dumping syndrome and diarrhea. (See Chapter 36.) Possible complications include bile reflux, marginal ulcers and obstruction.

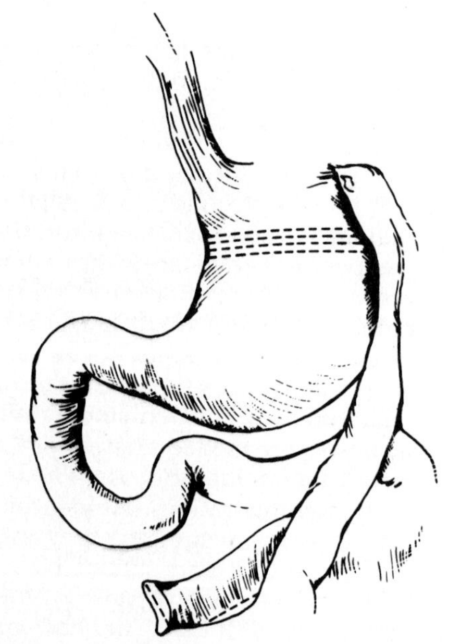

Figure 27–4. Gastric bypass. (From: Bothe, A., et al.: "Energy Regulation in Morbid Obesity by Multidisciplinary Therapy," *Surg. Clin. North. Am.*, **59**:1017–31, 1979. Used with permission.)

Failure to lose sufficient weight has been reported and a few cases of vitamin deficiencies have been documented. The frequency of metabolic problems, such as liver failure, is much less than that following intestinal bypass surgery. At 1 year postoperative, weight loss patterns are similar in the two groups.[29]

Dietary Considerations Following jejunoileal bypass surgery, diarrhea is a major problem once oral food intake is resumed. Excesses of dietary fat or fibrous foods aggravate the diarrhea. A low-oxalate, high-protein, low-fat, low-carbohydrate diet is given in six small feedings.[30] Fluids are permitted between meals rather than with the meal and may be restricted to less than 1 liter daily initially. Calcium, magnesium, and potassium losses may be substantial and good food sources of these minerals should be emphasized. Multivitamins are generally recommended. Vitamin B-12 injections are recommended unless evidence of normal B-12 absorption is obtained.[31]

Dietary considerations following gastric bypass are similar to those in the dumping syndrome. (See page 594.)

Dietary Counseling

Success in weight reduction is dependent upon effective motivation and suitable knowledge.

MOTIVATION AND PSYCHOLOGIC SUPPORT. A diet prescription is worthless unless the client has some motivation for losing weight, such as the maintenance or recovery of health, the ability to win friendship, admiration, and affection, or the importance of normal weight in being able to earn one's livelihood or in being considered for occupational advancement, as the case may be. The client must have the capacity for self-discipline, patience, and perseverance.

Although the motivation must come from within the client, the physician, nurse, and dietitian can be of immeasurable help toward initiating this motivation, and subsequently by providing encouragement and guidance at frequent follow-up visits. The client needs to understand that a calorie intake in excess of needs is the cause of overweight and that weight loss is accomplished only when the calorie intake is reduced below the client's needs. But this explanation is not enough. The client also needs to gain insight into the reasons he or she is overeating, and to work at correcting these.

Obesity is not a moral issue but a clinical problem and it is important that all who work with obese clients keep this in mind. Threatening the client with the dire consequences of failing to lose weight or chiding him or her for not adhering to the diet rarely accomplishes anything. On the contrary, each client must be helped to maintain self-esteem and deserves to be treated with dignity.

COUNSELING AND GROUP SESSIONS. Individual counseling is essential to determine the goals that are realistic for the client and to initiate a dietary regimen that is appropriate for the client's food habits and patterns of living. (See also Chapter 24.)

Group sessions are effective in that people compare their progress, share their problems in adhering to diets, and exchange ways to vary their diets. When groups are formed it is important that professional guidance be available from a physician, dietitian, or nurse. Each individual joining such a group should first be evaluated by the physician to determine his or her fitness for weight reduction.

ESSENTIAL KNOWLEDGE. The dieter needs to understand that weight loss is accompanied by a reduction in the metabolic rate. This may explain the decreased rate of weight loss with time that many persons experience in spite of careful adherence to a calorie-restricted diet. Further calorie restriction or increased energy expenditure will be required to continue weight loss. The importance of moderate regular exercise as an essential part of any weight reduction program should be pointed out to clients.

Most people are quite ignorant of the calorie values of foods. Each of the food exchange lists (Table A–4) provides a variety of foods that have approximately equal calorie values, and their consistent use helps to develop awareness of nutritive values. Many other tables of calorie values of foods are also available. Keeping a record of the daily calorie intake is useful, at least for a period of time. However, it is important that clear distinctions be made between the calorie values of foods that also supply protein, minerals, and vitamins and those foods that are principally carbohydrate and fat.

Portion control, taught by means of measuring cups, spoons, food models, or actual foods, is esential. Although a given diet is planned for a specific calorie level, it must be expected that the daily calorie intake may vary by as much as 200 to 300 kcal because of variations in food composition as well as in the precision of measurements.

Few dietetic foods are necessary. When fresh fruits are expensive or unavailable, water-packed canned fruits may be used. Artificial sweetening may be used if desired. Many low-calorie beverages currently available provide less than half the calories contained in regular beverages. The calorie information on the label should be checked if these beverages are used.

Some clients ask about including cocktails and wine in their diets. If the physician permits these beverages, the client needs to know that each gram of alcohol supplies 7 kcal and that the calorie value of the beverage must be taken into consideration. A glass of dry table wine provides fewer calories than a cocktail. Usually an alcoholic beverage is restricted to one serving daily, (See Table A–1 for caloric values of alcoholic beverages.)

A single dinner in a restaurant can nullify careful adherence given to a diet for several days. Usually it is possible to select a clear soup, broiled or roasted meat without sauces, vegetables without sauces, and salad without dressing. Meat portions are likely to be larger than those allowed and the dieter will need to restrict intake to that allowed. The diet will not be exceeded too much if one foregoes the rolls, butter, and dessert.

What does the dieter do when he or she has many dinner invitations? For every dieter there are occasions when the limitations of the diet are exceeded, and such breaks in the dieting pattern should be anticipated. Each day gives an opportunity to begin again toward the goal of desired weight. Nevertheless, the person who has many social engagements will find it difficult to make the progress he or she would like to make. Occasionally, when one knows that the social event will make it difficult to keep within dietary restrictions, the intake at the preceding meal can be kept especially light. Most hostesses are very understanding about a guest who is on a diet and is therefore restricting the size of portions or letting some of the foods pass by without partaking of them.

MAINTENANCE OF WEIGHT To lose weight is not easy; to maintain the desirable level of weight is even more difficult. The calorie-restricted diet planned with regard for the client's pattern of living also provides the basis for building a maintenance diet. The client must learn that a change in food habits is essential not only for losing weight but to maintain desirable weight. Thus, additions of foods should be made judiciously until weight is being kept constant at the desired level. It is important for the client to weigh himself or herself at weekly intervals or so in order to be sure that the foods added are in appropriate amounts.

If foods added for maintenance are also selected from the Daily Food Guide, the quality of the diet with respect to protein, minerals, and vitamins is thereby enhanced. On the other hand, the additions of concentrated high-calorie foods may be more difficult to control in amounts suitable for maintenance. For example, the sedentary person of middle age must continue to forego rich desserts and sweets except on rare occasions.

Problems and Review

1. What are the hazards of obesity to health?
2. List eight situations that may account for obesity.
3. Mr. Reese's calorie requirement is 2,600, but he is restricting his diet to 1,800 kcal. How much weight might he expect to lose in a month?
   a. As part of his weight reduction program, Mr. Reese has increased his activity by walking each day. If he uses 285 kcal per hour, how many hours will it take him to lose 1 pound of adipose tissue?
   b. The physician has indicated that Mr. Reese may include alcoholic beverages not to exceed 150 kcal each day. By consulting Table A–1 prepare a list of several choices that come within this allowance. What adjustments would be necessary in the 1,500-kcal diet in Table 27–3 to include the beverage?
   c. What are some important factors to consider in order that maximum cooperation of this patient may be achieved?
4. Mrs. Aston has adhered to her 1,500-kcal diet for the past 3 weeks but has lost no weight. What possible explanations may there be for her failure to lose weight?
   a. Write menus for 2 days for the 1,500-kcal moderate-fat diet listed in Table 27–3.
   b. Mrs. Aston has brought her weight to the desired level. What measures are now important so that this weight level will be maintained?

Cited References

1. Van Itallie, T. B.: "Obesity: Adverse Effects on Health and Longevity," *Am. J. Clin. Nutr.*, **32**:2723–33, 1979.
2. Sorlie, P. et al.: "Body Build and Mortality: The Framingham Study," *JAMA*, **243**:1828–31, 1980.
3. Drenick, E. J. et al.: "Excessive Mortality and Causes of Death in Morbidly Obese Men," *JAMA*, **243**:443–45, 1980.
4. Bray, G. A. et al.: "Evaluation of the Obese Patient. 1. An Algorithm," *JAMA*, **235**:1487–91, 1976.
5. Baker, G. L.: "Human Adipose Tissue Composition and Age," *Am. J. Clin. Nutr.*, **22**:829–35, 1969.
6. Stuart, R. B. et al.: "Weight Loss Over Time," *J. Am. Diet. Assoc.*, **75**:258–61, 1979.
7. Yang, M. U., and Van Itallie, T. B.: "Composition of Weight Lost During Short-Term Weight Reduction. Metabolic Responses of Obese Subjects to Starvation and Low Calorie Ketogenic and Non-ketogenic Diets," *J. Clin. Invest.*, **58**:722–30, 1976.
8. Bray, G. A. ed.: *Obesity in America*, NIH Publication No. 79–359, U.S. Department of Health, Education, and Welfare, Public Health Service, 1979.
9. Neumann, C. G.: "Obesity in Pediatric Practice: Obesity in the Preschool and School-Age Child," *Pediatr. Clin. North Am.*, **24**:117–22, 1977.
10. Abraham, S., and Johnson, C. L.: "Prevalence of Severe Obesity in Adults in the United States," *Am. J. Clin. Nutr.*, **33**:364–69, 1980.
11. Garn, S. M., and Clark, D. C.: "Trends in Fatness and the Origins of Obesity," *Pediatrics*, **57**:443–56, 1976.
12. Mayer, J.: "Obesity: Causes and Treatment," *Am. J. Nurs.*, **59**:1732–36, 1959.
13. Mayer, J.: *Overweight: Causes, Cost, and Control*, Prentice-Hall, Englewood Cliffs, N.J., 1968.
14. Mayer, J.: "Obesity," in *Modern Nutrition in Health and Disease*, 6th ed., R. S. Goodhart and M. E. Shils, eds. Lea & Febiger, Philadelphia, 1980, p. 724.
15. Stalonas, P. M. et al.: "Behavior Modification for Obesity: The Evaluation of Exercise,

Contingency Management, and Program Adherence," *J. Consult. Clin. Psychol.*, **46**:463–69, 1978.
16. Kingsley, R. G., and Wilson, G. T.: "Behavior Therapy for Obesity: A Comparative Investigation of Long-Term Efficacy," *J. Consult. Clin. Psychol.*, **45**:288, 1977.
17. Stunkard, A. J. et al.: "Controlled Trial of Behavior Therapy, Pharmacotherapy and Their Combination in the Treatment of Obesity," *Lancet*, **2**:1045–47, 1980.
18. Stunkard, A., and McLaren-Hume, M.: "The Results of Treatment for Obesity," *Arch. Intern. Med.*, **103**:79–85, 1959.
19. Merritt, R. J. et al.: "Consequences of Modified Fasting in Obese Pediatric and Adolescent Patients. I. Protein-Sparing Modified Fast," *J. Pediatrics*, **96**:13–19, 1980.
20. Bistrian, B. R.: "Clinical Use of a Protein-Sparing Modified Fast," *JAMA*, **240**:2299–2302, 1978.
21. DeHaven, J. et al.: "Nitrogen and Sodium Balance and Sympathetic-Nervous System Activity in Obese Subjects Treated with a Low Calorie-Protein or Mixed Diet," *New Engl. J. Med.*, **302**:477–82, 1980.
22. Lantigua, R. A. et al.: "Cardiac Arrhythmias Associated with a Liquid Protein Diet for the Treatment of Obesity," *New Engl. J. Med.*, **303**:735–38, 1980.
23. Van Itallie, T. B.: "Liquid Protein Mayhem," *New Engl. J. Med.*, **240**:144–45, 1978.
24. Council on Foods and Nutrition: "A Critique of Low-Carbohydrate Ketogenic Weight Reduction Regimens," *JAMA*, **224**:1415–19, 1973.
25. Franklin, B. A., and Rubenfire, M.: "Losing Weight Through Exercise," *JAMA*, **244**:377–79, 1980.
26. Weltman, A. et al.: "Caloric Restriction and/or Mild Exercise: Effects on Serum Lipids and Body Composition," *Am. J. Clin. Nutr.*, **33**:1002–1009, 1980.
27. Leon, A. S. et al.: "Effects of a Vigorous Walking Program on Body Composition and Carbohydrate and Lipid Metabolism of Obese Young Men," *Am. J. Clin. Nutr.*, **33**:1776–87, 1979.
28. *FDA Drug Bulletin*, Rockville, Md., Food and Drug Administration, December 1972.
29. Griffen, W. O. et al.: "A Prospective Comparison of Gastric and Jejunoileal Bypass Procedures for Morbid Obesity," *Ann. Surg.*, **186**:500–9, 1977.
30. Swenson, S. A., and Oberst, B.: "Pre- and Postoperative Care of the Patient with Intestinal Bypass for Obesity," *Am. J. Surg.*, **129**:225–28, 1975.
31. Coyle, J. J. et al.: "Vitamin B_{12} Absorption Following Human Intestinal Bypass Surgery," *Am. J. Digest. Dis.*, **22**:1069–71, 1977.

Additional References

Ball, M. F. et al.: "Comparative Effects of Caloric Restriction and Total Starvation on Body Composition in Obesity," *Am. J. Clin. Nutr.*, **67**:60–67, 1967.

Bernstein, R. S., and Van Itallie, T. B.: "An Overview of Therapy for Morbid Obesity," *Surg. Clin. North Am.*, **59**:985–94, 1979.

Bloom, W. L.: "Obesity: Medical and Surgical Management and Mismanagement," *South. Med. J.*, **72**:1189–92, 1979.

Bray, G. A. et al.: "Use of Anthropometric Measures to Assess Weight Loss," *Am. J. Clin. Nutr.*, **31**:769–73, 1978.

Condon, S. C. et al.: "Role of Caloric Intake in the Weight Loss Following Jejunoileal Bypass for Obesity," *Gastroenterology*, **74**:34–37, 1978.

Golden, M. P.: "An Approach to the Management of Obesity in Childhood," *Pediatr. Clin. North Am.*, **26**:187–97, 1979.

Kannel, W. B. et al.: "Obesity, Lipids, and Glucose Intolerance. The Framingham Study," *Am. J. Clin. Nutr.*, **32**:1238–45, 1979.

MASON, E. E. et al.: "Gastric Bypass in Morbid Obesity," *Am. J. Clin. Nutr.*, **33**:395–405, 1980.

STRAW, W. E., and SONNE, A. C.: "The Obese Patient," *J. Fam. Practice*, **9**:317–23, 1979.

ZACK, P. M. et al.: "A Longitudinal Study of Body Fatness in Childhood and Adolescence," *J. Pediatr.*, **95**:126–30, 1979.

28 *Undernutrition and Protein Deficiency: High-Calorie Diet; High-Protein Diet*

CASUAL observation of most segments of society in the United States and Canada reveals that undernutrition and protein deficiency are not major problems in North America; in fact, quite the opposite appears to be true—overnutrition appears to be much more common than undernutrition. Nevertheless, persons affected by these conditions, especially the poor and elderly, enjoy less than optimal health because of fatigue, weight loss, and lowered resistance to infection.

To some extent, undernutrition and protein deficiency go hand in hand; those who are visibly undernourished are often found to be deficient in protein. On the other hand, some persons who do not appear to be undernourished, are, in fact, deficient in protein. With the availability of various types of nutritional support, both conditions are potentially reversible.

Underweight

Causes Failure to ingest sufficient calories to meet the energy requirement results in underweight. Not infrequently this occurs in people who are very active, tense, and nervous, and who obtain too little rest. Sometimes irregular habits of eating and poor selection of foods are responsible for an inadequate caloric intake.

Just as psychologic factors have been noted as contributing to overeating, so they may contribute to eating too little food. Some patients with mental illness reject food to such an extent that severe weight loss results; this condition is referred to as *anorexia nervosa.* (See Chapter 42.)

Underweight also occurs in many pathologic conditions such as fevers in which the appetite is poor and the energy requirements are increased; gastrointestinal disturbances characterized by nausea, vomiting, and diarrhea; cancer; and hyperthyroidism in which the metabolic rate is greatly accelerated.

Changes in Body Tissue Compartments The extent of changes in body tissue compartments depends somewhat on the severity of the nutritional deprivation. In moderate undernutrition, losses occur primarily in visceral protein and muscle cell mass, while body fat is not affected. In severe undernutrition significant losses of both muscle cell mass and body fat occur.[1] Prediction of the extent of changes in body tissue compartments can be made from knowledge of anthropometric measures and laboratory determinations of protein status as discussed in Chapter 24.

Modifications of the Diet Before weight gain can be effected, the direct cause for the inadequate caloric intake must be sought. As in obesity, these causes in relation to the individual must be removed and a high calorie diet provided.

Energy. Approximately 500 kcal in excess of the daily needs will result in a weekly gain of about 0.5 kg (1 pound). For moderately active individuals diets containing 3,000 to 3,500 kcal will bring about effective weight gain. Somewhat higher levels are required when fever is high, or gastrointestinal disturbances are interfering with absorption, or metabolism is greatly increased.

Protein. A daily intake of 100 gm protein or more is usually desirable since body protein as well as body fat must be replaced.

Minerals and vitamins. If the quality of the diet resulting in weight loss was poor, considerable body deficits of minerals and vitamins may likewise have occurred. Usually the high-calorie diet will provide liberal levels of all these nutrients. When supplements are prescribed, it is important that the patient understand that they are in no way a substitute for the calories and protein provided by food.

Planning the Daily Diet A patient cannot always adjust immediately to a higher caloric intake. It is better to begin with the patient's present intake and to improve the diet both qualitatively and quantitatively day by day until the desired caloric level is reached. Nothing is more conducive to loss of appetite than the appearance of an overloaded tray of food.

The caloric intake may be increased by using additional amounts of foods from the Daily Food Guide, thus increasing the intake of protein, minerals, and vitamins. For example, 500 kcal might be added to the patient's present intake as follows:

1 glass milk, ½ cup ice cream, 1 small potato, 1 small banana; *or*
2 slices bread, 2 ounces meat, 1 ounce cheese, ½ cup Lima beans.

The judicious use of cream, butter, jelly or jam, and sugars will quickly increase the caloric level, but excessive use may provoke nausea and loss of appetite.

Some patients make better progress if given small, frequent feedings; but for many patients midmorning and midafternoon feedings have been found to interfere with the appetite for the following meal. Bedtime snacks, however, may be planned to provide 300 to 800 kcal, thus making it possible to follow a normal pattern for the three meals.

The following list of foods illustrates one way in which the Daily Food Guide may be adapted to a high-calorie level. The meal patterns outlined for the high-protein diet (page 499) suggest suitable arrangements of these foods.

3 to 4 cups milk
1 cup light cream
5 to 7 ounces meat, fish, poultry, or cheese
1 egg
4 servings vegetables including:
  1 serving green or yellow vegetable
  2 servings white or sweet potato, corn, or beans
  1 serving other vegetable
2 to 3 servings fruit, including one citrus fruit
1 serving whole-grain or enriched cereal
3 to 6 slices whole-grain or enriched bread
4 tablespoons or more butter or margarine
High-calorie foods to complete the caloric requirement: cereals such as macaroni, rice, noodles, spaghetti; honey, molasses, syrups; hard candies; glucose; salad dressings; cakes, cookies, and pastry in moderation; ice cream, puddings, sauces

Protein Deficiency

Incidence and Etiology Findings from both the Ten-State Nutrition Survey and the Health and Nutrition Examination Survey (HANES) indicate that the vast majority of Americans receive sufficient protein, and severe protein deficiency is rare. The intake of protein may be inadequate under certain conditions. Strict weight reduction diets, especially those that require fasting, can lead to depletion of tissue proteins. Chronic alcoholism and drug addiction also interfere with a satisfactory food intake, in part because the cost of the habit often leaves insufficient money for the purchase of an adequate diet. Ignorance of the essentials of an adequate diet and child neglect are contributing factors to malnutrition in children. Protein-calorie malnutrition as a principal world health problem in children has been discussed in Chapter 23.

Many pathologic conditions are aggravated by nutritional deficiency, and, conversely, an existing deficiency is likely to become more severe during illness.

1. Disturbances of the gastrointestinal tract frequently initiate nutritional deficiency because of interference with intake, digestion, or absorption of foods. Anorexia, nausea, vomiting, the discomfort of ulcers, the abdominal distension present in many illnesses, and the cramping associated with diarrhea preclude a satisfactory food intake. Many patients are afraid to eat and restrict their choice to a few foods that do not meet nutritional requirements.

Even though the food intake may be adequate under normal circumstances, increased motility that accompanies some disturbances does not permit sufficient time for digestion and absorption so that excessive amounts of nutrients are lost. In the malabsorption syndrome—sprue, for example—a reduction in the digestive enzymes and in the absorptive surfaces leads to great losses of all nutrients from the bowel.

2. Excessive protein losses result from proteinuria in certain renal diseases, from hemorrhage, from increased nitrogen losses in the urine during the catabolic phase accompanying injury and immobilization, and from exudates of burned surfaces or draining wounds. The increased catabolism that follows immobilization is not fully understood, but is related, at least in part, to an increased production of adrenocortical hormones. Following an injury healthy individuals show greater nitrogen losses than do persons who have more limited reserves. During the acute stage of catabolism high-protein high-calorie diets seem to have little effect on reducing the losses. Eventually, of course, such losses must be replaced.

3. An increased metabolic rate in fevers and in thyrotoxicosis is accompanied by increased destruction of tissue proteins.

4. In diseases of the liver the synthesis of plasma proteins may be reduced even though the supply of amino acids is satisfactory.

Clinical and Biochemical Signs of Protein Undernutrition Fatigue, loss of weight, and lower resistance to infection are among the symptoms presented by patients with protein deficiency. Because these are common to many pathologic conditions they are of little diagnostic value.

Underweight together with a history of recent weight loss is of particular concern in many disease conditions. Weight loss entails loss of tissue proteins as well as adipose tissue. Recovery from illness is often slow, and wound healing is prolonged because the essential amino acids for tissue repair are lacking. Anemia is sometimes observed because of a reduced synthesis of the protein globin. The immune response is impaired as patients become protein depleted.

Following prolonged protein deficiency the concentration of the plasma proteins and the circulating blood volume are decreased. Low albumin levels indicate visceral protein deficit. Moreover, since plasma albumin is particularly important for the maintenance of oncotic pressure, severe hypoalbuminemia may result in nutritional edema. When edema occurs it is necessary to rule out impaired circulation and excretion that occur in cardiac or renal failure. Edema is a rather inconstant finding that is not directly related to the plasma protein level. Thus, an individual may be severely depleted of proteins and show no signs of edema. The serum transferrin level is a more sensitive indicator of visceral protein deficit than is albumin. Because of the shorter half-life of transferrin, 5 to 7 days, compared to a half-life of approximately 20 days for albumin, a decrease in transferrin levels can occur before a significant fall in albumin.[1] Low levels of serum albumin and transferrin are associated with an increased incidence of anergy. Anergic patients are more susceptible to increased morbidity and mortality from infectious diseases.

Although the liver has an amazing ability to carry out its functions even under adverse conditions, a prolonged nutritional deficiency gradually reduces the regeneration of liver cells as well as the synthesis of many regulatory compounds. A deficit in the lipotropic factors and of the lipoproteins leads to a decreased mobilization of fats from the liver, and thus fatty infiltration reduces the efficiency of the organ. The liver is less able to neutralize the effects of toxic substances and its cells may be damaged—sometimes beyond repair.

Nutritional Considerations Protein and energy requirements are increased in stress, infection, and trauma. Under these conditions, skeletal proteins are mobilized to provide substrates for gluconeogenesis to meet energy needs. Protein repletion cannot be accomplished by giving a patient a high protein diet for a few days. A diet adequate in calories and somewhat liberalized in protein is essential for several weeks to several months. The levels of protein and calories are equally important in achieving satisfactory tissue synthesis. If the calorie intake is insufficient, protein will be utilized to meet energy needs. On the other hand, protein intake beyond the body's need for essential amino acids will be wasted since the body has no capacity to store protein in the sense that it stores carbohydrate as glycogen or fat as adipose tissue.

Protein. A nitrogen-to-calorie ratio of 1 to 300 is satisfactory for maintenance; for anabolism the ratio is adjusted to 1:150.[3] In stress, protein utilization is less efficient than during convalescence, thus, provision of 16 per cent of the calculated energy needs as protein has been recommended.[3] Most pre- and postoperative patients probably experience mild stress, whereas those with severe burns or multiple trauma would be described as severely stressed. During infection optimal protein intake is 1.5 to 2.0 gm protein per kilogram per day.[4]

Energy. Several approaches are used to estimate energy needs, depending somewhat on personnel available. Some estimate the basal energy expenditure (BEE) on the basis of the patient's height, weight, age, and sex.[2] Others calculate the basal energy expenditure using the Harris-Benedict formula shown inside the back cover of this text.[5] The calorie requirement for anabolism is expressed as a multiple of the basal energy expenditure. Feedings given by way of the enteral route are used more efficiently than those administered parenterally; thus, the energy requirement is greater when intravenous feeding is used. Oral intakes of 35 kcal per kilogram per day result in positive nitrogen balance whereas 40 kcal per kilogram daily are needed if parenteral feeding is used.[5]

Management of the Diet A high-protein diet furnishes 100 to 125 gm protein and includes at least 2,500 kcal. To consume these amounts is not difficult for an individual with a good appetite. Most patients who require these liberal diets have had an impaired appetite for some time, and only the continuous and determined effort on the part of the nurse and others working with the patient can help the patient toward the goal of adequate intake. Some patients prefer small meals with between-meal feedings whereas for others three meals and an evening snack are more suitable. High-protein beverages aid in achieving maximum protein intake with a minimum increase in volume. They may be prepared by combining milk, nonfat dry milk, and eggs and using a variety of flavorings. A number of palatable, inexpensive, and convenient proprietary compounds using nonfat dry milk and casein as the principal sources of protein are also available.

For emaciated patients the amount of food and the concentration of protein are increased gradually until the gastrointestinal tract again becomes accustomed to handling more food, and until the heart and circulatory system can cope with the additional demands made on it. When the food intake by these patients is rapidly increased, circulatory failure and even death can occur.

Tube feedings are used for those patients who are unable to consume sufficient calories and protein. A regimen for gradual introduction of enteral feedings for patients with chronic diarrhea secondary to protein calorie malnutrition has been described. A tube feeding mixture composed of calcium caseinate and medium-chain triglycerides is used initially, with gradual introduction of small amounts of carbohydrate into the formula. After 10 days on this formula a high-protein milkshake is given orally. If this is tolerated, the patient progresses to small bland feedings gradually increasing in volume and variety of foods permitted.[6]

Dietary Counseling

Dietary counseling is initiated by an evaluation of the patient's present meal pattern and food intake. The patient needs to know why adequate calorie and protein intakes are essential. Practical suggestions are given for increasing the calorie intake (see page 495) and the protein intake. With a list of protein equivalents from which to choose, the patient is guided toward developing a meal pattern that more nearly meets his or her needs.

PROTEIN EQUIVALENTS (6–8 gm protein per unit)

1 cup milk or buttermilk
⅓ cup nonfat dry milk
1 ounce American type cheese
¼ cup cottage cheese
1 egg
1 ounce meat, fish, or poultry
2 tablespoons peanut butter
8 ounces ice cream
⅔ cup milk pudding

From such a list patients select a combination that will be acceptable to them. Some will prefer additional amounts of milk, whereas others find larger portions of meat to be more acceptable. A high-protein diet need not strain the food budget since nonfat dry milk can be used in substantial amounts. Most patients, and those who cook for them, need practical suggestions, including recipes, for incorporating dry milk into eggnogs, milk shakes, custards, puddings, cream soups, and other prepared foods.

The individual who requires a high-protein high-calorie diet is likely to be one who finds it difficult to consume a large volume of food. One who has a daily intake of 55 gm protein and 1,600 kcal does not readily consume 120 gm protein and 2,500 kcal. The physician, nurse, and dietitian can help the patient to recognize his or her needs, but only the patient can set goals that are realistic. Perhaps a regular meal pattern requires emphasis; skipping breakfast, for example, makes it difficult to consume enough food for the rest of the day. Possibly a high-protein high-calorie beverage can be substituted for a low-calorie beverage, or an additional portion of dessert can be eaten at bedtime.

Patients need to know whether their efforts are successful. Probably one of the better guides for the patient is gradual weight gain—1 to 2 pounds per week being a reasonable expectation. With improvement in the state of protein nutrition the patient will experience a greater sense of well-being.

High-Protein Diet

Characteristics and General Rules

Select ½ to ⅔ of the day's protein allowance from complete protein foods. Include some complete protein at each meal.
Divide the protein allowance as evenly as practical among the meals of the day.
To increase the protein content of liquid milk add 2 to 4 tablespoons nonfat dry milk to each cup of milk.
For a soft high-protein diet consult the list of foods for a soft diet, page 466.

Include These Foods, or Their Nutritive Equivalents, Daily:
4 cups (1 quart) milk
7–8 ounces (cooked weight) meat, fish, poultry, or beans
2 eggs
6 servings vegetables and fruits including:
  1 serving green or yellow vegetable
  1 to 2 servings potato
  1 to 2 servings other vegetable
  One vegetable to be eaten raw daily
  1 serving citrus fruit—or other good source of ascorbic acid
  1 serving other fruit
6 servings bread and cereals including:
  1 serving whole-grain or enriched cereal
  5 slices whole-grain or enriched bread
Additional foods from the Fats-Sweets group including butter or margarine, sugars, desserts, or more of the listed foods to meet caloric needs.

Nutritive value: On the basis of specified amounts of foods above: protein, 125 gm; kcal, 2,500. All vitamins and minerals in excess of normal diet—see page 461.

Meal Pattern	Sample Menu
BREAKFAST	
Fruit	Half grapefruit
Cereal	Oatmeal
Egg—1	Fried egg
Bread, whole-grain or enriched	Whole-wheat toast
Butter or margarine	Butter
Milk to drink and for cereal	Milk
Beverage	Coffee
LUNCHEON OR SUPPER	
Meat or substitute of egg, cheese, fish or poultry—large serving	Chicken soufflé Mushroom sauce
Potato, macaroni, spaghetti, noodles or vegetable	Buttered green beans
Salad with dressing	Shredded carrot and raisin salad
Bread with butter or margarine	Whole-wheat roll and butter
Fruit	Fresh peaches
Milk—1 glass	Milk
DINNER	
Meat, fish, or poultry—large serving	Broiled trout with parsley garnish
Potato	Creamed potato
Vegetable	Buttered spinach
Bread with butter or margarine	Rye bread with butter
Dessert	Lemon-flake ice cream Brownies
Milk	Milk
Beverage	Tea with lemon
EVENING NOURISHMENT	
Eggnog—1 glass	Chocolate eggnog
Sandwich with cheese or equivalent	American cheese and tomato sandwich

High-Protein Fluid Diet

Characteristics and General Rules

From 2 to 4 tablespoons nonfat dry milk may be added to each cup of milk or it may be used in custards or cream soups.

Eggs are sometimes contaminated with *Salmonella.* Pasteurized eggnogs may be purchased and are preferable to those made with raw eggs.

The calorie intake is increased by adding butter to gruels and cream soups; adding sugar to beverages; and substituting light cream for part of the milk allowance.

Include These Foods or Their Nutritive Equivalents Daily:

6 cups milk
⅔ cup nonfat dry milk
4 eggs
1–2 ounces strained meat
½ cup strained cereal for gruel
1 cup citrus juice
½ cup tomato juice
¼ cup vegetable purée for cream soup
2 servings plain dessert—gelatin, Junket, custard, cornstarch pudding, ice cream, sherbet
2–3 tablespoons sugar
1–2 tablespoons butter or margarine
Cream for coffee, for gruel, and in milk
Tea, coffee, decaffeinated coffee, cocoa powder, carbonated beverages
Flavoring extracts

Nutritive value: Protein, 110 gm; kcal, 2,100.

Meal Pattern

BREAKFAST
Citrus fruit juice
Cereal gruel with milk and sugar
Poached or soft-cooked egg
Hot beverage with cream, sugar

MIDMORNING
High-protein beverage

LUNCHEON OR SUPPER
Cream soup with butter
Tomato juice
High-protein milk, plain or flavored
Fruit-juice gelatin, cornstarch pudding, ice cream, or custard

MIDAFTERNOON
Malted milk or eggnog

DINNER
Broth with strained meat
Strained fruit juice
Milk, high-protein milk, or eggnog
Ice cream, Junket, custard, gelatin or plain pudding

EVENING
Eggnog, milk shake, or plain milk
Ice cream, gelatin, or custard

Problems and Review

1. When the availability of protein for tissue synthesis is reduced, what functions of protein will be affected? What clinical and biochemical changes result?
2. In what pathologic conditions is protein deficiency likely to be a problem? Why?

3. Why is a liberal calorie intake essential for effective use of a high-protein diet?
4. *Problem.* The normal diet (page 461) furnishes about 94 gm protein and 2,100 kcal. Develop three plans whereby this pattern could be supplemented with 25 gm protein and 500 kcal.
5. *Problem.* Plan a meal pattern for a 17-year-old boy who is allergic to eggs and who needs 150 gm protein and 4,000 kcal.
6. A patient's food intake averages 50 gm protein and 1,700 kcal. What are some things you need to know about this patient before you can give him guidance for a high-protein high-calorie diet?
7. A teenage girl is 25 pounds underweight and needs some help in planning a diet to bring about weight gain. She is now averaging 55 gm protein and 1,800 kcal daily.
   a. Plan some additions to her diet that would increase calories to about 2,600 with a minimum of bulk.
   b. What are some factors that may contribute to underweight?
   c. Using the food exchange lists, calculate the protein, fat, and carbohydrate value of the list of foods suggested for weight gain on page 495. How many calories are provided?
   d. Plan three bedtime snacks that will each provide 500 kcal.

Cited References

1. Barac-Nieto, M. et al.: "Body Composition in Chronic Undernutrition," *Am. J. Clin. Nutr.*, **31**:23–40, 1978.
2. Wright, R. A.: "Nutritional Assessment," *JAMA*, **244**:559–60, 1980.
3. Blackburn, G. L. et al.: "Nutrition in the Critically Ill Patient," *Anesthesiology*, **47**:181–94, 1977.
4. Blackburn, G. L.: "Nutritional Assessment and Support During Infection," *Am. J. Clin. Nutr.*, **30**:1493–97, 1977.
5. Blackburn, G. L. et al.: "Nutritional and Metabolic Assessment of the Hospitalized Patient," *J.P.E.N.*, **1**.11–22, 1977.
6. Coale, M. S. and Robson, J. R. K.: "Dietary Management of Intractable Diarrhea in Malnourished Patients," *J. Am. Diet. Assoc.*, **76**:444–50, 1980.

Additional References

BISTRIAN, B. R. et al.: "Protein Status of General Surgical Patients," *JAMA*, **230**:858–60, 1974.

LONG, C. L., and BLAKEMORE, W. S.: "Energy and Protein Requirements in the Hospitalized Patient," *J.P.E.N.*, **3**:69–71, 1979.

STEFFEE, W. P.: "Malnutrition in Hospitalized Patients," *JAMA*, **244**:2630–35, 1980.

29 *Immunity, Infections, and Fevers*

POOR nutritional status adversely affects the body's ability to cope with the stress of infections, fever, trauma, surgery, and disease. In this chapter is presented a brief discussion of some aspects of immune function, the influence of infection on nutrient utilization, and nutritional needs in fevers.

The Immune Response The body has a number of nonspecific and specific defense mechanisms that contribute to resistance in infection. Both types of defenses are impaired in malnutrition.

Among the nonspecific factors are anatomic barriers, such as the skin and mucous membranes, collagen, secretions, and so on; fever; intestinal flora; hormonal influences; iron-binding protein; and certain nutrients. Deficiencies of protein, vitamin A, B-complex, ascorbic acid, and zinc lead to characteristic skin lesions which serve as entry points for bacteria and subsequent infections. Protein and vitamin A deficiencies lead to damage to the intestinal mucosa with alterations in the number and type of flora. A review of the effect of nutrient deficiencies on the various nonspecific host factors is included in the references at the end of this chapter.[1]

Specific defense mechanisms include *cell-mediated immunity,* which involves T-lymphocytes, and *humoral immunity,* involving B-lymphocytes. Plasma accessory (A) cells are also involved. Each of these types of cells has several subgroups that have important roles in different phases of the immune response. T-lymphocytes are derived from the thymus after maturation from stem cells produced by the bone marrow, and they play a major role in protection against viral and bacterial infections. B-cells are derived from plasma cells and originate in the bursa equivalent. (See Figure 29–1.) The B-cells produce specific antibodies that protect against pyogenic bacteria. A-cells are composed of a heterogenous group of leukocytes which are involved in initiation and regulation of the immune response and destruction of bacteria. Interactions among these three types of leukocytes in immune activities are dependent on adequate protein synthesis. Decreased immunocompetence is often seen in nutritionally depleted individuals or in

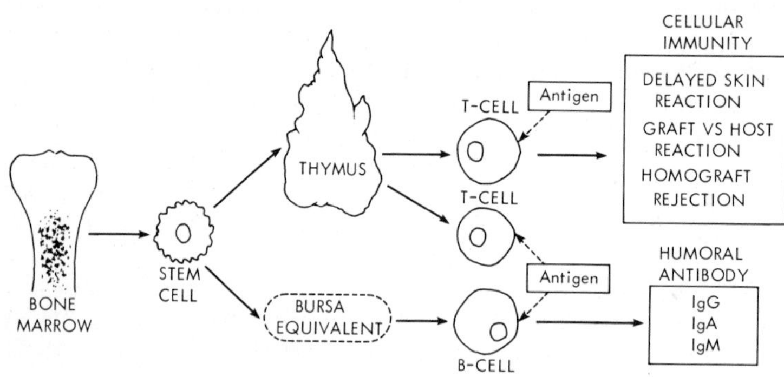

Figure 29–1. Origins of T-cells and B-cells and their role in immunity. (From: O'Loughlin, J. M.: "Infections in the Immunosuppressed Patient," *Med. Clin. North Am.*, **59**:495–501, 1975. Used with permission.)

those in whom protein catabolism exceeds protein synthesis.

Infections

Incidence Each year community acquired infections account for more than 3 million persons being hospitalized in the United States. Another 2 million acquire infections while in the hospital. Together these account for about 10 per cent of total patient days in acute care hospitals at an estimated cost of nearly $5 billion yearly.[2] According to data from the National Center for Health Statistics, some 123,000 deaths in the United States each year are due to infections or their sequelae. Infection ranked fourth among causes of death in 1976, surpassed only by ischemic heart disease, malignant neoplasms, and cerebrovascular disease.[3]

Nutrition and Infection The interaction between nutrition and infection is synergistic, that is, nutritional deficiency lowers resistance to infection, and infection aggravates existing malnutrition. Persons who are chronically undernourished not only succumb to infections more readily but have a longer period of recovery than do the well nourished. In the United States the vulnerable groups are the elderly who are poor or who lack incentive to eat properly, the chronically ill who have poor appetites, the young child living in a low-income area, and the teenager who follows a poor pattern of food intake. In the developing countries infants and preschool children are the most vulnerable.

Infection may have significant effects on nutritional status. The extent of the changes depends upon the nature and severity of the infectious disease, its duration, the presence of fever, and the previous nutritional status of the individual. Nutrient needs are generally increased during infection by the following mechanisms: (1) the stress reaction induces a catabolic response with increased losses of nitrogen, magnesium, potassium, phosphate, and zinc; (2) in severe infections or if fever is present, the increased metabolic rate raises energy needs; (3) anorexia decreases food intake; (4) nutrient losses may be increased due to increased perspiration, vomiting, or diarrhea; and (5) malabsorption, in enteric infections, may interfere with nutrient utilization.

Table 29–1. **Some Hormone-Induced Catabolic Effects of Infections**

Effect	Mechanism
↑ Blood glucose	Insulin resistance
↑ Gluconeogenesis	↑ Catacholamines (epinephrine) ↑ Glucagon
↑ Glycogenolysis	↑ Glucagon
↑ Free fatty acids	↑ Growth hormone ↑ Insulin resistance
↑ Skeletal protein catabolism	↑ Glucocorticoids
↑ Plasma amino acids	Insulin resistance
↓ Ketogenesis	Insulin resistance

Metabolic Consequences of Infection A number of hormonal responses favor catabolism during infections, namely, increased levels of growth hormone, glucagon, glucocorticoids, and insulin resistance. (See Table 29–1.)

Profound alterations in carbohydrate metabolism occur during the acute phase of an infection and result in release of amino acids, primarily from catabolism of skeletal muscle, in order to meet energy needs. This sequence occurs even though fat stores may be adequate. Following the acute phase there is an adaptation period in which hormonal levels revert to normal; the blood glucose falls, blood ketones are elevated, and nitrogen excretion is reduced. In this phase the body utilizes ketones in place of keto derivatives of the branched chain amino acids for energy substrates, thereby lessening the need for skeletal muscle breakdown.

Nutritional Considerations Perhaps the most important nutritional consequence of infection is the catabolic effect on protein metabolism. Even in mild infections some protein depletion occurs whether or not fever is present. Restoration of body cell mass is thus the primary goal of nutritional therapy. Depending upon the nature and severity of the infection, the net loss of protein is from 0.6 to 1.2 gm per kilogram body weight daily.[4] Assuming the anabolic period of recovery lasts three times as long as the catabolic period, and a mean loss of 0.9 gm per kilogram daily, an additional allowance of 0.3 gm per kilogram per day of high-quality protein for adults would be needed during the period of recovery from acute infectious diseases.[4]

Energy needs during and after acute infections may be increased 10 to 30 per cent depending on the degree of physical activity and whether or not fever is present.[4] Generally, 30 to 40 kcal per kilogram per day for adults, or 100 to 150 kcal per kilogram per day for children are needed.[5]

Energy and protein needs for recovery from mild infections in previously well-nourished persons can usually be met by supplements to the regular diet. A variety of proprietary products is available, most providing about 1 kcal per milliliter. The carbohydrate sources in these products should be considered because those high in mono- and disaccharides present a high osmolar load to the intestine, and those high in lactose may not be well tolerated. (See Chapter 33.)

Individuals with marginal nutritional status with regard to vitamins are at increased risk for deficiencies of these vitamins during infectious disease. For these individuals, liberal intakes, 2 to 3 times the minimum daily requirements, are needed.[6] No advantage of increased vitamin intake during simple infection has been demonstrated for those whose previous intake has been satisfactory.[7] Vitamin requirements are increased if infection is accompanied by inflammation and necrosis of tissue.

Losses of potassium, magnesium, and phosphorus during acute infections accompany nitrogen losses. Retention of salt and water occur due to the influence of mineralocorticoid and antidiuretic hormones. Shifts in plasma levels of certain minerals occur. For example, plasma zinc and iron levels fall while copper increases.[8] These appear to be protective mechanisms. Both zinc and iron are believed to be involved in the immune process, altering phagocytosis and bactericidal activity. Zinc is also needed for globulin synthesis and repair of tissue damage. Microorganisms require iron for growth; during infection leukocytes secrete lactoferrin, an iron-binding protein, thus making iron less available for promotion of bacterial growth.[9] During the acute phase of an infection provision of large amounts of iron may be detrimental.

Fevers

Classification of fevers FEVER is an elevation in body temperature above the normal which may occur in response to infection, inflammation, or unknown causes. It may be due to exogenous agents, such as bacteria or fungi, or to endogenous factors, such as antigen-antibody reactions, malignancy, or graft rejection. Exogenous factors produce fever through activation of phagocytes in bone marrow to release a fever-inducing hormone, endogenous pyrogen.[10] This hormone, in turn, is believed to induce synthesis of prostaglandins which act as mediators in the initiation of fever by somehow influencing the thermoregulatory center in the anterior hypothalamus to increase its normal "set point" for body temperature. Drugs such as aspirin are effective in reducing fever because they inhibit prostaglandin synthesis.[11]

The duration of fever may be (1) short as in acute fevers of colds, tonsillitis, influenza, and so on or (2) chronic as in long-standing tuberculosis, or it may be intermittent as in malaria.

Metabolism in fevers The metabolic effects of fevers, proportional to the elevation of body temperature and the duration, include the following:

1. An increase in the metabolic rate amounting to 13 per cent for every degree Celsius rise in body temperature (7 per cent for each degree Farenheit); an increase also in the restlessness and hence a greatly increased calorie need.
2. Decreased glycogen stores and decreased stores of adipose tissue.
3. Increased catabolism of proteins, especially in typhoid fever, malaria, typhus fever, poliomyelitis, and others; the increased nitrogen wastes place an additional burden upon the kidneys.
4. Accelerated loss of body water owing to increased perspiration and the excretion of body wastes.
5. Increased excretion of sodium and potassium.

General Dietary Considerations The diet in fevers depends upon the nature and severity of the pathologic conditions and upon the length of the convalescence. In general it should meet the following requirements:

Energy. The caloric requirement may be increased as much as 50 per cent if the temperature is high and the tissue destruction is great. Restlessness also increases the caloric requirement. Initially, the patient may be able to ingest only 600 to 1,200 kcal daily, but this should be increased as rapidly as possible.

Protein. About 100 gm protein or more is prescribed for the adult when a fever is prolonged. This will be most efficiently utilized when the calorie intake is liberal (see Chapter 28). High-protein beverages may be used as supplements to the regular meals.

Carbohydrates. Glycogen stores are replenished by a liberal intake of carbohydrates. Any sugars such as glucose, corn syrup, and cane sugar may be used. However, glucose is less sweet than some other sugars and consequently more of it can be used. Furthermore, it is a simple sugar which is absorbed into the bloodstream without the necessity for enzyme action. Lactose, in some individuals, may increase fermentation in the small intestine resulting in diarrhea.

Fats. The energy intake may be rapidly increased through the judicious use of fats, but fried foods and rich pastries may retard digestion unduly.

Minerals. A sufficient intake of sodium chloride is accomplished by the use of salty broth and soups and by liberal sprinklings of salt on food. Generally speaking, foods are a good source of potassium, but a limited food intake might result in potassium depletion whenever fever is high and prolonged. Fruit juices and milk are relatively good sources of this element.

Vitamins. Fevers apparently increase the requirements for vitamin A and ascorbic acid, just as the B-complex vitamins are needed at increased levels proportionate to the increase in calories; that is, 0.5 mg thiamin, 0.6 mg riboflavin, and 6.6 mg niacin equivalents per 1,000 additional kcal. Oral therapy with antibiotics and drugs interferes with synthesis of some B-complex vitamins by intestinal bacteria, thus necessitating a prescription for vitamin supplements for a short time.

Fluid. The fluid intake must be liberal to compensate for the losses from the skin and to permit adequate volume of urine for excreting the wastes. From 2,500 to 5,000 ml daily are necessary, including beverages, soups, fruit juices, and water.

Ease of digestion. Bland, readily digested foods should be used to facilitate digestion and rapid absorption. The food may be soft or of regular consistency. Although fluid diets may be used initially there are some disadvantages: (1) most fluid diets occupy bulk out of all proportion to their caloric and nutrient values, so that reinforcement of liquids is essential; (2) a liquid diet sometimes increases abdominal distension to the point of acute discomfort, whereas solid foods may be better tolerated; (3) many patients experience less anorexia, nausea, and vomiting when they are taking solid foods.

Intervals of feeding. Small quantities of food at intervals of 2 to 3 hours will permit adequate nutrition without overtaxing the digestive system at any one time. With improvement, many patients consume more food if given three meals and a bedtime feeding.

Diet in fevers of short duration The duration of many fevers has been shortened by antibiotic and drug therapy, and nutritional needs are usually met without difficulty. During an acute fever the patient's appetite is often very poor, and small feedings of soft or liquid foods as desired should be offered at frequent intervals. (See Chapter 25.) Sufficient intake of fluids and salt is essential. If the illness persists for more than a few days, high-protein, high-calorie foods will need to be emphasized. See High-Protein Diet (Chapter 28).

Diet in Typhoid Fever Improved sanitation has greatly reduced the incidence of typhoid fever. In the United States, typhoid is unusual. The reported incidence has decreased from 4 per 100,000 population in 1942 to 0.2 cases per 100,000 in 1975. About one third of the reported cases are associated with international travel.[12] Antibiotic therapy has dramatically shortened the acute stage of the disease so that the fever subsides within a few days. Nevertheless, short and uneventful convalescence is determined to an important degree by adequate nutrition.

The febrile period may cause loss of tissue protein amounting to as much as ½ to ¾ pound of muscle a day. The body store of glycogen is quickly depleted, and a probable upset in water balance occurs.

The intestinal tract becomes highly inflamed and irritable, and diarrhea, which is a frequent complication, interferes with the absorption of nutrients. The ulceration may be so severe that hemorrhage and even perforation of the intestines may occur.

The dietary considerations outlined on page 505 apply as in other fevers. Special emphasis must be placed upon a caloric intake of 3,500 or more and a protein intake in excess of 100 gm. Because of the intestinal inflammation, great care must be exercised to eliminate all irritating fibers. The high-protein fluid diet may be used as a basis in dietary planning. In addition, low-fiber foods including white breads and crackers, refined cooked and dry cereals, eggs, cheese, tender meat, fish, and poultry, potato, and plain desserts may be used. A representative meal pattern is as follows:

BREAKFAST
Orange juice with glucose
Cream of Wheat with cream and sugar
Poached egg on
Buttered white toast
Cocoa

MIDMORNING
Eggnog made with cream

LUNCHEON OR SUPPER
Cream of tomato soup
Roast chicken
Baked potato (no skin) with butter
Buttered white toast
Vanilla ice cream
High-protein milk

MIDAFTERNOON
Orange juice
Baked custard

DINNER
Consommé with gelatin
Soft-cooked egg
Boiled rice with sugar and cream
Buttered white toast
Tapioca cream
Milk

BEDTIME
Chocolate malted milk
Cream cheese sandwich on white bread

Diet in Rheumatic Fever Accurate epidemiologic data on the incidence of rheumatic fever are lacking; however, it appears to be decreasing. The crude death rate from acute rheumatic fever and rheumatic heart disease in the United States was 6.8 per 100,000 in 1972 compared with 14.5 per 100,000 in 1950.[13] Development of rheumatic fever follows *Streptococcus* infections of the upper respiratory tract. It is more common among the poor; however, no specific nutrient deficiencies have been identified. An autoimmune or toxic reaction has been proposed in the etiology.

Carditis is a common feature of juvenile rheumatic fever whereas arthritis is more frequent in adults.[14] Antibiotics, to eliminate the streptococcal infection, and antiinflammatory agents, such as salicylates, are used to treat manifestations of carditis and arthritis. Corticosteroids are prescribed if congestive heart failure or cardiomegaly develop.[15] When there is cardiac involvement, bedrest is essential to relieve the workload of the heart. For arthritis manifestations, activity is restricted until pain and swelling subside.

During the acute phase, the soft and liquid diets described in Chapter 25 are suitable. Because the appetite may be poor, sweets should probably be limited as a means of ensuring adequate intake of important foods. The diet is planned according to the principles of the normal diet described in Chapter 25. Mild sodium restriction (see Chapter 40) is needed in order to avoid sodium retention and edema formation if steroids are prescribed.

Diet in Tuberculosis Tuberculosis is an infectious disease caused by the bacillus *Mycobacterium tuberculosis.* It affects the lungs most often but may also be localized in other organs, such as the lymph nodes or kidneys, or it may be generalized. The initial infection is believed to be a rather benign process in which the tubercle bacilli enter the body but are kept in check by the body's cell-mediated immune system, and the disease heals spontaneously. The presence of the organisms constitutes a potential risk of active disease which often occurs years after the initial attack in susceptible persons.

Tuberculosis is a major cause of illness and death worldwide. The incidence in the United States has declined sharply since the turn of the century. From 1960 to 1977, the case rate per 100,000 fell from 30.8 to 13.9.[16] The reduced incidence has been attributed to more effective chemotherapeutic agents, better housing, and improved nutrition; yet there is still concern among the elderly and those with increased susceptibility to disease, and in areas where inadequate housing, poverty, and poor sanitation prevail.

Pulmonary tuberculosis is accompanied by wasting of tissues, exhaustion, cough, expectoration, and fever. The acute phase resembles pneumonia, with high fever, and increased circulation and respiration. The chronic phase is accompanied by low-grade fever and the metabolic rate is lower than in acute fevers. Because of the protracted illness, wasting may be considerable.

The individual with chronic tuberculosis often has increased energy needs in order to achieve desirable weight. From 2,500 to 3,000 kcal daily is usually satisfactory. A protein intake of 75 to 100 gm helps to regenerate the serum albumin levels which are often low. Calcium is needed to promote healing of the tuberculous lesions. At least a quart of milk, or its equivalent, should be taken daily. Iron supplementation may be necessary if there has been hemorrhage. Carotene appears to be poorly converted to vitamin A so that the diet should provide as much preformed vitamin A as possible. In addition, a vitamin A supplement may be necessary. Ascorbic acid deficiency is frequently present, and additional amounts of citrus fruits or ascorbic acid supplementation are essential.

Prolonged administration of chemotherapeutic agents used in treatment of tuberculosis may have an adverse effect on certain of the B-complex vitamins. Isoniazid is an antagonist of vitamin B-6 and may inhibit the folate-dependent interconversion of glycine and serine. Low serum folate and megaloblastic anemia have been noted in patients receiving this therapy. Supplements of vitamin B-6 are indicated to prevent the peripheral neuritis characteristic of B-6 deficiency. See Chapter 24 for side effects of other chemotherapeutic agents.

Selection of foods. During the acute stage of the illness, a high-protein high-calorie fluid diet may be given as in other acute fevers, progressing to the soft and regular diets when improvement occurs. Most patients have very poor appetites. For some a six-meal routine is best, whereas others eat better if they receive three meals and a bedtime feeding. The individuals responsible for planning meals should respect the patient's food idiosyncrasies. To this end, a selective menu from which the patient chooses foods each day is helpful. Other patients may eat better when they are not consulted in advance about their diets, thus introducing an element of surprise. Needless to say, every attention must be given to making meals as appetizing in appearance and taste as possible. The high-protein and high-calorie diets described in Chapter 28 may be adapted to the individual patient's needs.

Dietary Counseling

Failure of the patient to follow the prescribed drug regimen leads to great increase in recurrence and repeated hospitalization. Good nutrition is likewise important in preventing recurrence. The characteristics of a normal diet, with special emphasis on a liberal milk intake, protein-rich foods, fruits, and vegetables, must be pointed out. To increase the calcium and protein intake, 3 to 5 tablespoons of nonfat dry milk may be added to each 8 ounces of whole milk. If desired, fruit flavors or chocolate syrup may be added. This beverage supplementation is conveniently prepared, provides substantial nutritive value at minimum bulk, and is low in cost.

Because many of the patients with tuberculosis have low incomes, some assistance is necessary in providing practical measures to purchase the necessary foods. This entails not only additional welfare allowances in some instances but guidance in budgeting the food money. In families with low incomes it may not be practical to improve the diet of the patient alone, for additional allowances of money may be spent for the children's diet rather than for the patient. In such situations the best prophylaxis may well be the improvement of the diet of all members of the family.

Emphysema This is a lung disorder characterized by enlargement of the air spaces beyond the terminal bronchioles and pathologic changes in the walls of the alveoli.[17] It occurs primarily in men over 40 years of age who have a long history of cigarette smoking and bronchitis. Other possible causes are air pollution and respiratory infections. Exertional dyspnea is often the first symptom and may be accompanied by chronic cough, wheezing, and fatigue. The course of the disease may be slow over many years or it may progress rapidly to the terminal stage in a few years. In early stages some patients may be obese, and the distress in breathing is further accentuated. Some improvement is noted when weight is brought within desirable levels.

Shortness of breath places a severe limitation upon the ability to ingest an adequate diet, with the result that weight loss and tissue wasting are common. Chewing and swallowing require further effort and the patient often stops short of satisfactory intake. Not infrequently the purchase and preparation of food, or seeking a place to eat a meal, require more effort than the patient can expend. Because the patient is unable to work, there may be insufficient income to purchase adequate food.

A soft high-calorie diet is usually indicated. Patients are especially short of breath after a night's sleep and experience difficulty in eating breakfast. Small, frequent feedings of concentrated foods should be used. High-protein commercial supplements are useful because they are concentrated, palatable, easy to prepare, and easy to ingest. Too many fibrous fruits and vegetables or meats requiring much chewing may necessitate an energy expenditure beyond that justified by the nutrient values obtained. The patient will eat very slowly, and should refrain from talking while eating since the swallowing of air is responsible for much of the discomfort.

For a discussion of infectious hepatitis, see page 564; for a discussion of infections from food poisoning, see page 300.

Problems and Review

1. How does infection influence metabolism?
2. What is the effect of nutritional status on the incidence of infections?
3. How great is the increase in energy metabolism brought about by fever? What other changes in metabolism of nutrients take place during fever? In view of these changes how do you view the widely held belief in "starving a fever"?
4. Give examples of foods that can be used to reinforce the protein and calorie level of the diet.
5. *Problem.* Plan a fluid diet in six meals that eliminates milk. Calculate the calorie value.
6. *Problem.* Plan a full fluid diet in six meals to include 80 gm protein and 2,500 kcal.
7. *Problem.* Plan a diet for a 12-year-old boy with rheumatic fever. What techniques can you use to help the boy accept the diet?
8. What are the principles of dietary management in typhoid fever?
9. Outline a plan of dietary counseling for a 34-year-old woman with healed tuberculosis. She has three children under the age of 10 years and is receiving welfare assistance. You will need to determine the amount of money available through welfare in your community to this family of four.
10. *Problem.* Keep a record of the food intake for 2 days by a patient with an infection. What factors enter into this patient's acceptance of food? Develop recommendations for any improvement that may be required.
11. What are the problems encountered in feeding a patient with emphysema? How would you try to solve them?

Cited References

1. Neumann, C. G.: "Nonspecific Host Factors and Infection in Malnutrition—A Review," in *Malnutrition and the Immune Response,* R. M. Suskind, ed. Raven Press, New York, 1977.
2. Dixon, R. W.: "Effect of Infections on Hospital Care," *Ann. Intern. Med.,* **89**:749–53, 1978.
3. Bennett, J. V.: "Human Infections: Economic Implications and Prevention," *Ann. Intern. Med.,* **89**:761–63, 1978.
4. Scrimshaw, N. S.: "Effect of Infection on Nutrient Requirements," *Am. J. Clin. Nutr.,* **30**:1536–44, 1977.
5. Beisel, W. R.: "Impact of Infection on Nutritional Status: Concluding Comments and Summary," *Am. J. Clin. Nutr.,* **30**:1564–66, 1977.
6. Dionigi, R. et al.: "Nutrition and Infection," *J.P.E.N.,* **3**:62–68, 1979.
7. Vitale, J. J.: "The Impact of Infection on Vitamin Metabolism: An Unexplored Area," *Am. J. Clin. Nutr.,* **30**:1473–77, 1977.

8. Powanda, M. C.: "Changes in Body Balances of Nitrogen and Other Key Nutrients: Description and Underlying Mechanisms," *Am. J. Clin. Nutr.*, **30**:1254–68, 1977.
9. Weinberg, E. D.: "Infection and Iron Metabolism," *Am. J. Clin. Nutr.*, **30**:1485–90, 1977.
10. Bernheim, H. A. et al.: "Fever: Pathogenesis, Pathophysiology, and Purpose. A Review," *Ann. Intern. Med.*, **91**:261–70, 1979.
11. Dinarello, C. A., and Wolff, S. M.: "Pathogenesis of Fever in Man," *New Engl. J. Med.*, **298**:607–12, 1978.
12. Ryder, R. W., and Blake, P. A.: "Typhoid Fever in the United States, 1975 and 1976," *J. Infect. Dis.*, **139**:124–26, 1979.
13. Mortimer, E. A.: "Control of Rheumatic Fever: How Are We Doing?" *JAMA*, **237**:1720, 1977.
14. McDanald, E. C., and Wersman, M. H.: "Articular Manifestations of Rheumatic Fever in Adults," *Ann. Intern. Med.*, **89**:917–20, 1978.
15. Kaplan, E. L.: "Acute Rheumatic Fever," *Pediatr. Clin. North Am.*, **25**:817–29, 1978.
16. Leff, A. et al.: "Tuberculosis. A Chemotherapeutic Triumph But a Persistent Socio-economic Problem," *Arch. Intern. Med.*, **139**:1375–77, 1979.
17. Meneely, G. R. et al.: "Definition and Classification of Chronic Bronchitis, Asthma and Pulmonary Emphysema," *Am. Rev. Resp. Dis.*, **85**:762–68, 1962.

Additional References

BISTRIAN, B. R.: "Interaction of Nutrition and Infection in the Hospital Setting," *Am. J. Clin. Nutr.*, **30**:1228–32, 1977.

BROWN, R. E.: "Interaction of Nutrition and Infection in Clinical Practice," *Pediatr. Clin. North Am.*, **24**:241–52, 1977.

CHANDRA, R. K.: "Interactions of Nutrition, Infection, and Immune Response," *Acta Paediatr. Scand.*, **68**:137–44, 1979.

Committee on Nutrition: "Relationship Between Iron Status and Incidence of Infection in Infancy," *Pediatrics*, **62**:246–50, 1978.

DAVIS-SHARTS, J.: "Mechanisms and Manifestations of Fever," *Am. J. Nurs.*, **78**:1874–78, 1978.

GLASSROTH, J. et al.: "Tuberculosis in the 1980s," *New Engl. J. Med.*, **302**:1441–50, 1980.

HUGH-JONES, P., and WHIMSTER, W.: "The Etiology and Management of Disabling Emphysema," *Am. Rev. Resp. Dis.*, **117**:343–78, 1978.

KENDIG, E. L.: "Tuberculosis Among Children in the United States: 1978," *Pediatrics*, **62**:269–71, 1978.

PEKAREK, R. S. et al.: "Abnormal Cellular Immune Responses During Acquired Zinc Deficiency," *Am. J. Clin. Nutr.*, **32**:1466–71, 1979.

STIEHM, E. R.: "Humoral Immunity in Malnutrition," *Fed. Proc.*, **39**:3093–97, 1980.

VITALE, J. J.: *Impact of Nutrition on Immune Function.* Nutrition in Disease, Ross Laboratories, 1979.

Anemias 30

BLOOD is a constantly changing, highly complex tissue which is concerned with the transport of cell nutrients, the elimination of wastes, and the maintenance of chemical equilibrium. Its intricate function and composition suggest the need for a considerable variety of nutrients, and these have been discussed especially in Part One. This chapter is concerned with some of the more common deficiencies that arise in the framework of the red blood cells and in the hemoglobin within these cells.

Synthesis of Erythrocytes and Hemoglobin The red blood cells are synthesized in the bone marrow and proceed through a number of stages before they are released into the circulation as nonnucleated fully mature cells. For their synthesis many nutrients are required, including the amino acids. Vitamin B-12 and folinic acid are required for the synthesis of DNA, which is essential for the growth and normal division of cells. When either or both of these vitamins are deficient, fewer cells can be produced, and they are released into the circulation as large, nucleated cells called megaloblasts. (See also Chapter 12, pages 235 and 237.)

Hemoglobin synthesis requires a constant source of iron for the formation of heme and of protein for the formation of globin. The rate of synthesis can be no more rapid than the supply of iron. The iron is made available to the erythroid marrow by the plasma, which in turn is supplied by the reserves held in the liver and by the absorption from the intestinal tract. (See page 143 for discussion of iron metabolism.)

The normal red cell count is about 5 million per cubic millimeter for males and 4.5 million for females. Normal hemoglobin levels range from 14 to 17 gm per 100 ml for males, and from 12 to 15 gm per 100 ml for females. Hemoglobin concentrations in blacks are about 0.5 to 1.0 gm per 100 ml less than that of whites.[1] The normal packed-cell volume (hematocrit) is about 45 per cent; for men the lower limit of normal is 42 per cent, for women, 36 per cent, and for pregnant women, 33 per cent.[2]

Anemia

ANEMIA is a condition in which there is a reduction in the total circulating hemoglobin. Anemias may be described biochemically in terms of lowered hemoglobin levels, number of red blood cells, and hematocrit. They are also differentiated on the basis of appearance of red cells: normocytic, macrocytic, or microcytic; nucleated or nonnucleated; normochromic, hyperchromic, or hypochromic. Other diagnostic aids include measurements of plasma iron levels, iron-binding capacity, and transferrin saturation.

Etiology Anemias may be caused by several factors:

1. Blood loss.
2. Decreased production of blood. Failure to provide essential nutrients due to inadequate intake or defective utilization may lead to anemias. The anemias of nutritional origin may be microcytic or macrocytic, depending

on the specific nutrient lacking. Exposure to x-ray or radium, bone tumors, cirrhosis of the liver, carcinoma, and leukemias are examples of conditions that may interfere with red cell formation within the bone marrow.

3. Increased destruction of blood. This may be the result of the action of intestinal parasites, hemolytic bacteria, chemical agents such as coal tar products and sulfonamide compounds, or abnormal red cell structure (sickle cells).
4. Drug-induced anemias. A number of drugs may interfere with vitamin B-12 absorption and lead to anemia. Included are para-aminosalicylic acid, neomycin, colchicine, and ethanol. (See also Chapter 24.)

Decreased serum vitamin B-12 levels have been observed in women taking oral contraceptives although the significance of this is not yet known.[3] Impaired metabolism of folate polyglutamate has also been noted in some of these women. The mechanism involved is not clear, but is believed by some to occur only in women who have an underlying defect in absorption or whose diet is marginal in folate.[4]

Impaired utilization of folic acid also occurs in persons receiving anticonvulsants. Many drugs used in cancer chemotherapy induce anemias by interfering with DNA synthesis. (See Chapters 24 and 35.)

Chronic diseases such as severe infections, malignancies, alcoholism, uremia, rheumatoid arthritis, liver disease, myxedema, and malabsorptive states following ileal resection or bypass are also associated with anemias.

Symptoms Mild anemias diagnosed by laboratory studies are not closely associated with clinical symptoms or with changes in cardiorespiratory functions. When anemias become more severe, however, the symptoms are more consistent and include skin pallor, weakness, easy fatigability, headaches, dizziness, sensitivity to cold, paresthesia, and reduced physical work capacity as determined by treadmill testing.[5] Cheilosis, glossitis, loss of appetite, and loss of gastrointestinal tone with accompanying symptoms of distress are seen in severe anemias. Concave "spoon" fingernails (koilonychia) with longitudinal ridging of the nails is sometimes present. With increasing severity of anemia, the oxygenation of tissues is reduced—hence the feeling of fatigue. The heart rate increases, palpitation occurs, and there is shortness of breath.

Treatment The treatment of anemias is dependent upon determination of the cause and eliminating it whenever possible. Nutritionally, specific supplements may be required to improve the formation of red cells and hemoglobin. A normal diet to restore good nutrition is usually emphasized to support the specific therapy.

Iron-Deficiency Anemia

Incidence Iron-deficiency anemias are widely prevalent throughout the world. Incidence in the various countries ranges from about 5 to 15 per cent in males, 10 to 50 per cent in women, and 15 to 92 per cent in children.[6] This type accounts for 30 per cent of the anemias in the United States.[7] Data from both the Ten-State Nutrition Survey and the Health and Nutrition Examination Survey (HANES) indicated widespread iron deficiency based on dietary intakes and biochemical data.[8,9] Generally, the incidence is high in preschool children, adolescents, and women in the childbearing years. It occurs more frequently among persons of low economic status, although it is by no means limited to this group. (See Figure 30–1.)

Blood Studies for Diagnosis Iron deficiency follows a specific sequence. First, the iron reserves drop to lower levels, the transferrin level of the blood increases slightly, and the hematocrit and plasma iron levels remain normal. Then the iron reserves are used up, the transferrin level increases fur-

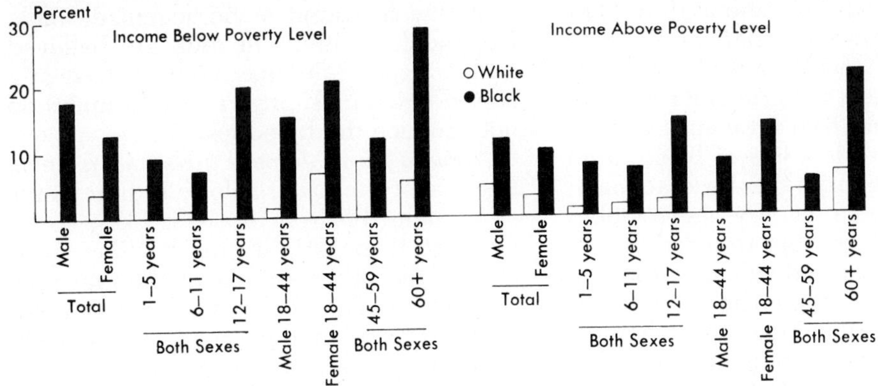

Figure 30–1. Percentage of persons with low hemoglobin values by age, sex, and race for income levels, United States, 1971–1972. (From Abraham, S., et al.: *Preliminary Findings of the First Health and Nutrition Examination Survey, United States, 1971–1972: Dietary Intake and Biochemical Findings.* Pub. (HRA) 74–1219–1. U.S. Department of Health, Education, and Welfare, Health Services Administration, Rockville, Md. 1974.)

ther, the hematocrit and plasma iron are reduced, and fewer red blood cells are produced. Finally, with no remaining iron reserves, the hematocrit and plasma iron continue to fall, and the cells are pale and reduced in size. Thus, the designation for the anemia is microcytic, hypochromic.

Laboratory values associated with severe iron-deficiency anemia are as follows:[10]

serum iron, less than 50 μg per 100 ml
iron-binding capacity, more than 400 mg per 100 ml
transferrin saturation, less than 15 per cent
serum ferritin, less than 10 μg per 100 ml

In mild iron-deficiency anemia serum ferritin is usually diminished but changes in the other constituents are not necessarily seen. In this stage, microcytic, hypochromic cells are not characteristic.

Etiology Among the factors to be considered as initiating iron-deficiency anemia are these:

1. Blood loss (most common cause in adults)
   a. Accidental hemorrhage
   b. Chronic diseases, such as tuberculosis, ulcers or intestinal disorders, when accompanied by hemorrhage
   c. Excessive menstrual losses
   d. Excessive blood donation
   e. Parasites such as hookworm
2. Deficiency of iron in the diet during period of accelerated demand
   a. Infancy—rapidly expanding blood volume
   b. Adolescence—rapid growth, and onset of menses in girls
   c. Pregnancy and lactation
3. Inadequate absorption of iron
   a. Diarrhea, as in sprue, pellagra
   b. Lack of acid secretion by the stomach
   c. Antacid therapy in chronic renal disease[11]
4. Nutrition deficiencies such as severe protein depletion
   a. Protein-calorie malnutrition

Blood loss. Whenever hypochromic anemia occurs in adult males or in women past the menopause, blood loss, as from a bleeding ulcer or other cause, must always be suspected. Menstrual losses by some women may be sufficiently great to result in anemia, especially if the diet is poorly selected. Losses of iron in menses average about 0.5 mg per day, or about 15 mg per month. The repeated donation of blood likewise could be a significant factor in anemia causation unless a liberal diet relatively rich in protein and iron is taken.

Whenever there is a loss of blood, fluid is quickly drawn in from the tissues to maintain the blood volume. The hemoglobin level and red cells are thus reduced in concentration, but the individual with adequate stores quickly replenishes the levels so that anemia is not evident unless hemorrhage is prolonged or repeated. From 3 weeks to 3 months may be required to replenish the losses from the donation of 1 pint of blood.

Infants and preschool children. The full-term infant born of a well-nourished mother has sufficient iron stores for the first 4 to 6 months of life.[12] Many babies, however, are not born with this endowment. Infants of low birth weight, those who are multiple births, and those whose mothers have had several previous pregnancies are least likely to have adequate reserves.

The Committee on Nutrition of the American Academy of Pediatrics has recommended introduction of a variety of foods by 4 to 6 months of age and has suggested that iron-fortified cereals are a good early choice.[13] Many infants from low socioeconomic groups are anemic because mothers are unaware of the importance of using iron-fortified cereals or because they cannot afford to purchase them. Many pediatricians recommend that an iron-fortified formula be continued throughout the first year. Some advocate limiting the volume of formula to 1 quart daily in order to encourage use of iron-rich foods and to increase the variety of foods eaten.[14]

Iron fortification or supplementation during the first 4 months of life for term infants, or 2 months for preterm infants, is not indicated.[15] The percentage of iron absorbed is lower at these periods than at a later age.

A cause of anemia in certain infants has been gastrointestinal bleeding resulting from the ingestion of homogenized milk. Heat-labile proteins in milk are believed to be responsible inasmuch as heat-processed cow's milk proprietary formulas do not produce the blood loss.[16]

Anemia in adolescent girls and women. Because of the lower calorie requirements of women, the iron intake is likely to be no more than 10 to 12 mg per day, even though the other aspects of the diet may be fully adequate. For women whose menstrual losses are high these intakes are likely to be inadequate to cover the losses and to build up iron reserves. Adolescent girls, in addition, must have iron to meet their growth requirements; yet, during these years their diets are often of generally poor quality.

Pregnancy imposes substantial additional demands upon the iron supply. The woman who has had repeated pregnancies and the young girl who is still maturing are most likely to become anemic and to bear infants who have little or no reserves.

Treatment For iron-deficiency anemia the primary emphasis in treatment is a supplement of iron salts such as ferrous sulfate, gluconate, or fumarate. Oral therapy is as effective as parenteral therapy except where there is severe interference with absorption as in ulcerative colitis or regional enteritis. Some individuals have an initial intolerance to iron salts, but usually become adjusted to the medication. It is helpful to take the salts after meals.

Dietary Counseling

Although the specific therapy for iron-deficiency anemia is iron medication, the patient needs guidance in the selection of an adequate diet. The diet history will establish the previous pattern of food intake and will indicate the corrections that are to be recommended. Frequently, the choice of foods has been poor with respect to sources of iron. With special emphasis on the inclusion of liver every week, if possible, and on the liberal use of dried fruits, dark green leafy vegetables, and enriched breads and cereals, the daily iron intake for women will be approximately 12 to 15 mg. A good source of ascorbic acid at each meal improves the absorption of iron. The heme iron in red meat is more available than is the iron in plant foods. For many women, the importance of continuing to use a prophylactic supplement even after the anemia has been corrected may need to be emphasized.

In moderately severe anemias the regeneration of hemoglobin is improved if protein intakes are increased to 80 to 100 gm daily. The diets of many women and girls are low in protein, and suggestions for increasing the protein content of the diet should be given. When cost is an important factor, simple recipes for dishes that use non-fat dry milk, poultry, fish, and less expensive cuts of meat are useful if food is prepared in the home.

Megaloblastic Anemias

Both folic acid and vitamin B-12 are needed for the synthesis and maturation of red blood cells. The interrelationship of these two vitamins in DNA synthesis is shown in Figure 30–2.

Vitamin B-12 Deficiency Vitamin B-12 must be bound to intrinsic factor, produced by the parietal cells of the stomach, before it is absorbed in the terminal ileum. Inability to produce intrinsic factor results in *pernicious anemia.* The red cell count is often less than 2.5 million and a large proportion of the cells are macrocytic. The anemia occurs chiefly in middle-aged and elderly persons and may be a genetic defect. Onset in black women is at a younger age and is associated with a high prevalence of circulating antibodies to intrinsic factor.[17]

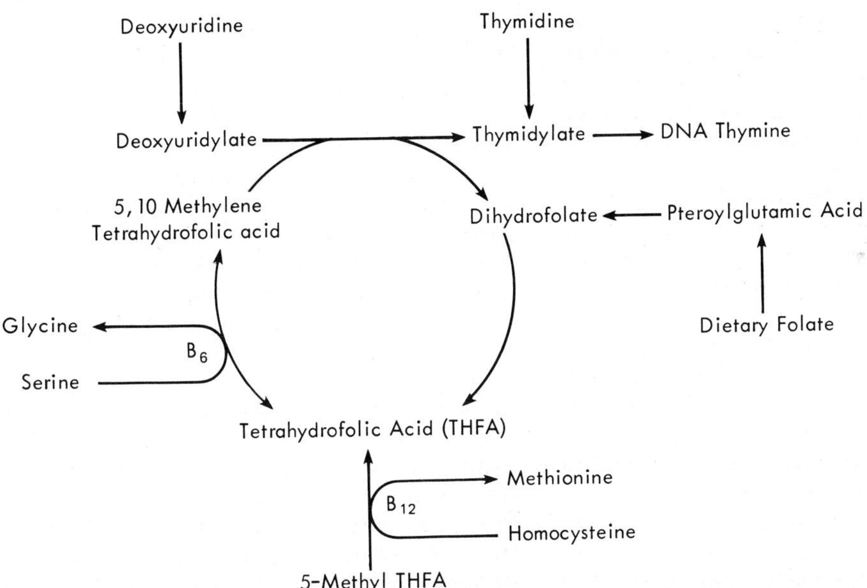

Figure 30–2. Interrelationship of folic acid and vitamin B-12 in DNA synthesis. Continuous regeneration of tetrahydrofolic acid (THFA) requires vitamin B-12. The vitamin acts as a coenzyme by taking a methyl group from 5 methyl THFA and donating it to homocysteine to form methionine. The THFA that remains is then converted to 5,10-methylene THFA which is needed for thymine formation. Deficiency of either vitamin B-12 or folic acid interferes with the cycle.

Pernicious anemia also occurs following total gastrectomy or removal of the terminal ileum. In these situations pernicious anemia does not become evident for 3 to 5 years postoperatively, depending on the body's reserves of the vitamin. The prolonged used of a strict vegetarian diet (vegan) has led to vitamin B-12 deficiency in a few cases. (See Chapter 15.)

Patients with pernicious anemia have a lemon-yellow pallor, anorexia, glossitis, achlorhydria, abdominal discomfort, frequent diarrhea, weight loss, and general weakness. Numbness of the limbs, coldness of the extremities, and difficulty in walking are manifestations of neurologic changes. Pernicious anemia is associated with an increased risk of gastric cancer.[18]

Tests used to determine the ability to absorb vitamin B-12 are (1) the plasma uptake test, in which the radioactivity of isotope-labeled vitamin B-12 is measured in plasma after an oral loading dose, and (2) the Schilling test. In the latter test, radioactive vitamin B-12 is given orally and is followed by a parenteral injection of the nonradioactive vitamin. Excretion of the radioactive vitamin in a 24-hour urine sample is monitored; low excretion implies vitamin B-12 deficiency. The test is then repeated with an oral dose of intrinsic facor in addition to the vitamin B-12. Improved absorption when intrinsic factor is added indicates pernicious anemia.

Treatment Parenteral doses as small as 1 μg of vitamin B-12 produce a marked hematopoietic response. Oral administration of massive doses, 1 mg daily, is reported to be as effective as intermittent parenteral injections of vitamin B-12.[19]

Although folic acid brings about correction of the hematologic picture in pernicious anemia, it has no effect on the associated neurologic symptoms. Folic acid should never be used in place of vitamin B-12 for the treatment of these patients, lest the neurologic symptoms become progressively worse.

Dietary Considerations Poor appetite, sore mouth, and gastrointestinal discomfort seriously interfere with an adequate food intake so that patients often present a picture of general nutritional deficiency. Their diets must be corrected for adequate calories and for protein. Because of the achlorhydria in pernicious anemia the rate of digestion is retarded. Hence, the fat content of the diet should be kept to moderate levels, restricting especially fried foods that may further delay gastric emptying.

A soft, or even liquid, diet is preferable until the glossitis disappears. Tart and spicy foods should especially be avoided. (See Soft Diet, page 466 and Full-Fluid Diet, page 468.) Supplementation with ascorbic acid is essential if citrus fruits and other rich sources of the vitamin are not ingested. One practical way to supplement the usual diet is to use high-protein high-calorie beverages two or three times daily. They may be prepared from milk, nonfat dry milk, and flavorings, or one of several relatively inexpensive proprietary preparations may be used.

Folic Acid Deficiency

This is probably the most common vitamin deficiency in the United States[20] and is observed in a variety of circumstances.

Elderly patients. A high incidence of folic acid deficiency has been noted in elderly patients, correlated with a poor intake of milk, fresh fruits, and vegetables.[21] The dietary fault results from lack of knowledge concerning the needs for foods in later life, insufficient income to purchase the essential foods, and organic diseases that interfere with food intake and further aggravate the deficiency. Malignancies, malabsorption, loss of blood, and certain drug therapies also reduce the serum folate levels. Additional folate therapy is recommended especially during acute stages of illness, but the blood levels of vitamin B-12 should also be monitored.

Pregnancy. Megaloblastic anemia occurs with lesser frequency than iron-deficiency anemia. It is usually caused by inadequate diet and is corrected by folic acid therapy.

Infancy. Macrocytic anemia in babies is more frequent in those born to mothers who also have a folic acid deficiency. Anemia is present in infants who have scurvy, because lack of ascorbic acid reduces the conversion of folic acid to its active form folinic acid.

Disorders of absorption. Macrocytic anemia, often severe in tropical sprue, improves dramatically with folic acid therapy. Some improvement is often seen in the anemia of nontropical sprue and celiac disease with folic acid therapy. (See Chapter 33.)

Dietary Considerations Folic acid therapy brings about rapid remission of symptoms. Nevertheless, most patients will benefit from improvement in diet. Guidance in selection of economical sources of the vitamin whould be given. Liver and dark green leafy vegetables are excellent sources. Lean beef, eggs, peanut butter, and whole-grain products provide moderate amounts. For some, instruction in proper cooking methods is desirable since the vitamin is easily destroyed in cooking.

Sickle Cell Anemia

This is a hemolytic anemia of genetic origin occurring primarily in blacks. An abnormal hemoglobin causes the red cells to assume a crescent or sickle shape when deoxygenated. The distorted shape of the red cells prevents their passage through capillaries and leads to thrombosis and infarction. The sickle cells have a shortened life span, and the individual becomes anemic because the red cells are destroyed more quickly than they can be replaced. In the United States, about 1 in 10 blacks are heterozygotes (carry one defective gene) for the sickle cell trait; these individuals usually do not have clinical manifestations.

Sickle cell crises occur periodically following even minor infections and are accompanied by severe bone pain, abdominal tenderness, fever, and so on. The frequency and severity of crises decrease as the child grows older. In older patients degenerative changes are seen in the retina, lungs, heart, kidneys, liver and spleen, bone, brain, and other tissues.

Dietary Considerations Although nutritional requirements for the child with sickle cell disease are the same as for any growing child, careful attention should be given to providing adequate calories and protein. Intakes of iron and folic acid may be less than desirable. The parents should be encouraged to have available foods enjoyed by the child which are good sources of these nutrients. Liquids may be preferred during crises. Recommendations made for older children and adults should include those considerations indicated in the sections on dietary counseling in iron and folic acid deficiencies.

Problems and Review

1. What nutrients are essential for the production of hemoglobin and red blood cells?
2. What are some of the etiologic agents that cause anemia? Which anemias originate because of a faulty diet? Which anemias may be classified as secondary nutritional deficiencies?
3. What are the laboratory findings and clinical symptoms of iron-deficiency anemia? Which groups are especially vulnerable?
4. What factors may interfere with the efficient use of iron in the body? Why is a so-called "high-iron" diet impractical in the treatment of iron-deficiency anemia?
5. What iron preparations are commonly provided for patients with iron-deficiency anemia? What dietary modification may be indicated?

6. List important steps that can be taken to prevent iron-deficiency anemia; folic-acid-deficiency anemia.
7. What problems may be encountered in the dietary intake by patients with pernicious anemia? How can these be controlled?
8. *Problem.* Plan a diet for a young woman who has iron-deficiency anemia to include 80 gm protein, 15 mg iron, and not more than 2,000 kcal.

Cited References

1. Garn, S. M. et al.: "The Magnitude and the Implications of Apparent Race Differences in Hemoglobin Values," *Am. J. Clin. Nutr.*, **28**:563–68, 1975.
2. Committee on Iron Deficiency, Council on Foods and Nutrition: "Iron Deficiency in the United States," *JAMA*, **203**:407–14, 1968.
3. Stebbins, R., and Bertino, J. R.: "Megaloblastic Anemia Produced by Drugs," *Clin. Haemat.*, **5**:619–30, 1976.
4. Shojania, A. M., and Hornady, G. J.: "Oral Contraceptives and Folate Absorption," *J. Lab. Clin. Med.*, **82**:869–75, 1973.
5. Gardner, G. W. et al.: "Physical Work Capacity and Metabolic Stress in Subjects with Iron-Deficiency Anemia," *Am. J. Clin. Nutr.*, **30**:910–17, 1977.
6. FAO/WHO Expert Group: *Requirements of Ascorbic Acid, Vitamin D, Vitamin B_{12}, Folate and Iron. WHO Tech. Rep. Series* No. 452, Geneva, 1970.
7. Brunning, R. D.: "Differential Diagnosis of Anemia," *Geriatrics*, **29**:52–60, February 1974.
8. "Highlights from the Ten-State Nutrition Survey," *Nutr. Today*, **7**:4–11, July–August 1972.
9. Abraham, S. et al.: *Preliminary Findings of the First Health and Nutrition Examination Survey, United States, 1971–1972: Dietary Intake and Biochemical Findings.* Pub. (HRA) 74–1219–1. U.S. Public Health Service, Department of Health, Education, and Welfare, Health Services Administration, Rockville, Md., 1974.
10. Pisciotta, A. V.: "The Anemic Patient," *Am. Fam. Physician*, **18**:144–52, November 1978.
11. Fried, W.: "Hematologic Complications of Chronic Renal Failure," *Med. Clin. North Am.*, **62**:1363–79, 1978.
12. Committee on Nutrition: "Iron Supplementation for Infants," *Pediatrics*, **58**:765–68, 1976.
13. Committee on Nutrition: "On the Feeding of Supplemental Foods to Infants," *Pediatrics*, **65**:1178–81, 1980.
14. Dallman, P. R. et al.: "Iron Deficiency in Infancy and Childhood," *Am. J. Clin. Nutr.*, **33**:86–118, 1980.
15. Picciano, M. F., and Deering, R. H.: "The Influence of Feeding Regimens on Iron Status During Infancy," *Am. J. Clin. Nutr.*, **33**:746–53, 1980.
16. Wilson, J. F. et al.: "Studies on Iron Metabolism. V. Further Observations on Cow's Milk-Induced Gastrointestinal Bleeding in Infants with Iron-Deficiency Anemia," *J. Pediatr.*, **84**:335–44, 1974.
17. Carmel, R., and Johnson, C. S.: "Early Age at Onset and Increased Frequency of Intrinsic Factor-Antibodies in Black Women," *New Engl. J. Med.*, **298**:647–50, 1978.
18. Elsborg, L., and Mosbech, J.: "Pernicious Anemia as a Risk Factor in Gastric Cancer," *Acta Med. Scand.*, **206**:315–18, 1979.
19. Berlin, R. et al.: "Vitamin B_{12} Body Stores During Oral and Parenteral Treatment of Pernicious Anemia," *Acta Med. Scand.*, **204**:81–84, 1978.
20. Bleich, H. L., and Boro, E. S.: "Folate Absorption and Malabsorption," *New Engl. J. Med.*, **293**:1303–8, 1975.

21. Meindok, H., and Dvorsky, R.: "Serum Folate and Vitamin B_{12} Levels in the Elderly," *J. Am. Geriatr. Soc.,* **18**:317–26, 1970.

Additional References

ADLER, S. S.: "Anemia in the Aged: Causes and Considerations," *Geriatrics,* **35**:49–59, April 1980.
DUFFY, T. P.: "Anemia in Adolescence," *Med. Clin. North Am.,* **59**:1481–88, 1975.
GREEN, J. B.: "Macrocytic Anemias," *Postgrad. Med.,* **61**:155–61, June 1977.
MCCURDY, P. R.: "Microcytic Hypochromic Anemias," *Postgrad. Med.,* **61**:147–51, June 1977.
MUSS, H. B., and WHITE, D. R.: "Iron-Deficiency Anemia in Adults," *Am. Fam. Physician,* **17**:174–85, February 1978.
OSKI, F. A., and STOCKMAN, J. A.: "Anemia Due to Inadequate Iron Sources or Poor Iron Utilization," *Pediatr. Clin. North Am.,* **27**:237–52, 1980.
SEARS, D. A.: "The Morbidity of Sickle Cell Trait. A Review of the Literature," *Am. J. Med.,* **64**:1021–36, 1978.
VICHINSKY, E. P., and LUBIN, B. H.: "Sickle Cell Anemia and Related Hemoglobinopathies," *Pediatr. Clin. North Am.,* **27**:429–47, 1980.

31 Diet in Diseases of the Esophagus, Stomach, and Duodenum:

BLAND FIBER-RESTRICTED DIET IN THREE STAGES

APPROXIMATELY 10 per cent of the United States population, or some 18 million persons, have chronic digestive disease. These diseases account for about 15 per cent of all absences from work in the 17-to-64-year-old age group, thus representing an important economic loss to both employers and employees.[1]

Modified diets are commonly prescribed for many digestive diseases, including hiatal hernia, peptic ulcer, gastritis, diarrhea, constipation, malabsorption syndrome, cirrhosis of the liver, cholecystitis, and pancreatitis, among others. Much controversy exists over the role of diet in the treatment of gastrointestinal disturbances. In certain conditions there is a physiologic basis for dietary modification; in others, a sound rationale is lacking and diets traditionally used are of unproven value. For the latter more objective evidence is needed before sound conclusions can be reached in regard to beneficial effects of dietary modification.

Diagnostic Tests in Gastrointestinal Disease

Disorders of the gastrointestinal tract are classified as *functional* or *organic* in nature. Functional disturbances involve no alterations in structure. In organic diseases, on the other hand, pathologic lesions are seen in tissue, as in ulcers or carcinoma. Both types of disorders are characterized by changes in secretory activity and motility. A number of factors including diet are believed to influence these changes. (See Table 31–1.)

Studies of motility and secretion, together with radiologic evidence and, in some instances, biopsy specimens of the affected mucosa, are used in the diagnosis of gastrointestinal disease.

Measurement of Motility Fluoroscopic and x-ray examinations are widely used to determine the emptying time and motility of the intestinal tract, and to locate the site of the disturbance. Following an overnight fast the patient is given a "barium swallow" consisting of a pint of buttermilk or malted milk in which barium sulfate has been mixed. The progress of this opaque "meal" along the intestinal tract can then be visualized by means of fluoroscopy. X-rays taken before and after the meal are studied for filling defects and other abnormalities. (See Figure 31–1.)

In GASTRIC ATONY, due to lack of normal muscle tone of the stomach, contractions are not of sufficient strength to move the food mass out of the stomach at a normal rate. Larger pieces or fragments of food are not adequately disintegrated and mixed with the stomach juices.

Increased action of the musculature of the stomach and intestine is known as HYPERPERISTALSIS. It may be brought on by excessive amounts of fibrous foods, psychological factors such as worry or fear, or nervous stimulation.

Measurement of Gastric Acidity Tests of gastric secretory function per se are of limited diagnostic value and are most useful in patients in whom a lesion has been demonstrated by x-ray or gastroscopy.

Various test meals were formerly used to stimulate gastric secretion. At present, drugs such as caffeine, histamine, or hista-

Table 31-1. **Factors That Modify Acid Secretion and Gastrointestinal Motility and Tone**

Increased Flow of Acid and Enzyme Production	Decreased Flow of Acid and Enzyme Production
1. Chemical stimulation—meat extractives, seasonings, certain spices, alcohol, acid foods	1. Large amounts of fat, especially as fried foods, pastries, nuts, etc.
2. Attractive, appetizing, well-liked foods	2. Large meals
3. State of happiness and contentment	3. Poor mastication of food
4. Pleasant surroundings for meals	4. Foods of poor appearance, flavor, or texture
	5. Foods acutely disliked
	6. Worry, anger, fear, pain*
Increased Tone and Motility	**Decreased Tone and Motility**
1. Warm foods	1. Cold foods
2. Liquid and soft foods	2. Dry, solid foods
3. Fibrous foods, as in certain fruits and vegetables	3. Low-fiber foods
4. High-carbohydrate low-fat intake	4. High-fat intake, especially as fried foods, pastries, etc.
5. Seasonings; concentrated sweets	5. Vitamin B complex deficiency, especially thiamin
6. Fear, anger, worry, nervous tension	6. Sedentary habits
	7. Fatigue
	8. Worry, anger, fear, pain

*In certain individuals these emotional disturbances may stimulate the flow of gastric juice.

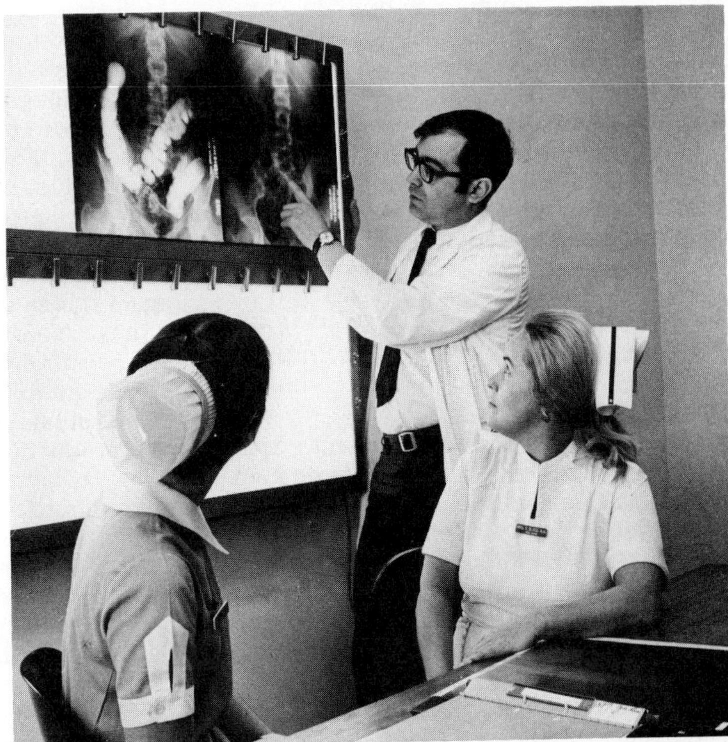

Figure 31–1. Patient care conference. The physician points out the site of intestinal lesion to nurse and student nurse. (Courtesy, Yale–New Haven Medical Center.)

log, which are vigorous stimulants to gastric secretion, are used to determine the amount of acid produced.

Basal acid secretion is measured by collecting gastric juice for a timed period after an overnight fast. Pharmacologic agents such as histamine are then administered to stimulate maximal acid secretion, and collections of gastric juice are again made for a specified period. Results are reported in terms of maximal acid output or peak acid output. Excess acid secretion is known as HYPERCHLORHYDRIA and is often accompanied by gastric distress. It may be associated with emotional or nervous upsets, or it may accompany organic disease such as peptic ulcer or cholecystitis.

HYPOCHLORHYDRIA denotes a diminished amount of free acid and may be present indefinitely in otherwise healthy persons. The cause should be determined, if possible, since hypochlorhydria also accompanies diseases such as pernicious anemia and is a common finding in sprue, chronic gastritis, and pellagra. It occurs occasionally in cancer, nephritis, cholecystitis, and diabetes. In ACHLORHYDRIA no free acid is present although there is some peptic activity; this finding suggests pernicious anemia and malignant gastric ulcer. ACHYLIA GASTRICA refers to the absence of both acid and enzyme activity.

General Dietary Considerations in Diseases of the Gastrointestinal Tract

Factors in Dietary Management Many dietary recommendations have been made for the management of gastrointestinal diseases; yet actual knowledge of the specific effects of various foods on the digestive tract is rather limited. Any proposed dietary modifications should take into consideration the possible effects of ingested food upon (1) the secretory activity of the stomach, small intestine, pancreas, liver, and gallbladder; (2) motility of the tract; (3) the bacterial flora; (4) the comfort and ease of digestion; and (5) the maintenance and repair of the mucosal structures. In addition, some disorders interfere with the completeness of digestion or the absorption of one or more nutrients so that the nutrient intake must be modified in order to meet the net requirements of the body.

Influence of Foods on Gastric Acidity Most foods have a pH between 5 and 7, thus are considerably less acid than gastric juice. No food is sufficiently acid to have an adverse effect on a gastric lesion, although citrus juices and fruits might cause some discomfort to a lesion of the mouth, esophagus, or the achlorhydric stomach.

Gastric secretion is initiated by the sight, smell, and taste of food. As food enters the stomach, the secretion continues and reaches its height sometime later. Protein foods stimulate more acid secretion than carbohydrates and fats.

Protein foods initially have a temporary buffering effect; hence there is less free acid immediately available to erode tissue when protein is fed. Milk has some buffering effect, although this may be outweighed by its ability to stimulate acid secretion. Nevertheless, most patients with active peptic ulcer have progressed well on diets in which frequent milk feedings were used for their neutralizing effect. Regardless of buffering activity, the amount of free acid again is high within ½ to 2 hours following a meal. No diet alone will maintain a 24-hour neutralization of gastric contents.

Fats inhibit gastric secretion. The entrance of fats into the duodenum stimulates the production of enterogastrone, a hormone, which retards gastric secretion and delays gastric emptying.

Meat extractives, tannins, caffeine, and alcohol are well known for their effect in stimulating the flow of acid. Chili powder, cloves, mustard seeds, nutmeg, and black pepper have been shown to be irritating to the gastric mucosa;[2] thus, these spices should be used with discretion by persons with ulcer disease. Black pepper is usually excluded from diets used in treatment of ulcers. Most other commonly used spices exert no harmful effects and need not be contraindicated.

Influence of Foods on Motility The rate of gastric emptying is related to the caloric density of the food given and is independent of the volume given; that is, isocaloric amounts of carbohydrate and triglyceride are equally effective in slowing gastric emptying.[3] This finding is consistent with the long-held belief that foods high in fiber increase peristaltic action, and low-fiber foods reduce such motility.

Fiber and Residue Defined DIETARY FIBER is defined as the plant polysaccharides resistant to hydrolysis by the digestive enzymes in the human intestinal tract. It includes (1) structural polysaccharides of the plant cell wall such as cellulose and hemicellulose, and lignin, a noncarbohydrate structural material; and (2) nonstructural polysaccharides such as pectins, gums, and mucilages. These components of dietary fiber are discussed in more detail in Chapter 5.

Tables of food composition commonly list values for *crude* fiber in foods. Crude fiber comprises only one fifth to one half of the total dietary fiber. (See Table 31–2.) Thus, such tables should not be relied upon for fiber content of foods. Values for dietary fiber are shown in Table A-3.

The effects of fiber on the intestinal tract vary with the type of fiber and its components. These were discussed in Chapter 5. In general, foods containing large amounts of cellulose and hemicellulose absorb water, thereby decreasing (shortening) transit time, and increasing both fecal weight and the number of stools. Lignin adsorbs organic materials such as bile acids and increases the rate at which they are excreted. Pectin, on the other hand, increases excretion of fecal lipids and bile acids, but does not significantly influence fecal weight or transit time.[4,5] Much of the dietary fiber is degraded by intestinal bacteria to volatile fatty acids such as acetic, proprionic, and butyric acids. These stimulate intestinal motility and act as a mild cathartic.[6]

RESIDUE refers to the volume of materials remaining after the digestive processes are completed, and includes indigestible fiber, bacterial residues, and desquamated cells from the mucosa. Foods high in dietary fiber are considered to be high-residue foods.

Table 31–2. **Comparison of Crude Fiber and Dietary Fiber Content in Some Common Foods.***

	Crude Fiber	Total Dietary Fiber
	(gm per 100 gm edible portion)	
Apple without skin	0.6	1.42
Banana	0.5	1.75
Peach, fresh	0.6	2.28
Lettuce	0.6	1.53
Tomato, fresh	0.5	1.40
Green beans, boiled	1.0	3.35
Peas, garden canned	2.3	6.28
All-bran cereal	7.8	26.70
Cornflakes	0.7	11.00
Puffed wheat	2.0	15.41
White bread	0.2	2.72
Wholewheat bread	1.6	8.50

*Adapted from USDA Handbook No. 8, *Composition of Foods,* 1963, and *Am. J. Clin. Nutr.,* **31**: S281–S284, 1978.

Influence of Foods on Bacterial Flora Experimental studies indicate that increased dietary fiber does not significantly alter the concentration or composition of major groups of fecal bacteria. However, the total output of fecal bacteria is increased as dietary fiber increases.[7]

Foods and Their Effect on Lesions Fibrous foods have often been omitted from diets for diseases of the gastrointestinal tract in the belief that they might mechanically injure or retard the healing of a lesion such as an ulcer. However, it is unlikely that fibrous foods, when sufficiently chewed, would be injurious to a peptic ulcer. Patients should be instructed to chew foods properly. Puréeing of foods is not necessary unless the teeth are poor or absent. The individual can best determine tolerance for specific foods by trial and error.

Influence of Foods upon Digestive Comfort Ingestion of certain foods has long been associated with symptoms of belching, distension, epigastric distress, flatulence, constipation, or diarrhea in some persons with digestive disorders. Among these foods are baked beans, cabbage, fried foods, onions, and spicy foods. Tolerance to these and other foods is a highly individual matter. Not all patients react to foods in the same way, nor does the same patient always react to a specific food in the same way.

Traditional Diets Clinicians who favor a conservative approach to the dietary management of gastrointestinal disease generally use diets based on recommendations made early in the century for treatment of peptic ulcer by Sippy (1915) and Meulengracht (1935).[8,9] Such diets are based on the principle that the presence of some food in the stomach at all times will dilute and neutralize excess acid and consequently lessen pain. In most of these, milk forms the basis of the diet with small feedings of "bland" foods being given at frequent intervals. Generally speaking, foods allowed are limited to those considered to be *chemically, mechanically,* and *thermally* nonirritating; other foods are rigidly excluded.

Foods believed to be *chemically* irritating because of their stimulatory effect on gastric secretion include meat extractives, caffeine, alcohol, citrus fruits and juices, and some spicy foods. (See page 521.) *Mechanically* irritating foods include those with indigestible carbohydrate, such as whole grains and most raw fruits and vegetables. Foods believed to be *thermally* irritating are those ordinarily served at extremes of temperature, such as very hot or iced liquids. In addition, certain foods traditionally forbidden include strongly flavored vegetables (Brussels sprouts, cabbage, cauliflower, onions, turnips, and others), baked beans, pork, and fried foods. Restriction of these foods is based on subjective evidence from patients who experienced distress following ingestion of these items.

Over the years, the practice of recommending or restricting certain foods in the management of ulcer disease has been carried over to treatment of other gastrointestinal disorders as well. Foods customarily allowed are described as bland, nonirritating, smooth, low fiber, or nonstimulating; those contraindicated are considered to be distending, gaseous, indigestible, stimulating, and so on. The soft diet, fiber-restricted diet, or stage 3 of the bland diet is appropriate for most gastrointestinal conditions; these diets are all very similar. The details of the soft diet are discussed in Chapter 25. The bland, fiber-restricted diet is on page 529.

Trend to More Liberal Diets Current opinion among liberal clinicians is that strict diets are no longer appropriate for the majority of patients with gastrointestinal disease. Liberalization of foods used in diets for gastrointestinal disease has come about gradually as a result of (1) the realization that many of the dietary recommendations made in these diseases are not backed by scientific evidence; (2) evidence that traditional diets do not influence the rate of healing of ulcers; (3) concern for the nutritional adequacy and patient acceptance of the diets; and (4) availability of potent drugs that are effective in promoting healing of lesions.

Disorders of the Esophagus and Stomach

Esophagitis This is an acute or chronic inflammation of the esophageal wall. *Acute* esophagitis is usually characterized by substernal pain brought on by swallowing. It may be a consequence of upper respiratory infections, extensive burns, prolonged gastric intubation, excessive vomiting, ingestion of poisonous substances such as lye, or diseases such as scarlet fever or diphtheria.

Most cases of *chronic* esophagitis are attributed to a sliding hernia that permits the reflux of gastric juice into the esophagus. Mucosal erosions and narrowing of the lumen occur. The disorder occurs most frequently in persons with high gastric acidity, many of whom have a history of duodenal ulcer.

Symptoms. Heartburn, intermittent at first, but becoming progressively worse, is often the chief complaint in esophagitis. Pain following ingestion of very hot or cold foods and spicy or acid foods and eventual dysphagia occur as the disease progresses.

Treatment. The objectives of therapy are to protect the esophagus, to reduce gastric acidity, and to reduce reflux of gastric contents into the esophagus. Antacid preparations are usually prescribed.

Dietary management consists of weight reduction (see Chapter 27) for obese individuals since excess abdominal fat is believed to increase gastric herniation and reflux. Large meals should be avoided in favor of more frequent small meals. A bland, fiber-restricted diet is desirable for most individuals. (See page 529.)

Hiatus Hernia A common disorder affecting the esophagus is the herniation of a portion of the stomach through the esophageal hiatus of the diaphragm. This disorder, known as HIATAL HERNIA, occurs most frequently in persons over 45 years of age. The incidence is greater in persons of stocky build and in overweight persons. Loss of muscle tone weakens muscles around the diaphragm and increased abdominal pressure helps push the stomach through the diaphragm. Symptoms occur when the herniated portion is irritated or injured or is large enough to affect other organs. Tight garments or belts appear to provoke symptoms and should be avoided. Substernal pain, belching, or hiccoughing occurs following meals or while lying down.

A bland, fiber-restricted diet with between-meal snacks is usually recommended. (See page 529.) Of equal importance are eating small amounts at any one time and omitting food for several hours before bedtime. Weight reduction is essential for obese individuals. (See Chapter 27.)

Esophageal Reflux The lower esophageal sphincter normally maintains a pressure greater than that in the stomach thereby preventing reflux of gastric contents into the esophagus. Incompetence of the sphincter permits postural reflux and may cause esophagitis. Heartburn and dysphagia also occur. Inadequate release of gastrin following a meal, and diseased sphincter muscle have been postulated as causes of the sphincter incompetence.[10] Esophageal reflux is not synonymous with histal hernia although both may occur together.

Diagnostic tests for esophageal reflux include an x-ray series following a barium swallow, an acid perfusion test, esophagoscopy, esophageal biopsy, and measurement of lower esophageal sphincter pressure. In the acid perfusion test, a weak solution of acid is given, alternating with saline, to provoke symptoms of gastroesophageal reflux. A combination of two or more of these tests is often used in the diagnosis.

Factors that decrease lower esophageal sphincter pressure include alcohol, caffeine, chocolate, fatty meals, peppermint, and smoking. Proteins and antacids increase sphincter pressure. Carbohydrates appear to have little effect on sphincter pressure.

Dietary recommendations include a high-protein diet, restriction of fat, avoidance of substances that lower esophageal sphincter pressure and those that might be irritating to an inflamed mucosa, for example, citrus or tomato juice, and frequent small meals.[11] Weight reduction for overweight persons is encouraged. Lying down after meals should be avoided. Other measures include antacid therapy, avoidance of tight clothing, and elevation of the head of the bed.

Achalasia This is a disorder of esophageal motility in which the lower esophageal sphincter fails to relax normally upon swallowing so that food can enter the stomach. Loss or absence of ganglion cells is believed to be involved. The resting lower esophageal pressure is twice the normal level.[12] Long-continued intraesophageal pressure may lead to dilatation above the point of stricture. The primary symptom is dysphagia with possible vomiting and eventual weight loss.

Treatment consists of dilatation of the stricture. Drug therapy is used to lower esophageal sphincter pressure. Dietary considerations include avoidance of excessively hot or iced beverages and any foods that may be irritating to the esophagus. If weight loss has been considerable, increased calories and protein are needed. (See Chapter 28.) Some individuals tolerate several small feedings better than larger ones.

Esophageal obstruction This may result from a number of causes including pressure from adjacent organs, hiatal hernia, scar tissue formation, foreign bodies, diverticula, and neoplasms. Swallowed foods do not progress beyond the point of stricture owing to narrowing of the lumen, and if the condition is untreated, death from starvation follows. Measures to restore the normal passageway include dilatation, irradiation, or surgical intervention, depending on the nature of the obstruction.

Dietary management is the same for obstruction from any cause. Efforts are directed toward providing foods in suitable form and sufficient amounts to meet the patient's needs. In partial obstruction, liquids should be offered with progression to low-fiber foods (see page 529) as tolerated. Small amounts of food at frequent intervals are preferable. When it is not possible or desirable for food to pass through the esophagus, the patient is fed by means of a gastrostomy. Food is administered through a tube inserted directly into the stomach. (See Chapter 36 for characteristics of tube feedings.)

Indigestion Indigestion, or dyspepsia, is a functional or organic disease manifested by symptoms of heartburn, acid regurgitation, epigastric pain, "fullness" or bloating especially after meals, flatulence, nausea, or vomiting.

The majority of cases of indigestion are of functional origin and are usually due to faulty dietary habits or emotional factors. The organic type is associated with diseases affecting the digestive organs; it may also be a symptom of generalized disease as in uremia. Treatment in organic types consists of treating the underlying disease.

Persons with functional dyspepsia need individualized dietary counseling in the essentials of a nutritionally adequate diet. Specific instructions should be given with emphasis on selection of foods from each group in the Daily Food Guide and the importance of regular mealtimes, sufficient time to eat in a relaxed atmosphere, rest after meals, and avoidance of emotional tension.

Gastritis This is an inflammation of the mucosa of the stomach, occurring as an acute or chronic lesion with atrophy or hypertrophy in some persons. Causes are toxins of bacterial or metabolic origin (*Salmonella, Staphylococcus,* uremia, syphilis); irritation of the gastric mucosa by ingestion of ethyl alcohol, certain drugs (digitalis, glucogenic steroids, salicylates, and others), gastric irradiation, heavy metals, strong alkali or acid; or faulty dietary habits, such as excessive intake of highly seasoned foods. The diagnosis of gastritis is based on biopsies of the gastric mucosa.

ACUTE gastritis is characterized by a general inflammatory reaction of the mucosa with hyperemia, edema, and exudation; in more severe cases, erosion of localized areas and hemorrhages occur. Symptoms vary from anorexia, vague epigastric discomfort, or heartburn, to severe vomiting.

Since acute gastritis usually heals within 3 or 4 days, nutritional management is not the primary concern. Treatment is directed toward removal or neutralization of the offending agent by gastric lavage, antibiotics, withholding of food for 24 to 48 hours to allow the stomach to rest, and replacement of water and electrolyte losses due to severe vomiting. After 1 or 2 days small amounts of clear fluids (100 ml per hour) are administered with gradual progression to soft, easily digested foods. (See page 466.)

CHRONIC gastritis is characterized by altered resistance of the gastric mucosal barrier to hydrogen ions. The resulting tissue damage may be induced by bile reflux or salicylates.[13] Recurrent inflammation leads to glandular atrophy and changes in enzyme activities of the gastric mucosal cells. Complete atrophy results in the inability to absorb vitamin B-12 and in pernicious anemia. Symptoms include epigastric distress, nausea, and vomiting. Chronic gastritis is often directly attributed to dietary indiscretion or indirectly to toxic substances; nevertheless, it may also occur in the absence of any known cause. Gastritis may be the cause of persistent symptoms in patients in whom peptic ulcer has seemingly healed.

Dietary treatment of chronic gastritis consists in correcting faulty dietary habits, providing a relaxed atmosphere at mealtime, and emphasizing adequate caloric intake of soft or bland foods. (See page 529.) Arrangement of meals in four or six small feedings is sometimes preferred. Iron supplements may be desirable. Once symptoms have abated, progression to a normal diet may be made.

Peptic Ulcer

The term *peptic ulcer* is used to describe any localized erosion of the mucosal lining of those portions of the alimentary tract that come in contact with gastric juice. The majority of ulcers are found in the duodenum, although they also occur in the esophagus, stomach, or jejunum. Similar symptoms are produced by the ulcer regardless of its location, and response to treatment is essentially the same. The same principles of dietary treatment apply to all regardless of etiology.

Some 3 million persons in the United States suffer from peptic ulcer each year. Of these, 80 per cent have duodenal ulcer and the remainder have gastric ulcers. Within the past decade both hospital admissions and death rates for peptic ulcer have declined markedly in the United States. Nevertheless, the cost in terms of economic losses is over $3 billion annually.[14,15] Males were formerly more likely than females to develop peptic ulcer, but the sex ratio is now nearly equal.

Etiology In spite of extensive literature on the subject, the exact cause of peptic ulcer has not been determined. In duodenal ulcer, hypersecretion of acid is found although tissue resistance is normal. Acid hypersecretion is attributed to an increased number of parietal cells, impaired inhibition of gastrin release, and possibly more rapid gastric emptying with loss of buffering effect.[16] In gastric ulcer, both a back diffusion of hydrogen ions into the mucosa and reflux of bile are believed to be involved. An abnormality in the mucosa permits penetration of hydrogen ions. Drugs such as aspirin and indomethacin (used in rheumatoid arthritis) can alter the gastric mucosal barrier by increasing back diffusion of hydrogen. Bile acids can destroy the gastric mucosal barrier. Reflux of bile acids from the duodenum due to an incompetent pyloric sphincter leads to chronic gastritis and subsequent ulceration. In both gastric and duodenal ulcers, then, the net effect is an excess of acid and pepsin for the amount of local tissue resistance.

Personality type plays a role—highly nervous and emotional individuals seem to be more susceptible to the disease. Anxiety, worry, and strain may cause hypersecretion of acid and hypermotility. A positive family history of recurrent pain is not uncommon.

Symptoms and Clinical Findings Epigastric pain occurring as deep hunger contractions 1 to 3 hours after meals is often the chief complaint. The pain may be described as dull, piercing, burning, or gnawing and is usually relieved by the taking of food or alkalies. The basis for the pain may be the action of unneutralized hydrochloric acid on exposed nerve fibers at the site of the ulcer. Pain is also associated with hypermotility of the stomach or gastric distention following ingestion of large amounts of food or liquids.

Low plasma protein levels are often present and delay rapid and complete healing of the ulcer. Weight loss and iron-deficiency anemia are common. The intake of iron, ascorbic acid, and the B-complex vitamins, particularly thiamin, may be less than desirable because of self-imposed limitation of leafy green vegetables and other food sources of these nutrients. (See Chapters 8, 11, and 12.)

In some instances, hemorrhage is the first indication of an ulcer and requires surgical intervention. Other complications such as intractability, obstruction, perforation, and carcinoma of gastric ulcer are treated surgically.

Rationale for Treatment Individualized attention to the whole person rather than to the ulcer per se is extremely important in the management of persons with ulcer disease. The patient must be taught to accept responsibility for progress since medical and dietary therapies produce only symptomatic improvement. In general, treatment consists of drugs, rest, and diet therapy.

Drugs. A histamine hydrogen receptor antagonist, cimetidine, inhibits basal and stimulated acid secretion and increases the rate of ulcer healing.[17] *Antacid* preparations are prescribed to neutalize excess acid, but usual dosages do not influence the rate of healing. *Anticholinergic* drugs inhibit acid secretion, and *antispasmodics* delay gastric emptying. Nutritional side effects of these drugs are listed in Table 24–1.

Rest. Good physical and mental hygiene is basic if the person is to learn to cope with his or her problems constructively. Mental and physical rest is important; modification of living and work habits is needed when overwork and physical stress cause exacerbations of the disease. Control of emotional stress is equally important.

Diet. The development of potent drugs, such as cimetidine, has renewed the controversy over the role of diet in treatment of peptic ulcer. Most clinicians agree that diet does not influence the rate of healing of an ulcer, that regularity of mealtimes is essential, and that individualization of the diet is important. On other aspects of the diet there is less agreement. Liberal proponents favor three meals a day with few food restrictions. Frequent feedings are discouraged because of their repeated stimulation of acid.[16,18] A bedtime snack, in particular, is not recommended because of its stimulatory effect on acid secretion during the night.[19] An intermediate approach recommends frequent feedings and fiber restriction. Conservatives favor a strict diet such as that described in the section on traditional diets on page 524.

For the majority of patients hospitalized for an active peptic ulcer, some type of bland diet is commonly used, although there is much variation in nomenclature and composition of these diets. Milk is a very important part of most of these diets. Individualization of the diet is essential, especially since large amounts of milk may produce symptoms in patients with lactose malabsorption. (See Chapter 33.) The diet must be nutritionally adequate in order to correct any preexisting deficiencies and to promote healing. In some instances, intakes of nutrients in excess of the recommended dietary allowances are desirable, with emphasis on high quality protein, ascorbic acid and iron. The student is encouraged to compare the three stages of the bland fiber-restricted diet listed here.

Bland Fiber-Restricted Diet in Three Stages

Characteristics and General Rules

The stages of diet are set up for gradual progression in quantity of food eaten at a meal, in fiber content, and in selection of foods.

The selection of foods includes those mild in flavor, and which infrequently bring forth complaints of intolerance. The lists should not be considered as restrictive, inasmuch as food tolerance is a highly individual matter. Additions or subtractions should be made according to individual need.

For many patients with peptic ulcer, frequent feedings are desirable. The six-meal sample menus listed here could be arranged for 2-hourly feedings of smaller size, if the physician believes this to be necessary.

Food Selection for Three Stages of Diet

Stages I and II	Stage III
	All foods of stages I and II plus the following:
Beverages—milk and fruit juices	*Beverages*—decaffeinated coffee; 1 cup regular coffee with half milk, if desired; weak tea
Breads—enriched white bread or toast; saltines; soda crackers; Melba toast; zwieback	*Breads*—rye without seeds; fine whole-wheat
Cereals—cornflakes, cornmeal, farina, hominy grits, oatmeal, Puffed Rice, rice flakes; macaroni, noodles, rice, spaghetti	*Cereals*—all except coarse bran
Cheese—mild American in sauces; cream; cottage	*Cheeses*—all
Desserts—plain cake and cookies; custard; fruit whip; gelatin; plain ice cream; bread, cornstarch, rice, or tapioca puddings without raisins or nuts	
Eggs—any way except fried	*Eggs*—including fried
Fats—butter, cream, margarine, smooth peanut butter, cooking fat, vegetable oils	*Fats*—mayonnaise and salad dressings
Fruits—fruit juices; avocado, banana, grapefruit and orange sections; baked apple without skin, applesauce; canned apricots, cherries, peaches, pears	*Fruits*—raw apple, cherries, peaches, pears, plums; stewed apricots and prunes
Meat—tender or ground. Baked, broiled, creamed, roasted, stewed: beef, chicken, fish, lamb, liver, pork, sweetbreads, turkey, veal	

Stages I and II

Milk—in all forms

Seasonings—salt, sugar, flavoring extracts

Soups—cream

Vegetables—cooked; asparagus tips, green and wax beans, beets, carrots, white potato, winter squash, spinach, sweet potato

Stage III

Seasonings—allspice, cinnamon, mace, paprika, sage, thyme

Soups—fish chowders

Vegetables—lettuce and other tender salad greens; celery; tomatoes; any others as tolerated

Meal Patterns for Stages I and II

Stage I

(10–12 oz per meal)

On Awaking

Milk—8 oz

Breakfast

Cereal—4 oz

Milk—4 oz

Sugar

Egg—1

White toast—1 slice

Butter or margarine

Midmorning

Milk beverage—8 oz

Crackers, custard, plain pudding, gelatin—3 oz

Luncheon

Cream soup—4 oz

Crackers—2

Egg—1; or mild cheese—1 oz; or tender meat—1 oz

White bread or toast—1 slice

Butter or margarine

Dessert—3 to 4 oz

Citrus juice—3 oz

Midafternoon

Milk beverage—8 oz

Crackers, custard, plain pudding, gelatin—3 oz

Dinner

Egg, soft cheese, or tender meat—1 oz

Potato or substitute—3 oz

Toast or bread—1 slice

Butter or margarine

Fruit—3 oz

Milk or cream soup—4 oz

Stage II

(approximately 12–16 oz)

Milk—8 oz

Cooked or dry cereal

Milk

Sugar

Egg

Enriched toast

Butter or margarine

Fruit juice or fruit

Milk beverage—8 oz

Crackers, custard, plain pudding, gelatin

Cream soup

Crackers

Meat, fish, poultry, eggs, or cheese—2 to 3 oz

Potato or substitute

White bread or toast

Butter or margarine

Dessert

Fruit

Milk

Milk beverage or small meat sandwich

Plain dessert

Meat, fish, poultry, eggs, or cheese—3 oz

Potato or substitute

Cooked vegetable

Bread or roll

Butter or margarine

Fruit or dessert

Milk

Stage I

EVENING
Milk beverage—8 oz
Crackers or dessert—3 oz

Stage II

Milk beverage or small meat sandwich
Crackers or plain dessert

A Typical Day's Menu for Stage III

BREAKFAST
Stewed apricots
Oatmeal with milk and sugar
Soft-cooked egg
Enriched toast with butter
Coffee with half milk—1 cup

MIDMORNING
Milk—8 oz
Saltines—4

LUNCHEON
Cream of asparagus soup
Baked rice with cheese
Peas with butter
Lettuce and sliced tomatoes with mayonnaise
Rye bread and butter
Vanilla ice cream
Milk

MIDAFTERNOON
Chicken sandwich
Gelatin dessert

DINNER
Broiled lamb chop
Mashed potato
Diced buttered beets
Dinner roll with butter
Sliced peaches (fresh, frozen, or canned)
Milk

EVENING NOURISHMENT
Malted milk
Sugar cookies

Dietary Counseling

According to one survey, about half the patients with peptic ulcer who are given dietary instructions prior to discharge from the hospital or as outpatients are instructed on a bland diet; the remainder on a regular or modified regular diet.[18] Regardless of the type of diet used, emphasis should be on positive rather than negative aspects of the diet. The patient needs to know which foods are needed for a nutritionally adequate diet and the importance of including these daily. He or she should be taught to select an essentially normal diet from a wide variety of foods, omitting those foods known to be distressing to the patient. Moderate use of seasonings is permitted and may greatly enhance the flavor of foods. The patient should be instructed to establish regularity of mealtimes, to include between-meal snacks—preferably of some protein foods—and to use moderation in amounts eaten. If the diet to be used at home is planned with the patient, giving consideration to his or her cultural pattern, the patient is more likely to follow recommendations made. Meals eaten in restaurants should pose no particular problems if the individual uses good judgment in food selection.

Dietitians or nurses should stress the importance of eating meals in a relaxed atmosphere with a happy frame of mind and advise the patient to try to forget personal or family problems while eating. A short rest before and after meals may be conducive to greater enjoyment of meals.

Ulcers frequently recur even after complete healing is believed to have taken place. To prevent recurrence of symptoms prompt treatment is advisable following great stress. In periods of great emotional strain careful compliance with medical therapy is especially important. Taking of food every few hours may be desirable.

Modification of Diet in Bleeding Ulcer The degree of dietary modification in bleeding ulcer depends on the peculiarities of the individual case. In severe hemorrhage, it is customary to give no food until the bleeding has been controlled and the patient's condition is stabilized. If hemorrhage is not severe, and if nausea and vomiting are not a problem, the patient may desire food and tolerate it well. In many hospitals initial dietary treatment consists of milk alternated at 2-hour intervals with small feedings of easily digested foods, such as egg, custards or simple puddings, toast, crackers, and tender cooked fruits and vegetables. Gradual progression in amounts and types of foods is made as the patient improves.

Problems and Review

1. List some of the nutritional disturbances which may develop when the stomach and intestinal tract are impaired.
2. Miss B. is a 28-year-old file clerk who is about 20 pounds overweight and has a hiatal hernia. Her physician has recommended a diet with small frequent feedings for her but she is afraid she will gain weight if she follows the diet. What suggestions could you offer to assist her in planning her diet?
3. Mrs. D. is a 33-year-old housewife who complains of indigestion. Name five dietary factors which could lead to development of this condition. What recommendations would you make concerning her diet?
4. Mrs. G. and Mrs. F. are discussing their husbands' recent hospitalizations for peptic ulcer. Mr. G.'s physician recommended a traditional bland diet; Mr. F. was advised to follow a regular diet.
   a. In what respects would you expect their diets to be similar? How would you expect them to differ?
   b. Mr. G. will soon return to his teaching position and he plans to carry his lunch to school. Plan a day's menu for him.
   c. List five food combinations suitable for between-meal feedings for Mr. G.
   d. Mr. F. eats lunch in a restaurant. Plan a day's menu for him.
5. Mrs. G. does not understand the reasons for some of the recommendations made concerning her husband's diet. Explain the principle involved in each of the following:
   a. Milk.
   b. Those foods that depress acid secretion.
   c. Foods that are most effective in acid neutralization.
   d. Feedings at 2-hour intervals.
   e. Omission of coffee and tea.
6. Mrs. F. has asked whether it makes any difference what foods her husband eats as long as he takes his medications. What would you tell her in regard to:
   a. Effects of foods on acid secretion.
   b. Effects of foods on acid neutralization.
   c. Effects of foods on motility of the gastrointestinal tract.
7. Mr. F. is concerned that his ulcer will recur when he returns to his job and his very demanding boss. What prophylactic measures can he take to prevent recurrence?

Cited References

1. Almy, T. P. et al.: "Prevalence and Significance of Digestive Disease," *Gastroenterology*, **68**:1351–71, 1975.

2. Schneider, M. A. et al.: "The Effect of Spice Ingestion Upon the Stomach," *Am. J. Gastroenterology,* **26:**722–32, 1956.
3. Hunt, J. N., and Stubbs, D. F.: "The Volume and Energy Content of Meals as Determinants of Gastric Emptying," *J. Physiol.,* **245:**209–25, 1975.
4. Kelsay, J. L.: "A Review of Research on Effects of Fiber Intake on Man," *Am. J. Clin. Nutr.,* **31:**142–59, 1978.
5. Stasse-Wolthuis, M. et al.: "Influence of Dietary Fiber from Vegetables and Fruits, Bran or Citrus Pectin on Serum Lipids, Fecal Lipids, and Colonic Function," *Am. J. Clin. Nutr.,* **33:**1745–56, 1980.
6. Achord, J. L.: "Irritable Bowel Syndrome and Dietary Fiber," *J. Am. Diet. Assoc.,* **75:**452–53, 1979.
7. Bornside, G. H.: "Stability of Human Fecal Flora," *Am. J. Clin. Nutr.,* **31:**S141–S144, 1978.
8. Sippy, B. W.: "Gastric and Duodenal Ulcers. Medical Care by an Efficient Removal of Gastric Juice Corrosion," *JAMA,* **64:**1625–30, 1915.
9. Meulengracht, E.: "Treatment of Haematemesis and Melaena with Food," *Lancet,* **2:**1220–22, 1935.
10. Cohen, S., and Snape, W. J.: "The Pathophysiology and Treatment of Gastroesophageal Reflux Disease," *Arch. Intern. Med.,* **138:**1398–1401, 1978.
11. Castell, D. O.: "Medical Measures that Influence the Gastroesophageal Junction," *South. Med. J.,* **71:** (Suppl.) 26–28, January 1978.
12. Cohen, S.: "Motor Disorders of the Esophagus," *New Engl. J. Med.,* **301:**184–92, 1979.
13. Ivey, K. J.: "Gastritis," *Med. Clin. North Am.,* **58:**1289–1304, 1974.
14. Elashoff, J. D., and Grossman, M. I.: "Trends in Hospital Admissions and Death Rates for Peptic Ulcer in the United States from 1970 to 1978," *Gastroenterology,* **78:**280–85, 1980.
15. Almy, T. P.: "Clinical Strategy in Peptic Ulcer," *Hosp. Practice,* **14:**11 ff., November 1979.
16. Chapman, M. L.: "Peptic Ulcer: A Medical Perspective," *Med. Clin. North Am.,* **62:**39–51, 1978.
17. Binder, H. J., et al.: "Cimetidine in the Treatment of Duodenal Ulcer. A Multi-Center Double Blind Study," *Gastroenterology,* **74:**380–88, 1978.
18. Welsh, J. D.: "Diet Therapy of Peptic Ulcer Disease," *Gastroenterology,* **72:**740–45, 1977.
19. Richardson, C. T.: "Pharmacotherapy: A Perspective," *South. Med. J.,* **72:**260–62, 1979.

Additional References

American Dietetic Association: "Position Paper on Bland Diet in the Treatment of Chronic Duodenal Ulcer Disease," *J. Am. Diet. Assoc.,* **59:**244–45, 1971.

BRUNNER, L. S.: "What to Do (And What to Teach) Your Patient About Peptic Ulcer," *Nursing,* **6:**27–34, November 1976.

CHERNOW, B., and CASTELL, D. O.: "Diet and Heartburn," *JAMA,* **241:**2307–8, 1979.

EASTWOOD, M. A., and KAY, R. M.: "An Hypothesis for the Action of Dietary Fiber Along the Gastrointestinal Tract," *Am. J. Clin. Nutr.,* **32:**364–67, 1979.

GRIFFIN, J. W., and TOLLISON, J. W.: "Dysphagia," *Am. Fam. Physician,* **22:**154–60, November 1980.

KELSAY, J. L. et al.: "Effect of Fiber from Fruits and Vegetables on Metabolic Responses of Human Subjects. I. Bowel Transit Time, Number of Defecations, Fecal Weight,

Urinary Excretions of Energy and Nitrogen and Apparent Digestibilities of Energy, Nitrogen, and Fat," *Am. J. Clin. Nutr.*, **31**:1149–53, 1978.

LEVIN, B., and HORWITZ, D.: "Dietary Fiber," *Med. Clin. North Am.*, **63**:1043–55, 1979.

SAMBORSKY, V.: "Drug Therapy for Peptic Ulcer," *Am. J. Nurs.*, **78**:2064–66, 1978.

SANDSTEAD, H. H. et al.: "Influence of Dietary Fiber on Trace Element Balance," *Am. J. Clin. Nutr.*, **31**:S180–S184, 1980.

SPILLER, G. A., and KAY, R. M.: "Recommendations and Conclusions of the Dietary Fiber Workshop of the XI International Congress of Nutrition, Rio de Janeiro, 1978," *Am. J. Clin. Nutr.*, **32**:2102–3, 1979.

Diet in Disturbances of the Small Intestine and Colon 32

VERY LOW RESIDUE DIET; HIGH-FIBER DIET

THE functions of the small intestine may be unfavorably influenced by diseases affecting the tract itself or those organs closely related to the digestive process—the liver, gallbladder, and pancreas. In addition, many seemingly unrelated pathologic conditions to be discussed in chapters that follow have profound effects on the functioning of the gastrointestinal tract, for example, renal diseases. Depending upon the nature of the disease, there may be disturbances in motility, adequacy of enzyme production or release, hydrolytic activity, integrity of the mucosal surfaces, transport mechanisms, and so on. Any of these abnormalities interferes with the efficiency and completeness of absorption and hence the nutritional status of the individual. This chapter includes a discussion of alterations in bowel motility and inflammatory diseases of the mucosa. The malabsorption syndrome will be discussed in Chapter 33 and diseases of the liver, gallbladder, and pancreas in Chapter 34.

Alterations in Bowel Motility

Diarrhea This is the passage of stools with increased frequency, fluidity, or volume compared to the usual for a given individual. A reduction in segmental activity of the sigmoid colon lowers intraluminal pressure and peripheral resistance, permitting more rapid passage of intestinal contents.[1] The number of stools varies from several per day to one every few minutes.

Diarrhea is a symptom of underlying functional or organic disease and is acute or chronic in nature. Some causes of diarrhea are shown in Table 32–1.

Acute diarrhea is characterized by the sudden onset of frequent stools of watery consistency, abdominal pain, cramping, weakness, and sometimes fever and vomiting. Since the duration is usually 24 to 48 hours, nutritional losses are not a prime concern. Acute diarrhea may be the presenting symptom of systemic infection or chronic gastrointestinal disease such as regional enteritis or ulcerative colitis.

Diarrhea is chronic when it persists for 2 weeks or longer. Nutritional deficiencies eventually develop because the rapid passage of the intestinal contents does not

Table 32–1. **Some Causes of Diarrhea**

Acute Types	Chronic Types
1. Chemical toxins, such as arsenic, lead, mercury, or cadmium	1. Malabsorptive lesions of anatomic, mucosal, or enzymatic origin
2. Bacterial toxins, such as *Salmonella* or staphylococcal food poisoning	2. Metabolic diseases, such as diabetic neuropathy, uremia, or Addison's disease
3. Bacterial infections, such as *Streptococcus, E. coli,* or *Shigella*	3. Alcoholism
4. Drugs, such as quinidine, colchicine, or neomycin	4. Carcinoma of small bowel or colon
5. Psychogenic factors, such as emotional instability	5. Postirradiation to small bowel or colon
6. Dietary factors, such as food sensitivity or allergy	6. Cirrhosis
	7. Laxative abuse

allow sufficient time for absorption. Mechanisms that increase fluid loss are (1) osmotic, as when poorly absorbed water-soluble molecules remain in the intestinal lumen and retain water, for example, lactase deficiency or laxative abuse; (2) secretory, in which the mucosa of the large intestine is stimulated to secrete, rather than absorb fluids, as in cholera; and (3) exudative, which is caused by the outpouring of serum proteins, blood, or mucus from sites of inflammation, as in inflammatory bowel disease.

Nutritional Considerations in Diarrheas Fluid, electrolyte, and tissue protein losses are usually severe if diarrhea is prolonged.

Fluids. Losses of fluids should be replaced by a liberal intake to prevent dehydration, especially in susceptible age groups such as the very young or elderly persons. Parenteral fluids are often administered to these individuals.

Electrolytes. Losses of sodium, potassium, and other electrolytes account for the profound weakness associated with severe diarrhea. Potassium loss, in particular, is detrimental as potassium is necessary for normal muscle tone of the gastrointestinal tract. Anorexia, vomiting, listlessness, and muscle weakness may occur unless losses are replaced by a liberal intake of fluids such as fruit juices that are high in potassium (see Chapter 41.)

Nutrient malabsorption. Long-continued diarrhea may result in depletion of tissue proteins and decreased serum protein levels. Fat losses are considerable in certain disorders with consequent loss of calories and fat-soluble vitamins. Intake of calories must be great enough to replace losses and may need to be as high as 3,000, with 100 to 150 gm protein, 100 to 120 gm fat, and the remainder as carbohydrate (see Chapter 28.)

Vitamin deficiencies frequently seen in chronic diarrheas are related to the decreased intake of vitamins and the increased requirements because of losses in the stools. A temporary reduction of synthesis of some B-complex vitamins also occurs when antibiotic therapy is used. Vitamin B-12, folic acid, and niacin deficiencies have been observed in various diarrheas.

Iron deficiency is a prominent finding in patients with chronic diarrhea owing to the increased losses of iron in the feces, the occasional blood losses, and the reduced intake of iron-rich foods because of fear that some foods might aggravate an existing lesion. Patients often show remarkable improvement when given supplemental iron therapy.

Diet in diarrheal states. Any dietary modification in diarrheal states depends on the nature of the underlying defect. In acute diarrhea, current recommendations include ad libitum oral intake of glucose-electrolyte solutions for those able to drink, with progression to foods as tolerated in small frequent feedings, as appetite improves.[2]

Many patients with chronic diarrhea of a functional or organic nature do not tolerate milk or foods high in fat or fiber content. Generally speaking, however, the need is for a diet high in protein (see Chapter 28) and calories, with adequate amounts of vitamins and minerals, and liberal amounts of fluids.

Constipation In this condition, hypermotility of the sigmoid colon increases resistance to movement of intestinal contents; consequently, there is distention and infrequent or difficult evacuation of feces from the intestine. An accurate definition is related to personal habits since the frequency of bowel movements varies greatly among individuals. For some, daily elimination is normal; in other equally healthy persons, regular evacuation occurs every second or third day.

Infrequent or insufficient emptying of the bowel may lead to malaise, headache, coated tongue, foul breath, and lack of appetite. These symptoms usually disappear after satisfactory evacuation has taken place.

Temporary or chronic constipation can

be due to any one of a number of factors such as: (1) failure to establish regular times for eating, adequate rest, and elimination; (2) faulty dietary habits, such as inadequate fluid intake or use of highly refined and concentrated foods that leave little residue in the colon; (3) interference with the urge to defecate brought on by poor personal hygiene or injury to the nervous mechanism; (4) changes in one's usual routine brought on by illness, nervous tension, or a trip away from home; (5) chronic use of laxatives and cathartics; (6) difficult or painful defecation due to hemorrhoids or fissures; (7) poor muscle tone of the intestine and stasis due to lack of exercise occurring especially in bedridden patients, invalids such as arthritics, the aged, and others; (8) organic disorders, such as diverticulosis or obstruction from adhesions or neoplasms; (9) ingestion of drugs, large amounts of sedatives, ganglionic blocking agents, or opiates; and (10) spasm of the intestine due to presence of irritating material, psychogenic influences, or others.

Determination of the cause is important so that proper treatment can be given. Correction of constipation depends in large measure on establishing regularity in habits—eating, rest, exercise, and elimination.

Dietary considerations. Attention to diet may be beneficial in *atonic* and *spastic* constipation. (See Irritable Colon Syndrome, following.) In the atonic type the diet should contain sufficient fiber to induce peristalsis and to contribute bulk to the intestine. A regular diet with an abundance of both raw and cooked fruits and vegetables is suitable for such patients. Wholegrain breads and cereals should be substituted for refined ones. Bran is useful for some patients but excesses are to be avoided since it may act as an irritant to sensitive intestinal tracts. Fat-containing foods such as bacon, butter, cream, and oils are useful for some because of the stimulating effect of the fatty acids on the mucous membranes. Excesses may cause diarrhea and should be avoided. Mineral oil if used should not be taken at mealtime because of its interference with the absorption of fat-soluble vitamins.

A fluid intake of 8 to 10 glasses a day is useful in keeping the intestinal contents in a semisolid state for easier passage along the tract. Some individuals find that 1 or 2 glasses of hot or cold water, plain or with lemon, are helpful in initiating peristalsis when taken before breakfast.

Irritable Colon Syndrome This condition, also known as *spastic colon,* is a functional disorder involving a disturbance in normal motor activity of the colon. This disorder probably accounts for 50 to 70 per cent of all gastrointestinal complaints. It is considered by some to be a forerunner of diverticular disease.

Etiology. Many factors contribute to this functional disorder. Included are excessive use of laxatives or cathartics; antibiotic therapy; food allergy; inadequate dietary fiber; poor hygiene in regard to rest, work, fluid intake, and elimination; and emotional upsets. Nervous, tense individuals are especially sensitive to gastrointestinal neurosis.

Symptoms. The most frequent symptom is pain, due to gaseous distension or to vigorous contractions of the colon. Pain is described as dull aching, cramping, or sharp and intermittent and may be accompanied by anorexia, nausea, and vomiting. Headache, palpitation, and heartburn sometimes occur. Constipation, or diarrhea, or both may occur in the same individual. Weight loss is uncommon.

Treatment. The underlying causes should be determined and corrected. Most patients need help in developing good personal and mental hygiene. Through counseling the individual will hopefully gain insight into the relationship between tension and the symptoms. Faulty eating habits must be corrected and the use of laxatives forbidden.

Dietary treatment for those patients with irritable colon syndrome who are constipated should consist of foods that increase intestinal residue enough to aid in evacuation.[3] Increased amounts of fruits, vegetables, and whole-grain cereals provide additional bulk. Some persons experience relief of symptoms when unprocessed bran is added to the diet.[4]

In recurrent diarrhea, a diet restricted in fiber and residue allows the colon the most rest. (See page 539.)

Intestinal Obstruction The movement of the intestinal contents is impaired or prevented by many causes such as tumors, impaction of material in the intestine, or paralytic ileus following surgery. As a rule, the obstruction must be removed by surgical intervention before an adequate diet can be administered. The postoperative diet should be fiber free (see page 539) for a period of time, following which a soft diet is usually ordered.

Inflammatory Disease of the Mucosa

Regional Enteritis *(Crohn's disease).* This is a chronic, nonspecific inflammatory disease involving chiefly the terminal ileum, but which affects any part of the intestine. The cause is unknown, although genetic and environmental factors have been implicated. The incidence and prevalence of the disease appear to be increasing throughout the world.[5] It occurs most frequently in young adults; nevertheless, 15 to 20 per cent of patients have symptoms before the age of 15 years.[6] The onset may be acute or insidious; the latter is typical in children.

The inflammatory reaction extends through the entire intestinal wall causing edema and fibrosis. It may be confined to one segment or involve multiple segments with normal areas in between.

Symptoms and clinical findings. Characteristic symptoms include abdominal pain, cramping, diarrhea, steatorrhea, weight loss, fever, and weakness. Systemic complications, malnutrition, and fistula formation are common. Intestinal protein loss, negative nitrogen balance, and anemia occur in a high proportion of patients. Deficiencies of a number of vitamins and minerals are frequent as a consequence of inadequate intake, increased losses, interference with absorption by drugs, or increased requirements.[7] Growth failure in children is usually secondary to insufficient calorie intake.

Conservative management is used unless obstruction or other complications make surgical intervention (ileal resection) necessary.

Dietary considerations. The importance of adequate nutritional support must be recognized. The diet should provide 1 to 1.5 gm of protein and 40 to 50 kcal per kilogram of ideal body weight to overcome losses due to exudation and malabsorption.[7] (See Chapter 28.) Medium-chain-triglyceride therapy (see Chapter 33) is effective in reducing steatorrhea and electrolyte losses in some patients. Foods high in potassium should be given in cases of prolonged diarrhea. (See Chapter 41.) During acute attacks, diets very low in residue (see following) are given initially in order to eliminate foods known to stimulate peristalsis and to prevent danger of obstruction. Supplements of iron, folic acid, and vitamin B-12 are needed to overcome deficiencies. Alternatively, semisynthetic fiber-free diets (Chapter 36) or total parenteral nutrition (Chapter 36) are sometimes used to restore nutrition while permitting the bowel to rest. Progression to a regular diet is made, eliminating only those foods known by the patient to aggravate symptoms.[8] For selected patients with extensive disease and malnutrition home parenteral nutrition provides additional nutritional support.

Diverticulosis In this condition, many small mucosal sacs, called DIVERTICULA, protrude through the intestinal wall. Most diverticula are found in the sigmoid colon, although they have been demonstrated throughout the length of the gastrointestinal tract. Diverticulosis is fairly common and the incidence increases with age.

The underlying defect is attributed to ab-

Very Low Residue Diet

Characteristics and General Rules

This diet is essentially fiber free and leaves a minimum of residue in the intestinal tract. See discussion on page 523.

If the diet is used for more than a few days, it should be supplemented with calcium, iron, and multivitamin concentrates.

As improvement takes place, the diet is liberalized by gradually adding tender cooked vegetables and fruits, and milk.

Foods Allowed

Beverages—coffee in limited amounts, tea
Breads—enriched bread or toast, crackers, plain rolls, Melba toast, zwieback
Cereals—cornmeal, farina, strained oatmeal; cornflakes, Puffed Rice, rice flakes; macaroni, noodles, rice, spaghetti
Cheese—cottage, cream, mild American in sauces
Desserts—plain cake, cookies, custard, gelatin, ice cream, puddings, rennet desserts
Eggs—cooked any way except fried
Fats—butter, cream, margarine, vegetable oils
Fruits—strained juices only. Occasionally applesauce is given to patients with diarrhea because of its pectin content.
Meats—tender or minced lean meat, fish, or poultry
Soups—clear: bouillon or broth without fat
Sweets—hard candy, honey, jelly, syrup, sugar in moderation
Vegetables—tomato juice; white potato
Miscellaneous—salt; spices in moderation

Foods to Avoid

Beverages—milk and milk drinks
Breads—whole-grain breads or crackers
Cereals—whole-grain such as wheat flakes, wheat meal, granola type
Cheese—sharp
Desserts—with fruit or nuts; pies and pastries. Note: milk desserts are occasionally omitted.
Fruits—all except juices
Meats—tough; fried; fatty meats, fish, or poultry such as pork, mackerel, goose
Soups—fatty; cream; spicy
Sweets—with fruit or nuts; jam, marmalade
Vegetables—all except tomato juice and potato
Miscellaneous—nuts, popcorn, pickles, excessive seasonings

Meal Pattern

BREAKFAST
Strained fruit juice
Refined cereal with cream and sugar
Egg
White toast with margarine
Coffee with cream and sugar

LUNCHEON
Broth
Tender meat, fowl, fish, or cheese
Potato, rice, macaroni, or noodles
White bread with margarine
Plain dessert
Coffee or tea

DINNER
Strained citrus juice
Tender meat, poultry, or fish
Potato or substitute
White bread with margarine
Plain dessert
Coffee or tea

normal thickening of the muscle layers of the sigmoid colon resulting in narrowing of the lumen and increased intraluminal pressure.[9] Contraction of the colon further increases pressure within the lumen and leads to herniation of the mucosa through the intestinal wall at points where it is weakened by penetration of blood vessels. Intraluminal pressure is greater when the diet is low in residue. On the other hand, foods that leave a high residue increase the volume and weight of materials reaching the sigmoid colon, and, by distending the colon, may prevent development of high-pressure segments. For this reason, foods high in fiber (see following) have been recommended for use in diverticulosis.[10] Low-residue diets formerly used in this disorder are now considered to be contraindicated.

DIVERTICULITIS occurs when one or more diverticula become inflamed and perforate. Inflammation usually results from accumulation of food particles or residues in the sacs and subsequent bacterial action. Symptoms include steady pain in the lower left abdomen, abdominal distension, changes in bowel habits—usually as constipation, colonic spasm, and occasionally fever. Steatorrhea and megaloblastic anemia, often associated with small bowel diverticula, are due to stasis.

The management of acute attacks of diverticulitis includes bedrest, antibiotics, and clear liquids with progression to a very low residue diet. (See page 539.) In recurrent or persistent attacks, surgical resection of the involved portion of colon may be necessary. Complications, such as obstruction, perforation, or fistula formation, also necessitate surgical intervention.

Dietary Counseling

Persons with diverticular disease who are placed on high-fiber diets need careful counseling in regard to the purpose of the diet. Those accustomed to restricting fiber intake may be especially apprehensive about such a drastic change in their diets and need frequent reassurance from the dietitian and the nurse. For most patients, increasing the fiber content of the diet should be made gradually. Whole-grain cereals should be used, and breads and other baked goods made with 100 per cent whole wheat or whole rye flour substituted for those made with white flour. Generous amounts of fruits and vegetables such as raw carrots, apples, oranges, and lettuce, stewed fruits, potatoes cooked in skins, and so on should be encouraged. Some physicians may recommend the use of bran, the amount depending on the fiber content of the rest of the diet. It is usually best to start with 1 tablespoon of bran per day in a liquid such as milk or juice, gradually increasing the amount of bran until one soft stool is produced daily or until symptoms are relieved. Some patients experience flatulence and distension at first but the diet should not be discontinued because of these. Coarsely ground bran is preferable to finely ground wheat bran.[11] Bran can be mixed with foods such as cereals, soups, or puddings or added to homemade breads, muffins, and cakes.

Ulcerative Colitis This is a diffuse inflammatory and ulcerative disease of unknown etiology involving the mucosa and submucosa of the large intestine. No single etiologic factor has been identified, although genetic and autoimmune factors are thought to be involved.

Symptoms and clinical findings. Ulcerative colitis may occur at any age but predominates in young adults. The onset is insidious in the majority of cases with mild abdominal discomfort, an urgent need to defecate several times a day, and diarrhea accompanied by rectal bleeding. Loss of water, electrolytes, blood, and protein from the colon produces systemic symptoms such as weight loss, dehydration, fever, anemia, and general debility. In early stages the mucosa is edematous and hyperemic. In more severe disease, necrosis and frank

High-Fiber Diet

Characteristics

This diet is essentially a regular diet with fiber content increased as follows:

1. Substitute at least four servings whole-grain bread and cereals for refined breads and cereals.
2. Emphasize raw fruits and vegetables that are high in fiber.
3. Add 1 to 2 tablespoons bran each day.

The substitution of fibrous foods should be made gradually; for example, whole-grain breads and cereals are added first, then fibrous cooked fruits and vegetables followed by raw fruits and vegetables.

Foods Allowed

Beverages—all
Breads—breads, muffins, or rolls made from 100 per cent whole-wheat or whole-rye flour; graham, wheat, or rye crackers; Ry-Krisp
Cereals—whole-grain such as oatmeal, rolled oats; bran flakes, granola; grapenuts; Shredded Wheat, wheat flakes; brown rice; bran, in moderation
Cheese—all
Desserts—all, with fruit and nuts, if tolerated
Eggs—all
Fats—all
Fruits—all, including dried; preferably raw
Meats—all
Soups—all, preferably vegetable
Sweets—jam, marmalade, preserves
Vegetables—all, especially raw; potatoes in skin
Miscellaneous—condiments and seasonings in moderation

Sample Menu

BREAKFAST
Orange sections
Oatmeal with milk and brown sugar
Poached egg
Bran muffins
Butter or margarine
Marmalade
Coffee

LUNCHEON
Vegetable soup
Club sandwich:
  Sliced turkey
  Bacon
  Whole-wheat bread
  Lettuce and tomato
  Mayonnaise
Baked apple with raisin stuffing
Milk

DINNER
Brown beef stew
  Onions
  Carrots
Oven-browned potato
Coleslaw with pineapple
Rye bread
Butter or margarine
Apricot fruit crisp
Tea with lemon and sugar

BEDTIME SNACK
Milk
Fresh pear
Graham crackers

ulceration of the mucosa occur. The severity of the symptoms does not necessarily correlate with the extent of the disease. Patients with localized disease can be very seriously ill; on the other hand, persons with very troublesome symptoms may have mild disease.

Dietary considerations. One of the most important factors in the dietary management of this disorder is the individual attention given to the patient. Frequent visits by the dietitian and the nurse can do much toward convincing the patient of a sincere interest in his or her welfare. Many individuals with this disease are extremely apprehensive about what they can eat and seem to need constant reassurance. Mealtime visits provide an excellent opportunity to give encouragement and support.

Much patience and understanding are needed in helping ulcerative colitis patients with dietary problems. The diet must be highly individualized and yet be nutritionally adequate. Genuine efforts to meet the patient's requests must be made; the patient must never be made to feel that numerous questions and frequent demands are troublesome. On the other hand, gentle, but firm guidance must be given in helping the patient select a nutritionally

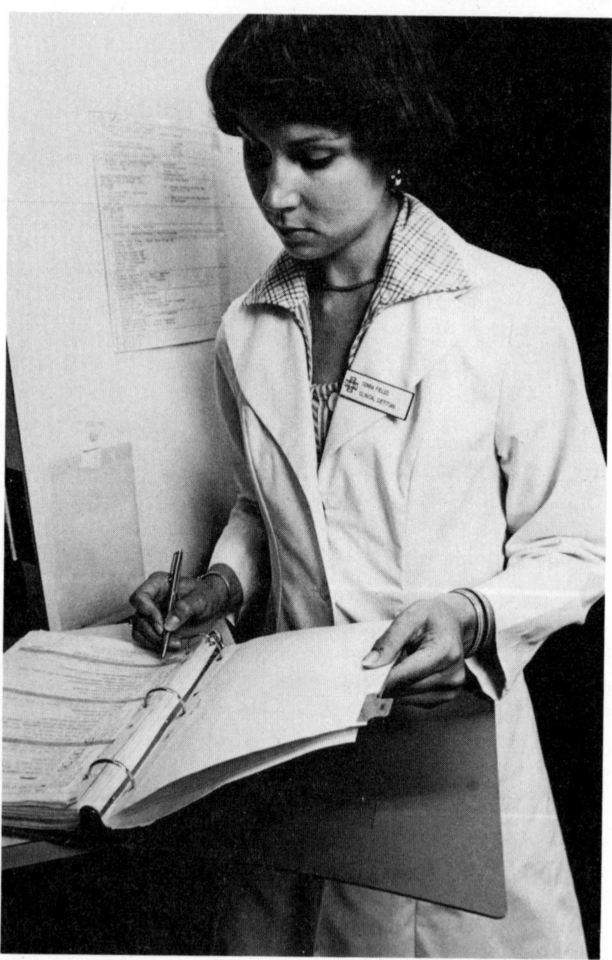

Figure 32–1. The patient's chart provides important information that must be considered in planning nutritional care. The chart should include progress notes concerning the patient's acceptance of his diet and any problems of nutritional adequacy that may be present. Sometimes the intake of specific nutrients is calculated and charted. Also included are recommendations for action that needs to be taken. (Courtesy, Metropolital Medical Center, Minneapolis.)

adequate diet. It must be understood that he or she is expected to eat the entire meal. Many patients have poor appetites, and it may be preferable to provide six or eight small feedings; for others, however, having less frequent meal intervals is a more satisfactory approach. (See Figure 32–1.)

Liberal amounts of high-quality protein (1 to 1.5 gm per kilogram of desirable body weight) are needed since nitrogen losses from the bowel may be considerable. (See Chapter 28.) Emphasis should be on tender meats, fish, poultry, and eggs for those patients who are allergic or intolerant to milk. Intakes of 40 to 50 kcal per kilogram desirable body weight are necessary to replace losses due to steatorrhea, and to promote weight gain. The very low residue diet may be used at first; thereafter, some degree of fiber restriction is usually needed as many ulcerative colitis patients do not tolerate raw fruits or vegetables, and further damage to an already inflamed mucosa must be prevented. Supplementary vitamins and minerals are usually indicated to compensate for gastrointestinal losses and inadequate dietary intake. Especially important are iron salts when anemia is present, and calcium salts if milk is not tolerated.

Problems and Review

1. Discuss the role of diet in the incidence of diseases of the small intestine and colon.
2. What is the relationship of psychologic factors to the occurrence of gastrointestinal disorders? Cite examples.
3. List some causes of malnutrition in inflammatory bowel disease.
4. Mrs. K. is troubled with chronic diarrhea, although her physician has ruled out organic disease. What other factors might provoke diarrhea? In what ways would you expect her diet to be modified? What are the reasons for each modification?
5. Mrs. L. complains of constipation. List five possible causes.
   a. What type of person is likely to develop atonic constipation?
   b. What factors should be considered in treating constipation?
   c. What dietary recommendations would you make for Mrs. L.?
6. Mrs. R., now 75 years of age, has been troubled with diverticulosis for 20 years. For much of this time she has been on a low-residue diet. Her physician has recently recommended that she start eating whole-grain breads and cereals daily and that she add 2 tablespoons of bran to her diet daily.
   a. Mrs. R. is afraid to change her eating habits after all these years. How would you advise her in regard to the diet?
   b. What is the first change you would suggest Mrs. R. make in her diet?
   c. Mrs. R. states that she cannot afford to purchase the bran and fruits and vegetables. What suggestions would you make?
   d. Mrs. R. asks if a popular laxative, "nature's own," which is frequently advertised on TV, would serve the same purpose as the bran which her physician has recommended. What would you tell her?
   e. Show how you would modify Mrs. R.'s present very low residue diet for a soft-low-fiber diet; for a diet with increased residue, but omitting raw fruits and vegetables; for a high-fiber diet.
7. List the recommendations you would make for a person with irritable colon.
8. Mr. P., a 16-year-old student, is hospitalized with ulcerative colitis. His doctor has ordered a 3,500-kcal, 150-gm protein diet for him.
   a. Plan a day's menu for him. He has many food intolerances, does not eat raw fruits or vegetables, and dislikes milk. He is especially fond of pizza and carbonated beverages.

b. Mr. P. will be going home soon but is somewhat apprehensive about this as he does not get along well with his parents. What advice would you give him concerning his diet?
c. What suggestions could you offer Mr. P.'s mother to help her win her son's cooperation at mealtime?

Cited References

1. Parks, T. G.: "Colonic Motility in Man," *Postgrad. Med. J.*, **49**:90–99, 1973.
2. Hirschhorn, N.: "The Treatment of Acute Diarrhea in Children. An Historical and Physiological Perspective," *Am. J. Clin. Nutr.*, **33**:637–63, 1980.
3. Burns, T. W.: "Colonic Motility in the Irritable Bowel Syndrome," *Arch. Intern. Med.*, **140**:247–51, 1980.
4. Piepmeyer, J. L.: "Use of Unprocessed Bran in Treatment of Irritable Bowel Syndrome," *Am. J. Clin. Nutr.*, **27**:106–107, 1974.
5. Kirsner, J. B.: "Inflammatory Bowel Disease. Considerations of Etiology and Pathogenesis," *Am. J. Gastroent.*, **69**:253–71, 1978.
6. Fonkalsrud, E. W. et al.: "Surgical Management of Crohn's Disease in Children," *Am. J. Surg.*, **138**:15–21, 1979.
7. Driscoll, R. H., and Rosenberg, I. H.: "Total Parenteral Nutrition in Inflammatory Bowel Disease," *Med. Clin. North Am.*, **62**:185–201, 1978.
8. Poley, J. R.: "Chronic Inflammatory Bowel Disease in Children and Adolescents," *South. Med. J.*, **71**:935–48, 1978.
9. Morson, B. C.: "Pathology of Diverticular Disease of the Colon," *Clin. Gastroenterol.*, **4**:37–52, 1975.
10. Painter, N. S. et al.: "Unprocessed Bran in Treatment of Diverticular Disease of the Colon," *Brit. Med. J.*, **2**:137–40, 1972.
11. Heller, S. N., et al.: "Dietary Fiber: The Effect of Particle Size of Wheat Bran on Colonic Function in Young Adult Men," *Am. J. Clin. Nutr.*, **33**:1734–44, 1980.

Additional References

BASS, L.: "More Fiber—Less Constipation," *Am. J. Nurs.*, **77**:254–55, 1977.

BAYLESS, T. M. et al.: "Crohn's Disease," *South. Med. J.*, **71**:825–30, 1978.

BUHAC, I., and BALINT, J. A.: "Diarrhea and Constipation," *Am. Fam. Physician*, **12**:149–59, November 1975.

CHERNOFF, R., and DEAN, J. A.: "Medical and Nutritional Aspects of Intractable Diarrhea," *J. Am. Diet. Assoc.*, **76**:161–69, 1980.

HEATON, K. W. et al.: "Treatment of Crohn's Disease with an Unrefined Carbohydrate, Fibre-Rich Diet," *Brit. Med. J.*, **2**:764–66, 1979.

KELTS, D. G. et al.: "Nutritional Basis of Growth Failure in Children and Adolescents with Crohn's Disease," *Gastroenterology*, **76**:720–27, 1979.

KEWENTER, J. et al.: "Cancer Risk in Extensive Ulcerative Colitis," *Ann. Surg.*, **188**:824–28, 1978.

KRONER, K.: "Are You Prepared for Your Ulcerative Colitis Patient?" *Nursing*, **10**:43–45 ff., April 1980.

MATSESHE, J. W., and PHILLIPS, S. F.: "Chronic Diarrhea. A Practical Approach," *Med. Clin. North Am.*, **62**:141–54, 1978.

NETCHVOLODOFF, C. V., and HARGROVE, M. D.: "Recent Advances in the Treatment of Diarrhea," *Arch. Intern. Med.*, **139**:813–16, 1979.

NISHI, Y. et al.: "Zinc Status and Its Relation to Growth Retardation in Children with Chronic Inflammatory Bowel Disease," *Am. J. Clin. Nutr.*, **33**:2613–21, 1980.

SANDSTEAD, H. H. et al.: "Influence of Dietary Fiber on Trace Element Balance," *Am. J. Clin. Nutr.*, **31**:S180–S184, 1978.

SITRIN, M. D. et al.: "Nutritional and Metabolic Complications in a Patient with Crohn's Disease and Ileal Resection," *Gastroenterology*, **78**:1069–79, 1980.

33 Malabsorption Syndrome

MEDIUM-CHAIN-TRIGLYCERIDE DIET; LACTOSE-RESTRICTED DIET; SUCROSE-RESTRICTED DIET; GLUTEN-RESTRICTED DIET

General Characteristics and Treatment

The term *malabsorption syndrome* is used to describe a number of disorders that are characterized by steatorrhea and multiple abnormalities in absorption of nutrients. Malabsorption in these disorders may be due to defects in (1) the intestinal lumen, resulting in inadequate fat hydrolysis or altered bile salt metabolism; (2) the mucosal epithelial cells, affecting absorbing surfaces and interfering with transport functions; or (3) intestinal lymphatics. (See Table 33–1.) Malabsorption is also often associated with infectious disease, as in tropical sprue, or with certain metabolic and endocrine disorders.

Symptoms and Laboratory Findings Symptoms present to a variable degree in most persons with this syndrome include (1) pale, bulky, frothy, and offensive stools due to abnormally high fat content; (2) muscle wasting and progressive weight loss due to steatorrhea, diarrhea, and anorexia; (3) abdominal distension in children, less marked in adults; (4) evidence of vitamin and mineral deficiencies, such as macrocytic anemia due to inadequate absorption of folic acid and vitamin B-12, iron deficiency anemia, hypocalcemic tetany, glossitis, and so on.

Laboratory findings include decreases in serum concentrations of electrolytes, albumin, and carotene; impaired absorption of *d*-xylose, glucose, folic acid, and vitamin B-12; and increased fecal fat and nitrogen.

Diagnostic Tests The diagnosis of malabsorption syndrome is based upon findings from absorption tests, intestinal mucosal biopsy, and radiologic studies.

Direct tests of absorption involve measurement of *fecal fat.* The balance study method is widely used and involves the chemical analysis of a 72-hour stool collec-

Table 33–1. **Some Malabsorptive Disorders Responsive to Dietary Modification**

Abnormalities in the Intestinal Lumen	Abnormalities in the Mucosa
Inadequate lipid hydrolysis*	Specific defects
1. Pancreatic insufficiency	1. Lactase insufficiency
2. Gastric resection	2. Sucrase-isomaltase deficiency
	3. Glucose-galactase deficiency
	4. A-beta-lipoproteinemia
Alteration of bile salt metabolism*	Nonspecific defects*
1. Hepatobiliary disease	1. Short-bowel syndrome
2. Intestinal resection	2. Gluten enteropathy
3. Bacterial overgrowth	3. Radiation enteritis
4. Drug therapy	Intestinal lymphatic obstruction*
	Lymphangiectasia

*MCT therapy effective in disorders in this group.

tion. The patient is fed a diet containing a known amount of fat, usually 50 to 100 gm, for several days before and during the collection period. Stools are then analyzed for fat. Normal excretion is less than 5 gm per 24 hours. Stool collections are also used to measure fecal radioactivity following administration of a test dose of ^{131}I-labeled triolein. The triolein is mixed with a marker and stools are collected until the marker is no longer visible. Normal fecal radioactivity is less than 7 per cent of the test dose.

The *serum carotene* level is a useful screening test, and malabsorption is suspected if levels of less than 60 micrograms per 100 ml are found.

Oral tolerance tests provide indirect evidence of malabsorption. Most commonly used are d-*xylose* and *lactose.* Urinary excretion of *d*-xylose following ingestion of a 25-gm load is used as an indication of carbohydrate absorption. Excretion of less than 4.5 gm in 5 hours in patients with normal renal function indicates decreased absorptive capacity. The *lactose tolerance test* is used in suspected lactase deficiency. Administration of lactose, 2 gm per kilogram body weight, or a maximum of 50 gm, is followed by determination of blood glucose levels for 2 hours.[1] *Lactose malabsorption* is indicated if the blood glucose rises less than 26 mg per 100 ml. Symptoms of abdominal distension, cramping, and diarrhea may occur following ingestion of the lactose in persons with *lactose intolerance.*[1]

Measurement of breath hydrogen following a lactose load is a more sensitive test for lactose malabsorption. Unabsorbed lactose undergoes bacterial fermentation in the colon with production of hydrogen gas, part of which is excreted through the lungs. An increase in breath hydrogen in expired air samples collected at specified intervals indicates lactose malabsorption.[2] In another breath test, excretion of carbon dioxide following administration of certain fats labeled with stable isotopes is used as a screening test for fat malabsorption.[3,4] Other screening tests for malabsorption involve measurement of urinary excretion of 4-hydroxyphenylacetic acid[5] or determination of urinary oxalate following administration of sodium oxalate.[6]

The *Schilling test* is frequently used as an index of vitamin B-12 absorption; an oral dose of radioactive vitamin B-12 is administered followed at 2 hours by an intramuscular injection of nonradioactive B-12. Urinary excretion of less than 5 to 8 per cent of the radioactive dose indicates malabsorption.

The *folic acid test* consists of assaying urine for 24 hours following injection of the vitamin and again after it is given orally 48 hours later. In malabsorption, excretion of folic acid is less after an oral dose than after injection.

Biopsy specimens of the jejunal mucosa showing villous atrophy provide nonspecific evidence of disturbances in absorptive function. Radiologic evidence of intestinal dilatation, altered motility, and bone demineralization may also be seen in malabsorption.

Treatment Therapy is directed toward alleviation of symptoms by correction of the basic defect insofar as possible, dietary modification in accordance with the nature of the defect, vitamin and mineral supplements, and prevention or correction of complications by administration of appropriate agents.

Dietary Modification Generally speaking, the diet in malabsorption syndrome should be high in protein and calories. (See Chapter 28.) In a few of the disorders elimination of specific carbohydrates or proteins is necessary and the dietary management is outlined in the sections that follow. Modification of fat intake is often indicated. Vitamin and mineral supplementation is usually needed. A soft or fiber-restricted diet is useful for patients with persistent diarrhea. (See Chapter 25.)

Fat absorption can be improved in some malabsorptive disorders by changing the type of fat ingested. Food fats are composed principally of fatty acids containing 12 to

18 carbon atoms (long-chain triglycerides). In contrast, fats composed almost entirely of fatty acids containing 8 and 10 carbon atoms (medium-chain triglycerides) have been synthesized. Substitution of medium-chain triglycerides (MCT) for longer chain fats (LCT) is associated with reduced steatorrhea and decreased losses of calcium, sodium, and potassium in many of the disorders comprising the malabsorption syndrome. (See Table 33–1.)

The effectiveness of MCT over long-chain fats appears to be due to differences in the rate of hydrolysis, absorption, and route of transport. Medium-chain fats are hydrolyzed much more rapidly than long chain fats by intestinal and pancreatic lipases. A mucosal enzyme system, specific for medium-chain-triglyceride hydrolysis, has been described. Medium-chain triglycerides are transported by way of the portal vein as free fatty acids bound to albumin whereas long-chain fats must undergo esterification and chylomicron formation and are transported by way of the lymph.

Side effects of nausea, abdominal distension or cramps, and diarrhea have been noted in about 10 per cent of patients receiving MCT supplements. Symptoms are attributed to the hyperosmolar load produced by rapid hydrolysis of MCT and possible irritating effects of high levels of free fatty acids in the stomach and intestine. These symptoms can be overcome by slow ingestion of small amounts of the supplement.

Medium-chain triglycerides are available commercially as an oil preparation* or as a powdered formula.† A number of recipes have been developed for incorporating these products into the diet.** The oil provides a concentrated source of calories, and can be used in frying and in recipes such as salad dressings, hot breads, and desserts. It is a clear, odorless oil with a bland taste. The powder, on the other hand, is useful as a calorie-protein supplement to an otherwise very low fat diet. A proprietary formula containing MCT is available for infants.‡

Dietary management From 50 to 70 per cent of the fat is supplied as MCT and the remainder as foods containing long-chain triglycerides. To maintain this ratio, foods containing LCT are limited to

4 ounces meat, fish, or poultry
1 egg
3 teaspoons butter

This provides about 25 gm LCT daily.

The following diet is adapted from the plan described by Schizas et al.[7]

* MCT® from fractionated coconut oil, by Mead Johnson & Co., Evansville, Indiana. Provides 8.3 kcal per gram, or approximately 225 kcal per 30 ml.

† Portagen® by Mead Johnson & Co., Evansville, Indiana. An 8-ounce glass of the product reconstituted to 20 kcal per ounce provides 5.6 gm protein from sodium caseinate, 18.4 gm carbohydrate from corn syrup solids and sucrose, and 7.75 gm fat from MCT and corn oil.

** Available from Mead Johnson & Co., Evansville, Indiana.

‡ Pregestimil® by Mead Johnson & Co., Evansville, Indiana.

Medium-Chain-Triglyceride (MCT) Diet

Characteristics and General Rules

This diet provides for a reduction in long-chain triglycerides by substituting an oil containing medium-chain triglycerides as a source of fat. The diet is adjusted to provide 50 to 70 per cent of the fat calories as MCT.

The protein intake may be increased by adding nonfat dry milk to fluid skim milk, skim cottage cheese, egg whites, and cereal products.

The caloric level may be increased by adding high-carbohydrate foods such as fruits, sugar, jelly, and fat-free desserts.

Modifications in fiber and consistency may be made by applying restrictions concerning the soft diet (see Chapter 25) to the following listed foods.

Initially, small amounts of MCT should be taken with meals and gradually increased according to individual tolerance. Between-meal feedings may be desirable if large amounts of food are not tolerated.

Include These Foods Daily:

2 or more cups skim milk
4 ounces (cooked weight) lean meat, poultry, or fish
1 egg
3 or more fruits including:
  1–2 servings citrus fruit or other good source of ascorbic acid
  1–2 other fruits
3–4 servings vegetables including:
  1 dark green or deep yellow
  1 potato
  1–2 other vegetables, raw or cooked, as tolerated
5 servings bread and cereals
3 teaspoons butter
MCT oil in amounts prescribed (usually 2 ounces)

Nutritive value: On the basis of these specified amounts of foods: protein, 75 gm (13 per cent of calories); fat, 35 gm (13 per cent of calories); carbohydrate, 315 gm (53 per cent of calories); MCT, 60 gm (21 per cent of calories); 2,400 kcal.

Foods Allowed	**Foods to Avoid**
Beverages—cereal beverages, coffee, tea, soft drinks	
Breads and substitutes—hamburger rolls, hard rolls, white enriched, whole-wheat, pumpernickel, or rye bread. Bread products contain some LCT but are permitted to add palatability and variety to the diet. Cooked or dry cereals, macaroni, noodles, rice, spaghetti	Commercial biscuits, coffeecake, corn bread, crackers, doughnuts, muffins, sweet rolls
Cheese—skim cottage cheese	Cheese made from whole milk
Desserts—angel cake, gelatin, meringues, any made from MCT special recipes	Commercial cakes, pies, cookies, pastries, puddings and custards; mixes allowed only if they contain no LCT
Egg—egg whites as desired; whole eggs and egg yolks only in prescribed amounts	Whole eggs and egg yolks except as prescribed
Fats—butter in prescribed amounts, gravies made from clear soups and MCT oil	Oils and shortenings of all types, sauces and gravies except those made with MCT oil
Fruits—all except avocado	Avocado
Meats—lean meat, fish, and poultry only in prescribed amounts	Fatty meats, fish, frankfurters, cold cuts, sausages
Milk—skim milk	Buttermilk, partially skim milk, whole milk, light, heavy, or sour cream
Soups—fat-free broth, bouillon, consommé	Cream soups, others
Sweets—jelly, syrups, sugars	Butter, chocolate, coconut, or cream candies
Vegetables—all to which no fat is added except MCT	Creamed vegetables, or those with fats other than MCT added

Foods Allowed	Foods to Avoid
Miscellaneous—any special recipe in which MCT is substituted for long-chain fats	Creamed dishes; commercial popcorn; frozen dinners; homemade products containing eggs, whole milk, and fats; mixes for biscuits, muffins, and cakes; olives

Sample Menu

BREAKFAST
Fresh grapefruit—1 half
MCT waffle—1
Butter—1 teaspoon
Maple syrup—2 tablespoons
Sugar—1 teaspoon
Coffee or tea

LUNCHEON OR SUPPER
Chicken sandwich
Chicken—2 ounces
MCT mayonnaise—1 tablespoon
Whole-wheat bread—2 slices
Lettuce and tomato
Fresh fruit cup—½ cup
MCT brownie—1
Skim milk—1 cup

DINNER
Veal chop—2 ounces
MCT scalloped potatoes—½ cup
Carrots—½ cup
With lemon butter—2 teaspoons
Mixed green salad—1 serving
MCT Italian dressing—2 teaspoons
Angel cake—1/16 of 8 inch diameter
Fresh strawberries—1 cup
Coffee or tea

EVENING SNACK
Skim milk—1 cup
MCT sugar cookies—2

Dietary Counseling

The patient must understand the importance of using the recommended amounts of MCT in the diet. He or she should be cautioned to take the oil slowly in small amounts; no more than 1 tablespoon of MCT should be taken at any given feeding. The diet to be used at home should be planned with consideration given to the individual's cultural background and usual meal pattern. The patient must be taught to use cuts of meat that are low in fat and to select only lean meats. Suggestions for incorporating the MCT oil into meals should be offered and suitable recipes supplied. Some persons prefer to take the oil mixed in fruit juice or as a "milkshake" composed of skim milk, fruit ice, and the oil. Others prefer to add the oil to solid foods such as cooked cereals, mashed potatoes, or sauces. The oil imparts a golden color to foods when used in frying; care should be taken to see that all the oil is removed from the frying pan, however, and actually consumed. Meals eaten away from home need not be a problem if the individual orders clear soups, lean meats trimmed of all visible fat, vegetables without cream sauces or other added fat, and so on. Desserts such as fruits, angel cake, and gelatin are suitable and usually available.

Abnormalities in the Intestinal Lumen

Inadequate Digestion Any condition that interferes with normal secretion or activity of pancreatic lipase causes inadequate hydrolysis of lipids in the intestinal lumen and results in malabsorption.

Pancreatic insufficiency. Inadequate production of lipase occurs in pancreatic insufficiency. This disorder may result from chronic pancreatitis, cystic fibrosis, carcinoma, pancreatectomy, or destruction of exocrine function by ligation of the duct. Steatorrhea and symptoms of generalized malabsorption occur due to poor utilization of fats and protein. Weight loss may be significant in spite of a good appetite.

The diet is designed to prevent further weight loss and to control gastrointestinal symptoms. From 2,500 to 4,000 kcal are required. The protein intake should be 100 to 150 gm. Carbohydrate (400 gm or more) is the chief source of calories since fat is poorly tolerated. Generally, long-chain fatty acids should be restricted to 30 to 60 gm daily. Pancreatic enzymes are given with meals to aid in fat absorption. MCT can be used to increase the calorie intake.[8] (See page 548.)

Gastric resection. Steatorrhea sometimes follows gastric resection because of inadequate mixing of food with pancreatic juice and bile or bacterial overgrowth in an afferent loop of intestine. In addition, anemia is frequently seen because of limited intake or impaired absorption of iron, vitamin B-12, and folic acid. Weight loss is common and persistent. Improved absorption of fats may be achieved by supplementing the diet with MCT. Other dietary considerations are described on page 592.

Altered Bile Salt Metabolism Steatorrhea occurs if adequate amounts of conjugated bile salts are not available for micelle formation and is frequently associated with the following conditions.

Hepatobiliary disease. Decreased amounts of bile salts in the lumen in hepatobiliary disease are due to impaired synthesis of bile acids or biliary stasis.

Ileal resection. Removal of the ileum reduces the bile salt pool thereby lowering the concentration of conjugated bile salts in the jejunum available for hydrolysis of fats. Unabsorbed fatty acids and bile salts may provoke diarrhea. Parenteral administration of vitamin B-12 is indicated if the distal ileum is not functional.

Bacterial overgrowth (blind loop syndrome). Intestinal stasis is associated with changes in the bacterial flora. Deconjugation of bile salts by bacteria prevents adequate micelle formation. In some instances steatorrhea can be corrected by feeding conjugated bile salts. Bacteria also bind vitamin B-12 so that it is unavailable for absorption, and replacement therapy is needed.

Effects of drug therapy. Certain drugs bind ionized fatty acids and bile salts in the proximal intestine with subsequent fat malabsorption. Other mechanisms involved in drug-induced malabsorption are decreased disaccharidase activity, interference with absorption of nutrients and increased fecal losses of nutrients.[9,10] Drugs exerting this multifactorial influence on absorption include neomycin, cholestyramine, colchicine, and *p*-aminosalicylic acid, among others.[9]

Abnormalities in Mucosal Cell Transport—Specific Disorders

Absence or deficiency of specific enzymes or failure of proper regulation of enzyme activity in the cell interferes with the absorption of certain nutrients and produces symptoms of malabsorption.

Lactose Intolerance Inability to utilize lactose may be due to lactase deficiency or may be secondary to conditions that produce alterations in absorptive surfaces. In the absence of lactase lactose is not hydrolyzed to glucose and galactose. The accumulation of lactose in the intestine causes fermentation, abdominal pain, cramping, and diarrhea. Failure to gain weight is an important symptom in infants.

Congenital lactose intolerance is a rare disorder characterized by absent brush border lactase activity. Symptoms occur following ingestion of milk by the infant. A strict lactose-free formula is used, several commercial products being available.* All

* Isomil, by Ross Laboratories, Columbus, Ohio; MBF (Meat-base formula) by Gerber Products Company, Fremont, Michigan; Neomullsoy® by Syntex Laboratories, Inc., Palo Alto, California. Nutramigen® and ProSobee® by Mead Johnson and Company, Evansville, Indiana.

products containing lactose in any form whatsoever are rigidly excluded.

Intestinal lactase activity is normally high during infancy but declines after weaning to low levels in adults. Throughout most of the world the majority of adults are unable to digest lactose, and they develop symptoms of distension, cramping, and diarrhea following its ingestion. These individuals who have no history of gastrointestinal disease or childhood intolerance to milk, are described as having *primary* lactose intolerance. In the United States, from 60 to 95 per cent of adult blacks, American Indians, Jews, Mexican-Americans, and Orientals are lactose malabsorbers compared to 5 to 15 per cent for whites.[11]

Several hypotheses have been proposed to explain the differences in ability to utilize lactose among various ethnic groups. One theory holds that a genetic mutation occurring as a result of some selective advantage may permit high levels of lactase to persist into the adult years in certain populations.[12]

Adults with primary lactose intolerance can usually tolerate the amounts of milk in many prepared foods such as breads, lunch meats, and even cream soups and cream sauces providing that the lactose source is spaced throughout the day. Those who experience classical symptoms following excessive milk or lactose ingestion, can be kept asymptomatic by limiting their intake of milk products. A controlled lactose diet that restricts only obvious sources of lactose is used. The quantity of lactose allowed is a matter of individual tolerance.

Several studies with lactose malabsorbers indicate that subjects experience significantly fewer symptoms following ingestion of lactose-hydrolyzed milk than regular milk. A commercially available enzyme,* when added to milk, hydrolyzes about 75 per cent of the lactose, thus permitting intake of a larger quantity of milk without provoking symptoms.

* Lact-Aid®, SugarLo Company, Atlantic City, New Jersey.

Secondary lactose intolerance is often observed following gastrectomy or extensive small bowel resection, and in celiac disease, sprue, colitis, enteritis, cystic fibrosis, kwashiorkor, and malnutrition. In these conditions it may be necessary to omit obvious sources of lactose initially, but a strict lactose-free diet is usually not required.

Dietary Counseling

Adults who become symptomatic after excess lactose ingestion should be advised to limit intake of milk, cream soups, puddings, custards, ice cream, and so on. Some find that milk is better tolerated if taken in small amounts several times daily, especially with meals, and at room temperature rather than cold. Many persons remain symptom free by limiting their intake of milk to one glass per day. Chocolate milk is sometimes tolerated better than plain milk; this may be related to a slower rate of emptying from the stomach.[11] Individuals failing to respond to a lactose-controlled diet may need to further restrict lactose intake. When improvement is noted small amounts of lactose-containing foods are tested, one at a time (for example, one-fourth cup of milk at a meal) to determine levels that may be tolerated. Fermented dairy products such as yogurt, buttermilk, and many cheeses may be included if tolerated.

Persons on lactose-free diets should be advised to carefully check labels on all commercial products. Foods containing milk in any form, butter, and margarine are to be avoided. Typical sources of lactose include breads, candies, cold cuts, mixes of all types, powdered soft drinks, preserves, soups, and so on. Fruit juices or water can be substituted for milk in many recipes. Meals eaten away from home should include foods prepared without breading, cream sauces, gravies, and so on. Broiled or roasted meats, baked potato, vegetables without added fat, salads, and desserts such as plain angel cake, fresh fruit, and gelatin are good choices. Kosher-style foods are suitable.

Lactose-Free Diet

Characteristics and General Rules

This diet is designed to eliminate all sources of lactose.

All milk and milk products must be eliminated.

Lactose is used in the manufacture of many foods and medicines. It is essential to read labels of commercial products before use.

The diet is inadequate in calcium and riboflavin. Supplements of these nutrients should be prescribed.

The protein intake may be increased by adding meat, fish, poultry, or eggs, lactose-free milk substitutes, or breads and cereals from those allowed.

The caloric level may be increased by adding high-carbohydrate foods such as fruits, sugar, jelly, and desserts free of lactose.

Modifications in fiber and consistency may be made by applying restrictions concerning the soft diet (see Chapter 25) to the foods listed here.

Include the Following Foods Daily:

- 7 ounces meat, fish, or poultry
- 1 egg
- 3 or more fruits including:
  - 1–2 servings citrus fruit or other good source of ascorbic acid
  - 1–2 other fruits
- 3–4 servings vegetables including:
  - 1 dark green or deep yellow
  - 1 potato
  - 1–2 other vegetables, raw or cooked, as tolerated
- 6 servings enriched bread or cereals
- 6 teaspoons fortified milk-free margarine

Other foods as needed to provide calories

Foods Allowed	Foods to Avoid
Beverages—carbonated drinks, fruit drinks, coffee, tea	Cereal beverages, cocoa, instant coffee (check label)
Breads and cereals—breads and rolls made without milk, cooked cereals, some prepared cereals (check labels), macaroni, spaghetti, soda crackers	Bread with milk added, crackers made with butter or margarine, French toast, mixes of all types, pancakes, some dry cereals (read labels), waffles, zwieback
Cheese—none	All types
Desserts—angel cake, cakes made with vegetable oils, gelatin, puddings made with fruit juices, water, or allowed milk substitutes, water ices	Cakes, cookies, pies, puddings or other desserts made with milk and butter or margarine, commercial fruit fillings, commercial sweet rolls, custards, custard and cream pies, ice cream, pie crust made with butter or margarine, sherbets
Eggs—prepared any way except with milk or cheese	Any prepared with milk or cheese
Fats—lard, peanut butter, pure mayonnaise, vegetable oils, margarines without milk or butter added, some cream substitutes (check labels)	Butter, cream substitutes, cream, sweet and sour, margarine with butter or milk added, salad dressings
Fruits—all except canned and frozen to which lactose is added	Canned or frozen prepared with lactose

Foods Allowed	**Foods to Avoid**
Milk—none	All types, infant food formulas, simulated mother's milk, yogurt
Meat, fish, or poultry—all kinds, cold cuts (check labels for added nonfat dry milk), kosher frankfurters	Breaded or creamed dishes, cold cuts and frankfurters containing nonfat dry milk, liver sausage
Vegetables—fresh, canned, or frozen—plain or with milk-free margarine (check labels of canned or frozen	Canned or frozen vegetables prepared with lactose, commercial french-fried potatoes, corn curls, creamed vegetables, instant or mashed potatoes, any seasoned with butter or margarine
Soups—meat and vegetable only (check labels)	All others
Miscellaneous—corn syrup, honey, nuts, nut butters, olives, pickles, pure seasonings and spices, pure jams and jellies, pure sugar candies, some cream substitutes, sugar	Ascorbic acid and citric acid mixtures, butterscotch, caramels, chewing gum, chocolate candy, cream sauces, cream soups, diabetic and dietetic preparations, dried soups, frozen cultures, frozen desserts, gravy, health and geriatric foods, monosodium glutamate extender, party dips, peppermints, powdered soft drinks, spice blends, starter cultures, sweetness reducers in candies, fruit pie fillings, icings, and preserves, toffee

Sample Menu

BREAKFAST

Orange juice
Cornflakes with cream substitute and sugar
Soft-cooked egg
French bread, toasted enriched
Margarine—milk free
Coffee with cream substitute and sugar

LUNCH

Baked chicken breast
Parslied potato
Asparagus tips
Sliced tomato and lettuce
French or Italian bread, enriched
Margarine—milk free
Grape jelly
Canned peach halves
Tea with lemon and sugar

DINNER

Roast beef sirloin
Baked potato
Diced carrots
French or Italian bread, enriched
Margarine—milk free
Apple jelly
Fresh fruit cup
Tea with lemon and sugar

Sucrase-Isomaltase Deficiency Deficiencies of these enzymes lead to symptoms similar to those seen in lactase insufficiency following ingestion of significant amounts of sucrose and isomaltose. A sucrose tolerance test is used to confirm the diagnosis.

Sucrose is added to many foods during processing and preparation. In addition, naturally occurring sucrose is present in a number of foods, making a strict sucrose-

Table 33–2. **Foods Containing More Than 5 gm Sucrose per 100 gm Edible Portion***

Apricots	Jams and jellies	Puddings
Bananas	Macadamia nuts	Syrups
Candy	Mangoes	Sorghum
Cane sugar	Milk chocolate	Soybeans
Cake	Molasses	Soybean flour or meal
Chestnuts, Va.	Oranges	Sugar beets
Chocolate, sweet	Pastries	Sweet breads and rolls
Condensed milk	Peaches	Sweet pickles
Cookies	Peanuts	Sweet potatoes
Dates	Peas	Tangerine
Honeydew melon	Pineapple	Watermelon
Ice cream	Prune plums, Italian	Wheat germ

*Adapted from Hardinge, M. G. et al.: "Carbohydrates in Foods," *J. Am. Diet. Assoc.*, **46**:197–204, 1965.

free diet impractical. Nevertheless, elimination of foods containing relatively large amounts of sucrose should be made (see Table 33–2). Glucose is substituted as a sweetening agent. Products containing wheat and potato starches should be avoided as these yield more isomaltose upon hydrolysis than do other starches such as rice and corn.

Increased sucrase activity following fructose feeding has been reported in this disorder, thus permitting ingestion of small amounts of sucrose without provoking symptoms. Infants with the disorder have responded to a strict sucrose-free diet within 24 hours, and after about 1 week are permitted gradual additions of foods low in sucrose.[13]

Glucose-Galactase Deficiency This rare disease is characterized by inability to absorb any carbohydrate that yields glucose or galactose upon hydrolysis. Substitution of fructose as the sole source of carbohydrate in the diet leads to improvement in symptoms. A special formula containing 4 to 8 per cent fructose has been devised for infants.[14] This formula is used almost exclusively for the first few months, after which it is gradually decreased and addition of foods low in starch is begun. By the age of three, a regular diet for age is usually tolerated with limited amounts of milk and starch-containing foods. Some degree of dietary restriction is necessary throughout life in order to prevent recurrence of symptoms of diarrhea. If a galactose-free diet is ordered, the lactose-free diet (see page 553) is used; sugar beets, peas, and Lima beans must also be avoided. Liver, brains, and sweetbreads store galactose and are usually avoided.

A-Beta-Lipoproteinemia This is a rare congenital disorder which is believed to involve a defect in the release or synthesis of β-lipoprotein. As a result fat is not transported from the intestinal cells into the lacteals. Total β-lipoprotein deficiency is manifested by steatorrhea and failure to thrive among other symptoms in infants. The malabsorption of fats is associated with extremely low serum concentrations of β-lipoprotein, cholesterol, vitamin A, and phospholipids.

Substitution of medium-chain triglycerides for long-chain fats in the diet results in improved fat absorption since the shorter chain fats are absorbed by way of the portal vein rather than by lymph.

Abnormalities in Mucosal Cell Transport—Nonspecific Disorders

Reduction in the absorptive surface area by massive intestinal resection or by damage to the villi produced by disease may

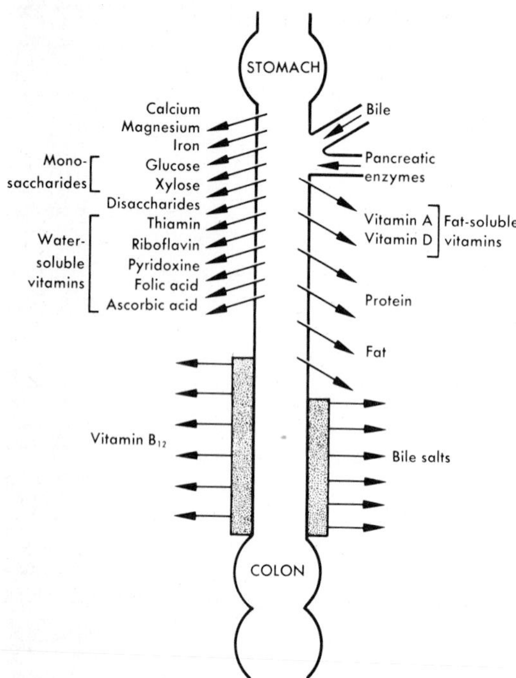

Figure 33–1. Sites of absorption in the small bowel. Most nutrients are absorbed from the proximal portion of the small intestine. (Adapted from Booth, C. C.: "Effect of Location Along Small Intestine on Absorption of Nutrients," Chapter 76 in *Handbook of Physiology. Alimentary Canal,* Vol. 1, American Physiological Society, Washington, D.C., 1967.)

have profound effects on nutrient uptake and absorption.

Short-Bowel Syndrome This term is used to describe those patients who are in metabolic imbalance as a consequence of massive resection of the small intestine. Removal of large portions of the bowel shortens the transit time of the contents through the intestine, thereby reducing the time for absorption. Attempts to increase absorption by delaying transit time include dietary modification and drug therapy. In this syndrome, the length of the remaining bowel is generally less than 8 feet. The amount of bowel left intact and the site of resection have an important bearing on the patient's nutritional status.

Nutrients normally absorbed in the proximal intestine are shown in Figure 33–1. Following removal of the jejunum, some absorption of these nutrients may take place in the ileum by virtue of its ability to act as a functional intestinal reserve. On the other hand, the jejunum has a limited capacity to absorb water and electrolytes and cannot compensate for the massive losses that occur when the ileum is removed. Following ileal resection, steatorrhea occurs because of bile salt deficiency.

Typically, the patient goes through three stages after massive resection of the bowel. In the immediate postoperative period, diarrhea and fluid and electrolyte imbalance may be so severe as to be life threatening. Total parenteral nutrition is used as the sole source of nutrients for 1 or 2 months. The patient surviving this period enters the second stage when nutritional concerns are of prime importance. Steady weight loss occurs as a result of anorexia, diarrhea, and steatorrhea. Osteomalacia may develop. Oral intake during this period usually is not sufficient, and supplemental calories are provided by intravenous feedings. Carbohydrates low in fiber are the first foods added since they are well absorbed by the remaining intestine. From 50 to 100 gm per day are used initially. After the patient tolerates carbohydrates and proteins, small amounts of fat are gradually introduced. For many patients a maximum of 40 gm fat is tolerated. Amounts greater than this increase steatorrhea. Finally after 3 months or more, the patient's condition stabilizes, usually at a substantially lower weight. The fat intake can usually be increased to 50 to 60 gm daily.

The extreme losses of all nutrients in this syndrome require greatly increased intakes of calories, protein, vitamins, and minerals. Up to 5,000 kcal and175 gm of protein may be needed to prevent further weight loss. Substitution of medium-chain triglycerides for long-chain fats has led to decreased diarrhea and electrolyte losses and improvement in nutritional status. Frequent small meals are tolerated best. Dietary oxalate is restricted together with fat to compensate for enhanced oxalate absorption by colonic mucosa.[15]

Semisynthetic fiber-free diets have been useful in this and other malabsorptive disorders. These diets are designed to provide complete nutritional support for extended periods in patients in whom it is desirable to reduce gastrointestinal residue to a minimum. Semisynthetic fiber-free diets, composed of purified amino acids, simple carbohydrates, fats, vitamins, and minerals, have no indigestible bulk, hence require minimum digestion, and are rapidly absorbed from the upper intestinal tract. Both frequency and volume of stools are decreased. Commercial powdered preparations, available in several flavors, when diluted with water may be used for tube feeding, beverages, or frozen as popsicles. Home parenteral nutrition is also used in selected cases.

Gluten Enteropathy This is a disease of genetic origin characterized by intolerance to the gliadin fraction of gluten with consequent malabsorption. The disorder is known as *celiac disease* in childhood and as *adult celiac disease* or *nontropical sprue* in later life. The mechanism of the sensitivity to gluten is not understood. Current hypotheses hold that a primary mucosal defect permits gluten to exert a toxic effect in genetically predisposed individuals[16] or that immune factors are involved. According to the latter theory, gluten binds to cell-surface receptors and interacts with lymphocytes to produce antibodies and other immune products which damage the cell.[17] The diagnosis is made by intestinal biopsies initially, after 3 months of a gluten-free diet and after a gluten challenge.[17]

The onset of this disease is insidious and is manifested by diarrhea, steatorrhea, weight loss, and other symptoms of the malabsorption syndrome. Stools are characteristically loose, pale, and frothy (due to fermentation of undigested carbohydrate) and contain excessive amounts of fat. Biopsy specimens of the mucosal surface have a flattened appearance; the villi become shorter and club shaped and appear to be fused. A marked decrease in the number of microvilli in the brush border drastically reduces the absorptive surface. Laboratory findings are consistent with those of the malabsorption syndrome. (See page 546).

Exacerbations and remissions are common in this disorder. Symptoms are provoked by ingestion of gluten from wheat, rye, barley, buckwheat, and, in some instances, oats. Gluten from rice and potato has no deleterious effect.

Elimination of gluten from the diet (see Gluten-Restricted Diet) should be given a trial of at least 6 weeks. Regeneration of villi and return of enzyme activity occur in most cases following strict adherence to a gluten-restricted diet. Lack of response to the diet in some cases may be due to failure to follow the diet or to secondary lactose intolerance resulting from mucosal damage. In this case, a gluten-restricted, lactose-free diet leads to improved fat and carbohydrate absorption.

The diet should provide 100 gm or more protein to replace wasted tissue. Some moderation in fiber content and fat intake may be needed initially as these are usually poorly tolerated. Improved fat absorption can be achieved through the use of MCT. Supplementary vitamins and minerals are needed to overcome nutritional deficiencies resulting from excessive losses in the stools.

Dietary Counseling

Proteins from lean meats, poultry, fish, cottage cheese, egg white, and skim milk are well utilized and should be encouraged. Individual tolerance for fibrous foods and strongly

Gluten-Restricted Diet

Characteristics and General Rules

This diet excludes all products containing wheat, rye, oats, and barley. Read all labels carefully.

Aqueous multivitamins are usually prescribed in addition to the diet.

The diet may be progressed gradually; that is, small amounts of unsaturated fats may be used at first, adding harder fats later. Fiber may be reduced initially by using only cooked fruits and vegetables. Strongly flavored vegetables may be poorly tolerated at first.

Include These Foods, or Their Nutritive Equivalents, Daily:

4 cups milk
6–8 ounces (cooked weight) lean meat, fish, or poultry
1 egg
4 vegetables including:
  1 dark green or deep yellow
  1 potato
  2 other vegetables
  Other to be served raw, if tolerated
3 fruits including:
  1–2 servings citrus fruit or other good source ascorbic acid
  1–2 other fruits
4 servings bread and cereals: corn, rice, soybean
NO WHEAT, RYE, OATS, BARLEY
2 tablespoons fat

Additional calories are provided by using more of the foods listed, dessert, soups, sweets

Nutritive value of listed foods: Protein, 105 gm; fat, 110 gm; carbohydrate, 200 gm; 2,200 kcal. Minerals and vitamins in excess of recommended allowances.

Foods Allowed	Foods to Avoid
Beverages—carbonated, cocoa, coffee, fruit juices, milk, tea	*Beverages*—ale, beer, instant coffee containing cereal, malted milk, Postum, products containing cereal
Breads—corn bread, muffins, and pone with no wheat flour; breads made with cornmeal, cornstarch, potato, rice, soybean, wheat starch flour	*Breads*—all containing any wheat, rye, oats, or barley; bread crumbs, muffins, pancakes, rolls, rusks, waffles, zwieback; all commercial yeast and quick bread mixes; all crackers, pretzels, Ry-Krisp
Cereals—cooked cornmeal, Cream of Rice, hominy or grits, rice; ready to eat: corn or rice cereals such as cornflakes, rice flakes, Puffed Rice	*Cereals*—cooked or ready-to-eat breakfast cereals containing wheat, oats; barley, macaroni, noodles, pasta, spaghetti, wheat germ
Cheese—cottage; later, cream cheese	
Desserts—custard, fruit ice, fruit whips, plain or fruit ice cream (homemade), plain or fruit gelatin, meringues; homemade puddings—cornstarch, rice, tapioca; rennet desserts; sherbet; cakes and cookies made with allowed flours	*Desserts*—cake, cookies, doughnuts, pastries, pie; bisques, commercial ice cream, ice cream cones; prepared mixes containing wheat, rye, oats, or barley; puddings thickened with wheat flour

Foods Allowed	**Foods to Avoid**
Eggs—as desired	
Fats—oil: corn, cottonseed, olive, sesame, soybean; French dressing, pure mayonnaise, salad dressing with cornstarch thickening Later additions: butter, cream, margarine, peanut oil, vegetable shortening	*Fats*—bacon, lard, suet, salad dressing with flour thickening
Flour—cornmeal, potato, rice, soybean	*Flour*—barley, oat, rye, wheat—bread, cake, entire wheat, graham, self-rising, whole wheat, wheat germ
Fruits—all cooked, canned, and juices; fresh and frozen as tolerated, avoiding skin and seeds initially	*Fruits*—prunes, plums, and their juices; those with skins and seeds at first
Meat—all lean meats, poultry, fish: baked, broiled, roasted, stewed	*Meat*—breaded, creamed, croquettes, luncheon meats unless pure meat, meat loaf, stuffings with bread, scrapple, thickened stew Fat meats such as corned beef, duck, frankfurters, goose, ham, luncheon meats, pork, sausage Fatty fish such as herring, mackerel, sardines, swordfish, or canned in heavy oil
Milk—all kinds	
Soups—broth, bouillon, cream if thickened with cornstarch, vegetable	*Soups*—thickened with flour; containing barley, noodles, etc.
Sweets—candy, honey, jam, jelly, marmalade, marshmallows, molasses, syrup, sugar	*Sweets*—candies with high fat content, nuts; candies containing wheat products
Vegetables—cooked or canned: buttered; fresh as tolerated	*Vegetables*—creamed if thickened with wheat, oat, rye, or barley products. Strongly flavored if they produce discomfort: baked beans, broccoli, Brussels sprouts, cabbage, cauliflower, corn, cucumber, lentils, onions, peppers, radishes, turnips
Miscellaneous—gravy and sauces thickened with cornstarch; olives, peanut butter, pickles, popcorn, potato chips	*Miscellaneous*—gravies and sauces thickened with flours not permitted

Sample Menu

BREAKFAST

Tomato juice
Rice Krispies
Milk, sugar
Southern corn muffins
Butter or margarine
Currant jelly
Scrambled eggs
Coffee, with cream, sugar

LUNCH

Beef stew (not thickened)
  Beef cubes
  Potato
  Carrots
  Onions
Tossed green salad
French dressing
Rice-flour bread
Butter or margarine
Milk
Vanilla cornstarch pudding with sliced frozen peaches

DINNER

Broiled lamb patties (all meat)
Mint jelly
Rice with saffron seasoning

Sample Menu
DINNER

Buttered asparagus
Celery and olives
Milk
Lemon meringue pudding (thickened with cornstarch)
Coffee with cream, sugar

flavored vegetables should determine whether or not these foods are included. The patient should be advised to read labels on all commercial food products in order to avoid any foods containing wheat, rye, oats, or barley. Besides cereals and breads as obvious sources, many other foods contain wheat or other flour as a thickener. Canned soups, cheese spreads, cooked salad dressings, cold cuts, breaded meats, mixes of all kinds, catsup, ice cream, and pastries are but a few of the many foods that contain cereal products. Information on prepared and packaged foods known to be gluten free is available for patients.* Many standard cookbooks contain suitable recipes utilizing cornstarch, cornmeal, potato, rice, or tapioca instead of flour. Sources of special recipes utilizing arrowroot starch or wheat starch (from which the gluten is removed) should be supplied to the patient.* However, patients should be cautioned that mere substitution of other flours for wheat will not produce satisfactory results; other adjustments in mixing technique, baking time, and temperature are also needed. When meals are eaten away from home, plain foods, without breading, gravies, cream sauces, and so on, should be selected. Persons who are not intolerant to oats should be permitted to add this cereal to the diet.

Radiation Enteritis Radiation to the abdomen damages the intestinal mucosa resulting in flattened villi and depressed enzyme activities, thus interfering with absorption of many nutrients. (See also Chapter 35.)

* Available from companies such as General Foods, General Mills, and others.

Abnormality of Intestinal Lymphatics

Intestinal Lymphangiectasia This is a congenital defect in which obstruction of intestinal lymphatics is associated with leakage of chylomicron fat and plasma proteins into the intestinal lumen. In addition to decreased serum protein levels and associated edema and ascites formation, steatorrhea occurs. Protein losses are reduced considerably by use of medium-chain triglycerides or a fat-restricted diet. (See page 572.)

Tropical Sprue This disorder is a form of the malabsorption syndrome that occurs chiefly in the West Indies, Central America, and the Far East. In some respects it is similar to nontropical sprue, but the onset is more acute and it responds to different therapy. Both disorders are characterized by steatorrhea and secondary enzyme deficiencies in the intestinal mucosa. In tropical sprue there is also ileal involvement. Hypocalcemia with tetany and osteomalacia do not occur as commonly as in nontropical sprue; however, nutritional deficiencies of folic acid and vitamin B-12 do occur and are manifested as macrocytic anemia. Dramatic improvement in symptoms is often shown following administration of folic acid and vitamin B-12.

The diet in tropical sprue should be high in protein and calories and restricted in fiber and in fat. The substitution of medium-chain triglycerides for some of the fat has resulted in weight gain and disappearance of steatorrhea. The restriction of gluten for patients with tropical sprue does not usually lead to further improvement.

Problems and Review

1. What symptoms are characteristic of the malabsorption syndrome? In what ways is the diet modified?
2. What information is provided by each of the following tests:
   a. Serum carotene level
   b. Schilling test
   c. *d*-Xylose test
3. Plan a lactose-free diet for Mr. R., a single graduate student, who lives alone in an apartment with adequate cooking facilities. He enjoys Italian and Mexican foods. His caloric needs are estimated to be 2,500 per day.
   a. List at least 10 foods that may contain lactose.
   b. Give suggestions for increasing calories in this diet.
   c. In which nutrients would this diet be inadequate?
   d. Which foods could be added if the diet is changed to controlled lactose?
   e. Mr. R. sometimes eats his lunch in a cafeteria. Give suggestions for suitable food choices.
4. Mrs. W. is a 45-year-old housewife and mother of four who was recently diagnosed as having adult celiac disease. The doctor prescribed a gluten-restricted diet for her.
   a. Explain what gluten is, and why it must be restricted in her diet.
   b. What are typical sources of gluten in the diet? Name some other less obvious foods that may contain gluten. What cereal grains can be substituted for those containing gluten?
   c. Mrs. W. is quite apprehensive about her diet. She states that she does not have time to bake special products for herself because her husband is a diabetic and one child has severe asthma. Give suggestions to help her in planning her diet. She wants to gain 10 pounds.
5. How could you change the diet you ate yesterday to make it free of gluten? To make it lactose free? To eliminate both lactose and gluten?
6. Mr. N. had a massive bowel resection. Which nutrients are likely to be poorly absorbed? Would MCT be useful in this disorder? Why?
7. Compare the dietary modifications used in nontropical and tropical sprue.

Cited References

1. Committee on Nutrition: "The Practical Significance of Lactose Intolerance in Children," *Pediatrics,* **62**:240–45, 1978.
2. Solomons, N. W. et al.: "Hydrogen Breath Test of Lactose Absorption in Adults: The Application of Physiological Doses and Whole Cow's Milk Sources," *Am. J. Clin. Nutr.,* **33**:545–54, 1980.
3. Newcomer, A. D. et al.: "Triolein Breath Test. A Sensitive and Specific Test for Fat Malabsorption," *Gastroenterology,* **76**:6–13, 1980.
4. Meeker, H. E. et al.: "Clinical Experience in ^{14}C-Tripalmitin Breath Test for Fat Malabsorption," *Am. J. Gastroenterology,* **73**:227–31, 1980.
5. Chalmers, R. A. et al.: "Measurement of 4-Hydroxyphenylacetic Aciduria as a Screening Test for Small Bowel Disease," *Clin. Chem.,* **25**:1791–94, 1979.
6. Rampton, D. S. et al.: "Oxalate Loading Test: A Screening Test for Steatorrhoea," *Gut,* **20**:1089–94, 1979.
7. Schizas, A. A. et al.: "Medium-Chain Triglycerides—Use in Food Preparation," *J. Am. Diet. Assoc.,* **51**:228–32, 1967.

8. Regan, P. T., and DiMagno, E. P.: "The Medical Management of Malabsorption," *Mayo Clin. Proc.*, **54**:267–74, 1979.
9. Mueller, J. F.: "Drug-Nutrient Interrelationships," in *Human Nutrition. A Comprehensive Treatise. 3B. Nutrition and the Adult: Micronutrients.* Alfin-Slater, R. B., and Kritchevsky, D., eds. Plenum Press, New York, 1980.
10. Green, P. H. R., and Tall, A. R.: "Drugs, Alcohol and Malabsorption," *Am. J. Med.*, **67**:1066–76, 1979.
11. Welsh, J. D.: "Diet Therapy in Adult Lactose Malabsorption: Present Practices," *Am. J. Clin. Nutr.*, **31**:592–96, 1978.
12. Johnson, J. D. et al.: "Lactose Malabsorption. Its Biology and History," *Adv. Pediatrics*, **21**:197–237, 1974.
13. Ament, M. E. et al.: "Sucrase-isomaltase Deficiency—A Frequently Misdiagnosed Disease," *J. Pediatr.*, **83**:721–27, 1973.
14. Lindquist, B., and Meeuwisse, G.: "Diets in Disaccharidase Deficiency and Defective Monosaccharide Absorption," *J. Am. Diet. Assoc.*, **48**:307–10, 1966.
15. Greenberger, N. J.: "State of the Art: The Management of the Patient with Short Bowel Syndrome," *Am. J. Gastroenterology*, **70**:528–40, 1978.
16. Cornell, H. J., and Rolles, C. J.: "Further Evidence of a Primary Mucosal Defect in Coeliac Disease," *Gut*, **19**:253–59, 1978.
17. Falchuk, Z. M.: "Update on Gluten-Sensitive Enteropathy," *Am. J. Med.*, **67**:1085–96, 1979.

Additional References

BARR, R. G. et al.: "Breath Tests in Pediatric Gastrointestinal Disorders: New Diagnostic Opportunities," *Pediatrics*, **62**:393–401, 1978.

CHENG, A. H. R. et al.: "Long-Term Acceptance of Low-Lactose Milk," *Am. J. Clin. Nutr.*, **32**:1989–93, 1979.

DISSANAYAKE, A. S. et al.: "Lack of Harmful Effect of Oats on Small-Intestinal Mucosa in Coeliac Disease," *Brit. Med. J.*, **4**:189–91, 1974.

DODGE, J. A.: "Gluten Intolerance, Gluten Enteropathy, and Coeliac Disease," *Arch. Dis. Child.*, **55**:143–45, 1980.

JONES, D. V. et al.: "Symptom Response to Lactose-Reduced Milk in Lactose-Intolerant Adults," *Am. J. Clin. Nutr.*, **29**:633–38, 1976.

KORETZ, R. L., and MEYER, J. H.: "Elemental Diets—Facts and Fantasies," *Gastroenterology*, **78**:393–410, 1980.

MCNEISH, A. S.: "Coeliac Disease: Duration of Gluten-Free Diet," *Arch. Dis. Child.*, **55**:110–111, 1980.

MILNE, D.: "Oats and Coeliac Disease," *Brit. Med. J.*, **1**:152, 1975.

Riley, J. W., and Glickman, R. M.: "Fat Malabsorption—Advances in Our Understanding," *Am. J. Med.*, **67**:980–88, 1979.

ROSENBERG, F. H.: "Lactose Intolerance," *Am. J. Nurs.*, **77**:823–24, 1977.

ROSENSWEIG, N. S.: "On-Lactose-Hydrolyzed Milk," *Am. J. Clin. Nutr.*, **32**:1979, 1979.

SIMOONS, F. J.: "The Geographic Hypothesis and Lactose Malabsorption," *Am. J. Digest. Dis.*, **23**:963–80, 1978.

SIMOONS, F. J. et al.: "Perspective on Milk-Drinking and Malabsorption of Lactose," *Pediatrics*, **59**:98–108, 1977.

WESER, E.: "Nutrition Aspects of Malabsorption. Short Gut Adaptation," *Am. J. Med.*, **67**:1014–20, 1979.

Diet in 34 Disturbances of the Liver, Gallbladder, and Pancreas

HIGH-PROTEIN, HIGH-CARBOHYDRATE, MODERATE-FAT DIET; FAT-RESTRICTED DIET

Diseases of the Liver— General Considerations

The liver is the largest and most complex organ in the body. It performs many functions that have an important bearing on one's nutritional state. Diseases of this organ may therefore markedly affect health.

Functions The role of the liver in intermediary metabolism with reference to proteins, fats, and carbohydrates has been described in Chapters 4, 5, and 6 and is briefly summarized as follows:

1. Protein metabolism (Chapter 4)—synthesis of plasma proteins; deamination of amino acids; formation of urea.
2. Carbohydrate metabolism (Chapter 5)—synthesis, storage, and release of glycogen; synthesis of heparin.
3. Lipid metabolism (Chapter 6)—synthesis of lipoproteins, phospholipids, cholesterol; formation of bile; conjugation of bile salts; oxidation of fatty acids.
4. Mineral metabolism (Chapter 8)—storage of iron, copper and other minerals.
5. Vitamin metabolism (Chapter 10)—storage of vitamins A and D; some conversion of carotene to vitamin A, and of vitamin K to prothrombin.
6. Detoxification of bacterial decomposition products, mineral poisons, and certain drugs and dyes.

Etiology Liver diseases may have a number of causes: infectious agents, toxins, metabolic or nutritional factors, biliary obstruction, and carcinoma. The pathologic changes in the liver parenchymal cells are similar regardless of the etiology of the disease. Basic changes include atrophy, fatty infiltration, fibrosis, and necrosis.

Symptoms and Clinical Findings *Jaundice* is a symptom common to many diseases of the liver and biliary tract and consists of a yellow pigmentation of the skin and body tissues because of the accumulation of bile pigments in the blood. *Obstructive jaundice* results from the interference of the flow of bile by stones, tumors, or inflammation of the mucosa of the ducts. *Hemolytic jaundice* results from an abnormally large destruction of blood cells such as occurs in yellow fever, pernicious anemia, and so forth. *Toxic jaundice* originates from poisons, drugs, or virus infections.

Other symptoms commonly seen in liver diseases include lassitude, weakness, fatigue, fever, anorexia, and weight loss; abdominal pain, flatulence, nausea, and vomiting; hepatomegaly; ascites and edema; and portal hypertension.

Nutritional Considerations in Liver Disease Protection of the parenchymal cells is the foremost consideration in all types of liver injury. Since the liver is so intimately involved in the metabolism of foodstuffs, a nutritious diet is an important part of therapy and should be designed to protect the liver from stress and to enable it to function as efficiently as possible. With the exception of hepatic coma, generous amounts of high-quality protein should be provided for tissue repair and for prevention of fatty infiltration and degeneration of liver cells. A high-carbohydrate intake ensures an adequate reserve of glycogen, which, together with adequate protein stores, has a protective effect. Moderate amounts of fat are indicated for many persons. Signs of nutritional deficiency such as glossitis, nutritional anemia, or peripheral neuropathy are not uncommon in patients with liver disease. Generous amounts of vitamins, especially of the B complex, must be provided to compensate for deficiencies. If edema and ascites are present, sodium restriction may be necessary.

Hepatitis

Etiology and Symptoms This is an infectious disease characterized by inflammatory and degenerative changes of the liver. Two classes are recognized, *viral* and *drug-induced*. The viral type is more common and occurs as *Type A* (formerly called *infectious*), *Type B (serum)*, or *Type C* (posttransfusion). Specific viruses have been identified for Types A and B. Type A is transmitted either by fecal contamination of water or food or parenterally. Epidemics occur from time to time in young people and are usually traced to a breakdown in sanitation. Type B is transmitted chiefly by the parenteral route through improperly sterilized needles. Type C accounts for a high percentage of cases of posttransfusion hepatitis in hospitalized patients. Type A viral hepatitis is usually mild and rarely progresses to chronic hepatitis whereas Type B is often more severe and more likely to progress to a potentially serious liver disorder, chronic active hepatitis, which is associated with a number of pathologic lesions.

Drug-induced hepatitis may be due to alcohol, heroin, marihuana, or hashish, or to hypersensitivity to sulfa compounds or penicillin, or to a direct toxic effect on the liver by agents such as carbon tetrachloride.

Aside from mode of transmission and period of incubation, the two classes of hepatitis are similar. Nonspecific symptoms such

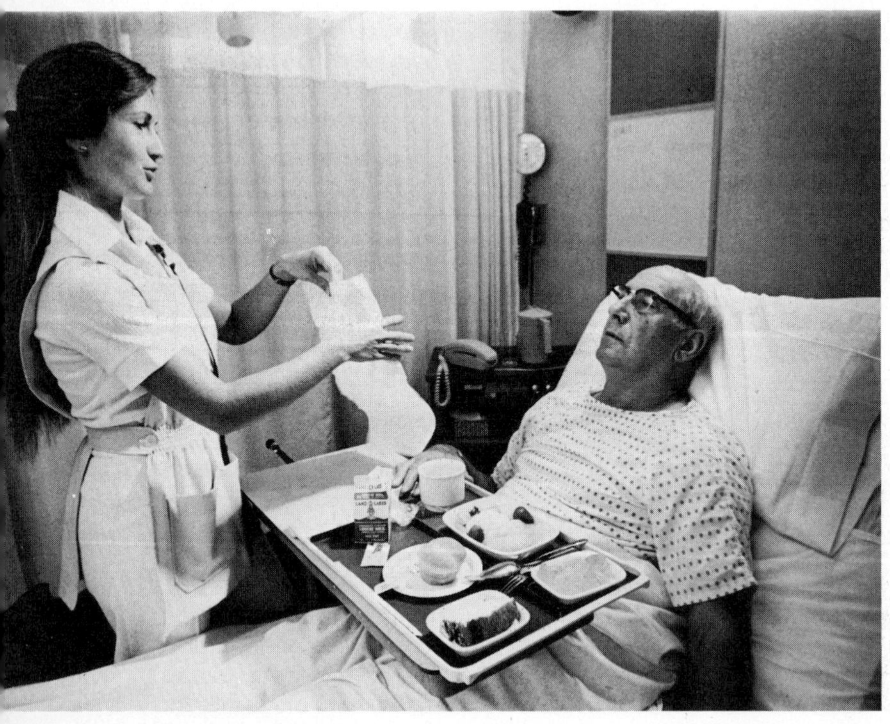

Figure 34–1. Many patients with diseases of the liver have poor appetites. The nurse encourages the patient to eat and helps him as needed. (Courtesy, Metropolitan Medical Center, Minneapolis.)

as anorexia, fatigue, nausea and vomiting, diarrhea, fever, weight loss, and abdominal discomfort usually precede the development of jaundice, which ordinarily subsides after 1 or 2 weeks. Complete recovery may take several months. Treatment consists of adequate rest, nutritious diet, and avoidance of further damage to the liver.

Dietary Modification The objectives of dietary treatment are to aid in the regeneration of liver tissue and to prevent further liver damage. This can be accomplished by providing a nutritious diet and enticing the patient to eat it. The patient must be convinced of the importance of the diet in promoting recovery and preventing relapses. Anorexia is frequently a problem; hence every effort must be made to encourage the patient to eat. Foods must be well prepared and attractively served with consideration given to the individual's food preferences (See Figure 34–1.)

Initially, foods of liquid-to-soft consistency (see Chapter 25) may be preferable if there is anorexia in the acute stages of the illness, progressing to a wider selection of foods with convalescence. Sufficient calories should be provided to maintain weight, or to bring about weight gain, if needed. A liberal intake of carbohydrate and fat as tolerated is required to reduce protein catabolism. At least 1 gm protein or more per kilogram of body weight daily is needed to overcome negative nitrogen balance, to promote regeneration of parenchymal cells, and to prevent fatty infiltration of the liver. Judicious use of spices and condiments may help to stimulate the appetite. Small to moderate portions at mealtime with between-meal supplements of high-protein beverages are frequently more acceptable than larger meals. Some individuals need assistance in feeding themselves and should be allowed adequate time to eat at a leisurely pace. The following high-protein, moderate-fat, high-carbohydrate diet is appropriate to meet the nutritional goals for patients whose appetite has returned.

High-Protein, Moderate-Fat, High-Carbohydrate Diet

Characteristics and General Rules

The caloric level may be increased by adding high-carbohydrate foods. Small amounts of cream and ice cream may be used when tolerated.

The protein intake may be increased by adding nonfat dry milk to liquid milk.

Modifications in fiber and consistency may be made by applying restrictions concerning the soft diet (Chapter 25) to the foods listed here.

Six or more small feedings may be preferred when there is lack of appetite.

When sodium restriction is ordered, all food must be prepared without salt. Low-sodium milk should replace part or all of the prescribed milk. See Sodium-Restricted Diets, Chapter 40.

Include These Foods Daily:

1 quart milk
8 ounces lean meat, poultry, or fish
1 egg
4 servings vegetables including:
- 2 servings potato or substitute
- 1 serving green leafy or yellow vegetable
- 1–2 servings other vegetable
- One vegetable to be raw each day

3 servings fruit including:
  1 serving citrus fruit or other good source of ascorbic acid
  2 servings other fruit
1 serving enriched or whole-grain cereal
6 slices enriched or whole-grain bread
2 tablespoons butter or margarine
4 tablespoons sugar, jelly, marmalade, or jam
Additional foods to further increase the carbohydrate as the patient is able to take them

Nutritive value of basic pattern on page 565: Protein, 135 gm; fat, 106 gm; carbohydrate, 236 gm; kcal, 2,590; calcium, 2.53 gm; iron, 18.3 mg; vitamin A, 18,770 I.U.; thiamin, 2.11 mg; riboflavin, 3.39 mg; niacin, 27.6 mg; ascorbic acid, 159 mg.

Typical Food Selection

Beverages—carbonated beverages, milk and milk drinks, coffee, tea, fruit juices, cocoa flavoring
Breads and cereals—all kinds
Cheese—cottage, cream, mild Cheddar
Desserts—angel cake, plain cake and cookies, custard, plain or fruit gelatin, fruit whip, fruit pudding, Junket, milk and cereal desserts, sherbets, ices, plain ice cream
Eggs—any way
Fat—butter, margarine, cream, cooking fat, vegetable oils
Fruits—all
Meat—lean beef, chicken, fish, lamb, liver, pork, turkey
Potato or substitute—hominy, macaroni, noodles, rice, spaghetti, sweet potato
Seasonings—salt, spices, vinegar (in moderation)
Soups—clear and cream
Sweets—honey, jam, jelly, sugar, sugar candy, syrups
Vegetables—all

Foods to Avoid

No foods are specifically contraindicated. Many patients complain of intolerance to the following groups of foods: strongly flavored vegetables; rich desserts; fried and fatty foods; chocolate; nuts; and highly seasoned foods. Although such complaints cannot always be explained on a physiologic basis, nothing is gained by giving the offending foods to the patient.

Meal Pattern	**Sample Menu**
BREAKFAST	
Fruit	Half grapefruit
Cereal with milk and sugar	Wheatena with milk and sugar
Egg	Scrambled egg
Whole-grain or enriched toast—2 slices	Whole-wheat toast
Butter or margarine—2 teaspoons	Margarine
Marmalade—1 tablespoon	Orange marmalade
Beverage with cream and sugar	Coffee with cream and sugar

Meal Pattern	Sample Menu
LUNCHEON OR SUPPER	
Lean meat, fish, or poultry—4 ounces	Broiled whitefish
Potato or substitute	Escalloped potatoes
Cooked vegetable	Asparagus with margarine
Salad	Celery and carrot strips
Whole-grain or enriched bread—2 slices	Whole-wheat bread
Butter or margarine—2 teaspoons	Margarine
Jelly—1 tablespoon	Grape jelly
Fruit	Sliced banana
Milk	Milk
MIDAFTERNOON	
Milk with nonfat dry milk	High-protein milk with strawberry flavor
DINNER	
Lean meat, fish, or fowl—4 ounces	Roast beef
Potato	Mashed potato
Vegetable	Baked acorn squash
Whole-grain or enriched bread—2 slices	Dinner rolls
Butter or margarine—2 teaspoons	Margarine
Jelly—1 tablespoon	Apple jelly
Fruit, or dessert	Raspberry sherbet
Milk—1 glass	Milk
Tea, if desired	
EVENING NOURISHMENT	
Milk beverage	High-protein milk flavored with caramel Bread-and-jelly sandwich

Cirrhosis

Etiology This chronic disease of the liver is characterized by diffuse degenerative changes, fibrosis, and nodular regeneration of the remaining cells. The causes include infectious hepatitis in a small percentage of patients, chronic alcoholism in association with malnutrition, underlying metabolic disturbances such as hemochromatosis or Wilson's disease, hepatotoxins derived from certain plants and fungi, and prolonged biliary stasis.

Laennec's cirrhosis. The most common type of cirrhosis in the United States is Laennec's (*alcoholic, portal*) cirrhosis. The exact etiology has not been established although alcohol and relative or absolute malnutrition are implicated in the majority of patients. Alcohol has a direct toxic effect on the liver but the extent to which malnutrition promotes this effect is not clear.[1] Only about 10 per cent of alcoholics develop cirrhosis, and it occurs after years of excessive alcohol intake in individuals whose diets are less than optimal in a number of nutrients. Pathologic changes include fatty infiltration, necrosis, and proliferation of fibrous tissue.

Symptoms and Clinical Findings The onset of cirrhosis may be gradual with gastrointestinal disturbances such as anorexia, nausea, vomiting, pain, and distension. As the disease progresses, jaundice and other serious changes occur.

Ascites. Ascites is the accumulation of abnormal amounts of fluid in the abdomen. It may develop as a consequence of portal vein hypertension, obstruction of the hepatic vein, a fall in plasma colloid osmotic pressure due to impaired albumin synthesis, increased sodium retention, or impaired water excretion.

Esophageal varices (varicose veins). Varices in the esophagus and upper part of the stomach may develop as a complication of portal hypertension. Hemorrhage is then an ever-present danger and may be provoked by roughage of any kind. The hemorrhage itself may be fatal, or the blood may provide for the accumulation of ammonia and subsequent hepatic coma.

Modification of the Diet Regeneration of parenchymal cells occurs if appropriate diet therapy is initiated before the disease is well advanced. The high-protein, high-carbohydrate diet outlined for infectious hepatitis is satisfactory. In advanced cirrhosis, however, further dietary modification is needed.

Protein. Individual requirements for protein must be considered and intake must be adjusted as the disease progresses or improves. Most clinicians recommend an initial protein intake high enough to maintain nitrogen equilibrium, but low enough to prevent hepatic coma (approximately 35 to 50 gm per day).[2] Lieber recommends a protein intake that does not exceed the recommended dietary allowances or the individual's tolerance, whichever is lower.[1] Intakes greater than this risk hepatic coma. Protein intake is restricted to less than 35 gm daily if signs of impending coma develop.

Fats. Malabsorption of fats occurs in many cirrhotics. For some patients the substitution of medium-chain triglycerides for part of the dietary fat is effective in reducing steatorrhea. (See Chapter 33.)

Vitamins and minerals. Malabsorption of fat-soluble and B-complex vitamins occurs in alcoholic and biliary cirrhosis. Serum calcium, magnesium, and zinc are decreased. Potassium supplements are sometimes needed to correct deficiency resulting from nausea, vomiting, diarrhea, antibiotic therapy, or a reduced protein intake. Vitamin supplements may be advisable to replenish liver stores and repair tissue damage, especially if there is anorexia.

Sodium. Sodium restriction is prescribed if edema and ascites are present. Severe restriction of sodium for many months is often necessary for effective removal of excess fluid accumulation. Diets restricted to 200–300 mg sodium daily are not uncommon in this disorder. On such very low sodium diets, all food used must be naturally low in sodium and prepared without sodium-containing compounds. Low-sodium milk is substituted for regular milk. Close attention to food selection is needed in order to provide an adequate protein intake without exceeding the sodium allowance. (See Chapter 40.)

Consistency. Reduction in fiber content of the diet is necessary in advanced cirrhosis when there is danger of hemorrhage from esophageal varices. A liquid or soft diet with small meals is used. (See Chapter 25.)

Hepatic Coma

Etiology This is a complex syndrome characterized by neurologic disturbances which may develop as a complication of severe liver disease. It usually results from entrance of certain nitrogen-containing substances such as ammonia into the cerebral circulation without being metabolized by the liver. It may be a consequence of shunting of the portal blood into the systemic circulation in cirrhosis, or of severe damage to liver cells in hepatitis. Precipitating factors include gastrointestinal bleeding, severe infections, surgical procedures, excessive dietary protein, and sedatives. Plasma aromatic amino acid levels (phenylalanine and tyrosine), and methionine are elevated while branched-chain amino acids (isoleucine, leucine, and valine) are lowered. It has been postulated that alterations in the plasma amino acid pattern may be causally related to the encephalopathy.[3]

Symptoms Signs of impending coma include confusion, restlessness, irritability, inappropriate behavior, delirium, and drowsiness. There may also be incoordination and a flapping tremor of the arms and legs when extended. Electrolyte imbalance occurs. The patient may go into coma and may have convulsions. The breath has a fecal odor *(fetor hepaticus)*. Prompt treatment is imperative or death occurs.

Treatment Treatment consists of dietary protein restriction, cleansing of the bowel with enemas or laxatives to reduce the nitrogenous load, or antibiotics to suppress bacterial growth. Lactulose is sometimes used to increase motility. This is a synthetic disaccharide containing galactose and fructose, which is metabolized by colonic bacteria to acetic and lactic acids and which lowers the pH of the colon thereby favoring diffusion of ammonia from blood to the colon. Oral or intravenous administration of branched-chain amino acids,* or their keto analogs, have reportedly improved both the plasma amino acid pattern and the encephalopathy.[3,4] Branched-chain amino acids are believed to decrease the transport of aromatic amino acids into the brain and also serve as an energy source in muscle thereby lessening efflux of amino acids into the circulation.[3]

Dietary Modification The fundamental principle in the dietary management of hepatic coma is to reduce the protein intake to a minimum, thus decreasing the amount of ammonia produced. Catabolism of tissue proteins must also be avoided.

Calories. About 1,500 to 2,000 kcal are needed to prevent breakdown of tissue proteins for energy and are provided chiefly in the form of carbohydrates and fats. Although anorexia may occur, attempts should be made to keep the caloric intake as high as is practical to minimize tissue breakdown.

Protein. Some clinicians omit protein completely for 2 or 3 days and others permit 20 to 30 gm daily. As the patient improves, the protein intake is gradually increased by 10 to 15 gm at a time until a maximum of 1 gm per kilogram of body weight is reached. The patient must be carefully watched following each increment lest signs of coma recur.

Levels of 40 to 50 gm protein daily may be used for long periods of time without detriment to nutritional status provided the diet supplies sufficient calories to maintain weight. Nitrogen balance can be achieved on protein intakes as low as 35 gm daily[2] if high-quality protein is used and caloric intake is adequate. Some advocate use of diets composed of vegetable protein, 40 gm, because these are lower in certain amino acids and other compounds implicated in the etiology of encephalopathy.[5]

Dietary Management These patients pose problems in feeding because of anorexia and behavioral patterns ranging from apathy, drowsiness, and confusion to irritability and hyperexcitability. The protein-free diet consisting of commercial sugar-fat emulsions, a butter-sugar mixture, or glucose in beverages or fruit juices may be used initially through oral or tube feeding. (See Chapter 41.) With improvements, the diets providing 20, 40, and 60 gm protein (see page 668) may be gradually introduced.

Diseases of the Gallbladder

Incidence Gallbladder disease affects some 15 to 20 million adults in the United States. The exact prevalence is not known because many persons have asymptomatic gallbladder disease and never seek medical care. However, gallbladder disease is the fifth leading cause of hospitalization in the United States, and cholecystectomy is one of the most frequently performed surgical procedures. Gallstones are frequently found at autopsy in persons who were not known to have gallbladder disease. The in-

* Hepatic-aid (TM) McGaw Laboratories, Irvine, California.

cidence of gallbladder disease is higher in northern Europe and North and South America than in the Orient and other parts of the world. The American Indian, in particular, is at increased risk for the disease, and a genetic predisposition has been postulated.[6] Studies among the Pima Indians in the Southwest indicate that 70 per cent of the women eventually develop gallstones; about half have gallstones by age 25.[7]

In most populations the incidence of gallbladder disease is higher in females than in males. Obesity correlates strongly with the disease, and the prevalence increases with age. Gastrointestinal disorders involving malabsorption of bile acids, such as ileal disease, resection, or bypass, are frequently associated with gallstone development. Certain drugs, such as clofibrate and estrogens, increase the risk for gallstone formation.

Function of the Gallbladder The gallbladder concentrates bile formed in the liver and stores it until needed for digestion of fats. The entrance of fat into the duodenum stimulates secretion of the hormone *cholecystokinin* by the intestinal mucosa. The hormone is carried by way of the bloodstream to the gallbladder and forces it to contract, thus releasing bile into the common duct, and then into the small intestine where it is needed for the emulsification of fats. Interference with the flow of bile occurring in gallbladder disease may cause impaired fat digestion.

Inflammation of the gallbladder is known as CHOLECYSTITIS. Gallstone formation, or CHOLELITHIASIS, occurs when cholesterol, bile pigments, bile salts, calcium, and other substances precipitate out of the bile. CHOLEDOCHOLITHIASIS refers to stones lodged in the common duct.

Diagnostic Tests The most widely used test for the diagnosis of gallbladder disease is oral cholecystography. This involves administration of an iodine contrast dye which is taken up and concentrated by the gallbladder. Presence of stones can then be visualized by x-ray. When a diseased gallbladder is not visualized, intravenous cholangiography is sometimes used. Injection of an iodine contrast medium permits visualization of the biliary ducts. Ultrasonography or computerized transaxial tomography (CAT scan) are also used to visualize the biliary tree and gallbladder.

Pathophysiology In the United States and Canada, the principal component of the vast majority of gallstones is cholesterol. Growth of the stones involves several stages, each of which is a prerequisite for the next: (1) a genetic and metabolic stage in a susceptible individual; (2) a chemical stage, in which bile becomes supersaturated with cholesterol; (3) a physical stage, in which the supersaturated bile is nucleated and growth of cholesterol crystals begins; (4) aggregation of microscopic crystals into stones; (5) a symptomatic stage occurring when stones initiate cholecystitis or block the cystic or common bile duct.[7]

Limited data suggest that enhanced activity of HMA-CoA reductase, the rate-limiting enzyme in hepatic cholesterol synthesis, occurs in individuals with cholesterol gallstones.[8] In obese persons there is increased hepatic cholesterol secretion. Conversion of cholesterol to bile acids is increased in these individuals but apparently not in sufficient amounts to solubilize the excess cholesterol. Persons of normal weight with cholesterol gallstones have a decreased bile acid pool size. It is not clear whether the decrease in bile acid pool size is a cause or consequence of cholelithiasis.[9]

In Western countries, about 10 per cent of gallstones are pigment stones. This type occurs more frequently in countries where malnutrition and parasitic infection are common. The chief pigment in these stones is bilirubin. Biliary tract infections and hemolytic disorders predispose to increased formation of free bilirubin, which complexes with calcium in bile to form insoluble stones.

Symptoms and Clinical Findings Acute cholecystitis is usually associated with a gallstone lodged in the cystic duct and is accompanied by mild to severe pain, abdominal distension, nausea and vomiting, and fever. The pain occurs whenever the gallbladder contracts. Ingestion of fatty foods may thus cause discomfort, and fat digestion may be impaired because of the diminished flow of bile. Intolerance to certain strongly flavored vegetables, legumes, melons, and berries occurs in many persons with gallbladder disease but the reason for this is not known.

Treatment of Gallbladder Disease Dietary, medical, or surgical intervention are used, depending on the individual case. Conservative treatment includes dietary management, although the importance of dietary factors in the etiology of gallbladder disease is not known. The principal aim is to reduce discomfort by providing a diet restricted in fat.

Energy. Excess caloric intake appears to be a risk factor for development of gallbladder disease. The disease is much more common among the obese than in persons of normal weight. Persons at increased risk for gallbladder disease should be encouraged to achieve and maintain normal weight through controlled dietary intake and a regular exercise program. For many, strict dieting is not needed if smaller portion sizes are used, and energy-dense snacks and desserts are replaced by low-calorie vegetables and fruits or other foods high in fiber. (See Chapter 27.)

Fat. The patient receives no food initially during acute attacks of cholecystitis. Progression to a 20- to 30-gm fat diet is then made. If this is tolerated, the fat can then be increased to 50 to 60 gm daily, thus improving palatability of the diet. In chronic cholecystitis some degree of fat restriction is usually necessary. With restriction of fats, carbohydrates are used more liberally.

Cholesterol. Several studies have found

Table 34-1. **Food Allowances for Two Levels of Fat Restriction** (Approximately 1,500 kcal)

	20 gm Fat	50 gm Fat
Milk, skim	2 cups	2 cups
Meat, fish, poultry (lean)	6 ounces*	6 ounces*
Eggs (3 per week)	½	½
Vegetables		
Dark green leafy or deep yellow	1 serving	1 serving
Potato	1 serving	1 serving
Other	1 or more servings	1 or more servings
Fruits		
Citrus	1 serving	1 serving
Other	3 servings	3 servings
Bread and cereals		
Cereals	1 serving	1 serving
Breads	6 slices	3 slices
Fats, vegetable	None	6 teaspoons
Sweets	3 tablespoons	2 tablespoons
Total fat, gm	20	50
Cholesterol, mg	270†	270†
Protein, gm	85	80
Kcal (approximate)	1,500	1,500

*Only lean cuts of meat, fish, poultry made be used. Each ounce is equivalent to 8 gm protein and 3 gm fat.

†Cholesterol level would be reduced to about half this level if eggs were not used. If butter is used instead of vegetable fat, the cholesterol level would be increased.

no relationship between serum cholesterol levels and gallstone formation. High-cholesterol diets increase biliary cholesterol; however, much more cholesterol is synthesized in the body from fragments of carbohydrates, amino acids, and fat metabolism. Dietary restriction of cholesterol, therefore, is probably not very effective in prevention of gallstones. If a reduction in cholesterol content of the diet is ordered, egg yolks, liver, and other organ meats are omitted, and skim milk and margarine are substituted for whole milk and butter. See Table A-5 for cholesterol content of foods. Food allowances for two levels of fat restriction are shown in Table 34–1.

Fiber. The association of gallbladder disease in populations consuming low-fiber diets and the relative lack of the disease in those populations that habitually consume diets high in fiber has led to speculation that fiber plays a role in prevention of the disease. Some evidence suggests that interactions among certain components of fiber, bile salts, and intestinal flora alter the composition of the bile acid pool, leading to increased chenodeoxycholic acid, which enhances solubility of biliary cholesterol.[10] More research is needed to determine whether dietary fiber has a sustained influence on biliary saturation.

Diet Following Cholecystectomy Some fat restriction is indicated for several weeks following removal of the gallbladder. Thereafter, most individuals can tolerate a regular diet.

Dissolution of Gallstones For selected patients, medical therapy provides an alternative to cholecystectomy. Oral administration of certain bile acids induces dissolution of gallstones. Chenodeoxycholic acid and its epimer, ursodeoxycholic acid, are effective in dissolving radiolucent stones after 6 to 24 months of continuous therapy.[11] A fat-restricted diet is not indicated for patients receiving this therapy. Some recommend substitution of high-fiber foods for those high in calories.[12]

Fat-Restricted Diet

Foods Allowed	Foods to Avoid
Beverages—skim milk as desired; coffee, coffee substitute, tea; fruit juices	*Beverages*—with cream; soda-fountain beverages with milk, cream, or ice cream; whole milk
Breads—all kinds except those with added fat	*Breads*—griddle cakes; sweet rolls with fat; French toast
Cereals—all cooked or dry breadfast cereals, except possibly bran; macaroni, noodles, rice, spaghetti	
Cheese—cottage only	*Cheese*—all whole-milk cheeses, both hard and soft
Desserts—angel cake; fruit whip; fruit pudding; gelatin; ices and sherbets; milk and cereal puddings using part of milk allowance	*Desserts*—any containing chocolate, cream, nuts, or fats: cookies, cake, doughnuts, ice cream, pastries, pies, rich puddings
Eggs—3 per week	*Eggs*—fried
Fats—vegetable oil or margarine	*Fats*—cooking fats, cream, salad dressings
Fruits—all kinds when tolerated	*Fruits*—avocado; raw apple, berries, melons may not be tolerated

Foods Allowed	Foods to Avoid
Meats—broiled, baked, roasted, or stewed without fat: lean beef, chicken, lamb, pork, veal, fish	*Meats*—fatty meats, poultry, or fish: bacon, corned beef, duck, goose, ham, fish canned in oil, mackerel, pork, sausage; organ meats Smoked and spiced meats if they are poorly tolerated
Seasonings—in moderation: salt, pepper, spices, herbs, flavoring extracts	*Seasonings*—sometimes not tolerated: pepper; curries; meat sauces; excessive spices; vinegar
Soups—clear	*Soups*—cream, unless made with milk and fat allowance
Sweets—all kinds: hard candy, jam, jelly, marmalade, sugars	*Sweets*—candy with chocolate and nuts
Vegetables—all kinds when well tolerated; cooked without added butter, or cream	*Vegetables*—strongly flavored may be poorly tolerated: broccoli, Brussels sprouts, cabbage, cauliflower, cucumber, onion, peppers, radish, turnips; dried cooked peas and beans
	Miscellaneous—fried foods; gravies; nuts; olives; peanut butter; pickles; popcorn; relishes

Meal Pattern (20 gm fat)	Sample Menu
BREAKFAST	BREAKFAST
Fruit	Stewed apricots
Cereal with skim milk and sugar	Cornflakes with skim milk and sugar
Egg—1 only (3 per week)	Poached egg
Enriched or whole-grain toast	Whole-wheat toast with jelly
Jelly	
Beverage with skim milk and sugar	Coffee with skim milk and sugar
LUNCHEON OR SUPPER	LUNCHEON OR SUPPER
	Tomato bouillon
Lean meat, fish, poultry, or cottage cheese	Fruit salad plate:
Potato or substitute	Cottage cheese
Vegetable	Sliced orange
Salad; no oil dressing	Tokay grapes
	Pear
	Romaine
Enriched or whole-grain bread	Whole-wheat roll
Dessert or fruit	Vanilla blanc mange (using milk allowance)
Milk, skim—½ cup	Tea with milk, sugar
DINNER	DINNER
Lean meat, poultry, or fish	Roast lamb, trimmed of fat
Potato or substitute	Boiled new potatoes; no added fat
Vegetable	Zucchini squash
Enriched or whole-grain bread	Parkerhouse roll
Jelly	Jelly
Dessert or fruit	Angel cake with sliced peaches
Milk, skim—1 glass	Milk, skim—1 glass

Dietary Counseling

Restriction of dietary fat influences the methods of food preparation permitted. The patient should be advised to prepare meats by baking, broiling, roasting, or stewing, and to use only lean meats trimmed of all visible fats. Meat drippings, cream sauces, and so on are not allowed, but spices and herbs in moderation can be used to enhance flavor of foods. Use of fortified skim milk and inclusion of green leafy or yellow vegetables is needed to help ensure adequate intake of vitamin A. The small amounts of fat permitted should be taken as butter or margarine. Any foods known to cause distension should be omitted. Most individuals need guidance in selecting suitable substitutes for desserts that are high in fat.

Pancreatic Disorders

Pancreatic disease may be due to congenital or inflammatory diseases, trauma, or tumors. Disorders of the pancreas usually involve inadequate production of enzymes needed for normal digestive processes. Interference with this process leads to impaired digestion and is manifested by the presence of excess fat and undigested protein in the stools. Some starch may also be present. Dietary treatment of pancreatic disorders depends on the nature and extent of digestive impairment rather than on the disease itself.

Acute Pancreatitis Acute inflammatory disease of the pancreas results from interference with the blood supply to the organ or from obstruction to the outflow of pancreatic juice. The usual causes are alcoholism and biliary tract disease; however, acute pancreatitis may also be due to trauma, virus infections, tumors, nutritional deficiency, certain vascular diseases, and a number of metabolic diseases. Gallstones cause about half the cases of acute pancreatitis in the United States.[13] Acute pancreatitis and severe fat intolerance are also seen in Types I and V hyperlipoproteinemias. (See Chapter 39.)

Acute pancreatitis may range from a mild inflammatory reaction to severe illness. The most predominant symptom is severe upper-abdominal pain radiating to the back and is aggravated by eating. Epigastric tenderness, distension, constipation, nausea, and vomiting occur.

Increased pressure in the ducts causes the activated pancreatic enzymes to escape into the interstitial tissues, thus leading to elevations in serum amylase and lipase. Other clinical findings include hyperlipemia and hypocalcemia. Alteration of structure or function of the pancreas or adjacent organs may be demonstrated radiographically. The islets of Langerhans are not necessarily involved.

Treatment. Conservative management is used. Aims are to alleviate pain, to keep pancreatic secretory activity at a minimum, and to replace fluids and electrolytes. Dietary management usually consists of giving the patient nothing by mouth during acute attacks. Progression from clear liquids or a semisynthetic fiber-free to a soft (see Chapter 25) or bland (Chapter 31) diet is made as tolerated.

Chronic Pancreatitis This disease may be described as relapsing, recurrent, or continuous in nature. As in acute pancreatitis, alcoholism is the most common cause of attacks but the basic defect is not known. Alcohol indirectly stimulates pancreatic secretions, and one popular theory holds that it also obstructs pancreatic outflow.[14] Obstruction of the ducts leads to chronic changes including destruction of the islets of Langerhans in some patients, fibrosis, pseudocyst, and pancreatic calcification. When enzyme secretion is only 10 per cent of normal, impaired digestion leads to steatorrhea, creatorrhea, and deficiency of the B-complex and fat-soluble vitamins.

The chronic form is characterized by recurrent attacks of burning epigastric pain, especially after meals containing alcohol and fat. Other symptoms include flatulence, anorexia, weight loss, nausea, and vomiting.

Treatment. Conservative management is used unless the patient has unremitting pain or complications necessitating partial or complete pancreatectomy. Medications to alleviate pain and to inhibit pancreatic secretion are used.

The aim of dietary treatment is to minimize gastric secretion because of its stimulating effect on secretin output. Diet during attacks is the same as in acute pancreatitis. Thereafter, a soft diet, high in protein and calories, and low in fat, should be used. Some recommend 3,000 to 6,000 kcal, 100 to 150 gm protein, at least 400 gm carbohydrate, and 30 to 60 gm fat.[15] Six small meals are better tolerated than large meals. Pancreatic extract is used to aid in fat absorption. Medium-chain triglycerides (MCT) and semisynthetic fiber-free diets have been useful in the disease.

Cystic Fibrosis This is a congenital disorder of unknown etiology in which there is generalized dysfunction of exocrine glands. The incidence is 1 per 2,000 live births. About 10 million persons in the United States are carriers of the gene. The median age of survival in the United States is 21 for males and 17 years for females.[16]

Characteristics of the disease include abnormalities in mucus secretion and in sweat sodium and chloride levels. Secretion of abnormally thick mucus by exocrine glands obstructs ducts in the pancreas, lungs, and liver. Blockage of the ducts in the pancreas leads to fibrosis and cyst formation, and pancreatic enzymes are not released into the duodenum, interfering seriously with the utilization of proteins, fat, and carbohydrates. As much as 50 per cent of the protein and fat of the diet may be present in the feces. Impaired absorption of all nutrients occurs in many cases. Osteoporosis may be demonstrated radiologically. Chronic pulmonary disease and bronchial obstruction develop, and in some instances, obstruction of hepatic biliary ducts leads to portal hypertension and cirrhosis. Elevated levels of sodium and chloride—up to 2½ times normal—are found in sweat. Massive salt loss in hot weather may cause heat stroke.

Symptoms. In the neonatal period, cystic fibrosis may present as meconium ileus, or there may be insidious onset of malnutrition in infants with good appetite but who nevertheless fail to grow and gain weight. Passage of foul-smelling, bulky, soft stools, haggard appearance, marked enlargement of the abdomen, and tissue wasting, especially about the buttocks, occur. Appetite is often decreased because of bloating, cramping, and diarrhea.

Treatment. General treatment consists of controlling pulmonary complications, maintaining good nutrition, and preventing abnormal salt loss. Measures designed to liquefy mucus, to minimize its formation, and to prevent obstruction are taken. Daily administration of pancreatic extract is prescribed.

Optimum nutrition should be maintained by careful attention to diet. A diet high in calories and protein with moderation in fat intake is needed in cases where fat is poorly tolerated. Calorie allowances must be sufficient to enable the individual to achieve desirable weight. The protein intake must be great enough to compensate for that lost in the stools. Protein hydrolysates may be useful in treating children who fail to grow. Medium-chain triglycerides are useful in this disorder and a proprietary formula containing these is available for infants.* Additional B-complex vitamins, ascorbic acid, and aqueous preparations of fat-soluble vitamins should be prescribed. Some recommend 2 to 4 gm of salt daily as a prophylactic measure. Distribution of foods into six small feedings may be advisable for some persons, especially in the younger age groups.

* Pregestimil® by Mead Johnson & Co., Evansville, Indiana.

Problems and Review

1. Mr. T. is a 70-year-old retired bricklayer whose physician has recommended a soft, fat-restricted diet. Mr. T. lives alone since the recent death of his wife. He does some light cooking but usually eats his evening meal in a restaurant. He states that he does not have much of an appetite. Plan a day's menu for him. What recommendations would you make for foods eaten away from home?
2. Mr. J. is a 20-year-old unemployed laborer who has Type A hepatitis. Ordinarily, he eats all foods, but has lost 18 pounds due to marked anorexia. He still enjoys milkshakes, however.
   a. What type of diet would you expect his doctor to order for him?
   b. Plan 2 days' menus for him.
   c. He has a history of very irregular eating habits. Will this affect the course of his disease at present?
3. Mr. V. has cirrhosis of the liver and his physician has prescribed a 2,500-kcal diet to help him regain some of the 22 pounds he has lost. The diet is to provide 75 gm protein, 80 gm fat, and 350 gm carbohydrate.
   a. Plan a day's menu for him.
   b. Show how you would modify this menu to reduce the sodium to 250 mg.
   c. Mr. and Mrs. V. depend on state aid for financial assistance. Because of their limited resources, they are accustomed to buying salt pork and other less expensive cuts of meat. How would you advise them in this regard?
   d. Mr. V.'s physician wants Mrs. V. to learn to adjust the protein intake at home so that she can adapt her husband's diet upon the physician's recommendation when signs of impending coma appear. How would you go about teaching her to do this?
   e. Mr. V. was later readmitted to the hospital in hepatic coma. The doctor has ordered a protein-free diet for him. Plan a day's menu that supplies 2,000 kcal. Adjust this menu to provide 10, 20, 30, and 40 gm protein.
4. Mrs. M. is a 56-year-old woman with cholelithiasis whose physician has ordered a 1,200-kcal fat-restricted diet. What factors are important in the dietary management of this woman?
   a. What problems might she face in preparing meals if fat is limited to 25 gm per day?
   b. Plan a day's menu for her with 25 gm fat; adjust to provide 50 gm fat.
5. Mr. H. has chronic pancreatitis. What type of diet would you expect his doctor to order? Plan a day's menu. Should he take vitamin supplements?

Cited References

1. Lieber, C. S.: "Alcohol, Protein Metabolism, and Liver Injury," *Gastroenterology,* **79**:373–90, 1980.
2. Gabuzda, G. J., and Shear, L.: "Metabolism of Dietary Protein in Hepatic Cirrhosis. Nutritional and Clinical Considerations," *Am. J. Clin. Nutr.,* **23**:479–87, 1970.
3. Freund, H. et al.: "Chronic Hepatic Encephalopathy. Long-term Therapy with a Branched-Chain Amino-Acid-Enriched Elemental Diet," *JAMA,* **242**:347–49, 1979.
4. Maddrey, W. C., and Weber, F. L.: "Chronic Hepatic Encephalopathy," *Med. Clin. North Am.,* **59**:937–44, 1975.
5. Greenberger, N. J. et al.: "Effect of Vegetable and Animal Protein Diets in Chronic Hepatic Encephalopathy," *Am. J. Digest. Dis.,* **22**:845–55, 1977.
6. Morris, D. L. et al.: "Gallbladder Disease and Gallbladder Cancer Among American Indians in Tricultural New Mexico," *Cancer,* **42**:2472–77, 1978.

7. Small, D. M. et al.: "Diseases of the Gallbladder and Biliary Passages," *Gastroenterology,* **69**:1121–30, 1975.
8. Redinger, R. N.: "Cholelithiasis," *Postgrad. Med.,* **65**:56–62, 66–71, June 1979.
9. Roslyn, J. J. et al.: "Chronic Cholelithiasis and Decreased Bile Salt Pool Size," *Am. J. Surg.,* **139**:119–24, 1980.
10. Story, J. A., and Kritchevsky, D.: "Bile Acid Metabolism and Fiber," *Am. J. Clin. Nutr.,* **31**:S199–S202, 1978.
11. Schoenfield, L. J.: "Stone Dissolution and the National Cooperative Gallstone Study," *Am. J. Digest. Dis.,* **22**:1115–16, 1977.
12. Tangedahl, T.: "Dissolution of Gallstones—When and How?" *Surg. Clin. North Am.,* **59**:797–809, 1979.
13. Tucker, L., and Tangedahl, T. N.: "Manifestations of Gallstone Disease," *Postgrad. Med.,* **66**:179–84, October 1979.
14. Sarles, H.: "Alcohol and the Pancreas," *Ann. N.Y. Acad. Sci.,* **252**:171–82, 1975.
15. Regan, P. T., and DiMagno, E. P.: "The Medical Management of Malabsorption," *Mayo Clin. Proc.,* **54**:267–74, 1979.
16. Gurwitz, D. et al: "Perspectives in Cystic Fibrosis," *Pediatr. Clin. North Am.,* **26**:603–15, 1979.

Additional References

ALTSCHULER, A., and HILDEN, D.: "The Patient with Portal Hypertension," *Nurs. Clin. North Am.,* **12**:317–29, 1977.

ARVANITAKIS, C.: "Diet Therapy in Gastrointestinal Disease: A Commentary," *J. Am. Diet. Assoc.,* **75**:449–52, 1979.

BAKER, A. L.: "Amino Acids in Liver Disease: Cause of Hepatic Encephalopathy?" *JAMA* **242**:355–56, 1979.

BECKER, C. E.: "Medical Consequences of Alcohol Abuse," *Postgrad. Med.,* **64**:88–93, December 1978.

BRYAN, J. A.: "Viral Hepatitis. I. Clinical and Laboratory Aspects and Epidemiology," *Postgrad. Med.,* **68**:66–69 ff., November 1980.

CHASE, H. P., and LAVIN, M. H.: "Cystic Fibrosis and Malnutrition," *J. Pediatr.,* **95**:337–47, 1979.

DIMAGNO, E. P.: "Medical Treatment of Pancreatic Insufficiency," *Mayo Clin. Proc.,* **54**:435–47, 1979.

HOYUMPA, A. et al.: "Hepatic Encephalopathy," *Gastroenterology,* **76**:184–95, 1979.

MEZEY, E.: "Alcoholic Liver Disease: Roles of Alcohol and Malnutrition," *Am. J. Clin. Nutr.,* **33**:2709–18, 1980.

SHAHINPOUR, N.: "The Adult Patient with Bleeding Esophageal Varices," *Nurs. Clin. North Am.,* **12**:331–43, 1977.

THORPE, C. J., and CAPRINI, J. A.: "Gallbladder Disease: Current Trends and Treatments," *Am. J. Nurs.,* **80**:2181–85, 1980.

WOOD, R. E.: "Cystic Fibrosis: Diagnosis, Treatment, and Prognosis," *South. Med. J.,* **72**:189–202, 1979.

35 *Nutrition for the Cancer Patient*

CANCER is the second leading cause of death in the United States, exceeded only by ischemic heart disease, and accounting for 20 per cent of all deaths.[1] Some 80 to 90 per cent of the cancer cases in the United States are believed to be due to environmental factors; one such factor is diet. The role of diet in the etiology of malignant disease is not clear. Epidemiologic evidence suggests a possible indirect role for dietary factors in certain types of cancer.

Nutritional status is adversely affected by cancer. A high proportion of patients exhibit protein-calorie malnutrition, characterized by depletion of visceral protein stores. Loss of visceral protein is associated with increased morbidity and mortality in cancer patients. The malnutrition affects tissue function and repair, immune status, and metabolism of drugs.

The discussion in this chapter is limited to dietary factors associated with increased risk for cancer in humans, some metabolic effects of cancer, the influence of cancer therapy on nutritional status, and dietary management for patients with cancer.

Role of Dietary Factors in Cancer Incidence

A number of dietary factors have been implicated in the etiology of cancer, based on experimental research in animals and on epidemiologic studies. Animal studies often involve drastic dietary manipulations; furthermore, experimentally induced tumors in animals may not be comparable to spontaneous tumors in humans. Extrapolation of data from animal studies to humans should be made with great caution. Epidemiologic studies suggest possible relationships between diet and cancer but do not prove a cause and effect relationship.

Epidemiologic Studies Compared to the incidence in the United States, the incidence of colon and breast cancer in Japan is low whereas that of stomach cancer is high. Studies of Japanese who have migrated to the United States show that within two or three generations the cancer incidence patterns in Japanese Americans resemble those prevalent in the United States. This shift has been correlated with adoption of a Westernized diet high in calories and fat.[2] Homogeneous population groups, such as Seventh Day Adventists in California, have a lower incidence of colon cancer than the general population. This has been attributed to a difference in lifestyle—the Adventists are a nonsmoking vegetarian population whose diet is lower in animal protein and fat and higher in dietary fiber than that of most Americans.[3] Lower cancer incidence has also been reported in Mormons in Utah[4] but cannot be attributed solely to diet because dietary habits of this group do not differ markedly from those of the rest of the population. Worldwide correlations have shown higher mortality from breast and colon cancer in countries with a high habitual dietary fat intake. The studies are based on food disappearance data, and may not be indicative of actual consumption. Nevertheless, the United States is among the highest in the world for fat intake and mortality from these cancer types. The correlations are stronger for total fat than for type of fat intake.[5,6]

Dietary Factors Hypotheses proposed to explain the role of several dietary factors in development of cancer follow.

Calories. Animal studies have shown that severe calorie restriction inhibits growth of most types of tumors, possibly because insufficient energy is available for tumor formation or for replication of malignant cells. Calorie restriction, however, is not a means of preventing tumor formation in humans.

An excess of calories in humans is associated with increased risk for endometrial and possibly for breast cancer and has been attributed to increased conversion of androgens to estrogens in adipose tissue.[7]

Protein. Cancer of the colon occurs with greater frequency in the industrialized nations. Some have related this to the higher meat consumption in these countries.[8,9] In the United States lower rates of colon cancer have been reported in vegetarian Seventh Day Adventists. It is not known which of several dietary factors might be most important in this regard: lower intakes of meat and fat or increased dietary fiber. Insufficient evidence is available at present to conclude that a high meat intake increases risk for colon cancer or that a vegetarian diet lowers risk.

Fat. Both the type and amount of fat are believed to influence tumor formation in animals. A high per capita fat intake in humans has been epidemiologically linked to increased risk for breast and colon cancer. One theory relates a high fat intake to increases in intestinal anaerobic bacteria and biliary steroid secretion. Anaerobic bacteria are capable of synthesizing estrogens, which are believed to be potential carcinogens in mammary tissue, from biliary steroids.[10] In addition, bile acids are degraded by intestinal bacteria to the secondary bile acids, deoxycholate and lithocholate; these may act as carcinogens in the colon. One study reported an increased incidence of cancer in men who had consumed a high polyunsaturated fat diet for a prolonged period.[11] Another theory holds that *trans* fatty acids are more carcinogenic than *cis* conformations.[12]

Fiber. Dietary fiber is postulated to exert a protective effect against colon cancer by several mechanisms: shortening intestinal transit time, thereby reducing the exposure time of epithelial surfaces to potential carcinogens; influencing bile acid metabolism, resulting in decreased formation or enhanced excretion of potential carcinogens; influencing intestinal flora with decreased degradation of bile acids and neutral sterols; and diluting potential carcinogens in the bowel.[13-15] The effects of dietary fiber on colonic function vary with the nature and quantity of fiber, and other components of the diet, especially fat. Diets high in fat are often low in fiber. Underdeveloped countries have a low incidence of cancer of the colon, and the diet in these countries is generally high in dietary fiber compared with that in the United States. Differences in other aspects of the diet or life-style must also be considered before concluding that dietary fiber accounts for the differences in cancer incidence between underdeveloped countries and Western nations.

Alcohol. The incidence of cancers of the mouth, pharynx, larynx, and esophagus is significantly increased in heavy smokers who consume large amounts of alcohol. In nonsmokers use of alcohol is not associated with increased risk for these cancers. Alcohol may enhance the carcinogenic effects of smoking by modifying microsomal enzyme activities.[16]

Other nutritional factors. Other factors associated with increased risk for various cancers in humans include low serum retinol levels; intake of pickled foods and dried salted fish; nitrites; dietary cholesterol; low levels of serum cholesterol; and increased high-density lipoproteins.[17-22]

Metabolic Effects of Cancer

Cancer Cachexia In advanced disease, this complex metabolic syndrome is a major cause of morbidity and mortality. Anorexia, early satiety, weight loss, wasting, and weakness characterize the syndrome. The etiology is uncertain but according to one theory may be due to the systemic effects of peptides and other small metabolites produced by the cancer.[23] Alterations in energy, carbohydrate, protein, and fat metabolism, acid-base balance, enzyme activities, endocrine homeostasis, and immunologic status are seen. The metabolic rate is increased, especially in Hodgkin's disease and leukemia. There are impaired glucose tolerance, decreased insulin production, and insulin resistance. Marked loss of body fat due to mobilization of free fatty acids from adipose tissue is seen. Skeletal muscle mass is reduced and hypoalbuminemia is common. Negative nitrogen balance occurs in spite of sufficient intake. Fluid retention may mask true weight loss; urinary excretion of sodium and potassium is increased. Enzyme changes in liver and muscle occur. The marked wasting in the syndrome is due to inadequate energy intake, which may be secondary to altered metabolism, anorexia, impaired digestion and absorption, tumor-host competition for nutrients, and increased energy expenditure by the host.[23]

Anorexia A frequent but poorly understood finding in advanced cancer is anorexia. It may be related to the disease process, to adverse effects of cancer therapy, or to emotional and psychologic reactions to cancer. The weight loss experienced by many patients with cancer is often due to reduction in food intake associated with anorexia.

Alterations in taste and smell are common in advanced cancer. Some patients have an increased threshold for sweet or sour tastes. Addition of sugar or other sweeteners, or lemon can make food more acceptable to these patients. Some patients experience a reduction in threshold for bitter tastes. Most meats, but especially red meats, are associated with a bitter taste. Substitution of other protein sources (eggs, fish, milk, legumes) should be made so that protein intake is not compromised.

Insulin stimulates appetite. The reduction in insulin secretion in cancer patients may thus have an adverse effect on appetite. Lactic acid and products of anaerobic metabolism of glucose cause anorexia and nausea. Amino acid imbalance can suppress appetite. Anorexia is often due to radiation therapy or to various chemotherapeutic agents. It is likely that the anorexia of most cancer patients is multifactorial.

Nutritional Effects of Cancer Therapy

Obstruction by a tumor may interfere with nutritional intake or digestive or absorptive functions. Nutritional status may be further compromised by surgery, radiation therapy, chemotherapy, or immunotherapy.

Surgery The site and extent of surgery determine the nutritional consequences. For example, interference with chewing and swallowing mechanisms follow surgery of the head and neck regions; impaired absorption of nutrients, especially of fat, follows gastrointestinal surgery; and diabetes mellitus may occur secondary to pancreatectomy.[24]

Radiation therapy The nutritional problems associated with radiation therapy depend on the site and dose of irradiation. Adverse effects of irradiation to the upper alimentary tract include xerostomia (dry mouth) due to impaired salivary secretion, dental caries, loss of teeth, altered taste sensations, loss of appetite, dysphagia, sore mouth and throat, and esophageal irritation. Patients receiving radiation to the abdominal and pelvic areas commonly experience nausea and vomiting.[25] Gastric ulcer, enteritis, malabsorption, and weight loss are other consequences of radiation.

Chemotherapy Virtually all chemotherapeutic agents cause nausea and vomiting. Reduced food intake, generalized weakness, fluid and electrolyte imbalance, and weight loss ensue. Mucosal damage may be manifested as mucositis, stomatitis, glossitis, cheilosis, and esophagitis. Constipation or diarrhea are associated with some agents. Weight loss may be severe in prolonged therapy. Appetite suppression, malabsorption syndromes, and vitamin deficiencies occur with some drugs. Hormonal therapy may lead to fluid and electrolyte disturbances.[25, 26]

Immunotherapy This is used to stimulate the immune system, and may induce a flulike syndrome, with chills, fever, malaise, nausea, and body aches.

Nutritional Considerations

The various modes of cancer therapy—surgery, radiation, and chemotherapy—all have nutritional consequences. Assessment of nutritional status of cancer patients is, therefore, essential in order to determine those patients who are likely to be at increased risk for nutritional problems during treatment, and to provide a basis for planning appropriate nutritional support. Periodic monitoring of nutritional status should continue during therapy.

Appropriate nutritional support can help reduce weight loss, provide an improved sense of well-being, and improve immunocompetence. Well-nourished patients tolerate cancer therapy better than the malnourished.[27] Improved nutrition of the host causes an increased rate of tumor growth; thus, nutritional support should be accompanied by appropriate antitumor therapy.[28] The goals of nutritional therapy are to minimize weight loss and to correct nutrient imbalances and deficiencies. When oral feedings are contraindicated, tube feedings or parenteral feeding are used. These are discussed in the chapter that follows.

Little is known of nutrient requirements in cancer. One group estimates the requirement for protein to be 1.2 to 1.5 gm per kilogram body weight, whereas that for energy is 30 to 35 kcal per kilogram per day when enteral feeding is used, and 35 to 45 kcal per kilogram using parenteral feeding.[29] Others suggest that energy and protein requirements are increased by approximately 20 per cent in cancer patients and can be estimated as follows:[27]

Protein: desirable weight in pounds × 0.77
Calories: desirable weight in pounds × 20 (males) or 18 (females)

Vitamin deficiencies are not uncommon in cancer patients; however, the therapeutic use of vitamins in treatment has been controversial. Concern has been expressed that therapeutic doses of vitamins might accelerate tumor growth. The prevailing opinion now seems to be that additional vitamins probably do not appreciably influence growth of most tumors. An exception is the tumor that requires folic acid for growth. Rapid depletion of folate is desirable in order to inhibit cell growth. A folic acid antagonist, methotrexate, is used for a defined period to inhibit replication of tumor cells.[30] Deficiency of minerals, especially trace minerals, is likely in any patient whose dietary intake is inadequate in other respects.

Dietary Counseling

Most cancer patients need a good deal of guidance and encouragement in order to cope with the nutritional problems that arise during and following cancer therapy. Initially, the diagnosis of cancer may so overwhelm the patient and family that the importance of maintaining good nutritional status is not appreciated. Most have no understanding of the devastating effects that cancer therapy has on one's ability and willingness to eat. The dietitian and nurse can provide invaluable assistance to patients and their families by offering suggestions to make dietary management easier.

Before cancer therapy is started, guidance in the essentials of a nutritionally adequate diet should be given. The patient also needs to know what to expect from the various forms of cancer therapy, and should be informed of typical dietary problems experienced by others undergoing similar therapy. Some nutritional side effects of cancer therapy and suggested means for coping with them are shown in Table 35–1. Omitting food for several hours before radiation or chemotherapy treatments may prevent some of the nausea and food aversions that develop in many patients.

Table 35-1. **Some Side Effects of Cancer Therapy and Suggested Dietary Management**

Nausea and vomiting	Clear, cold, and carbonated beverages with added Polycose Sipping beverages slowly through a straw Small, frequent meals low in fat Dry crackers or toast before arising Tart or salty foods Cold foods—meat plates, fruit plates, cottage cheese, popsicles, gelatin desserts Liquids 30 to 60 minutes before eating
Dry mouth	Drinking at least 2 quarts of liquid daily High-calorie beverages are preferable to water Sauces, gravies, broth to moisten foods, and to make them easier to swallow Chewing sugar-free gum or sugar-free candy to stimulate salivation Artificial saliva
Taste alterations	Experimenting with different flavors and seasonings Substitution of other proteins for red meats Marinating meats in wine, fruit juices, etc.
Loss of appetite	Small, frequent feedings High-calorie, high-protein snacks and beverages
Sore mouth and throat	Soft, nonacid foods Blended or liquefied foods Foods and beverages at room temperature Using straw with liquids Avoiding highly seasoned foods
Swallowing problems	Liquid feedings or puréed foods Frequent feedings Tube feedings may be needed in some cases Adding butter and sauces to foods Finely chopped foods or foods cut into small pieces
Early satiety	Small frequent meals Chewing foods well and eating slowly Avoiding foods excessively high in fat, rich sauces Liquids 30 to 60 minutes before meals, not at meals

The importance of weight maintenance should be stressed. Patients should be encouraged to take advantage of times when they are feeling well to prepare foods that can be frozen for later use. Convenience foods, mixes, casseroles, and snack items prepared in advance are useful for those times when nausea and fatigue limit ability and desire to prepare meals.

The atmosphere at mealtimes should be conducive to enjoyment of food. An attractively set table, relaxing music, pleasant conversation, and perhaps a glass of wine before dinner can help turn the patient's thoughts away from how he or she is feeling. Families should encourage, but not pressure, the patient to eat. Appropriate use of antiemetics and pain medication before meals permits eating to be more pleasant. Zinc supplements may improve taste acuity.

The diet is modified in texture and composition as needed. For example, for a patient who has had a laryngectomy, custards and puréed fruits and vegetables are tolerated better than more coarse foods. One who is undergoing radiation to the abdomen may need foods low in lactose, fiber, and fat. Constipation is sometimes a problem and may be due to emotional stress, pain medications, or chemotherapeutic drugs. Dietary fiber can easily be increased by use of bran cereals, whole-grain breads, fruits and vegetables, and use of snack foods such as granola bars, date bars, oatmeal cookies, and so on. (See Chapter 32.) For some patients, diarrhea may necessitate reduction in fibrous foods (see Chapter 31) and provision of those high in potassium.

Most patients fare better with small, frequent meals. Nutritious snacks should be readily available. A compromise must be reached between the need for high-protein, high-calorie foods and avoidance of excessive amounts of sugars and fats. A number of proprietary balanced formulas are suitable. Some patients find certain of these to be too sweet; thus, it is important to try a variety of formulas to find those acceptable to the patient. Taste preferences often change during therapy, and it may be preferable to keep on hand a supply of bland-tasting formulas which can be easily flavored with coffee, brandy, lemon, chocolate, and so on as the patient desires. Beverages kept on ice in a place readily accessible to the patient are more likely to be consumed. Ingenuity in varying the form and texture of supplements (for example, beverages, puddings, soups) will enhance their appeal to the patient.

The protein content of the diet can be increased by adding skim milk powder to soups, gravies, and sauces; using milk in place of water for canned cream soups, and instant cocoa; adding diced meat to soups and casseroles; adding grated cheese to sauces, vegetables, soups, and so on. Calories can be increased by adding butter or margarine to soups, vegetables, or cooked cereals; adding honey to tea or cooked cereal, adding brown sugar and raisins to cooked cereals, and so on. (See also Chapter 28.) The National Cancer Institute has compiled a booklet of recipes and tips for better nutrition for cancer patients.[31] Similar booklets are available from local and regional cancer referral centers.

Problems and Review

1. Mrs. S. will soon begin radiation therapy treatments. Her physician has requested that you do a preliminary assessment of her nutritional status. What criteria would you use? What additional information would be of use?
2. Various dietary factors have been implicated in the etiology of cancer. How important are these, in your opinion? Is there any point in modifying dietary intake as a means of preventing cancer? If so, what modifications would be practical? If not, why not?
3. What are some of the problems involved in the nutritional rehabilitation of cancer patients?

4. Outline points to emphasize in counseling an ambulatory cancer patient regarding his or her diet.
   a. For a patient in remission, and receiving no therapy
   b. For a patient who is receiving radiation therapy
   c. For an individual undergoing chemotherapy
5. Look up several drugs used in the treatment of cancer and list their nutritional side effects. How could these problems be overcome?

Cited References

1. Silverberg, E.: "Cancer Statistics, 1980," *Ca—A Cancer Journal for Clinicians*, **30**:23–38, January/February 1980.
2. Gori, G. B.: "Dietary and Nutritional Implications in the Multifactorial Etiology of Certain Prevalent Human Cancers," *Cancer*, **43**:2151–61, 1979.
3. Phillips, R. L.: "Role of Life-Style and Dietary Habits in Risk of Cancer Among Seventh-Day Adventists," *Cancer Research*, **35**:3513–22, 1975.
4. Lyon, J. L., and Sorenson, A. W.: "Colon Cancer in a Low-Risk Population," *Am. J. Clin. Nutr.*, **31**:S227–S230, 1978.
5. Carroll, K. K.: "Experimental Evidence of Dietary Factors and Hormone Dependent Cancers," *Cancer Res.*, **35**:3374–83, 1975.
6. Wynder, E. L.: "The Epidemiology of Large Bowel Cancer," *Cancer Res.*, **35**:3388–94, 1975.
7. Van Itallie, T. B., and Hirsch, J.: "Appraisal of Excess Calories as a Factor in the Causation of Disease," *Am. J. Clin. Nutr.*, **32**:2648–53, 1979.
8. Vitale, J. J.: "Possible Role of Nutrients in Neoplasia," *Cancer Res.*, **35**:3320–25, 1975.
9. Mendeloff, A. I.: "A Critique of 'Fiber Deficiency,'" *Am. J. Digest. Dis.*, **21**:109–12, 1976.
10. Hankin, J. H., and Rawlings, V.: "Diet and Breast Cancer: A Review," *Am. J. Clin. Nutr.*, **31**:2005–16, 1978.
11. Pearce, M. L., and Dayton, S.: "Incidence of Cancer in Men on a Diet High in Polyunsaturated Fat," *Lancet*, **1**:464–67, 1971.
12. Enig, M. G., et al.: "Dietary Fat and Cancer Trends—A Critique," *Fed. Proc.*, **37**:2215–20, 1978.
13. Burkitt, D. P.: "Workshop V—Fiber and Cancer. Summary and Recommendations," *Am. J. Clin. Nutr.*, **31**:S213–S215, 1978.
14. Huang, C. T. L. et al.: "Fiber, Intestinal Sterols, and Colon Cancer," *Am. J. Clin. Nutr.*, **31**:516–26, 1978.
15. Lipkin, M.: "Dietary, Environmental, and Hereditary Factors in the Development of Colorectal Cancer," *Ca—A Cancer Journal for Clinicians*, **29**:292–99, 1979.
16. Wynder, E. L.: "Dietary Habits and Cancer Epidemiology," *Cancer*, **43**:1955–61, 1979.
17. Wald, N. et al.: "Low Serum Vitamin A and Subsequent Risk of Cancer," *Lancet*, **2**:813–15, 1980.
18. Dunn, J. E.: "Cancer Epidemiology in Populations of the United States—with Emphasis on Hawaii and California—And Japan," *Cancer Res.*, **35**:3240–45, 1975.
19. Editorial: "Nitrate and Human Cancer," *Lancet*, **2**:281, 1977.
20. Liu, K. et al.: "Dietary Cholesterol, Fat, and Fibre, and Colon-Cancer Mortality. An Analysis of International Data," *Lancet*, **2**:782–85, 1979.
21. Diet/Heart Disease Commentaries: "Eruption Reaction," *Nutr. Today*, **15**:4, 5, 7–9, July/August 1980.

22. Keys, A.: "Alpha Lipoprotein (HDL) Cholesterol in the Serum and the Risk of Coronary Heart Disease and Death," *Lancet*, **2**:603–6, 1980.
23. Theologides, A.: "Cancer Cachexia," *Cancer*, **43**:2004–12, 1979.
24. Lawrence, W.: "Nutritional Consequences of Surgical Resection of the Gastrointestinal Tract for Cancer," *Cancer Res.*, **37**:2379–86, 1977.
25. Ohnuma, T., and Holland, J. F.: "Nutritional Consequences of Cancer Chemotherapy and Immunotherapy," *Cancer Res.*, **37**:2395–2406, 1977.
26. Driever, C. W.: "Food and Drug Interactions in the Cancer Patient," in *Nutritional Management of the Cancer Patient*, J. Wollard, ed., Raven Press, New York, 1979, pp. 13–19.
27. Rosenbaum, E. H., and Rosenbaum, I. R.: "Principles of Home Care for the Patient with Advanced Cancer," *JAMA* **244**:1484–87, 1980.
28. Shils, M. E.: "Principles of Nutritional Support," *Nutr. Today*, **13**:25, September/October 1978.
29. Harvey, K. B. et al.: "Nutritional Assessment and Patient Outcome During Oncological Therapy," *Cancer*, **43**:2065–69, 1979.
30. Bertino, J. R.: "Nutrients, Vitamins, and Minerals as Therapy," *Nutr. Today*, **13**:28, September/October 1978.
31. *Eating Hints. Recipes and Tips for Better Nutrition During Treatment.* NIH Publ. No. 80–2079, U.S. Department of Health, Education, and Welfare. PHS. 1980.

Additional References

AKER, S. N.: "Oral Feedings in the Cancer Patient," *Cancer* **43**:2103–7, 1979.

BECK, J.: "Nutritional Assessment of the Adult Cancer Patient," in *Nutritional Management of the Cancer Patient.* (See Reference 26.)

BLACKBURN, G. L. et al.: "The Effect of Cancer on Nitrogen, Electrolyte, and Mineral Metabolism," *Cancer Res.*, **37**:2348–53, 1977.

BLUMBERG, B. D., and FLAHERTY, M.: "Services Available to Persons with Cancer, National and Regional Organizations," *JAMA*, **244**:1715–17, 1980.

COSTA, G., and DONALDSON, S. S.: "Effects of Cancer and Cancer Treatment on the Nutrition of the Host," *New Engl. J. Med.*, **300**:1471–74, 1979.

DEWYS, W. D.: "Nutritional Care of the Cancer Patient," *JAMA*, **244**:374–76, 1980.

DWYER, J. T.: "Dietetic Assessment of Ambulatory Cancer Patients," *Cancer*, **43**:2077–86, 1979.

FLEMING, S. M. et al.: "The Patient with Cancer Affecting the Head and Neck: Problems in Nutrition," *J. Am. Diet. Assoc.*, **70**:391–94, 1977.

HERBERT, V.: "Laetrile: The Cult of Cyanide. Promoting Poison for Profit," *Am. J. Clin. Nutr.*, **32**:1121–58, 1979.

LAWRENCE, W.: "Effects of Cancer on Nutrition," *Cancer*, **43**:2020–29, 1979.

SHILS, M. E.: "Nutritional Problems Associated with Gastrointestinal and Genitourinary Cancer," *Cancer Res.*, **37**:2366–72, 1977.

SOBOL, S. M. et al.: "Nutritional Concepts in the Management of the Head and Neck Cancer Patient. II. Management Concepts," *Laryngoscope*, **89**:962–79, 1979.

THORNTON, C.: "Nutritional Management with Radiotherapy," in *Nutritional Management of the Cancer Patient.* (See Reference 26.)

36 Nutrition in Surgical Conditions

TUBE FEEDINGS; HIGH-PROTEIN, HIGH-FAT, LOW-CARBOHYDRATE DIET

SIGNIFICANT advances have been made in the area of surgical nutrition within the past decade. A better understanding of the effects of stress on metabolism, together with the development of numerous preparations suitable for oral, intravenous, or tube feeding, has made possible substantial improvement in the nutritional status of patients both before and after surgery. Moreover, the report that approximately 50 per cent of surgical patients in one study suffered moderate to severe protein malnutrition[1] has given new impetus to the nutritional assessment of surgical patients.

Effects of Surgery on the Nutritive Requirements Good nutrition prior to and following surgery ensures fewer postoperative complications, better wound healing, shorter convalescence, and lower mortality. The patient whose preoperative nutritional state is poor is at increased risk when undergoing major surgery. Persons with chronic diseases are especially likely to have less than optimal nutriture. Hyperthyroidism or chronic infection as in bronchiectasis increases requirements. Serious malabsorption of nutrients may occur especially in liver diseases and those involving the gastrointestinal tract. Extensive losses of nutrients and fluids may have occurred through hemorrhage, vomiting, or diarrhea.

The extent of the deficiency is manifested by weight loss, poor wound healing, decreased intestinal motility, anemia, edema, or dehydration, and the presence of decubitus ulcers. The circulating blood volume and the concentration of the serum proteins, hemoglobin, and electrolytes may be reduced.

Following surgery or injury the need for nutrients is greatly increased as a result of loss of blood, plasma, or pus from the wound surface; hemorrhage from the gastrointestinal or pulmonary tract; vomiting; and fever. During immobilization, the loss of some nutrients such as protein is accelerated.

A fairly simple operation often involves moderate deficiency in food intake for a few days following the operation. Some nutrients may be supplied by parenteral fluids, but the full needs of the body usually are not met by that means alone. Provided that adequate oral intake is rapidly resumed, the metabolic losses are not of serious consequence. On the other hand, adequate oral intake is often delayed for a considerable period following cardiac or gastrointestinal surgery. Metabolic losses are great and alternative methods of nutritional support are needed.

Preoperative Nutritional Assessment Evaluation of nutritional status should be a routine part of preoperative assessment. A brief dietary history and clinical observations, together with anthropometric and biochemical measurements identify those likely to be at increased risk for complications. One group has developed a formula based on serum albumin and transferrin levels, triceps skinfold, and delayed hypersensitivity skin testing measurements to predict risk of complications in individuals undergoing gastrointestinal surgery.[2] Actual morbidity and mortality increase significantly as predicted risk increases.

Nutritional Considerations The objectives in the dietary management of surgical conditions are (1) to improve the preoperative nutrition whenever the operation is not of an emergency nature, (2) to maintain correct nutrition after operation or injury insofar as possible, and (3) to avoid harm from injudicious choice of foods.

Protein. A satisfactory state of protein nutrition ensures rapid wound healing by providing the correct assortment and quantity of essential amino acids, increases the resistance to infection, exerts a protective action upon the liver against the toxic effects of anesthesia, and reduces the possibility of edema at the site of the wound. The presence of edema is a hindrance to wound healing and, in operations on the gastrointestinal tract, may reduce motility thus leading to distension.

The protein status of surgical patients is of special concern because the postoperative complication rate is increased in patients who are protein depleted.[3] It is not always realistic to fully replace protein losses prior to surgery because the disease process itself may be such as to preclude a satisfactory intake of food. For selected patients, parenteral administration of amino acids and adequate calories is useful. The extent to which surgery should be delayed in order to improve the nutritional state is obviously a highly individual matter.

Protein catabolism is increased for several days immediately following surgery or injury; patients are characteristically in negative nitrogen balance even though the protein intake may be appreciable. Well-nourished persons lose more nitrogen than poorly nourished persons whose labile protein stores are already depleted. The degree of negative balance can be reduced at higher intakes of protein and calories.

The level of protein to be used in preoperative and postoperative diets depends upon the previous state of nutrition, the nature of the operation, and the extent of the postoperative losses. Intakes of 1.0 to 1.5 gm per kilogram, or about 100 gm protein, are necessary as a rule.

Energy. The weight status is an important pre- and postoperative consideration, for it serves as a guide to the caloric level to be recommended. Without sufficient caloric intake, tissue proteins cannot be synthesized. Excessive metabolism of body fat may lead to acidosis, whereas depletion of the liver glycogen may increase the likelihood of damage to the liver. Some recommend 35 to 45 kcal per kilogram daily for maximal utilization of amino acids for protein synthesis.[4]

In hyperthyroidism or fever, as much as 4,000 kcal daily may be essential to bring about weight gain. Other patients will make satisfactory progress at 2,500 to 3,000 kcal.

Obesity constitutes a hazard in surgery. Whenever possible, it should be corrected, at least in part, by using one of the calorie-restricted diets. (See page 482.) Rapid weight loss results in loss of lean body mass and should be avoided.

Minerals. Phosphorus and potassium are lost in proportion to the breakdown of body tissue. In addition, derangements of sodium and chloride metabolism may occur subsequent to vomiting, diarrhea, perspiration, drainage, anorexia, and diuresis or renal failure. The detection of electrolyte imbalance and appropriate parenteral fluid therapy requires careful study of clinical signs and biochemical evaluation.

Iron-deficiency anemia occurs in association with malabsorption or excessive blood loss. Diet alone is ineffective in correction of anemia, but a liberal intake of protein and ascorbic acid, together with administration of iron salts, is of value in convalescence. Transfusions are usually required to overcome severe reduction in hemoglobin level.

Fluids. The sources of water and the large amounts of fluids lost daily by the normal individual are outlined on page 164. The fluid balance may be upset prior to and following surgery owing to failure to ingest normal quantities of fluids and to increased losses from vomiting, exudates, hemorrhage, diuresis, and fever. A patient should not go to operation in a state of dehydration since the subsequent dangers of acidosis are great. When dehydration exists prior to operation, parenteral fluids are administered if the patient is unable to ingest sufficient liquid by mouth. Following major surgery the fluid balance is maintained by parenteral fluids until satisfactory oral intake can be established.

Vitamins. Ascorbic acid is especially important for wound healing and should be provided in increased amounts prior to and following surgery. Vitamin K is of concern to the surgeon since the failure to synthesize vitamin K in the small intestine, the inability to absorb it, or the defect in conversion to prothrombin is likely to result in bleeding. Hemorrhage is especially likely to occur in patients who have diseases of the liver.

Planning the Preoperative Diet Patients who have lost much weight prior to surgery benefit considerably by ingesting a high-protein, high-calorie diet (see page 495) for even a week or two prior to surgery. The diet may be of liquid, soft, or regular consistency depending upon the nature of the pathologic condition. Parenteral nutrition or semisynthetic fiber-free diets are sometimes used. In addition, the maintenance of metabolic equilibrium as in diabetes or other diseases must not be overlooked.

When surgery is delayed in order to improve the nutritional status, each day's intake should represent such improvement in nutrition that the delay is justified. This necessitates constant encouragement by the nurse and dietitian; it likewise requires imagination in varying the foods offered to the patient and ingenuity in getting the patient to eat. Foods which provide a maximum amount of nutrients in a minimum volume are essential. Small feedings at frequent intervals are likely to be better accepted than large meals which cannot be fully consumed.

For additional protein, milk beverages may be fortified with nonfat dry milk or commercial protein supplements. Strained meat in broth may be used when patients are unable to eat other meats. Fruit juices fortified with glucose, high-carbohydrate lemonade, jelly with crackers and bread, and hard candy may be used to increase the carbohydrate intake and to facilitate storage of glycogen. Butter incorporated into foods and light cream mixed with equal amounts of milk are also useful for increasing the caloric intake. The excessive use of sugars and fats may provoke nausea, however.

Food and fluids are generally allowed until midnight just preceding the day of operation, although a light breakfast may be given when the operation is scheduled for afternoon and local anesthesia is to be used. It is essential that the stomach be empty prior to administering the anesthesia so as to reduce the incidence of vomiting and the subsequent danger of aspiration of vomitus. When an operation is to be performed on the gastrointestinal tract, a diet very low in residue (page 539) may be ordered 2 to 3 days prior to operation. In acute abdominal conditions such as appendicitis and cholecystitis, no food is allowed by mouth until nausea, vomiting, pain, and distension have passed in order to prevent the danger of peritonitis.

Planning the Postoperative Diet Resumption of oral intake depends upon the nature of the surgery and the individual's progress. Following minor surgery, liquids are often tolerated within a few hours and rapid progression to a normal diet is made. After major surgery, however, oral intake may be delayed for days. Alternative methods for partial or complete nutritional support are provided by conventional intravenous feedings, catheter jejunostomy, total parenteral nutrition, tube feedings, or semisynthetic fiber-free diets.

Parenteral feedings. During the interval when the patient is unable to ingest food or fluid by mouth, intravenous feedings are used for maintenance or restoration of fluid and electrolyte balance. These feedings furnish primarily fluids and salts. Some contain glucose, which serves to prevent ketosis and to minimize tissue catabolism. Amino acid solutions are sometimes used in place of glucose because of their nitrogen-sparing effects but are more costly. None of these intravenous fluids can meet nutritional needs completely.

Total parenteral nutrition. For severely debilitated patients, TOTAL PARENTERAL NUTRITION is useful in providing complete nutritional support for extended periods. This method requires a careful consideration of the nature of the illness, physical examination to evaluate subjective changes, and laboratory analyses for blood glucose, electrolytes, pH, and proteins. The precise nutritional contributions made by such feedings and the details of management are beyond the scope of this text but have been reviewed elsewhere.[5] The method involves passage of an indwelling catheter into the superior vena cava with continuous infusion of a hypertonic solution of 20 to 25 per cent glucose, 3 to 5 per cent protein hydrolysate or amino acids, vitamins, and minerals. Essential fatty acid deficiency has been reported in adult patients who received no source of linoleic acid.[6] Likewise, deficiencies of zinc, copper, and chromium have been reported in patients maintained on total parenteral nutrition for prolonged periods without supplements.[7,8] The energy requirements associated with positive nitrogen balance in adults is 1.2 times the basal energy requirement for noncatabolic patients; this is increased to 1.76 for catabolic patients. Utilization of nitrogen is maximized when nonprotein calories are given in a ratio of 150 per gram of nitrogen.[9] The energy and nitrogen requirements for children receiving total parenteral nutrition are greater than those for adults and are described in detail elsewhere.[10]

Peripheral administration of intravenous fat emulsions makes possible a substantial increase in caloric intake, provides a source of essential fatty acids, and permits positive nitrogen balance. Products available in the United States include emulsions of soy (Intralipid®) or safflower (Liposyn®) oil.*

Progression of oral feeding. Motility of the gastrointestinal tract is diminished following abdominal surgery. Small intestine motility recovers rapidly but return of gastric motility may take 24 hours or longer, and colonic motility 3 to 5 days.[11] Patients are given nothing by mouth for the first 24 hours following surgery. Oral feeding is begun after gastrointestinal secretions are being produced and peristalsis resumes. Feeding should not be delayed once such function has returned. The accumulation of gastrointestinal secretions may result in a feeling of fullness. Moreover, the wound strength is sufficient to permit digestion of food.

Progression from ice chips to sips of water, then clear liquids and full liquids is made in accordance with the patient's tolerance. Patients usually respond better once they are given solid foods. Initially, the feedings are small and may be restricted to a low-residue diet. (See also Chapter 31.) Foods which are high in protein and fat are believed to be less distending than those which are high in carbohydrate. Perhaps of greater importance is the emphasis upon eating slowly and in small amounts to reduce the amount of air which is swallowed. As the patient improves, the selection of foods is that of a soft or regular diet, depending upon the nature of the surgery.

Tube Feedings

Feeding by tube may be required for a short period of time or indefinitely in a variety of circumstances: surgery of the head and neck; esophageal obstruction; gastrointestinal surgery; in severe burns; in anorexia nervosa; and in the comatose pa-

* Intralipid® by Cutter Laboratories, Berkeley, California; Liposyn® by Abbott Laboratories, North Chicago, Illinois.

tient. For short-term use the feedings are ordinarily given by nasogastric tube, but for long-term use, the feeding is administered through a tube inserted into a new opening (*"-ostomy"*) made in the esophagus (esophagostomy), stomach (gastrostomy), or intestine (enterostomy).

Characteristics of Tube Feedings A satisfactory tube feeding must be (1) nutritionally adequate; (2) well tolerated by the patient so that vomiting is not induced; (3) easily digested with no unfavorable reactions such as distension, diarrhea, or constipation; (4) easily prepared; and (5) inexpensive.

The concentration of the feeding may be adjusted from about ⅔ to 1⅓ kcal per milliliter. Lesser concentrations increase the volume which must be given to meet nutrient and energy needs, and greater concentrations are more likely to produce diarrhea and may be too thick to pass through a nasogastric tube. A concentration of about 1 kcal per milliliter is satisfactory. Two liters per 24 hours is a customary volume. The proportion of protein, fat, and carbohydrate should approximate that of the normal diet. Adverse effects of tube feedings include nausea, dehydration, diarrhea, and coma. Adequate fluid intake is essential to prevent salt or protein overload.

Types of Tube Feedings Three types of tube feedings are in common use: milk-base, blended, and semisynthetic fiber-free formulas. Several commercial preparations are available for each of these types. Likewise, recipes are available for the preparation of milk-based and blended feedings within the hospital or home. Most of these recipes use whole or skim milk, eggs, and vitamin supplements together with some form of carbohydrate such as strained cooked cereals, sugar, or molasses. Vegetable oil or cream and nonfat dry milk are also incorporated to increase the calorie and protein levels, respectively.

Tube feedings prepared from the ordinary foods of a normal diet by using a high-

Table 36-1. **Composition of Some Products Suitable for Tube Feeding***

	Brand A Blenderized	Brand B Lactose-Free	Brand C Semisynthetic Fiber-Free	Brand D Milk-based
	per 1,000 ml			
Kcal	1,000	1,000	1,000	1,000
Protein, gm	40	35	20	38
Fat, gm	40	35	1	52
Carbohydrate, gm	120	137	226	96
Nutrient source:				
Protein	Beef Nonfat milk	Soy protein Casein	Crystalline amino acids	Skim milk Casein
Fat	Corn oil	Corn oil	Safflower oil	Corn oil
Carbohydrate	Sucrose Maltodextrin Vegetables Fruit Orange juice	Corn syrup solids Sucrose	Glucose oligosaccharides	Sucrose Corn syrup solids
Lactose, gm	24	0	0	50
mOsm/kg	390	450	550	500
Volume needed to meet 100% of RDAs	1,600	1,887	1,800	1,920

*Brand A: Compleat B (in cans), Doyle Pharmaceutical Company, Minneapolis, Minnesota; Brand B: Ensure, Ross Laboratories, Columbus, Ohio; Brand C: Vivonex, Eaton Laboratories, Norwich, New York; Brand D: Nutri-1000, Cutter Laboratories, Berkeley, California.

speed blender are generally preferred to other types of formulas. Strained baby meats, fruits, and vegetables are used in addition to the foods listed previously. Blenderized tube feedings are well tolerated and are only infrequently associated with diarrhea. They permit flexibility in meeting specific nutrient needs and are less expensive than commercial formulas. On the other hand, the commercial preparations possess the advantages of convenience, constant composition, presterilization, minimal preparation time, and ease of administration. The nutrient composition of several of these preparations is shown in Table 36–1.

Administration of Tube Feedings Depending upon its nature, the feeding may be heated over hot water to body temperature, taking care that curdling does not occur with certain mixtures. Initially, small amounts of a dilute formula (50 ml) are given at hourly intervals. It is important that the feeding be given at a slow constant rate. A food pump is recommended for use with blenderized feedings. In patients who do not have an adequate swallowing mechanism or who are comatose, special care must be taken to avoid vomiting and aspiration of the vomitus. The patient should be positioned to prevent aspiration, and suction should be readily available at the bedside if vomiting occurs. Close attention to individual water needs is essential. (See Figure 36–1.)

When the small feedings are satisfactorily tolerated, the concentration and amount of the formula is gradually increased, with feedings not exceeding 12 ounces per 3- to 4-hour interval.

Semisynthetic fiber-free diets. Mixtures of hydrolyzed protein, egg albumen, or amino acids, sugars, oil, vitamins, and minerals, are used in both preoperative and postoperative patients. They are given orally or by tube and have been used for extended periods. Palatability is a problem when the feedings are given orally. Frequent determinations of blood glucose and electrolytes and of urinary sugar and acetone are needed. The precautions needed in administration of tube feedings apply to use of these formulas as well.

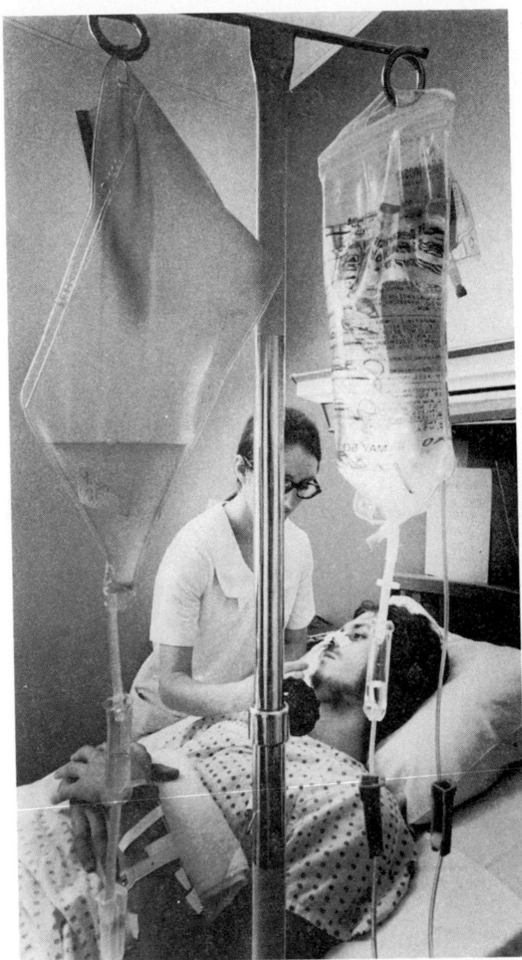

Figure 36–1. The nurse closely monitors the administration of the tube feeding, including position of the patient, the rate of flow, and the total intake. (Courtesy, Hennepin County Medical Center, Minneapolis.)

Diet in Specified Surgical Conditions

Diet Following Operations on the Mouth, Throat, or Esophagus The period between full extraction of teeth and satisfactory adjustment to new dentures may take several weeks. For 1 or 2 days following the surgery, it may be necessary to restrict the diet to liquids taken through a drinking tube. Thereafter, any soft foods which require little if any chewing may be used for 3 weeks or longer.

Radical surgery of the mouth necessitates the use of full fluids or puréed foods, but immediately after surgery one of the regimens for tube feeding described in the previous section may be used. Following an operation on the esophagus, a gastrostomy tube feeding is used.

After tonsillectomy the patient is given cold fluids including milk, bland fruit juices, ginger ale, plain ice cream, and sherbets. Tart fruit juices and fibrous foods must be avoided. On the second day, soft foods such as custard, plain puddings, soft eggs, warm but not hot cereals, strained cream soups, mashed potatoes, and fruit and vegetable purées may be tolerated. As a rule, the regular diet is swallowed without difficulty within the week.

Diet Following Gastrectomy A number of problems arise following gastrectomy, and their treatment should be anticipated. Weight loss is common, and studies undertaken up to 20 years following surgery indicate that most patients fail to regain weight to desirable levels.[12] The loss of a reservoir for food means that small feedings given at frequent intervals must be used if sufficient nutrients are to be ingested. Moreover, the absence of pepsin and hydrochloric acid entails the entire digestion of protein by the enzymes of the small intestine. Fat utilization is often impaired because of inadequate biliary and pancreatic secretions or defective mixing of food with the digestive juices. Intestinal motility is frequently increased. After total gastrectomy the lack of gastric acidity may permit bacterial overgrowth that disrupts the vitamin B-12-intrinsic factor complex and deconjugates bile salts, resulting in malabsorption. This was discussed in Chapter 33.

Iron is less readily absorbed and hypochromic microcytic anemia is common. After total gastrectomy the absence of intrinsic factor eventually leads to macrocytic anemia unless injections of vitamin B-12 are given. Decreased levels of vitamin D and calcium have been reported following gastrectomy.[13]

Proximal gastric vagotomy inhibits gastric secretion but leaves the pylorus intact so that gastric emptying is nearly normal. Nutritional consequences are thus minimized.

Dietary progression. Oral feedings vary widely from one patient to another. The usual sequence consists of hourly feedings of 60 to 90 ml fluids for several days with progression from water to full liquids by the third day. Thereafter, the diet increases from day to day according to the individual's tolerance for food. By the fourth or fifth day, soft low-fiber foods are used. Eggs, custards, thickened soups, cereals, crackers, milk, and fruit purées are suitable. Tender meats, cottage cheese, and puréed vegetables are the next foods added. Meals are divided into five or six small feedings daily with emphasis on foods high in protein and fat; carbohydrate is kept relatively low. The selection of foods allowed for the first stage of the Bland Low-Fiber Diet (Chapter 31) or the Very Low Residue Diet (Chapter 32) may be used initially. Many patients progress more satisfactorily if no liquids are taken with meals, and if the diet continues to be low in carbohydrate, especially the simple sugars. Patients who have had proximal gastric vagotomy usually need not restrict their diet.[14]

Diet Following Intestinal Surgery Obstruction, persistent ileitis or diverticulitis, perforation, and malignancy are among the reasons for removal of a section of the ileum (ILEECTOMY) or colon (COLECTOMY). A permanent opening is made in the abdominal wall for elimination of wastes. Following removal of part of the ileum and colon, the proximal end of the ileum is attached to the opening (ILEOSTOMY). Because the absorptive function of the colon has been eliminated by the surgery, the waste material is fluid and continuous. Fluid, sodium, and potassium losses may be considerable, fat absorption is often poor, and vitamin B-12 absorption is reduced or absent.

A COLOSTOMY consists in attaching the proximal end of the resected colon to the opening in the abdominal wall. Some ability to absorb water is retained so that feces are more or less formed, and bowel regularity can be reestablished.

Following any operation upon the small intestine or colon, the initial oral intake is restricted to clear fluids and followed with a low-residue diet as a rule. Patients with an ileostomy are usually young and require a good deal of guidance and support from the nurse and dietitian. Gradually, they may add foods moderately low in fiber, but each food should be tested for tolerance before introducing a second. Weight loss may be considerable, and a high-protein, high-calorie diet is generally required. Vitamin B-12 injections are required to prevent the occurrence of macrocytic anemia in later years.

Colostomy is performed more frequently on elderly persons. In time they may resume an essentially normal diet, but usually they require some counseling concerning the foods required for nutritive adequacy. They too require emotional support as well as assurance that foods will not be harmful.

Small intestinal bypass is used in treating selected persons with massive obesity. By means of a JEJUNOILEOSTOMY a short segment of the jejunum is joined to the terminal ileum, effectively bypassing about 90 per cent of the small bowel. Weight loss follows as a result of the shortened transit time and reduced surface area for absorption of nutrients. A number of serious metabolic consequences have been described, including diarrhea, electrolyte imbalance, anemia, calcium oxalate urinary calculi, hyperuricemia, osteoporosis, beriberi, fatty infiltration of the liver, cirrhosis, and death. The fatty changes in the liver usually improve by 1 year postoperatively. Average weight loss after 1 year is about 30 per cent; in some instances loss of an excessive amount of weight or failure to lose sufficiently has necessitated revision of the shunt.

Diarrhea and electrolyte imbalance are severe in the immediate postoperative period. Diarrhea is worsened by the ingestion of foods high in fat, fiber, or lactose, or by excessive fluids. In severe diarrhea fluids are restricted to 1,000 to 1,200 ml per 24 hours, and are given between meals rather than at meals. A high-protein, low-fat, low-carbohydrate diet is given in six small feedings.[15] Multivitamins are usually recommended. Losses of potassium, calcium, and magnesium may be substantial and provision of good food sources of these minerals should be made.

Diet Following Other Abdominal Operations The principles outlined on page 588 pertain to the planning of diet following appendectomy, cholecystectomy, and other abdominal operations. Adynamic ileus is present longer following cholecystectomy and hysterectomy than after removal of the appendix. Patients who have had the gallbladder removed may require a fat-restricted diet for several weeks after which a regular diet is used.

Following peritonitis and intestinal obstruction, nothing whatever is given by mouth until gastrointestinal function has been resumed. Drainage of the stomach and upper intestine is essential until there is reduction of distension and passage of gas. This may require several days, during which time nutrition is maintained by intravenous therapy. When the patient shows tolerance for water, broth, and weak tea, a very low residue diet is introduced cautiously.

See Chapters 39 and 41 for nutritional considerations following coronary bypass surgery for advanced coronary artery disease and renal transplantation, respectively.

Diet Following Burns Tremendous losses of protein, salts, and fluid take place when large areas of the body have been burned. Energy expenditure following major burns is increased up to 200 per cent above basal needs and the greatly increased nutritive requirements exist for weeks or months.[16] One formula[17] for estimating calorie requirements for burns covering more than 20 per cent of the body surface is

(Adults) 25 kcal(preburn weight in kilograms) + 40 kcal(per cent burn)
(Children) 40–60 kcal(preburn weight in kilograms) + 40 kcal(per cent burn)

Thus, a patient weighing 70 kg with a 40 per cent burn would require 25(70) + 40(40) = 3,350 kcal. Severe hypoproteinemia, edema at the site of injury, failure to obtain satisfactory skin growth, gastric atony, and weight loss are among the nutritional problems encountered. In patients with serious weight loss and inadequate oral intake, total parenteral nutrition or tube feeding, or both, may be needed to establish caloric equilibrium.[17] At least 150 gm protein, and often much more, are required daily together with 3,500 to 5,000 kcal. When oral feedings are tolerated, high-protein meals supplemented with high-protein beverages are used. (See Chapter 28.) The need for as much as 1.0 gm ascorbic acid has been definitely established, and additional B-complex vitamins are also considered essential. Pharmacologic doses of vitamin A are sometimes used to prevent occurrence of stress ulcers.[4]

Diet Following Fractures Following fractures there is a tremendous catabolism of protein, which may not be reversed for several weeks. Nitrogen loss is accompanied by loss of phosphorus, potassium, and sulfur. Fever and infection may further accentuate such losses.

Calcium loss is also great but calcium therapy may lead to the formation of renal calculi and should not be attempted until the cast is removed and some mobilization is possible.

A liberal intake of protein is essential to permit restoration of the protein matrix of the bone so that calcium can be deposited. Sufficient calories to permit maximum use of the protein for synthesis should be provided.

Dumping Syndrome

Nature of the Dumping Syndrome Following convalescence from gastric surgery a relatively high proportion of patients experience distressing symptoms about 10 to 15 minutes after eating. There is a sense of fullness in the epigastrium with weakness, nausea, pallor, sweating, and dizziness. The pulse rate increases and the patient seeks to obtain relief by lying down for a few minutes. Vomiting and diarrhea are infrequently present. Weight loss is common because of insufficient intake and malabsorption. A small percentage of patients who develop this syndrome continue to have severe symptoms as long as 10 years after the surgery. The late postprandial dumping syndrome, occuring 1½ to 3 hours after eating, is less common and is characterized by symptoms of reactive hypoglycemia.

The exact etiology of the dumping has not been established but may be partly explained as follows: Ingestion of large amounts of easily hydrolyzed carbohydrates following loss of the pylorus rapidly introduces a hyperosmolar mixture into the proximal intestine. Fluid withdrawn from the extracellular space to dilute this mixture leads to distension and the cardiovascular symptoms. Both the gastrointestinal and the vasomotor symptoms have been attributed to release of vasoactive hormones from the small intestine.[18,19] Newer operative procedures such as proximal gastric vagotomy are usually not accompanied by symptoms of dumping.[14]

Modification of the Diet Dietary regimens developed to alleviate the symptoms of the dumping syndrome emphasize the following: (1) avoidance of sugar and concentrated forms of carbohydrate, (2) liberal protein, (3) small frequent feedings, and (4) dry meals with fluids taken only between meals.

To control early postprandial symptoms, carbohydrate is limited to 100 to 120 gm per day.[20] With carbohydrate restriction dietary fat is increased to provide needed calories and to retard gastric emptying. Six small meals are given daily; meals must be eaten regularly without omission. Liquids low in carbohydrate are taken 30 to 60 minutes after meals. Foods and beverages should be of moderate temperature. The diet is individualized in accordance with the patient's food tolerances; many do not tolerate milk. Meals should be eaten slowly and followed by a short rest.

In the late dumping syndrome, carbohydrate is initially limited to 50 gm per day and gradually increased to 60 to 80 gm daily for the first year following surgery. Thereafter, up to 100 gm carbohydrate daily is permitted. Frquent small feedings are needed to prevent symptoms of hypoglycemia. Fluids at meals need not be restricted.[21]

High-Protein, High-Fat, Low-Carbohydrate Diet

Characteristics and General Rules:

1. Initially, the amount of carbohydrate permitted is severely restricted; it is gradually increased as the patient's condition warrants. Carbohydrates must be measured accurately.
2. Liberal portions of proteins and fats are used.
3. Six small meals are given daily.
4. Liquids are taken 30 to 60 minutes after meals.
5. Multiple vitamin and mineral supplements are prescribed.
6. Rest before and after meals, eating slowly, and chewing well are essential.
7. Foods to avoid include milk, ice cream and other frozen desserts; sugars, sweets, candy, syrup, chocolate; gravies and rich sauces.
8. The composition of the two routines is approximately:

	Routine I	Routine II
Carbohydrate, gm	95	125
Protein, gm	95	125
Fat, gm	83	110
Kcal	1,500	2,000

Foods Allowed:

Meat, fish, poultry—all kinds: broiled, baked, poached, stewed, grilled; luncheon meats without cereal filler

Eggs—2 to 3; poached, scrambled, coddled, shirred, hard cooked

Bread—enriched toast, zwieback, Melba toast; only one slice with each feeding

Bread substitutes—Lima beans, sweet corn, cooked dried beans and peas, saltines, soda crackers, grits, noodles, macaroni, rice, spaghetti, parsnips, boiled potato, mashed potato, sweet potato. See Table A-4, Bread List, for equivalents.

Cereals—thick, cooked, only one serving

Vegetables—all kinds, not more than one serving per meal

Fruits—fresh, canned, or frozen without sugar. Drained of all liquid. Fruit juices may be taken 30 to 60 minutes after meals.

Fats—butter or margarine, crisp bacon, cream cheese, whipping cream

Nuts—when tolerated, plain or salted. Chew thoroughly.

Miscellaneous—olives, pimiento, salt, lemon or lime juice on fish, etc.

Sample Menu Plans for Patients with Dumping Syndrome

Routine I	Routine II
MORNING	
2 eggs, poached	Same
1 slice toast with	Same
1 teaspoon butter or margarine	Same
MIDMORNING	
2 tablespoons smooth peanut butter	Same
3 saltines	6 saltines
NOON	
3 ounces ground round	4 ounces ground round
¼ cup noodles with	½ cup noodles
1 teaspoon butter or margarine	Same
2 halves unsweetened peaches	Same
	½ cup asparagus with
	1 teaspoon butter or margarine
MIDAFTERNOON	
¼ cup tuna with	½ cup tuna with
1 teaspoon mayonnaise on	2 teaspoons mayonnaise
1 slice bread	Same
EVENING	
3 ounces roast leg of lamb	4 ounces roast leg of lamb
½ cup mashed potato with	Same
1 teaspoon butter or margarine	Same
½ cup carrots with	Same
1 teaspoon butter or margarine	Same
1 half unsweetened pear	½ cup unsweetened applesauce
BEDTIME	
2 ounces cold chicken on	2 ounces cold chicken on
1 slice bread	1 slice bread with
	1 teaspoon mayonnaise
	1 half unsweetened pear

Problems and Review

1. Mrs. N. needs to undergo major surgery but her physician has recommended that the surgery be delayed for 2 weeks in order to improve her nutritional status.
   a. List some symptoms and laboratory findings that indicate the need for specific attention to dietary management before surgery.
   b. Which nutrients will be especially important in Mrs. N.'s diet?
   c. Is a high-carbohydrate diet advantageous prior to surgery? Why?
   d. List several high-protein beverages which could be used to supplement Mrs. N.'s protein intake.

e. Which fluids should be emphasized in the diet if a high potassium intake is ordered?

2. Study the charts of six postoperative patients and prepare a chart showing the following: nature of the surgery; orders for parenteral fluids; orders for diet. Indicate the length of time each diet was used, and explain the variations which were found.
3. Prepare a list of parenteral feedings, tube feedings, and semisynthetic fiber-free diets used in your hospital and enumerate the chief nutritive contributions made by each.
4. Mr. E.'s physician ordered a tube feeding for him following surgery.
   a. Compare advantages and disadvantages of blenderized and commercial formula feedings.
   b. What adjustments might be made to correct diarrhea in patients receiving tube feedings?
   c. List several precautions that must be considered in administration of tube feedings?
5. List the factors important to consider in the dietary management of persons with a gastrostomy; an ileostomy; a colostomy.
6. Mrs. Q. recently underwent a subtotal gastrectomy.
   a. List some of the nutritional problems she may develop.
   b. What type of diet would you expect Mrs. Q.'s physician to order?
   c. Mrs. Q. has symptoms of the early dumping syndrome; list some of these. What steps can she take to prevent occurrence of symptoms?
   d. What dietary modifications should be made for persons with this condition? For the late dumping syndrome? Explain the rationale for each change. Plan a day's menu for Mrs. Q.

Cited References

1. Bistrian, B. R. et al.: "Protein Status of General Surgical Patients," *JAMA*, **230**:858–60, 1974.
2. Buzby, G. P. et al.: "Prognostic Nutritional Index in Gastrointestinal Surgery," *Am. J. Surg.*, **139**:160–67, 1980.
3. Mullen, J. L. et al.: "Implications of Malnutrition in the Surgical Patient," *Arch. Surg.*, **114**:121–25, 1979.
4. Wolfe, B. M. et al.: "Evaluation and Management of Nutritional Status Before Surgery," *Med. Clin. North Am.*, **63**:1257–69, 1979.
5. Shils, M. E.: "Parenteral Nutrition," in *Modern Nutrition in Health and Disease*, 6th ed., R. S. Goodhart and M. E. Shils, eds. Lea & Febiger, Philadelphia, 1980, pp. 1125–52.
6. Richardson, T. J., and Sgoutas, D.: "Essential Fatty Acid Deficiency in Four Adult Patients During Total Parenteral Nutrition," *Am. J. Clin. Nutr.*, **28**:258–63, 1975.
7. McCarthy, D. M. et al.: "Trace Metal and Essential Fatty Acid Deficiencies During Total Parenteral Nutrition," *Am. J. Digest. Dis.*, **23**:1009–16, 1978.
8. Jeejeebhoy, K. N. et al.: "Chromium Deficiency, Glucose Intolerance, and Neuropathy Reversed by Chromium Supplementation, in a Patient Receiving Long-Term Total Parenteral Nutrition," *Am. J. Clin. Nutr.*, **30**:531–38, 1977.
9. Rutten, P. et al.: "Determination of Optimal Hyperalimentation Infusion Rate," *J. Surg. Research*, **18**:477–83, 1975.
10. Renner, L. L. et al.: "Nutritional Support of the Critically Ill Child," *Pediatr. Clin. North Am.*, **27**:647–60, 1980.

11. Nachlas, M. M. et al.: "Gastrointestinal Motility Studies as a Guide to Postoperative Management," *Ann. Surg.*, **175**:510–22, 1972.
12. Glober, G. A. et al.: "Long Term Results of Gastrectomy with Respect to Blood Lipids, Blood Pressure, Weight, and Living Habits," *Ann. Surg.*, **179**:896–901, 1974.
13. Imawari, M. et al.: "Serum 25-Hydroxyvitamin D and Vitamin D-Binding Protein Levels and Mineral Metabolism After Partial and Total Gastrectomy," *Gastroenterology*, **79**:255–58, 1980.
14. Sawyers, J. L.: "Proximal Gastric Vagotomy Without Drainage. A Promising Operation for Duodenal Ulcer," *Postgrad. Med.*, **63**:115–21, April 1978.
15. Swenson, S. A., and Oberst, B.: "Pre- and Postoperative Care of the Patient with Intestinal Bypass for Obesity," *Am. J. Surg.*, **129**:225–28, 1975.
16. Fischer, J. E.: "Nutritional Support in the Seriously Ill Patient," *Current Prob. Surg.*, **17**:469–531, 1980.
17. Curreri, P. W., and Luterman, A.: "Nutritional Support of the Burned Patient," *Surg. Clin. North Am.* **58**:1151–56, 1978.
18. Woodward, E. R.: "The Early Postprandial Dumping Syndrome: Clinical Manifestations and Pathogenesis," *Major Prob. Clin. Surg.*, **20**:1–13, 1976.
19. Woodward, E. R.: "The Late Postprandial Dumping Syndrome," *Major Prob. Clin. Surg.*, **20**:28–33, 1976.
20. Unser, H. L.: "Principles of Diet Therapy for Postgastrectomy Dumping Syndrome," *Major Prob. Clin. Surg.*, **20**:159–62, 1976.
21. Harris, A. I., and Janowitz, H. D.: "Medical Management of Problems Following Peptic Ulcer Surgery," *Postgrad. Med.*, **63**:127–32, April 1978.

Additional References

BOUCHER, M.: "Broken Jaw Guide and Cookbook," *Am. J. Nurs.*, **77**:831–33, 1977.

BUSH, J.: "Cervical Esophagostomy to Provide Nutrition," *Am. J. Nurs.*, **79**:107–9, 1979.

COLLINS, J. P. et al.: "Assessment of Protein Nutrition in Surgical Patients—The Value of Anthropometrics," *Am. J. Clin. Nutr.*, **32**:1527–30, 1979.

FISCHER, J. E.: "Hyperalimentation," *Med. Clin. North Am.*, **63**:973–83, 1979.

GAZZARD, B. G. et al.: "Diets and Stoma Function," *Brit. J. Surg.*, **65**:642–44, 1978.

GRIGGS, B. A., and HOPPE, M. C.: "Nasogastric Tube Feeding," *Am. J. Nurs.*, **79**:481–85, 1979.

HOOVER, H. C. et al.: "Nutritional Benefits of Immediate Postoperative Jejunal Feeding of an Elemental Diet," *Am. J. Surg.*, **139**:153–59, 1980.

KLIDJIAN, A. M. et al.: "Relation of Anthropometric and Dynamometric Variables to Serious Postoperative Complications," *Brit. Med. J.*, **281**:899–901, 1980.

KORETZ, R. L., and MEYER, J. H.: "Elemental Diets—Facts and Fantasies," *Gastroenterology*, **78**:393–410, 1980.

LAMANSKE, J.: "Helping the Ileostomy Patient to Help Himself," *Nursing*, **7**:34–39, January 1977.

MONCRIEF, J. A.: "Burns. I. Assessment," *JAMA*, **242**:72–74, 1979.

PETERS, C., and FISCHER, J. E.: "Studies on Calorie to Nitrogen Ratio for Total Parenteral Nutrition," *Surg. Gynec. Obstet.*, **151**:1–8, 1980.

SHIZGAL, H. M., and FORSE, R. A.: "Protein and Calorie Requirements with Total Parenteral Nutrition," *Ann. Surg.*, **191**:562–68, 1980.

Diabetes Mellitus 37

DIABETES mellitus is a chronic disease that has affected humankind throughout the world. The records of the ancient civilizations of Egypt, India, Japan, Greece, and Rome describe the symptoms of the disease and usually include recommendations for treatment. The wasting away of flesh, copious urination, and the sweet taste of the urine were frequently noted by the ancient medical writers. Aretaeus of Cappadocia, who lived between A.D. 30 and 90, not only named the disease *diabetes,* which means "to run through or to siphon," but also recommended milk, cereals, starch, autumn fruits, and sweet wines.[1] The term *mellitus,* which means honeylike, was added by a London physician, Willis, in 1675.

The Nature of Diabetes

Insulin and Metabolic Defects Diabetes has been defined as a genetically and clinically heterogeneous group of disorders all of which show glucose intolerance.[2] It is characterized by a partial or total lack of functioning insulin and alterations in carbohydrate, protein, and fat metabolism.

The insulin defect may be a failure in its formation, liberation, or action. Since insulin is produced by the beta cells of the islets of Langerhans, any reduction in the number of functioning cells will decrease the amount of insulin that can be synthesized. Many diabetics can produce sufficient insulin, but some stimulus to the islet tissue is needed in order that secretion can take place. Especially in the early stages of the disease the insulinlike activity (ILA) of the blood is often increased, but most of this insulin appears to be bound to protein and is not available for transport across the cell membrane and action within the cell.

The hormones of the anterior pituitary, adrenal cortex, thyroid, and alpha cells of the islets of Langerhans are glucogenic; that is, they increase the supply of glucose. Just how these hormones are involved in the etiology of diabetes is not fully understood. Possibly they could increase the demand, decrease the secretion, or antagonize and inhibit the action of insulin.

Scope of the Problem Diabetes mellitus is an important public health problem in the United States. Although the exact prevalence is not known, various surveys indicate that about 2 per cent of the population, or some 4 million persons, have the disease. Another 5.5 million will eventually develop diabetes.[3] About 400,000 cases are diagnosed annually, most of whom are over 40 years of age and are also affected by one or more chronic conditions of the vascular system including heart disease, high blood pressure, neuropathy, nephropathy, and retinopathy.

During the 1970s the age-adjusted mortality rate from diabetes fell in both men and women in the United States to about 10.4 deaths per 100,000 population.[4] In spite of this, the life span of diabetics is shorter than that of nondiabetics at nearly all ages. About 38,000 deaths from diabetes are reported annually, placing it as the sixth leading cause of death. Diabetes is a major socioeconomic ill costing some $5 billion annually in loss of earnings and costs of hospitalization, physicians' fees, medication, and rehabilitation. The disease is much more prevalent in lower economic groups, with the rate in families with annual incomes below $4,000 being more than double that in families with incomes over $4,000.

Classes of Diabetes Three distinct classes, each of which has subtypes, have been identified.

1. DIABETES MELLITUS characterized by fasting hyperglycemia or elevated plasma glucose levels during an oral glucose tolerance test. Three subtypes are known:

Type I, insulin-dependent diabetes mellitus. Various genetic and environmental or acquired factors have been implicated in the etiology: altered frequency of certain human lymphocyte antigens (HLA) on chromosome 6, abnormal immune responses, autoimmunity, and islet cell antibodies. In some cases viral infectious diseases such as measles or mumps may trigger the autoimmune response.[5]

Type II, noninsulin-dependent diabetes mellitus. Genetic factors include familial aggregation of cases and autosomal dominant inheritance in some cases. Environmental factors, such as obesity, superimposed on a genetic susceptibility, may precipitate the disease.

Diabetes secondary to other conditions, such as pancreatic disease; endocrine disorders, such as acromegaly, Cushing's syndrome, primary aldosteronism, and others; certain drug therapy including diuretics, oral contraceptives, thyroid hormones, antidepressants, or catecholamines. This subtype may also be associated with abnormalities in insulin receptors or certain genetic syndromes.

2. IMPAIRED GLUCOSE TOLERANCE. In this class hyperglycemia occurs but the fasting plasma glucose level is less than that seen in classical diabetes (140 mg per deciliter) and the plasma glucose level during an oral glucose tolerance test is intermediate between normal and diabetic. This type may be a stage in the development of Type I or Type II diabetes, although many do not go on to develop clinical diabetes.

3. GESTATIONAL DIABETES. This class includes women who develop glucose intolerance during pregnancy. Known diabetics who become pregnant are excluded from this class. Complex hormonal and metabolic changes are probably involved in the etiology, and insulin resistance may play a part.

Factors Influencing the Risk of Diabetes Two additional classes identify those who are known to be at increased risk for diabetes. (1) *Previous abnormality of glucose tolerance.* Individuals who now have normal glucose tolerance but who have a history of impaired glucose tolerance are included. Such persons were formerly described as being prediabetic or latent diabetics. Women who have had gestational diabetes and formerly obese diabetics whose weight has returned to normal are included in this group. (2) *Potential abnormality of glucose tolerance.* Persons in this group have never had abnormal glucose tolerance but are at greatly increased risk for development of diabetes. They include persons who are identical twins, siblings, or children of diabetics; mothers of infants weighing more than 9 pounds at birth; obese individuals; or certain racial or ethnic groups with a high prevalence of diabetes, such as American Indians. The Pima tribe has an especially high incidence.

Clinical Characteristics *Insulin-dependent diabetes (Type I)* is characterized by an absolute deficiency of endogenous insulin, and proneness to ketosis. The onset is usually abrupt and is seen most frequently in juveniles, but may occur at any age. Most patients are of normal weight or underweight. They manifest the classic symptoms of diabetes.

POLYURIA, or frequent urination and an abnormally large volume of urine
POLYDIPSIA, or excessive thirst
POLYPHAGIA, or increased appetite
Loss of weight
KETOSIS is sometimes the abnormality that brings the patient to the physician. It is a condition in which the accumulation of lower

fatty acids in the blood leads to the excretion of ketones in the urine. The ketonuria is accompanied by loss of base, acidosis, dehydration, and eventually coma.

Exogenous administration of insulin is necessary to control symptoms. In the early stages after metabolic control has been restored, endogenous insulin secretion appears to be restored and symptoms abate. This period, often called the "honeymoon" phase, is only temporary and is followed by a period of exacerbation in which symptoms are difficult to control, and finally by lifelong dependence on exogenous insulin. The extent to which residual insulin secretory ability is maintained is important in stability of diabetes control. Individuals with a severe insulin secretory defect are often termed "brittle" diabetics because their blood sugar levels are difficult to control and they fluctuate between diabetic coma and hypoglycemia.

The insulin secretory defect is less severe in *Type II diabetes mellitus.* Basal insulin levels are usually normal or increased while glucose-stimulated insulin is diminished. Individuals with this type often do not present with the classic symptoms, usually are not dependent on exogenous insulin, and are not ketosis prone. Those whose hyperglycemia is not controlled with diet or oral hypoglycemic agents require insulin. Onset is generally after the age of 40. About 80 per cent of patients are obese. In most of these diabetes is brought about by failure of the beta cells to keep up with the increased demand for insulin that accompanies obesity. Insulin resistance increases the demand for insulin and is associated with defective binding of insulin to receptors on cells of liver, muscle, and adipose tissue. In some patients insulin resistance occurs even though obesity is not a factor. The prevalence of diabetes in women over the age of 30 who are 50 per cent above desirable weight is increased two to threefold.[6] Many obese adult diabetics have Type IV hyperlipidemia. (See Chapter 39.)

Laboratory Studies Several tests are used in the diagnosis of diabetes.

Glycosuria, or the presence of an abnormal amount of sugar in the urine, should be regarded as evidence of diabetes until proved otherwise. Sugar is present in the urine in many other conditions including pentosuria as a result of the body's failure to use the 5-carbon sugars; lactosuria in nursing mothers; alimentary glycosuria from excessive dietary loads of carbohydrate; fructosuria and galactosuria, resulting from enzyme deficiencies; and renal glycosuria because of a reduced ability of the tubules to reabsorb glucose.

Hyperglycemia, a high blood sugar, may be detected after a fast of 12 hours. A fasting plasma glucose of more than 140 mg per deciliter is suggestive of diabetes. Many older persons have slightly elevated blood sugar levels without having diabetes.

The ORAL GLUCOSE TOLERANCE TEST measures the body's ability to utilize a known amount of glucose. The test is done in the morning after 3 days of a diet containing at least 150 gm of carbohydrate daily. The subject must have nothing to eat or drink, except water, for 10 to 16 hours preceding the test. A fasting blood sample is drawn, after which a solution containing a weighed amount of glucose is given. The glucose dose for nonpregnant adults is 75 gm. For children, 1.75 gm per kilogram of ideal body weight, up to a maximum of 75 gm, is used. A flavored commercial preparation is given* or the glucose is dissolved in flavored water, 25 gm glucose per deciliter. Blood samples are taken at ½, 1, 1½, and 2 hours after the ingestion of glucose. Under the conditions of the test, according to the National Diabetes Data Group criteria,[2] diabetes is present if both the 2-hour glucose concentration and an intermediate value exceed the values shown in Table 37–1 on more than one occasion. In children the fasting level must also be greater

* Trutol®, by Sherwood Medical Industries, St. Louis, Missouri.

Table 37-1. **Plasma and Blood Glucose Concentrations During Oral Glucose Tolerance Test for Nonpregnant Adults***

	Normal	Impaired Glucose Tolerance	Diabetes
		mg per deciliter	
Fasting			
Whole blood	< 100	< 120	⩾ 120
Plasma	< 115	< 140	⩾ 140
½, 1, or 1½ hours			
Whole blood	< 180	⩾ 180	⩾ 180
Plasma	< 200	⩾ 200	⩾ 200
2 hours			
Whole blood	< 120	120–180	⩾ 180
Plasma	< 140	140–200	⩾ 200

*Adapted from Reference 2 at the end of this chapter.

than those indicated. Typical glucose tolerance curves are shown in Fig. 37–1.

Ketonuria, or excretion of ketones, occurs when fatty acids are incompletely oxidized in the body.

Diagnostic Criteria The oral glucose tolerance test is not always needed to establish the diagnosis. In adults, the diagnosis of diabetes is based on the presence of any one of the following: classic symptoms of diabetes and unequivocal elevation of plasma glucose; elevated fasting plasma glucose levels (140 mg per deciliter) on more than one occasion; sustained plasma glucose elevation during an oral glucose tolerance test on more than one occasion. Values at 2 hours after the ingestion of glucose and at some other time between 0 and 2 hours must be 200 mg per deciliter or greater.[2] In children, presence of the classic symptoms and a random plasma glucose greater than 200 mg per deciliter is diagnostic. In asymptomatic children there must be fasting plasma glucose of 140 mg per deciliter and sustained plasma glucose elevation during an oral glucose tolerance test on more than one occasion using the same criteria as described above for adults.[2] The criteria for impaired glucose tolerance are indicated in Table 37–1.

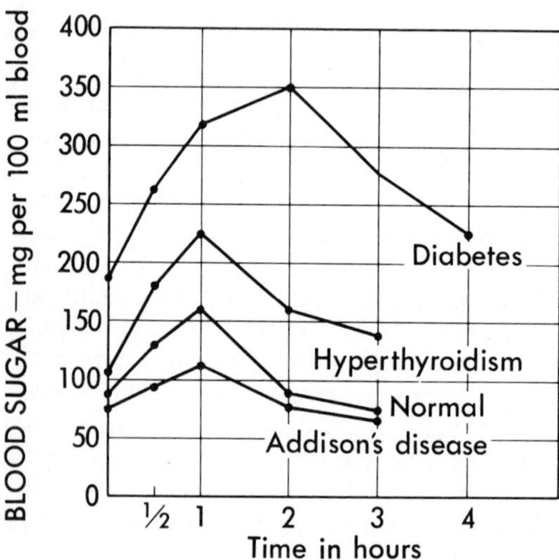

Figure 37–1. Glucose tolerance curves in various metabolic disorders.

Metabolism in Diabetes To understand the changes in metabolism that occur in diabetes, the student should first review the normal metabolism of proteins, carbohydrates, and fats (see Chapters 4, 5, and 6). A deficient supply of functioning insulin affects the metabolism of carbohydrates, fats, proteins, electrolytes, and water, and the consequences of the impairments are complex. (See Table 37–2.)

When insulin is not being produced or

Table 37-2. **Some Metabolic Effects of Insulin Deficiency**

Clinical Effect	Mechanism
Hyperglycemia	↓ uptake of glucose by liver, muscle, adipose tissue ↑ glucose production by liver due to glycogenolysis and gluconeogenesis ↑ release of substrate by muscle: ↑ glycogenolysis, ↑ amino acid release
Hypertriglyceridemia	↓ triglyceride uptake by adipose tissue
Ketonemia	↑ fatty acid mobilization by adipose tissue ↑ conversion of fatty acids to ketones by the liver ↓ uptake by muscle of ketones produced in liver
Hyperaminoacidemia	↓ hepatic uptake of branched-chain amino acids

is ineffective, the formation of glycogen is decreased, and the utilization of glucose in the peripheral tissues is reduced. As a consequence the glucose that enters the circulation from various sources is removed more slowly and hyperglycemia follows. This is further accentuated by gluconeogenesis through which about 58 per cent of the protein molecule and 10 per cent of the fat molecule can yield glucose. When the blood glucose level exceeds the renal threshold (about 160 to 180 mg per 100 ml), glycosuria occurs. The loss of glucose in the urine represents a wastage of energy and entails an increased elimination of water and sodium. Ordinarily thirst and the increased ingestion of liquids compensate for the water loss, but interference with the intake such as occurs in nausea or through vomiting could lead to rapid dehydration.

With a deficiency of insulin lipogenesis decreases and lipolysis is greatly increased, these effects being of both immediate and long-range consequence. The fatty acids released from adipose tissue or available by absorption from the intestinal tract are oxidized by the liver to form "ketone bodies" including acetoacetic acid, β-hydroxybutyric acid, and acetone. The liver utilizes only limited quantities of the ketones and releases them to the circulation. Normally the peripheral tissues metabolize the ketones at a rate equal to their production by the liver so that the blood level at any given time is minimal. In diabetes mellitus the ketones are produced at a rate that far exceeds the ability of the tissues to utilize them and the concentration in the blood is greatly increased (KETONEMIA). Acetone is excreted by the lungs and gives the characteristic fruity odor to the breath. Acetoacetic acid and β-hydroxybutyric acid are excreted in the urine (KETONURIA). Being fairly strong organic acids, these ketones combine with base so that the alkaline reserve is depleted, and acidosis results. The accompanying dehydration leads to circulatory failure, renal failure, and coma if not corrected. (See page 612.)

The rapid release of fatty acids into the blood circulation often results in a hyperlipemia and the blood serum may have a milky opalescent appearance. The blood levels of cholesterol are usually increased either because of increased synthesis or because of decreased destruction by the liver. The development of atherosclerosis in diabetic individuals occurs at an earlier age than in the nondiabetic and is more pronounced. (See page 630.)

Muscle protein catabolism is accelerated

Table 37-3. **Types of Insulin and Their Action***

Type	Onset	Peak Action	Duration
	hours		
Rapid action—short duration			
Regular crystalline	½	2–4	6–8
Semilente	½	2–4	10–12
Intermediate action and duration			
Lente	2	8–10	20–26
NPH	2	8–10	28–30
Delayed action—prolonged duration			
Protamine zinc	4–8	14–20	24–36
Ultralente	4–8	14–24	36+

*Adapted from Nelson, W. E. et al, eds.: *Textbook of Pediatrics,* W. B. Saunders Company, Philadelphia, 1979.

in uncontrolled diabetes; thus, amino acids, especially alanine, are released to the liver for gluconeogenesis. Protein catabolism also increases the amount of nitrogen that must be excreted as a result of deaminization. The catabolism of protein tissues is accompanied by the release of cellular potassium and its excretion in the urine.

Treatment for Diabetes Mellitus

Dietary control is central to success in treatment of diabetes. It is accompanied, when necessary, by insulin or oral hypoglycemic drugs. A regulated program of exercise and attention to personal hygiene are important to the total program. The many aspects of therapy require a continuing program of education for the patient together with periodic evaluation by the physician, nutritionist, and other specialists in health care.

Insulin When the islets of Langerhans are unable to produce insulin it must be supplied by injection. It cannot be taken orally because the insulin molecule, being protein in nature, would be hydrolyzed in the digestive tract and thus inactivated.

Specific circumstances vary the insulin requirement considerably. Exercise reduces the need and infections increase the need. Emotional upsets may also modify the utilization of insulin. The types of insulin and their action are listed in Table 37–3.

Oral Hypoglycemic Drugs Sulfonylurea compounds increase the release of insulin from the beta cells of the pancreas. Some have suggested that these drugs may act by increasing the activity of insulin receptors on the cell surface of target organs.[7] These agents are sometimes used in the management of noninsulin-dependent diabetes that cannot be controlled by diet alone. Since function of the beta cells is required for these compounds to be effective, they are not used in Type I, insulin-dependent diabetes. Several preparations are available,* which differ from one another chiefly in potency and duration of action. These drugs may produce hypoglycemia if food intake is delayed; thus, regularity of meals is important.

Rationale for Dietary Management The American Diabetes Association lists several goals for the dietary management of diabetes: (1) to improve the overall health of the patient by attaining and main-

* Tolbutamide (Orinase®), The Upjohn Company, Kalamazoo, Michigan; Chlorpropamide (Diabinese®), Charles Pfizer & Co., Inc., New York, New York; Acetohexamide (Dymelor®), Eli Lilly Company, Indianapolis, Indiana; Tolazamide (Tolinase®), The Upjohn Company, Kalamazoo, Michigan.

taining optimum nutrition; (2) to attain and maintain an ideal body weight; (3) to provide for normal physical growth in the child, and for adequate nutrition during pregnancy and lactation; (4) to maintain plasma glucose as near the normal physiologic range as possible; (5) to prevent or delay the development of chronic complications of diabetes: cardiovascular, renal, retinal, and neurologic; (6) to modify the diet as needed for complications of diabetes and for associated diseases; (7) to make the diet prescription as attractive and realistic as possible.[8] There are three points of view concerning the degree of dietary control needed.

Chemical control. A measured diet and insulin dosage are carefully regulated so that the blood sugar is kept within normal limits and the urine is free or nearly free of sugar at all times. Such control is believed to reduce the incidence and severity of degenerative complications. One criticism sometimes leveled against it is that the treatment may tend to be directed to the diabetes and not to the person as a whole.

Clinical control. Hyperglycemia and glycosuria are disregarded, and insulin is used to control ketosis. The diet differs little if any from that of normal persons and is controlled only to the point of maintenance of normal weight. Some physicians use these so-called free diets in the most liberal sense, but others restrict concentrated carbohydrate foods, especially those from sources contributing no other nutrients. Those who favor clinical control believe that the patient has an increased sense of well-being and that the degenerative complications are not more frequent.

Intermediate control. The majority of physicians adopt a regimen that falls between the preceding two. The objectives are: (1) to treat the patient as an individual and not on the basis of the diabetes alone; (2) to provide adequate nutrition for the maintenance of normal weight, a sense of well-being, and a life of usefulness; (3) to keep the blood sugar almost at normal levels for a large part of the day by using insulin as needed and by avoiding hypoglycemia; (4) to keep the urine sugar free or with only traces of sugar for most of the day.

Nutritional Needs Dietary control is an integral part of management for the diabetic. The diet should always provide the essentials for good nutrition and adjustments must be made from time to time for changing metabolic needs, for example, during growth, pregnancy, or modified activity.

Energy. Control of calorie intake to achieve normal weight is a primary objective for all diabetics. The calorie allowance is essentially the same as that for normal individuals of the same activity, size, and sex. Obese individuals should be placed on a calorie-restricted diet until the desirable weight for height and age is attained. Such weight loss in middle-aged obese patients very often leads to return of normal glucose tolerance. From 30 to 40 per cent of diabetics do not need insulin if their diets are controlled.

One approach to planning the calorie level is to determine the patient's present food intake and to use it as a guide for the calculated diet. The patient's continuing weight status determines whether the diet, in fact, is satisfactory in its calorie level—assuming, of course, that the patient is adhering to it. A convenient guide for planning the energy level is as follows:

	Kcal per kg (Desirable Weight)	Kcal per pound (Desirable Weight)
For weight loss	20	9
For a bed patient	25	11
For light work	30	14
For medium work	35	16
For heavy work	40	18

Protein. The recommended dietary allowance for protein for each age and sex category is satisfactory for the diabetic individual. From 12 to 20 per cent of calories should be from protein.[8]

Carbohydrate. A level of 100 gm carbohydrate will prevent ketosis. Several studies have shown that raising the carbohydrate intake does not adversely affect fasting blood glucose levels, glucose tolerance, or insulin requirements, provided that total calories are not increased. Insulin needs are more closely correlated with total calorie intake than with the carbohydrate level in the diet. Consequently, liberalization of the carbohydrate intake to more closely approximate that of the typical diet in the United States has been recommended. For the majority of diabetics, 50 to 60 per cent of calories as carbohydrate, mostly of the complex type, is recommended.[8] For the 20 per cent or so of adult diabetics with hypertriglyceridemia, carbohydrate should be limited to 35 per cent of calories.[9]

Fat. After protein and carbohydrate levels have been established, the fat allowance makes up the remaining calories. For most diets, 30 to 35 per cent of the calories as fat is satisfactory. Foods high in saturated fat and cholesterol should be limited.[8] The level of saturated fat recommended is less than 10 per cent of total calories, with polyunsaturated fat providing up to 10 per cent of total calories. This entails use of skim milk, low-fat meats, and polyunsaturated fats in calculating the diet and planning the daily meals. (See Table A-4.) Fat intake should be appropriately reduced when alcohol is ingested so that the energy intake will not be excessive. Carbohydrate intake should also be reduced to compensate for any carbohydrate in the alcoholic beverage.

Fiber Trowell has postulated that fiber-deficient diets may be involved in the etiology of diabetes mellitus.[10] Diets providing 20 gm or more of plant fiber have been associated with reductions in postprandial plasma glucose, LDL-cholesterol, and total cholesterol, and insulin requirements.[11] The American Diabetes Association recommends substitution of foods containing unrefined carbohydrate with fiber for highly refined carbohydrate foods that are low in fiber.[8]

Regularity of Meals Day-to-day consistency in amounts and distribution of carbohydrate, protein, and fat is needed especially for persons taking insulin or oral hypoglycemic agents. Meals should be spaced to coincide with the availability of insulin. A delay in eating may produce hypoglycemia. On the other hand, hyperglycemia, brought on by eating an excess of rapidly hydrolyzed carbohydrate, is to be avoided. Physical activity influences insulin requirements and adjustments in the diet may be needed as well. Many patients are advised to have a carbohydrate-rich snack before participating in vigorous physical exercise.

Calculation of the diabetic diet prescription A number of procedures may be used to arrive at the diet prescription. This is the responsibility of the physician, but the nurse and dietitian should have an understanding of the basis for the calculation. Following is described one of the methods often used.

Let us assume that a diet is to be planned for a secretary who is 25 years old and 170 cm (67 inches) tall. According to the table of heights and weights (Table A-10), her desirable weight is 60 kg (132 pounds) (medium frame).

1. Calories: 30 kcal per kilogram (14 per pound) of desirable body weight
   $60 \times 30 = 1{,}800$ kcal per day
2. Protein: 12 to 20 per cent of total calories
   $1{,}800 \times 15\% = 270$ kcal
   270 kcal $\div 4 = 67.5$ gm protein daily
3. Carbohydrate: 50 to 60 per cent of total calories
   $1{,}800 \times 55\% = 990$ kcal
   $990 \div 4 = 247.5$ gm carbohydrate per day
4. Fat calories: Total calories minus calories from protein and carbohydrate
   $1{,}800 - (270 + 990) = 540$ kcal
5. Fat: fat calories divided by 9
   $540 \div 9 = 60$ gm fat per day

By rounding off the numbers, the prescription is: protein, 65–70 gm; carbohydrate, 245–250 gm; fat, 60 gm.

Distribution of Calories Calories, especially those from carbohydrate, are distributed so as to coincide with the type of insulin being used and modified according to each patient's needs in order to achieve the best possible regulation of carbohydrate utilization. When intermediate or long-acting insulins are used, a portion of the carbohydrate—usually 20 to 40 gm—is reserved for a midafternoon or bedtime feeding or both. This carbohydrate must be in slowly available form and should be accompanied by a portion of the day's protein. For example, a patient receiving an intermediate-acting insulin such as NPH, might receive 1/7, 2/7, 1/7, 2/7, 1/7 of the total carbohydrate and calories for breakfast, lunch, afternoon snack, dinner, and evening snack, respectively. See Table 37–4. Some prefer to have a distribution in tenths, thus 2/10, 3/10, 1/10, 3/10, 1/10 for the previous example.[9]

Planning the Meal Pattern The dietitian and the nurse must translate the prescription into terms of common foods, keeping the following points especially in mind.

1. The diet should be planned with the patient so that it can be adjusted to his or her pattern of living. This requires consideration of the patient's economic status, the availability and cost of food, national, religious, and social customs, personal idiosyncrasies, occupation, facilities for preparing or obtaining meals, and so on.

The diabetic diet need not be an expensive one, and, ideally, it should be so planned that it fits in with the menus of the rest of the family. However, if the family diet is a poor one, the entire family will benefit when the basic food groups become the center about which meals are planned. The diet for the diabetic person does not require many special foods; thus, the rest of the family should not be deprived.

2. The adequacy of the diet for minerals and vitamins is most easily ensured if one includes basic amounts of foods from the Daily Food Guide.

3. Including some of the protein and fat in each meal helps to provide satiety and balance of food selection.

4. The food exchange lists (Table A-4) permit reasonable dietary constancy from day to day and considerable flexibility in meal planning. The method for dietary calculation using these lists has been described in Chapter 26 and is illustrated in Table 26–2.

5. The meal distribution of the carbohydrate can be adjusted to within 7 or 8 gm without using fractions of exchanges. The protein and fat should be adjusted within meals so that maximum flexibility is possible in meal planning. For example, the inclu-

Table 37–4. **Typical Meal Distribution of Calories and Carbohydrate**

Type of Insulin	Breakfast	Noon	Midafternoon	Evening	Bedtime
None	1/3 1/5	1/3 2/5		1/3 2/5	Usually none
Short-acting (before breakfast and dinner)	2/5	1/5		2/5	Usually none
Intermediate-acting NPH	1/7	2/7	1/7	2/7	1/7
Long-acting	1/5	2/5		2/5	20–40 gm carbohydrate
With regular insulin at breakfast	1/3	1/3		1/3	20–40 gm carbohydrate

Table 37-5. **Meal Pattern and Sample Menu**
Calorie and carbohydrate division: breakfast, 1/7; luncheon, 2/7; midafternoon, 1/7; dinner, 2/7; bedtime, 1/7

Meal Pattern	Exchange	C gm	P gm	F gm		Sample Menu
Breakfast						
Milk, list 1	½	6	4	–		Skim milk–½ cup
Fruit, list 3	1	10	–	–		Orange–1
Bread, list 4	1	15	2	–		Whole-wheat toast–1 slice
Fat, list 6	2	–	–	10		Margarine–2 teaspoons
Coffee or tea						
		31	6	10	=	238 kcal = 13%
Luncheon						
Meat, list 5	2	–	14	6		Sliced chicken–2 ounces
Bread, list 4	3	45	6	–		Whole-wheat bread–2 slices Broth/saltines–6
Vegetables, list 2	1	5	2	–		Sliced tomato/lettuce
Fat, list 6	2	–	–	10		Mayonnaise–2 teaspoons
Fruit, list 3	2	20	–	–		Banana–1 small
Coffee or tea						
		70	22	16	=	512 kcal = 28%
Midafternoon						
Bread, list 4	1	15	2	–		Graham crackers–2 squares
Fat, list 6	1	–	–	5		Margarine–1 teaspoon
Fruit, list 3	1	10	–	–		Grapes–12
Milk, list 1	1	12	8	–		Skim milk–1 cup
		37	10	5	=	233 kcal = 13%
Dinner						
Meat, list 5	2	–	14	10		Chopped beef–2 ounces
Bread, list 4	3	45	6	–		Rice–1 cup Dinner roll–1
Vegetables, list 2	2	10	4	–		Wax beans–½ cup Sliced cucumbers–½ cup
Fat, list 6	2	–	–	10		Margarine–2 teaspoons
Fruit, list 3	2	20	–	–		Cantaloupe–¼ small Strawberries–¾ cup
Coffee or tea						
		75	24	20	=	579 kcal = 32%
Evening snack						
Bread, list 4	1	15	2	–		Popcorn–3 cups
Fat, list 6	2	–	–	10		Margarine–2 teaspoons
Fruit, list 3	1	10	–	–		Apple–1 small
Milk, list 1	½	6	4	–		Skim milk–½ cup
		31	6	10	=	238 kcal = 13%
Totals, gm		244	68	61	=	1,797 kcal = 99%
Per cent of kcal		54	15	31		

sion of milk at breakfast permits either cereal or bread to be selected from the bread exchanges; meat exchanges are wisely divided among the three meals with somewhat larger amounts being allocated to dinner. An example of the distribution of food exchanges into meal patterns is shown in Table 37–5 for the diet calculation illustrated on page 474.

Dietary Counseling

ESSENTIAL KNOWLEDGE The diabetic patient needs to know about (1) the nature of diabetes and the reasons for the measures that will be recommended, (2) the importance of weight control, (3) the details of the dietary program, (4) the amounts, time intervals, and method of administration of insulin or oral drugs, if needed, (5) skin care and personal hygiene, (6) procedures for testing the urine, (7) signs of hypoglycemia or acidosis and what steps to take in the event they occur, (8) emergency measures to take during infection and illness until medical help is available, and (9) the importance of periodic visits to the physician. (See Figure 37–2.)

Insofar as diet is concerned, the patient needs to be taught the amount of food exchanges to use at each meal, how to use the food exchange lists in daily meal planning, how to interpret labels when purchasing food, and how to prepare food for meals. (See Figure 37–3.)

RESPONSIBILITY FOR EDUCATION The physician, nurse, and dietitian share the responsibility for counseling the patient. The physician explains the nature of diabetes and the factors of importance in maintaining control. He or she also makes referrals to the dietitian and nurse for detailed aspects of education. In the hospital or outpatient clinic the dietitian usually initiates dietary instruction and arranges for a continuing program of education. The nurse instructs the patient regarding insulin administration, urine testing, and hygiene. The nurse is a valuable assistant for dietary counseling and may be fully responsible for dietary instruction in some situations where no dietitian is available.

Experience has shown that the majority of diabetics fail to understand their diets. Some of the reasons for failure have been outlined

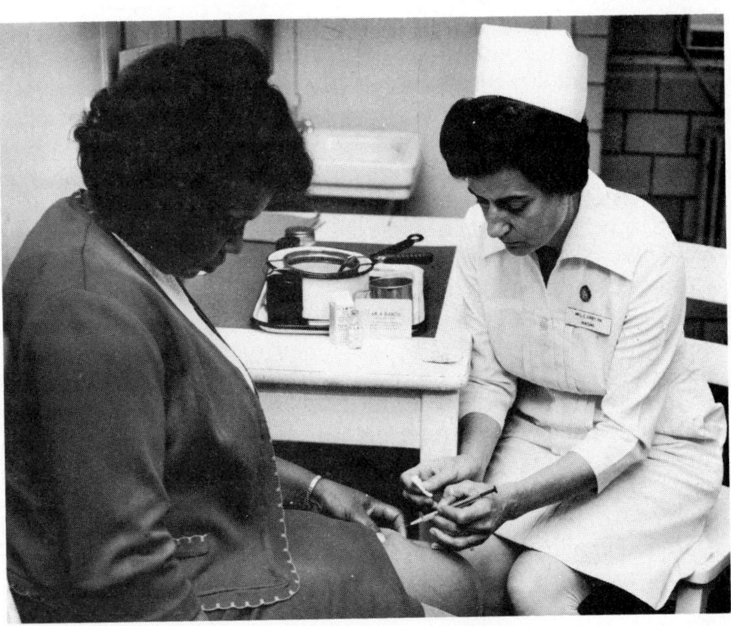

Figure 37–2. Nurse teaching patient how to administer insulin. (Courtesy, Medical College of Virginia, Health Sciences Division, Virginia Commonwealth University, Richmond.)

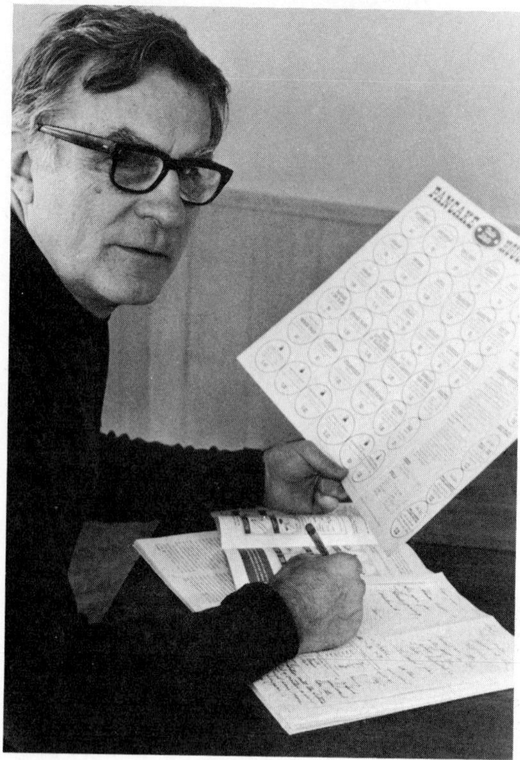

Figure 37–3. Ability to select appropriate foods for meals eaten away from home is an important part of the learning process for the diabetic. (Courtesy, Diabetes Education Center, Minneapolis.)

with suggestions for successful counseling.[12]

Satisfactory counseling of the patient includes individualized instruction which may be supplemented by group instruction. The patient must be involved throughout in order to fully understand and adopt the program necessary. Frequent follow-up visits with the dietitian or public health nurse are essential to reinforce motivation, to answer questions, and to give added information.

Not only the patient but members of the family must be included in the counseling sessions. Each member of the family needs to understand that the diet for the diabetic patient is essentially a normal one, but that a regulated routine of meals and of the quantities of food is a vital aspect of the program. Members of the family also need to be aware of the complications that could arise and should know what to do in emergencies.

TEACHING AIDS Many books and pamphlets pertaining to diabetes have been prepared by health agencies, pharmaceutical firms, and physicians for the guidance of the patient. When these are selected at a reading level appropriate for the patient, these printed materials are useful for further study and reference. They should never be regarded as a substitute for personal counseling.

The patient's tray at each meal constitutes one of the best visual aids if the dietitian and nurse take the opportunity to so use it. If the patient has been introduced to the food exchange lists, the foods on the tray can be located in these lists and the amounts served identified in number of exchanges. Needless to say, careful checking of the tray before it is brought to the patient is important to emphasize dietary control. Measuring cups, measuring spoons, and various sizes of glasses and cups used for table service should be demonstrated during the instruction of the patient. Paper and plastic food models are useful in demonstrating menu planning and may be used by the patient for practice sessions in planning his or her own diet. In a relatively short time most patients can learn to estimate the portion sizes allowed on their diets. (See Figure 37–4.)

Programmed instruction, when available, can be an important teaching aid. Slides, filmstrips, and movies pertaining to the many aspects of diabetic care are especially useful for group instruction. Each patient should be encouraged to participate in some group events not only for their instructional value, but to afford the opportunity to share experiences with others.

Some Problems in Education of the Diabetic Patient Lack of education, inability to read English, and failing vision are among the problems encountered in the use of printed materials. Sometimes a member of the family can assist in using printed materials. Posters, tapes, films, and food models may be used. The nurse and dietitian must expect to spend more time with patients who present these problems, but repeated verbal instruction can be successful.

About half the diabetic patients are from families with very limited incomes. Although the diabetic diet need not be more expensive than a normal diet, the daily meal pattern must be carefully planned to make the best use of inexpensive foods. Most patients and their families can profit by advice in the wise purchase of foods.

Patients often ask about the use of dietetic foods. Water-packed fruits are available in most supermarkets at costs only slightly above that of regular packs and are useful when fresh fruits are out of season. Many water-packed fruits are sweetened with artificial sweeteners.

Dietetic foods such as cookies, candies, ice cream, and gluten breads are not needed since most diabetic diets are sufficiently liberal to include a wide choice of foods. Some of the specialty products are expensive. Although low in carbohydrate, most of them contain protein and fat, thus contributing available glucose and calories. Short-term studies suggest that fructose or sorbitol does not elevate fasting plasma glucose, but long-term studies are needed.[13] Products contain-

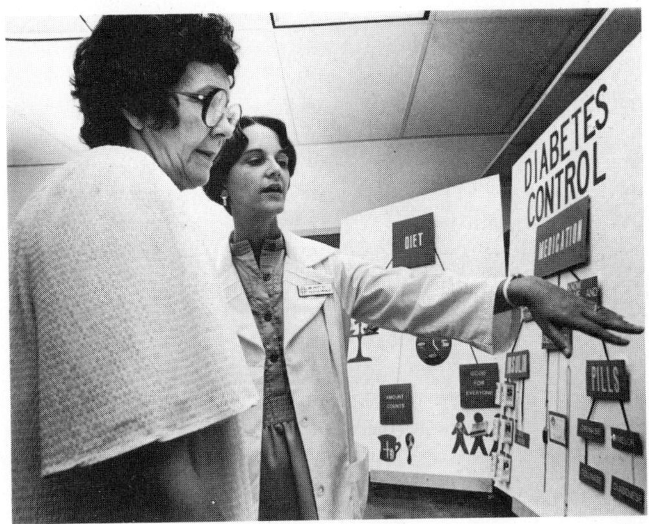

Figure 37–4. These visual aids help the patient to understand the several aspects of diabetic control. Each treatment program is individualized according to the patient's life-style, nutritional requirements, and the clinical and biochemical findings. (Courtesy, Metropolitan Medical Center, Minneapolis.)

ing fructose or sorbitol should not be used freely as the calorie value of these sugars is equivalent to that of glucose. The patient who wishes to use such products should be advised about the specific changes which need to be made in his or her meal pattern.

Some patients ask about the use of alcoholic beverages. If the physician permits their use, the caloric equivalent of the beverage, as fat, is first subtracted from the day's allowance, and the balance of the diet is calculated accordingly.

Initially the patient should become thoroughly familiar with the kinds and amounts of foods allowed from the exchange lists. Once confidence has been developed in the use of these lists, the patient needs to be given some assistance in the use of food mixtures. A number of cookbooks have been prepared specifically for diabetic patients and include calculations of nutritive values. Some food processors have developed tables showing how their products can fit into the food exchanges. Patients usually need some assistance in the interpretation of these printed materials.

Acute Complications of Diabetes

Hypoglycemia INSULIN SHOCK or hypoglycemia is caused by an overdose of insulin, a decrease in the available glucose because of delay in eating, omission of food, or loss of food by vomiting and diarrhea, or an increase in exercise without accompanying modification of the insulin dosage.

The patient going into insulin shock becomes uneasy, nervous, weak, and hungry. He or she is pale, the skin is moist, and perspiration is excessive. There may be trembling, dizziness, faintness, headache, and double vision. Movements may be uncoordinated. Emotional instability may be indicated by crying, by hilarious behavior, or by belligerency. Occasionally, there may be nausea and vomiting or convulsions. Without treatment coma follows and death is impending. Laboratory studies show a blood sugar below 50 mg per 100 ml.[14]

Orange juice or other fruit juices, sugar, candy, syrup, honey, a carbonated beverage, or any readily available carbohydrate may be given. If absorption is normal, recovery follows in a few minutes. If there is stupor, intravenous glucose is necessary. Some patients are now using one or another of the slowly acting insulins, in which case reactions may recur after a few hours. To avoid such subsequent reactions, it is necessary to follow the initial carbohydrate therapy in 1 or 2 hours and at later intervals with foods containing carbohydrate which is slowly absorbed—such as in milk and bread.

The patient must be impressed with the importance of balance between diet and insulin dosage and the importance of close adherence to the physician's orders. The patient should always carry some sugar or hard candy to avert symptoms when they are still mild.

Diabetic Acidosis and Coma Diabetic ketoacidosis is a state of severe insulin deficiency which is characterized by hyperglycemia, acidosis, and elevated blood ketones, and which may progress to coma. Coma often originates because the patient consumed additional foods for which the insulin did not provide, or because he failed to take the correct amount of insulin or omitted it entirely. The presence of diabetes is first detected in some persons who were not aware of the disease until coma occurred. Infection is an especially sinister influence since even a mild infection reduces the carbohydrate tolerance and severe acidosis may sometimes occur before the insulin dosage has been appropriately increased. Trauma of any kind, whether an injury or surgery, aggravates the diabetes so that acidosis is more likely.

Some of the signs of diabetic acidosis and coma are similar to those of insulin shock, and a differentiation cannot be made without information concerning the patient prior to the onset of the symptoms, together with blood and urine studies. The patient complains of feeling ill and weak; he or she may have a headache, anorexia, nausea and vomiting, abdominal pain, and aches and pains elsewhere. The skin is hot, flushed, and dry; the mouth is dry and the patient is thirsty. An acetone odor on the breath, painful, rapid breathing, and drowsiness are typical signs. Symptoms of shock, unconsciousness, and death follow unless prompt measures are taken. Sugar, acetone, and acetoacetic acid are present in the urine, the blood glucose is elevated to very high levels, and the blood carbon dioxide content is decreased.

When early signs of ketosis are present, small repeated doses of insulin are given together with small carbohydrate feedings. Diabetic coma, however, is a medical emergency best treated in a hospital where close nursing care can be given. The physician directs the therapy, which includes large doses of regular insulin with smaller doses repeated as needed every hour or so until the urine sugar is reduced and the blood sugar is lowered to less than 200 mg per 100 ml; saline infusions for the correction of dehydration; gastric lavage if the patient has been vomiting; and alkali therapy for the correction of the severe acidosis.

When the urine sugar decreases and the blood sugar begins to fall, glucose is given by infusion in order to avoid subsequent hypoglycemic reactions. As soon as fluids can be taken orally, the patient is given fruit juices, gruels, ginger ale, tea, and broth. All of these are useful for their fluid content; fruit juice, ginger ale, and gruels provide carbohydrate; broth and gruels contain sodium chloride; and fruit juices, broth and gruels contribute potassium. These fluids may be given in amounts of 100 ml, more or less, every hour or so during the first day. By the second day, the patient is usually able to take a soft diet which is calculated to contain 100 to 200 gm carbohydrate, and by the third day the patient may take the diet which meets his or her particular requirements.

Chronic Complications of Diabetes

Large Vessel Disease Atherosclerosis of the coronary, cerebral, and lower extremity arteries is accelerated in all age groups. The likelihood of cardiovascular disease is two to three times greater, with higher morbidity and mortality than in nondiabetics. Obese women with diabetes are at especially high risk for cardiovascular disease.[15]

Small Vessel Disease Generalized thickening of the capillary basement membranes occurs in long-standing diabetes and precedes the development of retinopathy and nephropathy.

Changes in vessels of the retina may lead to cataracts, retinopathy, or blindness. Diabetes is the leading cause of new cases of blindness in the United States.[16] Retinopathy is seen in about 20 per cent of those who have had the disease for 10 years and in nearly half of those with diabetes for 25 years or more.[5]

Renal disease accounts for about half the deaths in persons with insulin-dependent diabetes of many years' duration. Glomerulosclerosis, vascular changes, hypertension, albuminuria and edema are characteristically seen in Kimmelstiel-Wilson's disease, a syndrome occurring in diabetes.

Neuropathy Peripheral nerve dysfunction is a common finding in diabetes. Several hypotheses have been proposed to explain the etiology: (1) ischemic vascular disease; (2) biochemical changes in nerves and structural changes in Schwann cells, leading to demyelination. Loss of myelin could slow the rate of nerve conduction; (3) damage to the neurons followed by degeneration of axons and eventual nerve demyelination.[17] Because of the sensory impairment good foot care is essential. Even minor trauma can lead to infection and gangrene.

It is not known how important the control of blood glucose levels is in preventing or delaying development of chronic complications of diabetes. Some investigators believe that large vessel changes are related primarily to obesity and abnormal lipid metabolism whereas small vessel disease and neuropathy are more closely related to hyperglycemia. Control of blood glucose levels may have a favorable effect in decreasing the latter type of complications.[18]

Special Situations

Surgery Ideally, the diabetic patient who is having surgery should have a normal blood sugar, no glycosuria, and no ketosis. A glycogen reserve is essential and can be ensured only if sufficient carbohydrate is included up to 12 hours prior to the operation and if insulin is supplied in great enough amounts for the utilization of the carbohydrate. Fluids in abundance are indicated. When emergency surgery is needed, parenteral glucose is usually ordered.

Carbohydrate feedings should begin within 3 hours after operation, as a rule. Initially glucose may be given parenterally. When liquids can be taken by mouth, tea with sugar, orange juice, and ginger ale may be used. When a full fluid or soft diet can be tolerated, the diet can be calculated to provide the protein and fat as well as the carbohydrate allowances.

Infection The guidance of a physician is important when a diabetic patient has an infection. An infection lowers the carbohydrate tolerance and increases the insulin requirement. A mild diabetic may become a severe case, and infections may precipitate coma. The physician sometimes orders insulin for patients who are not ordinarily required to use insulin.

Pregnancy Diabetes increases the hazards of pregnancy because of the dangers of glycogen depletion, hypoglycemia, acidosis, and infection. Despite the increased hazards the diabetic woman can have an uneventful pregnancy and a healthy baby. She should have medical guidance throughout her pregnancy with emphasis on control of the rate of weight gain and the prevention of edema. The nutritional requirements are similar to those of the nondiabetic pregnant woman. The insulin requirements are usually increased. Most diabetic women are unable to produce enough milk for the baby and should not be encouraged to nurse their infants.

Problems and Review

1. List some possible reasons for increased prevalence of diabetes in older persons.
2. What factors may account for the declining mortality rate from diabetes?
3. Mr. White is an overweight 45-year-old factory worker who has just been diagnosed as a diabetic. Answer the following questions in relation to this patient.
   a. List the important predisposing factors in diabetes mellitus.
   b. Explain how insulin deficiency affects the metabolism of carbohydrate; protein; fat; sodium; potassium; water.
   c. Explain the typical symptoms of diabetes on the basis of the metabolic changes.
   d. What advice might be appropriate for Mr. White's children in order to delay or avoid the onset of diabetes mellitus?
   e. State the important objectives to be achieved in the therapy of this patient. What factors may influence the realization of these objectives?
   f. What information do you need in order to plan a satisfactory dietary program for Mr. White?
4. The following diet prescription was ordered for Mr. White: protein, 60 gm; carbohydrate, 230 gm; fat, 55 gm. The carbohydrate and calories should be distributed in thirds as Mr. White is taking tolbutamide. The fat allowance is to be chosen from foods low in saturated fat, and that are good sources of polyunsaturated fat. Mr. White carries his lunch to work.

a. Calculate the daily meal plan.
b. Plan one day's menu for Mr. White on a work day.
c. Explain the basis for the low saturated fat and increased polyunsaturated fat prescription.

5. Show how each of the following combinations could be used in the dinner pattern for Mr. White:
   a. Tuna-noodle casserole
   b. Beef stew with carrots, onion, potatoes, and celery
   c. A picnic supper including ham and potato salad
6. Mr. White believes that he can eat as he pleases because the tolbutamide he takes will control his diabetes. Explain why this thinking is incorrect.
7. Mr. White is not feeling well and would prefer to have liquids at lunch. Calculate a full fluid diet to provide: protein, 20 gm; carbohydrate, 75 gm; fat, 20 gm.
8. Mr. Johnson, the patient in the next bed, is an insulin-dependent diabetic who has refused to eat the following foods on his tray: ½ slice bread, ½ cup carrots, 1½ ounces meat, and 1 small potato. He has agreed to take a carbohydrate replacement as orange juice.
   a. On the basis of the carbohydrate content of the foods refused, how much orange juice would be required?
   b. If the amount of orange juice given was kept to ½ cup, how much sugar would you need to add to the juice to cover the carbohydrate replacement?
   c. List two other juices and the appropriate amounts of each that could be used if Mr. Johnson had not expressed a preference for orange juice.
   d. If the replacement were based on the total glucose available from the foods refused, what changes would you need to make in items *a* and *b*?

Cited References

1. Stowers, J. M.: "Nutrition in Diabetes," *Nutr. Abstr. Rev.*, **33**:1–15, 1963.
2. National Diabetes Data Group: "Classification and Diagnosis of Diabetes Mellitus and Other Categories of Glucose Intolerance," *Diabetes*, **28**:1039–57, 1979.
3. Knowles, H. C. et al.: "Diabetes Mellitus: The Overall Problem and Its Impact on the Public," in *Diabetes Mellitus*, S. S. Fajans, ed., Publ. No. (NIH) 76–854, U.S. Department of Health, Education, and Welfare, 1976, pp. 11–32.
4. Metropolitan Life Insurance Company: "Life Expectancy Among Diabetics. II," *Statistical Bull.*, **60**:11–13, October–December 1979.
5. Sperling, M. A.: "Diabetes Mellitus," *Pediatr. Clin. North Am.*, **26**:149–69, 1979.
6. Rimm, A. A. et al.: "Relationship of Obesity and Disease in 73,532 Weight-Conscious Women," *Publ. Health Reports*, **90**:44–51, 1975.
7. Khachadurian, A. K., et al.: "Management of Noninsulin-dependent Diabetes Mellitus," *Am. Fam. Physician*, **21**:154–60, February 1980.
8. American Diabetes Association: "Principles of Nutrition and Dietary Recommendations for Individuals with Diabetes Mellitus: 1979," *Diabetes*, **28**:1027–30, 1979.
9. Arky, R. A.: "Current Principles of Dietary Therapy of Diabetes Mellitus," *Med. Clin. North Am.*, **62**:655–62, 1978.
10. Trowell, H. C.: "Dietary-Fiber Hypothesis of the Etiology of Diabetes Mellitus," *Diabetes*, **24**:762–65, 1975.
11. Anderson, J. W. and Chen, W-J. L.: "Plant Fiber. Carbohydrate and Lipid Metabolism," *Am. J. Clin. Nutr.*, **32**:346–63, 1979.
12. West, K. M.: "Diet Therapy of Diabetes: An Analysis of Failure," *Ann. Intern. Med.*, **79**:425–34, 1973.

13. Brunzell, J. D.: "Use of Fructose, Sorbitol, or Xylitol as a Sweetener in Diabetes Mellitus," *J. Am. Diet. Assoc.*, **73**:499–506, 1978.
14. Newmark, S. R., et al.: "Hyperglycemic and Hypoglycemic Crises," *JAMA*, **231**:185–87, 1975.
15. Gordon, T. et al.: "Diabetes, Blood Lipids, and the Role of Obesity in Coronary Heart Disease Risk for Women. The Framingham Study," *Ann. Intern. Med.*, **87**:393–97, 1977.
16. Ellenberg, M.: "Chronic Complications of Diabetes Mellitus," *N.Y. State J. Med.*, **79**:2005–14, 1979.
17. Clements, R. S.: "Diabetic Neuropathy—New Concepts of Its Etiology," *Diabetes*, **28**:604–11, 1979.
18. Cahill, G. F. et al.: "Blood Glucose Control in Diabetes," *Diabetes*, **25**:237–39, 1976.

Additional References

ALBRINK, M. J.: "Dietary and Drug Treatment of Hyperlipidemia in Diabetes," *Diabetes*, **23**:913–18, 1974.

ANDERSON, J. W., and SIELING, B.: "High Fiber Diets for Obese Diabetic Patients," *Obesity/Bariatric Med.*, **9**:109–13, 1980.

KEYES, M.: "The Somogyi Phenomenon in Insulin-Dependent Diabetics," *Nurs. Clin. North Am.*, **12**:439–45, 1977.

KOIVISTO, V. A., and SHERWIN, R. S.: "Exercise in Diabetes," *Postgrad. Med.*, **66**:87–96, November 1979.

KRALL, L. P., and CHABOT, V. A.: "Oral Hypoglycemic Agent Update," *Med. Clin. North Am.*, **62**:681–94, 1978.

REAVEN, G. M. et al.: "Nutritional Management of Diabetes," *Med. Clin. North Am.*, **63**:927–43, 1979.

SAUDEK, C. D., and EDER, H. A.: "Lipid Metabolism in Diabetes Mellitus," *Am. J. Med.*, **66**:843–52, 1979.

SHERWIN, R., and FELIG, P.: "Pathophysiology of Diabetes Mellitus," *Med. Clin. North Am.*, **62**:695–711, 1978.

SLATER, N. L.: "Insulin Reactions vs. Ketoacidosis: Guidelines for Diagnosis and Intervention," *Am. J. Nurs.*, **78**:875–77, 1978.

THOMAS, K. P.: "Diabetes Mellitus in Elderly Persons," *Nurs. Clin. North Am.*, **11**:157–68, 1976.

VRANIC, M., and BERGER, M.: "Exercise and Diabetes Mellitus," *Diabetes*, **28**:147–63, 1979.

WALESKY, M. E.: "Diabetic Ketoacidosis," *Am. J. Nurs.*, **78**:872–74, 1978.

WEST, K. M.: "Diabetes in American Indians and Other Native Populations of the New World," *Diabetes*, **23**:841–55, 1974.

38 Various Metabolic Disorders

PURINE-RESTRICTED DIET

MANY diseases for which dietary modification is an effective part of treatment are deviations of normal metabolic pathways in the body. They occur because of abnormal production of one or more hormones, a deficiency of an enzyme, or a modification of excretion. Those which are discussed in this chapter fall into one or another of these categories but otherwise bear little, if any, relation to each other.

Hypoglycemia

Hypoglycemia refers to an abnormally low blood glucose level and may be of organic or functional origin. Organic causes include the following: (1) hyperinsulinism due to tumors or hyperplasia of islet cells; surgery rather than dietary management is essential; (2) hepatic diseases involving enzyme defects (see Chapter 44), alcoholism, or cirrhosis; and (3) endocrine disorders such as hypothyroidism and adrenocortical or pituitary insufficiency. Functional hypoglycemias are more common and may produce symptoms in the fasting state (spontaneous type) or, more frequently, in response to food intake (reactive type). An example of the latter is functional hyperinsulinism, in which there is oversecretion of insulin following carbohydrate ingestion, with the following effects on the blood glucose level: (1) a normal fasting blood sugar; (2) hypoglycemia 2 to 4 hours after meals, especially in the forenoon and late afternoon; (3) no hypoglycemia following fasting or the omission of meals; and (4) a glucose tolerance curve (see Figure 37–1) which shows a normal fasting sugar, initially elevated glucose level after taking the glucose, and a sharp fall to very low sugar levels.

Functional hypoglycemia may occur following gastrectomy or gastroenterostomy when nutrients are absorbed at an extremely rapid rate. In such situations the food reaches the small intestine much more rapidly than is normal, is very quickly absorbed, and the sudden elevation of the blood sugar serves as an extra stimulus to the islet cells and a subsequent hypoglycemia. See Chapter 36 for description of the dumping syndrome. Functional hypoglycemia may also be a manifestation of early noninsulin-dependent diabetes or may be idiopathic in nature.

Symptoms Rapid fall of the blood glucose level causes release of catecholamines and produces symptoms of weakness, nervousness, trembling, perspiring freely, rapid heartbeat, hunger, or nausea and vomiting. As a result of inadequate delivery of glucose to the brain, the person with chronic, severe hypoglycemia may experience headache, incoordination, irritability, confusion, emotional instability, and even coma.

Contrary to popular belief, occurrence of these symptoms does not necessarily indicate hypoglycemia. Criteria for the diagnosis include occurrence of symptoms when the blood glucose is at its lowest point (nadir) during a 5 hour glucose tolerance test, and relief of symptoms by glucose ingestion. In addition a significant rise in plasma cortisol must follow the glucose nadir.[1] A symptomatic response without true hypoglycemia during the test has been attributed to emotional disturbances.[2]

Modification of the Diet A diet prescription to meet each patient's needs is planned.

Carbohydrate. In hypoglycemias associated with some hepatic enzyme deficiencies or liver diseases, carbohydrate supplements are needed. In postprandial hypoglycemias the carbohydrate serves as a stimulus to further insulin secretion and is provocative of the hypoglycemic attack; thus, it is usually restricted to 100 gm or less. Refined carbohydrates are eliminated and complex carbohydrates are substituted. Some evidence suggests that certain patients benefit from a more liberal carbohydrate intake, providing 45 to 55 per cent of total calories as complex carbohydrate and fiber, and avoiding rapidly absorbed sugars.[3,4]

Protein. A high-protein diet, 120 to 140 gm, is essential, since there is no appreciable increase in the blood sugar level following high-protein meals even though protein furnishes approximately 50 per cent of its weight in available glucose. This available glucose is released to the bloodstream so gradually that there is little stimulation to the islets of Langerhans.

Fat. When the levels of carbohydrate and protein have been established, the remaining calories are obtained from fat. Because the carbohydrate is so severely restricted, the fat level is, of necessity, high.

Dietary Counseling

The exchange lists (see Table A-4) may be used for calculation of the diet prescription. Since carbohydrates are drastically restricted, it becomes apparent that the bread exchanges will usually be omitted. In order to include adequate amounts of fruits and vegetables, milk is limited to 2 or 3 cups; children should receive calcium supplements.

In order that absorption from the intestine will be gradual, the daily allowances of protein and fat, as well as carbohydrate, are divided into three approximately equal parts. Midmorning, midafternoon, and bedtime feedings are often desirable, in which case part of the food planned for the preceding meal can be used for the interval feeding. Carbohydrate-containing foods must be carefully measured.

Adrenocortical Insufficiency

Addison's disease is a comparatively rare condition resulting from an impairment of the functioning of the adrenal cortex because of atrophy of unknown origin, or, in some instances, because of tuberculosis. Some patients with idiopathic adrenal atrophy have circulating adrenal and thyroid antibodies, suggesting an autoimmune mechanism.

Sometimes adrenalectomy is necessary because of cancer, in which event the resultant metabolic effects are those of Addison's disease. Since the pituitary governs the activity of the adrenal cortex, hypophysectomy will also lead to characteristic symptoms of adrenal insufficiency.

Metabolic Effects and Related Symptoms Clinical manifestations usually do not occur until 90 per cent of the adrenal cortex has been destroyed. The symptoms of insufficiency are directly related to the absence of hormones produced by the adrenal cortex.

Glucocorticoids. The principal action of these hormones, chiefly cortisol, is upon the regulation of the metabolism of carbohydrate, protein, and fat. Upon stimulation of cortisol, the liver forms glycogen from the amino acids supplied by the tissues. The hormone increases the rate of protein catabolism and decreases the permeability of the muscle cells to amino acids. On the other hand, the permeability of the liver cells is increased and the amino acids released as a result of protein catabolism are transported to the liver and may be used for synthesis of new protein. The glucocorticoids also influence the deposition of fatty tissue or the mobilization of fats.

In the absence of glucocorticoids rapid glycogen depletion occurs, followed by hypoglycemia a few hours after meals. Such hypoglycemia may be severe in a patient who has had no food for 10 or 12 hours. A glucose tolerance test shows a lower maximum blood sugar and a more rapid return to normal fasting levels than is obtained in normal individuals (see Figure 37–1.)

The production of glucocorticoids by the adrenal gland is governed by the adrenocorticotropic hormone (ACTH) of the pituitary. In the event hypophysectomy is performed, the adrenal cortex atrophies and glucocorticoids are not produced, just as they are not elaborated in Addison's disease.

Mineralocorticoids. Mineralocorticoids, of which aldosterone is of primary importance, are concerned with maintaining electrolyte homeostasis, especially for sodium and potassium. The production is regulated by the levels of sodium and potassium in the circulation. Aldosterone production leads to increased retention of sodium and greater excretion of potassium. Unlike the glucocorticoids, aldosterone production is not influenced by the pituitary. A deficiency of aldosterone, as seen in Addison's disease, leads to excessive excretion of sodium and increased retention of potassium. With the large salt loss much water is also excreted, thus leading to dehydration, hemoconcentration, reduced blood volume, and hypotension. In severe deficiency the patient experiences profound weakness and may have a craving for salt.

Androgenic hormones. These stimulate protein synthesis. In their absence tissue wasting, weight loss, reduction of muscle strength, and fatigue are present.

Patients with adrenal insufficiency frequently experience anorexia, nausea, vomiting, abdominal discomfort, and diarrhea. Most of the patients have an increased pigmentation of the skin, often that of a deep tan or bronze. This results from the excessive production of *melanophore-stimulating hormone* by the pituitary when the adrenal steroids are lacking to exert an inhibitory effect.

Diagnostic tests An ACTH stimulation test is done to determine the adrenal reserve capacity for steroid production. A test dose of ACTH is administered intravenously over an 8-hour period and urine is collected for determination of 17-hydroxycorticoids and 17-ketosteroids. Patients with Addison's disease show little or no rise in urinary steroid excretion.

Treatment Replacement of glucocorticoids and mineralocorticoids is necessary. Cortisone (or hydrocortisone) is the primary drug; however, supplementary mineralocorticoid as fludrocortisone is sometimes needed. A liberal salt intake is needed especially during periods of excessive physical exercise, very hot weather, or gastrointestinal upsets.

Dietary Counseling

A diet high in protein and relatively low in carbohydrate reduces the stimulation of insulin and helps to avoid the episodes of hypoglycemia. Meals should be given at frequent intervals—allowing between-meal feedings and a late bedtime feeding. Each of the feedings should include protein in order to reduce the rate of carbohydrate absorption. Simple carbohydrates—candy, sugar, and other sweets—are best avoided because of their rapid digestion and absorption and their stimulation of excessive insulin production. Patients should be advised to take cortisone with meals or with milk to prevent irritation of the gastric mucosa by the drug.

Metabolic Effects of Adrenocortical Therapy

The adrenocorticotropic hormone of the anterior pituitary gland (ACTH) and the steroids of the adrenal cortex are used for the treatment of a wide variety of diseases such as arthritis, allergies, skin disturbances, adrenal insufficiency, many gastrointestinal diseases, and others. Although the various products used may vary somewhat in the degree of their effects on metabolism, it is important to be aware of possible nutritional implications of long-continued use of these hormones.

Water and Electrolyte Metabolism Adrenocortical steroids in excess lead to retention of sodium and water and loss of potassium, as seen in Cushing's syndrome. Some sodium restriction is necessary for many patients. Usually, it is sufficient to avoid salty foods and to use no salt at the table, but a 1,000-mg-sodium diet may occasionally be required (see Chapter 40). When the patient is eating well, the amounts of potassium in the diet are liberal. Foods especially high in potassium include broth, fruit juices, vegetables, whole-grain cereals, and meats.

Protein Metabolism A negative nitrogen balance may result when large doses of cortisone are used. This can be prevented when the diet is sufficiently liberal in carbohydrate to exert maximum protein-sparing effect and when high protein intakes are emphasized.

Carbohydrate Metabolism Cortisone therapy increases the storage of glycogen by increasing the amount of glycogen formation from protein. There also appears to be an insensitivity to insulin, as indicated by hyperglycemia and glycosuria. In diabetic patients who are also receiving cortisone, additional insulin may be required.

Gastrointestinal System Hydrochloric acid secretion is increased following adrenocortical steroid therapy, and peptic ulceration may develop. In such a situation, the dietary modification described for peptic ulcer should be used. (See Chapter 31.)

Hyperthyroidism

Symptoms and Clinical Findings Hyperthyroidism is a disturbance in which there is an excessive secretion of the thyroid gland with a consequent increase in the metabolic rate. The disease is also known as exophthalmic goiter, thyrotoxicosis, Graves' disease, or Basedow's disease. The chief symptoms are weight loss sometimes to the point of emaciation, excessive nervousness, prominence of the eyes, and a generally enlarged thyroid gland. The appetite is often increased, weakness may be marked, and signs of cardiac failure may be present.

Metabolism All of the metabolic processes in the body are accelerated in hyperthyroidism. Serum protein-bound iodine values are elevated. The basal metabolic rate may be increased 50 per cent or more in severe cases. Moreover, the patient tends to be restless so that the total energy metabolism is further increased. When the level of calories is insufficient, the liver store of glycogen is rapidly depleted. This is especially serious just prior to surgery since postoperative shock is more likely.

The increased level of nitrogen metabolism leads to destruction of tissue proteins. Unless both protein and caloric levels are adequate, loss of weight may be rapid.

The excretion of calcium and phosphorus is greatly increased in hyperthyroidism. Osteoporosis and bone fractures are associated with severe losses. The increased level of energy metabolism increases the requirement for B-complex vitamins. For reasons not fully understood, the utilization of vitamin A and ascorbic acid is also speeded up.

Treatment Hyperthyroidism is treated by radioactive iodine, antithyroid drugs, or surgery. Antithyroid drugs reduce the basal metabolic rate to normal, but a liberal diet is still indicated because patients have usually experienced severe malnutrition prior to therapy.

Dietary Counseling

Until normal nutrition is restored, approximately 4,000 to 5,000 kcal and 100 to 125 gm protein should be allowed. (See High-Calorie Diet, Chapter 28.) Frequent feedings will help satisfy hunger. A liberal calcium intake is desirable and may be provided as calcium salts in addition to the liberal use of milk. The diet itself will include generous allowances of vitamin A, the B complex, and ascorbic acid, but supplements are often prescribed.

Hypothyroidism

Hypothyroidism, or decreased production of the thyroid hormone, is known as myxedema when severe in the adult, or cretinism when its symptoms become apparent shortly after birth. (See Chapter 8.) Myxedema is characterized by a lowered rate of energy metabolism—often 30 to 40 per cent below normal, muscular flabbiness, puffy face, eyelids, and hands, sensitivity to cold, marked fatigue with slight exertion, and a personality change including apathy and dullness. Constipation is a frequent finding. The patient frequently responds to therapy with thyroid hormone.

Obesity is an occasional problem in patients with hypothyroidism since they may continue in their earlier patterns of eating even though the energy metabolism has been significantly reduced. In other patients, the appetite may be so poor that undernutrition results. For overweight persons, reduction of calories is necessary. (See Chapter 27.) Adequate fluids and foods high in dietary fiber are needed to overcome constipation.

Joint Diseases

Incidence Arthritis is the principal crippler in the United States. It affects about 20 million Americans, of whom some 3 million persons are limited in their usual activity. The incidence is higher in women, in people with low incomes, in the later years of life, and among residents of rural areas.

Eighty-three per cent of all cases of arthritis occur in persons over 45 years of age.[5]

Symptoms and Clinical Findings The terms *arthritis* and *rheumatism* are applied to many joint diseases. Rheumatic fever is a special threat to the child or young adult because inadequate treatment may permanently damage the heart. (See page 507.) Gout, another of the joint diseases, is an error of uric acid metabolism and is discussed on page 622.

The most common form of arthritis is *osteoarthritis* or *degenerative* arthritis. Theories regarding etiology hold that it is (1) primarily a degenerative disease of cartilage which leads to subsequent changes in bone, or (2) due to pathologic changes in bone which increase stress on cartilage and lead to its breakdown. The earliest pathologic changes occur in joint cartilage and subsequent new bone spurs develop at the edges. Joint stiffness is characteristic. Pain is confined to joints and is associated with motion or weight bearing. Joints of the fingers, knees, hip, and spine are frequently involved. Degenerative joint disease may also occur secondary to obesity, trauma, and metabolic and endocrine diseases, among others.[5]

Rheumatoid arthritis is a highly inflammatory and very painful condition having its onset in young adults, especially women. Autoimmunity and an infectious process have been proposed as etiologic factors. Rheumatoid arthritis is characterized by fatigue, pain, stiffness, deformity which may be severe, and limited function. The disease is progressive but the symptoms may spontaneously disappear only to reappear again at a later time. With early diagnosis the disabling effects can be delayed but there is no known cure.

Treatment Probably few diseases have had more theories offered concerning therapy. Arthritics spend over $435 million annually on phony diets and devices. None of the claims made by promoters have been supported by research. Over the years numerous diets have been tried by clinicians, but none has been effective in modifying the course of the disease. These trials have included diets high or low in protein, fat, and carbohydrate; modified for acid or alkaline ash; or supplemented with vitamins, especially ascorbic acid and vitamin D.

A number of drugs beginning with aspirin bring relief to the arthritic patient. Steroid therapy and gold salts have been effective for many. Since these drugs may bring about undesirable side effects, their use for each patient must be carefully evaluated.

Patients whose deformities limit their activities can be helped by physical and occupational therapy. The occupational therapist, home economist, dietitian, and nurse can help patients to greater independence by teaching them how to use many self-help devices that have been designed (See Figure 38–1.) Homemakers need counseling on ways to accomplish their housekeeping activities with less effort. Sometimes a rearrangement of kitchen equipment is sufficient; in other instances some modification of the design of the kitchen itself is needed. (See also pages 454 to 457.)

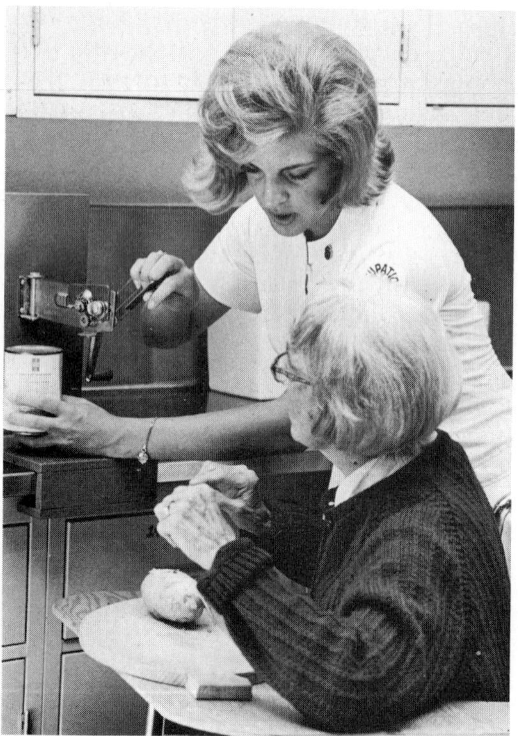

Figure 38–1. An occupational therapist shows a handicapped homemaker how to modify food preparation procedures for her physical limitations. (Courtesy, The Arthritis Foundation.)

Dietary Counseling

Arthritic patients require the same foods for health that other persons need. When patients are of normal weight and in good nutritional status, the normal diet is suitable.

Obesity is a common problem in osteoarthritis, and weight loss should be brought about in order to reduce the added stress on weight-bearing joints. (See Chapter 27 for low-calorie diets.)

Many patients with rheumatoid arthritis have lost weight and are in poor nutritional status. For them a high-calorie high-protein diet is indicated until good nutritional status has been achieved. (See pages 495 and 498.)

Some individuals experience gastric irritation or even ulceration from aspirin or steroid therapy. These effects can be prevented by taking these medications with meals and with a bedtime snack containing protein foods for their buffering capacity. Steroid therapy also leads to sodium retention in some in which case mild sodium restriction is indicated. Usually it is sufficient to omit salty foods and the use of salt at the table; sometimes, a 1,000-mg-sodium diet may be required. Continued steroid therapy adversely affects the calcium balance, leading to gradual bone demineralization. A liberal intake of milk, contrary to popular opinion, is desirable.

Gout

Primary gout is a disorder of purine metabolism occurring principally in middle-aged and older men. Women are more susceptible after the menopause. It is a hereditary disease characterized by hyperuricemia, recurrent attacks of acute inflammatory arthritis, and deposits of sodium urate (tophi) in joints, cartilage, and kidneys. Uric acid nephrolithiasis occurs in many patients. Secondary gout develops as a complication of some other acquired condition. The majority of cases of gout are due to impaired ability of the kidney to excrete the normal urate load presented to it, with a consequent rise in serum uric acid. A smaller percentage of cases are attributed to overproduction of uric acid.[6]

Nature and Occurrence of Uric Acid Cellular material of both plant and animal origin contains *nucleoproteins.* Glandular organs such as liver, pancreas, and kidney are among the richest sources; meats and the embryo or germ of grains and legumes, together with the growing parts of young plants, also furnish appreciable amounts. During digestion nucleoproteins are first split into proteins and nucleic acid. Further cleavage of nucleic acid leads to several products, one group of which are the purines. The latter in turn are oxidized to uric acid, probably by the liver.

In addition to the uric acid available from the metabolism of nucleic acid, the body can synthesize purines from the simplest carbon and nitrogen compounds such as carbon dioxide, acetic acid, and glycine. Thus any substances from which these materials originate, namely carbohydrate, fat, and protein, give rise to a considerable production of uric acid. Even in the fasting state there is a constant production of uric acid from cellular breakdown.

The liver and tissues store uric acid and its precursors for variable lengths of time and release them later. As a normal constituent of urine, uric acid represents a part of the daily nitrogenous excretion. Some uric acid is also excreted via the bile into the intestinal tract.

Symptoms and Clinical Findings The range of plasma uric acid in normal individuals is 2 to 5 mg per cent, whereas in those with susceptibility to gout the concentration is above 7 mg per cent and may reach as high as 20 mg per cent. A large percentage of individuals with hyperuricemia sooner or later will have acute attacks of gout characterized by sudden inflammation and swelling accompanied by severe pain of the joints, especially the metatarsal, knee, and toe joints. The acute attack usually responds dramatically in 24 to 48 hours to treatment with colchicine.

Acute attacks may be precipitated by rapid weight loss, overindulgence in food or alcohol, high fat diets, ketoacidosis, and drugs, such as thiazide diuretics. Both lactic acid, resulting from heavy alcohol use, and keto acids favor urate retention by the kidney and hyperuricemia.

Treatment A number of drugs are effective in the treatment of gout, and diet is considered to be an adjunct to drug therapy. Colchicine and a number of other drugs provide effective relief from the pain that accompanies the acute attack. In addition, these drugs reduce the frequency of attacks when they are also used as interval therapy.

Uricosuric drugs (probenecid and others) increase the excretion of uric acid, thereby bringing plasma levels within a normal range. With the lowering of the plasma uric acid levels, sodium urate deposits in the joints are gradually dissolved out. These drugs are not effective in reducing the pain of the acute attack and may exacerbate the symptoms during an attack. Therefore, they are used during the quiescent periods of the disease.

Allopurinol is a drug that inhibits the action of the enzyme *xanthine oxidase,* which is responsible for the formation of uric acid from xanthine and hypoxanthine. Therefore, the excretion of uric acid is diminished and that of xanthine is increased. Inasmuch as xanthine can precipitate out to form kidney stones, it is essential that the patient have a liberal fluid intake and excrete a urine that is neutral or slightly alkaline.

Modification of the Diet During the acute attacks a low-purine diet is often ordered in addition to drug therapy. Some physicians also recommend moderate restriction of purines as interval therapy for patients receiving uricosuric drugs.

Dietary Counseling

Data on the purine content of foods are limited. Foods have been grouped into three categories in Table 38–1. As may be seen from this classification, all flesh foods and extractives from them such as gravies and soups must be eliminated for the low-purine diet. If purine restriction is also prescribed for interval therapy, the allowance of meat, poultry, and fish is limited to 2 to 3 ounces on each of 3 to 5 days.

Energy. Since obesity has adverse effects on general health as well as on gout, the overweight individual should gradually lose weight. Patients should not be placed on low-calorie diets during acute attacks of gout since the catabolism of adipose tissue reduces the excretion of uric acid. Rapid weight loss effected by starvation or by extremely low-calorie diets can precipitate an attack of gout. Usually, men can lose weight satisfactorily when their diets are restricted to 1,200 to 1,600 kcal. (See Chapter 27.)

Protein, fat, and carbohydrate. Because the nitrogen of the purine nucleus is supplied by protein, the intake is restricted to about 1 gm per kilogram. Fat is often restricted to about 60 gm daily. When the food intake is poor because of illness, it is essential that high-carbohydrate fluids be given so that adipose tissue is not excessively catabolized.

Table 38–1. **Purine Content of Foods per 100 gm**

Group I (0–15 mg)	Group II (50–150 mg)	Group III (150 mg and over)
Breads and cereals	Beans, dry	Anchovies
Butter and other fats*	Fish	Asparagus*
Caviar*	Lentils	Brains*
Cheese	Meats	Gravies*
Eggs	Oatmeal*	Kidney
Fish roe*	Peas, dry	Liver
Fruits	Poultry*	Meat extracts
Gelatin*	Seafood	Mincemeat*
Milk	Spinach	Mushrooms*
Nuts*		Sardines
Sugar, sweets*		Sweetbreads
Vegetables		

*Adapted from Turner, D.: *Handbook of Diet Therapy*, 5th ed. University of Chicago Press, Chicago, 1970, p. 117. Starred items are additions to Turner's list.

Fluid. The daily intake of fluids should be at least 3 liters. Coffee and tea may be used in moderate amounts. These beverages contain methylated purines, which are oxidized to methyl uric acid. The latter is excreted in the urine and is not deposited in the tissues. Hence, the customary omission of coffee and tea may impose an unnecessary hardship. Some clinicians forbid use of alcohol whereas other permit small amounts occasionally.

To effect a neutral or slightly alkaline urine when allopurinol is prescribed, the diet should be liberal in its content of fruits and vegetables. In addition, the physician usually prescribes small amounts of sodium bicarbonate or sodium citrate.

Purine-Restricted Diet

General Rules

For a diet essentially free of exogenous purines, use foods only from group 1, Table 38–1.

For a low-purine level, allow 3 to 5 small servings of lean meat, poultry, and fish from group II each week.

If a low-fat regimen is ordered, the butter is omitted, and skim milk is substituted for the whole milk.

Include These Foods Daily:
3–4 cups milk; 1–2 ounces cheese
2 eggs; allow 2 to 3 ounces lean beef, veal, lamb, poultry, or fish 3 to 5 times a week during interval therapy
3–4 servings vegetables including:
1 medium potato
1–2 servings green leafy or yellow vegetable
1 serving other vegetable
2–3 servings fruit including:
1 serving citrus fruit
1–2 servings other fruits
1 serving enriched cereal
4–6 slices enriched bread
2 tablespoons margarine or butter
Additional calories are provided as needed by increasing the amount of potato, potato substitutes such as macaroni, rice, noodles, bread, sugars, sweets, fruits, and vegetables.

Nutritive value of basic foods above: Calories, 1,850; protein, 68 gm; fat, 80 gm; carbohydrate, 220 gm; calcium, 1,400 mg; iron, 11.3 mg; vitamin A, 11,350 I.U.; thiamin, 1.3 mg; riboflavin, 2.3 mg; niacin, 10 mg; ascorbic acid, 145 mg.

Foods to Avoid
All foods high in purines (see group III, Table 38–1)
Alcohol
For low-fat diets:
Pastries and rich desserts
Cream and ice cream
Fried foods
Eggs not to exceed 2 daily; hard cheese not to exceed 1 ounce. Severe restriction may require the omission of eggs, whole milk, cheese, and butter. Skim milk and cottage cheese must then be used in ample amounts to provide the necessary protein.

Sample Menu

BREAKFAST
Half grapefruit
Rice Krispies with milk and sugar
Buttered toast
Scrambled egg
Coffee with milk and sugar

LUNCHEON OR SUPPER
Jelly omelet
Boiled rice
Broiled tomato
Half peach with cottage cheese on lettuce
Bread with 1 teaspoon butter
Milk—1 glass

DINNER
Cheese soufflé
Baked potato
Beets
Green celery strips
Bread with 1 teaspoon butter
Apple snow
Milk—1 glass

BEDTIME
Milk—1 glass

Osteoporosis

Osteoporosis is a disorder characterized by a decrease in total bone mass without a change in chemical composition. It occurs when the rate of bone resorption exceeds the rate of formation. Because of the reduction in the number of cells, there is a decrease in the thickness of the cortex, a thinning of the trabeculae, and an increased porosity of bone. As a result, fractures occur with greater frequency. Common fracture sites include the vertebrae, femur, and radius, and often these occur in spite of little or no trauma. The rate of femoral fractures alone doubles for each decade after age 50 at an annual cost of nearly $1 billion in the United States.[7] The disease occurs four times as frequently in women as in men.

Etiology The etiology of osteoporosis is multifactorial and includes the following age-related changes: decreased estrogen production associated with menopause, decreases in intestinal absorption of calcium, and production of vitamin D, reduced physical activity, and increased parathyroid hormone secretion. Some factors that increase risk include gastrectomy, hyperthyroidism, rheumatoid arthritis, immobilization, and chronic inadequate calcium intake.

The role of dietary factors is not clear. Older persons may require more calcium to achieve balance. Some studies indicate that those with the disorder have lower calcium intakes than persons without osteoporosis. Not all persons with low calcium intakes develop osteoporosis, however. Some believe a high intake of phosphorus in relation to calcium is a critical factor.[8] Excessive nitrogen intake is associated with increased calcium excretion and negative calcium balance, but it is unlikely that this is a common cause of the disorder in the elderly. Excessive fluoride intake may cause osteoporosis unless the calcium intake is also high.

Clinical Manifestations The disorder is seen primarily in postmenopausal Caucasians of small stature. Approximately one fourth of women over the age of 50 are afflicted. The principal symptoms are low back pain, sometimes severe, and often a history of vertebral fractures. Over a period of years the individual may have lost height—sometimes several inches. Roentgenographic changes are not diagnosed until as much as 30 per cent of the bone mass has been lost.

Treatment The factors which may have initiated the osteoporosis must be determined before effective therapy can be instituted. Low dose cyclic estrogen therapy has been used to prevent bone loss and for those with recurring fractures. Some clinicians recommend calcium intakes of 1 to 1.5 gm daily as a means of slowing bone loss and restoring bone mass. Since most diets do not supply this amount, supplements, such as calcium gluconate or calcium lactate, are usually needed. As much as 36 months of calcium therapy may be required before bone density improves.[9] Some also advocate vitamin D, 25 μg (1,000 I.U.), daily.[10] For patients with severe bone loss and frequent fractures, a carefully monitored program of calcium, fluoride, and vitamin D has been suggested.[10] Because of serious side effects and inconclusive evidence of a beneficial effect of fluoride therapy, this therapy remains investigational.[11]

The primary effort should be directed early in life to the prevention of bone loss. A diet adequate in calcium and protein is important for maintenance of bone structure; however, until more is known of the etiology of this disease the most effective prophylaxis as well as treatment cannot be prescribed.

Problems and Review

1. Mrs. H. is admitted to the hospital with the chief complaint of "hypoglycemia." She will undergo diagnostic tests to determine the cause of her symptoms.

a. Differentiate between the hypoglycemia in functional hyperinsulinism, Addison's disease, and liver disease. What modification of carbohydrate level of the diet is required for each?
b. What is the advantage of a high protein and high fat intake in hyperinsulinism?
c. The tests revealed Mrs. H. has functional hyperinsulinism. Calculate a diet for her to provide: 2,000 kcal, 125 gm protein, and 225 gm carbohydrate. Use the exchange lists for the calculation. Divide the day's allowance into three equal meals.
d. Draw a typical glucose tolerance curve for a person who has functional hyperinsulinism, Addison's disease, hyperthyroidism, diabetes mellitus.

2. You are assigned to care for Mr. J., a 58-year-old patient with Addison's disease.
   a. What modifications of mineral and water metabolism are present in Addison's disease? In what way is this corrected by hormone therapy?
   b. Why is a sodium-restricted diet occasionally ordered for a patient receiving hormone therapy in Addison's disease? Under what circumstances would an increase in sodium intake be used?
   c. On the basis of your understanding of the metabolism in Addison's disease, what are some of the functions of the adrenal gland in the normal individual? What is the effect of the activity of the pituitary?
   d. What are the characteristic symptoms of hyperthyroidism?
3. A patient with hyperthyroidism was seen in the metabolism clinic and was asked to return in 1 month for surgery. The nutritionist instructed the patient on a diet to provide 5,000 kcal and 125 gm protein.
   a. What are some of the characteristic symptoms of hyperthyroidism; of hypothyroidism?
   b. Compare the diet which might be used in a hyperthyroid patient who is well controlled with antithyroid drugs and one who has an elevated metabolic rate.
   c. Suggest five ways in which the calories of a diet for a patient with hyperthyroidism might be increased.
   d. Why does a surgeon so frequently insist that a patient gain weight before an operation on the thyroid?
   e. What is myxedema? What is its chief cause? How can you explain the frequent occurrence of overweight?
4. Your grandmother shows you an ad for a booklet with a diet "guaranteed" to cure arthritis and aid in weight reduction.
   a. What would you tell her about the role of diet in arthritis?
   b. Outline briefly the dietary considerations in arthritis.
   c. What are the dietary implications of long-term use of cortisone in this disease or in other conditions?
5. You are asked to teach Mr. O. about his diet for gout. Consider the following questions in planning your remarks:
   a. What are the sources of uric acid in the body? In what ways is uric acid metabolism disturbed in gout?
   b. How can you explain the fact that a person who has gout may have an acute attack following surgery or during an acute infection?
   c. What is the basis for restricting the protein intake to 1 gm per kilogram in the dietary planning for a patient with gout?
   d. What problems are entailed when a purine-free diet is ordered for a patient, insofar as nutritional adequacy is concerned?
   e. Plan a menu for 1 day for a low-purine diet.
6. What is the role of each of these hormones on protein and mineral metabolism: thyroxine; parathormone; androgen; cortisone?
7. What role do dietary factors play in the etiology of osteoporosis? In treatment?

Cited References

1. Hofeldt, F. D.: "Reactive Hypoglycemia," *Metabolism,* **24:**1193–1208, 1975.
2. Johnson, D. D. et al.: "Reactive Hypoglycemia," *JAMA,* **243:**1151–55, 1980.
3. Anderson, J. W., and Herman, R. H.: "Effects of Carbohydrate Restriction on Glucose Tolerance of Normal Men and Reactive Hypoglycemia Patients," *Am. J. Clin. Nutr.,* **28:**748–55, 1975.
4. Leichter, S. B.: "Alimentary Hypoglycemia: A New Appraisal," *Am. J. Clin. Nutr.,* **32:**2104–14, 1979.
5. *Arthritis, Prevention, Treatment, and Rehabilitation.* Hearing before the Subcommittee on Public Health and Environment. Committee on Interstate and Foreign Commerce. House of Representatives. 93rd Congress, 2nd Session, November 15, 1974. Serial No. 93–109. U.S. Government Printing Office, Washington, D.C., 1975.
6. Boss, G. R., and Seegmiller, J. E.: "Hyperuricemia and Gout. Classification, Complications, and Management," *New Engl. J. Med.,* **300:**1459–68, 1979.
7. Gallagher, J. C., et al.: "Epidemiology of Fractures of the Proximal Femur in Rochester, Minnesota," *Clin. Orthop.,* **150:**163–71, 1980.
8. Jowsey, J.: "Osteoporosis. Its Nature and the Role of Diet," *Postgrad. Med.,* **60:**75–79, August 1976.
9. Albanese, A. A.: "Osteoporosis: Effects of Calcium," *Am. Fam. Physician,* **18:**160–67, October 1978.
10. Thomson, D. L., and Frame, B.: "Involutional Osteopenia: Current Concepts," *Ann. Intern. Med.,* **85:**789–803, 1976.
11. Riggs, B. L. et al.: "Treatment of Primary Osteoporosis with Fluoride and Calcium," *JAMA.,* **243:**446–49, 1980.

Additional References

FAJANS, S. S. et al.: "Fasting Hypoglycemia in Adults," *New Engl. J. Med.,* **294:**766–72, 1976.

HALLAL, J. C.: "Hyperthyroidism," *Am. J. Nurs.,* **77:**419–27, 1977.

HALLAL, J. C.: "Hypothyroidism," *Am. J. Nurs.,* **77:**427–32, 1977.

HUSKISSO, E. C.: "Osteoarthritis: Changing Concepts in Pathogenesis and Treatment," *Postgrad. Med.,* **65:**97–104, March 1979.

KOZAK, G. P.: "Primary Adrenocortical Insufficiency (Addison's Disease)," *Am. Fam. Physician,* **15:**124–35, May 1977.

MARX, J. L.: "Osteoporosis: New Help for Thinning Bones," *Science,* **207:**628–30, 1980.

NERUP, J.: "Addison's Disease—A Review of Some Clinical, Pathological and Immunological Features," *Danish Medical Bulletin,* **21:**201–17, 1974.

PERMUTT, M. A.: "Postprandial Hypoglycemia," *Diabetes,* **25:**719–33, 1976.

SIMKIN, P. A.: "Management of Gout," *Ann. Intern. Med.,* **90:**812–16, 1979.

SKILLMAN, T. G.: "Can Osteoporosis Be Prevented?" *Geriatrics,* **35:**95–102, February 1980.

TALBOTT, J. H.: "Gouty Arthritis: A Disease for All Ages," *Geriatrics,* **35:**69–71ff., May 1980.

Hyperlipidemia and Atherosclerosis 39

FAT-CONTROLLED DIETS; DIETS FOR HYPERLIPOPROTEINEMIAS

Cardiovascular Disease, a Major Public Health Problem Cardiovascular diseases represent an enormous medical, social, and economic burden to the American public. Some statistics illustrate this point.

Some 30 million Americans have some form of cardiovascular disease.

Each year some 25,000 children are born with congenital heart disease.

More than 100,000 children and 1.6 million adults have rheumatic heart disease.

Over 4 million have clinical manifestations of atherosclerosis.

Each year 1.5 million Americans experience a heart attack, and another 500,000 suffer a stroke. An adult male has about 1 chance in 3 of developing coronary heart disease before age 60, usually in the form of a heart attack. The probability of succumbing to heart disease within 5 years is five times greater in these men than in those with no history of coronary disease.

The economic cost of cardiovascular diseases in this country is over $40 billion annually for medical expenses, lost wages, and lost productivity.

Cardiovascular diseases are the leading cause of Social Security disability. They account for more hospital bed days than any other cause, some 48 million per year, and rank second only to respiratory diseases in terms of bed disability.[1, 2]

The mortality rates from cardiovascular diseases in the United States are among the highest in the world. The leading cause of death in this country is coronary (ischemic) heart disease which accounts for about two thirds of cardiovascular deaths and for one third of deaths from all causes.[3, 4] Each year more than 640,000 deaths are attributed to ischemic heart disease, and some 200,000 more are due to atherosclerosis of other major vessels.

Since the mid-1960s the mortality rate from major cardiovascular diseases has been decreasing in the United States and Canada while that in most of the rest of the world is unchanged or increasing. From 1950 to 1976 the age-adjusted death rates for cardiovascular diseases fell from 425.6 to 284.4 per 100,000 population, with most of the decline occurring in the latter part of this period. From 1968 to 1976, age-adjusted death rates from ischemic heart disease fell 20 per cent in black and white men and women of all age groups.[5] (See Table 39–1.) The precise reasons for the declining mortality rates have not been identified. It is likely that both prevention, through reduction of risk factors, and improved medical care have contributed. Whether the frequency of nonfatal coronary events is also decreasing is not yet clear.

Ischemic heart disease may occur at any age, but it is not common until middle age at which time it assumes practically epidemic proportions. Males over 45 years of age are highly susceptible. Except for those who have hypertension or diabetes mellitus, ischemic heart disease is not common in women until after the menopause. A disturbed hormonal balance is believed by some to be the key factor underlying ischemic heart disease.[6, 7]

Table 39-1. **Age-adjusted Death Rates for Major Cardiovascular Diseases, United States, 1968-76***

	Number of Deaths, 1976	Rates per 100,000, 1976	Per Cent Change, 1968-76
Major cardiovascular diseases	974,429	284.4	-21.4
Diseases of the heart	723,878	216.7	-19.3
Active rheumatic fever and chronic rheumatic heart disease	13,110	4.7	-34.7
Hypertensive heart disease	10,690	3.0	-50.8
Ischemic heart disease	646,073	191.6	-20.7
Acute myocardial infarction	319,477	102.9	-26.5
Chronic ischemic heart disease	322,382	87.3	-12.4
Chronic disease of endocardium and other myocardial insufficiency	4,195	1.3	-53.6
All other forms of heart disease	49,810	16.1	+47.7
Hypertension	6,130	1.8	-45.5
Cerebrovascular diseases	188,623	51.4	-27.9
Arteriosclerosis	29,366	6.4	-33.3
Other diseases of arteries, arterioles, and capillaries	26,432	8.0	-11.1

*Adapted from *Proceedings of the Conference on the Decline in Coronary Heart Disease Mortality*. NIH Publ. No. 79-7610, U.S. Department of Health, Education, and Welfare. PHS, May 1979.

Multiple Risk Factors in Coronary Disease No single factor is an absolute cause either of atherosclerosis or of coronary disease. Many factors are interrelated and to the extent that they are present they increase the risk of disease. Major risk factors are elevated serum cholesterol, hypertension, and cigarette smoking. Presence of one of these factors doubles the risk of coronary disease. If all three are present, the risk of coronary disease is ten times greater than if none is present. (See Figure 39–1.) Other risk factors include a family history of early heart disease, other lipid abnormal-

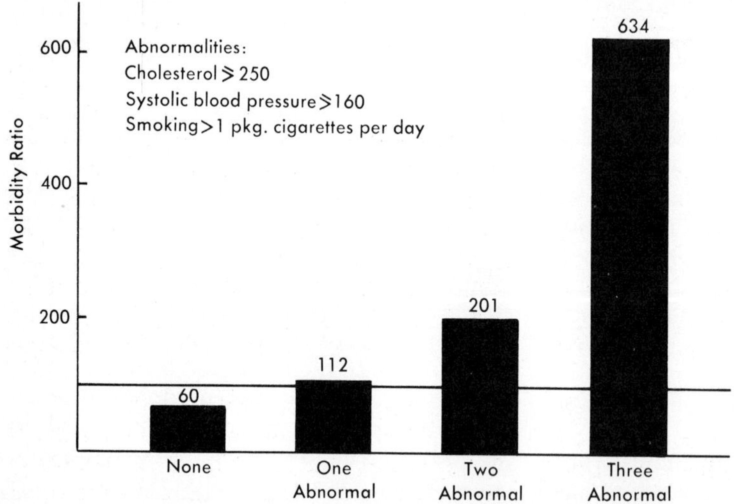

Figure 39–1. The presence of a single risk factor doubles the risk of heart disease. If the three abnormalities listed in this chart are present, the risk is ten times as high. (Courtesy, The Framingham Heart Study and National Heart, Lung, and Blood Institute.)

ities, glucose intolerance, obesity, certain personality-behavior patterns, lack of physical activity, and stress. At least one group holds that testosterones constitute a risk factor for men.[8]

Coronary Disease and the Role of Diet

The discussion in this chapter is concerned with (1) the rationale for dietary modification to reduce the incidence of atherosclerosis and coronary disease, (2) the fat-controlled diet, and (3) diets for five types of hyperlipoproteinemia. The dietary management of acute episodes of illness is discussed in the chapter that follows. The student should review normal fat and carbohydrate metabolism in order to understand the effects of altered physiology and biochemistry in coronary disease. (See Chapters 5 and 6.)

Ischemic Heart Disease MYOCARDIAL ISCHEMIA is a cardiac disability resulting from an inadequacy of the coronary arterial system to meet the needs of the heart muscle for oxygen and nutrients. It may be manifested as sudden death, myocardial infarction, or angina pectoris.

An *infarct* is a localized area of necrosis that results when the supply of blood to that area is inadequate for cellular survival. An infarct of the heart is known as a MYOCARDIAL INFARCTION (heart attack), and one in the brain as a CEREBROVASCULAR ACCIDENT (stroke). If the infarct is small, the remainder of the organ can function and healing takes place with the formation of scar tissue. The functional capacity of the organ is curtailed to the extent that tissue has been lost. Thus, repeated myocardial infarctions continue to reduce the functional capacity of the heart.

ANGINA PECTORIS refers to the tight, pressing, burning, and sometimes severe pain across the chest that follows exertion and that is a result of inadequate oxygen to the myocardium. As the coronary arteries become increasingly occluded, the pain develops with less and less exertion.

ATHEROSCLEROSIS is a disease of the blood vessels resulting from the interaction of multiple factors such as heredity and the individual's environment (diet, activity, smoking, life-style, etc.). Atheromatous plaques begin as soft, mushy accumulations of lipid material in the intima of the blood vessels. These plaques consist of a proliferation of the blood vessel wall of connective tissue into which lipids are deposited. The lipids include free cholesterol, cholesterol esters, and triglycerides in proportions that approximate those of the circulating blood lipids.

Atherosclerosis begins in the first decades of life and is almost universally present in people who live in affluent, highly developed countries. It develops gradually with increasing thickening of the arterial wall, loss of elasticity, and narrowing of the lumen. Finally, some event brings about occlusion of the vessel and ischemia of the affected part. (See Figure 39–2.)

Most myocardial infarctions are due to atherosclerosis of the major coronary arteries, but many people with atherosclerosis do not develop clinical disease. The conditions that bring about occlusion are not well understood. In some instances ulceration of the atheroma and hemorrhage into the lumen with clot formation occur. The anatomic location of the atheroma, the extent to which the lumen has been narrowed, the changes in the clearing of the blood lipids, and decrease in fibrinolytic activity are probably involved in the process.

Blood Studies Related to Coronary Disease Measurements of various blood constituents can be used not only to determine the presence of abnormal concentrations but also to evaluate the effects of changes in diet and other therapy on the levels of these components. HYPERLIPIDEMIA is a general term that denotes an elevation of one or more lipids in the blood. HYPERCHOLESTEROLEMIA refers to an elevation of se-

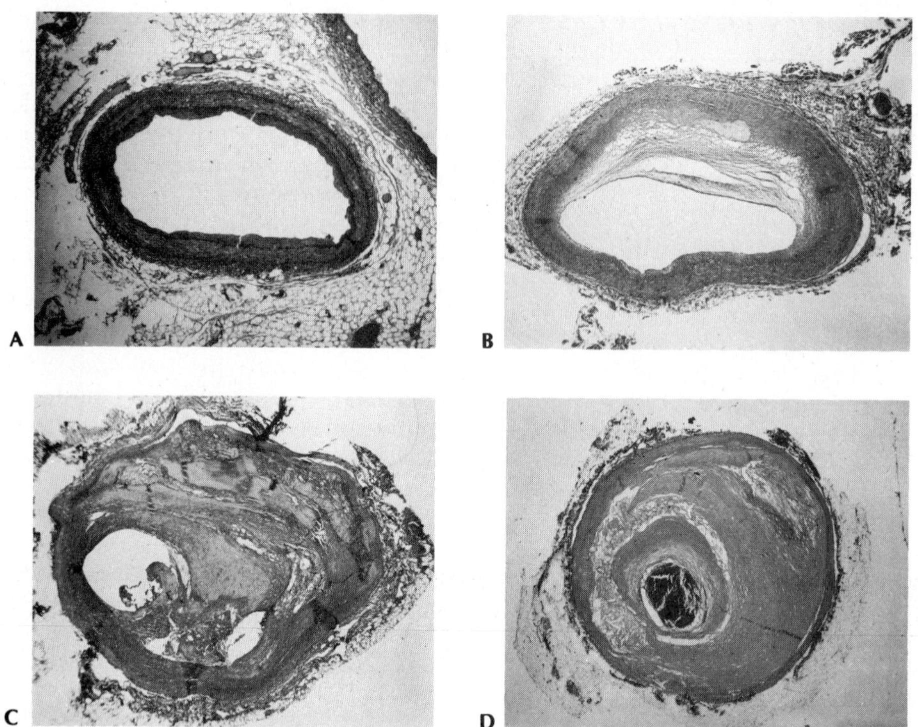

Figure 39–2. Gradual development of atherosclerosis in a coronary artery, leading to a heart attack. **A.** Normal artery. **B.** Deposits formed in inner lining of artery. **C.** Deposits harden. **D.** Channel is blocked by a blood clot. (Courtesy, American Heart Association.)

rum cholesterol and HYPERTRIGLYCERIDEMIA to increased triglycerides. Although the specific levels separating normal from abnormal have not been determined, the National Heart, Lung, and Blood Institute recommends treatment for all persons under 55 years of age whose serum cholesterol concentration is in excess of 220 mg per cent or whose fasting triglycerides are more than 150 mg per cent.[9] HYPERLIPOPROTEINEMIA refers to elevation of any one of the classes of lipoproteins. (See Chapter 6). HYPERTENSION, or elevated blood pressure, is generally considered to be present when the systolic pressure is 160 mm Hg or greater and the diastolic pressure is 95 mm Hg. Readings of 140/90 represent borderline hypertension.[10] (See Chapter 40.)

Determination of serum cholesterol is considered by some to be the best single measurement for estimating risk of atherosclerosis.[11] Data from the Framingham Study indicate that total cholesterol is a useful predictor of risk for persons less than 50 years of age, but for those over 50, measurement of high-density lipoprotein (HDL) cholesterol is the best indicator.[12] However, at any given plasma cholesterol level, the ratio of total or low-density lipoprotein (LDL) cholesterol to HDL-cholesterol is more important than the absolute values.[12, 13] The hypothesis linking elevated serum cholesterol levels to atherosclerosis and premature coronary heart disease may be summed up as follows: (1) Elevated levels of serum total and LDL-cholesterol are associated with increased risk for coronary disease. Low levels of HDL-cholesterol also appear to increase risk. This does not mean, however, that all persons with these alterations in serum cholesterol levels will develop coronary disease. (2) Serum LDL-cholesterol levels can be altered by dietary changes, particularly in cholesterol and saturated fat intake. (3) There is insufficient evidence at present to state unequivocally that the serum LDL-cholesterol level is the direct cause of coronary disease. However, extensive epidemiologic data indicate that habitual consumption of a diet high in cholesterol and saturated fat is a key factor. (4) Further data are needed to confirm the assumption that returning serum cholesterol levels to normal will reduce the risk of coronary heart disease.

In some individuals hyperlipidemia is induced by carbohydrates, especially sucrose and fructose.[14] Serum triglyceride levels are increased in these persons.

Fredrickson and his associates have described five types of hyperlipoproteinemia.[15] The differentiation is based upon the appearance of the serum, the concentrations of cholesterol and triglyceride, and the classes of lipoproteins that serve as the vehicles for the lipids. The distinctions are important in determining whether the disorders are fat induced or carbohydrate induced so that appropriate diet therapy can be instituted. (See pages 635 to 637.)

Long-Term Studies on Modified Diets Numerous studies have established that serum cholesterol can be lowered by dietary modification. Many investigators have sought to determine whether dietary modification could also lessen morbidity and mortality from coronary disease. In these studies, the ages and health characteristics of the subjects assigned to control and experimental groups were similar. The control groups ate their customary diets while the experimental groups consumed diets in which cholesterol was reduced and polyunsaturated fat was substituted for part of the saturated fats.

Well-known primary prevention studies include the Anti-coronary Club Project in New York,[16] the Los Angeles Veterans Study,[17] and the Helsinki study of patients in two mental hospitals.[18] A Norwegian study aimed at secondary prevention in subjects with established heart disease.[19] In all of these, sustained reduction of serum cholesterol by long-term dietary modification was associated with a decline in morbidity and mortality from coronary disease although the results were not statistically significant in all of the studies.

The National Heart, Lung, and Blood Institute of the National Institutes of Health undertook three long-term studies in the 1970s. (1) The Lipid Research Clinics Program is studying the relationship between diet and blood lipid/lipoprotein levels and between these levels and ischemic heart disease. (2) The Lipid Research Clinics Coronary Prevention Trial is a 10-year study of 4,000 men, aged 35 to 59, designed to determine whether drug-induced reduction of elevated serum cholesterol levels in otherwise healthy men will prevent development of heart disease. (3) The Multiple Risk Factor Intervention Trial (MRFIT) is studying 12,000 men, aged 35 to 55 years, who are at increased risk for coronary heart disease because of elevated serum cholesterol, high blood pressure, and cigarette smoking. Investigators hope to determine whether intervention to decrease these risk factors can significantly reduce mortality from coronary heart disease.[1, 20]

Dietary Adjustments for Hyperlipidemias Health professionals are not in unanimous agreement concerning dietary recommendations for prevention of coronary heart disease. Most believe that persons *at increased risk* should make specific dietary changes as outlined below to lower fat and cholesterol intake. The American Heart Association has stated that such dietary modifications are appropriate for the general population.[21] Others are of the opinion that drastic changes in the diet are not necessary for the general public.[22] See page 42 for discussion of the Dietary Guidelines for Americans. The rationale for dietary adjustments in hyperlipidemias follows.

Calorie balance. Obesity has long been recognized as one of the risk factors in cardiovascular disease. In the Framingham Heart Study overweight was considered to constitute only a slight risk. However, the Framingham Offspring Study suggested that obesity may be a more important risk factor than was previously believed. In this study nearly all obese subjects were found to have a higher ratio of total cholesterol to HDL-cholesterol than subjects of normal weight.[23] When overweight is associated with diabetes mellitus, the serum cholesterol and triglyceride levels are customarily high, thereby increasing risk. Reduction in body weight and blood lipids is accomplished by lowering calorie intake and substituting polyunsaturated fats for part of the saturated fats in the diet.

Increased body weight probably has its greatest effect by increasing the work load of the heart. A mild stenosis associated with obesity can be critical in a situation of added stress.

Normal weight is maintained only when energy intake and output are equal. Therefore, early in life it is important to develop a program of regular exercise that can be continued throughout the years. (See Chapter 27.) A regular program of modest exercise is also effective in raising serum HDL-cholesterol levels.[24, 25]

Fats. Dietary fat is the single most important factor requiring adjustment in programs of prevention and control. (See also Figure 1–2.) The typical American diet furnishes about 42 per cent of the calories from fat. The saturated fat in the diet is about twice as high as the polyunsaturated fat.[26]

For the prevention of hyperlipidemia the total fat content should be reduced to about 30 to 35 per cent of calories. The content of polyunsaturated fat should be increased and that of saturated fat strictly limited. Ratios of polyunsaturated fat to saturated fat (P/S ratio) range from 1 : 1 to 2 : 1. Some concern has been expressed about the safety of high intakes of polyunsaturated fats. In a study at a Veterans Administration Hospital, autopsy records revealed increased frequency of gallstones in men, especially those who were overweight, who had participated in a long-term study involving use of a diet high in polyunsaturated fats.[27] This has not been confirmed in other studies.

Cholesterol. The cholesterol content of American diets ranges from 500 to 1,000 mg daily, depending largely upon the number of eggs that are consumed. (See Table 6–3.) Increasing the dietary cholesterol from 0 to 600 mg daily without other dietary change results in a progressive increase in the blood cholesterol.[28] Thus, even the addition of one or two eggs a day can in part nullify the effects of a diet high in polyunsaturated fat. Most dietary regimens now restrict the cholesterol intake to 300 mg daily when hypercholesterolemia is present.

Carbohydrate. In the United States a marked decline has taken place in the consumption of breads and cereals, and the use of sugars and sugar-containing foods has increased considerably. Some investigators believe that the increase in sugars in the diet is as important in the elevation of blood lipids as is the increase in saturated fats.[29, 30] A high-carbohydrate low-fat diet brings about an elevation in serum triglycerides even in normal individuals, although the effect is a temporary one.

For hyperglyceridemias that are carbohydrate-induced the most important adjustment in diet is a reduction of the total carbohydrate and an elimination, insofar as possible, of sugars. This entails not only the elimination of sugar and sugar-containing foods, but control of the amounts of fruits and vegetables that are sources of fructose and sucrose. (See also pages 75 and 555.)

Dietary Fiber Pectins, gums, and soluble fibers have a serum cholesterol lowering effect. Wheat bran and cellulose have little influence on serum cholesterol levels; however, hard red spring wheat bran lowers both total cholesterol and LDL-cholesterol.[31] Mechanisms proposed to explain the hypocholesterolemic effect of these fibers include (1) altered intestinal absorption, metabolism, and release of cholesterol, through an influence on bile acids; (2) altered hepatic metabolism and release of cholesterol. Increased excretion of bile acids reduces the size of the bile acid pool; thus less cholesterol is available for incorporation into lipoproteins and subsequent release into the circulation; (3) altered peripheral metabolism of lipoproteins. Fiber may alter the proportion of cholesterol incorporated into chylomicrons and lipoproteins.[32]

Other Dietary Factors Soy protein has a hypocholesterolemic effect compared with animal protein in both normal and hypercholesterolemic subjects.[33,34] Habitual high salt intake increases risk for hypertension in susceptible persons. Lowering salt intake has been proposed to reduce risk. The American Medical Association has stated that moderation in salt intake is desirable for the entire population.[35] The role of minerals in cardiovascular disease is uncertain. The mortality rate from cardiovascular diseases is significantly lower in areas where the drinking water is hard than in those areas where the water is soft. Sufficient evidence is lacking to incriminate specific minerals; however, some data suggest that higher concentrations of calcium and magnesium in hard water may have a protective effect.[36,37] Patients dying suddenly from ischemic heart disease have been found to have lower concentrations of magnesium and potassium in myocardial tissue than patients dying of causes unrelated to heart disease.[38] Interactions of copper and zinc have been proposed.[39] In a well-controlled metabolic study a healthy young man on a copper-deficient diet showed a significant increase in plasma cholesterol; plasma cholesterol reverted to normal during copper repletion.[40] Alterations of copper balance are also associated with irregularities in electrocardiograms and respond to administration of copper salts.[40,41] Pharmacologic doses of zinc lowered HDL-cholesterol levels by 25 per cent in healthy men in one study.[42] Ascorbic acid is needed for sulfation of intercellular substance in the arterial wall. Accumulation of nonsulfated substance in ascorbate deficiency is associated with increased binding of plasma lipids and fibrinogen in the arterial wall.[43]

Fat-Controlled Diets

Diet Plans The plans for fat-controlled meals at 1,200 and 1,800 kcal and for 2,000 to 2,600 kcal have been presented in two booklets published by the American Heart Association.[44] The principal characteristics of these diets are summarized in the following.

1. About 30 to 35 per cent of the calories are supplied by fat.
2. Less than 10 per cent of the calories are furnished by saturated fat. Only skim milk and very lean meats, fish, and poultry may be used. Beef, lamb, and pork are restricted to three 3-ounce portions per week. Butter, cream, and whole-milk cheeses are not used.
3. Up to 10 per cent of the calories are supplied by polyunsaturated fats. The P/S ratio of the diets ranges from 1:1 to 2:1. The polyunsaturated fat content is increased principally by the use of safflower, corn, soy, or cottonseed oils. Limited amounts of special margarines may be included. (See Figure 39–3.)
4. Cholesterol is restricted to 300 mg daily or less. No more than three egg yolks per week may be used. Liver is used only as a substitute for egg yolk. Shellfish except shrimp are permitted as a substitute for meat.
5. Calorie adjustments may be made in the diet plans by including some sweets and desserts. These lists are not

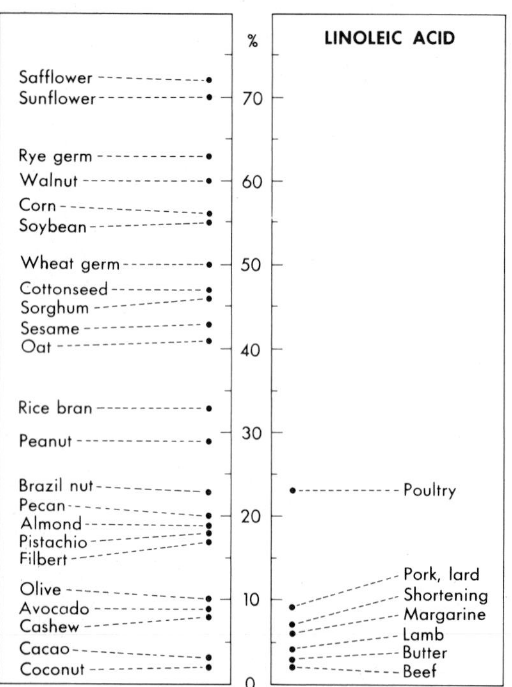

Figure 39–3. Percentage of linoleic acid in fats and oils of plant and animal origin. (Courtesy, Dr. Callie M. Coons and the *Journal of the American Dietetic Association.*)

used when the hyperlipidemia is carbohydrate induced.

The dietary plans are adequate for men in all nutritional essentials, but for women the level of iron does not meet the recommended allowances.

Food Lists The food lists for fat-controlled diets are similar but not identical to the food exchange lists used for diabetic and other calculated diets. (See Table A-4.) The detailed listings of foods for fat-controlled diets appear on pages 638 to 640.

Hyperlipoproteinemia

Types I to V Some hyperlipoproteinemias are induced by an excess of endogenous or exogenous fat, others by an intolerance to carbohydrates, especially sugars, and still others are influenced by dietary cholesterol. These disorders of lipid metabolism may be hereditary or they may be caused by an intake of an abnormal diet. They are frequently associated with diabetes mellitus. Some types predispose to early atherosclerosis. Xanthomas are frequent, and in Types I and V abdominal pain and acute pancreatitis may occur. In all types diet is the primary therapy. When diet alone is ineffective, drug therapy is used, except in Type I.

Type I. An extremely high triglyceride concentration in the serum is characteristic of this type, with the serum cholesterol being normal to high. There is an inability to clear chylomicrons (dietary fat) from the blood, probably as a result of a genetic deficiency of lipoprotein lipase. The condition is rare, usually familial, and seen early in life. It may be associated with diabetes mellitus.

The diet must be very low in fat—25 to 35 gm daily for adults and about 15 gm for children. Cholesterol is not restricted. The carbohydrate is necessarily high in order to supply the needed calories. Alcohol is contraindicated because it increases the serum triglyceride levels when it is metabolized. The elimination of table spreads, cooking fats, and oils results in a dry diet. Medium-chain triglycerides are sometimes prescribed by the physician since they increase the calorie intake and may be used in food preparation. (See page 548.)

Types IIa and IIb. Decreased clearance of low-density lipoprotein (LDL) causes increased serum cholesterol levels. Very low density lipoprotein (VLDL) and triglycerides are normal in Type IIa. This type is a common hereditary disorder, often detectable as early as the first year of life. It may also be associated with an excessive cholesterol intake or with nephrosis, myxedema, or liver disease. Xanthomas and vascular disease are often seen early in adult life. In Type IIb cholesterol and triglycerides are both elevated.

Calories are not restricted in Type IIa, but weight reduction is often indicated in Type IIb. The cholesterol content of the diet is restricted to less than 300 mg daily. Egg yolks are not permitted. The only source of cholesterol is the meat. Protein is not restricted. Saturated fats are decreased and polyunsaturated fats increased so that a high P/S ratio is achieved. Carbohydrate may be limited in Type IIb. Alcohol may be used with discretion.

Type III. This relatively uncommon disorder is characterized by an increase in intermediate-density lipoprotein (IDL). The defect is not clear but may involve overproduction of VLDL or inhibition of its conversion to LDL. Both serum cholesterol and triglycerides are elevated. The incidence of vascular diseases is increased. Lesions on the elbows, knees, and buttocks are common.

Overweight is frequent, and a calorie-restricted diet is indicated until the desirable weight is attained. The fat and carbohydrate are each limited to not more than 40 per cent of the calories. Concentrated sweets are eliminated and polyunsaturated fats are substituted for saturated fats. Cholesterol is restricted to 300 mg per day. Alcohol may be substituted for up to two servings bread or cereal.

Type IV. This is a very common pattern characterized by an increase in VLDL. The abnormality is attributed to overproduction and impaired clearance of VLDL. Triglycerides are elevated but the serum cholesterol is often normal. Many patients in this group have an abnormal glucose tolerance and some have hyperuricemia. This disorder may be hereditary or associated with diabetes mellitus or another metabolic disorder. Obesity and the complications of atherosclerosis are frequent.

Initially the calories are restricted until desirable weight is achieved. Weight loss alone usually lowers the serum lipids, sometimes to normal. The maintenance diet provides not more than 45 per cent of the calories from carbohydrates and eliminates concentrated sweets. A P/S ratio of about 1 is maintained by substituting polyunsaturated fats for saturated fats. Cholesterol is restricted to 300 to 500 mg daily. Alcohol may be used at the physician's discretion.

Type V. Chylomicrons and VLDL are elevated in this type, indicating intolerance to both endogenous and exogenous sources of fat. As with Type IV, glucose tolerance and blood uric acid levels are often abnormal. This disorder is commonly associated with diabetic acidosis, nephrosis, alcoholism, and obesity. The liver and spleen may be enlarged, and abdominal pain is relatively common.

Calorie restriction is emphasized until the desired weight is achieved. The fat in the maintenance diet is kept as low as practical, but not more than 25 to 30 per cent of the calories. The P/S ratio, although not important, is somewhat higher than in typical diets because polyunsaturated fats are substituted for saturated fats. Cholesterol is restricted to 300 to 500 mg daily. The carbohydrate intake is not more than 50 per cent of the calories, thus necessitating a protein intake of 20 to 25 per cent of calories. Concentrated sweets and alcohol are contraindicated.

Dietary Plans A committee of the Heart, Lung, and Blood Institute, National Institutes of Health, has developed detailed dietary plans for the five types of hyperlipoproteinemia described here. These are available in separate booklets for the patient, including individualized dietary plans for the patient, food lists, guidelines for the purchase and preparation of food, and suggestions for eating out. The daily food allowances for the five diets are summarized in Table 39–2. Although the food lists for these diet plans differ in some details, the lists for the fat-controlled diet (page 638) may be used with complete confidence. The sample menus for diets for Type I, Type IIa, and Type IV hyperlipoproteinemia are shown in Table 39–3 to illustrate the variations that are applicable for a given menu.

Table 39-2. **Food Allowances for Types I to V Hyperlipoproteinemia***

Food	Type I	Type IIa	IIb Type III	Type IV	Type V
Skim milk, cups	4	2	2	2	4
Meat, poultry, fish, ounces	5	6–9	6	6	6
Egg yolks as substitute for 1 ounce meat	3/week	None	None	3/week	3/week
Bread, cereals	6+	7+	7	3	10
Potato or other starchy vegetable	1+	1+	1	2	1
Vegetables Dark green or yellow, daily	5 (vegetables and fruit)	5 (vegetables and fruit)	2	2	Ad lib.
Fruit, servings Citrus, daily			3	3	3
Fat, teaspoons	None	6–9	12	10	9
Sugar, sweets	Ad lib.	Ad lib.	None	None	None
Low-fat dessert	Ad lib.	Ad lib.	None	None	None
Alcohol	None	With discretion	Subst.†	Subst.†	None

*Adapted from Fredrickson, D. S. et al.: *Dietary Management of Hyperlipoproteinemia.* Publ. No. (NIH) 76-110. U.S. Department of Health, Education, and Welfare, Washington, D.C., 1975.

†In these diets up to two servings of alcoholic beverages may be substituted for 2 slices bread. One slice of bread is equal to 1 ounce gin, rum, vodka, or whiskey; 1½ ounces sweet or dessert wine; 2½ ounces dry wine; or 5 ounces beer.

Food Lists for Fat-Controlled Diets*

Foods to Use	Foods to Avoid
MILK LIST Skim milk Nonfat dry milk Buttermilk	Whole milk, homogenized milk, canned milk; sweet cream, powdered cream; ice cream unless homemade with nonfat dry milk; sour cream; whole-milk buttermilk and whole-milk yogurt; cheese made from whole milk
VEGETABLES See list 2, Table A-4	
FRUITS See list 3, Table A-4	Avocados Olives
BREADS, CEREALS LIST Breads: biscuits, corn bread, or muffins (all homemade); bread crumbs, bread sticks, rolls; griddlecakes (made with skim milk and fat from day's allowance); matso, melba toast, popcorn, pretzels, rye wafers; cereals: cooked or dry; barley, buckwheat groats, grits, hominy, rice; macaroni, noodles, spaghetti, cornmeal; flour; dried beans, peas, lentils, chickpeas; corn, kernel or cream style; potato, white or sweet	Commercial biscuits, muffins, corn breads, waffles, griddle cakes, cookies, crackers; mixes for biscuits, muffins, and cakes; coffee cakes, cakes (except angel food), pies, sweet rolls, doughnuts, and pastries Potato chips, french-fried potatoes

Foods to Use	**Foods to Avoid**
MEAT, FISH, AND POULTRY LIST	
Make selections from this group for 11 of the 14 main meals	
Poultry without skin—chicken, Cornish hens, squab, turkey	Skin of chicken or turkey; duck or goose; fish roe; caviar; fish canned in olive oil; shrimp
Fish—any but shrimp; veal—any lean cut; meat substitutes—cottage cheese (uncreamed), yogurt from partially skimmed milk; dried peas or beans, peanut butter, nuts (especially walnuts)	Coconut; macadamia nuts
Make selections from this group for 3 of the 14 main meals	
Beef: hamburger—round or chuck; roasts, pot roasts, stew meats—sirloin tip, round, rump, chuck, arm; steaks—flank, sirloin, T bone, porterhouse, tenderloin, round, cube; soup meats—shank or shin; other—dried chipped beef; lamb: roast or steak—leg; chops, loin, rib, shoulder; pork: roast—loin, center cut ham; chops—loin; tenderloin; ham: baked, center cut steaks, picnic, butt, Canadian bacon	Meats high in fat or marbled: beef, lamb, pork; bacon, salt pork, spareribs; frankfurters, sausage, cold cuts; canned meats and meat mixtures: stew, hash; organ meats such as kidney, brain, sweetbread, liver (Note: 2 ounces liver, sweetbreads or heart may be substituted for 1 egg); any visible fat on meat; commercially fried meats, chicken, or fish; frozen or packaged casseroles or dinners
FAT LIST	
Oils: corn, cottonseed, sesame, safflower, soybean, sunflower; mayonnaise, French dressing made with allowed oil, special margarine	Butter, ordinary margarines and solid shortenings, lard, salt pork, chicken fat, coconut oil, olive oil, chocolate
SUGARS AND SWEET LIST	
Sugar: white, brown or maple; syrup—corn or maple; honey, molasses; jelly, jam, marmalade	
DESSERT LIST	
Cakes made from allowed fat, skim milk, and eggs: chiffon, quick yellow or white, angel; candies: gum drops, marshmallows, hard fruit drops, mint patties (no chocolate); cookies: sugar; gelatin desserts; fruits, fruit whips; nut meringues; fruit pies; puddings made with fruit and fruit juice or with skim milk: cornstarch, tapioca; sherbet, preferably water ice	Cookies unless made with allowed fat or oil and egg; custards, puddings, and ice creams unless made with skim milk or nonfat dry milk; whipped cream desserts; candies made with butter, chocolate, cream, or coconut
MISCELLANEOUS	
Cocoa (not chocolate) made with skim milk	Sauces and gravies unless made with allowed fat or oil or made with skim milk; cream soups, creamed dishes un-
Coffee, coffee substitutes, tea, carbon-	

Foods to Use	Foods to Avoid
ated beverages, artificial sweeteners, egg white, sugar, lemons and lemon juice, fat-free consommé and bouillon, pickles, relishes, catsup, vinegar, prepared mustard, herbs, spices	less made with skim milk and allowed oil; foods containing egg yolk except from day's allowance; commercial popcorn; substitutes for coffee cream

* Adapted from food lists and text in *Planning Fat-Controlled Meals for 1200 and 1800 Calories*, revised 1966, and *Planning Fat-Controlled Meals for Approximately 2000–2600 Calories*, revised 1967, American Heart Association, New York.

Table 39-3. **Sample Menus for Three 1,800-Kcal Diets***

Fat-Controlled Diet (Type IIa)	Very Low Fat Diet (Type I)	Carbohydrate-Restricted Diet (Type IV)
Breakfast		
Orange slices—½ cup	Same	Same
Whole-wheat cooked cereal—½ cup	Same	Same
Brown sugar—1 teaspoon	Same	None
Skim milk—1 cup	Same	Same
Homemade muffin—2	Toast—2 slices	Toast—2 slices
Special margarine—2 teaspoons	None; use jelly—2 teaspoons	Margarine—2 teaspoons
Coffee	Same	Same
Sugar for coffee—2 teaspoons	Same	None
Luncheon or Supper		
Roast chicken—3 ounces	Roast chicken—2 ounces; no fat	Broiled chicken—3 ounces; brushed with 1 teaspoon oil
Mashed potato with 1 teaspoon special margarine	Mashed potato; no fat	Mashed potato—with 1 teaspoon margarine
Ripe tomato wedges	Tomato wedges; no fat	Tomato wedges
Tossed green salad	Same	Same
French dressing—1 tablespoon	None	French dressing—1 tablespoon
Rye bread—1 slice	Same	Bread—2 slices
Special margarine—1 teaspoon	None; add jelly—1 teaspoon	Margarine—1 teaspoon
Skim milk—1 cup	Same	Same
Baked apple with 1 tablespoon sugar	Same	Fresh apple
Dinner		
Veal—3 ounces, baked in tomato sauce with oil—1 teaspoon	Same	Veal—3 ounces baked in sauce with oil—2 teaspoons
Rice—½ cup	Same	Same
Asparagus with pimiento	Same	Same; add 1 teaspoon oil
Dinner roll	Hard roll	Dinner roll
Special margarine—1 teaspoon	None; use jelly—1 teaspoon	Margarine—2 teaspoons
Skim milk—1 cup	Same	Same
Fresh peach	Gelatin, ⅔ cup	Fresh peach
Angel cake—small slice	Same	None
Tea or coffee	Same	Same
Snack		
None	Skim milk—1 cup Fresh peach Bread; jelly—1 teaspoon	None

*See Table 39-2 for food allowances.

Dietary Counseling

Dietary modification for the correction of hyperlipidemia requires substantial changes in food selection and preparation for many individuals. Nevertheless, the diet is a palatable one that fits into family menus, the foods are readily available in any food market, and numerous recipes are available for meal planning. The diet need not cost more than conventional diets.

FOOD LISTS The food lists must be meticulously followed with respect to the kinds and amounts of food that may be used and also those that must be avoided. Once the patient is familiar with the lists a great deal of flexibility is both possible and desirable. The food habits must be permanently changed if the diet is to be effective.

MOTIVATION Because the serum lipids generally respond within a few weeks following dietary modification, the lowering of lipid levels usually encourages dietary adherence. On the other hand, the patient needs to know that the full benefits of diet on the incidence of clinical disease may not become apparent for up to 2 or even 3 years.

Usually the patient who has had a heart attack is more highly motivated to adhere to a modified diet than is the coronary-prone individual. Periodic visits to the physician and the dietitian or nurse are helpful in giving support to the patient as well as in giving greater depth to the level of instruction. (See Fig. 39–4.)

SOME SPECIAL PROBLEMS Some patients find it difficult for one reason or another to restrict beef, lamb, and pork to three meals a week. The market supply of fish and veal in some locations is limited, and some people dislike fish and poultry. When beef, lamb, and pork are used more often, the use of safflower oil in preference to other oils helps to counteract the effect of the higher saturated fatty acid content of these meats.

Food preparation. More food preparation "from scratch" is a key rule for these modified diets. Frozen dinners, casseroles, baked foods, and cake, bread, and pudding mixes usually contain more saturated fat than is permitted. Although home preparation implies that more time must be spent in the kitchen, the results can be rewarding by creating numerous dishes that are delicious and lower in cost than the convenience foods of comparable quality. The person responsible for food preparation often needs some guidance in adapting recipes to the needs of the diet. Home economists for processors of fats and oils have developed many excellent recipes,

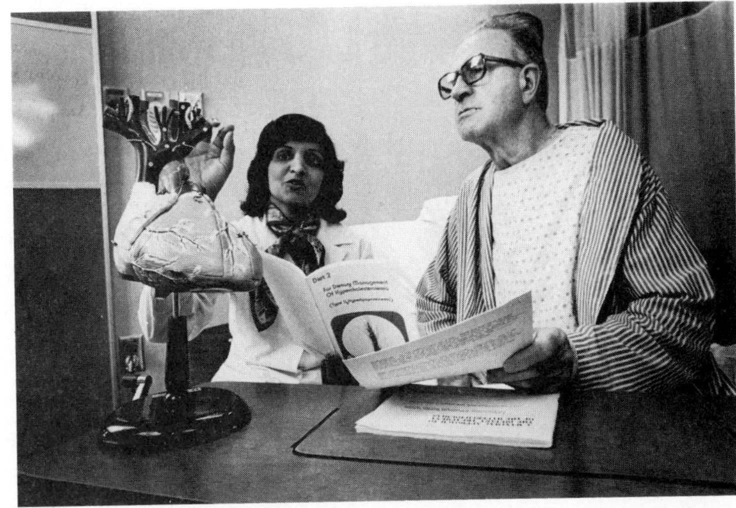

Figure 39–4. Patient with Type IIa hyperlipoproteinemia must understand the principles on which his diet is based, what results can reasonably be expected by adherence to the diet, and what choices are available for his daily meal plan. (Courtesy, Metropolitan Medical Center, Minneapolis.)

and the dietitian or nurse should give the homemaker guidance in using those that are appropriate for the diet prescription. The following guidelines may be helpful:

1. Select only lean cuts of meat. Cut off any visible fat. Use only skim milk.
2. Meat, fish, and poultry may be cooked in any way. If calories are restricted, frying should not be used. Part of the daily oil allowance may be used in meat preparation.
3. When including soups or stews prepare them a day before use. Chill them thoroughly and remove the fat when it is hardened.
4. The oil allowance may be used in these ways:
   a. Substitute oil for an equivalent amount of solid fat in recipes for muffins, griddle cakes, waffles, yeast breads. Special recipes are also available for pie crust, cake, and cookies made with oil.
   b. Brush meat, poultry, or fish with oil before broiling. Put drippings as a sauce over the food before serving.
   c. Make cream sauces by using oil instead of solid fat, flour, and skim milk; season with herbs.
   d. Marinate meat, poultry, or fish in a mixture of oil, lemon juice or vinegar, and herb seasonings. Use the marinade for basting meat when broiling.
   e. Cook vegetables in a tightly covered pan, using a minimum amount of water, and adding oil and seasonings for flavor. Remove the vegetables when cooked; reduce the volume of liquid and pour over the vegetables as a sauce.
5. Special soft margarines may be substituted for part of the oil allowance.

Eating away from home. Adhering to a fat- or carbohydrate-controlled diet is more difficult in a restaurant, partly because the composition of foods is unknown and partly because the varied menu may be too tempting for the dieter. Nevertheless, an occasional meal away from home should be enjoyed. Those who must eat all their meals in a restaurant will need to determine which ones can best meet their dietary requirements. Some restaurants may be able to give a regular customer some special consideration if his or her needs are made known. The dieter can safely choose from these foods: fruit, fruit juice, or clear soup; roasted or broiled meat, fish or poultry without gravy; plain vegetables (many restaurants do not add much seasoning); tossed or fruit salad with or without dressing (no cheese dressing); hard rolls; fruit, plain gelatin, or fruit ice. Sauces, cream soups, butter, cream, ice cream, pastries, and puddings should be avoided.

Surgery for Coronary Artery Disease

Surgical intervention is sometimes undertaken when severe atherosclerosis of the coronary arteries produces myocardial ischemia and disabling angina. The occluded vessels are bypassed by constructing new sources of blood supply to the heart by using portions of a vein or artery grafted from elsewhere in the body. In the immediate postoperative period fluids and sodium are restricted to prevent development of pulmonary edema or congestive heart failure. (See Chapter 40.) Thereafter, restriction of calories and a diet low in saturated fat and cholesterol are usually recommended to prevent recurrence or progression of the coronary artery disease.[45]

Problems and Review

1. List some possible reasons for the recent decline in mortality from coronary (ischemic) heart disease in the United States and Canada.

2. List at least eight factors that have a bearing on the serum cholesterol level.
3. What relationship exists between the amount and nature of the dietary fat and the serum cholesterol level?
4. In what circumstances is a carbohydrate-restricted diet recommended?
5. *Problem.* Plan a normal diet for 1 day. Calculate the total fat, the saturated fat, and the linoleic acid content. Revise the diet so that the linoleic acid level is two times as high as the saturated fat. What measures can you suggest for making such a change acceptable to the patient?
6. Examine several pieces of advertising for food fats. Evaluate the statements made according to your understanding of the relationship of fat to the change in blood lipid levels.
7. *Problem.* Look up recipes for escalloped potatoes; fish chowder; waffles. How could you adjust these so that they are suitable for a fat-controlled diet?
8. What are some of the problems that the patient might encounter when restricted to a very low fat diet for Type I hyperlipoproteinemia?
9. Plan a week's lunches for a patient with Type IIa hyperlipoproteinemia who carries his lunch to work.

Cited References

1. Levy, R. I.: Statement before the Senate Subcommittee on Agriculture and Related Agencies, Committee on Appropriations, United States Senate, July 16, 1980, in "Nutrition and Your Health—Dietary Guidelines for Americans," Department of Health and Human Services, Nutrition Coordinating Office, Washington, D.C.
2. Levy, R. I.: "Prevalence and Epidemiology of Cardiovascular Disease," in Cecil: *Textbook of Medicine,* 15th ed. P. B. Beeson et al., eds., W. B. Saunders Company, Philadelphia, 1979, pp. 1059–63.
3. Metropolitan Life Insurance Co.: "Recent Trends in Mortality from Cardiovascular Disease," *Statistical Bull.,* **60**:2–8, April–June 1979.
4. Rosenberg, H. M., and Klebba, A. J.: "Trends in Cardiovascular Mortality with a Focus on Ischemic Heart Disease: United States, 1950–76," in *Proceedings of the Conference on the Decline in Coronary Heart Disease Mortality,* (NIH) Publ. No. 79–1610, U.S. Department of Health, Education, and Welfare, PHS, May 1979.
5. Summary, in *Proceedings of the Conference on the Decline in Coronary Heart Disease Mortality,* U.S. Department of Health, Education, and Welfare, (NIH) Publ. No. 79–1610, PHS, May 1979, pp. xxiii–xxvii.
6. Yudkin, J.: "Dietary Factors in Atherosclerosis: Sucrose," *Lipids,* **13**:270–72, 1978.
7. Lewis, L. A., and Naito, H. K.: "Relation of Hypertension, Lipids, and Lipoproteins to Atherosclerosis," *Clin. Chem.,* **24**:2081–98, 1978.
8. Heller, R. F., and Jacobs, H. S.: "Coronary Heart Disease in Relation to Age, Sex, and the Menopause," *Brit. Med. J.,* **1**:472–74, 1978.
9. *Dietary Management of Hyperlipoproteinemia.* A Handbook for Physicians and Dietitians. National Heart and Lung Institute, Bethesda, Md., 1973.
10. Kannel, W. B.: "Role of Blood Pressure in Cardiovascular Disease: The Framingham Study," *Angiology,* **26**:1–14, 1975.
11. Stamler, J.: "Dietary and Serum Lipids in the Multifactorial Etiology of Atherosclerosis," *Arch. Surg.,* **113**:21–25, 1978.
12. Kannel, W. B. et al.: "Cholesterol in the Prediction of Atherosclerotic Disease," *Ann. Intern. Med.,* **90**:85–91, 1979.
13. Witztum, J., and Schonfeld, G.: "High Density Lipoproteins," *Diabetes,* **28**:326–33, 1979.

14. Reiser, S. et al.: "Isocaloric Exchange of Dietary Starch and Sucrose in Humans. I. Effects on Levels of Fasting Blood Lipids," *Am. J. Clin. Nutr.*, **32**:1659–69, 1979.
15. Fredrickson, D. S. et al.: "Fat Transport in Lipoproteins—An Integrated Approach to Mechanisms and Disorders," *N. Engl. J. Med.*, **276**:34–44; 94–103; 148–56; 215–26; 273–81, 1967.
16. Christakis, G. et al.: "The Anti-Coronary Club. A Dietary Approach to the Prevention of Coronary Heart Disease—A Seven-Year Report," *Am. J. Public Health*, **56**:299–314, 1966.
17. Review: "Los Angeles Veterans Administration Diet Study," *Nutr. Rev.*, **27**:311–16, 1969.
18. Turpeinen, O. et al.: "Dietary Prevention of Coronary Heart Disease: Long Term Experiment. I. Observations on Male Subjects," *Am. J. Clin. Nutr.*, **21**:255–76, 1968.
19. Leren, P.: "Effect of Plasma Cholesterol Lowering Diet in Male Survivors of Myocardial Infarction," *Bull. N.Y. Acad. Med.*, **44**:1012–20, 1968.
20. Farrand, M. E., and Mojonnier, L.: "Nutrition in the MRFIT," *J. Am. Diet. Assoc.*, **76**:347–51, 1980.
21. American Heart Association Committee Report: "Risk Factors and Coronary Heart Disease," *Circulation*, **62**:449A–455A, 1980.
22. Reiser, R.: "Oversimplification of Diet: Coronary Heart Disease Relationships and Exaggerated Diet Recommendations," *Am. J. Clin. Nutr.*, **31**:865–75, 1978.
23. Garrison, R. J. et al.: "Obesity and Lipoprotein Cholesterol in the Framingham Offspring Study," *Metabolism*, **29**:1053–60, 1980.
24. Streja, D., and Mymin, D.: "Moderate Exercise and High-Density Lipoprotein-Cholesterol," *JAMA*, **242**:2190–92, 1979.
25. Erkelens, D. W. et al.: "High-Density Lipoprotein-Cholesterol in Survivors of Myocardial Infarction," *JAMA*, **242**:2185–89, 1979.
26. Page, L., and Marston, R. M.: "Food Consumption Patterns: U.S. Diet," *Proceedings of the Conference on the Decline in Coronary Heart Disease Mortality*, U. S. Department of Health, Education, and Welfare, PHS, (NIH) Publ. No. 79–1610, May 1979, pp. 236–43.
27. Sturdevant, R. A. L. et al.: "Increased Prevalence of Cholelithiasis in Men Ingesting a Serum-Cholesterol-Lowering Diet," *N. Engl. J. Med.*, **288**:24–27, 1973.
28. McGill, H. C.: "Appraisal of Cholesterol as a Causative Factor in Atherogenesis," *Am. J. Clin. Nutr.*, **32**:2632–36, 1979.
29. Albrink, M. J.: "Triglyceridemia," *J. Am. Diet. Assoc.*, **62**:626–30, 1973.
30. Ahrens, R. A.: "Sucrose, Hypertension and Heart Disease: An Historical Perspective," *Am. J. Clin. Nutr.*, **27**:403–22, 1974.
31. Munoz, J. M. et al.: "Effects of Some Cereal Brans and Textured Vegetable Protein on Plasma Lipids," *Am. J. Clin. Nutr.*, **32**:580–92, 1979.
32. Anderson, J. W., and Chen, W-J. L.: "Plant Fiber. Carbohydrate and Lipid Metabolism," *Am. J. Clin. Nutr.*, **32**:346–63, 1979.
33. Carroll, K. K. et al.: "Hypocholesterolemic Effect of Substituting Soybean Protein for Animal Protein in the Diet of Healthy Young Women," *Am. J. Clin. Nutr.*, **31**:1312–21, 1978.
34. Descovich, G. C. et al.: "Multicentre Study of Soybean Protein Diet for Outpatient Hypercholesterolaemic Patients," *Lancet*, **2**:709–12, 1980.
35. Council on Scientific Affairs: "American Medical Association Concepts of Nutrition and Health," *JAMA*, **242**:2335–38, 1979.
36. Dawson, E. B. et al.: "Relationship of Metal Metabolism to Vascular Disease Mortality Rates in Texas," *Am. J. Clin. Nutr.*, **31**:1188–97, 1978.
37. Punsar, S. et al.: "Coronary Heart Disease and Drinking Water," *J. Chronic Dis.*, **28**:259–87, 1975.
38. Johnson, C. J. et al.: "Myocardial Tissue Concentrations of Magnesium and Potassium

in Men Dying Suddenly from Ischemic Heart Disease," *Am. J. Clin. Nutr.*, **32**:967–70, 1979.

39. Klevay, L. M.: "Interactions of Copper and Zinc in Cardiovascular Disease," *Ann. N.Y. Acad. Sci.*, **355**:140–51, 1981.
40. Klevay, L. M., et al.: "Effects of a Diet Low in Copper on a Healthy Man," *Clin. Res.*, **28**:758A, 1980.
41. Spencer, J. C.: "Direct Relationship Between the Body's Copper/Zinc Ratio, Ventricular Premature Beats, and Sudden Coronary Death," *Am. J. Clin. Nutr.*, **32**:1184–85, 1979.
42. Hooper, P. L. et al.: "Zinc Lowers High-Density Lipoprotein-Cholesterol Levels," *JAMA*, **244**:1960–61, 1980.
43. Krumdieck, C., and Butterworth, C. E.: "Ascorbate-Cholesterol-Lecithin Interactions: Factors of Potential Importance in the Pathogenesis of Atherosclerosis," *Am. J. Clin. Nutr.*, **27**:866–76, 1974.
44. Zukel, M. C.: "Revising Booklets on Fat-Controlled Meals," *J. Am. Diet. Assoc.*, **54**:20–24, 1969.
45. Peterson, C. R.: "Dietary Counseling for Patients Admitted for Coronary Artery Bypass Graft," *J. Am. Diet. Assoc.*, **68**:158–59, 1976.

Additional References

BRESLOW, J. L.: "Pediatric Aspects of Hyperlipidemia," *Pediatrics*, **62**:510–20, 1978.

BRUNNER, D. et al.: "Serum Cholesterol and HDL-Cholesterol in Coronary Patients and Healthy Persons," *Atherosclerosis*, **33**:9–16, 1979.

EATON, R. P.: "High Density Lipoprotein—Key to Anti-Atherogenesis," *J. Chronic Dis.*, **31**:131–35, 1978.

FEINLEIB, M. et al.: "A Comparison of Blood Pressure, Total Cholesterol and Cigarette Smoking in Parents in 1950 and Their Children in 1970," *Am. J. Epidemiol.*, **110**:291–303, 1979.

GLUECK, C. J., and CONNOR, W. E.: "Diet-Coronary Heart Disease Relationships Reconnoitered," *Am. J. Clin. Nutr.*, **31**:727–37, 1978.

GORDON, T. et al.: "Diabetes, Blood Lipids, and the Role of Obesity in Coronary Heart Disease Risk for Women," *Ann. Intern. Med.*, **87**:393–97, 1977.

GOTTO, A. M.: "Is Atherosclerosis Reversible?" *J. Am. Diet. Assoc.*, **74**:551–57, 1979.

HAVEL, R. J.: "High-Density Lipoproteins, Cholesterol Transport, and Coronary Heart Disease," *Circulation*, **60**:1–3, 1979.

KEYS, A.: "Alpha Lipoprotein (HDL) Cholesterol in the Serum and the Risk of Coronary Heart Disease and Death," *Lancet*, **2**:603–6, 1980.

KUMMEROW, F. A.: "Nutrition Imbalance and Angiotoxins as Dietary Risk Factors in Coronary Heart Disease," *Am. J. Clin. Nutr.*, **32**:58–83, 1979.

RIFKIND, B. M. et al.: "Current Status of the Role of Dietary Treatment in the Prevention and Management of Coronary Heart Disease," *Med. Clin. North Am.*, **63**:911–25, 1979.

SCOTT, L. W. et al.: "Are Low-Cholesterol Diets Expensive?" *J. Am. Diet. Assoc.*, **74**:558–61, 1979.

40 Dietary Management of Acute and Chronic Diseases of the Heart

SODIUM-RESTRICTED DIET

Clinical Findings Related to Dietary Management Heart disease affects people of all ages, but it is most frequent in those of middle age and is most often caused by atherosclerosis. (See Chapter 39.) Diseases of the heart may affect (1) the pericardium or outer covering of the organ, (2) the endocardium or membranes lining the heart, or (3) the myocardium or the heart muscle. In addition, the blood vessels within the heart or those leaving the heart or the heart valves may be diseased. Heart disease may be acute with no prior warning, as in a coronary occlusion, or chronic with progressively decreasing ability to maintain the circulation.

The heart may be only slightly damaged so that nearly normal circulation is maintained to all parts of the body; this is a period of *compensation.* The patient is able to continue normal activities with perhaps some restriction of vigorous activity. On the other hand, in severe damage, or *decompensation,* the heart is no longer able to maintain the normal circulation to supply nutrients and oxygen to the tissues, or to dispose of carbon dioxide and other wastes. Prompt measures including bedrest, oxygen, and drug therapy are essential to relieve the strain.

Impairment of the heart is manifested by dyspnea on exertion, weakness, and pain in the chest. In severe failure there is a marked dilation of the heart with enlargement of the liver. The circulation to the tissues and through the kidney is so impaired that sodium and water are held in the tissue spaces. Edema fluid collects first in the extremities and, with increasing failure, in the abdominal and chest cavities. This is referred to as CONGESTIVE HEART FAILURE.

Infections, obesity, hypertension, and constipation complicate and make the treatment of diseases of the heart more difficult. Moreover, the heart is located close to several other organs, especially the stomach and intestines, and distension taking place in either of these organs is likely to press against and interfere with the functioning of the heart. Loss of appetite, nausea, vomiting, and other digestive disorders are common symptoms of heart disease.

Modification of the Diet Objectives in the dietary management of cardiac patients include (1) maximum rest for the heart, (2) prevention or elimination of edema, (3) maintenance of good nutrition, and (4) acceptability of the program by the patient. The following modifications of the diet are necessary to achieve these goals.

Energy. Loss of weight by the obese leads to considerable reduction in the work of the heart because the imbalance between body mass and strength of the heart muscle is corrected. There are a slowing of the heart rate, a drop in blood pressure, and thereby improved cardiac efficiency. Some physicians recommend a mild degree of weight loss even for the cardiac patient of normal weight. Usually a 1,000- to 1,200-kcal diet is suitable for an obese patient in bed; rarely is it necessary to reduce calories to a level below this.

Those patients whose weight is at a desirable level are permitted a maintenance level of calories during convalescence and their return to activity. Usually 1,600 to 2,000 kcal will suffice, with slight increases as the activity becomes greater.

Nutritive adequacy. Normal allowances

of protein, minerals, and vitamins are recommended. The proportions and kinds of fat and carbohydrate may be modified so that polyunsaturated fatty acids and/or complex carbohydrates predominate. (See Chapter 39.) When sodium is restricted, other sources of iodine should be prescribed especially for pregnant women and children. A severe restriction of sodium also reduces the intake of vitamin A because carrots and some of the deep green leafy vegetables that are high in sodium must be omitted.

Sodium. A sodium-restricted diet is indicated when there is retention of fluid and sodium. Usually a restriction of sodium to 1,600 to 2,300 mg (70 to 100 mEq) is satisfactory in patients with congestive heart failure who are receiving diuretics, but occasionally sodium needs to be reduced further.[1] Some patients who have associated renal disease are unable to reabsorb sodium in a normal fashion; these "salt wasters" become depleted of sodium on a severely restricted diet.

Fluid. The restriction of fluid is not required as long as the sodium is restricted. Less work is required by the kidney when ample fluid is available for the excretion of wastes. Because of the homeostatic mechanisms afforded by adrenal and pituitary hormones, water is retained only when there is sufficient sodium to maintain physiologic concentrations. (See also page 174.) An intake of 2 liters of fluid daily is usually permitted.

In advanced congestive failure, especially with excessive use of diuretics, water may be retained even though the sodium intake is low. The hormonal controls are no longer balanced, and the sodium concentration of extracellular fluid is low even though the total body content of sodium is high. Such a circumstance necessitates the restriction of fluid as well as sodium.

Amount of food. Small amounts of food given in five or six meals are preferable to bulky, large meals that place an excessive burden upon the heart during digestion. Part of the food normally allowed at mealtime may be saved for between-meal feedings.

Consistency. When decompensation occurs, liquid or soft, easily digested foods that require little chewing should be used. During the early stages of illness, the patient may need to be fed. When the patient's condition improves, he or she should be given foods that are easy to chew and to digest.

Choice of food. Abdominal distension must be avoided. Until the patient's food tolerances are known, it is best to omit vegetables of the cabbage family, onions, turnips, legumes, and melons. Occasionally a patient may complain that milk is distending. Because of its relaxing effect, the physician may prescribe small amounts of alcohol.

Constipation must be avoided by the judicious use of fruits and vegetables, prune juice, and a sufficient fluid intake.

Progression of the Diet During severe decompensation, as in coronary occlusion, rest is the primary consideration, and all attempts to feed the patient are avoided for the first few days. Liquids are then used for 2 or 3 days. All liquids are served at room temperature. Extremes of temperature such as very hot or iced beverages are contraindicated because they may induce arrhythmias. Beverages containing caffeine are omitted because of their stimulating effect on the heart rate.[2] When the acute phase has passed, more solid foods are permitted and small feedings of easily digested foods are given as tolerated. The foods may be selected from those permitted for the Soft Diet, page 466, giving only small amounts at each of five or six feedings. Mild sodium restriction (2 gm) is usually prescribed. During this phase calories are usually limited to 1,000 to 1,200 daily, with the distribution being 45, 20, and 35 per cent from carbohydrate, protein, and fat, respectively.[3] Cholesterol and saturated fat are restricted. (See Chapter 39 for adjustments made in hyperlipoproteinemias.) In the rehabilitative stage, calories are adjusted as necessary to bring about weight change if needed. The fat-controlled diet (see Chapter 39) is used with sodium restriction if needed. If decompensation is severe, sodium may be restricted to 500 mg or less daily.

Sodium-Restricted Diets

Levels of Sodium Restriction Sodium-restricted diets are used for the prevention, control, and elimination of edema in many pathologic conditions, and occasionally for the alleviation of hypertension. Since sodium is the ion of importance, it is incorrect to designate a diet as "salt free," "salt poor," or "low salt." Moreover, to call a diet "low sodium" or "sodium-restricted" is misleading, since any amount of sodium below the normal sodium intake would satisfy such a description, but would not necessarily be at therapeutic levels. Sodium-restricted diets should be prescribed in terms of milligrams of sodium, for example, 500–700-mg-sodium diet.

Because of the wide range of sodium in single foods, precision in determining actual sodium intake is not possible in the usual clinical situation. For most patients sodium restriction entails major changes in life-style because of the extra care required in shopping and in preparing meals that are appealing yet sufficiently low in sodium to meet the therapeutic goal. The Food and Nutrition Board has stated that the level of sodium used should involve the least amount of restriction necessary to achieve the desired clinical response.[1] Four levels of sodium restriction are used.

The normal diet contains about 3 to 6 gm of sodium daily, although a liberal intake of salty food results in considerably higher sodium levels. The normal diet is modified for its sodium content as described in the following paragraphs.

200 to 300 mg (9 to 13 mEq*; *extreme* sodium restriction). No salt used in cooking; careful selection of foods low in sodium; low-sodium milk substituted for regular milk. This diet is used in conditions such as cirrhosis of the liver with ascites to induce a diuresis, and in congestive heart failure if severe sodium restriction is ineffective.[1]

500 to 700 mg (22 to 30 mEq; *severe* sodium restriction). No salt used in cooking; careful selection of foods in measured amounts; regular milk. This level is used for severe congestive heart failure; occasionally in severe renal disease with edema if patients are not being dialyzed, or in cirrhosis with ascites.[1]

1,000 to 1,500 (43 to 65 mEq; *moderate* sodium restriction). No salt in cooking; careful selection of foods low in sodium, but may include measured amounts of salt, or salted bread and butter. This level is suggested for those with a strong family history of hypertension or patients with borderline hypertension.[1]

2,000 to 3,000 mg (87 to 130 mEq; *mild* sodium restriction.) Some salt may be used in cooking, but no salty foods are permitted; no salt is used at the table. This level is used as a maintenance diet in cardiac and renal diseases.

Sources of Sodium The sodium-restricted diet must be planned with respect to the amount of naturally occurring sodium in foods and the sodium added in food preparation and processing. Sodium values for common foods are given in Table A-2. Most prepared foods show wide variations in sodium content, depending upon conditions of growth and processing of the food, sodium content of water used in preparation, and others. The values listed in any table should not be considered absolute, but they do give reasonable approximations of foods which may be used and which should be avoided.

Naturally occurring sodium in foods. The natural sodium content of animal foods is relatively high and reasonably constant. Thus, meat, poultry, fish, eggs, milk, and

* One milliequivalent of sodium is 23 mg; thus, 100 mg ÷ 23 = 9 mEq.

cheese are the foods which, although nutritionally essential, must be used in measured amounts. Organ meats contain somewhat more sodium than muscle meats. Shellfish of all kinds are especially high in sodium, but other saltwater fish contain no more sodium than freshwater fish. A few plant foods, especially greens like spinach, chard, and kale, contain significant amounts of sodium and are omitted in the more severely restricted diets.

Fruits, cereals, and most vegetables are insignificant sources of sodium. Likewise, sugars, oils, shortenings, and unsalted butter and margarine are negligible sources of sodium.

The drinking water in many localities contains appreciable quantities of sodium, either naturally or through the use of water softeners. When the sodium content is in excess of 20 mg per liter, the daily intake from water alone may be appreciable.[1]

Sodium added to foods. Table salt is by far the most important source of sodium in the diet. Each gram of salt contains about 400 mg sodium; thus, a teaspoon of salt would furnish 2,000 mg sodium. Salt is not only used in cooking and at the table but it also finds its way into many products through manufacturing processes: as in the preservation of ham, bacon, frozen and dried fish; in the brining of pickles, corned beef, and sauerkraut; in koshering of meat; as a rinse to prevent discoloration of fruits in canning; as a means of separating peas and Lima beans for quality before freezing or canning. Canned foods (except fruits), frozen casseroles, dinners, and baked foods, biscuit, bread, cookie, dessert, and sauce mixes contain high levels of salt.

Baking powder and baking soda are widely used in food preparation. Potassium bicarbonate may be used in place of sodium bicarbonate, and sodium-free baking powder may be substituted for regular baking powder.

Numerous sodium compounds other than sodium chloride, baking soda, and baking powder are used in food manufacture: sodium benzoate as a preservative in relishes, sauces, margarine; disodium phosphate to shorten the cooking time of cereals; sodium citrate to enhance the flavor of gelatin desserts and beverages; monosodium glutamate (MSG) as a widely used seasoning in restaurants and in food processing; sodium propionate in cheeses, breads, and cakes to retard mold growth; sodium alginate for smooth texture in chocolate milk and ice cream; and sodium sulfite as a bleach in the preparation of maraschino cherries and to prevent discoloration of dried fruits. (See Figure 40–1.)

Label information. Standards of identity have been established for many food products by the Food and Drug Administration. Such products do not need to carry a listing of ingredients. Thus, the fact that salt is not listed is no guarantee that it is a low-sodium product. Mayonnaise, catsup, and canned vegetables are examples of foods ordinarily prepared with salt but which belong in the category of foods for which a standard of identity has been set up.

Foods specially produced for sodium-restricted diets must be labeled according to regulations set up by the Food and Drug Administration. The label must indicate the sodium content in an average serving and also in 100 gm of the food. (See Figure 40–2.) Although foods may have been pro-

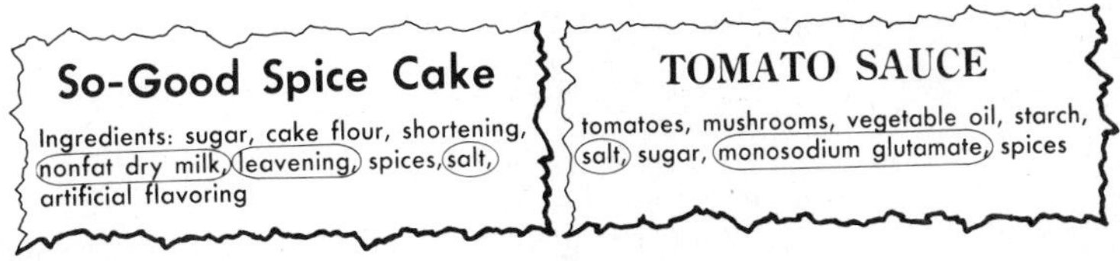

Figure 40–1. Watch for the words *salt* and *sodium* on labels when selecting foods for sodium-restricted diets. Leavenings and nonfat dry milk also contain significant amounts of sodium.

cessed without added sodium compounds, some of them may exceed the limits allowed for a given category. For example, a vegetable that contains 50 mg sodium per serving is much higher than the average sodium content of vegetables. (See Table 40–1.)

Sodium in drugs. Many laxatives, antibiotics, alkalizers, cough medicines, and sedatives contain sodium, and the physician needs to determine whether the amount of a given drug will nullify the effects of a prescribed diet. Patients need to be especially warned against self-medication with sodium bicarbonate or antacids.

Unit Lists for Sodium-Restricted Diets A joint committee of the American Dietetic Association, the American Heart Association, and the U.S. Public Health Service has grouped foods for sodium-restricted diets in *Unit Lists.* Each list corresponds closely to the meal exchange lists (Table A-4, Appendix), but foods which are not to be used are also listed. The group C vegetables of the unit lists are those included in the bread exchange lists. (See Table 40–1.)

Meal Planning with Unit Lists A 500-mg sodium diet at three caloric levels is shown in Table 40–2.

DIETETIC PEACHES

Nutritional Information per ½ cup serving

Calories	40
Protein	1 gm
Carbohydrate	14 gm
Fat	0 gm
Sodium	3.5 mg

(Less than 2.7 in 100 gm)

Percentage of U.S. Recommended Daily Allowances (U.S.R.D.A.)

Protein	*
Vitamin A	4
Vitamin C	2
Thiamin	*
Riboflavin	*
Niacin	4
Calcium	*
Iron	*

*Contains less than 2% of U.S.R.D.A. of these nutrients

Ingredients: Peaches, Pear, Apple, and Grape Juices from Concentrates

Figure 40–2. Foods intended for therapeutic diets must be labeled with information concerning nutritive values. The sodium content per 100 gm and per average serving is included.

Table 40–1. **Nutritive Values of Food Lists for Planning Sodium-Restricted Diets***

List	Amount	Energy kcal	Protein gm	Fat gm	Carbohydrate gm	Sodium mg
1. Milk, whole	1 cup, regular	170	8	10	12	120
	1 cup, low sodium	170	8	10	12	7
Milk, nonfat	1 cup, regular	85	8	—	12	120
	1 cup, low sodium	85	8	—	12	7
2. Vegetables						
List 2	½ cup	25	2	—	5	9
Starchy vegetables	Varies with choice	70	2	—	15	5
3. Fruits	Varies with choice	40	—	—	10	2
4. Low-sodium breads, cereals	Varies with choice	70	2	—	15	5
5. Meat, poultry, fish, eggs, or cheese	1 ounce meat or equivalent	75	7	5	—	25
6. Fats	1 teaspoon butter or equivalent	45	—	5	—	tr

*Arranged from *Your 500 Milligram Sodium Diet,* American Heart Association, New York, 1970.

Table 40-2. **Food Allowances for 500-mg Sodium Diet***

Food List	1,200 Kcal units	1,800 Kcal units	Unrestricted Calories units
Milk	2 (skim)	2 (2% fat)	2 (whole)
Vegetables, List 2	2	2	2 or more
Starchy vegetables	1	1	1 or more
Fruit	4	6	2 or more
Bread	4	8	4 or more
Meat	5	5	5 only
Fat	4	7	as desired
Distribution of Kcal:			
Protein, %	21	16	
Fat, %	30	33	
Carbohydrate, %	49	51	

*Adapted from *Your 500 Milligram Sodium Diet,* American Heart Association, New York, 1970. Allowances calculated to provide less than 500 mg sodium in order to allow for sodium in water used for cooking and drinking. Sodium content of water assumed to be 5 mg per deciliter.

Food Lists for Sodium-Restricted Diets*

See Table A-4, pages 780–784, for food groupings and portion sizes. For each list, note the following items that must be avoided.

Foods Allowed	Foods to Avoid
LIST 1. MILK Skim, whole, evaporated, low sodium	Commercial foods made with milk—chocolate milk, condensed milk, ice cream, malted milk, milk mixes, milk shakes, sherbet
LIST 2. VEGETABLES Fresh, frozen, or dietetic canned with no salt or other sodium compounds	Canned vegetables or juices except low-sodium dietetic
(See list 2, page 781)	Artichoke, beet greens, celery, chard (Swiss), dandelion greens, kale, mustard greens, sauerkraut, spinach Beets, carrots, frozen peas if processed with salt, white turnips
Starchy vegetables (see Bread list, pages 781–782)	Frozen Lima beans if processed with salt, hominy, potato chips
LIST 3. FRUITS Fresh, frozen, canned, or dried (See list 3, page 781.)	Crystallized or glazed fruit, maraschino cherries, dried fruit with sodium sulfite added

Foods Allowed	**Foods to Avoid**
LIST 4. BREAD	
Low-sodium breads, cereals, and cereal products	
Breads and rolls (yeast) made without salt; quick breads made with sodium-free baking powder or potassium bicarbonate and without salt, or made from low-sodium dietetic mix	Yeast bread, rolls, or Melba toast made with salt or from commercial mixes; quick breads made with baking powder, baking soda, salt or MSG or made from commercial mixes
Cereals, cooked, unsalted; dry cereals: Puffed Rice, Puffed Wheat, Shredded Wheat	Quick-cooking and enriched cereals which contain a sodium compound. Read the label. Dry cereals except as listed
Barley; cornmeal; cornstarch; crackers, low sodium; matzo, plain, unsalted; waffle, yeast	Graham crackers or any other except low-sodium dietetic; salted popcorn; self-rising flour; pretzels; waffles containing salt, baking powder, baking soda, or egg white
LIST 5. MEAT	
Meat, poultry, fish, eggs, and low-sodium cheese and peanut butter	
Meat or poultry: fresh, frozen, or canned low sodium	Brains or kidneys
Liver (only once in 2 weeks)	Canned, salted, or smoked meat: bacon, bologna, chipped or corned beef, frankfurters, ham, kosher meats, luncheon meat, salt pork, sausage, smoked tongue, etc.
Tongue, fresh	
Fish or fish fillets, fresh only	Frozen fish fillets
Bass, bluefish, catfish, cod, eels, flounder, halibut, rockfish, salmon, sole, trout, tuna	Canned, salted, or smoked fish: anchovies, caviar, salted and dried cod, herring, canned salmon (except low-sodium dietetic), sardines, canned tuna (except low-sodium dietetic)
Salmon, canned low-sodium dietetic	
Tuna, canned low-sodium dietetic	
	Shellfish: clams, crabs, lobsters, oysters, scallops, shrimp, etc.
Cheese, cottage, unsalted	Cheese, except low-sodium dietetic
Cheese, processed, low-sodium dietetic	
Egg (limit 1 per day)	Egg substitutes, frozen or powdered
Peanut butter, low-sodium dietetic	Peanut butter unless low-sodium dietetic
LIST 6. FAT	
Spreads, oils, cooking fats unsalted	Salted butter or margarine, bacon and bacon fat; salt pork; olives; commercial French or other dressing except low sodium; commercial mayonnaise, except low sodium; salted nuts
MISCELLANEOUS FOODS	
Beverages	
Alcoholic with doctor's permission	Fountain beverages; instant cocoa mixes; prepared beverage mixes, including fruit-flavored powders
Cocoa made with milk from diet	
Coffee, instant, freeze dried, or regular; coffee substitutes	

Foods Allowed	Foods to Avoid
Lemonade; Postum; tea *Candy,* homemade, salt free, or special low sodium *Gelatin,* plain unflavored	Commericial candies, cakes, cookies Commercial sweetened gelatin desserts Mixes of all types Pastries
Leavening agents Cream of tartar; sodium-free baking powder; potassium bicarbonate; yeast *Rennet dessert powder* (not tablets)	Regular baking powder; baking soda (sodium bicarbonate) Rennet tablets; pudding mixes; molasses

Flavoring Aids Allowed

Allspice
Almond extract
Anise seed
Basil
Bay leaf
Bouillon cube (low sodium)
Caraway seed
Cardamom
Chives
Cinnamon
Cloves
Cocoa (1–2 teaspoons)
Cumin
Curry
Dill
Fennel
Garlic
Ginger
Horseradish (prepared without salt)
Juniper
Lemon juice or extract
Mace
Maple extract
Marjoram
Mint
Mustard, dry
Nutmeg
Onion, fresh, juice or sliced
Orange extract
Oregano
Paprika
Parsley
Pepper
Peppermint extract
Poppy seed
Poultry seasoning
Purslane
Rosemary
Saccharin
Saffron
Sage
Salt substitutes (with physician's approval)
Savory
Sesame seeds
Sorrel
Sugar
Tarragon
Thyme
Turmeric
Vanilla extract
Vinegar
Wine, if allowed by physician
Walnut extract

Flavoring Aids to Avoid

Barbecue sauce
Bouillon cube, regular
Catsup
Celery salt, seed, leaves
Chili sauce
Cyclamates
Garlic salt
Horseradish prepared with salt
Meat extracts, sauces tenderizers
Monosodium glutamate
Mustard, prepared
Olives
Onion salt
Pickles
Relishes
Salt
Soy sauce
Sugar substitutes containing sodium
Worcestershire sauce

* Adapted from *Your 500 Milligram Sodium Diet,* American Heart Association, New York, 1970.

Adjustments for Sodium Level The 500-mg sodium diet in Table 40–2 may be adjusted for lower or higher levels of sodium as follows:

200 to 300 mg (9 to 13 mEq): substitute low-sodium milk for regular milk

1000 to 1500 mg (43 to 65 mEq): substitute limited amounts of ordinary salted bread (contains 100 to 125 mg sodium per slice) and salted butter or margarine (contains 50 mg sodium per teaspoon); or a carefully measured amount of salt placed in a shaker and used for cooking or at table (¼ teaspoon salt contains approximately 500 mg sodium).

2,000 to 3,000 mg (87 to 130 mEq): At

1,200 kcal use lightly salted food and allow ordinary salted bread and regular milk. When 1,800 kcal or more are allowed, it is possible to keep the sodium level around 2,000 to 3,000 mg only by omitting salt in food preparation. Omit salting of food at the table. Omit salty foods such as potato chips, salted popcorn, and nuts, olives, pickles, relishes, meat sauces, smoked and salted meats.

Dangers of Sodium Restriction Diets that are very low in sodium must be used with caution since there is occasional danger of depletion of body sodium. Hot weather may bring about great losses of sodium through the skin, and vomiting, diarrhea, surgery, renal damage, or the use of mercurial diuretics also increases the amounts of sodium lost from the body. Sodium depletion is characterized by weakness, abdominal cramps, lethargy, oliguria, azotemia, and disturbances in the acid-base balance. Patients must be instructed to recognize the symptoms of danger and to consult a physician immediately when they occur.

Sample Menu for 500-mg Sodium Diet

1,200 kcal	1,800 kcal
BREAKFAST	
Honeydew melon, ⅛ medium	Same
Shredded Wheat, 1 biscuit	Same
Low-sodium corn muffin, 1	2
Unsalted margarine, 1 teaspoon	2
Milk, 1 cup skim	1 cup 2%
Coffee or tea, no sugar	Same
LUNCHEON OR SUPPER	
Toasted sandwich:	
Low-sodium bread, 2 slices	Same
Low-sodium tuna fish, 2 ounces	Same
Low-sodium mayonnaise, none; use lemon juice	Same
Lettuce	Same
Tomato	Same
Mixed green salad	Same
Low-sodium, low-calorie dressing, 1 tablespoon	Same
Fresh apple, medium	Baked apple with stuffing: Raisins, 2 tablespoons; Brown sugar, 2 teaspoons
Milk, skim, 1 cup	1 cup 2%
DINNER	
Broiled pork chop, 3 ounces	Same
Baked potato, small	Same
Baked acorn squash, ½ cup	Same
Low-sodium dinner roll, none	2
Low-sodium margarine, 2 teaspoons	3 teaspoons
Fruit cup:	
Fresh pineapple, ¼ cup	½ cup
Fresh strawberries, ½ cup	1 cup
Coffee or tea, no sugar	Same

Dietary Counseling

Perhaps no diet provides greater obstacles with respect to acceptance for taste appeal and understanding of the permissible food choices than does the sodium-restricted diet. Skilled counseling of the patient by dietitian, nurse, and physician is essential from the time the diet is first prescribed. Far too many patients have assumed that the omission of salt merely represented poor cookery and have eaten forbidden foods brought in by well-meaning but uninformed relatives and friends.

When a sodium-restricted diet is to be continued in the home, the patient should be given some understanding of the purposes of the diet and some indication regarding the length of time it needs to be used. The patient needs information on the foods that are permitted on the diet, what foods are contraindicated, where foods may be purchased, and how to prepare palatable foods with flavoring aids. He or she should not expect foods to taste the same as those that are salted, but in time most patients learn to adjust to the change in flavors.

The individual responsible for meal preparation must be included in all phases of dietary counseling so that he or she understands the importance of the diet and learns what modifications in planning, purchasing, and preparation are required.

The American Heart Association has published detailed booklets concerning three levels of sodium restriction and low-calorie and maintenance energy allowances. For patients who find the details confusing, concise leaflets have also been prepared. Neither of these teaching aids should take the place of individualized instruction, nor should the patient be expected to comprehend all the information in one or two counseling sessions.

Cultural patterns must be considered, inasmuch as favorite dishes are often high in sodium. Usually, these dishes may be adapted within the sodium restriction rather than omitting them entirely.

The patient and the homemaker must be taught to read labels of food products, looking especially for the words *salt* and *sodium*. (See Figure 40–1.)

PREPARATION OF FOOD Ingenuity is required in the preparation of foods for sodium-restricted diets so that they will be accepted by the patient. A number of salt substitutes are available, but they should be used only upon the recommendation of the physician since many of them contain substantial amounts of potassium, which may be contraindicated when there is renal damage.

Numerous flavoring aids are available (see page 653 for list) to provide taste appeal. Herbs and spices are especially useful, but they should be used with a light touch.

Delicious yeast breads, muffins, waffles, and doughnuts may be prepared using part of the milk and egg allowance of the diet. Low-sodium baking powder must be substituted for regular baking powder. When low-sodium milk is required in the diet, recipes may be successfully prepared by substituting low-sodium milk for regular milk. The calcium value of low-sodium milk is about 80 per cent of that of whole milk, the thiamin content is about half as great, and the potassium level is almost twice as high. In other nutrients low-sodium milk compares favorably with whole milk.[4]

The sodium content of kosher meats is too high for sodium-restricted diets. Orthodox Jewish patients should salt their meats lightly and allow them to stand for a minimum length of time to draw out the blood. Thoroughly washing with water will remove much of the salt. Then meats are simmered in a large volume of water, and the cooking liquid is discarded. The leaching is more effective if the meat is cut into pieces before cookery.[5]

RESTAURANT MEALS Meals eaten in restaurants and fast-food chains contribute substantially to the sodium intake. For persons on mild sodium-restricted diets, occasional meals in fast-food chains are permissible if discretion is used in choice of foods. Items such as beef or chicken on a bun (without ketchup or barbeque sauce), coleslaw or lettuce and tomato, milk, juice, coffee, or tea could be ordered. French fries, onion rings, milkshakes, and pastries should be avoided. Foods that might be ordered in more traditional restaurants could include broiled meat or fish except shellfish, baked potato, plain vegetables, salads without dressing, juice, fruit, or sherbet. Broth-based soups, cheeses, crackers with salted tops, and most bakery products should be omitted.

Hypertension

Hypertension, or elevation of the blood pressure above normal, is a symptom that accompanies many cardiovascular and renal diseases. In the Framingham study, hypertension was found to be the most important of the major risk factors that influence morbidity and mortality from cardiovascular disease.[6] Even mild hypertension (diastolic pressure, 90–104 mm Hg) is associated with a twofold increase in risk for cardiovascular disease.[7] However, at least two large studies have shown that mortality, including that from congestive heart failure, retinopathy, and stroke, can be reduced with systematic control of blood pressure.[8,9]

Some 24 million Americans are estimated to have hypertension. The prevalence in adult blacks is nearly twice that in whites.[10] In children, such racial differences in blood pressure are not seen.[11] Hypertension occurs at any age, but is found most frequently in those over 40 years of age. About 85 to 90 percent have ESSENTIAL HYPERTENSION for which the cause is unknown. Emotional disturbances, excessive smoking, certain kidney diseases, and adrenal tumors account for a small proportion of cases.

Prevention Some epidemiologic evidence indicates that areas with low habitual salt intakes have low prevalence of hypertension. Prolonged very high salt intakes are associated with elevations in blood pressure even in normal subjects.[12] Some recommend lifelong modest sodium restriction as a means of delaying onset of the disorder and preventing its complications in persons who are genetically susceptible to hypertension.[13,14] Some 10 to 30 per cent of the U.S. population is genetically predisposed to hypertension.[14] The Food and Nutrition Board recommends that those with a family history of hypertension or who have borderline hypertension should limit sodium intake to *less* than 1,600 to 2,300 mg (70 to 100 mEq) per day.[1] The Dietary Guidelines for Americans propose a reduction in daily salt intake as a preventive measure.[15]

Dietary Modification Hypertension is often lowered with weight loss in the obese patient. Even a 5 to 6 percent weight loss is sufficient to produce a substantial fall in blood pressure in overweight persons with mild hypertension.[16] Sodium restriction is also effective in lowering blood pressure; when used alone, however, except for patients with mild hypertension, the level of sodium permitted is so low as to be impractical for most. The primary means of treating hypertension is through use of diuretics. Some evidence suggests that excessive intake of sodium may block the antihypertensive effects of these drugs. For this reason the Committee on Sodium-Restricted Diets of the Food and Nutrition Board recommends use of sodium-restricted diets in combination with diuretics in the treatment of hypertension. The suggested intake is 1,600 to 2,300 mg (70 to 100 mEq).[1] Sodium restriction also enhances the effects of diuretic therapy and permits smaller doses of such drugs.[17] The Joint National Committee on Detection, Evaluation, and Treatment of High Blood Pressure has recommended mild sodium restriction, 2 gm, for all patients as adjunctive therapy in the management of hypertension.[7]

Dietary Counseling

Failure to comply with therapy is a major problem in management of hypertension. In addition to the considerations described on pages 648–54, the importance of weight control should be stressed at regular follow-up visits. Good food sources of potassium should be recommended to patients receiving diuretics such as thiazides, furosemide, and ethacrynic acid. A few examples of potassium-rich foods that are also low in sodium are apricots, bananas, prunes, raisins, broccoli, Brussels sprouts, baked squash, and baked potato. Dried fruits and legumes are especially good sources for those who are not on calorie-restricted diets. The amount of potassium needed has not been determined but a reasonable goal is 100 mEq (3,900 mg) daily.[1] Potassium supplements such as potassium chloride may be necessary to achieve this level of intake. Most salt substitutes contain approximately 60 mEq (2,350 mg) of potassium per teaspoon.[18] Some physicians may approve use of these for patients without renal disease.

Problems and Reviews

1. Explain the rationale for the various dietary restrictions used for patients in the coronary care unit.
2. When is an extremely low sodium diet likely to be ordered? A severe low-sodium diet? A moderately restricted sodium diet? A mildly restricted sodium diet? Outline the important differences in food allowances for each of these levels.
3. *Problem.* Plan a menu for 1 day that furnishes moderate sodium restriction and 1,500 kcal, with 30 to 35 per cent of calories as fat.
4. Examine the labeling on five food products to find examples of different sodium compounds used in processing. Could any of these be used on a sodium-restricted diet? Explain.
5. *Problem.* A 60-year-old man is being discharged from the hospital. A moderately restricted sodium diet has been prescribed. Neither the patient nor his wife has had much education and they read with difficulty. Their income is low. Outline the steps you would take to provide guidance for them in the management of the diet at home.
6. *Problem.* Determine the sodium content of the local water supply. If a patient drinks 2 quarts of this water daily, how much sodium will be ingested? If the sodium content of the water is high, what recommendations would you make to a patient? Compare the sodium content of the local water supply to that of some bottled waters available in the supermarket.
7. What is the rationale for sodium restriction in essential hypertension?
8. What foods might present problems in planning sodium-restricted diets for the following ethnic groups: Jewish, Chinese, Italian, black Americans who enjoy soul food.

Cited References

1. Committee on Sodium-Restricted Diets, Food and Nutrition Board, National Research Council: *Sodium-Restricted Diets and the Use of Diuretics. Rationale, Complications, and Practical Aspects of Their Use.* National Academy of Sciences, Washington, D.C., 1979.
2. Wenger, N. K.: "Guidelines for Dietary Management After Myocardial Infarction," *Geriatrics*, **34**:75–83, August 1979.
3. Stegemann, N.: "Dietary Management in the Coronary Care Unit," *JAMA*, **238**:1913, 1977.
4. Council on Foods and Nutrition: "Low-Sodium Milk," *JAMA*, **163**:739, 1967.
5. Kaufman, M.: "Adapting Therapeutic Diets to Jewish Food Customs," *Am. J. Clin. Nutr.*, **5**:676–81, 1957.
6. Kannel, W. B.: "Hypertension, Blood Lipids, and Cigarette Smoking as Co-Risk Factors for Coronary Heart Disease," *Ann. N.Y. Acad. Sci.*, **304**:128–39, 1978.

7. Joint National Committee Report: "The 1980 Report of the Joint National Committee on Detection, Evaluation, and Treatment of High Blood Pressure," *Arch. Intern. Med.*, **140**:1280–85, 1980.
8. Frohlich, E. D.: "Mild Essential Hypertension: Benefit of Treatment," *Ann. N.Y. Acad. Sci.*, **304**:68–73, 1978.
9. Hypertension Detection and Follow-Up Program Cooperative Group: "Five-Year Findings of the Hypertension Detection and Follow-Up Program," *JAMA* **242**:2562–71, 1979.
10. Hypertension Detection and Follow-up Program Cooperative Group: "Race, Education, and Prevalence of Hypertension," *Am. J. Epidemiol.*, **106**:351–61, 1977.
11. Morrison, J. A. et al.: "Studies of Blood Pressure in School Children (Ages 6–19) and Their Parents in an Integrated Suburban School District," *Am. J. Epidemiol.*, **111**:156–65, 1980.
12. Calabrese, E. J., and Tuthill, R. W.: "Elevated Blood Pressure and High Sodium Levels in the Public Drinking Water," *Arch. Environ. Health*, **32**:300–2, 1977.
13. Tobian, L.: "The Relationship of Salt to Hypertension," *Am. J. Clin. Nutr.*, **32**:2739–48, 1979.
14. Freis, E. D.: "Salt, Volume, and the Prevention of Hypertension," *Circulation*, **53**:589–95, 1976.
15. "Nutrition and Your Health. Dietary Guidelines for Americans," *Nutr. Today*, **15**:14–18, March/April, 1980.
16. Stamler, J. et al.: "Prevention and Control of Hypertension by Nutritional-Hygienic Means," *JAMA*, **243**:1819–23, 1980.
17. Gifford, R. W.: "The Hypertension Detection and Follow-Up Program, the Joint National Committee, and Non-pharmacologic Management of Hypertension," *Mayo Clin. Proc.*, **55**:651–52, 1980.
18. Sopko, J. A., and Freeman, R. M.: "Salt Substitutes as a Source of Potassium," *JAMA*, **238**:608–10, 1977.

Additional References

BECKSON, D. M. et al.: "Changing Trends in Hypertension Detection and Control: The Chicago Experience," *Am. J. Public Health*, **70**:389–93, 1980.

FEDERSPIEL, B.: "Renin and Blood Pressure," *Am. J. Nurs.*, **75**:1462–64, 1975.

FUJITA, T. et al.: "Factors Influencing Blood Pressure in Salt-Sensitive Patients with Hypertension," *Am. J. Med.*, **69**:334–44, 1980.

HADDY, F. J.: "Mechanism, Prevention and Therapy of Sodium-Dependent Hypertension," *Am. J. Med.*, **69**:746–58, 1980.

HILL, M.: "Helping the Hypertensive Patient Control Sodium Intake," *Am. J. Nurs.*, **79**:906–9, 1979.

JONES, R. J.: "Dietary Management in the Coronary Care Unit," *JAMA*, **237**:2645, 1977.

Maloney, R.: "Helping Your Hypertensive Patients Live Longer," *Nursing*, **8**:26–35, October 1978.

MARCINEK, M. B.: "What Hypertension Does to the Body," *Am. J. Nurs.*, **80**:928–32, 1980.

MOSER, M.: "How Hypertensive Therapy Works," *Am. J. Nurs.*, **80**:937–41, 1980.

National High Blood Pressure Education Program: *Statement on the Role of Dietary Management in Hypertension Control*, U.S. Department of Health and Human Services, PHS, NIH, Publ. No. 0–311-201/3129, U.S. Government Printing Office, Washington, D.C., 1980.

NIES, A. S.: "Clinical Pharmacology of Antihypertensive Drugs," *Med. Clin. North. Am.*, **61**:675–98, 1977.

TANNER, G.: "Heart Failure in the MI Patient," *Am. J. Nurs.*, **77**:230–34, 1977.

Diet in Diseases of the Kidney 41

CONTROLLED PROTEIN, SODIUM, POTASSIUM, AND PHOSPHORUS DIET; CALCIUM-RESTRICTED DIET

Renal Function and Disease The important function of the kidneys is to maintain the normal composition and volume of the blood. They accomplish this by the excretion of nitrogenous and other metabolic wastes, by regulation of electrolyte and fluid excretion so that water balance is maintained, by making the final adjustment of acid-base balance, and by the synthesis of enzymes and other substances that influence metabolic activities. In view of the central role of the kidneys in maintaining the constant internal environment it is not surprising that renal disease and eventually renal failure affect every system and tissue in the body. A review of the functions of the normal kidney (see pages 170 to 173) is recommended before the student begins the study of dietary management in renal diseases. (See Figure 41–1.)

Disease may affect the glomeruli, the tubules, or both. NEPHRITIS means literally an inflammation of the nephrons. Although GLOMERULONEPHRITIS indicates that the glomeruli are particularly affected, the functioning of the tubules will also be disturbed. Renal disease may be acute, subacute or latent, or chronic. The majority of patients with acute glomerulonephritis recover completely but a small group progress to chronic nephritis. In some patients disease may be in a latent stage for months or even years during which the individual is asymptomatic. Obviously, for each patient a careful evaluation must be made of the etiology, the presenting symptoms, and the level of renal function before any treatment including dietary control can be initiated.

Acute Glomerulonephritis

Symptoms and Clinical Findings Acute glomerulonephritis, also known as *hemorrhagic nephritis,* is primarily confined to the glomeruli. It occurs mostly in children and young adults as a frequent sequel to steptococcic infections such as scarlet fever, tonsillitis, pneumonia, and respiratory infections. In some patients the renal infection is so mild that there is no awareness of the disease until symptoms resulting from permanent damage appear much later. Others notice some swelling of the ankles and puffiness around the eyes and complain of headache, anorexia, nausea, and vomiting. Varying degrees of hypertension, dimness of vision, and even convulsions may occur. Usually there is a diminished urinary volume, hematuria, some albuminuria, and some nitrogen retention.

The acute phase of the illness lasts from several days to a week, but renal function returns to normal much more slowly. Full recovery is the rule, provided that treatment is prompt and appropriate. The recovery time varies from 2 or 3 weeks to several months, as determined by renal function tests.

Modification of the Diet During the acute phase of illness when nausea and vomiting are present it is unrealistic to provide a diet that fully meets nutritional requirements. An effort should be made to maintain fluid balance and to provide nonprotein calories, either orally or parenterally, to minimize the catabolism of tissue

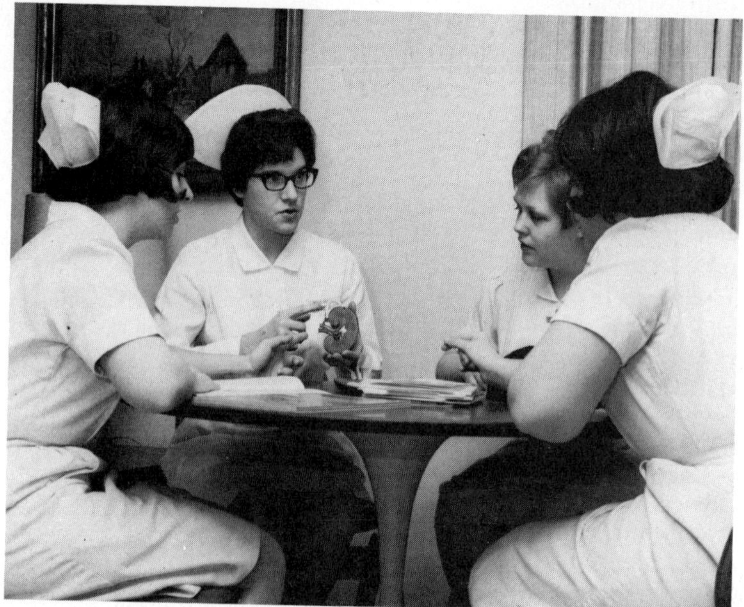

Figure 41–1. An understanding of the structure and function of the normal kidney is an essential foundation for developing the rationale for nutritional care in renal failure. (Courtesy, School of Nursing, Thomas Jefferson University, Philadelphia.)

proteins. High-carbohydrate, low-electrolyte supplements,* fruit juices sweetened with glucose, sweetened tea, ginger ale, fruit ices, and hard candy contribute to the carbohydrate intake. Excessive amounts of sweet foods, however, may contribute to the nausea.

As the patient improves and the appetite returns, the following dietary modifications are appropriate:

Energy. The recommended dietary allowances (page 35) provide a general guide to the caloric requirement for persons of various ages and body size. In the absence of fever and at bedrest, these allowances can be reduced somewhat if there is not a previous condition of malnutrition.

Protein. Unless oliguria or renal failure develops, protein is not restricted. If it is determined that protein restriction is necessary, a diet not exceeding 40 gm protein daily is used initially.[1] Gradual increases are made over the next 2 weeks in accordance with individual tolerance. When there is marked albuminuria, the protein intake should be increased by the amount of protein lost in the urine.

Sodium. If there is edema or hypertension, sodium restriction to 500 or 1,000 mg may be prescribed. Sodium restriction is also used if there is danger of congestive failure and pulmonary edema.[2]

Fluid. In the presence of oliguria, fluids are restricted to prevent further edema. The volume permitted depends on the previous day's output. Usually 500 to 1,000 ml more fluid than the previous day's output is allowed. Larger amounts of fluid are given to replace losses by vomiting, diarrhea, or excessive perspiration.

Selection of foods The food allowances for 20 gm-, 40 gm-, and 60-gm-protein diets listed in Table 41–2 (page 668) are used as the basis for meal planning. The emphasis is upon protein foods of high biologic value, especially eggs and milk; however, the amounts of each must be carefully con-

* Polycose® by Ross Laboratories, Columbus, Ohio; Controlyte® by Doyle Pharmaceutical Co., Minneapolis, Minnesota; Hy-Cal® by Beecham-Massengill Pharmaceuticals, Melrose, Massachusetts; Sumacal® Plus by Organon, Inc., West Orange, New Jersey; Cal-Power Dietary Specialties, Henkel Corporation, Minneapolis, Minnesota.

trolled. Peas, Lima beans, dried beans and peas, nuts, peanut butter, and gelatin are high in protein of poor biologic value and they should be omitted.

Achieving a satisfactory caloric intake is doubly difficult; the limitations placed upon protein intake necessitate restriction of breads, cereals, potatoes, and similar foods that are good sources of calories, and poor appetite often interferes with food intake. The caloric intake can be increased by using appropriate supplements, low-protein desserts, sugars, jellies, hard candy, butter or margarine, vegetable oils, and carbonated beverages. Cream may be substituted for part of the milk allowance.

When sodium restriction is ordered, the food lists on pages 651 to 653 should be consulted. Regular milk can be used in the amounts listed, but all foods must be prepared without salt or other sodium-containing compounds for any restriction of 1,000 mg or less.

Chronic Glomerulonephritis

Clinical Findings. The majority of cases of chronic glomerulonephritis have an immunologic basis of unknown etiology. Patients may be asymptomatic for months or even years. The nephritis may be detected only by laboratory studies. As the disease progresses there is gradually increasing involvement: proteinuria, hematuria, hypertension, and vascular changes in the retina. The kidneys are unable to concentrate urine and there are both frequent urination and nocturia. Although the specific gravity of the urine is low, the large volume of urine makes possible the excretion of the metabolic wastes. In some patients the nephrotic syndrome (see following) characterized by massive edema and severe proteinuria develops. Hypoproteinemia and anemia are sometimes encountered. Eventually the symptoms of renal failure occur (see following).

Modification of the Diet The objectives of dietary management are (1) to maintain a state of good nutrition; (2) to control or correct protein deficiency; (3) to prevent edema; and (4) to provide palatable, easily digested meals adjusted to the individual patient's needs.

During the period when the kidneys are able to excrete wastes adequately the normal daily allowance of protein plus the amount of protein lost in the urine is allowed. With progression of the disease, elevated blood urea nitrogen levels may necessitate restriction of protein to 40 gm or less daily.

Sufficient carbohydrate and fat should be provided so that the energy needs of the body can be met without the breakdown of body protein. The daily caloric needs for the adult will usually range from 2,000 to 3,000 kcal.

Sodium restriction to 500 or 1,000 mg is indicated only when edema is present. Some clinicians recommend a mild level of sodium restriction (see page 648) even when there is no edema. During the diuretic phase of nephritis increased amounts of sodium may be excreted because of the kidneys' inability to reabsorb the ion. Thus, a markedly restricted sodium diet could lead to body depletion with its attendant weakness, nausea, and symptoms of shock.

Nephrotic Syndrome

Glomerular injury from a number of causes may lead to massive proteinuria, hypoalbuminemia, and edema. Hypercholesterolemia is often marked but the mechanism involved is not clear. Large urinary losses of albumin and other plasma proteins lead to tissue wastage, malnutrition, fatty liver, edema, and increased susceptibility to infection. Besides a fall in plasma oncotic pressure that accompanies loss of albumin, other factors contribute to the edema, including reductions in plasma volume and renal blood flow. Consequently, enhanced renal renin production leads to increased aldosterone secretion. Aldosterone favors sodium reabsorption and further contributes to the edema.

Sodium. Diuretics and sodium restriction are used to prevent further accumulation of edema fluid. The level of sodium permitted is usually less than 2 gm daily, and even as low as 500 mg daily. The sodium intake is liberalized when edema is corrected. Modest restriction may be used to prevent recurrence of edema.

Protein and energy. Studies in patients with prolonged proteinuria have shown that positive nitrogen balance is associated with use of high protein intake, which suggests that a general body protein deficit is involved.[2] The reduced serum protein level is one manifestation of this deficit.

Protein, 120 gm daily, and a high calorie intake (50 to 60 kcal per kilogram) are needed for tissue repletion. High-protein supplements are useful for some patients provided the sodium content does not exceed the permitted intake.* In some areas palatable low-sodium milk is available and can be used to increase the protein intake.

Fat. Types IIa, IIb, and V hyperlipoproteinemia have been observed in nephrotic syndrome. Dietary measures to reduce plasma lipids in these disorders are appropriate and were discussed in Chapter 39.

Nephrosclerosis

Nephrosclerosis, or hardening of the renal arteries, occurs in adults after 35 years of age, as a rule, and is associated with arteriosclerosis. The disease may run a benign course for many years. During late stages some albuminuria, nitrogen retention, and retinal changes develop. Death usually results from circulatory failure. In a small number of younger persons nephrosclerosis runs a stormy, rapid course leading to uremia and death. This is called *malignant hypertension.*

Modification of the diet Weight reduction of the obese is desirable. A 200-mg-sodium diet has been used successfully in some instances. The protein intake is kept at a normal level until marked nitrogen retention indicates that the kidney is no longer able to eliminate wastes satisfactorily. The diet on page 668, Table 41–2, may be used with or without sodium restriction when a lower level of protein becomes necessary.

Renal Failure

Symptoms and Biochemical Findings Chronic glomerulonephritis, nephrosclerosis, and chronic pyelonephritis are the principal diseases of the kidney leading to renal failure. This is a condition in which the kidneys are no longer able to maintain the normal composition of the blood. UREMIA, a general term applied to the syndrome arising from the failing function of the kidney, refers to the retention of urea and other urinary constituents in the blood. It is accompanied by nausea and vomiting, hyperkalemia, azotemia, oliguria, and bone disease. AZOTEMIA is a more specific term for the accumulation of nitrogenous constituents in the blood. OLIGURIA denotes a scanty output of urine (less than 500 ml), and ANURIA is the minimal production or absence of urine (less than 100 ml per day).

Acute Renal Failure This is characterized by a rapid fall in glomerular filtration rate and a progressive rise in serum creatinine and urea concentrations. Oliguria or even anuria occur. Acute renal failure occurs in extensive burns, severe acute glomerulonephritis, following inhalation or ingestion of poisons such as carbon tetrachloride or mercury, crushing injuries, or shock from surgery. The mortality rate is nearly 50 per cent. Dialysis is often employed until the kidney again resumes its function.

* Casec by Mead Johnson and Company, Evansville, Indiana; Gevral Protein, by Lederle Laboratories, American Cyanamid Co., Pearl River, New York.

Dietary treatment is directed toward correction of fluid and electrolyte imbalances and maintenance of adequate nutritional status in order to minimize endogenous protein catabolism and subsequent uremia.

Energy. In the initial period when vomiting and diarrhea preclude oral intake, intravenous glucose, 100 gm per 24 hours, is administered to reduce protein catabolism. In some cases, total parenteral nutrition, using hypertonic glucose and amino acids is appropriate. When oral intake is permitted a high calorie intake is needed to prevent catabolism of proteins to meet energy needs.

Protein. Traditionally, severe protein restriction has been used in acute renal failure, but in recent years use of dialysis to remove accumulated nitrogen wastes has permitted a more liberal protein intake. Initially a protein-free diet is used in the nondialyzed patient. Intravenous glucose with the essential amino acids added has also been used successfully. In the diuretic phase, 20 to 40 gm protein is permitted, with gradual increases to a normal intake as renal function improves.[1] Losses into the dialysate must be replaced for those on peritoneal or hemodialysis.[3]

Fluid. The fluid allowance is regulated in accordance with the urinary output, any additional losses from vomiting or diarrhea, and an allowance for insensible water losses. During the oliguric phase, the fluid permitted is less than 600 ml daily for nondialyzed patients.[4] In the diuretic phase that follows accurate measurement of urinary output is essential so that appropriate fluid replacement can be made.

Potassium. The potassium allowance is individualized in accordance with serum levels and whether or not the patient is being dialyzed.

Sodium. The dietary sodium allowance is based on frequent measurements of the ion in serum and urine. For the nondialyzed patient in the oliguric phase, restriction of sodium to 500 to 1,000 mg daily is usually necessary. Patients on dialysis are permitted a more liberal sodium intake, 1,500 to 2,000 mg daily.

Chronic Renal Failure In chronic renal failure symptoms appear when the glomerular filtration rate (GFR) is inadequate to excrete nitrogenous wastes. When the GFR is less than 10 ml per minute (normal 120 ml per minute) and the blood urea nitrogen (BUN) is more than 80 mg per 100 ml (normal 8 to 18 mg per cent), dietary modifications usually bring about improvement in symptoms. Patients in whom the BUN is only mildly elevated usually do not experience symptoms and, therefore, dietary restrictions may not be needed. When the GFR falls to less than 3 ml per minute, dietary control alone is inadequate and dialysis is necessary.

Symptoms involving the gastrointestinal tract are often present in chronic renal failure and are especially trying because of the discomfort associated with them and the constant interference with food intake. The sight or smell of food may bring about nausea or vomiting. The breath has an ammoniacal odor that interferes with the taste of food. Ulcerations of the mouth and hiccups also interfere with food intake.

The nervous system is usually affected. Patients are irritable or drowsy and eventually sink into coma. Headache, dizziness, muscular twitchings, neuritis, and even failing vision occur, especially if there is also hypertension.

The functioning of the heart is seriously disturbed. Congestive failure occurs when the heart failure is associated with retention of sodium and water. Death results when HYPERKALEMIA (elevated serum potassium) blocks the contraction of the heart.

Many alterations in metabolic and endocrine function occur in end-stage renal disease. Patients with terminal uremia have a progressively worsening anemia. There is interference with the clotting mechanism, the capillaries are fragile, ulcerations in the gastrointestinal tract may lead to bleeding, the life span of the red cells is reduced, hemolysis occurs readily, and hematopoiesis is reduced. Because the anemia reduces the effective exchange of oxygen and carbon dioxide at the tissues and in the lungs, fatigue and weakness are ever present.

When the GFR falls to 25 ml per minute, the serum phosphorus level is elevated and hypocalcemia occurs. Parathyroid hormone secretion is increased to compensate for the elevated phosphorus. This hormone decreases the reabsorption of phosphorus by the kidney and increases calcium resorption from bone. In spite of elevated parathyroid hormone production phosphorus accumulates and hypocalcemia results. Besides the secondary hyperparathyroidism induced by the disturbed calcium and phosphorus metabolism, there is RENAL OSTEODYSTROPHY. This term is used to encompass osteomalacia, other bone deformities, and deposition of calcium in soft tissues. The kidney is unable to convert 25-hydroxy vitamin D-3 to its active form, 1,25-dihydroxy vitamin D-3, so that calcium absorption from the intestine is decreased. (See Chapter 10 and Figure 10–6.) Excess fluoride may also play a role in the bone demineralization seen in uremia.[5] Hyperglycemia and impaired glucose tolerance occur possibly due to peripheral insulin insensitivity and an increase in hormones antagonistic to insulin.[6] Elevation of serum triglycerides (Type IV hyperlipoproteinemia) is frequent and may increase the risk of premature cardiovascular disease. About half of all deaths in patients on long-term hemodialysis are due to atherosclerotic vascular disease.[7] Excessive hepatic synthesis of triglycerides may be a consequence of insulin resistance. Deficient lipolysis may also be a factor in the hypertriglyceridemia. As the function of the kidneys further deteriorates, hyperkalemia and acidosis become increasingly severe, and edema is marked. Progressive weakness, itching, and jaundice occur. Mental disorientation, severe gastrointestinal symptoms, bleeding, and coma are characteristic of the final stages.

Nutritional Assessment Ongoing assessment of nutritional status is essential in patients with chronic renal failure because of the wasting and malnutrition seen in many patients. In addition to the usual anthropometric and biochemical parameters discussed in Chapters 22 and 24, determinations of the serum urea nitrogen to serum creatinine ratio and the urinary urea nitrogen excretion are useful in determining optimal protein intake.

Dialysis

In the management of end-stage renal disease, whether acute or chronic, dialysis is often used on a temporary or permanent basis. In *hemodialysis* the patient's blood circulates outside the body through coils or sheets of semipermeable membranes that are constantly bathed by a hypotonic dialyzing fluid so that the nitrogenous wastes are removed into the dialysate. The membranes do not permit bacteria to enter the blood nor can proteins escape from the blood. However, some amino acids are lost into the dialysate.

Although hemodialysis is a lifesaving measure, the patient does not return to a full normal life. He or she must be attached to a dialyzer for perhaps 18 hours each week. With dialysis for 4 to 6 hours three times weekly, blood urea levels that range from 100 to 170 mg per 100 ml fall to 20 to 40 mg per 100 ml. Dialysis does not eliminate the need for dietary control, however. Between dialyses nitrogenous end products, potassium, and sodium accumulate. If the diet is uncontrolled, dialysis will need to be more frequent. Since the artificial kidney does not correct the endocrine failure of the kidneys, most of the patients have severe anemia and hypertensive disease.

Dialysis and the associated diet require a great deal of the patient in terms of emotional stability, motivation, and intelligence. Those who are under 21 years especially resent the program, and those between 21 and 41 years seem to adapt best to the program. If home dialysis is used, the husband or wife, father or mother, or other relative or friend is trained to operate the dialyzer, and must also be able to provide moral support to the patient. Other considerations such as the scarcity of the equipment and the great cost limit the program to only a small number of those who could benefit.

Peritoneal dialysis. This consists of introducing 1 to 2 liters of dialysis fluid into the peritoneal cavity and 30 to 90 minutes later withdrawing the fluid. The process is repeated until the blood urea level drops to tolerable levels.

Some blood proteins (10 to 44 gm per dialysis period) as well as amino acids are lost through peritoneal dialysis and compensation must be made for this loss in order to avoid severe hypoproteinemia.

In 1972, Medicare coverage became available for more than 90 per cent of patients with end-stage renal disease. By 1979, approximately 50,000 patients were participating in the program at a cost exceeding $1 billion.[8]

General Dietary Considerations in Chronic Renal Failure

Present-day management of the diet in chronic renal disease is based on the principles outlined by Giordano[9] and Giovannetti[10] in the early 1960s. These investigators found that essential amino acid requirements could be met by providing diets containing limited amounts of high-biologic-value protein such as egg and milk. Other protein-containing foods were sharply restricted. Such a diet provides a minimum of nonessential amino acids, theoretically enabling the patient to utilize accumulated urea nitrogen for protein synthesis. Subsequent studies by others have shown that recycling of urea is only a minor source of nitrogen for protein synthesis.[11] Nevertheless, such diets are accompanied by lowering of the blood urea nitrogen level and symptomatic improvement. Simultaneous provision of adequate nonprotein calories is essential to enhance protein utilization and to prevent endogenous protein catabolism. Restriction of fluids, sodium, potassium, and phosphorus are also employed.

A number of suitable diets have been developed utilizing the principles just described. In general, all of these aim for provision of adequate calories, regulation of protein, sodium, potassium, and fluid intake, restriction of phosphate, and supplements of calcium, iron, trace minerals, ascorbic acid, and the B vitamins.

Energy. The importance of adequate calories cannot be overemphasized, for without an adequate calorie intake body tissues will be rapidly catabolized, thus increasing the blood urea and potassium levels beyond the capacity of the kidney to excrete them. For adults, caloric needs range from 35 to 45 kcal per kilogram of ideal body weight,[1] or about 2,000 to 3,000 kcal per day. Carbohydrates are the main source of calories and should be ingested simultaneously with the protein so that the protein will not be utilized for energy. High-carbohydrate supplements that are protein free and low in electrolytes can greatly increase caloric intake if accepted by the patient.* In addition, a high-calorie supplement containing the essential amino acids plus histidine is available.† Many products made from low-protein wheat starch are suitable.‡

Protein. The optimal level of protein intake in advanced renal failure is not known. Some evidence indicates that 0.6 gm protein per kilogram of body weight is associ-

* Controlyte® by Doyle Pharmaceutical Co., Minneapolis, Minnesota; Cal-Power by General Mills, Inc., Minneapolis, Minnesota; Hycal by Beecham-Massengill Pharmaceuticals, Melrose, Massachusetts.

† Amin-aid by McGaw Laboratories, Santa Ana, California.

‡ Aproten Pasta by Henkel Corporation, Minneapolis, Minnesota.

ated with improved nitrogen balance and a greater sense of well-being in nondialyzed uremic patients than are more restricted intakes.[12] Use of a low-protein diet (less than 30 gm) plus essential amino acids is associated with improved nitrogen utilization in renal failure.[13] Hemodialysis patients need at least 1.0 gm protein per kilogram body weight daily to compensate for losses of amino acids in the dialysate. Some recommend 1.2 gm protein per kilogram with additional supplements during complications such as bleeding or infection; or 1.0 gm protein per kilogram plus 0.2 gm per kilogram of high biological value protein or essential amino acids per dialysis.[14] In peritoneal dialysis greater protein losses into the dialysate increase the protein requirement to 1.0–1.5 gm per kilogram.[15] Children on dialysis need 1.5 to 2.0 gm high biologic value protein per kilogram per day.[16] Generally, the aim is to provide about three fourths of the protein allowance as high-biologic-value protein.

Carbohydrate and fat. Type IV hyperlipoproteinemia is common in patients with chronic renal disease. Elevated serum triglycerides can be lowered by controlling carbohydrate intake, restriction of dietary cholesterol, and increasing the intake of polyunsaturated fat. (See Chapter 39.) In two studies with renal patients, effective lowering of serum lipids was achieved with diets that differed substantially in carbohydrate and fat content but which had a polyunsaturated to saturated fat ratio of 1.1 or more, 300 mg or less of cholesterol, and carbohydrate not more than 50 per cent of calories.[17,18]

Potassium. Excess or deficiency of potassium is detrimental to the patient, but in chronic renal failure hyperkalemia is the rule. The potassium allowance is individualized in accordance with the patient's blood chemistries, urinary output, and the amount of potassium in the dialysate. For nondialyzed patients, potassium intake is generally limited to 1,500 to 2,000 mg, depending somewhat on the protein allowance. The upper limit permitted for hemodialysis patients is 2,700 mg, or 70 mEq.[3] In peritoneal dialysis, 75 to 90 mEq or 3.0 to 3.5 gm is used.[15] Foods high in animal protein are usually high in potassium and many fruits and vegetables must be sharply limited or excluded from the diet because of their high potassium content. Kayexalate,* a potassium-binding agent is often prescribed in addition to dietary potassium restriction.

Sodium. Dietary sodium intake depends on amounts in serum and urine. Restriction is often needed because of edema, hypertension, and threat of congestive heart failure. Nondialyzed patients who are hypertensive may be permitted less than 1 gm sodium, 40 mEq, daily; those who are depleted of sodium need to increase their intake to about 2 gm daily (90 mEq).[19] Patients on hemodialysis are usually permitted intakes of 1.5 to 2.0 gm (65 to 85 mEq), whereas those on peritoneal dialysis receive 2 to 3 gm (85 to 130 mEq).[1,15] The sodium allowance in children is 50 mg per kilogram per day.[16]

Other minerals. Blood levels of phosphorus gradually increase in the uremic patient, thus contributing to the acidosis and also to metastatic calcification. Early restriction of phosphorus to 600 to 750 mg per day, calcium supplements, 1.5 to 2.0 gm daily, along with vitamin D supplements, 300,000 to 600,000 I.U. twice weekly, are used to prevent hyperparathyroidism.[20] Dairy products are restricted because of their high phosphorus content, thereby lowering the calcium content of the diet. Aluminum hydroxide gel is often prescribed to bind some of the phosphate in the intestinal tract, thereby reducing the absorption. Concern over use of this drug has arisen because aluminum is absorbed and is believed to contribute to dialysis dementia, a lethal degeneration of the central nervous system.[8] Diet alone cannot meet

* Kayexalate, by Winthrop Laboratories, New York, New York.

the iron and trace mineral requirements; supplements should be prescribed.

Vitamins. Losses of ascorbic acid and many of the B vitamins occur during dialysis. In addition, intake of these vitamins is likely to be low because raw fruits and vegetables are restricted and because foods may be cooked in large volumes of water to reduce the potassium content. Folic acid and pyridoxine requirements may be increased because of antagonistic effects of drug therapy. Impaired vitamin D metabolism occurs because the nonfunctioning kidney cannot convert the vitamin into its active form. Supplements of all of these vitamins are needed.

Fluids. Rigid control of fluid intake is necessary to prevent excess fluid retention. The daily allowance is usually 400 to 600 ml for nondialyzed patients and less than 1,000 ml for those on dialysis. Weight gain of about 1 pound per day for patients on dialysis is permitted.

Controlled Protein, Sodium, Potassium and Phosphorus Diet

Food Lists A number of dietary regimens have been described for the control of protein, potassium, and sodium. Each of these is based upon food groupings in which the foods within a given list are of approximately the same protein, potassium, and sodium value. Food choices for daily menus can therefore be made from a given group in the amounts specified. Generally speaking, the broad food groupings used in the various regimens are similar, but they differ in the specific foods included and the portion sizes, depending upon the criteria used in setting them up. For example, oranges are relatively high in potassium and are omitted from some lists; they are included in other lists in controlled amounts because of their popular appeal, their relatively low cost, and their content of ascorbic acid. Potatoes are excluded in some lists but included in others, provided that they are prepared by methods to minimize their potassium content. When the directions for the use of any of these regimens are explicitly followed any one of them will lead to satisfactory results.

Dietitians, nurses, and physicians must be aware of the many factors that modify the sodium and potassium content of foods. Actual diet contents may be higher or lower than published values. The methods of food preparation significantly modify the electrolyte levels. Those factors that enter into

Table 41-1. **Protein, Sodium, Potassium, and Phosphorus Values for Food Lists**

Food List	Household Measure	Weight gm	Protein gm	Sodium* mg	Potassium mg	Phosphorus mg
Milk	1 cup	240	8	120	350	245
Meat or substitute	1 ounce	30	7	25	100	65
Vegetables						
Group I	½ cup	100	1	5–10	110–190	15–20
Group II	½ cup	100	2	2–10	120–185	30–35
Group III	½ cup	100	3	15	175	50
Fruits						
Group I	½ cup	100	tr	1–3	100–185	10–15
Group II	½ cup	100	1	2	115–210	15–20
Bread or substitute	Varies	Varies	2		30	30
Fats	Varies	Varies	—	—	—	—

*Except for milk, the values listed for sodium are those that apply when no salt is used in processing or preparation of the food. Also, certain high-sodium items in the meat and vegetable lists would be omitted for diets restricted in sodium.

Table 41–2. **Food Selection for Controlled Protein, Sodium, Potassium, and Phosphorus Diets**

Food List	Measure	Protein			
		20 gm	40 gm	60 gm	70 gm
Milk, whole or skim	1 cup	3/4	1	1	1
Meat or substitute	1 ounce	1	3	5	6
Vegetable, Group I	1/2 cup	2	2	2	3
Fruit, Group I	1/2 cup	3	3	3	3
Group II	1/2 cup	—	—	—	1
Bread or substitute	Exchange	1	3	5	6
Low-protein bread	Slice	5	—	—	—
Low-protein beverage	1 cup	1	1	1	1
Low-protein cookies	Each	2	2	2	2
Fat	Exchange	Ad lib	Ad lib	Ad lib	Ad lib
Jelly, sweets	Varies	Ad lib	Ad lib	Ad lib	Ad lib

the sodium content of foods have been discussed in Chapter 40. With respect to potassium, considerable leaching out occurs when foods are cooked in large volumes of water. The amount lost to the water is greater if food is cut into small pieces.

One dietary regimen for these controlled diets is described in detail in the pages that follow. Table 41–1 lists the composition of the food groups that follow. Table 41–2 indicates the food allowances for four levels of protein. Each of these plans must be individualized according to the patient's caloric requirement, the nutritional status, and the level of biochemical control.

The 20-gm- and 40-gm-protein diets are used only for patients whose renal function has deteriorated so much that they are no longer able to avoid the gastrointestinal and other symptoms of renal failure, and who are not being dialyzed. These diets should be supplemented with B-complex vitamins, calcium, iron, vitamin D, and trace minerals.

Dietary Counseling

IMPORTANCE OF ADEQUATE GUIDANCE Dietary treatment in renal failure, with or without dialysis, is an integral part of therapy. Although the dietary modification cannot lead to improvement in kidney function, it can do much toward alleviation of uncomfortable symptoms that interfere with adequate food intake. The rigid controls required make this diet as complex as any that can be prescribed. Particularly at 20- and 40-gm-protein levels, the diet lacks much in palatability, especially if sodium restriction is also severe, and the level of motivation of the patient and those who care for him or her must be high.

Many hours of dietary instruction are required for the patient and for those who will prepare the food at home. The counseling started in the hospital must be continued either in the out-patient clinic or by home visitation.

WHAT THE PATIENT NEEDS TO KNOW Each patient needs to know why the diet is important, and what risks will be encountered if he or she fails to follow the diet. The patient must understand that it is important to include the exact amounts of high-quality protein foods that have been prescribed. Likewise he or she needs to know the importance of eating sufficient quantities of low-protein low-electrolyte foods so that body weight is maintained and tissue catabolism does not take place.

High-calorie foods such as sugars, jams, honey, hard candies, butter, or margarine should be used. Patients must be reminded frequently to make liberal use of these items. Growth failure is a common problem in children on dialysis whose calorie intake is inadequate.[21]

There must be a thorough familiarity with

the food lists and the amounts of foods that may be used from each. Some practice in planning the daily meals from these lists is essential. If special products such as wheat starch are needed, the patient must be told where they can be purchased, and how much they will cost. Recipes for the use of these special products are needed together with precautions to take in food preparation.

FOOD PREPARATION The extraction of gluten from wheat flour yields a low-protein wheat starch that is also practically electrolyte free. Several sources of recipes using wheat starch are listed at the end of this chapter. With sodium and potassium restriction yeast must be used as a leavening agent; regular leavening agents are too high in sodium, and low-sodium leavening agents are too high in potassium. Breads and other products made from wheat starch do not have the same texture as those made from wheat flour because of the absence of the elastic gluten. Some patients find the bread more acceptable when toasted, or served with butter and jelly or jam, or prepared as cinnamon toast or French toast.

If potatoes are allowed they should be cut into small pieces and boiled in a large volume of water. Following this they may be pan fried with some of the fat or mashed with part of the milk and fat allowance. Meats that are simmered in a large volume of water also lose some of their potassium to the cooking liquid. Of course, these cooking procedures also result in greater losses of the water-soluble vitamins and of some other mineral elements.

Canned fruits are used, for the most part, instead of fresh raw fruits. Since part of the potassium has leached out into the syrup, only the solid fruit should be used.

Salt substitutes containing potassium are prohibited since they contain as much as 60 mEq, or about 2,350 mg, per teaspoon.[22]

Food Lists for Controlled Protein, Sodium, Potassium, and Phosphorus Diets*

Milk List
1 cup equals 8 gm protein, 350 mg potassium, 245 mg phosphorus
Evaporated milk, reconstituted
Nonfat dry milk, reconstituted
Skim milk
Whole milk
Yogurt

Foods to Avoid
Commercial foods made of milk:
- Chocolate milk
- Condensed milk
- Ice cream
- Malted milk
- Milkshake
- Milk mixes
- Sherbet

Meat or Substitute List
1 ounce cooked equals 7 gm protein, 100 mg potassium, 65 mg phosphorus
Beef, chicken, duck, lamb, liver, pork, tongue (unsalted), turkey, veal

Cod, flatfish (flounder and sole), kingfish (whiting), haddock, perch; canned salmon and tuna (omit on sodium-restricted diet)
Clams, crab, lobster, oysters, scallops, shrimp (all omitted on sodium-restricted diet)

Foods to Avoid
Brains, kidneys
Canned, salted, or smoked meats as: bacon, bologna, chipped beef, corned beef, frankfurters, ham, kosher meats, luncheon meats, salt pork, sausage, smoked tongue
Frozen fish fillets
Canned, salted, or smoked fish: anchovies, caviar, cod (dried and salted), herring, halibut, sardines, salmon, tuna

Meat or Substitute List

Egg (1 egg equals 7 gm protein, 60 mg potassium, 90 mg phosphorus)

Cheese (1 ounce equals 7 gm protein, 25 mg potassium, 280 mg phosphorus), Cheddar, cottage, American, Swiss

Foods to Avoid

Omit on sodium-restricted diets

Vegetable List, Group I

1 gm protein, 110 mg potassium, 15 mg phosphorus per serving

½ cup servings of raw cabbage, cucumber, lettuce, onion, tomato

Vegetable List, Group IA

1 gm protein, 125 mg potassium, 25 mg phosphorus per serving

½ cup servings of canned green or wax beans, carrots (+), spinach (+); fresh cooked cabbage, eggplant, mustard greens, onion, summer squash

Foods to Avoid

All items marked (+) if diet is sodium restricted
Artichokes
Beans, baked
Beans, dried
Beans, Lima
Beet greens
Broccoli, fresh
Brussels sprouts
Carrot, raw
Celery, raw
Chard
Endive, raw
Parsnips
Peas
Potato in skin, or frozen
Sauerkraut
Spinach, fresh or frozen
Squash, baked winter

Vegetable List, Group 1B

The following may be used for diets with liberal potassium allowance:

1 gm protein, 190 mg potassium, 20 mg phosphorus per serving

½ cup servings of canned beets (+), rutabagas, tomatoes; fresh cooked carrots (+), turnips (+); frozen summer squash, winter squash

Vegetable List, Group II

2 gm protein, 120 mg potassium, 30 mg phosphorus per serving

½ cup servings of canned asparagus; fresh or frozen green or wax beans, okra

Vegetable List, Group IIA

The following may be used for diets with liberal potassium allowance:

2 gm protein, 185 mg potassium, 35 mg phosphorus per serving

½ cup servings of fresh or frozen cauliflower; cooked dandelion greens (+); potato, boiled (pared before cooking) or mashed

Vegetable List, Group III
3 gm protein, 175 mg potassium, 50 mg phosphorus per serving
½ cup servings of kale (+); frozen asparagus, broccoli, collards (+), mixed vegetables (+), whole kernel corn

Fruit List, Group I
Less than 0.5 gm protein, 100 mg potassium, 10 mg phosphorus per serving
Apple, raw, 1 small
Grapes, European, 12
½ cup servings of canned applesauce, pears, pineapple; watermelon (diced)
½ cup of these juices: apple, grape, peach nectar, pear nectar, orange-apricot, pineapple-grapefruit, pineapple-orange

Foods to Avoid
All dried and frozen fruits with sodium sulfite added
Apricots, fresh
Avocado
Bananas
Glazed fruits
Maraschino cherries
Nectarines
Prunes
Raisins

Fruit List, Group IA
The following may be used for diets with liberal potassium allowance:
Less than 0.5 gm protein, 185 mg potassium, 15 mg phosphorus per serving
½ cup servings of apricot nectar, pineapple juice; canned fruit cocktail, peaches, purple plums

Fruit List, Group II
1 gm protein, 115 mg potassium, 15 mg phosphorus per serving
Pear, raw, 1 small
Tangerine, 1 small
½ cup servings of fresh or frozen blackberries, blueberries, boysenberries; canned cherries, figs; canned or fresh grapefruit; frozen red raspberries

Fruit List, Group IIA
The following may be used for diets with liberal potassium allowance:
1 gm protein, 210 mg potassium, 20 mg phosphorus per serving
Orange, 1 small
Peach, raw, 1 small
Plums, fresh, 2 medium
Strawberries, fresh, ⅔ cup
½ cup servings of cantaloupe, honeydew, frozen melon balls, fresh or frozen rhubarb
½ cup of these juices: grapefruit, grapefruit-orange, orange, tomato

Avoid tomato juice if diet is sodium restricted

Breads and Substitutes

2 gm protein, 30 mg potassium, 30 mg phosphorus per serving

Bread, 1 slice

Cereals, dry, 1 cup

Cornflakes, Puffed Rice, Puffed Wheat, Shredded Wheat

Cereals, cooked, ½ cup

cornmeal, farina, oatmeal, rice, rolled wheat

Crackers, soda, 3 squares

Flour, 2 tablespoons

Grits, 1 cup

Macaroni, noodles, or spaghetti, ¼ cup

Rice, ½ cup

Foods to Avoid

Yeast breads or rolls or melba toast made with salt or from commercial mixes

Quick breads made with baking powder, baking soda, or salt, or made from commercial mixes

Commercial baked products

Dry cereals except as listed

Self-rising cornmeal

Graham or other crackers except low-sodium dietetic

Self-rising flour

Salted popcorn

Potato chips

Pretzels

Waffles containing salt, baking powder, baking soda, or egg white

Fats

Negligible protein, potassium, and phosphorus content

Butter

Cream, light or heavy (1 ounce contains 35 mg potassium, 20 mg phosphorus)

Fat or cooking oil

Margarine

Salad dressings: French or mayonnaise

Foods to Avoid

Salted fats on sodium-restricted diets

Avocado

Bacon, bacon fat

Olives

Nuts

Salt pork

Miscellaneous

Cornstarch

Flavoring extracts (see list, page 653)

Ginger ale

Hard candies

Herbs (see list, page 653)

Honey

Jam or jelly

Jellybeans

Rice starch

Spices (see list, page 653)

Sugar, white, confectioners'

Syrup

Tapioca, granulated

Vinegar

Wheat Starch

Foods to Avoid

Antacids, laxatives

Bouillon, broth

Canned, dried, frozen soups

Chocolate

Cocoa, instant cocoa mixes

Coconut

Consommé

Fruit-flavored powders and prepared beverage mixes

Fountain beverages

Commercial candies except as listed

Commercial gelatin desserts

Regular baking powder and soda

Rennet tablets

Molasses

Pudding mixes

Peanut butter

Most carbonated beverages

Seasonings to Avoid
Catsup, celery leaves, celery salt, chili sauce, garlic salt, prepared horseradish, meat extracts, meat sauces, meat tenderizers, monosodium glutamate, prepared mustard, onion salt, pickles, relishes, salt, and salt substitutes, soy sauce, Worcestershire sauce

* Adapted from *Nutrition Care Manual,* Yale-New Haven Medical Center; The Hospital of St. Raphael, New Haven, Conn.; West Haven Veteran's Administration Medical Center; and Waterbury Hospital Health Center, 1979.

Diet Following Renal Transplantation Following successful renal transplantation most of the previous dietary restrictions are no longer needed. Mild sodium restriction (see Chapter 40) is usually necessary because prolonged administration of steroids favors fluid retention. Other side effects of long-term immunosuppressive therapy such as obesity, diabetes mellitus, and atherosclerosis may make further dietary modifications necessary.

Hypokalemia

Occurrence Although the emphasis in the preceding discussion has been upon the problems of elevated levels of blood potassium, there are renal and extrarenal circumstances in which the plasma or serum level of potassium is below 3.3 mEq per liter. One situation in which this occurs is by dilution of the extracellular fluid volume. This results when the fluid intake exceeds the ability of the kidney to excrete it as in oliguria and anuria. The total amount of the ion in the extracellular fluid remains the same, but the concentration is lowered because of the expanded volume.

In the diuretic stage of nephritis, the kidneys do not conserve potassium as effectively as normal, and potassium depletion occurs, especially if the intake is low because of a poor appetite. Adrenocortical steroids and many diuretics are likely to accentuate the renal losses of potassium.

Hypokalemia also occurs when there is rapid uptake of potassium by the cells. Growth, cellular repair, cellular dehydration, glycogen formation, and administration of glucose and insulin in diabetic acidosis promote entrance of potassium into the cell. In dehydration and in the correction of diabetic acidosis emergency measures are required to replace the extracellular potassium.

Excessive losses of potassium occur with vomiting, diarrhea, and gastrointestinal drainage. Unless these losses are replaced the plasma levels are often lowered to dangerous levels.

Treatment If hypokalemia is severe, the correction will require the parenteral administration of potassium-containing fluids. This is followed by therapy with potassium-containing syrups and emphasis on foods that are rich in potassium. When the appetite is good, any varied diet will supply a considerable amount of potassium. A few foods that are especially good sources of potassium include orange juice, tomato juice, milk, baked potato, and banana. Most salt substitutes contain substantial amounts of potassium (10 to 12 mEq per gram) and can increase the potassium intake considerably.[22]

Urinary Calculi

Nature of Calculi Urinary CALCULI (kidney stones) may be found in the kidney, ureter, bladder, or urethra. They consist of an organic matrix with interspersed crystals and vary in size from fine gravel to large stones.

About 90 per cent of all stones contain calcium as the chief cation. More than half the stones are mixtures of calcium oxalate and magnesium ammonium phosphate. Uric acid stones account for about 10 per cent of renal stones in the United States.[23] Xanthine stones are extremely rare. Cystine stones are unique in that they are often pure and are a hereditary defect.

Incidence and Etiology The incidence of renal calculi in the United States is not known. One study reported annual rates of 36 per 100,000 in women from 1950 to 1974. In men the incidence during this period rose from 78.5 to 123.6 per 100,000 population.[24]

In Thailand, India, and Turkey (known as stone belts) bladder stones are a common occurrence in children, especially small boys. Most of these are urate and oxalate stones and their cause is unknown. The incidence of bladder stones in adults is high in Syria, Bulgaria, India, China, Madagascar, and Turkey, but low in Africa. The reasons for these geographic variations are not known.

Renal calculi are more prevalent in sedentary people than in those who are active. No dietary relationship has been established, but kidney dehydration may be a factor and more fluid intake and exercise are urged as prophylaxis.

The formation of stones is more probable in the presence of urinary tract infections, during periods of high urinary excretion of calcium, in certain gastrointestinal disorders, following intestinal bypass surgery, and in disorders of cystine, oxalate, or uric acid metabolism. High urinary excretion of calcium occurs in hyperparathyroidism, following overdosage with vitamin D, in long periods of immobilization, in osteoporosis, or following excessive ingestion of calcium and of absorbable alkalies. Ascorbic acid intakes in excess of 4 gm per day may induce formation of calcium oxalate stones.[23] In disorders involving fat malabsorption and especially after intestinal bypass surgery, an excess of fatty acids in the intestinal lumen binds available calcium, thereby decreasing the calcium available to bind oxalate. Increased absorption of oxalate from the bowel and subsequent hyperoxaluria may contribute to stone formation.

Rationale of Treatment When the cause of urinary calculi is known, the physician can effectively direct treatment toward the correction of the disorder. For example, this might entail the treatment of an infection, or modification of the regimen for peptic ulcer, or avoidance of long immobilization. However, in a large percentage of urinary calculi, the cause is not known or the disorder is not easily corrected.

The solubility of salts may be increased and the tendency to stone formation minimized by means of acidifying or alkalinizing agents which increase or decrease the pH of the urine. Such treatment implies that the nature of the stones has been determined by laboratory analyses of the stones themselves or by appropriate urine and blood studies.

Modification of urine pH. When stones are composed of calcium and magnesium phosphates and carbonates, therapy is directed toward maintaining an acid urine. On the other hand, if oxalate and uric acid stones are being formed, the urine should be kept alkaline. Acidifying or alkalinizing agents are more effective than dietary modification, although the diet should support the therapy by medications.

Binding agents are often used to reduce the absorption of calcium and phosphorus from the gastrointestinal tract. Aluminum hydroxide gel is sometimes prescribed since it combines with phosphate to form an insoluble aluminum phosphate and thus diminishes the absorption of phosphorus and the subsequent formation of insoluble precipitates in the urinary tract. Sodium acid phosphate or sodium phytate similarly reduces the absorption of calcium.

Modification of the Diet No diet of itself is effective in bringing about solution of stones already formed. However, for the predisposed individual it is thought that diet may be of some value in retarding the growth of stones or preventing their recurrence, although the effectiveness of such prophylaxis has not been fully established.

A liberal fluid intake is essential—3,000 ml or more daily—to prevent the production of a urine at a concentration where the salts precipitate out. The patient should be impressed with the importance of taking fluids throughout the day, so that the urine dilution is maintained.

Calcium restriction. Increased calcium excretion occurs in some patients who form calcium oxalate stones. For these patients, fluid intake of 2,500 ml per 24 hours and reduction of calcium intake to 600 mg or less daily reduces the hypercalciuria and may prevent stone formation.[25] (See Table 41-3.) Patients who form calcium oxalate stones but in whom there is not hypercalciuria probably are not benefitted by restriction of dietary calcium alone. Reduced calcium intake enhances oxalate absorption and increases the urinary oxalate level. Thus, if calcium is restricted, dietary oxalate should also be restricted.[26] Elemental phosphorus, 2 gm per day, is useful in inhibiting the growth of crystals.

Oxalate restriction. Oxalate restriction in combination with calcium supplements and a fat-restricted diet is useful in decreasing the hyperoxaluria and calcium oxalate stones associated with fat malabsorption in small bowel disorders.[26, 27] Oxalate-rich foods include green and wax beans, beets and beet greens, chard, endive, okra, spinach, sweet potatoes; currants, figs, gooseberries, Concord grapes, plums, rhubarb, raspberries; almonds, cashew nuts; chocolate, cocoa, tea.

Other dietary modifications. When an acid-ash diet is prescribed, acid producing

Table 41-3. **Calcium-Restricted Diet**

Include These Foods Daily*		Protein gm	Fat gm	Carbohydrate gm	Calcium mg
Milk	1 cup	8	10	12	290
Egg	1 whole	7	5	—	25
Meat, fish, poultry	6 ounces	42	30	—	20
Vegetables:					
Potato	1 small	2	—	15	15
Leafy or yellow	½ cup	2	—	5	25
Other	½ cup	2	—	5	25
Fruits:					
Citrus	½ cup	—	—	10	30
Other	2 servings	—	—	20	25
Cereal, refined, without added calcium	2 servings	4	—	30	5
Bread, refined, without added calcium	6 slices	12	—	90	20
Fats	2 tablespoons	—	30	—	—
Sugars, sweets	2 tablespoons	—	—	30	—
		79	75	217	480

*Protein, fat, and carbohydrate values on the basis of meal exchange lists, Table A-4. Calcium values have been rounded off to the nearest 5 mg. Values for vegetables, fruits, cereals, and breads are averages of those permitted. Individual selections vary somewhat from these averages.

Calcium-Restricted Diet

Characteristics and General Rules

The diet provides a maintenance level of calcium. Milk constitutes the main source of calcium in the diet. (See Table 41–3.)

When further restriction of calcium is desired, the milk and egg may be eliminated. The calcium level is then reduced to 165 mg and the protein level to 64 gm.

Foods Allowed	Foods to Avoid
Beverages—milk in allowed amounts; coffee, tea	*Beverages*—chocolate; cocoa; fountain beverages; proprietary beverages containing milk powder
Breads—French or Italian without added milk; pretzels; saltines, matzoth; water rolls	*Breads*—biscuits; breads: brown, corn, cracked wheat, raisin, rye, white with nonfat dry milk, whole-wheat; rye wafers; muffins; pancakes; waffles
Cereals—cornflakes, corn grits, farina, rice, rice flakes, Puffed Rice; macaroni, noodles, spaghetti; cornmeal, cornstarch, tapioca, white flour	*Cereals*—bran, bran flakes, corn and soy grits, oatmeal, wheat flakes, wheat germ, Puffed Wheat, Shredded Wheat; rye flour, soybean flour, self-rising flour, whole-wheat flour
Cheese—½ ounce Cheddar or Swiss cheese may be used instead of ½ cup milk	
Desserts—angel cake, white sugar cookies, gelatin, fruit pies, fruit tapioca, fruit whip, pudding with allowed milk and egg, shortbread, water ices	*Desserts*—cakes and cake mixes, custard, doughnuts, ice cream, Junket, pies with cream filling or milk and eggs, milk puddings—except when daily allowance is used
Eggs—1 whole. Whites as desired	
Fats—butter, cooking oils and fats, lard, margarine, French dressing	*Fats*—mayonnaise, sweet and sour cream
Fruits—all, but restricting dried fruits to dates (3), prunes (2), raisins (1 tbsp.)	
Meats—beef, ham, lamb, pork, veal; chicken, duck, turkey; bluefish, cod, haddock, halibut, scallops, shad, swordfish, tuna	*Meats*—clams, crab, herring, lobster, mackerel, oyster, fish roe, salmon, sardines, shrimp; brains, heart, kidney, liver, sweetbreads
Milk—1½ cups daily	
Soups—broth of allowed meats; consommé; cream soups using allowed milk	*Soups*—cream in excess of milk allowance; bean, lentil, split pea
Sweets—sugar, syrup, jam, jelly, preserves, hard candy, marshmallows, mints without chocolate	*Sweets*—caramels, fudge, milk chocolate, molasses, dark brown sugar
Vegetables—artichokes, asparagus, beans—green or wax, Brussels sprouts, cabbage, carrots, cauliflower, corn, cucumber, eggplant, escarole, lettuce, onions, peppers, potatoes—white and sweet, pumpkin, radishes, romaine, squash, tomatoes, turnips	*Vegetables*—dry beans: kidney, Lima, navy, pea, soybean; beet greens, broccoli, chard, collards, chickpeas, dandelion greens, kale, okra, parsnips, peas—fresh and dried—rutabagas, soybeans, soybean sprouts, spinach, turnip greens, watercress
Miscellaneous—pickles, mustard, salt, spices	*Miscellaneous*—chocolate, cocoa, nuts, olives, brewers' yeast

Sample Menu

BREAKFAST

Fresh raspberries
Cornflakes
Milk—½ cup
Soft-cooked egg
Toasted Italian bread
Butter or margarine
Apple jelly
Coffee

LUNCHEON OR SUPPER

Cold sliced turkey
Potato salad (potato, diced cucumber, minced green pepper and onion, French dressing) on lettuce; tomato wedges
Italian bread
Butter or margarine
Angel cake with fresh strawberries
Milk—1 cup only

DINNER

Roast pork
Buttered noodles
Zucchini squash
Hard rolls, made without milk
Butter or margarine
Fruit gelatin
Tea with lemon

foods (see Table 41–4) are emphasized. Only 1 pint of milk, two servings of fruit, and two servings of vegetables are permitted.

On the other hand, for an alkaline-ash diet fruits and vegetables are used liberally, and the acid-producing foods are restricted to the amounts necessary for satisfactory nutrition.

The formation of uric acid stones may

Table 41-4. Acid-Producing, Alkali-Producing, and Neutral Foods

Acid Producing	Alkali Producing	Neutral
Bread, especially whole-wheat	Milk	Butter
Cereals	Fruits	Candy, not chocolate
Cheese	Vegetables	Coffee
Corn		Cornstarch
Crackers	*Especially these*	Fats, cooking
Cranberries	Almonds	Honey
Eggs	Apricots, dried	Lard
Lentils	Beans, Lima, navy	Salad oils
Macaroni, spaghetti, noodles	Beet greens	Sugar
Meat, fish, poultry	Chard	Tapioca
Pastries	Dandelion greens	Tea
Peanuts	Dates	
Plums	Figs	
Prunes	Molasses	
Rice	Olives	
Walnuts	Parsnips	
	Peas, dried	
	Raisins	
	Spinach	
	Watercress	
	Foods prepared with baking powder or baking soda	

be minimized by using a purine-restricted diet (see Chapter 38) and restricting the protein intake to 1 gm per kilogram body weight.

A protein-restricted diet reduces the intake of sulfur-containing amino acids but has not been shown to be effective in the prevention of cystine stones.

Problems and Review

1. What are the parts of the nephron? How do these parts function?
2. What are the chief wastes excreted by the kidney?
3. In addition to excreting wastes, what other functions are performed by the kidney?
4. What are the characteristic symptoms of acute glomerulonephritis? In what way do these symptoms affect dietary planning?
5. In what way do the abnormal excretion products in renal diseases affect dietary planning?
6. *Problem.* Outline the principles for a dietary regimen for a patient with acute glomerulonephritis, showing the progression of diet from time to time.
7. *Problem.* On the basis of the principles outlined in problem 6, write a menu for a patient for 1 day. Assume that the diet order restricts protein to 40 gm and sodium to 1,000 mg.
8. What reasons can you give for using a protein-free, high-carbohydrate, high-fat diet in acute renal failure? Why are frequent small feedings preferable to three meals?
9. What is accomplished by dialysis with an artificial kidney? Why is a diet restricted in protein and potassium necessary?
10. What problems are you likely to encounter in planning a potassium-restricted diet?
11. *Problem.* Write a menu for 1 day for a 20-gm controlled protein, sodium, and potassium diet, using the plan in Table 41–2 and the food lists on pages 669 to 673. What foods can you suggest that would increase the caloric intake without increasing the protein and potassium levels?
12. What is meant by hypokalemia? Under what circumstances is it likely to occur? What foods could you suggest for increasing the potassium intake of a patient who has a poor appetite?
13. Why is a calcium-restricted diet often prescribed for certain patients with urinary calculi? What is the purpose of using a binding agent with such a diet?
14. Under what circumstances would an acid-ash diet be used? An alkaline-ash diet?
15. List some of the factors that contribute to hypocalcemia seen in chronic renal failure.

Cited References

1. Burton, B. T.: "Current Concepts of Nutrition and Diet in Diseases of the Kidney. II. Dietary Regimen in Specific Kidney Disorders," *J. Am. Diet. Assoc.*, **65**:627–33, 1974.
2. Kark, R. M., and Oyama, J. H.: "Nutrition, Hypertension and Kidney Diseases," in *Modern Nutrition in Health and Disease*, 6th ed., R. S. Goodhart and M. E. Shils, eds. Lea & Febiger, Philadelphia, 1980, pp. 998–1044.
3. Kopple, J. D.: "Nutritional Management of Chronic Renal Failure," *Postgrad. Med.*, **64**:135 ff., November 1978.
4. Lemann, J.: "Acute Renal Failure," *Am. Fam. Physician*, **18**:146–56, September 1978.

5. Rao, T. K. S., and Friedman, E. A.: "Fluoride and Bone Disease in Uremia," *Kidney Internatl.*, **7**:125–29, 1975.
6. Frohlich, J. et al.: "Carbohydrate Metabolism in Renal Failure," *Am. J. Clin. Nutr.*, **31**:1541–46, 1978.
7. Frank, W. M. et al.: "Relationship of Plasma Lipids to Renal Function and Length of Time on Maintenance Hemodialysis," *Am. J. Clin. Nutr.*, **31**:1886–92, 1978.
8. Kolata, G. B.: "Dialysis After Nearly a Decade," *Science*, **208**:473–76, 1980.
9. Giordano, C.: "Use of Exogenous and Endogenous Urea for Protein Synthesis in Normal and Uremic Subjects," *J. Lab. Clin. Med.*, **62**:231–46, 1963.
10. Giovannetti, S., and Maggiore, Q.: "A Low Nitrogen Diet with Proteins of High Biological Value for Severe Chronic Uremia," *Lancet*, **1**:1000–3, 1964.
11. Furst, P. et al.: "Principles of Essential Amino Acid Therapy in Uremia," *Am. J. Clin. Nutr.*, **31**:1744–55, 1978.
12. Ritz, E. et al.: "Protein Restriction in the Conservative Management of Uremia," *Am. J. Clin. Nutr.*, **31**:1703–11, 1978.
13. Bauerdick, H. et al.: "Therapy with Essential Amino Acids and Their Nitrogen-Free Analogues in Severe Renal Failure," *Am. J. Clin. Nutr.*, **31**:1793–96, 1978.
14. Kluthe, P. et al.: "Protein Requirements in Maintenance Hemodialysis," *Am. J. Clin. Nutr.*, **31**:1812–20, 1978.
15. Blumenkrantz, M. J. et al.: "Nutritional Management of the Adult Patient Undergoing Peritoneal Dialysis," *J. Am. Diet. Assoc.*, **73**:251–56, 1978.
16. Holliday, M. A. et al.: "Nutritional Management of Chronic Renal Disease," *Med. Clin. North Am.*, **63**:945–62, 1979.
17. Gokal, R. et al.: "Dietary Treatment of Hyperlipidemia in Chronic Hemodialysis Patients," *Am. J. Clin. Nutr.*, **31**:1915–18, 1978.
18. Sanfelippo, M. L. et al.: "Response of Plasma Triglycerides to Dietary Change in Patients on Hemodialysis," *Kidney Internatl.*, **14**:180–86, 1978.
19. Anderson, C. F. et al.: "Nutritional Therapy for Adults with Renal Disease," *JAMA*, **223**:68–72, 1973.
20. Maschio, G. et al.: "Early Dietary Phosphorus Restriction and Calcium Supplementation in the Prevention of Renal Osteodystrophy," *Am. J. Clin. Nutr.*, **33**:1546–54, 1980.
21. Holliday, M. A., and Chantler, C.: "Metabolic and Nutritional Factors in Children with Renal Insufficiency,"*Kidney Internatl.*, **14**:306–12, 1978.
22. Spoko, J. A., and Freeman, R. M.: "Salt Substitutes as a Source of Potassium," *JAMA*, **238**:608–10, 1977.
23. Bleich, H. L., and Boro, E. S.: "Metabolic Basis of Renal-Stone Disease," *New Engl. J. Med.*, **300**:839–45, 1979.
24. Johnson, C. M. et al.: "Renal Stone Epidemiology: A 25 Year Study in Rochester, Minnesota," *Kidney Internatl.*, **16**:624–31, 1979.
25. Smith, L. H. et al.: "Nutrition and Urolithiasis," *New Engl. J. Med.*, **298**:87–89, 1978.
26. Wilson, D. M.: "Medical Treatment of Urolithiasis," *Geriatrics*, **34**:65 ff., August 1979.
27. Miller, R. L., and O'Leary, J. P.: "Nephrolithiasis Following Small Bowel Bypass: Pathogenesis and Treatment," *Am. Surgeon*, **44**:779–84, 1978.

Additional References

BLUMENKRANTZ, M. J. et al.: "Methods for Assessing Nutritional Status of Patients with Renal Failure," *Am. J. Clin. Nutr.*, **33**:1567–85, 2765, 1980.

CHANTLER, C. et al.: "Nutritional Therapy in Children with Chronic Renal Failure," *Am. J. Clin. Nutr.*, **33**:1682–89, 1980.

DAVIS, M. et al.: "Dietary Management of Patients with Diabetes Treated by Hemodialysis," *J. Am. Diet. Assoc.*, **75**:265–69, 1979.

GUARNIERI, G. et al.: "Simple Methods for Nutritional Assessment in Hemodialyzed Patients," *Am. J. Clin. Nutr.*, **33**:1598–1607, 1980.

HARVEY, K. B. et al.: "Nutritional Assessment and Treatment of Chronic Renal Failure," *Am. J. Clin. Nutr.*, **33**:1586–97, 1980.

SANDSTEAD, H. H.: "Trace Elements in Uremia and Hemodialysis," *Am. J. Clin. Nutr.*, **33**:1501–8, 1980.

WALSER, M.: "Does Dietary Therapy Have a Role in the Predialysis Patient?" *Am. J. Clin. Nutr.*, **33**:1629–37, 1980.

Instructional Materials for the Patient

COST, J. S.: *Dietary Management of Renal Disease.* Charles B. Slack, Inc., Thorofare, N. J., 1975.

Diet Guide for Patients on Chronic Dialysis. National Institutes of Arthritis, Metabolism, and Digestive Diseases, Bethesda, Md., 1975.

MARGIE, J. D. et al.: *The Mayo Clinic Renal Diet Cookbook.* Golden Press, New York, 1975. (Distributed by the National Kidney Foundation.)

Recipes for Protein-Restricted Diets. The Doyle Pharmaceutical Company, Minneapolis.

42 Nutrition in Neurologic Disturbances

KETOGENIC DIET

Nutrition and the Nervous System

The nervous tissues, like other tissues of the body, require energy for metabolic functions, protein for cell synthesis, vitamins as components of the enzyme systems, and mineral elements as activators of metabolic reactions and to maintain homeostasis of the fluid environment. The following discussion presents a brief summary of the principal effects of nutrient lack upon the functioning of the nervous system.

Energy. The brain normally utilizes glucose exclusively as its source of energy. To shut off the supply of glucose and oxygen from the brain for even a few minutes leads to irreversible damage. The body at rest utilizes up to 25 per cent of its total oxygen consumption for the brain alone.[1]

Protein. The influence of amino acid imbalances on mental development are dramatically illustrated by the severe mental retardation that accompanies inborn errors of metabolism. These are fully discussed in Chapter 44.

In recent years much research on experimental animals and on humans has shown that severe protein deficiency during pregnancy and during the first year of life especially can lead to profound alterations in brain development. Severe undernutrition is associated with deficits in physical, psychological, and intellectual capacities and has long-lasting effects on behavior. The retardation of development is accentuated when infection is also present. Although much evidence has been presented that implicates nutrition, it is exceedingly difficult to separate the effects of malnutrition from the economic, educational, emotional, and social deprivation that are simultaneously present. See also pages 420 to 424 for further discussion of protein-calorie malnutrition.

Vitamins. Deficiencies of the water-soluble vitamins bring about serious changes in functioning of the nervous system. (See Chapter 12.) Thiamin deficiency is characterized by reduced tendon reflexes, peripheral neuritis, incoordination of gait, muscle pains, irritability, inability to concentrate, lack of interest in affairs, and personality deterioration including hypochondriasis, depression, and hysteria.[2]

Classic niacin deficiency, pellagra, is rarely seen in the United States. Its neurologic signs include poor memory, irritability, dizziness, hallucinations, delusions of persecution, and finally dementia.

Vitamin B-6 deficiency is characterized by weakness, ataxia, and convulsions. Pantothenic acid lack leads to mental depression, peripheral neuritis, sullenness, cramping pains in the arms and legs, and burning sensations of the feet. Irritability and forgetfulness are seen in folic acid deficiency. The inability to absorb vitamin B-12 because of lack of intrinsic factor is the condition known as pernicious anemia, which presents such symptoms as unsteady gait, depression, and mental deterioration. (See Chapter 30.)

Nutrition for the Mentally Ill

Feeding Older Persons in Nursing Homes

Weiner[3] has described four categories of pathologic-psychological reactions in aging persons in nursing homes: anxiety, depression, suspicion, and confusion. In some individuals all of these may be present to a varying degree or they may appear one after the other. Each type of reaction requires specific measures in feeding.

The anxious person requires assurance that everything is all right. This individual worries about the effects that foods may have on bowel function and often asks questions about which foods are constipating. Worry about food may increase gastrointestinal motility so that the person has cramps or may reduce motility so that he or she becomes distended. The anxious person needs to be comforted, to have someone around, to be made to feel secure, and to be given special consideration by being served favorite foods as often as possible.

The depressed individual feels that his or her situation is hopeless and has a conscious or unconscious desire to die. Reassurance only frightens the person more and he or she will continue to demand more and more of it until there seems to be no end to the demands. Such individuals need external control and should be told firmly exactly what they must do, that they must eat, that they will be taken care of, and that they will be helped to eat what they need for their nourishment. Sometimes spoon feeding is needed to get them started. It is not advisable for these individuals to choose their own menu.

The suspicious person is afraid of being hurt and often suspects that the food is poisoned. Such persons feel that they must constantly be on watch lest something happens to their security. Efforts to reassure them to the contrary only increase their suspicions. Matter-of-factly they should be told that there is nothing wrong with the food, but it may be necessary for the attendant to taste the food in their presence to show that it is not poisoned. The suspicious person, unlike the depressed person, must not be forced to eat. He or she should be allowed to eat or not to eat what is presented.

The confused person has usually had some brain damage as in a stroke, from diabetic or hepatic coma, or from head injury. This individual does not know what is happening around him or her and often becomes anxious, depressed, or suspicious. Such persons may not know where they are, and regardless of what they are told they believe themselves to be in their own home as adults or in their childhood home. They need help in understanding what is going on around them. With respect to feeding, they need to be told that it is mealtime, what meal it is, and what foods are on the tray. When a favorite food is served, it is a good idea to specially identify it.

Diet for Patients in the Mental Hospital The relationship of nutrition to mental disorders has intrigued some researchers for years—since the discovery early in the century that a substantial number of patients in mental hospitals suffered from pellagra-associated dementia which could be corrected with niacin. Out of this interest has grown the field of *orthomolecular psychiatry* which advocates use of pharmacologic doses of vitamins as an adjunct to traditional therapy in treatment of mental disorders. Megadoses of niacin along with other B vitamins, ascorbic acid, and certain minerals and specific drug therapy have been advocated for use in treatment of schizophrenia. However, controlled studies have failed to show significant clinical improvement with this treatment in schizophrenia.[4] Most traditional psychiatrists reject the hypothesis that megavitamins have therapeutic value in treatment of mental disorders.

An association between schizophrenia and celiac disease has been proposed based on the increased probability of celiac disease in schizophrenics and of schizophrenia in patients with celiac disease. Schizophrenic patients treated with a milk- and cereal-free diet have reportedly shown improvement of symptoms which was reversed when gluten was added to the diet.[5,6] Further controlled studies are needed to test this hypothesis.

Although a therapeutic role for specific

dietary factors has not been clearly established in psychiatric disorders, diet is nevertheless an important part of the total program of rehabilitation for the psychiatric patient. Aside from its nutritional necessity, food provides basic security and pleasurable satisfaction. The patient needs to feel that someone is genuinely concerned about his or her welfare and cares for him or her. The dietitian and nurse—through the care shown in meal planning, preparation, and service, and through their expressions of interest to the individual—are participants in the therapy.

Planning a nutritionally adequate diet is obviously not enough. The service of food that is attractive to the eye, tempting in aroma, and satisfying to the palate is just as important in the psychiatric hospital as in any other feeding situation. The mentally ill may express marked irritability when given foods they dislike. Food service in a cafeteria permits the patient to exercise some choice in food selection, and thus helps to eliminate some of the irritations. On the other hand, staff-shared family-style meal service is favored by some and permits opportunity for closer rapport between staff and patients.

Patients react favorably and are less destructive when an attractive dining environment is provided. A well-planned dining room with a cheerful color scheme, curtains or draperies at the windows, small attractive tables, and suitable background music is conducive to food acceptance and contributes to the therapy of the patient. Attention to birthdays, holidays, and other special events provides additional evidence that the patient is cared for.

Psychiatric patients frequently eat inadequate or excessive amounts of food. A regular schedule of weighing of patients—about once a month—will help to detect such changes, and correction can be started before marked weight change has occurred. Marked weight gain is not uncommon. It would seem easy to control this in a hospital by providing a diet designed for weight maintenance. However, the privileges of food purchases from a canteen and food gifts from relatives and friends must be taken into consideration. Patients are often known to eat food left by other patients.

Refusal to eat is a problem presented by other psychiatric patients. The nurse or attendant should note any patient who refuses more than half of a meal. A 4- or 5-day simple checklist helps to identify whether the refusal follows a pattern with respect to a particular food or meal. Refusal of food sometimes denotes an underlying physical illness about which the patient who is withdrawn or mute does not complain. Those who need to gain weight may require close supervision in taking small, frequent feedings; some may be helped if butter is spread on the bread, milk and sugar are put on the cereal, the milk container is opened, the meat is cut, and so on; sincere words of encouragement should be offered when progress is made. Tube feeding (see Chapter 36) may be resorted to when all attempts to achieve satisfactory intake of food fail.

Feeding the mentally retarded presents many problems which may be especially acute in the child. The management of the diet for these patients is discussed in Chapter 45.

Anorexia Nervosa

Anorexia nervosa is a psychiatric disorder seen primarily in females with onset usually occurring in early adolescence. Most patients are from middle- and upper-class families. Epidemiological studies suggest an increased incidence of the disorder in recent years.[7] It is characterized by extreme weight loss, even to the point of emaciation, as a consequence of refusal to eat. Some authorities specify a weight loss of at least 25 per cent for the diagnosis of anorexia nervosa.[8] Mortality rates in hospitalized patients range from 5 to 20 per cent in various series. The individual often has a history of being "chubby" as a youngster. An overriding desire to lose weight leads to self-imposed starvation, bizarre food habits, self-induced vomiting, hyperactivity, laxative abuse, and so on as means of preventing weight gain. The individual usually is able to carry on normal school and social activities while denying hunger and fatigue. Amenorrhea, constipation, cold intolerance, hypotension, and bradycardia are characteristic findings. Anemia is not a common feature; serum iron and folate levels are normal. Hypercarotenemia is common. Plasma zinc, copper, and total iron-binding capacity are reduced.[9] The clinical signs and symptoms are reversible with weight gain.

Treatment Ultimately, individual and family psychotherapy is needed to resolve the basic conflict. For some individuals, short-term intervention as tube feeding or total parenteral feeding is needed to prevent death by starvation. Various means have been used to induce the patient to eat. One approach uses a contract between patient and therapist, in which privileges accorded the patient depend on achievement of a predetermined weight gain each day. Failure to gain the expected amount of weight results in suspension of privileges and use of supplemental feedings or tube feedings until the desired weight gain is reached. Behavior modification is used in conjunction with other therapies.

Hyperkinesis

The relationship between hyperactivity in children and certain food dyes has been the subject of much controversy since the mid-1970s. The hypothesis relating hyperactivity to food intake holds that the behavior of a large proportion of learning disabled or hyperactive children will improve when artificial food colors or flavors are omitted from the diet.[10] Results of several short-term studies indicate that only a small proportion of such children show improvement in behavior when fed the modified diet. In the majority, stimulant medications are more effective in controlling behavior.[11] In most studies objective criteria for judging behavioral improvement are lacking, thus making interpretation of results more difficult. Nevertheless, most studies do not support the hypothesis that artificial food colors and flavors are the cause of the behavioral disturbance.

Alcoholism

For about 9 million Americans chronic alcoholism severely affects health, job security, and family life.[12] Only about one fourth of these seek any kind of treatment. In the United States from 10 to 15 per cent of hospitalized patients have alcohol-related illnesses. Alcohol is a significant factor in approximately half of the highway fatalities each year in this country.[13] The American Academy of Pediatrics has expressed concern over the trend toward increased consumption of alcohol, and its related problems, in adolescents. Lowering of the drinking age and use of alcohol as an alternative to hard drugs have been cited as factors contributing to increased use.[14] Clearly, alcohol abuse is a major public health problem that must be considered in its physiologic, psychological, economic, and social aspects.

Alcohol and Metabolism Alcohol is considered to be a food in that it yields 7 kcal per gram; however, it does not provide any nutrients to speak of. Alcohol is rapidly and almost completely absorbed. The presence of food in the stomach, as is well known, delays gastric absorption. However, from the small intestine absorption is rapid regardless of whether food is present or not.

Upon absorption alcohol is dispersed rapidly throughout the body water. Less than 10 per cent of the alcohol absorbed is eliminated by way of the kidneys and lungs; the rest is oxidized chiefly in the liver. When present, alcohol becomes the preferred fuel for the liver, displacing up to 90 per cent of other substrates normally utilized by the liver.[15] The products of oxidation in the liver are hydrogen and acetaldehyde. (See Chapter 5 for a description of the pathways of alcohol oxidation.) Chronic alcohol intake produces a functional disturbance of the mitochondria so that further oxidation of acetaldehyde is reduced. The increases in NADH/NAD ratio and acetaldehyde account for a number of alterations in carbohydrate, lipid, and protein metabolism: elevated levels of lactic acid which lead to acidosis and decreased renal excretion of uric acid, hypoglycemia resulting from impaired gluconeogenesis, triglyceride accumulation, fatty liver, impaired protein secretion, and in some instances, depressed protein synthesis.[15]

Effects of Alcohol on Nutrition In the stomach, alcohol disrupts the mucosal barrier, increases acid secretion, and delays emptying. Alcohol-induced chronic pancreatitis interferes with secretion of bicarbonate and enzymes, resulting in impaired digestion of protein and fats. Alcohol has a direct toxic effect on the liver and its profound effects on carbohydrate, protein, and lipid metabolism have already been described. Altered bile salt metabolism further interferes with fat digestion and may result in steatorrhea. Effects of alcohol on the small intestine include inhibition of mucosal enzyme activities, interference with absorption of actively transported substances, increased motility, impaired vitamin B-12 absorption, and interference with folate metabolism. Urinary losses of amino acids, magnesium, potassium, and zinc are increased during periods of drinking. Symptoms of *delirium tremens* have been associated with severe hypomagnesemia.

Alcohol also exerts indirect effects on nutritional status through altered intakes of calories, vitamins, and minerals. Excessive or deficient intake of these substances is manifested as obesity or wasting; hypervitaminosis A and niacin "intoxication" or deficiencies of folacin and thiamin; iron overload or chronic deficiencies of magnesium, zinc, and potassium.[16]

Only about 20 per cent of alcoholics develop liver damage. Fatty infiltration is the most common change. With subsequent damage to the liver cells, alcoholic hepatitis occurs. About half of these patients develop alcoholic cirrhosis. (See Chapter 34.)

Diet for Alcoholics Alcohol reduces the appetite so that the heavy drinker eats poorly. Moreover, the chronic alcoholic often does not have the money to purchase an adequate diet inasmuch as he or she may be out of a job and spends what money he or she has for alcohol. A diet that meets normal nutritional requirements will restore the nutritional status of the alcoholic. When there is evidence of vitamin deficiencies, a supplement, especially of water-soluble factors, is indicated. It is a fallacy, however, that vitamin deficiencies are an etiologic factor in alcoholism, or that the correction of these deficiencies will cure the alcoholic.

When hepatitis or cirrhosis is present, the dietary modifications described on pages 565 to 567 should be considered. The possibility of hepatic coma and the need for drastic protein restriction when it occurs must always be kept in mind.

Nurses and dietitians can help the alcoholic return to better health by considering food habits, by encouraging him or her to eat, and by providing dietary counseling. No useful purpose is served by assuming a critical, moralizing posture either by what one says or by one's attitude.

Wernicke's and Korsakoff's Syndromes Wernicke's syndrome and Korsakoff's psychoses are associated with alcoholism and appear to be different phases of the same disease. Wernicke's syndrome is characterized by ophthalmoplegia (paralysis of the eye muscles), ataxia (uncoordinated gait), and mental confusion. Nystagmus (rapid movement of the eyeballs) is a prominent feature. The patient is often unable to stand or walk without support. The eye changes are dramatically corrected, often within hours, by the administration of thiamin.

Korsakoff's syndrome may not be apparent until several weeks after the changes in the eye and gait have become evident. The chief defect is the disturbance in memory and the inability to learn new things so that only the most routine tasks can be performed. Moreover, there is failure to associate past events in their proper sequence. Patients may be confused, anxious, fearful, and even delirious. Vitamin therapy has produced marked effects in restoring the patient to being responsive, alert, and attentive. However, when memory defects are present, they appear to persist despite therapy, suggesting that structural changes in the brain may be irreversible.

Epilepsy

The Nature of Epilepsy Epilepsy is a disease of the central nervous system characterized by loss of consciousness which may last for only a few seconds, as in petit mal attacks, or which may be accompanied by convulsions, as in grand mal attacks. It occurs more frequently in children than in adults. The disease in no way affects the individual's mental ability, but unthinking relatives and friends sometimes attach an entirely unwarranted stigma to the disease and thus may increase the tension states in the individual.

Treatment Various drugs such as phenobarbital or phenytoin sodium or others have been employed with considerable success in the treatment of epilepsy and have largely replaced the ketogenic diet once so widely used. As a rule, a normal diet for the individual's age and activity is prescribed when drug therapy is used. Folate deficiency, anemia, and osteomalacia have been attributed to use of these drugs.[17] Gastric distress associated with valproic acid therapy can be minimized by giving the drug with meals.

Some individuals with minor motor seizures and petit mal epilepsy who do not respond to drug therapy have been successfully managed with a ketogenic diet. The purpose of the diet is to produce ketosis by limiting very severely the amount of available glucose and increasing markedly the intake of fat so that complete combustion of fats cannot take place. Plasma ketones (acetone, acetoacetic acid, and beta-hydroxybutyric acid) gradually rise as glycogen stores become depleted. The accumulation of ketone bodies has a favorable effect on the irritability and restlessness of the child and does not dull the mental function as some drugs do. Preschool-age children seem to benefit most, presumably because higher plasma ketone levels can be achieved with the diet in this age group than in older children.[18] A rapid reversal of the anticonvulsant effect occurs when even small amounts of carbohydrate are ingested, and leads to seizures as the plasma ketones fall.

Some of the difficult features of the diet are that it permits selection from only a very limited list of foods, is severely restricted in carbohydrate, is unpalatable, lacks bulk, deviates sharply from customary food patterns, and requires great care in planning and preparation. A careful evaluation of the probable success of the diet for each patient and the ability of the parents to understand and adhere to the regulations is essential.

Modification of the Diet Sufficient calories for normal weight and for the maintenance of normal growth are necessary. The allowances recommended by Mike[19] are

Age (years)	kcal per kg
2–3	100 to 80
3–5	80 to 60
5–10	79 to 55

Protein. An allowance of 1 gm protein per kilogram of body weight is sufficient, but may be increased to 1.5 gm per kilogram for the older child.

Carbohydrate and fat. The nonprotein calories are so divided that a ketogenic to antiketogenic ratio of approximately 3 to 1 or 4 to 1 is maintained. Ketogenic factors (fatty acids) in the diet include 90 per cent of the fat, and about 50 per cent of the protein. The antiketogenic factors in the diet (available glucose) are derived from 100 per cent of the carbohydrate, plus approximately 50 per cent of the protein and 10 per cent of the fat. Obviously, to achieve a 3-to-1 or 4-to-1 ratio, the carbohydrate must be sharply restricted and the fat intake greatly increased. The level of carbohydrate usually needs to be less than 30 gm if ketosis is to be produced, but should never be less than 10 gm daily.

The diet for a 5-year-old child weighing 25 kg illustrates the calculation of a diet prescription.

1. Kcal: $25 \times 70 = 1750$
2. Protein: $25 \times 1 = 25$ gm
3. Kcal from protein: $25 \times 4 = 100$
4. Kcal from carbohydrate and fat: $1750 - 100 = 1650$

If we allow 25 gm carbohydrate, the fat intake would need to be 172 gm as noted in the following calculations:

5. Kcal from carbohydrate: $25 \times 4 = 100$
6. Kcal from fat: $1{,}650 - 100 = 1{,}550$
7. Grams of fat: $1{,}550 \div 9 = 172$

The fatty acid to glucose ratio of this diet is as follows:

$$\frac{FA}{AG} = \frac{0.50(25) + 0.9(172)}{0.50(25) + 0.1(172) + 1.0(25)} = \frac{167}{55} = \frac{3}{1}$$

The maintenance of a constant acidosis requires that the protein, fat, and carbohydrate for the day be divided in three equal meals. The urine shows a positive test for acetoacetic acid when acidosis is being maintained.

Minerals and vitamins. Calcium gluconate or lactate is prescribed to furnish calcium. An iron supplement providing 7 to 10 mg elemental iron is also given. The vitamin needs are met by giving an aqueous multivitamin preparation.

Management of the Diet For the first 24 to 72 hours the child is given nothing but water, usually restricted to 500 to 1,000 ml. Hunger disappears as ketosis increases. When ketosis is marked the diet is initiated, but is not forced until the transition has been accomplished. During this period nausea and vomiting may occur.

The diet may be calculated by using the values for individual foods as in Table A-1, or by using food groupings such as those developed by Mike[19] or Lasser.[20] The meal exchange lists are not satisfactory for the calculation. The predominant foods in the diet are carefully restricted amounts of meat, cheese, and eggs; cream, butter, bacon, mayonnaise; restricted amounts of low-carbohydrate vegetables and fruits. Other foods are avoided: sugar-containing beverages; breads and cereals; desserts such as cake, cookies, ice cream, pastries, pie, puddings; milk; all sweets including sugar, jellies, candy, preserves; vegetables and fruits high in carbohydrate.

The diet must be weighed on a gram scale and all food must be consumed at each meal. Foods may not be saved for later consumption. If no improvement occurs within 6 weeks, there is nothing to be gained by further continuance of the diet. If improvement does occur, the diet must be continued for a year or longer. Gradually the diet is liberalized with very small increases in the carbohydrate and corresponding caloric decreases in the fat. Table 42–1 illustrates a sample calculation for the ketogenic diet.

Signore[21] has described a ketogenic diet using medium-chain triglycerides. Inasmuch as medium-chain triglycerides are more ketogenic than conventional food fats, more carbohydrate is permitted on this diet. Foods need not be weighed.

Table 42-1. **Sample Calculation for Ketogenic Diet***

Food	No. of Units	Household Measure	Weight gm	Protein gm	Fat gm	Carbohydrate gm
Breakfast						
Orange juice	4	⅙ cup	40	—	—	4.0
Canadian bacon	6	¾ slice	21	6.0	3.0	—
Whipping cream	2½	½ cup	115	2.5	42.5	3.8
Cellu wafers						
Butter	2	2¼ teaspoons	12	—	10.9	—
Apricot spread (Cellu)	½	1 teaspoon	5	—	—	0.5
				8.5	56.4	8.3
Luncheon or Supper						
Beef, lean	6	⅔ ounce	21	6.0	3.0	—
Tomato, raw	1	¼ small	25	0.2	—	1.0
Whipping cream	2½	½ cup	115	2.5	42.5	3.8
Peach, raw	3	⅓ small	30	—	—	3.0
Butter	2	2¼ teaspoons	12	—	10.9	—
Cellu wafers						
Blackberry jelly (Cellu)	½	1 teaspoon	5	—	—	0.5
				8.7	56.4	8.3
Dinner						
Cheddar cheese	5	⅔ ounce	20	5.0	5.0	—
Strawberries	4	4 large	40	—	—	4.0
Whipping cream	2½	½ cup	115	2.5	42.5	3.8
Butter	2	2¼ teaspoons	12	—	10.9	—
Cellu wafers						
Apricot spread (Cellu)	½	1 teaspoon	5	—	—	0.5
				7.5	58.4	8.3
Total for the day				(24.7)	(171.2)	(24.9)
(Prescribed order)				(25.0)	(172.0)	(25.0)

$$\frac{\text{Ketogenic factors}}{\text{Antiketogenic factors}} = \frac{166.4}{54.4} = 3.1$$

*Based on plan described by Lasser, J. L., and Brush, M. K.: "An Improved Ketogenic Diet for Treatment of Epilepsy," *J. Am. Diet. Assoc.*, **62**:281–85, 1973.

Problems and Review

1. Describe the development of the nervous system in relation to other factors in growth and development of the young child.
2. What is the principal source of energy for the brain? What proportion of oxygen consumption is required by the brain?
3. Why would you expect vitamin deficiencies to have an adverse effect on the functioning of the nervous system? Describe the changes that take place in deficiency of thiamin; of vitamin B-6.
4. What is the effect of alcoholism on the nutritional state of the individual? How can you explain some of the symptoms characteristic of Wernicke's syndrome?

5. What are some of the meanings of food that may have special relevance to the mentally ill? What recommendations could you make for the feeding of the mentally ill?
6. What is anorexia nervosa? What role does dietary therapy have in treatment?
7. What is epilepsy? What is the rationale for a ketogenic diet for the treatment of epilepsy? Why is the diet seldom used?
8. *Problem.* Modify the diet calculated in Table 42–1 so that it provides a ketogenic-antiketogenic ratio of 3.5 to 1.
9. *Problem.* List some ways in which the whipping cream and butter may be used in the ketogenic diet. What purpose is served by the Cellu wafers?

Cited References

1. Horwitt, M. K.: "Nutrition in Mental Health," *Nutr. Rev.*, **23**:289–91, 1965.
2. Brozek, J.: "Psychologic Effects of Thiamine Restriction and Deprivation in Normal Young Men," *Am. J. Clin. Nutr.*, **5**:109–18, 1957.
3. Weiner, M. F.: "A Practical Approach to Encouraging Geriatric Patients to Eat," *J. Am. Diet. Assoc.*, **55**:384–86, 1969.
4. Kety, S. S.: "Dietary Factors and Schizophrenia," *Ann. Intern. Med.*, **84**:745, 1976.
5. Singh, M. M., and Kay, S. R.: "Wheat Gluten as a Pathogenic Factor in Schizophrenia," *Science*, **191**:401–2, 1976.
6. Dohan, F. C. et al.: "Relapsed Schizophrenics: More Rapid Improvement on a Milk- and Cereal-free Diet," *Brit. J. Psychiatry*, **115**:595–96, 1969.
7. Rohde, J. et al.: "Diagnosis and Treatment of Anorexia Nervosa," *J. Fam. Pract.*, **10**:1007–12, 1980.
8. Feighner, J. P. et al.: "Diagnostic Criteria for Use in Psychiatric Research," *Arch. Gen. Psychiatry*, **26**:57–63, 1972.
9. Casper, R. C. et al.: "An Evaluation of Trace Metals, Vitamins, and Taste Function in Anorexia Nervosa," *Am. J. Clin. Nutr.*, **33**:1801–8, 1980.
10. Feingold, B. F.: "Hyperkinesis and Learning Disabilities Linked to Artificial Food Flavors and Colors," *Am. J. Nurs.*, **75**:797–803, 1975.
11. Williams, J. I. et al.: "Relative Effects of Drugs and Diet on Hyperactive Behavior: An Experimental Study," *Pediatrics*, **61**:811–17, 1978.
12. Comprehensive Alcohol Abuse and Alcoholism Prevention, Treatment and Rehabilitation Act Amendments, 1973. Hearings before Subcommittee on Alcoholism and Narcotics. 93rd Congress. 1st Session. March 13–16, 1973.
13. "Alcohol: A Growing Danger," *WHO Chronicle*, **29**:102–5, 1975.
14. American Academy of Pediatrics: "Alcohol Consumption: An Adolescent Problem," *Pediatrics*, **55**:557–59, 1975.
15. Lieber, C. S.: "Alcohol, Protein Metabolism, and Liver Injury," *Gastroenterology*, **79**:373–90, 1980.
16. Roe, D. A.: "Nutritional Concerns in the Alcoholic," *J. Am. Diet. Assoc.*, **78**:17–21, 1981.
17. Hooshmand, H.: "Toxic Effects of Anticonvulsants: General Principles," *Pediatrics*, **53**:551–56, 1974.
18. Huttenlocher, P. R.: "Ketonemia and Seizures: Metabolic and Anticonvulsant Effects of Two Ketogenic Diets in Childhood Epilepsy," *Pediatr. Res.*, **10**:536–40, 1976.
19. Mike, E. M.: "Practical Guide and Dietary Management of Children with Seizures Using the Ketogenic Diet," *Am. J. Clin. Nutr.*, **17**: 399–405, 1965.
20. Lasser, J. L., and Brush, M. K.: "An Improved Ketogenic Diet for Treatment of Epilepsy," *J. Am. Diet. Assoc.*, **62**:281–85, 1973.
21. Signore, J. M.: "Ketogenic Diet Containing Medium-Chain Triglycerides," *J. Am. Diet. Assoc.*, **62**:285–90, 1973.

Additional References

BRUYA, M. A., and BOLIN, R. H.: "Epilepsy: A Controllable Disease. Classification and Diagnosis of Seizures," *Am. J. Nurs.*, **76**:388–92, 1976.

CISEAUX, A.: "Anorexia Nervosa. A View from the Mirror," *Am. J. Nurs.*, **80**:1468–70, 1980.

CLAGGETT, M. S.: "Anorexia Nervosa. A Behavioral Approach," *Am. J. Nurs.*, **80**:1471–72, 1980.

COHEN, S.: "The Pharmacology of Alcohol," *Postgrad. Med.*, **64**:97–100, 102, December 1978.

COOPER, C. R.: "Anticonvulsant Drugs and the Epileptics Dilemma," *Nursing*, **6**:45–50, January 1976.

COULTER, D. et al.: "Valproic Acid Therapy in Childhood Epilepsy," *JAMA*, **244**:785–88, 1980.

HYLANDS, J.: "The Wernicke-Korsakoff Syndrome," *Nursing*, **9**:26–29, July 1979.

KORSTEN, M. A., and Lieber, C. S.: "Nutrition in the Alcoholic," *Med. Clin. North Am.*, **63**:963–72, 1979.

LINDENBAUM, J.: "Folate and Vitamin B_{12} Deficiencies in Alcoholism," *Semin. Hematol.*, **17**:119–29, 1980.

MASSEY, E. W. et al.: "Managing the Epileptic Patient," *Postgrad. Med.*, **67**:134–43, February 1980.

PATEK, A. J.: "Alcohol, Malnutrition, and Alcoholic Cirrhosis," *Am. J. Clin. Nutr.*, **32**:1304–12, 1979.

PENRY, J. K., and PORTER, R. J.: "Epilepsy: Mechanisms and Therapy," *Med. Clin. North Am.*, **63**:801–12, 1979.

DROSSMAN, D. A. et al.: "Anorexia Nervosa," *Gastroenterology*, **77**:1115–31, 1979.

RUSSELL, R. M.: "Vitamin and Mineral Supplements in the Management of Liver Disease," *Med. Clin. North Am.*, **63**:537–44, 1979.

43 Diet in Allergic and Skin Disturbances

ELIMINATION DIETS

MORE than one in six persons in the United States or some 35 million persons, suffer from some form of allergy. This high incidence of allergic diseases is an important health and economic problem in terms of days lost from work and school. Food allergies account for a relatively small proportion of all allergies, but allergies to major food groups present serious problems in meal planning and in adequate nutrition. Moreover, many people who suffer from nonfood allergies find it difficult to ingest an adequate diet—the individual with severe asthma, for example.

Definition Terms commonly used to describe an adverse reaction to foods include food allergy, hypersensitivity, sensitivity, and intolerance. Strictly speaking, these terms are not synonymous. Food ALLERGY or HYPERSENSITIVITY denotes an adverse immunologic response to a specific substance with characteristic symptoms whenever the food is ingested. Food SENSITIVITY is a slightly broader term applied to conditions in which an abnormal reaction occurs following ingestion of specific foods and in which an immunologic etiology is likely, but not proven. Food INTOLERANCE, on the other hand, does not involve an immunologic mechanism, and may be due to an enzyme deficiency or other factors.[1] In food allergy, symptoms are produced within minutes or a few hours following ingestion of the food and the reaction occurs whenever the food is ingested. In food sensitivity or intolerance symptoms may occur hours or days after ingestion of the food substance, and the condition tends to improve spontaneously or following a period of elimination of the food.

The substance responsible for initiation of the allergic reaction is an ALLERGEN or ANTIGEN. It is usually a protein, but may be a polysaccharide, or a substance that binds to a protein to form a complex which becomes the active allergen. The reaction may be brought about by (1) *ingestion* of food or drugs; (2) *contact* with foods, pesticides, drugs, adhesive, fur, hair, feathers, molds, fungi, and so on; (3) *inhalation* of pollens, dust, molds, fungi, cosmetics, perfumes; and (4) *injection* of vaccines, serums, antibiotics, and hormones.

In most individuals, food antigens are destroyed in the gastrointestinal tract; however, in *atopic* persons, those with a predisposition to allergy, after repeated exposure to the allergen, the antigen is absorbed from the gastrointestinal tract and enters the circulation. In infants and young children food allergy is usually attributed to an immature gastrointestinal tract which permits passage of the antigenically active substance into the circulation.

Immunological Aspects The body has two mechanisms for coping with the presence of the antigen: (1) HUMORAL IMMUNITY, in which protection is conferred by formation of antibodies specific for certain antigens; and (2) CELL-MEDIATED IMMUNITY, which does not depend on antibody formation. Antibodies are chiefly gamma globulins and belong to the group of substances known as immunoglobulins (Ig). Several classes of immunoglobulins are known: IgE, IgA, IgM, IgG, and IgD.

Types of reactions. Immune reactions are immediate or delayed. The *immediate* type, IgE-mediated, results from an interaction between antigen and target cells sensitized by IgE, with release of mediators such as histamine from mast cells and basophils. Mediators act on blood vessels, smooth muscle, and mucous glands to produce symptoms which appear within minutes to a few hours following exposure to a small quantity of the allergen, and usually clear up in 24 to 48 hours. IgE-mediated reactions are usually associated with respiratory tract symptoms such as hay fever and asthma due to inhalants. Foods less commonly cause this type of reaction. However, individuals who are highly sensitive to foods, such as eggs or nuts, experience immediate, violent symptoms following ingestion of even small amounts of the food. *Delayed* reactions are cellular in nature and do not involve circulating antibodies. The reaction occurs 24 to 72 hours following exposure to the allergen and lasts for several days. This type may be involved in some cases of gastrointestinal food sensitivity or intolerance. The reaction to milk is often delayed. The whole food protein is believed to be the allergen in the immediate type of reaction, and a breakdown product formed during digestion of the food in delayed reactions. The reaction time toward a given substance always remains the same in an individual; that is, if the reaction to eggs is immediate, it will always be so, and not delayed. An individual may have an immediate reaction toward one substance and a delayed response to another.

Etiology Heredity is important in the development of allergies. The incidence is increased in children whose parents have allergies, especially if both parents are affected. The child does not inherit a sensitivity to a specific substance or an identical manifestation of the allergy. The parent may be sensitive to wheat, for example, and the child to pollens.

Any kind of physical or emotional stress increases the severity of allergic reactions. However, stress situations do not cause the allergy. Other factors that may influence the allergic reaction include: the frequency of eating the food, the amount eaten, the physical state of the food, and the season.

Food allergens Any food may produce reactions, but the most frequent offenders are milk, eggs, wheat, citrus fruits, chocolate or cola, legumes, corn, fish, shellfish, and some spices.[2] The increasing incidence of food allergies due to use of soy products and food additives is of some concern.[3]

Foods unlike in flavor and structure but belonging to the same botanic group may result in allergic manifestations. For example, buckwheat is not of the cereal family but in a group which includes rhubarb. The sweet potato is not related to the white potato but is a member of the morning-glory family. Spinach, a frequent reactor, is in the same family with beets. The following botanic classification of a few common foods illustrates the relation of foods which at first appear to be dissimilar.

Cereal—wheat, rye, barley, rice, oats, malt, corn, sorghum, cane sugar
Lily—onion, garlic, asparagus, chives, leeks, shallots
Gourd—squash, pumpkin, cucumber, cantaloupe, watermelon
Cabbage and mustard—turnips, cabbage, collards, cauliflower, broccoli, kale, radish, horseradish, watercress, Brussels sprouts

Symptoms of Food Allergies Manifestations of allergy may occur in any part of the body. The tissues of these systems are frequently involved: cutaneous, gastrointestinal, respiratory, and neurologic. The symptoms are consequently varied depending upon the parts affected.

1. Skin manifestations may include canker sores, dermatitis, edema, fever blisters, pruritus, and urticaria (hives).
2. Common gastrointestinal manifestations include cheilitis, stomatitis, colic in infants, abdominal distension, constipation, diarrhea, dyspepsia, and

nausea and vomiting. The symptoms may be suggestive of appendicitis, colitis, gallbladder disease, or ulcers, and there may be confusion in diagnosis.

3. Respiratory symptoms include allergic rhinitis, asthma, bronchitis, and nasal polyps among others.
4. Neurologic symptoms such as migraine, neuralgias, and the tension-fatigue syndrome are sometimes due to food allergy. The latter syndrome is characterized by anxiety, fatigue, irritability, muscle and joint aching, restlessness, stomach pains, and so on.
5. Miscellaneous symptoms such as anaphylactic reactions, arthralgias, arthritis, edema, and so on have been attributed to food allergy.

Diagnosis of Food Allergies The procedures used include a complete history, skin testing, possibly other tests, and trials with restricted diets.

History. A complete history is the single most important diagnostic tool. When a severe reaction occurs immediately, the patient is usually aware of the circumstances leading up to it. However, when reactions are delayed or when allergies are multiple in nature, the elucidation of the offending factors is often exceedingly difficult. The history must include a complete evaluation of the physical status and the conditions and events preceding the attack.

The patient is asked to keep a detailed diary of all foods ingested and of the occurrence of any symptoms. Individual likes and dislikes must be taken into consideration. One patient may like a food well enough to risk an allergic reaction by eating it while another may claim to be allergic to a food he or she dislikes.

Skin tests. Skin tests are sometimes used to confirm presence of allergies but their usefulness in the case of food allergy is limited. Skin tests include (1) *scratch* tests, in which a small amount of solution containing the antigen is placed into a series of scratches made on the skin; (2) *patch* tests, in which the antigen is applied to filter paper which is then placed on a prepared skin site and covered; and (3) *intradermal* tests which involve injection of a small amount of dilute antigen extract beneath the skin. Reactions to skin tests are checked immediately and at specified intervals thereafter, usually 24 to 48 hours. Positive reactions are usually characterized by a small area of circumscribed edema surrounded by erythema at the test site. A positive skin test does not necessarily indicate that the individual is clinically sensitive to the material. It may represent past or potential sensitivity. On the other hand, a negative skin reaction does not necessarily eliminate the possibility of food allergy, for symptoms may be manifested in other tissues. Verification of results from skin tests is made by recurrence of symptoms following ingestion of the food in a symptom-free patient.

Other tests. In vitro measurements of specific antibodies are another means of diagnosing allergies. For example, elevated serum IgE levels have been reported in individuals allergic to milk.[4] The radioallergosorbent test (RAST) is used to detect specific IgE antibodies to a variety of antigens and is considered by some to be useful in diagnosis of IgE-mediated food allergy.[5,6] Other cellular tests, such as leukocyte histamine release, are not widely used.

Restricted diets. Many variants of restricted diets have been proposed as diagnostic aids. For infants and very young children it is relatively simple to determine whether allergic symptoms are due to foods by allowing only milk and crystalline vitamins. If a food other than milk is responsible, symptoms such as eczema will be relieved in a few days; but if milk or nonfood allergy is responsible, no improvement will occur and further testing will be necessary. An approach used for older children and adults is to restrict the patient to a list of foods to which no skin reactions were shown. The restricted diet may be tested for 1 to 3 weeks, after which new foods are added, one at a time, at 3-day intervals. If symptoms develop following addition of a food, it is eliminated for a time and reintroduced later.

A number of *elimination diets* have been developed, based upon the principle that only those foods that are seldom responsible for allergy are included in the trial diet. Many elimination diets are modifications of the regimen advocated by Rowe (see following diets), who recommends its use for a minimum of 3 months in the diagnosis of food allergy.[7]

Rowe's patients are first placed on a cereal-free elimination diet. This diet eliminates all cereal grains, milk, egg, beef, pork (except bacon), fish, and a number of fruits and vegetables. Soybean oil is the only oil permitted; milk-free margarine made from soy oil is used. Bakery products are made from soy, Lima, or potato starch. Soymilk or meat-based formulas are used for infants. Calcium and vitamin supplements are needed. When the patient is free of allergic symptoms, fruits and vegetables are added, one at a time, every 2 to 5 days. Cereals are added in the following order: rice, oats, corn, rye, and wheat. Beef is added after 1 to 2 months. Tolerance for condiments and spices is determined by challenge testing. Subsequent additions of specified oils and other foods are made upon recommendation by the physician.

A fruit-free cereal-free elimination diet is used for patients who are allergic to fruits, spices, or condiments. On this diet careful planning is needed to ensure adequate calories, vitamins, and minerals, especially ascorbic acid, calcium, potassium, magnesium, iron, and iodine. A number of recipes suitable for use on cereal-free or fruit-free elimination diets are available.

Cereal-Free Elimination Diet*

Beverages—fruit juices: apricot, grapefruit, peach, pineapple, prune, or tomato; Neo-Mullsoy
Breads—Lima-potato, soy-potato; muffins made from allowed flours; pancakes or waffles made from soy-potato flours; soy crackers
Desserts—cakes, cookies, cupcakes made from soy or potato flours; gelatin, plain; soy ice cream; puddings made from allowed flours; water ices made with allowed fruits
Flours and starches—Lima, potato, soy; pearl tapioca
Fruits—fresh, cooked, or canned apricots, grapefruit, peaches, pears, pineapple; lemon; prunes
Fats—sesame oil, soy oil, milk-free margarine made with soy oil
Gravy—thickened with potato starch
Meats—bacon; Canadian bacon; chicken (no hens); lamb; lamb liver
Soups—broth, chicken or lamb; Lima bean; split pea; tomato
Sweets—brown sugar, beet or cane sugar; jams, jellies, preserves made from allowed fruits; maple syrup; maple sugar candy, plain fondant
Vegetables—artichokes, asparagus, carrots, lettuce, Lima beans, peas, potatoes, spinach, squash, string beans, sweet potatoes, tomatoes, yams
Miscellaneous—baking powder (no cornstarch or tartaric acid); baking soda, cream of tartar, lemon extract, salt, vanilla extract, white vinegar

* Adapted from Rowe, A. H.: *Food Allergy. Its Manifestations and Control and the Elimination Diets. A Compendium.* Charles C Thomas, Publisher, Springfield, Ill., 1972.

Sample Menu for Cereal-Free Elimination Diet

BREAKFAST

Half grapefruit with brown sugar
Canadian bacon
Hashed brown potatoes
Muffins, using soy-potato flour
Milk-free soy margarine
Peach preserves
Hot lemonade, pineapple, apricot, or prune juice

LUNCHEON OR SUPPER

Tomato juice with lemon wedge
Fried chicken, using soy oil, potato flour
New potato, boiled
Peas
Mixed fruit cup with peach, pear, pineapple
Lemon gelatin salad with grated carrot and crushed pineapple
Soy-potato bread
Milk-free soy margarine
Jam or preserves from allowed fruits
Soy ice cream with caramel sauce
Soy cookies
Lemonade or apricot juice

DINNER

Broiled lamb chops
Baked potato
Mashed squash
Lettuce and tomato salad
Salad dressing, using soy oil, lemon juice, salt
Soy-potato bread
Milk-free soy margarine
Jam or preserves from allowed fruits
Pineapple upside-down cake, using soy-potato flour
Lemonade, apricot, or tomato juice

Fruit-Free Cereal—Free Elimination Diet*

Beverages—Neo-Mullsoy; tea, if permitted by physician
Breads—Lima-potato, soy-potato; muffins made from allowed flours, pancakes or waffles from potato or soy flour
Desserts—cakes, cookies, cupcakes made from soy or potato flours; gelatin, plain; soy ice cream; puddings made from allowed flours.
Fats—sesame oil; soy oil; milk-free soy margarine
Gravy—thickened with potato starch
Meats—bacon; Canadian bacon; chicken (no hens); lamb; lamb liver
Soups—broth, lamb or chicken; Lima bean, split pea
Flours and starches—Lima, potato, soy; pearl tapioca
Sweets—beet or cane sugar; brown sugar; syrup made with cane sugar
Vegetables—artichokes, carrots, Lima beans, peas, potatoes, string beans, squash, sweet potatoes, yams
Miscellaneous—corn-free tartaric acid baking powder; salt

Sample Menu for Fruit-Free Cereal-Free Elimination Diet

BREAKFAST

Waffles, using soy-potato flour
Bacon
Pearl tapioca cooked with water or Neo-Mullsoy and sugar
Milk-free soy margarine
Maple syrup
Tea, if permitted

* Adapted from Rowe, A. H.: *Food Allergy. Its Manifestations and Control and the Elimination Diets. A Compendium.* Charles C Thomas, Publisher, Springfield, Ill., 1972.

LUNCHEON OR SUPPER
Split pea soup with bacon crumbs
Soy crackers
Sliced chicken sandwich on soy-potato bread
Milk-free soy margarine
Gelatin salad with shredded carrots
Frosted soy cupcake
Tea, if permitted

DINNER
Chicken broth with carrots, peas, Lima beans
Soy crackers
Roast lamb
String beans
Mashed potato, using Neo-Mullsoy and milk-free soy margarine, salt
Gravy, thickened with potato starch
Soy-potato muffin
Milk-free soy margarine
Carrot marmalade
Soy ice cream
Butterscotch sauce, using Neo-Mullsoy and milk-free soy margarine
Tea, if permitted.

Milk Sensitivity A special problem in infants and young children is milk sensitivity. From 1 to 3 per cent of all children are sensitive to cow's milk.[8] In many instances this may be associated with infection and emotional stress; in others genetic factors may be a cause. (See Galactose Disease, Chapter 44 and Lactose Intolerance, Chapter 33.)

In infants with true milk allergy the response to the ingestion of milk is immediate and may lead to colic, spitting up of the feeding, irritability, diarrhea, and respiratory disorders. In others, a delayed reaction may occur hours to days following the ingestion of milk, and thus it becomes difficult to determine the exact cause.

The incidence of hypochromic anemia in some infants has been attributed to sensitivity to milk. Following the ingestion of milk by these sensitive infants, some blood is lost from the gastrointestinal tract. This may average several milliliters per day and may go unnoticed until the anemia becomes apparent months later. Some infants may have a sufficiently high intake of other iron-rich foods so that the anemic tendency is counteracted.

Each of the common proteins in milk has been found to be allergenic, but β-lactoglobulin is the most common.[9] Several hypoallergenic formulas are available, with a casein hydrolysate, meat, or soybean often used as the protein source.*

Dietary Treatment of Food Allergy Especially for children, it is always necessary to consider the relative importance of the allergic disturbance in relation to the diet. It is better management, for example, to treat a mild case of eczema locally than to subject the child to the dangers of an inadequate diet with its far more serious consequences.

If a single food such as strawberries or grapefruit is implicated, the food is easily omitted from the diet. If allergy involves more than one food, the initial diet contains only those foods that produce no reactions. Thus, if improvement has occurred on an elimination diet, simple, not mixed, foods are added, one at a time, to the allowed list of foods. Several days to a week must elapse between the addition of each new food. A given food should be tested on at least two, preferably three, occasions before it is permanently added to, or eliminated from, the diet. Because wheat, eggs, and milk are frequent allergens, these foods are added last.

* Nutramigen® by Mead Johnson and Co., Evansville, Indiana; MBF® (Meat-base formula) by Gerber Products Company, Fremont, Michigan; Neomull-soy® by Syntex Laboratories, Palo Alto, California.

Dietary adequacy becomes a matter of great concern when important foods are eliminated for a long period of time. This is especially true in infants and young children and care must be taken to ensure inclusion of acceptable foods similar in nutrient content to the one omitted.

In milk sensitivity changing the form of the milk sometimes improves tolerance—that is, boiled, powdered, acidulated, or evaporated milk may be satisfactory when fresh cow's milk is not. Some children will tolerate no milk whatsoever, and a hypoallergenic formula must be substituted. Many youngsters outgrow their sensitivity to milk but others need to continue a milk-free diet indefinitely.

Hyposensitization consists of decreasing the sensitivity to a given substance by giving minute doses of the allergen in gradually increasing amounts. It is a very tedious procedure and is seldom used in food allergy, and then only when a major food group is involved.

Dietary management for asthmatic patients. Those who have severe asthma often find it difficult to consume an adequate diet. The meals should be small and eaten slowly in an environment free from stress. Interval feedings are necessary to bolster the caloric intake. Fluid intake should be encouraged. Usually breakfast and lunch are the best meals of the day, and particular attention should be paid to their nutritional quality and attractiveness. A rest period after meals is helpful. Ordinarily, late-evening feedings are not advisable. Some clinicians routinely eliminate highly allergenic foods such as chocolate, nuts, shellfish, and so on. Milk products are sometimes omitted because of their tendency to form mucus.

Dietary Counseling

The diet counselor should stress the importance of reading labels on food products every time purchases are made. Formulations change periodically and current ingredients are listed on the label. However, even conscientious checking of labels is not always adequate protection for the individual with food allergy. Foods for which a standard of identity has been established by the Food and Drug Administration need not be labeled with a complete listing of ingredients; only optional ingredients must be listed. For example, mayonnaise contains small amounts of egg, but this is not indicated on the label. A number of breads have been included under standards of identity, and thus the label would not indicate that milk is an ingredient.

Many patients may not be aware of the great number of food mixtures containing milk, eggs, cereal, or soy products. The patient should be provided with detailed lists showing typical uses of these foods and should be encouraged to ask specific questions concerning ingredients used in foods when in doubt. Examples of foods to be omitted for wheat, egg, milk, corn, or soy-free diets follow.

Recipes and helpful hints on substitutions should be offered the patient. For example, water or fruit juices can usually be substituted in recipes using milk. Quick breads can be made from rice, potato, rye, or other flours, but adjustments in baking temperature and time must be made. The proportion of baking powder is increased because of the lack of gluten in these flours. The finished products differ in texture from those prepared from wheat. They should be stored in a freezer rather than in the refrigerator as they tend to dry out quickly. Sources of recipes are given at the end of this chapter.

Patients should be cautioned that improperly washed utensils or use of the same stirring or serving spoon in foods for allergic and nonallergic persons may be sources of prohibited foods for the food-sensitive individual.

Suggestions for ordering foods when eating away from home are useful for patients. Broiled meats, baked potato, plain vegetables without sauces, lettuce salads, and fruits for dessert are usually acceptable.

Diet Without Wheat—Foods to Avoid

Beverages—beer; Cocomalt; coffee substitutes; instant coffee unless 100 per cent coffee; gin; malted milk; whiskey
Breads, crackers, and rolls—all breads including pumpernickel, rye, oatmeal, and corn; baking powder biscuits; crackers; gluten bread; griddle cakes; hot breads and muffins; matzoth, pretzels; rusk; waffles; zwieback
Cereals—All-bran, bran flakes, Cheerios, Cream of Wheat, farina, Granola type, Grape-nuts, Grape-nuts flakes, Kix, Krumbles, Maltex, New oats, Pettijohn's, Puffed Wheat, Ralston cereals, Shredded Wheat, Special K, Total, Wheatena, Wheat flakes, wheat germ, Wheaties, Wheat Chex
Desserts—cake or cookies, homemade, from mixes, or bakery; doughnuts; ice cream, ice-cream cones; pies; popovers; puddings
Flour—all-purpose; graham, white, whole-wheat
Gravies and sauces—thickened with flour
Meats—canned meat dishes such as stews; chili; frankfurters, luncheon meats, or sausage in which wheat has been used as a filler; prepared with bread, cracker crumbs or flour, such as croquettes and meatloaf; stews thickened with flour or made with dumplings; stuffings and commercial stuffing mixes
Pastas—macaroni, noodles, spaghetti, vermicelli, and so on
Salad dressings—thickened with flour
Soups—bouillon cubes; commercially canned

Diet Without Eggs—Foods to Avoid

Eggs—or commercial egg substitutes in any form
Beverages—Cocomalt; eggnog; malted beverages; Ovaltine; root beer; wine
Bread and rolls—containing eggs; crust glazed with egg; French toast; griddle cakes; muffins; pretzels; sweet rolls; waffles; zwieback
Desserts—cake; cookies; cream-filled pies, coconut, cream, custard, lemon, pumpkin; custard; doughnuts; ice cream; meringue; puddings; sherbet
Meat—breaded meats dipped in egg; meat loaf
Noodles
Salad dressings—cooked dressings; mayonnaise
Sauces—Hollandaise, tartar
Soups—bouillon; broth, consommé
Sweets—many cake icings; candies; chocolate, cream, fondant, marshmallow, nougat; whips
Miscellaneous—baking mixes; baking powder; cake flour; dessert powders; fondue; fritters; pastries; soufflé

Diet Without Milk—Foods to Avoid

Milk—all forms: buttermilk; evaporated; fresh whole or skim; malted; yogurt
Beverages—chocolate; cocoa; Cocomalt; Ovaltine
Breads and rolls—any made with milk (most breads contain milk); bread mixes; griddle cakes; soda crackers; waffles; zwieback
Cereals—some dry (read labels)
Cheese—all kinds; cheese dips and spreads

Desserts—cakes; cookies; custard; doughnuts; ice cream; mixes of all types; pie crust made with butter or margarine; pies with cream fillings such as chocolate, coconut, cream, custard, lemon, pumpkin; puddings with milk; sherbets
Fats—butter, cream, margarine
Meat—frankfurters, luncheon meats, meat loaf—unless 100 per cent meat
Sauces—any made with butter, margarine, milk, or cream
Soups—bisques; chowders; cream
Sweets—caramels; chocolate candy
Vegetables—au gratin; mashed potatoes; seasoned with butter or margarine; scalloped; with cream sauces

Diet Without Corn—Foods to Avoid

Corn sugar (dextrose) and syrup are widely used in commercially prepared foods. Cornstarch is also used as a binder and thickening agent in many commercial products. Labels should be carefully checked.
Beverages—ale; beer; carbonated; coffee lighteners; gin; grape juice; instant tea; milk substitutes; soy milks; whiskey
Breads, crackers, and rolls—corn breads or muffins; enchiladas; English muffins; corn chips; tacos; tortillas; graham crackers
Cereals—cornmeal; hominy; ready-to-eat: cornflakes; Corn Chex, Grapenuts, Kix
Desserts—cakes; candied fruits; canned or frozen fruit or juices; cream pies; ice cream; pastries; pudding mixes; sherbet
Fats—corn oil; corn oil margarine; gravies, salad dressings thickened with cornstarch; mayonnaise, salad dressings, and shortenings unless source of oil is specified
Flours and thickeners—cornmeal; cornstarch
Meats—bacon; hams (cured, tenderized); luncheon; sausage
Soups—all commercial; homemade thickened with cornstarch
Sweets—candy; cane sugar; corn syrups, corn sugars; imitation maple syrups; imitation vanilla; jams, jellies, preserves
Vegetables—Harvard beets, (thickened with cornstarch); corn; mixed vegetables containing corn; succotash
Miscellaneous—baking powder; batters for frying; catsup; chewing gum; cheese spreads; Chinese foods; commercial mixes of all types: baking, cake, pancake, pie crust, pudding; confectioner's sugar; distilled vinegar; monosodium glutamate; peanut butter; popcorn; sandwich spreads; sauces; toppings; vitamin capsules; yeast

Diet Without Soy—Foods to Avoid

Soy products are widely used in commercial food preparations. Omit all products for which labels state: soy, soybean oil, soy flour, soy milk, soy curd; vegetable protein; protein isolate; lecithin. Look for these terms especially on the following:
Beverages—beer, chocolate or cocoa mixes, coffee whiteners, soy milk, wine
Breads, crackers, or rolls—many commercial breads; frankfurter or hamburger rolls; dinner rolls; English muffins; biscuit/pancake mixes; bread or cereal stuffings
Cereals—natural or Granola type; flavored rice mixes; macaroni, spaghetti, noodle, or pizza mixes (canned or dry)
Desserts—cake and cake mixes; prepared frostings; chocolate pudding mixes
Fats—cooking oils, margarines, mayonnaise, salad oil, salad dressings, shortenings in which the type of oil is not specified
Flour—soy
Meat—meat extenders; frankfurters; luncheon meats; pork sausage; fish canned in oil
Soups—bouillon cubes; canned, dried, instant soups

Sweets—candy; chocolate chips; semisweet chocolate; caramels; some pancake syrups
Vegetables—frozen in sauces; au gratin potato mixes; instant mashed potatoes; prepared fried potatoes; potato chips
Miscellaneous—Baco's; pretzels; seasoned sauces: mushroom, soy, steak, tabasco, Worcestershire; dip mixes; powdered seasonings

Diseases of the Skin

The quality of the diet is a determining factor in skin health. Deficiencies of one or more nutrients are known to produce various cutaneous disorders. For example, there are the dermatitis associated with pellagra and resulting from lack of niacin (see page 227), the eruptions which accompany severe vitamin A deficiency (see page 193), the cheilosis of riboflavin lack (see page 224), and the eczema that occurs in infants with essential fatty acid deficiency (see page 102).

Some individuals may be allergic to certain substances and thus manifest skin disorders such as eczema or urticaria. Whenever allergy is suspected, it is essential to determine the offending agent as described in the preceding part of this chapter. No single food or food group predominates in producing allergic skin disorders.

Acne vulgaris is a particular problem during adolescence, and many boys and girls try bizarre diets in an effort to correct the situation. High-fat and concentrated carbohydrate diets have been considered to be undesirable. Chocolate, milk, nuts, cola, and iodized salt are among foods commonly implicated in exacerbation of symptoms. However, controlled studies show that dietary restriction is less effective than other forms of therapy, such as antibiotics, benzoyl peroxide, or vitamin A acid therapy.[10]

Dietary emphasis in skin disorders should be placed on nutritional adequacy; that is, the diet should contain sufficient milk, meat, eggs, fruits, vegetables, and whole-grain or enriched cereals and breads. Attention should be directed to improving the general hygiene, including skin cleanliness, regular meal hours, sufficient fluid intake, adequate rest, proper elimination, and psychological support. There is no harm in excluding candies and sweets, fried foods, chocolate, and rich desserts, but such exclusion probably is most useful in that these foods are replaced by others that are more nutritionally satisfactory.

Problems and Review

1. Define the following: allergen; antigen; atopic; food allergy; food hypersensitivity; food intolerance; food sensitivity.
2. List some of the characteristic symptoms of allergy.
3. List five foods that cause a great number of allergies. Name some foods that rarely cause sensitivity.
4. What is meant by skin test? Elimination diet?
5. What are the principles for the construction of elimination diets? What are some of the problems associated with using these diets?
6. *Problem.* Plan a day's menu for a patient who is sensitive to wheat, corn, and grapefruit.
7. What recommendation could you make to a 15-year old girl who has acne vulgaris?
8. *Problem.* Prepare a table that shows the nature of skin disorders when a diet is markedly deficient in each of the following: protein, essential fatty acids, vitamin A, riboflavin, niacin, ascorbic acid. Under what circumstances would you expect

these changes in the skin to become apparent? What is the incidence of these disorders in the United States?

9. List the nutritional suggestions you would give to a patient who is severely asthmatic.
10. What problems of dietary inadequacy should you anticipate if an individual is allergic to milk? To wheat? To many fruits?
11. List some problems that might be anticipated in a child who has food allergies. How might these be prevented?
12. List several ways in which milk sensitivity may be manifested. What substances in milk have been shown to produce such sensitivity? List three products that may be used satisfactorily in place of a milk formula.

Cited References

1. Goldstein, G. B., and Heiner, D. C.: "Clinical and Immunological Perspectives in Food Sensitivity: A Review," *J. Allergy*, **46**:270–91, 1970.
2. Speer, F.: "Food Allergy: The Ten Common Offenders," *Am. Fam. Physician*, **13**:106–12, February 1976.
3. Halpin, T. C. et al.: "Colitis, Persistent Diarrhea, and Soy Protein Intolerance," *J. Ped.*, **91**:404–7, 1977.
4. Bahna, S. L.: "Control of Milk Allergy: A Challenge for Physicians, Mothers, and Industry," *Ann. Allergy*, **41**:1–12, 1978.
5. Dannaeus, A., and Johansson, S. G. O.: "A Follow-Up of Infants with Adverse Reactions to Cow's Milk. I. Serum IgE, Skin Test Reactions, and RAST in Relation to Clinical Course," *Acta Paediatr. Scand.*, **68**:377–82, 1979.
6. Johnstone, D. E.: "Diagnostic Methods in Food Allergy in Children," *Ann. Allergy*, **40**:110–3, 1978.
7. Rowe, A. H.: *Food Allergy. Its Manifestations and Control and the Elimination Diets. A Compendium.* Charles C Thomas, Publisher, Springfield, Ill., 1972.
8. American Academy of Pediatrics: "Should Milk Drinking by Children Be Discouraged?" *Pediatrics*, **53**:576–82, 1974.
9. Lebenthal, E.: "Cow's Milk Protein Allergy," *Pediatr. Clin. North Amer.*, **22**:827–33, 1975.
10. Hurwitz, S.: "Acne Vulgaris. Current Concepts of Pathogenesis and Treatment," *Am. J. Dis. Child.*, **133**:536–44, 1979.

Additional References

ADKINSON, N.F.: "The Radioallergosorbent Test: Uses and Abuses," *J. Allergy Clin. Immunol.*, **65**:1–4, 1980.

BRIDGEWATER, S. C. et al.: "Allergies in Children: Recognition," *Am. J. Nurs.*, **78**:614–16, 1978.

DEAMER, W. C. et al.: "Cow's Milk Allergy. A Critical Review," *J. Fam. Practice*, **9**:223–32, 1979.

JONES, H. et al.: "13-Cis Retinoic Acid and Acne," *Lancet*, **2**:1048–49, 1980.

MILLER, J. B.: "Hidden Food Ingredients, Chemical Food Additives and Incomplete Food Labels," *Ann. Allergy*, **41**:93–98, 1978.

PARKER, C.: "Food Allergies," *Am. J. Nurs.*, **80**:262–65, 1980.

VOIGNIER, R. R., and BRIDGEWATER, S. C.: "Allergies in Children: Testing and Treating," *Am. J. Nurs.*, **78**:617–19, 1978.

Instructional Materials for the Patient

Allergy Diets. Ralston Purina Company, Checkerboard Square, St. Louis, Mo.

Allergy Recipes. The American Dietetic Association, 430 North Michigan Ave., Chicago, Ill.

Baking for People with Food Allergies. Home and Garden Bulletin 147, U.S. Government Printing Office, Washington, D.C.

Celiac Disease Recipes. Hospital for Sick Children, Toronto, Ontario, Canada.

Easy, Appealing Milk-free Recipes. Mead Johnson and Company, Evansville, Ind.

FRAZIER, C. A.: *Coping with Food Allergy.* Quadrangle/The New York Times Book Co., New York, N.Y.

Good Recipes to Brighten the Allergy Diet. Best Foods, Division Corn Products Company, New York, N.Y.

JOSEPH, L.: *"A Doctor Discusses Allergy: Facts and Fiction,* Budlong Press Co., Chicago, Ill.

Low Gluten Diet with Tested Recipes. University of Michigan Hospitals, Clinical Research Unit, Ann Arbor, Mich.

125 Recipes for Allergy Diets. Good Housekeeping Institute, 959 Eighth Ave., New York, N.Y.

SHATTUCK, R. R.: *Creative Cooking Without Wheat, Milk and Eggs,* Barnes & Co., Inc., Cranbury, N.J.

Special Recipes and Allergy Aids, General Foods Consumer Center, White Plains, N.Y.

THOMAS, L. L.: *Caring and Cooking for the Allergic Child.* Drake Publishers, Inc., New York, N.Y.

Understanding Allergy, Ross Laboratories, Columbus, Ohio.

Wheat, Milk, and Egg-Free Recipes. Quaker Oats Co., Chicago, Ill.

44 Inborn Errors of Metabolism

MANY professional and lay groups have united in their efforts to understand the nature of the ever-growing number of inborn errors of metabolism and to seek methods of prevention and treatment. To the physician, the problems are those of diagnosis, of early detection before damage has occurred, and of effective treatment. To the biochemist falls the task of identifying the metabolic defect so that a possible rationale of therapy can be developed. To the nurse and dietitian fall the practical aspects of nursing care and of dietary planning and implementation. The problem of control through genetic counseling belongs to the geneticist. Most of all, to the parent of a child affected the problem is immediate and urgent; in some disorders treatment is effective, but in others no remedy is available.

Nature of Inborn Errors The term INBORN ERROR was coined at the beginning of this century by Sir Archibald E. Garrod who wrote a book in which he described four diseases of a hereditary nature.[1] These were alkaptonuria, a defect of phenylalanine metabolism in which a metabolite excreted into the urine becomes dark upon standing; albinism, also a defect in phenylalanine metabolism characterized by a lack of pigmentation; cystinuria, or an excessive excretion of cystine because of a defect in the renal tubules which prevents the reabsorption of the amino acid cystine; and pentosuria, characterizied by the presence of pentose in the urine owing to the lack of an enzyme in metabolism.

Inborn errors of metabolism include well over 100 disorders that originate in one or more mutations of the gene so that normal function is disrupted. These diseases are also referred to as *genetic diseases* or as *hereditary molecular diseases.* The effects of genetic mutation vary widely and may alter the metabolism of specific amino acids, carbohydrates, lipids, vitamins, or minerals. They may affect the synthesis of a body product; interfere with the transport of materials across a cell membrane; or produce toxic effects on tissues because of the accumulation of intermediate products.

Some errors of metabolism result in no serious limitations upon the individual; others lead to rapid changes in the central nervous system so that mental retardation is severe; still others may be lethal shortly after birth. Some become evident a few days after birth, whereas other hereditary diseases such as diabetes mellitus and gout may show no signs until adult life. Dietary management is effective in the control of many disorders but no known therapy is yet available for others.

Some of the inborn errors of metabolism are characterized by serious mental retardation if the condition is not treated promptly. During the first years of life the brain is developing so rapidly that any interference with its growth cannot be fully corrected at a later time. Thus, diagnosis at a very early age is important if effective treatment is to take place before serious damage has occurred. Inexpensive screening tests may be applied to some conditions during the first weeks of life.

Several conditions for which dietary treatment has been successful are discussed in this chapter. For some of these disorders the diet is built around specialized formulas that supply most of the energy, protein, and other nutrients needed, but which are designed to be low in specific amino acids in accordance with the metabolic defect. Small amounts of natural foods are also used to provide a controlled intake of protein and certain amino acids in addition to other required nutrients. For some disorders specialized food equivalency lists are available in which all foods within a given group provide approximately the same amount of particular amino acids and protein. The detailed lists are not included in this chapter but are cited in the references. The diet for phenylketonuria serves as an example of the considerations that must be kept in mind when planning highly specialized diets.

Children with inborn errors of metabolism such as phenylketonuria are treated primarily in specialty clinics of major medical centers where a team of highly skilled specialists monitor the child's progress on a regular basis. Since the numbers of patients are small, health team members learn to know the child and parents and their ability to cope with the problems involved in management of the disorder. Dietary management is a special challenge for the dietitian and family alike. The importance of accuracy in calculating amounts of various foods permitted cannot be overemphasized for, in some instances, excessive amounts can lead to neurological damage. On the other hand, insufficient amounts of specific nutrients can impair normal growth and development. The child's progress must be monitored closely and the diet adjusted in accordance with physical and biochemical changes. The diet must be nutritionally adequate for all nutrients except the one(s) which must be limited. The dietitian must be aware of new food products and their nutrient composition as they become available in order to adequately counsel patients and their families regarding their use. The nurse is usually not directly involved in the planning of highly specialized diets, but must be aware of the child's progress on the diet and any problems encountered. The nurse must understand the general principles of the diet and should be cognizant of food sources of the nutrients that are restricted in order to be able to answer questions and evaluate information relayed by the family concerning the diet. Day-to-day dietary management is every bit as challenging for the parents and family as the technical aspects of management are for the health professional. The family must ensure strict adherence to the diet by the child, plan special menus, and encourage the child to eat specialized products.

The information presented in this chapter is not sufficient to enable the dietitian or nurse to competently plan nutritional care for children with inborn errors of metabolism. The material presented is intended to give an overview of some conditions requiring highly complex diets, the importance of careful dietary planning in these disorders, and the need for continuing counseling of parents regarding the child's nutritional management.

Phenylketonuria

PHENYLKETONURIA (often abbreviated PKU) was first diagnosed by Asbjörn Fölling, a Norwegian biochemist, in 1934, and has been successfully treated with a phenylalanine-restricted diet since 1952. When the disorder is discovered early in infancy and is treated with the phenylalanine-restricted diet, mental development is normal.

Incidence About 1 child in each 10,000 births has phenylketonuria, although 1 person in 50 is a carrier of the trait. About 1 per cent of all patients in mental institutions are estimated to be phenylketonurics.

Phenylketonuria is transmitted by an autosomal recessive gene. Thus, each of the parents would have one defective gene and would be clinically normal. Each birth from the mating of two heterozygotes involves a one in four chance that the child will be phenylketonuric, two chances that he or she will be a heterozygote but clinically normal, and one chance that he or she will be entirely normal.

Biochemical Defect An enzyme, PHENYLALANINE HYDROXYLASE, is missing in the phenylketonuric individual. As a consequence the hydroxyl (OH) grouping cannot be incorporated into the phenylalanine molecule to form tyrosine. Tyrosine levels remain normal but phenylalanine and several metabolites accumulate in the blood circulation and are excreted in the urine. One of these, phenylpyruvic acid, is a ketone which accounts for the naming of the condition. It reacts with ferric chloride to give a vivid green color, thus forming the basis for the widely used "diaper" tests. Another intermediate product is phenylacetic acid, which accounts for the characteristic "wild," "gamey," or "mousy" odor from the skin and urine of these patients. (See Figure 44–1.)

Testing for phenylketonuria. Most states require the testing of newborn infants, using the "diaper" tests. To avoid false interpretations these should be followed by blood tests in 4 to 6 weeks. The acceptable range of phenylalanine in the blood serum is 3 to 7 mg per cent. In phenylketonuric infants the initial blood level is usually above 15 mg per cent and as high as 30 mg per cent by 10 days of age. In untreated persons with PKU, the serum level reaches as high as 75 mg per cent.

In some children phenylalanine hydroxylase is not missing but is present in reduced amounts and there is consequent elevation of serum phenylalanine levels. Neurologic development in these youngsters is usually normal.[2] Occasionally infants have an initial elevation of serum phenylalanine that later returns to normal.[3] Other infants, especially prematures, show a slight elevation of serum phenylalanine, and sometimes tyrosine, because of delayed maturation of the tyrosine-oxidizing system. Usually this is corrected by the administration of ascorbic acid. It is important to distinguish these conditions from true PKU so that children

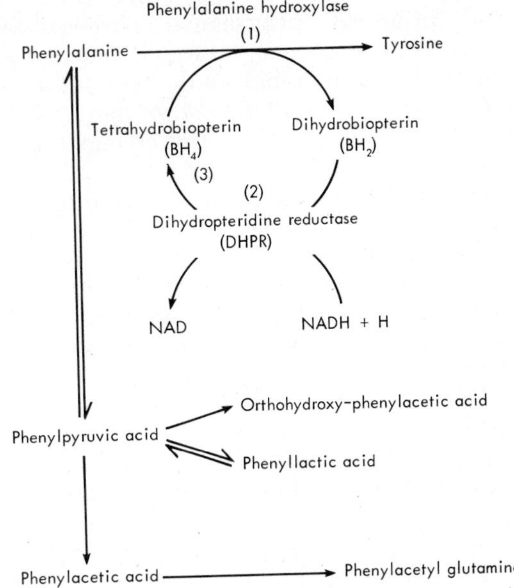

Figure 44–1. In classic phenylketonuria, there is a deficiency of phenylalanine hydroxylase *(1)*. Variant forms are due to deficiency of dihydropteridine reductase *(2)*, or deficiency of tetrahydrobiopterin or defective recycling of BH_4 due to DHPR deficiency *(3)*.

are not subjected to the phenylalanine-restricted diet unnecessarily.

Hyperphenylalaninemia may also occur due to deficiencies of two other components of the phenylalanine hydroxylase system, dihydropteridine reductase and tetrahydrobiopterin. (See Figure 44–1.) These cofactors are necessary for the synthesis of the neurotransmitters serotonin, dopamine, and norepinephrine. Deficiency of either component leads to elevated serum phenylalanine levels and neurological dysfunction.[4]

Clinical Changes Mental retardation in untreated subjects is usually severe with most patients having an intelligence quotient below 50. The child appears to be normal at birth but within the first few days or weeks of life the various intermediate products of faulty phenylalanine metabolism accumulate and can be detected in the blood and urine. If treatment is not initiated promptly progressive irreversible brain damage occurs. Although the faulty phenylalanine metabolism is clearly understood as the cause of the brain damage, it is not yet known just how this change takes place.

Because of the block in tyrosine formation, the production of pigments is reduced. Consequently, these children are usually blond, blue eyed, and have a fair skin, even though their parents may be of darker skin, eye, and hair coloring. Eczema is a common finding.

The behavior of untreated children is considerably altered. They are hyperactive, wave their arms, rock back and forth, and grind their teeth. They show poor coordination, are irritable, immature, and overdependent. At times they may have seizures. Their behavior can be extremely trying even to the most loving parents.

Treatment The successful treatment of PKU depends upon (1) early diagnosis; (2) restriction of phenylalanine intake to maintain an acceptable range of serum phenylalanine; (3) a nutritionally adequate diet adjusted from time to time to meet the requirements for normal growth and development; (4) continuing clinical and biochemical monitoring; and (5) a comprehensive program of education of the parents. Children for whom such treatment is begun within the first few weeks or months of life show apparently normal mental and physical development. The team approach is essential, including the physician, nurse, clinical chemist, social workers, dietitian, parents, and sometimes others. (See Figure 44–2.)

A delay in the initiation of the diet reduces the likelihood of satisfactory mental development. Once brain damage has occurred reversal does not take place. After 3 years of age, little improvement in mental development can be expected. However, even for the older child the phenylalanine-restricted diet is believed to be of some benefit in modifying the behavior characteristics.

Hyperphenylalaninemia due to deficiency of tetrahydrobiopterin is treated with neurotransmitter therapy, that is, DOPA and 5-hydroxytryptophan. Serum phenylalanine levels are controlled by diet or administration of tetrahydrobiopterin.[5]

Modification of the Diet The allowances for protein and for calories are essentially the same as those for normal children.

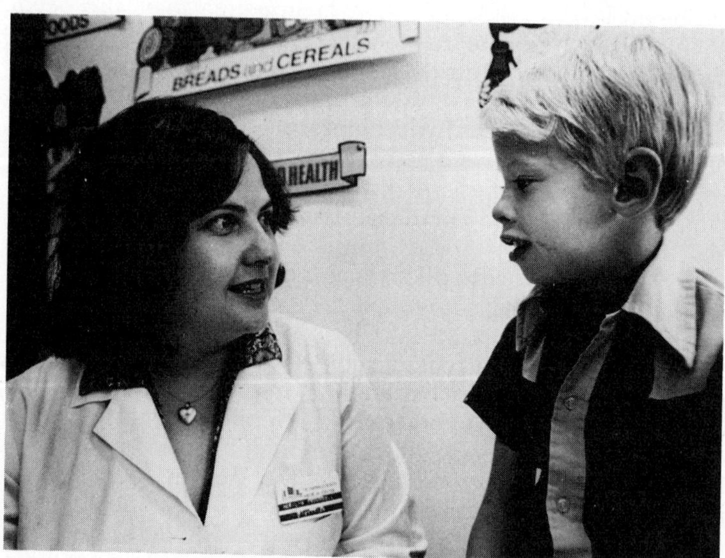

Figure 44–2. Nutritionist gains confidence of a young boy with PKU. She discusses his diet with him, as well as with his parents, and helps him to understand why he can have some foods and not others. (Courtesy, Hennepin County Medical Center, Minneapolis.)

Phenylalanine needs to be restricted but it cannot be totally eliminated from the diet since it is an essential amino acid. Proteins contain 4 to 6 per cent phenylalanine, which is excessive for the child with PKU. Several commercial preparations are available.* Lofenalac has 95 per cent of the phenylalanine removed and is designed for infants as the chief source of protein. Phenyl-free and PKU-AID, for older children, contain no phenylalanine, thus they permit the use of more natural foods containing phenylalanine.

Clinical experience has shown that a balance must be maintained between the amount of low-phenylalanine formula and the amount of natural foods that are fed. The formula supplies most of the energy, protein, and other nutrients, and if inadequate amounts are fed, the amino acid and other nutritional requirements of the child will not be met. On the other hand, if insufficient amounts of natural foods are given, the phenylalanine intake will be too low to meet growth requirements. Catabolism of tissue proteins then leads to a temporary increase in the serum phenylalanine level.

The signs of inadequate phenylalanine intake include anorexia, vomiting, listlessness, inconsistent growth or failure to grow, pallor, and skin rash.

Management of the Diet The diet is so unlike a normal diet that many problems are encountered in its administration. A skillful approach by physician, nurses, and nutritionist is required to achieve acceptance on the part of the parent as well as the child.

Considerations in planning the diet are as follows:

1. Estimate the daily protein, calorie, and phenylalanine requirements in accordance with the child's age and weight.
2. Calculate the amount of special formula required to meet the protein and calorie allowances.
3. Determine amounts of other foods needed to meet the phenylalanine allowance.

Lofenalac provides the basis for the diet in infants. Except for phenylalanine, this preparation is nutritionally complete, containing amino acids, unsaturated fat, carbohydrate, vitamins, and minerals. It is a satisfactory substitute for milk and other protein foods. Measured amounts are used to supply protein and calories for the young infant who is not yet receiving other foods, and to provide 85 per cent of the protein needs for the older child. To meet the phenylalanine requirement for the infant, from 1 to 2 ounces of milk are added to the Lofenalac formula. Milk contains about 55 mg per cent phenylalanine and should always be incorporated into the formula so that the infant does not develop a taste for milk. The diet should be progressed as for a normal infant and child. Appropriate amounts of fruits, vegetables, and cereal foods are introduced as the child grows, and Lofenalac may be incorporated into these and other allowed foods. A variety of recipes have been developed for such use. Planning the diet is made easier by the use of special serving lists in which all foods within a given group provide the same amount of phenylalanine, protein, and calories when given in the specified amounts.[6]

The optimal age for discontinuing the diet is not known. For psychologic reasons it is usually discontinued about the time the child enters school. A survey of phenylketonuria centers in the United States revealed varying results from centers that discontinued the diet. Some reported behavioral changes and deterioration of I.Q. in children taken off the diet.[7] Others have found no significant deterioration in I.Q. 3 years after termination of the diet at about 6 years of age.[8] Some recommend that until this issue is resolved, the diet should be

* Lofenalac®, by Mead Johnson and Company, Evansville, Indiana; Phenyl-free™, by Mead Johnson and Company; PKU-AID, available through Ross Laboratories, Columbus, Ohio. Manufactured in England.

maintained as long as possible and then a relaxed but still restricted low-phenylalanine diet should be used.[9] Phenylalanine restriction is often recommended during pregnancy of the phenylketonuric woman; however, one study has shown that such restriction may need to be in effect at the time of conception in these women in order to reduce the risk of infants with mental retardation, microcephaly, and congenital heart disease.[10]

Dietary Counseling

Eating problems are encountered frequently in the phenylketonuric children. These may be the result of great parental anxiety and feelings of guilt. The parent may overemphasize diet and allow it to dominate the relationships with the child. Initially, the acceptance of Lofenalac may be poor. If it is forced at first, or if the parent or brothers and sisters indicate dislike for the diet, the child may continue to refuse the formula. It is best to offer the formula at the beginning of the feeding when the child is hungry, and to avoid any show of concern if it is not fully accepted. When parents begin to see the improvement in the child, encouragement is provided for the considerable effort needed to maintain careful vigilance in its preparation.

Both parents must receive detailed information concerning the amounts of phenylalanine permitted daily and the amounts of foods that will provide them. They should be asked to demonstrate the measurement and preparation of the formula and to plan a series of daily menus showing the phenylalanine, protein, and calorie content. The diet must be continually monitored. A record of the child's daily intake should be kept and brought along each time the child is seen in the PKU clinic so that the physician and nutritionist can assess the child's progress in relation to the diet. A program of home services is invaluable in assuring that the diet is being used as planned. The public health nurse often supervises the home care and also consults with the dietitian or nutritionist in the planning and in problems of dietary management. Printed recipe materials should be carefully explained to the parent.

Tyrosinemia

Hereditary tyrosinemia is transmitted as an autosomal recessive gene. A deficiency of PARAHYDROXYPHENYLPYRUVIC ACID OXIDASE places a block upon the conversion of tyrosine to homogentisic acid. The plasma tyrosine, phenylalanine, and sometimes methionine levels are elevated, and increased amounts of tyrosine, *p*-hydroxyphenylpyruvic acid, methionine, other amino acids, and phosphates are excreted in the urine.

Patients with this deficiency show extensive liver and renal damage. Abdominal distension is present because of the enlarged liver and spleen. Liver disease may progress so rapidly that death results from liver failure. The reduced levels of blood phosphate are associated with vitamin-D-resistant rickets. Mental retardation is present.

Dietary Modification Initially a hydrolysate low in phenylalanine and tyrosine* is used with small amounts of milk added to provide these amino acids. If blood methionine levels are elevated, a synthetic mixture of amino acids without tyrosine, phenylalanine, and methionine is used together with a protein-free supplement† to provide carbohydrate, fat, vitamins, and minerals. A diet low in phenylalanine, tyrosine, and methionine has been described.[11]

Transient Tyrosinemia

Newborn infants sometimes have a transient form of tyrosinemia and tyrosyluria. These abnormalities occur especially in premature infants and are directly correla-

* Product 3200-AB, Mead Johnson & Company, Evansville, Indiana.

† Product 80056, Mead Johnson & Company, Evansville, Indiana.

ted with the level of protein intake. This appears to be a benign condition and is not associated with specific symptoms. The increased tyrosine levels in the blood and in the urine return to normal as the infant matures. The blood levels are reduced if adequate ascorbic acid is given early.

Maple Syrup Urine Disease

This inborn error of metabolism derives its name from the maple syrup odor of urine, a valuable clue in the diagnosis. The disease is also known as BRANCHED-CHAIN KETOACIDURIA, a term which relates to the biochemical defect. It was first recognized in the United States in 1954 and since then has been described in several other countries. It is transmitted as an autosomal recessive trait. The worldwide frequency is 1 per 224,000 newborns.[12]

Biochemical Defect and Clinical Changes

Three branched-chain amino acids, namely, leucine, isoleucine, and valine, are normally metabolized to keto acids and then further degraded through decarboxylation to simple acids. In maple syrup urine disease an OXIDATIVE DECARBOXYLASE in the white blood cells is missing. Because the carboxyl group cannot be removed, the amino acids and their keto acids accumulate in the blood and are excreted in excessive amounts in the urine. A metabolite related to isoleucine is believed to be responsible for the odor of the urine and of the sweat.

Infants appear normal at birth but begin to show symptoms within the first few days. They are unable to suck and swallow satisfactorily, respiration is irregular, and there are intermittent periods of rigidity and flaccidity. Seizures of the grand mal type may occur. If the infants survive, mental retardation is severe. Hypoglycemia has been observed in several patients and may be related to leucine sensitivity. Frequent infections lead to increased tissue catabolism and thus to a further accumulation of the offending metabolities in the circulation.

Dietary Treatment A diet restricted in leucine, isoleucine, and valine has given some encouraging results.[13] A special formula, consisting of one of several commercially available mixtures of amino acids without the branched-chain amino acids,* small amounts of milk, and a protein-free supplement,† has been described.[13] Fruits, vegetables, and cereals low in protein are added in controlled amounts as the child grows.[13,14] A variant form of the disorder responds to pharmacologic doses of thiamin.[15] The dietary modifications are needed permanently.

Homocystinuria

Biochemical and Clinical Findings This is a disorder of methionine metabolism. The enzyme CYSTATHIONINE SYNTHETASE is essential for the conversion of homocysteine to cystathionine, both of which are intermediate products formed in the metabolism of methionine. When the enzyme is lacking, increased amounts of methionine and homocystine are found in the plasma, and large amounts of homocystine are excreted in the urine. Lack of the enzyme is an autosomal recessive trait.

Homocystinuria may also be due to deranged vitamin B-12 metabolism or to low levels of the reductase enzyme involved in the remethylation of homocysteine to me-

* Gibco Amino Acid Mix minus Branched-Chain Amino Acids, Grand Island Biological Company, Grand Island, New York; MSUD Diet Powder, Mead Johnson & Company, Evansville, Indiana; MSUD-AID, available through Ross Laboratories, Columbus, Ohio. Manufactured in England. This product contains no carbohydrate or fat and should be used with an appropriate source, such as Product 80056.

† Product 80056, Mead Johnson & Company, Evansville, Indiana.

thionine. These disorders are characterized by low levels of methionine in serum. The optic lens is not dislocated in the latter type; otherwise symptoms are as in classic homocystinuria.

Homocystinuria occurs almost as frequently as phenylketonuria. Severe mental retardation is present in almost all patients. The optic lens is dislocated in all patients, and glaucoma and cataracts occur in some. There is a weakness of the muscles of the pelvic girdle and a shuffling gait. Skeletal abnormalities include long extremities, osteoporosis, and curvature of the spine. Pulmonary embolism, thrombosis, and cerebral accidents are common.

Dietary Modification Some patients respond to pyridoxine therapy. For these patients a normal, but not excessive, protein intake is recommended.[16] Low-methionine diets with adequate cysteine have been used for those patients who do not respond to pyridoxine therapy. Folic acid deficiency may occur in these patients. Methionine exchange lists and recipes have been described.[16] Commercial preparations low in methionine are available.*

Leucine-Induced Hypoglycemia

A relatively rare inborn error of metabolism, LEUCINE-INDUCED HYPOGLYCEMIA becomes apparent after about the fourth month of life. Convulsions may be the first indication of an abnormality. Infants with this disorder fail to thrive and show some evidence of delayed mental development. Signs typical of Cushing's syndrome—acne, hirsutism, obesity, and osteoporosis—are often present.

When L-leucine is given in a test dose to the infant, a profound lowering of the blood glucose occurs in the leucine-sensitive infant. The exact reason for the increased sensitivity is not known. Among the several theories suggested, the most likely one appears to be that leucine may act as a stimulus to insulin production or as an enhancement of insulin utilization.

Dietary Management A diet low in leucine is used,[17] but the minimum leucine requirement of 150 to 230 mg per kilogram must be included. Since all protein foods are sources of leucine, a restriction of this amino acid places restrictions upon the inclusion of protein-rich foods. The diet is planned to furnish the minimum requirements of protein for normal development. Fruits and vegetables are added to the diet according to the infant's normal feeding schedule. To counteract the hypoglycemic effects of the leucine, a carbohydrate feeding (equivalent to 10 gm) is given 30 to 40 minutes after each meal. By the age of 5 to 6 years the disease has run its course, and from that time on the child is able to tolerate a normal diet.

Galactosemia

Biochemical Defect Galactose disease is caused by the absence of an enzyme (GALACTOSE-1-PHOSPHATE URIDYL TRANSFERASE, sometimes abbreviated P-Gal-transferase) which is needed in the liver for the conversion of galactose to glucose. Galactose is derived from the hydrolysis of lactose in the intestine. It is absorbed normally in this inborn error, but in the absence of transferase, galactose, galactose-1-phosphate, and galactitol accumulate in the blood and tissues. Analysis of the red blood cells shows little or no transferase in those who have the disease, and only half the normal levels in carriers of the defect. Urine tests show the presence of galactose, albumin, and amino acids. A galactose tolerance test helps to establish the diagnosis. Mothers of galactosemic infants have a diminished ability to metabolize galactose. If they

* Product 3200-K, Mead Johnson & Company, Evansville, Indiana; Methionaid, available through Ross Laboratories, Columbus, Ohio. Manufactured in England. This product is devoid of methionine. Additional calories from carbohydrate and fat must be added.

drink unlimited amounts of milk during pregnancy, the possibility of damage to the fetus exists since galactose may pass the placenta. The enzyme defect is inherited as an autosomal recessive trait.

Clinical Changes The disease becomes apparent within a few days after birth by such symptoms as anorexia, vomiting, occasional diarrhea, drowsiness, jaundice, puffiness of the face, edema of the lower extremities, and weight loss. The spleen and liver enlarge, and in some there may be evidences of liver failure within a short time leading to ascites, bleeding, and early death. Mental retardation becomes evident very early in the course of the disease, and cataracts develop within the first year.

Dietary Treatment Milk is the important dietary source of lactose which in turn yields galactose. Human milk is especially high in galactose, and thus the breast-fed infant who lacks the necessary enzyme shows symptoms very early. The substitution of a nonmilk formula leads to rapid improvement as a rule. All of the symptoms disappear except that mental retardation which has already occurred is not reversible. Damage to the central nervous system is greatest during the first few weeks and months of life when growth is rapid. Therefore, the prompt initiation of therapy is essential.

A number of nonmilk formula products are available. These include Nutramigen,* ProSobee,* Neomullsoy,† and a meat-base formula.‡ Some pediatricians do not use the soybean preparations since STACHYOSE, a tetrasaccharide in soybeans, is believed to be hydrolyzed to galactose. Others have used such formulas with success. The maintenance of a galactose-free diet is monitored by testing red blood cells for their content of galactose-1-phosphate transferase.

The formulas are supplemented with calcium gluconate or chloride, iron, and vitamins. Since milk is the only food which supplies lactose, other foods may be introduced into the infant's diet at the appropriate times. These include breads, crackers, and cereals made without milk, eggs, meat, poultry, fish, fruits, vegetables, and gelatin desserts. All foods that contain milk must be rigidly excluded: most commercial breads, cookies, cakes, puddings, pudding mixes, some ready-to-eat cereals, all cheeses, cream, ice cream, butter, margarine churned with milk, chocolate, cold cuts, and others. See the list of foods to avoid for lactose-free diets, page 553. Liver, brains, and pancreas store galactose and are usually avoided. The stachyose present in soybeans, beets, Lima beans, and peas is not hydrolyzed to free galactose; thus, limited amounts of these foods are permitted.[18]

As with phenylketonuria, dietary counseling is of paramount importance. Infants accept the substitute formulas quite well, but older children may refuse them for a time. Parents must avoid showing too much anxiety about refusal of food. They need to become thoroughly familiar with lists of foods that contain milk and must learn to read labels with care. The diet is successful only when repeated opportunities are available for follow-up, whether in the clinic or in the home. Such follow-up visits not only reinforce dietary instruction but provide encouragement to the parents.

Complete elimination of galactose is necessary for the very young child but breads and other prepared foods containing milk are usually permitted when the child enters school.[18] Milk must be permanently excluded from the diet, however.

Fructosemia

This is an inborn error in which there is a deficiency of FRUCTOSE-1-PHOSPHATE AL-

* Nutramigen® and ProSobee® by Mead Johnson & Co., Evansville, Indiana.

† Neomullsoy by the Syntex Laboratories, Palo Alto, California.

‡ Meat-base formula by Gerber Products Company, Fremont, Michigan.

DOLASE which splits fructose-1-phosphate into glyceraldehyde and dihydroxyacetone phosphate. The introduction of sucrose or fructose in the infant's diet before 6 months of age results in anorexia, vomiting, failure to thrive, hypoglycemic convulsions, and dysfunction of the liver and kidney.[19] Older children with the defect are often asymptomatic or they may have spontaneous hypoglycemia. When an oral dose of fructose is given, the blood fructose and magnesium levels rise, but the levels of glucose and phosphate fall. The hypoglycemia that occurs is believed to be caused by reduced glycogenolysis and gluconeogenesis.

Treatment This condition is controlled by a diet that eliminates all sources of fructose from the diet. Most fruits contain some fructose, and the intestinal hydrolysis of sucrose also yields fructose. Sorbitol is oxidized to fructose; thus, foods containing this sugar should be avoided. Glucose should be used in place of sucrose, and starches are utilized normally. For the infant a formula is calculated to meet normal requirements, using glucose as the source of carbohydrate. Unsweetened cereals, egg yolk, strained meats, and strained vegetables are added at intervals as in normal infant feeding. Sugar beets, sweet potatoes, and peas contain appreciable amounts of sucrose.[20] (See also Table 33–2.) Most patients learn to avoid sweets.

Wilson's Disease

Hepatolenticular degeneration, or Wilson's disease, is a hereditary disorder transmitted by an autosomal recessive gene. The characteristic triad includes Kayser-Fleischer rings, a greenish brown discoloration in the eye, neurologic dysfunction, and low levels of ceruloplasmin, the copper-containing protein in blood. Increased deposits of copper in the brain, liver, and kidney are due to decreased biliary excretion. Because of renal intoxication by the copper, there is a marked aminoaciduria and a negative phosphate balance.

Clinical Findings In adults the disorder most often presents as neurologic disease while, in children, hepatic disease is seen. The onset of symptoms is correlated with the time required for sufficient copper to accumulate in the tissues to produce damage. They may appear as early as 4 or 5 years of age, or as late as the thirties. Signs and symptoms include splenomegaly, jaundice, liver enlargement, easy bruisability, and neurologic involvement. The common neurologic signs include indistinct speech, a fixed unblinking stare, hypertonus or rigidity, tremor, seizures, and dementia.

Treatment A chelating agent is used to increase the urinary excretion of copper. Patients are usually advised to avoid foods that are excessively high in copper such as organ meats, shellfish, mushrooms, legumes, whole-grain cereals, bran, chocolate, and nuts. (See Table A–2.) The normal copper intake is about 2 to 3 mg. To establish negative copper balance, a more restricted intake is necessary, usually 1.5 mg or less.[21] For such diets, distilled water must be used if the water supply contains more than 1 ppm copper. Cooking utensils made of copper cannot be used. A paucity of data on the copper content of foods introduces difficulty in planning a diet that is reliably low in copper. Because of the presence of copper in most foods, it is difficult to maintain a sufficiently high caloric intake.

Familial Hypercholesterolemia

This disorder involves a genetic defect in the catabolism of low-density lipoprotein (LDL). It is characterized by elevated plasma LDL-cholesterol levels, and deposits of LDL-cholesterol in tendons and arteries. It is inherited as an autosomal dominant trait. One of every 500 persons is a heterozygote for the disorder; the frequency of homozygotes is 1 per million population. The total plasma cholesterol for heterozygotes usually ranges from 300 to

600 mg per deciliter. The plasma cholesterol is moderately elevated from birth but the individual does not develop clinical symptoms until adulthood when tendon xanthomas and premature coronary disease develop. In homozygotes plasma cholesterol ranges from 650 to 1,000 mg per deciliter, and clinical symptoms occur in the very young child. Coronary disease is often fatal before adulthood is reached.[22]

Attempts to delay the atherosclerotic changes by dietary intervention in young children involve use of very low cholesterol intakes. Diets containing less than 150 mg cholesterol daily and a P/S ratio of 0.9:1 are effective in lowering serum cholesterol to normal levels in hypercholesterolemic 2-to-4-year-olds.[23] See Chapter 39 for diets restricted in cholesterol.

See Chapter 33 for discussion of the following genetic errors characterized by malabsorption: lactose intolerance; invertase-isomaltase deficiency; glucose-galactose malabsorption.

Problems and Review

1. A 1-month-old infant, weighing 4 kg, is diagnosed as having phenylketonuria.
   a. Why is prompt diet therapy essential for the treatment of this disorder and other errors of metabolism?
   b. What is phenylalanine? In what way is its function modified in phenylketonuria?
   c. What is Lofenalac? Why is it necessary to include some source of phenylalanine in the diet of the infant with phenylketonuria? What food source may be used?
   d. Outline the essential points to be covered in the counseling of the parents of this patient.
2. What is the principal defect in galactose disease?
   a. Examine the labels of a variety of packaged foods in a market, and prepare a list of those which contain milk.
   b. Plan a day's menu for a child with galactosemia.
   c. What points would you emphasize in counseling the parents of such a child?
3. Examine the labels of proprietary compounds such as Nutramigen, ProSobee, Neo-mullsoy, and Lofenalac. What supplements, if any, to these formulas are needed? What is the cost of any of these formulas for one day for a 3-month-old infant weighing 6 kg?
4. Why is carbohydrate given after meals to infants who are sensitive to leucine? What class of foods must be restricted when a leucine-restricted diet is used?
5. List some of the foods that would not be permitted for a patient who has Wilson's disease and who has been advised by his or her physician to omit foods high in copper.

Cited References

1. Garrod, A. E.: *Inborn Errors of Metabolism.* Frowde, Hodder & Stoughton, London, 1909.
2. Patel, M. S., and Arinze, I. J.: "Phenylketonuria: Metabolic Alterations Induced by Phenylalanine and Phenylpyruvate," *Am. J. Clin. Nutr.*, **28**:183–88, 1975.
3. O'Flynn, M. E. et al.: "The Diagnosis of Phenylketonuria," *Am. J. Dis. Child.*, **134**:769–74, 1980.
4. Kaufman, S.: "Differential Diagnosis of Variant Forms of Hyperphenylalaninemia," *Pediatrics,* **65**:840–41, 1980.

5. Danks, D. M., and Cotton, R. G. H.: "Early Diagnosis of Hyperphenylalaninemia Due to Tetrahydrobiopterin Deficiency (Malignant Hyperphenylalaninemia)," *J. Pediatr.*, **96**:854–56, 1980.
6. Acosta, P. B., and Wenz, E.: *Diet Management of PKU for Infants and Pre-School Children.* DHEW Publ. No. (HSA) 77–5209, U.S. Department of Health, Education, and Welfare, PHS, HSA, Bureau of Community Health Services. Rockville, Md., 1977.
7. Schuett, V. E., et al.: "Diet Discontinuation Policies and Procedures of PKU Clinics in the United States," *Am. J. Public Health,* **70**:498–503, 1980.
8. Koff, E. et al.: "Intelligence and Phenylketonuria: Effects of Diet Termination," *J. Pediatr.*, **94**:534–37, 1979.
9. Scriver, C. R., and Clow, C. L.: "Phenylketonuria: Epitome of Human Biochemical Genetics," *New Engl. J. Med.*, **303**:1394–1400, 1980.
10. Lenke, R. R., and Levy, H. L.: "Maternal Phenylketonuria and Hyperphenylalaninemia," *New Engl. J. Med.*, **303**:1202–8, 1980.
11. Michals, K. et al.: "Dietary Treatment of Tyrosinemia Type I," *J. Am. Diet. Assoc.*, **73**:507–14, 1978.
12. Naylor, E. W., and Guthrie, R.: "Newborn Screening for Maple Sirup Urine Disease (Branched Chain Ketoaciduria)," *Pediatrics,* **61**:262–66, 1978.
13. Bell, L. et al.: "Dietary Management of Maple-Sirup-Urine Disease: Extension of Equivalency Systems," *J. Am. Diet. Assoc.*, **74**:357–61, 1979.
14. Acosta, P. B., and Elsas, L. J.: "Dietary Treatment of Branched Chain Ketoaciduria (MSUD)," in *Dietary Management of Inherited Metabolic Disease: Phenylketonuria, Galactosemia, Tyrosinemia, Homocystinuria, Maple Sirup Urine Disease.* Atlanta: ACELMU Publishers, 1976.
15. Duran, M. et al.: "Effects of Thiamine in a Patient with a Variant Form of Branched-Chain Ketoaciduria," *Acta. Paediatr. Scand.*, **67**:367–72, 1978.
16. Carson, N. A. J.: "Homocystinuria," in *The Treatment of Inherited Metabolic Disease,* D. N. Raine, ed., MTP. Medical and Technical Publishing Co., Ltd., Lancaster, Lancs, Great Britain, 1975, Chap. 2.
17. Roth, H., and Segal, S.: "The Dietary Management of Leucine Sensitive Hypoglycemia with Report of a Case," *Pediatrics,* **34**:831–68, 1964.
18. Donnell, G. N., and Bergren, W. R.: "The Galactosaemias," in *The Treatment of Inherited Metabolic Disease,* D. N. Raine, ed., MTP. Medical and Technical Publishing Co., Ltd., Lancaster, Lancs, Great Britain, 1975, Chap. 4.
19. Froesch, E. R.: "Hereditary Fructose Intolerance and Fructose 1,6-Diphosphatase Deficiency," in *The Treatment of Inherited Metabolic Disease,* D. N. Raine, ed., MTP. Medical and Technical Publishing Co., Ltd., Lancaster, Lancs, Great Britain, 1975, Chap. 6.
20. Hardinge, M. G. et al.: "Carbohydrates in Foods," *J. Am. Diet. Assoc.*, **46**:197–204, 1965.
21. Goldstein, N. P., and Owen, C. A.: "Introduction: Symposium on Copper Metabolism and Wilson's Disease," *Mayo Clin. Proc.*, **49**:363–67, 1974.
22. Goldstein, J. L., and Brown, M. S.: "The LDL Receptor Locus and the Genetics of Familial Hypercholesterolemia," *Annu. Rev. Genet.*, **13**:259–89, 1979.
23. Larsen, R. et al.: "Special Diet for Familial Type II Hyperlipoproteinemia," *Am. J. Dis. Child.*, **128**:67–72, 1974.

Additional References

BERLOW, S.: "Progress in Phenylketonuria: Defects in the Metabolism of Biopterin," *Pediatrics,* **65**:837–39, 1980.

CARTWRIGHT, G. E.: "Diagnosis of Treatable Wilson's Disease," *New Engl. J. Med.*, **298**:1347–50, 1978.

Committee on Nutrition: "Special Diets for Infants with Inborn Errors of Amino Acid Metabolism" *Pediatrics*, **57**:783–92, 1976.

DOBYNS, W. B. et al.: "Clinical Spectrum of Wilson's Disease (Hepatolenticular Degeneration)," *Mayo Clin. Proc.*, **54**:35–42, 1979.

GRIECO, A. J.: "Homocystinuria: Pathogenetic Mechanisms," *Am. J. Med. Sci.*, **273**:120–32, 1977.

JUSTICE, P., and SMITH, G. F.: "Phenylketonuria," *Am. J. Nurs.*, **75**:1303–5, 1975.

Management of Newborn Infants with PKU. DHEW Publ. No. (HSA) 78–5211, U.S. Department of Health Education, and Welfare. PHS, HSA, Bureau of Community Health Services. Rockville, Md., 1978.

MARTIN, G. M., and NESTEL, P.: "Changes in Cholesterol Metabolism with Dietary Cholesterol in Children with Familial Hypercholesterolaemia," *Clin. Sci.*, **56**:377–80, 1979.

NAYMAN, R. et al.: "Observations on the Composition of Milk-Substitute Products for Treatment of Inborn Errors of Amino Acid Metabolism. Comparisons with Human Milk," *Am. J. Clin. Nutr.*, **32**:1279–89, 1979.

NOEL, M. B. et al.: "Dietary Treatment of Maple Sirup Urine Disease (Branched Chain Ketoaciduria)," *J. Am. Diet. Assoc.*, **69**:62–68, 1976.

ODIEVRE, M. et al.: "Hereditary Fructose Intolerance in Childhood," *Am. J. Dis. Child.*, **132**:605–8, 1978.

YUDKOFF, M. et al.: "Errors of Carbohydrate Metabolism in Infants and Children," *Clin. Pediatr.*, **17**:820–28, 1978.

45 Nutrition in Children's Diseases

ALTHOUGH the principles of normal and therapeutic nutrition that apply to the adult are also applicable to the sick child, additional factors that must be carefully considered for the child are (1) growth needs; (2) stage of physical, emotional, and social development; (3) the presence of physical handicaps in some; and (4) the more rapid nutritional deterioration which occurs.

The essentials of normal nutrition provide the base line for planning meals for the sick child. (See Chapters 19 and 20.) The factors affecting food acceptance must be considered (see Chapter 14), and the principles of nutritional care and counseling are similar to those for adults. (See Chapter 24.) The principles of dietary modification for many conditions are similar for adults and for children, and the preceding chapters pertaining to therapeutic nutrition should be consulted for specific regimens. The discussion that follows supplements the descriptive material set forth in the earlier chapters.

Feeding Problems of the Sick Child

Like adults, children face many obstacles in illness. Eating a satisfactory diet may be difficult because of fatigue, nausea, lack of appetite occasioned by the illness and by drugs, and pain. Children often regress to an earlier stage of feeding; for example, the child who has learned to accept chopped foods may refuse them, or the child who can feed himself or herself may refuse to eat unless someone feeds him or her. Older children especially may experience a sense of failure and express it by excessive eating or refusal to eat. Illness produces emotional tensions in the child as well as in the adult. The child who must be placed in a hospital is also faced with the separation from home and parents. The principles of feeding the normal child apply in even greater degree to the child who is ill.

Insofar as possible the feeding program should establish a pattern of continuity with that to which the child is accustomed. A record of the child's feeding history is a first requisite so that the normal or therapeutic diet makes allowances for individual likes and dislikes. The period of a child's illness is no time in which to introduce new foods or to provide equipment that the child does not know how to handle. (See Figure 45–1).

Even though careful menu planning takes into consideration the usual likes and dislikes of children and includes variations in both flavor and textures, foods may be refused. The illness itself and the strange environment are sufficient cause for such refusal; sometimes portions are a bit too large, or there may be a slight change in the flavoring or texture of a familiar food. Regardless of the reason for refusal, nothing can be gained by trying to force a child to eat.

Nurses and nutritionists must like children and must enjoy working with them if they expect to achieve good results in nutritional care. They must be observant of the child's behavior, of the acceptance or rejection of food, and of what the child says about the food. They have a special responsibility to communicate with the parents. From the parents they learn about the child's food habits at home, and about his or her attitudes toward food. In turn the parents are kept informed about the

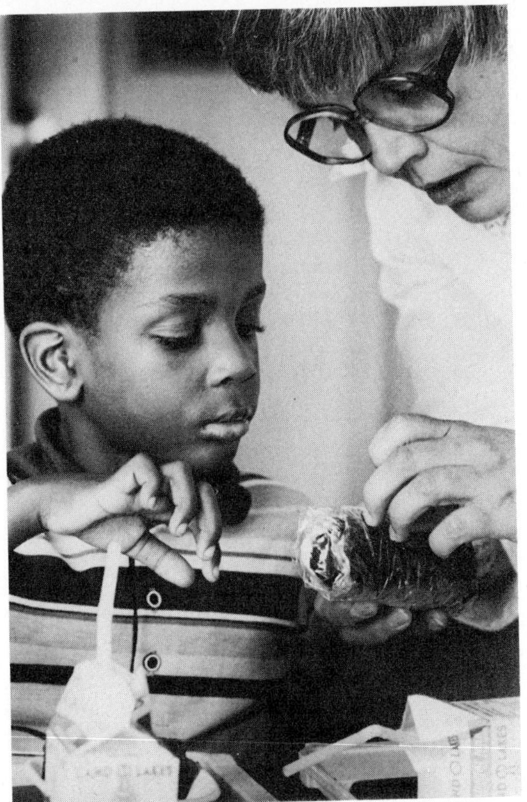

Figure 45–1. The child who is ill will usually eat better when he is given foods with which he is familiar. (Courtesy, Metropolitan Medical Center, Minneapolis.)

child's progress in food acceptance while in the hospital, and about changes that may be required after discharge.

Children often eat better when they are fed in groups. Family-style service in the pediatric ward to children who are well enough to sit up is more successful than individual tray service. Older children enjoy selecting their foods from a cafeteria arrangement whenever that is possible. Every advantage should be taken of birthdays and holidays to provide favorite foods and special treats. Many children are encouraged to eat when the mother can bring a favorite food, provided that it does not contradict the dietary regimen that has been ordered. Most hospitals now encourage parents to visit at any time they wish, and a young child fed by a parent may respond better than one who is fed by a stranger.

Dietary Counseling

Parents and children who are old enough to understand are jointly counseled regarding dietary modifications that will be required at home. Much less friction is likely to occur at home when the child is included in the interview. Parents assume the primary responsibility for nutritional care of the young child, but the child needs to know what is expected. As early as possible the child should begin to assume some responsibility for his or her care. Older children under parental guidance gradually assume full responsibility for their own diets. In counseling it is important to direct the interview and the instructions to the child rather than to the parent. (See Figure 45–2.)

One important aspect of counseling is to determine the attitudes of the parent toward the development of food habits, and likewise the child's attitudes not only toward the food but also toward his or her parents. Not infrequently the child uses food to achieve various ends.

If a modified diet will be required indefinitely as for diabetes mellitus, every effort must be made to plan this within the framework of the normal life pattern of the child; the diet must not become the dominating factor that interferes with the child's psychosocial development. Being like one's peers is very important to the child, and for many reasons the child may be reluctant to disclose that he or she is in any way different. Insofar as possible the diet should be planned so that it can include foods that are popular with other children. The child must be helped to understand that the condition does not make him or her abnormal in relations with others. Selecting foods from those offered by the school lunch would be better for the diabetic child, for example, than carrying a lunch.

Sometimes the hospital stay is sufficiently

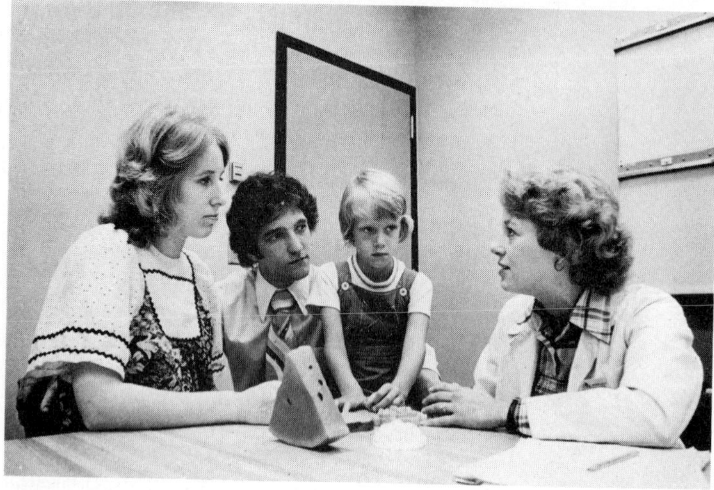

Figure 45–2. The dietitian consults with a young diabetic child and her parents. The child's meal plan is planned around the family pattern. The importance of snacks and avoidance of concentrated sweets is emphasized. (Courtesy, Metropolitan Medical Center, Minneapolis.)

long that some nutrition education can be included in a group situation. A number of movies appropriate for young children are available from the National Dairy Council and other sources. Other children often view movies with interest in the hospital playroom that they might consider to be boring in the school situation. The teacher assigned to the hospital schoolroom may also be involved in the dietary instruction. For example, children can learn to keep records, to score their diets, and to learn about their needs for basic foods. The calculation of a diet with meal exchanges may be used as an arithmetic assignment. Eye-catching fliers on patients' trays have been used to introduce new ideas about foods such as a food custom of an ethnic group or a simple recipe.

Weight Control

Obesity The problem of obesity is not limited to adults. From 10 to 20 per cent of children and teenagers are overweight and it is likely that many of these youngsters were overweight as infants. Excessive weight gain in the first year of life is highly correlated with development of obesity. Juvenile-onset obesity is characterized by increased number and size of adipose cells. Once formed, the excess number of adipose cells cannot be altered by dieting; only the size can be reduced. Since 80 per cent of youngsters who are obese remain so as adults, prevention, by regulation of food intake and activity patterns in childhood, has important implications for later years.

Some children overeat because the pattern of overfeeding established in infancy is carried over into childhood. An abundance of rich, high-calorie foods is readily available and, together with relative inactivity, becomes part of the family pattern.

In one study, several factors accounted for greater food intake by obese boys than their nonobese brothers both at home and at school: mothers tended to serve the obese boys larger portions; obese boys left less food on their plates; and they purchased more food at school or obtained it from their nonobese peers. Activity patterns also differed in the two groups. Compared with control subjects, the obese boys were less active at home but equally active at school. However, when oxygen consumption was measured, energy expenditure in the obese boys was greater than that of the nonobese. Thus, increased energy intake was more important than differences in energy output in maintaining the obese state in these boys.[1] Other studies have shown that obese children do not eat any more food than normal weight children and, in fact, may eat less, but their energy expenditure is considerably less.[2] They avoid active sports, and when they do participate they manage to become involved as little as possible. School health programs aimed at reducing obesity have emphasized increased physical exercise with or without nutrition education. In several of these, minimal weight reduction was achieved, but significant reductions in body fat as indicated by decreased triceps skinfold measurements were reported. In most, students were still overweight at the end of the treatment period and did not continue to exercise once the structured program ended.[3] Like adults, children may use food to cover up loneliness or lack of social relationships, or failure in everyday (school) activities.

Because the energy requirements of children are relatively high, their diets are usually less restricted than those for adults. About 1,200 to 1,800 kcal may be included, depending upon the stature and activity of the child. Liberal protein, mineral, and vitamin allowances are essential so that tissue and stature development are not adversely affected. Equally important is a program of regular physical activity with emphasis on increasing energy expenditure. Some recommend reducing caloric intake by 200 per day and increasing energy expenditure by the same amount.[4] The low-calorie diets described on page 482 may be used as a basis for planning the child's diet. One cup of milk should be added to these diets daily so that the child receives his or her quota of 1 quart. Favorite foods need not be omitted entirely but usually need to be limited. Learning to limit portion sizes and substituting low-calorie snacks are important concepts for the youngster to understand.

It is vital that the child (and parents) realize what a loss of weight may mean to him or her. This may mean improved appearance, poise, and gracefulness; greater participation in sports; or winning the approval of fellow playmates and schoolmates. The physician, nurse, and dietitian who are guiding the child's weight-reduction program must show understanding of the child's problems and must maintain interest through a careful follow-up of the progress being made.

Underweight Data from the Ten-State Nutrition Survey showed that a significant number of children are underweight and undersized.[5] Such children usually tire easily, are irritable and restless, and are more susceptible to infections. As in the correction of obesity, the cause for underweight must first be sought so that treatment may be properly directed. The diet is corrected with respect to its adequacy of the essential nutrients, after which increases in the level of kilocalories may be made gradually. A reasonable amount of outdoor exercise and regulated rest are important elements of the weight-gaining program. (For high-calorie diets, see Chapter 28.)

Growth Failure Infants sometimes fail to thrive when placed in institutions because they are deprived of the normal emotional environment of the home. Such growth failure also occurs in the home when parents reject their children, neglect them, or provide an otherwise hostile environment. Intellectual and neurologic development is impaired as well. Studies have shown that a disproportionately high number of children from such environments were low-birth-weight infants. Martin has suggested that the high incidence of brain damage in these children may be related to poor nutrition in utero. Postnatal undernutrition is also seen in many of these children. In a study of 42 abused and neglected children, 33 per cent were found to be undernourished. In children who were both undernourished and physically abused, the prognosis for normal intellectual development was much poorer.[6]

Gastrointestinal Disturbances in Infants and Children

Infant Feeding Problems Many babies regurgitate small amounts of food, and this is no cause for concern. Usually it can be avoided by more frequent "burping" of the infant. Vomiting is more serious and should receive the attention of the physician.

Some babies cry loudly and for long intervals following feeding. Usually they have swallowed excessive amounts of air and have been inadequately "burped." However, some babies continue to cry even with "burping" and parents are likely to become quite distraught. These "colicky" babies usually grow well, and the parents need reassurance that they are progressing satisfactorily and will usually outgrow the colic within a few months. Colic sometimes occurs because the baby is overfed, is tired, or is cold.

Constipation Formula-fed infants usually have but one bowel movement daily, whereas breast-fed infants have two or three. Only when the stools are hard and dry and eliminated with difficulty does constipation exist. Prune juice or strained prunes given daily usually suffice to correct the constipation.

In the young child, constipation is sometimes due to emotional upset arising out of conflict with the mother over toilet training. The child may learn to ignore the urge to defecate as a means of gaining attention. In time, delayed elimination weakens normal peristalsis and the stools become dry and hard and are difficult to evacuate.

The causes of constipation in older children are similar to those in adults. Corrective treatment includes emphasis upon regularity of habits, increased fluid intake, and a diet that includes raw and cooked vegetables and fruits and some whole-grain cereals and breads. (See Chapter 32) Milk may need to be limited for some persons.

Diarrhea Diarrhea occurring in infants and children may be functional or organic. It may be caused by the same factors as in adults or may be related to improper handling of the formula, or to its composition or concentration. Acute diarrhea can sometimes be traced to improper handling of foods or formulas. The incidence is several times higher in bottle-fed than in breast-fed infants and is greatly increased in the summer months when it is due to unsanitary preparation or inadequate refrigeration.

Serious consequences follow diarrhea in infants under 1 year of age if treatment is not prompt. The large loss of fluids and electrolytes quickly leads to dehydration, fever, loss of kidney function, and severe acidosis if electrolyte loss is chiefly through the intestinal tract. There may also be marked vomiting with loss of acid, in which case there may be no acidosis but a lowering of the total body anions and cations.

Modification of the diet. When mild diarrhea occurs in breast-fed infants, breast feeding may be continued but the baby is likely to take less milk for a few days. A 5 per cent glucose solution may also be offered at 3 or 4-hour intervals. Bottle-fed babies may be given a half-strength solution of skim milk or other fluids as directed by the physician. Both the volume of formula given and the concentration of the formula are increased gradually. Since it is important to maintain fluid balance, the formula may be supplemented with 5 per cent oral glucose solution.

In severe diarrhea, dehydration and acidosis are corrected by the intravenous administration of glucose and electrolyte solutions or through use of a semisynthetic fiber-free liquid diet by way of nasogastric tube. Many infants with moderate to severe diarrhea have a transient intolerance to lactose and sometimes to other carbohydrates as well. For these infants soy-isolate or casein hydrolysate formulas are sometimes used.* Convalescence may be prolonged

* Isomil® by Ross Laboratories, Columbus, Ohio. Mullsoy® and NeoMullsoy® by Syntex Laboratories,

and the increases in concentration and in volume of the formula must be made cautiously.

The treatment of diarrhea in older children is similar to that for adults, namely, the omission of food during the first day or two, the gradual introduction of low-residue foods (Chapter 32), and progression to a soft diet.

Celiac Disturbances The celiac syndrome includes several disturbances in which the symptoms, the disorders of absorption, and the nutritional deficiencies are similar. They are gluten-induced enteropathy also known as primary idiopathic steatorrhea, celiac disease (in children), or nontropical sprue (in adults); cystic fibrosis of the pancreas; and kwashiorkor. The symptoms, metabolic alterations, and dietary management for gluten enteropathy have been discussed in Chapter 33 and for cystic fibrosis in Chapter 34. However, some adaptations of the diet will need to be made for the infant and toddler according to their food requirements for growth and development.

Modification of the diet. A high caloric intake is mandatory in these diseases because up to 50 per cent of the calories may be excreted in the stools. The intake should be increased by 50 to 75 per cent above normal levels. For infants during the acute phase of illness this necessitates 120 to 200 kcal per kilogram. A high protein intake is also recommended initially. As improvement occurs the protein intake is gradually reduced to normal levels. Supplements of the fat-soluble and water-soluble vitamins are always indicated, and iron supplementation may also be needed.

In celiac disease and in cystic fibrosis large amounts of fat are excreted. This may persist for a long time after subjective improvement occurs. Although fat restriction was formerly used, most pediatricians now allow a moderate fat intake. The increased intake of fat leads to greater quantities of fat in the stool, but the total amount of fat absorbed is also increased, thereby increasing the caloric intake. Pancreatic enzymes are used for patients with cystic fibrosis of the pancreas and are taken with each meal. In hot weather the salt intake needs to be increased for patients with cystic fibrosis, but this is not necessary for celiac disease.

Children with cystic fibrosis vary widely in their tolerance to foods, and no single diet is appropriate for all patients. The levels of calories, protein, fat, and carbohydrate must be adjusted individually for each child. Some foods increase abdominal distension, pain, and steatorrhea in some children but not others.

For the young infant a high-protein formula such as *Probana** supplies two thirds to three fourths of total caloric intake. The remaining calories are furnished by glucose and/or banana flakes or banana powder added to the formula. At 2 to 4 months these foods are gradually introduced: cottage cheese, egg yolk, strained beef or liver, apple juice or applesauce, and banana or banana flakes.

With improvement, other foods are gradually added to include a wider variety of strained and then chopped meats, mild cheese, puréed and then chopped cooked vegetables and fruits, and plain gelatin. Wheat, rye, barley, and sometimes oat products must be excluded for the patient with gluten enteropathy, but these cereals may be gradually introduced into the diet for the patient with cystic fibrosis. (See also page 575.) The additions of food are made much more gradually than for normal infants and children. Strained foods are used for a somewhat longer period of time, and raw fruits and vegetables are introduced at a later time.

Some older children develop diabetes secondary to cystic fibrosis. In these chil-

---

Inc., Palo Alto, California. Nutramigen,® Pregestimil,® and ProSobee® by Mead Johnson & Company, Evansville, Indiana.

* *Probana*® by Mead Johnson and Company, Evansville, Indiana.

dren, the diabetes is usually mild and easily controlled with insulin injections. Ketoacidosis is uncommon in these youngsters.

Diabetes

The first patient treated with insulin prepared by Banting and Best in 1922 was a 14-year-old diabetic boy. Approximately 1 in every 2,500 children under 16 years is diabetic.[7]

Insulin-Dependent Diabetes The etiology, metabolic aberrations, diagnostic tests, and clinical characteristics of insulin-dependent (Type I) diabetes have been described in Chapter 37. The disease in children differs in a number of important respects from that in adults. The onset of symptoms is usually more abrupt and the disease usually increases in severity during the period of growth. A seasonal incidence has been noted, with an increase in new cases during the autumn and winter months. Some evidence suggests that viruses such as mumps or measles may precipitate the disease or may trigger an autoimmune response to some genetically predisposed children.[8] In contrast to the adult, obesity is uncommon; in fact, when first seen the diabetic child is likely to be underweight and not growing because he or she has not been metabolizing food adequately.

All diabetic children need insulin, since there appear to be few if any functioning cells of the islets of Langerhans. The maintenance of control between acidosis on the one hand and hypoglycemia on the other is often difficult because of the greater frequency of infections and the erratic physical activity and emotional control.

Psychologic Considerations Too often the child and parents feel that the child is different from other children and that there is a certain stigma attached to the diabetic state. If the child experiences insulin reactions, he or she will be afraid to participate in the activities of other children and may become more dependent upon parents. The diabetic adolescent is likely to be especially difficult to control. Like other adolescents he or she may rebel against authority, and may show independence by failure to keep the disease in good control.

The guidance of the child in all aspects of development, not only in the treatment of the diabetes, requires great patience, forbearance, and understanding on the part of the parent and physician. The child and the parent must recognize the interrelationship of diet, insulin, and activity and the importance of regulation. It is equally important that the child learn—and parents understand—that the child can take his or her place in the family and society just as the nondiabetic child.

Modification of the Diet The principles of dietary modification for the diabetic child are similar to those for the adult. (See Chapter 37.) The nutritive requirements are the same as those for the normal child of the same age, size, and activity. (See Chapter 20.) Briefly, these needs are as follows:

Calories. 48 to 100 kcal per kilogram (22 to 45 kcal per pound).

Protein. The recommended daily allowance is, for younger children, 1.5 gm per kilogram (0.68 gm per pound), and for older children, 1.0 gm per kilogram (0.45 gm per pound). The American Diabetes Association recommends that 12 to 20 per cent of total calories be provided as protein.[9]

Carbohydrate. From 50 to 60 per cent of calories are from carbohydrate. About 70 per cent of the carbohydrate is starch and the remainder is from lactose, fructose, or sucrose.

Fat. The remaining calories are from fat, with an emphasis on polyunsaturated fats and restriction of saturated fats and cholesterol. Some clinicians prefer a polyunsaturated to saturated fat ratio of 1.2, and cholesterol limited to 250 mg daily.[10]

Other. The additional calcium requirements are easily met when 3 to 4 cups of milk are included daily. Other minerals and vitamins are provided in satisfactory amounts when the exchange lists are used as the basis of meal planning. Children should receive vitamin D either in milk or as a supplement.

The diet prescription should be adjusted periodically to make allowances for satisfactory growth. Emphasis should be on day-to-day consistency in distribution of calories and carbohydrate for meals and snacks in accordance with the type and action of insulin and physical activity. Most children receive NPH insulin; thus, an appropriate division of calories and carbohydrate might be 2/10, 2/10, 3/10 for the three main meals and 1/10 at each of three snacks taken in the midmorning, midafternoon, and evening. Some clinicians favor regularity of calorie intake using a fixed dose of insulin,[11] whereas others prefer adjustment of insulin dosage without changing the basic meal pattern.[9] Children should receive a snack prior to exercise and should have available rapidly utilized carbohydrate such as juice, carbonated drinks, or candy to forestall the possibility of an insulin reaction during and after exercise.

Dietary Control Although the lifespan of diabetic children has improved greatly, the incidence of degenerative diseases is unusually high after 10 to 20 years. The possibilities of diminished vision and even blindness, of coronary artery disease, and of kidney disease during the prime of life are serious, and as yet unsolved, problems.

Retinopathy is present in about 20 per cent of diabetics after 10 years and in half of those with diabetes of 20 years' duration. Up to 40 per cent of those who have had the disease for 25 years have diabetic neuropathy. Renal disease accounts for half the deaths in insulin-dependent diabetics of many years.[11]

Measurement of A_1C hemoglobin is one means of assessing long-term control of hyperglycemia. The level of A_1C hemoglobin is normally less than 3 per cent but in persistent hyperglycemia may be 6 to 10 per cent.[12] Many investigators believe that the degenerative changes are related to persistent hyperglycemia.[7] Jackson believes that the changes can be delayed many years if the diabetes is well controlled.[7] Under such control the blood sugar is kept as nearly normal as possible and glycosuria is avoided for the most part.

Some pediatricians use a so-called *free diet*, allowing the child to eat all family foods but usually including snacks and restricting concentrated sweets and high-carbohydrate desserts. Enough insulin is given to metabolize food for normal growth and to avoid ketosis, but mild hyperglycemia and glycosuria are disregarded. At the other extreme are those pediatricians who maintain rigid chemical control and require weighed or carefully measured diets.

Insulin In early stages of juvenile diabetes the pancreas sometimes produces small amounts of insulin, but this rapidly diminishes. As growth accelerates the insulin requirement increases greatly and control becomes much more difficult.

Jackson recommends at least two doses of intermediate-acting insulin for the desirable three-meal-plus-snacks pattern. The morning dose is a mixture of regular and NPH insulin. A second dose of intermediate-acting insulin is given late in the afternoon (about 5:00 P.M.). With this program the blood sugar is maintained as nearly normal as possible throughout the 24-hour day. This regimen is intended to avoid glycosuria or insulin reactions.[7]

Dietary Counseling

Whenever possible, initial hospitalization is desirable not only to stabilize the diabetes in the child but especially to set up an adequate program of education. The child and parents must face the issue of diabetes squarely, but also recognize that the child can live a happy, useful life. Regardless of the opinions about chemical or clinical control, pediatricians agree that close adherence to the diet at the beginning provides security and guidance for the child and parent during the period of adjustment to the disease. The initial diet could be one that provides few substitutions until the patient is thoroughly accustomed to it; then gradually the diet is liberalized with respect to the food choices until the meal exchange lists are used with ease. On festive occasions, such as birthdays and holidays, allowance for special treats should be made.

Children, like adults, need to be taught the nature of the disease, how to administer insulin, how to select the daily diet from the plan set up, how to test the urine, and how to keep records. The importance of cleanliness and personal hygiene must be emphasized. The recognition of the signs of insulin reactions or of acidosis and what to do when these signs appear must be learned. See also pages 609 to 612 for further details on dietary counseling. (See Figure 45–3.)

Diabetic camps provide an unusual educational opportunity for children to learn more about the care of themselves and also to learn the important social adjustments with other children. Such camps are well staffed with recreational leaders, nurses, dietitians, physicians, and laboratory technicians.

Renal Disease

The causes of renal disease in children are similar to those in adults. The etiology, clinical manifestations, biochemical abnormalities, and principles of dietary modification are discussed in Chapter 41. These considerations hold for children as well, although quantitative differences must be taken into account. In this section nephrotic syndrome and chronic renal insufficiency in children are considered.

Nephrotic Syndrome

Symptoms and Clinical Findings The nephrotic syndrome includes so-called lipoid nephrosis and the nephrotic phase of glomerulonephritis. This rare syndrome occurs in young children at an average age of 2½ years. Its onset is usually insidious and is characterized by marked edema, heavy proteinuria (more than 4 gm in 24 hours), serious depletion of plasma proteins, especially the albumin fraction, and hypercholesterolemia. The edema is often so marked that it seems as if the skin would

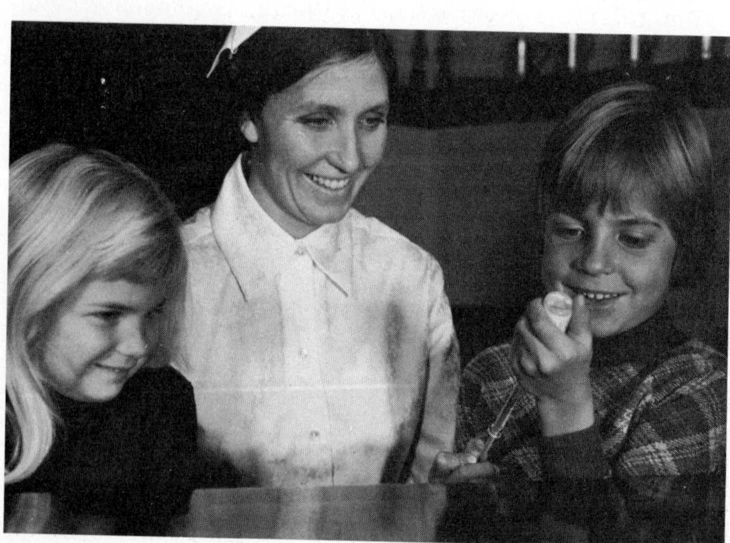

Figure 45–3. Success! Learning to measure his own insulin is an important first step toward independence for the young diabetic. (Courtesy, Diabetes Education Center, Minneapolis.)

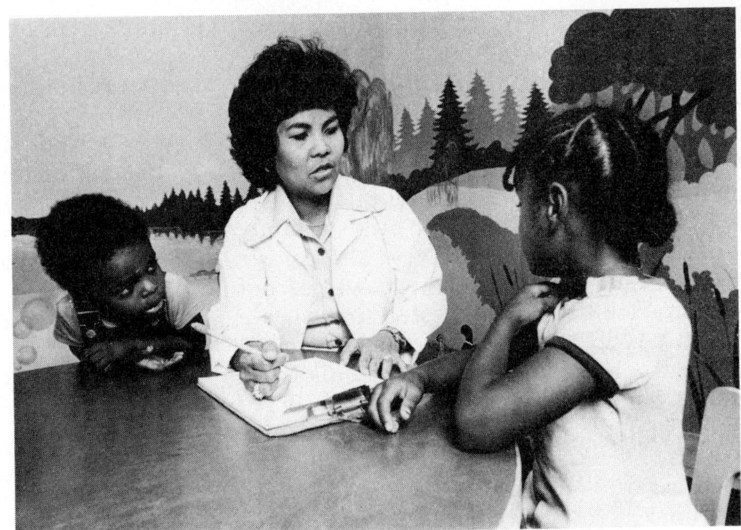

Figure 45–4. The dietitian talks with young child to determine what foods she likes. This is the first step in planning a diet that will meet the child's needs and that will be well accepted. (Courtesy, Hennepin County Medical Center, Minneapolis.)

burst. When diuresis occurs the severe depletion of tissue proteins and the accompanying undernutrition become fully apparent.

Excessive urinary wastage of ceruloplasmin, protein-bound iodine, iron-binding proteins, prothrombin, and complement also occur. Because of the loss of complement, the incidence of infections is high and is an important cause of death. Hematuria, hypertension, and azotemia are minimal or absent in lipoid nephrosis.

The aims of therapy include control of infections and edema and establishment of good nutrition. Corticosteroid therapy results in remission of clinical and biochemical aspects of the disease in the majority of patients. Others may progress to terminal stages of nephritis or succumb to infections.

Modification of the Diet Patients with nephrosis have a particularly poor appetite, and the high-calorie high-protein diets that are often ordered are not necessarily consumed. Much attention must be given to the selection of foods that are acceptable to the child. With the loss of edema fluid the appetite usually improves. (See Figure 45–4.)

The caloric intake should be based upon the desirable weight for the child's height and body build. Unless the caloric intake is adequate, effective tissue regeneration cannot take place. The protein intake is generally a little higher than normal; about 3 to 4 gm per kilogram is suitable for the preschool child and 2 to 3 gm per kilogram for school-age children.

Sodium restriction is prescribed in the presence of edema. Since unsalted foods are poorly accepted, prolonged restriction is undesirable. Diuretics may bring about such rapid diuresis that the blood levels of both sodium and potassium are reduced. In such instances the sodium content of the diet should be increased, and juices rich in potassium offered. See Chapter 40 for planning of sodium-restricted diets.

Chronic Renal Insufficiency

A major problem in most children on long-term dialysis for chronic renal disease is growth failure. The etiology is complex and inadequate caloric intake is just one of several factors involved. Poor appetite and multiple dietary restrictions make food less appealing.

Dietary Considerations A major difficulty with the diet is providing adequate calories without exceeding the protein, mineral, and fluid allowances. The calorie intake needed for optimal growth is not known. Holliday has suggested that prepubertal children with severe uremia need 60 kcal per kilogram in order to maintain nitrogen equilibrium, and from 35 to 40 gm protein.[13] Alternatively, a 20 gm protein diet supplemented with amino acids may be used. Improved nitrogen balance and better growth are achieved with amino acids than with the corresponding keto acid analogs.[14] The protein allowance for children on dialysis is 1.0 to 1.5 gm high-biologic value protein per kilogram of body weight. Sodium usually is not restricted unless there is hypertension, edema, or excessive weight gain between dialyses. The allowance is then limited to 50 mg per kilogram per day.[15] Hyperkalemia occurs and usually necessitates moderate potassium restriction.

The active form of vitamin D, 1,25-dihydroxycholecalciferol, is synthesized in the kidney. As renal function deteriorates, osteodystrophy becomes a serious metabolic problem. Hyperparathyroidism, defective absorption of calcium, and altered metabolism of vitamin D are involved. Small doses of synthetic 1,25-dihydroxycholecalciferol are used to correct the calcium and phosphorus imbalance. Phosphorus intake must also be restricted to less than 500 mg daily in renal osteodystrophy. Aluminum hydroxide gel is given to bind dietary phosphate. Restriction of milk to reduce the phosphorus intake also lowers the calcium intake, and supplements, 0.5 gm for younger children and 1.0 gm for older children, are needed. A number of suitable commercial products and recipes low in protein, sodium, and potassium are available, but monotony and lack of palatability limit their acceptance by many patients. Supplements of the B complex vitamins, folic acid, ascorbic acid, and trace minerals are needed, especially for patients on dialysis. Ferrous sulfate is recommended for patients who have iron-deficiency anemia.

Because of the many nutritional problems in this disease, parents of these children require much guidance in meal planning in order that they can provide appropriate foods which are acceptable to the child.

Allergy

The designation of allergy has been used frequently for those conditions resulting from a sensitivity to a food. With the increased understanding of hereditary diseases, it is now apparent that many so-called allergies are, in fact, the failure to metabolize a given nutrient because of the congenital deficiency of one or more enzymes. There remain, however, many diseases which are not yet explained on any such basis and which are classified as allergies.

Foods are responsible for the majority of allergies in children under 3 years of age. The chief offending foods are milk, eggs, chocolate, cola, citrus fruits, legumes, corn products, tomato, wheat, and pork. When the child is young, it is relatively simple to determine which food is responsible by allowing only milk and crystalline vitamins. If a food other than milk is responsible, the symptoms, such as eczema, will be relieved in a few days; but if milk or nonfood allergy is responsible for the disturbance, no improvement will take place.

When the symptoms of allergy are mild, it is always necessary to consider the relative importance of the allergic disturbance in relation to the diet of the child. It is better management, for example, to treat a mild case of eczema locally than to subject the child to the dangers of an inadequate diet with its far more serious consequences.

For older children, the diagnosis of allergy is determined by using an elimination diet and noting reappearance of symptoms after the food is reintroduced into the diet. The treatment is planned as for adults. (See Chapter 43.)

Milk Sensitivity About 2 per cent of all children are sensitive to milk, according to various estimates. In many instances this may be associated with infection and emotional stress; in others genetic factors may be a cause. (See Galactose Disease, Chapter 44, and Lactose Intolerance, Chapter 33.) The pediatric diagnostic tests for lactose intolerance have been discussed in Chapter 33.

The response to the ingestion of milk is almost immediate in some and may lead to colic, spitting up of the feeding, irritability, diarrhea, and respiratory disorders. A delayed reaction may occur hours to days following the ingestion of milk, and thus it becomes difficult to determine the exact cause. The incidence of hypochromic anemia in some infants has been attributed to sensitivity to milk. Following the ingestion of milk by these sensitive infants, some blood is lost from the gastrointestinal tract. This may average several milliliters per day and may go unnoticed until the anemia becomes apparent months later. Some infants may have a sufficiently high intake of other iron-rich foods so that the anemic tendency is counteracted.

Dietary treatment. Sometimes it is only necessary to change the form of the milk to improve tolerance—that is, boiled, powdered, acidulated, or evaporated milk may be satisfactory when fresh cow's milk is not. Some children will tolerate no milk whatsoever and it is necessary to substitute formulas in which the protein is derived from meat* or soybean. (See page 551.) The tolerance to milk improves in many infants, but others need to continue a milk-free diet indefinitely.

Feeding Handicapped Children

Cerebral Palsy This is a disorder in which motor control is disturbed due to brain damage. It affects some 300,000 children in the United States. A significant proportion weigh less than 2,500 gm at birth. Cerebral anoxia may be an etiologic factor in these infants. Feeding problems are common in children with cerebral palsy.

Reverse swallowing wave. When the motor system of the tongue and throat is affected, food is not pushed back to the throat, but the tongue motion pushes the food forward. Initially such children must be tube fed, but in time they learn to put food at the back of the tongue and by tilting the head backward learn to swallow. These children often become severely undernourished because feeding is such a prolonged process. Concentrated foods with maximum protein and calorie value should be emphasized to keep the volume to a minimum. Vitamin and mineral supplements are usually required.

Athetoids are those who are constantly in motion and who thus burn up a great deal of energy. Although they require a high-calorie high-protein diet, the ingestion of the necessary amounts of food is difficult because of the constant motion. Feeding is quite time consuming and emphasis should be placed upon concentrated foods of high caloric value. Children should be encouraged to feed themselves by giving them foods that they can pick up with their fingers such as pieces of fruit and sandwiches. Many devices have been developed as aids in feeding. (See page 456.)

Spastics are very limited in their activity, and they may also be indulged in eating by their parents. Consequently they gain excessive amounts of weight, and the obesity in turn further restricts their ability to get around. These individuals require

* MBF (Meat Base Formula) by Gerber Products Company, Fremont, Michigan.

marked restriction of caloric intake without jeopardizing the intake of protein, minerals, and vitamins.

Cleft palate The incidence of cleft palate is 1 in 2,500 births, and that of cleft lip is 1 per 1,000 births. Surgery for cleft palate is often not completed for several years. In addition to the needs for normal development, the infant and child must build up reserves for surgery, the promotion of healing, and the development of normal healthy gums and teeth. Several considerations should be borne in mind in feeding these children:

1. Infants may have difficulty in sucking, but most of them learn to use chewing movements to get the milk out of the nipple. An enlarged nipple opening is helpful. Some babies may be fed with a medicine dropper. Feeding in an upright position is helpful.
2. To counteract the tendency to choke, liquids should be taken in small amounts and swallowed slowly.
3. More frequent "burpings" are necessary because of the large amount of air which may be swallowed.
4. Spicy and acid foods often irritate the mouth and nose and should be avoided. If orange juice is not well taken, ascorbic acid supplement should be prescribed.
5. Among the foods which may get into the opening of the palate are peanut butter, peelings of raw fruit, nuts, leafy vegetables, and creamed dishes. Some children have no difficulty with any foods.
6. Puréed foods may be diluted with milk, fruit juice, or broth and given from a bottle with a large nipple opening. Some babies accept purées well if they are thickened with vanilla wafer or graham-cracker crumbs.
7. The time required for feeding may be long and requires much patience on the part of parent and nurse. For the older child, five or six small meals may be better than three.

When surgery has been performed, a liquid or puréed diet is offered until healing is complete.

Mental Retardation Some 3 per cent of persons in the United States are estimated to be mentally retarded. It is often difficult to distinguish the truly retarded child from one who functions at a retarded level because of environmental factors. From 85 to 90 per cent of the retarded are designated as mildly retarded (educable) and have an I.Q. between 50 and 75. This type tends to be associated with disadvantaged socioeconomic groups such as children of migrant farm workers who are deprived of opportunities for intellectual, cultural, or social development. Approximately 10 per cent of the mentally retarded are moderately retarded; that is, they have an I.Q. between 35 and 50 (trainable). The profoundly retarded individual with an I.Q. below 35 is believed to account for 5 per cent of the mentally retarded and presents the problems in feeding; however, even the profoundly retarded can be trained to eat properly and to use good table manners.[16]

The nutritional requirements of the mentally retarded child and adult are like those of the individual of normal mental development. The nurse can help parents to understand the problems of feeding by giving encouragement and support.

The mentally retarded child may be kept on the bottle too long, thus increasing the difficulties of introducing other foods. The child may eat very slowly, and feeding may be messy. Hand sucking and vomiting are not uncommon. To obtain adequate food intake for growth may require frequent, small feedings, and certainly an abundance of patience and ingenuity. One must strike a balance between overprotectiveness and lack of caring.

Retarded individuals, like normal persons, have an active emotional life. They feel the shunning of others and failure to achieve, but will respond to loving attention. They resist new foods, have definite likes and dislikes, and find it difficult to manage eating. They respond to the color of foods and like all children are fond of sweets.

When individuals are able to feed themselves, they should be permitted to do so even though feeding may be messy. Food must be presented in a form that can be easily managed. Foods may be eaten with the fingers for a long time until simple utensils can be managed. Children unable to support themselves should be held in a sitting position while they are being fed.

Problems and Review

1. What dietary problems may be anticipated in children who must be hospitalized? How can these problems be overcome?
2. How can a schoolchild be helped to adjust to a prolonged therapeutic diet?
3. *Problem.* List a number of ways in which you could encourage a boy with rheumatic fever to take an adequate diet.
4. What dietary considerations would apply for a 7-year-old child with scarlet fever?
5. *Problem.* Adjust a 1,500-kcal diet of an adult so that it will be suitable for a 12-year-old boy. In what ways would you try to effect acceptance of this diet?
6. *Problem.* Plan six high-calorie after-school and bedtime snacks which could be added to the regular diet of a teenage girl who is 20 pounds underweight.
7. What changes in diet might be indicated for an infant who is constipated? A 4-year-old child?
8. *Problem.* Plan a day's meals for a 3-year-old child with celiac disease for whom a gluten-restricted diet has been ordered. He is 34 inches tall and weighs 11 kg; he appears to be somewhat undernourished.
9. What are the similarities between celiac disease and cystic fibrosis? What differences are there?
10. A 10-year-old child has diabetes mellitus.
    a. List the differences between diabetes in children and in adults.
    b. What arguments can you give for, and against, chemical control in childhood diabetes?
    c. Enumerate the essential points in the instruction of the child and/or his parent with respect to diabetes.
    d. What is the effect of physical activity on the control of diabetes in the child?
    e. Prepare a plan for the organization of a diabetic club for children. Include suggestions for meetings for such a group.
    f. This child is invited to a birthday party. What plans can be made so that the child may eat at this party?
11. List several ways in which milk intolerance may be manifested. What substances in milk have been shown to produce such sensitivity? List three products that may be used satisfactorily in place of a milk formula.
12. *Problem.* For a 2-year-old child with nephrosis plan a suitable diet containing 50 gm protein and 1,200 kcal. How would you modify the diet for 500 mg sodium?
13. List some of the considerations to be kept in mind when planning the diet for a child undergoing chronic hemodialysis.

Cited References

1. Waxman, M., and Stunkard, A. J.: "Calorie Intake and Expenditure of Obese Boys," *J. Pediatr.*, **96**:187–93, 1980.
2. Huenemann, R. L.: "Food Habits of Obese and Non-obese Adolescents," *Postgrad. Med.*, **51**:99–105, May 1972.

3. Coates, T. J., and Thoresen, C. E.: "Treating Obesity in Children and Adolescents: A Review," *Am. J. Public Health,* **68**:143–51, 1978.
4. Dwyer, J. T. et al.: "Treating Obesity in Growing Children. 2. Specific Aspects. Activity and Diet," *Postgrad. Med.,* **51**:111–15, June 1972.
5. "Highlights from the Ten-State Nutrition Survey," *Nutr. Today,* **7**:4–11, July–August 1972.
6. Martin, H. P. et al.: "The Development of Abused Children," *Adv. Pediatr.,* **21**:25–73, 1974.
7. Jackson, R. L.: "Insulin-Dependent Diabetes in Children and Young Adults," *Nutr. Today,* **14**:26–32, November–December 1979.
8. Maclaren, N. K.: "Viral and Immunological Bases of Beta Cell Failure in Insulin-Dependent Diabetes," *Am. J. Dis. Child.,* **131**:1149–54, 1977.
9. American Diabetes Association: "Principles of Nutrition and Dietary Recommendations for Individuals with Diabetes Mellitus: 1979," *Diabetes,* **28**:1027–30, 1979.
10. Drash, A. C.: "Managing the Child with Diabetes Mellitus," *Postgrad. Med.,* **63**:85–92, June 1978.
11. Sperling, M.: "Diabetes Mellitus," *Pediatr. Clin. North Am.,* **26**:149–69, 1979.
12. Nelson, W. E. et al., eds.: *Textbook of Pediatrics,* W. B. Saunders Company, Philadelphia, 1979.
13. Holliday, M. A., and Chantler, C.: "Metabolic and Nutritional Factors in Children with Renal Insufficiency," *Kidney International,* **14**:306–12, 1978.
14. Giordano, C. et al.: "Amino Acid and Keto-Acid Diet in Uremic Children and Infants," Kidney International, **13** (Suppl. 8): S83–S85, 1978.
15. Holliday, M. A. et al.: "Nutritional Management of Chronic Renal Disease," *Med. Clin. North Am.,* **63**:945–62, 1979.
16. Azrin, N. H., and Armstrong, P. M.: "The 'Mini-Meal'—A Method for Teaching Eating Skills to the Profoundly Retarded," *Ment. Retard.,* **11**:9–13, February 1973.

Additional References

BARNESS, L. A. et al.: "The Practical Significance of Lactose Intolerance in Children," *Pediatrics,* **78**:240–45, 1978.

BARR, R. G. et al.: "Breath Tests in Pediatric Gastrointestinal Disorders. New Diagnostic Opportunities," *Pediatrics,* **62**:393–401, 1978.

BROWN, K. H. et al.: "Nutritional Consequences of Low-Dose Milk Supplements Consumed by Lactose-Malabsorbing Children," *Am. J. Clin. Nutr.,* **33**:1054–63, 1980.

CHASE, H. P., and LAVIN, M. H.: "Cystic Fibrosis and Malnutrition," *J. Pediatr.,* **95**:337–47, 1979.

COPELAND, L.: "Chronic Diarrhea in Infancy," *Am. J. Nurs.,* **77**:461–63, 1977.

DAVIS, G. T., and HILL, P. M.: "Cerebral Palsy," *Nurs. Clin. North Am.,* **15**:35–50, 1980.

GAMBLE, D. R.: "Relation of Antecedent Illness to Development of Diabetes in Children," *Brit. Med. J.,* **281**:99–101, 1980.

GOLDEN, M. P.: "An Approach to the Management of Obesity in Childhood," *Pediatr. Clin. North Am.,* **26**:187–97, 1979.

GRUPE, W. E.: "Childhood Nephrotic Syndrome," *Postgrad. Med.,* **65**:229–31, 234–36, May 1979.

GURWITZ, D. et al.: "Perspectives in Cystic Fibrosis," *Pediatr. Clin. North Am.,* **26**:603–15, 1979.

JACKSON, R. L.: "Management and Treatment of the Child with Diabetes," *Nutr. Today,* **15**:6–12 ff., March–April 1979.

LIEBMAN, W. M.: "Disorders of Defecation in Children," *Postgrad. Med.*, **66**:105–110, August 1979.

MERRITT, R. J. et al.: "Consequences of Modified Fasting in Obese Pediatric and Adolescent Patients. I. Protein-Sparing Modified Fast," *J. Pediatr.*, **96**:13–19, 1980.

PASHAYAN, H. M., and MCNAB, M.: "Simplified Method of Feeding Infants Born with Cleft Palate with or Without Cleft Lip," *Am. J. Dis. Child.*, **133**:145–47, 1979.

SCHMITT, B. D.: "An Argument for the Unmeasured Diet in Juvenile Diabetes Mellitus," *Clinical Pediatr.*, **14**:68–73, 1975.

Appendixes

Tabular Materials

TABLES

Tabular Materials

TABLE A–1 EXPLANATION

Table A–1 shows the food values in 730 commonly used foods. Foods are listed alphabetically under the following main headings: dairy products; eggs; fats and oils; fish, shellfish, meat, and poultry; fruits and fruit products; grain products; legumes (dry), nuts, and seeds; sugars and sweets; vegetables and vegetable products; and miscellaneous items. Part of the explanation offered in the bulletin is reproduced here:*

Most of the foods listed are in ready-to-eat form. Some are basic products widely used in food preparation, such as flour, fat, and cornmeal. . . .

The approximate measure shown for each food is in cups, ounces, pounds, some other well-known unit, or a piece of certain size. The cup measure refers to the standard measuring cup of 8 fluid ounces or one half pint of liquid. The ounce refers to one-sixteenth of a pound avoirdupois, unless fluid ounce is indicated. The weight of a fluid ounce varies according to the food measured. . . .

The values for food energy (calories) and nutrients shown in Table A–1 are the amounts present in the edible part of the item, that is, in only that portion customarily eaten—corn without cob, meat without bone, potatoes without skin, European-type grapes without seeds. If additional parts are eaten—the potato skin, for example—amounts of some nutrients obtained will be somewhat greater than shown. . . .

New fatty acid values are given for dairy products, eggs, meats, some grain products, nuts, and soups. The values are based on recent comprehensive research by USDA to update and extend tables for fatty acid content of foods.

Niacin values are for preformed niacin occurring naturally in foods. The values do not include additional niacin that the body may form from tryptophan, an essential amino acid in the protein of most foods. Among the better sources of tryptophan are milk, meat, eggs, legumes, and nuts.

Values have been calculated from the ingredients in typical recipes for many of the prepared items such as biscuits, corn muffins, macaroni and cheese, custard, and many dessert-type items.

Values for toast and cooked vegetables are without fat added, either during preparation or at the table. Some destruction of vitamins, especially ascorbic acid, may occur when vegetables are cut and shredded. Since such losses are variable, no deduction has been made.

For meat, values are for meat cooked and drained of the drippings. For many cuts, two sets of values are shown: meat including fat and meat from which the fat has been removed either in the kitchen or on the plate.

A variety of manufactured items—some of the milk products, ready-to-eat breakfast cereals,

* Adams, C. F., and Richardson, M.: *Nutritive Value of Foods.* Home and Garden Bulletin 72, Agricultural Research Service, U. S. Department of Agriculture, Washington, D. C., 1977.

imitation cream products, fruit drinks, and various mixes—are included in Table A–1. Frequently these foods are fortified with one or more nutrients. If nutrients are added, this information is on the label. Values shown here for these foods are usually based on products by several manufacturers and may differ somewhat from the values provided by any one source.

Table A-1. Nutritive Values of the Edible Parts of Foods

(Dashes (—) denote lack of reliable data for a constituent believed to be present in measurable amount)

Item No. (A)	Foods, approximate measures, units and weight (edible part unless footnotes indicate otherwise) (B)			Water (C)	Food Energy (D)	Protein (E)	Fat (F)	Fatty Acids: Saturated (total) (G)	Fatty Acids: Unsaturated: Oleic (H)	Fatty Acids: Unsaturated: Linoleic (I)	Carbohydrate (J)	Calcium (K)	Phosphorus (L)	Iron (M)	Potassium (N)	Vitamin A Value (O)	Thiamin (P)	Riboflavin (Q)	Niacin (R)	Ascorbic Acid (S)
			Grams	Per-cent	Cal-ories	Grams	Grams	Grams	Grams	Grams	Grams	Milli-grams	Milli-grams	Milli-grams	Milli-grams	I.U.	Milli-grams	Milli-grams	Milli-grams	Milli-grams
	DAIRY PRODUCTS (CHEESE, CREAM, IMITATION CREAM, MILK; RELATED PRODUCTS)																			
	Butter. See Fats, oils; related products, items 103–108.																			
	Cheese:																			
	Natural:																			
1	Blue	1 oz	28	42	100	6	8	5.3	1.9	0.2	1	150	110	0.1	73	200	0.01	0.11	0.3	0
2	Camembert (3 wedges per 4-oz container).	1 wedge	38	52	115	8	9	5.8	2.2	.2	Trace	147	132	.1	71	350	.01	.19	.2	0
	Cheddar:																			
3	Cut pieces	1 oz	28	37	115	7	9	6.1	2.1	.2	Trace	204	145	.2	28	300	.01	.11	Trace	0
4		1 cu in	17.2	37	70	4	6	3.7	1.3	.1	Trace	124	88	.1	17	180	Trace	.06	Trace	0
5	Shredded	1 cup	113	37	455	28	37	24.2	8.5	.7	1	815	579	.8	111	1,200	.03	.42	.1	0
	Cottage (curd not pressed down):																			
	Creamed (cottage cheese, 4% fat):																			
6	Large curd	1 cup	225	79	235	28	10	6.4	2.4	.2	6	135	297	.3	190	370	.05	.37	.3	Trace
7	Small curd	1 cup	210	79	220	26	9	6.0	2.2	.2	6	126	277	.3	177	340	.04	.34	.3	Trace
8	Low fat (2%)	1 cup	226	79	205	31	4	2.8	1.0	.1	8	155	340	.4	217	160	.05	.42	.3	Trace
9	Low fat (1%)	1 cup	226	82	165	28	2	1.5	.5	.1	6	138	302	.3	193	80	.05	.37	.3	Trace
10	Uncreamed (cottage cheese dry curd, less than ½% fat).	1 cup	145	80	125	25	1	.4	.1	Trace	3	46	151	.3	47	40	.04	.21	.2	0
11	Cream	1 oz	28	54	100	2	10	6.2	2.4	.2	1	23	30	.3	34	400	Trace	.06	Trace	0
	Mozzarella, made with—																			
12	Whole milk	1 oz	28	48	90	6	7	4.4	1.7	.2	1	163	117	.1	21	260	Trace	.08	Trace	0
13	Part skim milk	1 oz	28	49	80	8	5	3.1	1.2	.1	1	207	149	.1	27	180	.01	.10	Trace	0
	Parmesan, grated:																			
14	Cup, not pressed down	1 cup	100	18	455	42	30	19.1	7.7	.3	4	1,376	807	1.0	107	700	.05	.39	.3	0
15	Tablespoon	1 tbsp	5	18	25	2	2	1.0	.4	Trace	Trace	69	40	Trace	5	40	Trace	.02	Trace	0
16	Ounce	1 oz	28	18	130	12	9	5.4	2.2	.1	1	390	229	.3	30	200	.01	.11	.1	0
17	Provolone	1 oz	28	41	100	7	8	4.8	1.7	.1	1	214	141	.1	39	230	.01	.09	Trace	0
	Ricotta, made with—																			
18	Whole milk	1 cup	246	72	1,790	28	32	20.4	7.1	.7	7	509	389	.9	257	1,210	.03	.48	.3	0
19	Park skim milk	1 cup	246	74	340	28	19	12.1	4.7	.5	13	669	449	1.1	308	1,060	.05	.46	.2	0
20	Romano	1 oz	28	31	110	9	8	—	—	—	1	302	215	—	—	160	—	.11	Trace	0
21	Swiss	1oz	28	37	105	8	8	5.0	1.7	.2	1	272	171	Trace	31	240	.01	.10	Trace	0
	Pasteurized process cheese:																			
22	American	1 oz	28	39	105	6	9	5.6	2.1	.2	Trace	174	211	.1	46	340	.01	.10	Trace	0
23	Swiss	1 oz	28	42	95	7	7	4.5	1.7	.1	1	219	216	.2	61	230	Trace	.08	Trace	0
24	Pasteurized process cheese food, American.	1 oz	28	43	95	6	7	4.4	1.7	.1	2	163	130	.2	79	260	.01	.13	Trace	0
25	Pasteurized process cheese spread, American.	1 oz	28	48	82	5	6	3.8	1.5	.1	2	159	202	.1	69	220	.01	.12	Trace	0
	Cream, sweet:																			
26	Half-and-half (cream and milk)	1 cup	242	81	315	7	28	17.3	7.0	.6	10	254	230	.2	314	260	.08	.36	.2	2
27		1 tbsp	15	81	20	Trace	2	1.1	.4	Trace	1	16	14	Trace	19	20	.01	.02	Trace	Trace
28	Light, coffee, or table	1 cup	240	74	470	6	46	28.8	11.7	1.0	9	231	192	.1	292	1,730	.08	.36	.1	2

29		1 tbsp	15	74	30	Trace	3	1.8	.7	.1	1	14	12	Trace	18	110	Trace	.02	Trace	Trace
	Whipping, unwhipped (volume about double when whipped):																			
30	Light	1 cup	239	64	700	5	74	46.2	18.3	1.5	7	166	146	0.1	231	2,690	0.06	0.30	0.1	1
31		1 tbsp	15	64	45	Trace	5	2.9	1.1	.1	Trace	10	9	Trace	15	170	Trace	.02	Trace	Trace
32	Heavy	1 cup	238	58	820	5	88	54.8	22.2	2.0	7	154	149	.1	179	3,500	.05	.26	.1	1
33		1 tbsp	15	58	80	Trace	6	3.5	1.4	.1	Trace	10	9	Trace	11	220	Trace	.02	Trace	Trace
34	Whipped topping, (pressurized)	1 cup	60	61	155	2	13	8.3	3.4	.3	7	61	54	Trace	88	550	.02	.04	Trace	0
35		1 tbsp	3	61	10	Trace	1	.4	.2	Trace	Trace	3	3	Trace	4	30	Trace	Trace	Trace	0
36	Cream, sour	1 cup	230	71	495	7	48	30.0	12.1	1.1	10	268	195	.1	331	1,820	.08	.34	.2	2
37		1 tbsp	12	71	25	Trace	3	1.6	.6	.1	1	14	10	Trace	17	90	Trace	.02	Trace	Trace
	Cream products, imitation (made with vegetable fat):																			
	Sweet:																			
	Creamers:																			
38	Liquid (frozen)	1 cup	245	77	335	2	24	22.8	.3	Trace	28	23	157	.1	467	[1]220	0	0	0	0
39		1 tbsp	15	77	20	Trace	1	1.4	Trace	0	2	1	10	Trace	29	[1]10	0	0	0	0
40	Powdered	1 cup	94	2	515	5	33	30.6	.9	Trace	52	21	397	.1	763	[1]190	0	[1].16	0	0
41		1 tsp	2	2	10	Trace	1	.7	Trace	0	1	Trace	8	Trace	16	[1]Trace	0	[1]Trace	0	0
	Whipped topping:																			
42	Frozen	1 cup	75	50	240	1	19	16.3	1.0	.2	17	5	6	.1	14	[1]650	0	0	0	0
43		1 tbsp	4	50	15	Trace	1	.9	.1	Trace	1	Trace	Trace	Trace	1	[1]30	0	0	0	0
44	Powdered, made with whole milk.	1 cup	80	67	150	3	10	8.5	.6	.1	13	72	69	Trace	121	[1]290	.02	.09	Trace	1
45		1 tbsp	4	67	10	Trace	Trace	.4	Trace	Trace	1	4	3	Trace	6	[1]10	Trace	Trace	Trace	Trace
46	Pressurized	1 cup	70	60	185	1	16	13.2	1.4	.2	11	4	13	Trace	13	[1]330	0	0	0	0
47		1 tbsp	4	60	10	Trace	1	.8	.1	Trace	1	Trace	1	Trace	1	[1]20	0	0	0	0
48	Sour dressing (imitation sour cream) made with nonfat dry milk.	1 cup	235	75	415	8	39	31.2	4.4	1.1	11	266	205	.1	380	[1]20	.09	.38	.2	2
49		1 tbsp	12	75	20	Trace	2	1.6	.2	.1	1	14	10	Trace	19	[1]Trace	.01	.02	Trace	Trace
	Ice cream. See Milk desserts, frozen (items 75–80).																			
	Ice milk. See Milk desserts, frozen (items 81–83).																			
	Milk:																			
	Fluid:																			
50	Whole (3.3% fat)	1 cup	244	88	150	8	8	5.1	2.1	.2	11	291	228	.1	370	[2]310	.09	.40	.2	2
	Lowfat (2%):																			
51	No milk solids added	1 cup	244	89	120	8	5	2.9	1.2	.1	12	297	232	.1	377	500	.10	.40	.2	2
	Milk solids added:																			
52	Label claims less than 10 g of protein per cup.	1 cup	245	89	125	9	5	2.9	1.2	.1	12	313	245	.1	397	500	.10	.42	.2	2
53	Label claim 10 or more grams of protein per cup (protein fortified).	1 cup	246	88	135	10	5	3.0	1.2	.1	14	352	276	.1	447	500	.11	.48	.2	2
	Lowfat (1%):																			
54	No milk solids added	1 cup	244	90	100	8	3	1.6	.7	.1	12	300	235	.1	381	500	.10	.41	.2	2
	Milk solids added:																			
55	Label claim less than 10 g of protein per cup.	1 cup	245	90	105	9	2	1.5	.6	.1	12	313	245	.1	397	500	.10	.42	.2	2
56	Label claim 10 or more grams of protein per cup (protein fortified).	1 cup	246	89	120	10	3	1.8	.7	.1	14	349	273	.1	444	500	.11	.47	.2	2
	Nonfat (skim):																			
57	No milk solids added	1 cup	245	91	85	8	Trace	.3	.1	Trace	12	302	247	.1	406	500	.09	.37	.2	2

*Adams, C. F., and Richardson, M.: Nutritive Value of Foods. Home and Garden Bulletin 72, Agricultural Research Service, U.S. Department of Agriculture, Washington, D.C., revised 1977.

[1] Vitamin A value is largely from beta-carotene used for coloring. Riboflavin value for items 40–41 apply to product with added riboflavin.

[2] Applies to product without added vitamin A. With added vitamin A, value is 500 International Units (I.U.).

Table A-1. (Continued)

Item No. (A)	Foods, approximate measures, units, and weight (edible part unless footnotes indicate otherwise) (B)			Water (C)	Food Energy (D)	Protein (E)	Fat (F)	Fatty Acids: Saturated (total) (G)	Fatty Acids: Unsaturated: Oleic (H)	Fatty Acids: Unsaturated: Linoleic (I)	Carbohydrate (J)	Calcium (K)	Phosphorus (L)	Iron (M)	Potassium (N)	Vitamin A Value (O)	Thiamin (P)	Riboflavin (Q)	Niacin (R)	Ascorbic Acid (S)
			Grams	Percent	Calories	Grams	Grams	Grams	Grams	Grams	Grams	Milligrams	Milligrams	Milligrams	Milligrams	I.U.	Milligrams	Milligrams	Milligrams	Milligrams
	DAIRY PRODUCTS (CHEESE, CREAM, IMITATION CREAM, MILK; RELATED PRODUCTS; (CONTINUED)																			
	Milk: (cont.)																			
	Fluid: (cont.)																			
	Nonfat (skim): (cont.)																			
	Milk solids added:																			
58	Label claim less than 10 g of protein per cup.	1 cup	245	90	90	9	1	0.4	0.1	Trace	12	316	255	0.1	416	500	0.10	0.43	0.2	2
59	Label claim 10 or more grams of protein per cup (protein fortified).	1 cup	246	89	100	10	1	.4	.1	Trace	14	352	275	.1	446	500	.11	.48	.2	3
60	Buttermilk	1 cup	245	90	100	8	2	1.3	.5	Trace	12	285	219	.1	371	[3]80	.08	.38	.1	2
	Canned:																			
	Evaporated, unsweetened:																			
61	Whole milk	1 cup	252	74	340	17	19	11.6	5.3	0.4	25	657	510	.5	764	[3]610	.12	.80	.5	5
62	Skim milk	1 cup	255	79	200	19	1	.3	.1	Trace	29	738	497	.7	845	[4]1,000	.11	.79	.4	3
63	Sweetened, condensed	1 cup	306	27	980	24	27	16.8	6.7	.7	166	868	775	.6	1,136	[3]1,000	.28	1.27	.6	8
	Dried:																			
64	Buttermilk	1 cup	120	3	465	41	7	4.3	1.7	.2	59	1,421	1,119	.4	1,910	[3]260	.47	1.90	1.1	7
	Nonfat instant:																			
65	Envelope, net wt., 3.2 oz[5]	1 envelope	91	4	325	32	1	.4	.1	Trace	47	1,120	896	.3	1,552	[6]2,160	.38	1.59	.8	5
66	Cup[7]	1 cup	68	4	245	24	Trace	.3	.1	Trace	35	837	670	.2	1,160	[6]1,610	.28	1.19	.6	4
	Milk beverages:																			
	Chocolate milk (commercial):																			
67	Regular	1 cup	250	82	210	8	8	5.3	2.2	.2	26	280	251	.6	417	[3]300	.09	.41	.3	2
68	Lowfat (2%)	1 cup	250	84	180	8	5	3.1	1.3	.1	26	284	254	.6	422	500	.10	.42	.3	2
69	Lowfat (1%)	1 cup	250	85	160	8	3	1.5	.7	.1	26	287	257	.6	426	500	.10	.40	.2	2
70	Eggnog (commercial)	1 cup	254	74	340	10	19	11.3	5.0	.6	34	330	278	.5	420	890	.09	.48	.3	4
	Malted milk, home-prepared with 1 cup of whole milk and 2 to 3 heaping tsp of malted milk powder (about ¾ oz):																			
71	Chocolate	1 cup of milk plus ¾ oz of powder.	265	81	235	9	9	5.5	—	—	29	304	265	.5	500	330	.14	.43	.7	2
72	Natural	1 cup of milk plus ¾ oz of powder.	265	81	235	11	10	6.0	—	—	27	347	307	.3	529	380	.20	.54	1.3	2
	Shakes, thick:[8]																			
73	Chocolate, container, net wt., 10.6 oz.	1 container	300	72	355	9	8	5.0	2.0	.2	63	396	378	.9	672	260	.14	.67	.4	0
74	Vanilla, container, net wt., 11 oz.	1 container	313	74	350	12	9	5.9	2.4	.2	56	457	361	.3	572	360	.09	.61	.5	0
	Milk desserts, frozen:																			
	Ice cream:																			
	Regular (about 11% fat):																			
75	Hardened	½ gal	1,064	61	2,155	38	115	71.3	28.8	2.6	254	1,406	1,075	1.0	2,052	4,340	.42	2.63	1.1	6
76		1 cup	133	61	270	5	14	8.9	3.6	.3	32	176	134	.1	257	540	.05	.33	.1	1
77		3-fl oz container	50	61	100	2	5	3.4	1.4	.1	12	66	51	Trace	96	200	.02	.12	.1	Trace
78	Soft serve (frozen custard)	1 cup	173	60	375	7	23	13.5	5.9	.6	38	236	199	.4	338	790	.08	.45	.2	1

79	Rich (about 16% fat), hardened.	½ gal	1,188	59	2,805	33	190	118.3	47.8	4.3	256	1,213	927	.8	1,771	7,200	.36	2.27	.9	5
80		1 cup	148	59	350	4	24	14.7	6.0	.5	32	151	115	.1	221	900	.04	.28	.1	1
	Ice milk:																			
81	Hardened (about 4.3% fat)	½ gal	1,048	69	1,470	41	45	28.1	11.3	1.0	232	1,409	1,035	1.5	2,117	1,710	.61	2.78	.9	6
82		1 cup	131	69	185	5	6	3.5	1.4	.1	29	176	129	.1	265	210	.08	.35	.1	1
83	Soft serve (about 2.6% fat)	1 cup	175	70	225	8	5	2.9	1.2	0.1	38	274	202	0.3	412	180	0.12	0.54	0.2	1
84	Sherbet (about 2% fat)	½ gal	1,542	66	2,160	17	31	19.0	7.7	.7	469	827	594	2.5	1,585	1,480	.26	.71	1.0	31
85		1 cup	193	66	270	2	4	2.4	1.0	.1	59	103	74	.3	198	190	.03	.09	.1	4
	Milk desserts, other:																			
86	Custard, baked	1 cup	265	77	305	14	15	6.8	5.4	.7	29	297	310	1.1	387	930	.11	.50	.3	1
	Puddings:																			
	From home recipe:																			
	Starch base:																			
87	Chocolate	1 cup	260	66	385	8	12	7.6	3.3	.3	67	250	255	1.3	445	390	.05	.36	.3	1
88	Vanilla (blancmange)	1 cup	255	76	285	9	10	6.2	2.5	.2	41	298	232	Trace	352	410	.08	.41	.3	2
89	Tapioca cream	1 cup	165	72	220	8	8	4.1	2.5	.5	28	173	180	.7	223	480	.07	.30	.2	2
	From mix (chocolate) and milk:																			
90	Regular (cooked)	1 cup	260	70	320	9	8	4.3	2.6	.2	59	265	247	.8	354	340	.05	.39	.3	2
91	Instant	1 cup	260	69	325	8	7	3.6	2.2	.3	63	374	237	1.3	335	340	.08	.39	.3	2
	Yogurt																			
	With added milk solids:																			
	Made with lowfat milk:																			
92	Fruit-flavored[9]	1 container, net wt., 8 oz	227	75	230	10	3	1.8	.6	.1	42	343	269	.2	439	[10]120	.08	.40	.2	1
93	Plain	1 container, net wt., 8 oz	227	85	145	12	4	2.3	.8	.1	16	415	326	.2	531	[10]150	.10	.49	.3	2
94	Made with nonfat milk	1 container, net wt., 8 oz	227	85	125	13	Trace	.3	.1	Trace	17	452	355	.2	579	[10]20	.11	.53	.3	2
	Without added milk solids:																			
95	Made with whole milk	1 container, net wt., 8 oz	227	88	140	8	7	4.8	1.7	.1	11	274	215	.1	351	280	.07	.32	.2	1

EGGS

	Eggs, large (24 oz per dozen):																			
	Raw:																			
96	Whole, without shell	1 egg	50	75	80	6	6	1.7	2.0	.6	1	28	90	1.0	65	260	.04	.15	Trace	0
97	White	1 white	33	88	15	3	Trace	0	0	0	Trace	4	4	Trace	45	0	Trace	.09	Trace	0
98	Yolk	1 yolk	17	49	65	3	6	1.7	2.1	.6	Trace	26	86	.9	15	310	.04	.07	Trace	0
	Cooked:																			
99	Fried in butter	1 egg	46	72	85	5	6	2.4	2.2	.6	1	26	80	.9	58	290	.03	.13	Trace	0
100	Hard-cooked, shell removed	1 egg	50	75	80	6	6	1.7	2.0	.6	1	28	90	1.0	65	260	.04	.14	Trace	0
101	Poached	1 egg	50	74	80	6	6	1.7	2.0	.6	1	28	90	1.0	65	260	.04	.13	Trace	0
102	Scrambled (milk added) in butter. Also omelet.	1 egg	64	76	95	6	7	2.8	2.3	.6	1	47	97	.9	85	310	.04	.16	Trace	0

FATS, OILS; RELATED PRODUCTS

	Butter																			
	Regular (1 brick or 4 sticks per lb):																			
103	Stick (½ cup)	1 stick	113	16	815	1	92	57.3	23.1	2.1	Trace	27	26	.2	29	[11]3,470	.01	.04	Trace	0
104	Tablespoon (about ⅛ stick).	1 tbsp	14	16	100	Trace	12	7.2	2.9	.3	Trace	3	3	Trace	4	[11]430	Trace	Trace	Trace	0
105	Pat (1 in square, ⅓ in high, 90 per lb).	1 pat	5	16	35	Trace	4	2.5	1.0	.1	Trace	1	1	Trace	1	[11]150	Trace	Trace	Trace	0

[3] Applies to product without vitamin A added.
[4] Applies to product with added vitamin A. Without added vitamin A, value is 20 International Units (I.U.).
[5] Yields 1 qt of fluid milk when reconstituted according to package directions.
[6] Applies to product with added vitamin A.
[7] Weight applies to product with label claim of 1⅓ cups equal 3.2 oz.
[8] Applies to products made from thick shake mixes and that do not contain added ice cream. Products made from milk shake mixes are higher in fat and usually contain added ice cream.
[9] Content of fat, vitamin A, and carbohydrate varies. Consult the label when precise values are needed for special diets.
[10] Applies to product made with milk containing no added vitamin A.
[11] Based on year-round average.

Table A-1. (Continued)

Item No. (A)	Foods, approximate measures, units, and weight (edible part unless footnotes indicate otherwise) (B)			Water (C)	Food Energy (D)	Protein (E)	Fat (F)	Fatty Acids: Saturated (total) (G)	Fatty Acids: Unsaturated: Oleic (H)	Fatty Acids: Unsaturated: Linoleic (I)	Carbohydrate (J)	Calcium (K)	Phosphorus (L)	Iron (M)	Potassium (N)	Vitamin A Value (O)	Thiamin (P)	Riboflavin (Q)	Niacin (R)	Ascorbic Acid (S)
			Grams	Percent	Calories	Grams	Grams	Grams	Grams	Grams	Grams	Milligrams	Milligrams	Milligrams	Milligrams	I.U.	Milligrams	Milligrams	Milligrams	Milligrams
	FATS, OILS; RELATED PRODUCTS (CONTINUED)																			
	Butter (cont.)																			
	Whipped (6 sticks or two 8-oz containers per lb).																			
106	Stick (½ cup)	1 stick	76	16	540	1	61	38.2	15.4	1.4	Trace	18	17	.1	20	[11]2,310	Trace	.03	Trace	0
107	Tablespoon (about ⅛ stick).	1 tbsp	9	16	65	Trace	8	4.7	1.9	.2	Trace	2	2	Trace	2	[11]290	Trace	Trace	Trace	0
108	Pat (1¼ in square, ⅓ in high; 120 per lb).	1 pat	4	16	25	Trace	3	1.9	.8	.1	Trace	1	1	Trace	1	[11]120	0	Trace	Trace	0
109	Fats, cooking (vegetable shortenings).	1 cup	200	0	1,770	0	200	48.8	88.2	48.4	0	0	0	0	0	—	0	0	0	0
110		1 tbsp	13	0	110	0	13	3.2	5.7	3.1	0	0	0	0	0	—	0	0	0	0
111	Lard	1 cup	205	0	1,850	0	205	81.0	83.8	20.5	0	0	0	0	0	0	0	0	0	0
112		1 tbsp	13	0	115	0	13	5.1	5.3	1.3	0	0	0	0	0	0	0	0	0	0
	Margarine:																			
	Regular (1 brick or 4 sticks per 1lb):																			
113	Stick (½ cup)	1 stick	113	16	815	1	92	16.7	42.9	24.9	Trace	27	26	.2	29	[12]3,750	.01	.04	Trace	0
114	Tablespoon (about ⅛ stick)	1 tbsp	14	16	100	Trace	12	2.1	5.3	3.1	Trace	3	3	Trace	4	[12]470	Trace	Trace	Trace	0
115	Pat (1 in square, ⅓ in high; 90 per lb).	1 pat	5	16	35	Trace	4	.7	1.9	1.1	Trace	1	1	Trace	1	[12]170	Trace	Trace	Trace	0
116	Soft, two 8-oz containers per lb.	1 container	227	16	1,635	1	184	32.5	71.5	65.4	Trace	53	52	.4	59	[12]7,500	.01	.08	.1	0
117		1 tbsp	14	16	100	Trace	12	2.0	4.5	4.1	Trace	3	3	Trace	4	[12]470	Trace	Trace	Trace	0
	Whipped (6 sticks per lb):																			
118	Stick (½ cup)	1 stick	76	16	545	Trace	61	11.2	28.7	16.7	Trace	18	17	.1	20	[12]2,500	Trace	.03	Trace	0
119	Tablespoon (about ⅛ stick)	1 tbsp	9	16	70	Trace	8	1.4	3.6	2.1	Trace	2	2	Trace	2	[12]310	Trace	Trace	Trace	0
	Oils, salad or cooking:																			
120	Corn	1 cup	218	0	1,925	0	218	27.7	53.6	125.1	0	0	0	0	0	—	0	0	0	0
121		1 tbsp	14	0	120	0	14	1.7	3.3	7.8	0	0	0	0	0	—	0	0	0	0
122	Olive	1 cup	216	0	1,910	0	216	30.7	154.4	17.7	0	0	0	0	0	—	0	0	0	0
123		1 tbsp	14	0	120	0	14	1.9	9.7	1.1	0	0	0	0	0	—	0	0	0	0
124	Peanut	1 cup	216	0	1,910	0	216	37.4	98.5	67.0	0	0	0	0	0	—	0	0	0	0
125		1 tbsp	14	0	120	0	14	2.3	6.2	4.2	0	0	0	0	0	—	0	0	0	0
126	Safflower	1 cup	218	0	1,925	0	218	20.5	25.9	159.8	0	0	0	0	0	—	0	0	0	0
127		1 tbsp	14	0	120	0	14	1.3	1.6	10.0	0	0	0	0	0	—	0	0	0	0
128	Soybean oil, hydrogenated (partially hardened).	1 cup	218	0	1,925	0	218	31.8	93.1	75.6	0	0	0	0	0	—	0	0	0	0
129		1 tbsp	14	0	120	0	14	2.0	5.8	4.7	0	0	0	0	0	—	0	0	0	0
130	Soybean-cottonseed oil blend, hydrogenated.	1 cup	218	0	1,925	0	218	38.2	63.0	99.6	0	0	0	0	0	—	0	0	0	0
131		1 tbsp	14	0	120	0	14	2.4	3.9	6.2	0	0	0	0	0	—	0	0	0	0
	Salad dressings:																			
	Commercial:																			
	Blue cheese:																			
132	Regular	1 tbsp	15	32	75	1	8	1.6	1.7	3.8	1	12	11	Trace	6	30	Trace	.02	Trace	Trace
133	Low calorie (5 Cal per tsp)	1 tbsp	16	84	10	Trace	1	.5	.3	Trace	1	10	8	Trace	5	30	Trace	.01	Trace	Trace
	French:																			
134	Regular	1 tbsp	16	39	65	Trace	6	1.1	1.3	3.2	3	2	2	.1	13	—	—	—	—	—

135	Low calorie (5 Cal per tsp)	1 tbsp	16	77	15	Trace	1	.1	.1	.4	2	2	2	.1	13	—	—	—	—	—
	Italian:																			
136	Regular	1 tbsp	15	28	85	Trace	9	1.6	1.9	4.7	1	2	1	Trace	2	Trace	Trace	Trace	Trace	—
137	Low calorie (2 Cal per tsp)	1 tbsp	15	90	10	Trace	1	.1	.1	.4	Trace	Trace	1	Trace	2	Trace	Trace	Trace	Trace	—
138	Mayonnaise	1 tbsp	14	15	100	Trace	11	2.0	2.4	5.6	Trace	3	4	.1	5	40	Trace	.01	Trace	—
	Mayonnaise type:																			
139	Regular	1 tbsp	15	41	65	Trace	6	1.1	1.4	3.2	2	2	4	Trace	1	30	Trace	Trace	Trace	—
140	Low calorie (8 Cal per tsp)	1 tbsp	16	81	20	Trace	2	.4	.4	1.0	2	3	4	Trace	1	40	Trace	Trace	Trace	—
141	Tartar sauce, regular	1 tbsp	14	34	75	Trace	8	1.5	1.8	4.1	1	3	4	.1	11	30	Trace	Trace	Trace	Trace
	Thousand Island:																			
142	Regular	1 tbsp	16	32	80	Trace	8	1.4	1.7	4.0	2	2	3	.1	18	50	Trace	Trace	Trace	Trace
143	Low calorie (10 Cal per tsp)	1 tbsp	15	68	25	Trace	2	.4	.4	1.0	2	2	3	.1	17	50	Trace	Trace	Trace	Trace
	From home recipe:																			
144	Cooked type:[13]	1 tbsp	16	68	25	1	2	.5	.6	.3	2	14	15	.1	19	80	.01	.03	Trace	Trace
	FISH, SHELLFISH, MEAT, POULTRY; RELATED PRODUCTS																			
	Fish and shellfish:																			
145	Bluefish, baked with butter or margarine.	3 oz	85	68	135	22	4	—	—	—	0	25	244	0.6	—	40	0.09	0.08	1.6	—
	Clams:																			
146	Raw, meat only	3 oz	85	82	65	11	1	—	—	—	2	59	138	5.2	154	90	.08	.15	1.1	8
147	Canned, solids and liquid	3 oz	85	86	45	7	1	0.2	Trace	Trace	2	47	116	3.5	119	—	.01	.09	.9	—
148	Crabmeat (white or king), canned, not pressed down.	1 cup	135	77	135	24	3	.6	0.4	0.1	1	61	246	1.1	149	—	.11	.11	2.6	—
149	Fish sticks, breaded, cooked, frozen (stick, 4 by 1 by ½ in).	1 fish stick or 1 oz	28	66	50	5	3	—	—	—	2	3	47	.1	—	0	.01	.02	.5	—
150	Haddock, breaded, fried[14]	3 oz	85	66	140	17	5	1.4	2.2	1.2	5	34	210	1.0	296	—	.03	.06	2.7	2
151	Ocean perch, breaded, fried[14]	1 fillet	85	59	195	16	11	2.7	4.4	2.3	6	28	192	1.1	242	—	.10	.10	1.6	—
152	Oysters, raw, meat only (13–19 medium Selects).	1 cup	240	85	160	20	4	1.3	.2	.1	8	226	343	13.2	290	740	.34	.43	6.0	—
153	Salmon, pink, canned, solids and liquid.	3 oz	85	71	120	17	5	.9	.8	.1	0	[15]167	243	.7	307	60	.03	.16	6.8	—
154	Sardines, Atlantic, canned in oil, drained solids.	3 oz	85	62	175	20	9	3.0	2.5	.5	0	372	424	2.5	502	190	.02	.17	4.6	—
155	Scallops, frozen, breaded, fried, reheated.	6 scallops	90	60	175	16	8	—	—	—	9	—	—	—	—	—	—	—	—	—
156	Shad, baked with butter or margarine, bacon.	3 oz	85	64	170	20	10	—	—	—	0	20	266	.5	320	30	.11	.22	7.3	—
	Shrimp:																			
157	Canned meat	3 oz	85	70	100	21	1	.1	.1	Trace	1	98	224	2.6	104	50	.01	.03	1.5	—
158	French fried[16]	3 oz	85	57	190	17	9	2.3	3.7	2.0	9	61	162	1.7	195	—	.03	.07	2.3	—
159	Tuna, canned in oil, drained solids.	3 oz	85	61	170	24	7	1.7	1.7	.7	0	7	199	1.6	—	70	.04	.10	10.1	—
160	Tuna salad[17]	1 cup	205	70	350	30	22	4.3	6.3	6.7	7	41	291	2.7	—	590	.08	.23	10.3	2
	Meat and meat products:																			
161	Bacon, (20 slices per lb, raw), broiled or fried, crisp.	2 slices	15	8	85	4	8	2.5	3.7	.7	Trace	2	34	.5	35	0	.08	.05	.8	—
	Beef,[18] cooked:																			
	Cuts braised, simmered or pot roasted:																			
162	Lean and fat (piece, 2½ by 2½ by ¾ in).	3 oz	85	53	245	23	16	6.8	6.5	.4	0	10	114	2.9	184	30	.04	.18	3.6	—

[12] Based on average vitamin A content of fortified margarine. Federal specifications for fortified margarine require a minimum of 15,000 International Units (I.U.) of vitamin A per pound.
[13] Fatty acid values apply to product made with regular-type margarine.
[14] Dipped in egg, milk or water, and breadcrumbs; fried in vegetable shortening.
[15] If bones are discarded, value for calcium will be greatly reduced.
[16] Dipped in egg, breadcrumbs, and flour or batter.
[17] Prepared with tuna, celery, salad dressing (mayonnaise type), pickle, onion, and egg.
[18] Outer layer of fat on the cut was removed to within approximately ½ in of the lean. Deposits of fat within the cut were not removed.

Table A-1. (Continued)

Item No. (A)	Foods, approximate measures, units, and weight (edible part unless footnotes indicate otherwise) (B)			Water (C)	Food Energy (D)	Protein (E)	Fat (F)	Saturated (total) (G)	Oleic (H)	Linoleic (I)	Carbohydrate (J)	Calcium (K)	Phosphorus (L)	Iron (M)	Potassium (N)	Vitamin A Value (O)	Thiamin (P)	Riboflavin (Q)	Niacin (R)	Ascorbic Acid (S)
								Nutrients in Indicated Quantity; Fatty Acids	Unsaturated											
			Grams	Percent	Calories	Grams	Grams	Grams	Grams	Grams	Grams	Milligrams	Milligrams	Milligrams	Milligrams	I.U.	Milligrams	Milligrams	Milligrams	Milligrams
	FISH, SHELLFISH, MEAT, POULTRY; RELATED PRODUCTS (CONTINUED)																			
	Meat and meat products: (cont.)																			
	Beef,[18] cooked: (cont.)																			
	Cuts braised, simmered or pot roasted: (cont.)																			
163	Lean only from item 162	2.5 oz	72	62	140	22	5	2.1	1.8	.2	0	10	108	2.7	176	10	.04	.17	3.3	—
	Ground beef, broiled:																			
164	Lean with 10% fat	3 oz or patty 3 by 5/8 in	85	60	185	23	10	4.0	3.9	.3	0	10	196	3.0	261	20	.08	.20	5.1	—
165	Lean with 21% fat	2.9 oz or patty 3 by 5/8 in	82	54	235	20	17	7.0	6.7	.4	0	9	159	2.6	221	30	.07	.17	4.4	—
	Roast, oven cooked, no liquid added:																			
	Relatively fat, such as rib:																			
166	Lean and fat (2 pieces, 4 1/8 by 2 1/4 by 1/4 in).	3 oz	85	40	375	17	33	14.0	13.6	.8	0	8	158	2.2	189	70	.05	.13	3.1	—
167	Lean only from item 166	1.8 oz	51	57	125	14	7	3.0	2.5	.3	0	6	131	1.8	161	10	.04	.11	2.6	—
	Relatively lean, such as heel of round:																			
168	Lean and fat (2 pieces, 4 1/8 by 2 1/4 by 1/4 in).	3 oz	85	62	165	25	7	2.8	2.7	.2	0	11	208	3.2	279	10	.06	.19	4.5	—
169	Lean only from item 168	2.8 oz	78	65	125	24	3	1.2	1.0	0.1	0	10	199	3.0	268	Trace	0.06	0.18	4.3	—
	Steak:																			
	Relatively fat-sirloin, broiled:																			
170	Lean and fat (piece, 2 1/2 by 2 1/2 by 3/4 in).	3 oz	85	44	330	20	27	11.3	11.1	.6	0	9	162	2.5	220	50	.05	.15	4.0	—
171	Lean only from item 170	2.0 oz	56	59	115	18	4	1.8	1.6	.2	0	7	146	2.2	202	10	.05	.14	3.6	—
	Relatively lean-round, braised:																			
172	Lean and fat (piece, 4 1/8 by 2 1/4 by 1/2 in).	3 oz	85	55	220	24	13	5.5	5.2	.4	0	10	213	3.0	272	20	.07	.19	4.8	—
173	Lean only from item 172	2.4 oz	68	61	130	21	4	1.7	1.5	.2	0	9	182	2.5	238	10	.05	.16	4.1	—
	Beef, canned:																			
174	Corned beef	3 oz	85	59	185	22	10	4.9	4.5	.2	0	17	90	3.7	—	—	.01	.20	2.9	—
175	Corned beef, hash	1 cup	220	67	400	19	25	11.9	10.9	.5	24	29	147	4.4	440	—	.02	.20	4.6	—
176	Beef, dried, chipped	2 1/2-oz jar	71	48	145	24	4	2.1	2.0	.1	0	14	287	3.6	142	—	.05	.23	2.7	0
177	Beef and vegetable stew	1 cup	245	82	220	16	11	4.9	4.5	.2	15	29	184	2.9	613	2,400	.15	.17	4.7	17
178	Beef potpie (home recipe), baked[19] (piece, 1/3 of 9-in diam. pie).	1 piece	210	55	515	21	30	7.9	12.8	6.7	39	29	149	3.8	334	1,720	.30	.30	5.5	6
179	Chili con carne with beans, canned.	1 cup	255	72	340	19	16	7.5	6.8	.3	31	82	321	4.3	594	150	.08	.18	3.3	—
180	Chop suey with beef and pork (home recipe).	1 cup	250	75	300	26	17	8.5	6.2	.7	13	60	248	4.8	425	600	.28	.38	5.0	33
181	Heart, beef, lean, braised	3 oz	85	61	160	27	5	1.5	1.1	.6	1	5	154	5.0	197	20	.21	1.04	6.5	1

No.	Food	Measure																		
	Lamb, cooked:																			
	Chop, rib (3 per lb with bone), broiled:																			
182	Lean and fat	3.1 oz	89	43	360	18	32	14.8	12.1	1.2	0	8	139	1.0	200	—	.11	.19	4.1	—
183	Lean only from item 182	2 oz	57	60	120	16	6	2.5	2.1	.2	0	6	121	1.1	174	—	.09	.15	3.4	—
	Leg, roasted:																			
184	Lean and fat (2 pieces, 4⅛ by 2¼ by ¼ in).	3 oz	85	54	235	22	16	7.3	6.0	.6	0	9	177	1.4	241	—	.13	.23	4.7	—
185	Lean only from item 184	2.5 oz	71	62	130	20	5	2.1	1.8	.2	0	9	169	1.4	227	—	.12	.21	4.4	—
	Shoulder, roasted:																			
186	Lean and fat (3 pieces, 2½ by 2½ by ¼ in).	3 oz	85	50	285	18	23	10.8	8.8	.9	0	9	146	1.0	206	—	.11	.20	4.0	—
187	Lean only from item 186	2.3 oz	64	61	130	17	6	3.6	2.3	.2	0	8	140	1.0	193	—	.10	.18	3.7	—
188	Liver, beef, fried[20] (slice, 6½ by 2⅜ by ⅜ in).	3 oz	85	56	195	22	9	2.5	3.5	.9	5	9	405	7.5	323	[21]45,390	.22	3.56	14.0	23
	Pork, cured, cooked:																			
189	Ham, light cure, lean and fat, roasted (2 pieces, 4⅛ by 2¼ by ¼ in.)[22]	3 oz	85	54	245	18	19	6.8	7.9	1.7	0	8	146	2.2	199	0	.40	.15	3.1	—
	Luncheon meat:																			
190	Boiled ham, slice (8 per 8-oz pkg.).	1 oz	28	59	65	5	5	1.7	2.0	.4	0	3	47	.8	—	0	.12	.04	.7	—
	Canned, spiced or unspiced:																			
191	Slice, approx. 3 by 2 by ½ in.	1 slice	60	55	175	9	15	5.4	6.7	1.0	1	5	65	1.3	133	0	.19	.13	1.8	—
	Pork, fresh,[18] cooked:																			
	Chop, loin (cut 3 per lb with bone), broiled:																			
192	Lean and fat	2.7 oz	78	42	305	19	25	8.9	10.4	2.2	0	9	209	2.7	216	0	0.75	0.22	4.5	—
193	Lean only from item 192	2 oz	56	53	150	17	9	3.1	3.6	.8	0	7	181	2.2	192	0	.63	.18	3.8	—
	Roast, oven cooked, no liquid added:																			
194	Lean and fat (piece, 2½ by 2½ by ¾ in).	3 oz	85	46	310	21	24	8.7	10.2	2.2	0	9	218	2.7	233	0	.78	.22	4.8	—
195	Lean only from item 194	2.4 oz	68	55	175	20	10	3.5	4.1	.8	0	9	211	2.6	224	0	.73	.21	4.4	—
	Shoulder cut, simmered:																			
196	Lean and fat (3 pieces, 2½ by 2½ by ¼ in).	3 oz	85	46	320	20	26	9.3	10.9	2.3	0	9	118	2.6	158	0	.46	.21	4.1	—
197	Lean only from item 196	2.2 oz	63	60	135	18	6	2.2	2.6	.6	0	8	111	2.3	146	0	.42	.19	3.7	—
	Sausages (see also Luncheon meat—items 190–191):																			
198	Bologna, slice (8 per 8-oz pkg.).	1 slice	28	56	85	3	8	3.0	3.4	.5	Trace	2	36	.5	65	—	.05	.06	.7	—
199	Braunschweiger, slice (6 per 6-oz pkg.).	1 slice	28	53	90	4	8	2.6	3.4	.8	1	3	69	1.7	—	1,850	.05	.41	2.3	—
200	Brown and serve (10–11 per 8-oz pkg.), browned.	1 link	17	40	70	3	6	2.3	2.8	.7	Trace	—	—	—	—	—	—	—	—	—
201	Deviled ham, canned	1 tbsp	13	51	45	2	4	1.5	1.8	.4	0	1	12	.3	—	0	.02	.01	.2	—
202	Frankfurter (8 per 1-lb pkg.), cooked (reheated).	1 frankfurter	56	57	170	7	15	5.6	6.5	1.2	1	3	57	.8	—	—	.08	.11	1.4	—
203	Meat, potted (beef, chicken, turkey), canned.	1 tbsp	13	61	30	2	2	—	—	—	0	—	—	—	—	—	Trace	.03	.2	—
204	Pork link (16 per 1-lb pkg), cooked.	1 link	13	35	60	2	6	2.1	2.4	.5	Trace	1	21	.3	35	0	.10	.04	.5	—

[19]Crust made with vegetable shortening and enriched flour.
[20]Regular-type margarine used.
[21]Value varies widely.
[22]About one-fourth of the outer layer of fat on the cut was removed. Deposits of fat within the cut were not removed.

Table A-1. (Continued)

Item No. (A)	Foods, approximate measures, units, and weight (edible part unless footnotes indicate otherwise) (B)			Water (C)	Food energy (D)	Protein (E)	Fat (F)	Fatty Acids: Saturated (total) (G)	Fatty Acids: Unsaturated: Oleic (H)	Fatty Acids: Unsaturated: Linoleic (I)	Carbohydrate (J)	Calcium (K)	Phosphorus (L)	Iron (M)	Potassium (N)	Vitamin A value (O)	Thiamin (P)	Riboflavin (Q)	Niacin (R)	Ascorbic Acid (S)
			Grams	*Percent*	*Calories*	*Grams*	*Grams*	*Grams*	*Grams*	*Grams*	*Grams*	*Milligrams*	*Milligrams*	*Milligrams*	*Milligrams*	*I.U.*	*Milligrams*	*Milligrams*	*Milligrams*	*Milligrams*
	FISH, SHELLFISH, MEAT, POULTRY: RELATED PRODUCTS (CONTINUED)																			
	Meat and meat products: (cont.)																			
	Sausages (cont.)																			
	Salami:																			
205	Dry type, slice (12 per 4-oz pkg.).	1 slice	10	30	45	2	4	1.6	1.6	.1	Trace	1	28	.4	—	—	.04	.03	.5	—
206	Cooked type, slice (8 per 8-oz pkg.).	1 slice	28	51	90	5	7	3.1	3.0	.2	Trace	3	57	.7	—	—	.07	.07	1.2	—
207	Vienna sausage (7 per 4-oz can).	1 sausage	16	63	40	2	3	1.2	1.4	.2	Trace	1	24	.3	—	—	.01	.02	.4	—
	Veal, medium fat, cooked, bone removed:																			
208	Cutlet (4⅛ by 2¼ by ½ in), braised or broiled.	3 oz	85	60	185	23	9	4.0	3.4	.4	0	9	196	2.7	258	—	.06	.21	4.6	—
209	Rib (2 pieces, 4⅛ by 2¼ by ¼ in), roasted.	3 oz	85	55	230	23	14	6.1	5.1	.6	0	10	211	2.9	259	—	.11	.26	6.6	—
	Poultry and poultry products:																			
	Chicken, cooked:																			
210	Breast, fried,[23] bones removed, ½ breast (3.3 oz with bones).	2.8 oz	79	58	160	26	5	1.4	1.8	1.1	1	9	218	1.3	—	70	.04	.17	11.6	—
211	Drumstick, fried,[23] bones removed (2 oz with bones).	1.3 oz	38	55	90	12	4	1.1	1.3	.9	Trace	6	89	.9	—	50	.03	.15	2.7	—
212	Half broiler, broiled, bones removed (10.4 oz with bones).	6.2 oz	176	71	240	42	7	2.2	2.5	1.3	0	16	355	3.0	483	160	.09	.34	15.5	—
213	Chicken, canned, boneless	3 oz	85	65	170	18	10	3.2	3.8	2.0	0	18	210	1.3	117	200	.03	.11	3.7	3
214	Chicken a la king, cooked (home recipe).	1 cup	245	68	470	27	34	2.7	14.3	3.3	12	127	358	2.5	404	1,130	.10	.42	5.4	12
215	Chicken and noodles, cooked (home recipe).	1 cup	240	71	365	22	18	5.9	7.1	3.5	26	26	247	2.2	149	430	.05	.17	4.3	Trace
	Chicken chow mein:																			
216	Canned	1 cup	250	89	95	7	Trace	—	—	—	18	45	85	1.3	418	150	0.05	0.10	1.0	13
217	From home recipe	1 cup	250	78	255	31	10	2.4	3.4	3.1	10	58	293	2.5	473	280	.08	.23	4.3	10
218	Chicken potpie (home recipe), baked,[19] (piece, ⅓ of 9-in diam. pie).	1 piece	232	57	545	23	31	11.3	10.9	5.6	42	70	232	3.0	343	3,090	.34	.31	5.5	5
	Turkey, roasted, flesh without skin:																			
219	Dark meat, piece, 2½ by 1⅝ by ¼ in.	4 pieces	85	61	175	26	7	2.1	1.5	1.5	0	—	—	2.0	338	—	.03	.20	3.6	—
220	Light meat, piece, 4 by 2 by ¼ in.	2 pieces	85	62	150	28	3	.9	.6	.7	0	—	—	1.0	349	—	.04	.12	9.4	—
	Light and dark meat:																			
221	Chopped or diced	1 cup	140	61	265	44	9	2.5	1.7	1.8	0	11	351	2.5	514	—	.07	.25	10.8	—
222	Pieces (1 slice white meat, 4 by 2 by ¼ in with 2 slices dark meat, 2½ by 1⅝ by ¼ in).	3 pieces	85	61	160	27	5	1.5	1.0	1.1	0	7	213	1.5	312	—	.04	.15	6.5	—

FRUITS AND FRUIT PRODUCTS

	Apples, raw, unpeeled, without cores:																			
223	2¾-in diam. (about 3 per lb with cores).	1 apple	138	84	80	Trace	1	—	—	—	20	10	14	.4	152	120	.04	.03	.1	6
224	3¼ in diam. (about 2 per lb with cores).	1 apple	212	84	125	Trace	1	—	—	—	31	15	21	.6	223	190	.06	.04	.2	8
225	Applejuice, bottled or canned[24]	1 cup	248	88	120	Trace	Trace	—	—	—	30	15	22	1.5	250	—	.02	.05	.2	[25]2
	Applesauce, canned:																			
226	Sweetened	1 cup	255	76	230	1	Trace	—	—	—	61	10	13	1.3	166	100	.05	.03	.1	[25]3
227	Unsweetened	1 cup	244	89	100	Trace	Trace	—	—	—	26	10	12	1.2	190	100	.05	.02	.1	[25]2
	Apricots																			
228	Raw, without pits (about 12 per lb with pits).	3 apricots	107	85	55	1	Trace	—	—	—	14	18	25	.5	301	2,890	.03	.04	.6	11
229	Canned in heavy sirup (halves and sirup).	1 cup	258	77	220	2	Trace	—	—	—	57	28	39	.8	604	4,490	.05	.05	1.0	10
	Dried:																			
230	Uncooked (28 large or 37 medium halves per cup).	1 cup	130	25	340	7	1	—	—	—	86	87	140	7.2	1,273	14,170	.01	.21	4.3	16
231	Cooked, unsweetened, fruit and liquid.	1 cup	250	76	215	4	1	—	—	—	54	55	88	4.5	795	7,500	.01	.13	2.5	0
232	Apricot nectar, canned	1 cup	251	85	145	1	Trace	—	—	—	37	23	30	.5	379	2,380	.03	.03	.5	[26]36
	Avocados, raw, whole, without skins and seeds:																			
233	California, mid- and late-winter (with skin and seed, 3⅛-in diam.; wt., 10 oz).	1 avocado	216	74	370	5	37	5.5	22.0	3.7	13	22	91	1.3	1,303	630	.24	.43	3.5	30
234	Florida, late summer and fall (with skin and seed, 3⅝-in diam.; wt., 1 lb).	1 avocado	304	78	390	4	33	6.7	15.7	5.3	27	30	128	1.8	1,836	880	.33	.61	4.9	43
235	Banana without peel (about 2.6 per lb with peel).	1 banana	119	76	100	1	Trace	—	—	—	26	10	31	.8	440	230	.06	.07	.8	12
236	Banana flakes	1 tbsp	6	3	20	Trace	Trace	—	—	—	5	2	6	.2	92	50	.01	.01	.2	Trace
237	Blackberries, raw	1 cup	144	85	85	2	1	—	—	—	19	46	27	1.3	245	290	0.04	0.06	0.6	30
238	Blueberries, raw	1 cup	145	83	90	1	1	—	—	—	22	22	19	1.5	117	150	.04	.09	.7	20
	Cantaloup. See Muskmelons (item 271).																			
	Cherries:																			
239	Sour (tart), red, pitted, canned, water pack.	1 cup	244	88	105	2	Trace	—	—	—	26	37	32	.7	317	1,660	.07	.05	.5	12
240	Sweet, raw, without pits and stems.	10 cherries	68	80	45	1	Trace	—	—	—	12	15	13	.3	129	70	.03	.04	.3	7
241	Cranberry juice cocktail, bottled, sweetened.	1 cup	253	83	165	Trace	Trace	—	—	—	42	13	8	.8	25	Trace	.03	.03	.1	[27]81
242	Cranberry sauce, sweetened, canned, strained.	1 cup	277	62	405	Trace	1	—	—	—	104	17	11	.6	83	60	.03	.03	.1	6
	Dates:																			
243	Whole, without pits	10 dates	80	23	220	2	Trace	—	—	—	58	47	50	2.4	518	40	.07	.08	1.8	0
244	Chopped	1 cup	178	23	490	4	1	—	—	—	130	105	112	5.3	1,153	90	.16	.18	3.9	0
245	Fruit cocktail, canned, in heavy sirup.	1 cup	255	80	195	1	Trace	—	—	—	50	23	31	1.0	411	360	.05	.03	1.0	5
	Grapefruit:																			
	Raw, medium, 3¾-in diam. (about 1 lb 1 oz):																			
246	Pink or red	½ grapefruit with peel[28]	241	89	50	1	Trace	—	—	—	13	20	20	.5	166	540	.05	.02	.2	44
247	White	½ grapefruit with peel[28]	241	89	45	1	Trace	—	—	—	12	19	19	.5	159	10	.05	.02	.2	44
248	Canned, sections with sirup	1 cup	254	81	180	2	Trace	—	—	—	45	33	36	.8	343	30	.08	.05	.5	76
	Grapefruit juice:																			
249	Raw, pink, red, or white	1 cup	246	90	95	1	Trace	—	—	—	23	22	37	.5	399	([29])	.10	.05	.5	93
	Canned, white:																			
250	Unsweetened	1 cup	247	89	100	1	Trace	—	—		24	20	35	1.0	400	20	.07	.05	.5	84

[23] Vegetable shortening used.
[24] Also applies to pasteurized apple cider.
[25] Applies to product without added ascorbic acid. For value of product with added ascorbic acid, refer to label.
[26] Based on product with label claim of 45% of U.S. RDA in 6 fl oz.
[27] Based on product with label claim of 100% of U.S. RDA in 6 fl oz.

Table A-1. (Continued)

Item No. (A)	Foods, approximate measures, units, and weight (edible part unless footnotes indicate otherwise) (B)			Water (C)	Food Energy (D)	Protein (E)	Fat (F)	Fatty Acids: Saturated (total) (G)	Unsaturated: Oleic (H)	Unsaturated: Linoleic (I)	Carbohydrate (J)	Calcium (K)	Phosphorus (L)	Iron (M)	Potassium (N)	Vitamin A Value (O)	Thiamin (P)	Riboflavin (Q)	Niacin (R)	Ascorbic Acid (S)
			Grams	Percent	Calories	Grams	Grams	Grams	Grams	Grams	Grams	Milligrams	Milligrams	Milligrams	Milligrams	I.U.	Milligrams	Milligrams	Milligrams	Milligrams
	FRUITS AND FRUIT PRODUCTS (CONTINUED)																			
	Grapefruit: (cont.)																			
	Canned, white: (cont.)																			
251	Sweetened	1 cup	250	86	135	1	Trace	—	—	—	32	20	35	1.0	405	30	.08	.05	.5	78
	Frozen, concentrate, unsweetened:																			
252	Undiluted, 6-fl oz can	1 can	207	62	300	4	1	—	—	—	72	70	124	.8	1,250	60	.29	.12	1.4	286
253	Diluted with 3 parts water by volume.	1 cup	247	89	100	1	Trace	—	—	—	24	25	42	.2	420	20	.10	.04	.5	96
254	Dehydrated crystals, prepared with water (1 lb yields about 1 gal).	1 cup	247	90	100	1	Trace	—	—	—	24	22	40	.2	412	20	.10	.05	.5	91
	Grapes, European type (adherent skin), raw:																			
255	Thompson Seedless	10 grapes	50	81	35	Trace	Trace	—	—	—	9	6	10	.2	87	50	.03	.02	.2	2
256	Tokay and Emperor, seeded types	10 grapes[30]	60	81	40	Trace	Trace	—	—	—	10	7	11	.2	99	60	.03	.02	.2	2
	Grapejuice:																			
257	Canned or bottled	1 cup	253	83	165	1	Trace	—	—	—	42	28	30	.8	293	—	.10	.05	.5[25]	Trace
	Frozen concentrate, sweetened:																			
258	Undiluted, 6-fl oz can	1 can	216	53	395	1	Trace	—	—	—	100	22	32	.9	255	40	.13	.22	1.5	[31]32
259	Diluted with 3 parts water by volume.	1 cup	250	86	135	1	Trace	—	—	—	33	8	10	.3	85	10	.05	.08	.5	[31]10
260	Grape drink, canned	1 cup	250	86	135	Trace	Trace	—	—	—	35	8	10	.3	88	—	[32].03	[32].03	.3	([32])
261	Lemon, raw, size 165, without peel and seeds (about 4 per lb with peels and seeds).		74	90	20	1	Trace	—	—	—	6	19	12	.4	102	10	.03	.01	.1	39
	Lemon juice:																			
262	Raw	1 cup	244	91	60	1	Trace	—	—	—	20	17	24	.5	344	50	.07	.02	.2	112
263	Canned, or bottled, unsweetened	1 cup	244	92	55	1	Trace	—	—	—	19	17	24	.5	344	50	.07	.02	.2	102
264	Frozen, single strength, unsweetened, 6-fl oz can.	1 can	183	92	40	1	Trace	—	—	—	13	13	16	.5	258	40	.05	.02	.2	81
	Lemonade concentrate, frozen:																			
265	Undiluted, 6-fl oz can	1 can	219	49	425	Trace	Trace	—	—	—	112	9	13	.4	153	40	.05	.06	.7	66
266	Diluted with 4⅓ parts water by volume.	1 cup	248	89	105	Trace	Trace	—	—	—	28	2	3	.1	40	10	.01	.02	.2	17
	Limeade concentrate, frozen:																			
267	Undiluted, 6-fl oz can	1 can	218	50	410	Trace	Trace	—	—	—	108	11	13	0.2	129	Trace	0.02	0.02	0.2	26
268	Diluted with 4⅓ parts water by volume.	1 cup	247	89	100	Trace	Trace	—	—	—	27	3	3	Trace	32	Trace	Trace	Trace	Trace	6
	Limejuice:																			
269	Raw	1 cup	246	90	65	1	Trace	—	—	—	22	22	27	.5	256	20	.05	.02	.2	79
270	Canned, unsweetened	1 cup	246	90	65	1	Trace	—	—	—	22	22	27	.5	256	20	.05	.02	.2	52
	Muskmelons, raw, with rind, without seed cavity:																			
271	Cantaloup, orange-fleshed (with rind and seed cavity, 5-in diam., 2⅓ lb).	½ melon with rind[33]	477	91	80	2	Trace	—	—	—	20	38	44	1.1	682	9,240	.11	.08	1.6	90

272	Honeydew (with rind and seed cavity, 6½-in diam., 5¼ lb).	1/10 melon with rind[33]	226	91	50	1	Trace	—	—	—	11	21	24	.6	374	60	.06	.04	.9	34
	Oranges, all commercial varieties, raw:																			
273	Whole, 2⅝-in diam., without peel and seeds (about 2½ per lb with peel and seeds).	1 orange	131	86	65	1	Trace	—	—	—	16	54	26	.5	263	260	.13	.05	.5	66
274	Sections without membranes	1 cup	180	86	90	2	Trace	—	—	—	22	74	36	.7	360	360	.18	.07	.7	90
	Orange juice:																			
275	Raw, all varieties	1 cup	248	88	110	2	Trace	—	—	—	26	27	42	.5	496	500	.22	.07	1.0	124
276	Canned, unsweetened	1 cup	249	87	120	2	Trace	—	—	—	28	25	45	1.0	496	500	.17	.05	.7	100
	Frozen, concentrate:																			
277	Undiluted, 6-fl oz can	1 can	213	55	360	5	Trace	—	—	—	87	75	126	.9	1,500	1,620	.68	.11	2.8	360
278	Diluted with 3 parts water by volume.	1 cup	249	87	120	2	Trace	—	—	—	29	25	42	.2	503	540	.23	.03	.9	120
279	Dehydrated crystals, prepared with water (1 lb yields about 1 gal).	1 cup	248	88	115	1	Trace	—	—	—	27	25	40	.5	518	500	.20	.07	1.0	109
	Orange and grapefruit juice:																			
	Frozen concentrate:																			
280	Undiluted, 6-fl oz can	1 can	210	59	330	4	1	—	—	—	78	61	99	.8	1,308	800	.48	.06	2.3	302
281	Diluted with 3 parts water by volume.	1 cup	248	88	110	1	Trace	—	—	—	26	20	32	.2	439	270	.15	.02	.7	102
282	Papayas, raw, ½-in cubes	1 cup	140	89	55	1	Trace	—	—	—	14	28	22	.4	328	2,450	.06	.06	.4	78
	Peaches:																			
	Raw:																			
283	Whole, 2½-in diam., peeled, pitted (about 4 per lb with peels and pits).	1 peach	100	89	40	1	Trace	—	—	—	10	9	19	.5	202	[34]1,330	.02	.05	1.0	7
284	Sliced	1 cup	170	89	65	1	Trace	—	—	—	16	15	32	.9	343	[34]2,260	.03	.09	1.7	12
	Canned, yellow-fleshed, solids and liquid (halves or slices):																			
285	Sirup pack	1 cup	256	79	200	1	Trace	—	—	—	51	10	31	.8	333	1,100	.03	.05	1.5	8
286	Water pack	1 cup	244	91	75	1	Trace	—	—	—	20	10	32	.7	334	1,100	.02	.07	1.5	7
	Dried:																			
287	Uncooked	1 cup	160	25	420	5	1	—	—	—	109	77	187	9.6	1,520	6,240	.02	.30	8.5	29
288	Cooked, unsweetened, halves and juice.	1 cup	250	77	205	3	1	—	—	—	54	38	93	4.8	743	3,050	.01	.15	3.8	5
	Frozen, sliced, sweetened:																			
289	10-oz container	1 container	284	77	250	1	Trace	—	—	—	64	11	37	1.4	352	1,850	0.03	0.11	2.0	[35]116
290	Cup	1 cup	250	77	220	1	Trace	—	—	—	57	10	33	1.3	310	1,630	.03	.10	1.8	[35]103
	Pears:																			
	Raw, with skin, cored:																			
291	Bartlett, 2½-in. diam. (about 2½ per lb with cores and stems.)	1 pear	164	83	100	1	1	—	—	—	25	13	18	.5	213	30	.03	.07	.2	7
292	Bosc, 2½-in diam. (about 3 per lb with cores and stems).	1 pear	141	83	85	1	1	—	—	—	22	11	16	.4	83	30	.03	.06	.1	6
293	D'Anjou, 3-in diam. (about 2 per lb with cores and stems).	1 pear	200	83	120	1	1	—	—	—	31	16	22	.6	260	40	.04	.08	.2	8

[28] Weight includes peel and membranes between sections. Without these parts, the weight of the edible portion is 123 g for item 246 and 118 g for item 247.

[29] For white-fleshed varieties, value is about 20 International Units (I.U.) per cup; for red-fleshed varieties, 1,080 I.U.

[30] Weight includes seeds. Without seeds, weight of the edible portion is 57 g.

[31] Applies to product without added ascorbic acid. With added ascorbic acid, based on claim that 6 fl oz of reconstituted juice contain 45% or 50% of the U.S. RDA, value in milligrams is 108 or 120 for a 6-fl oz can (item 258), 36 or 40 for 1 cup of diluted juice (item 259).

[32] For products with added thiamin and riboflavin but without added ascorbic acid, values in milligrams would be 0.60 for thiamin, 0.80 for riboflavin, and trace for ascorbic acid. For products with only ascorbic acid added, value varies with the brand. Consult the label.

[33] Weight includes rind. Without rind, the weight of the edible portion is 272 g for item 271 and 149 g for item 272.

[34] Represents yellow-fleshed varieties. For white-fleshed varieties, value is 50 International Units (I.U.) for 1 peach, 90 I.U. for 1 cup of slices.

[35] Value represents products with added ascorbic acid. For products without added ascorbic acid, value in milligrams is 116 for a 10-oz container, 103 for 1 cup.

Table A-1. (Continued)

Item No. (A)	Foods, approximate measures, units, and weight (edible part unless footnotes indicate otherwise) (B)			Water (C)	Food Energy (D)	Protein (E)	Fat (F)	Fatty Acids: Saturated (total) (G)	Fatty Acids: Unsaturated: Oleic (H)	Fatty Acids: Unsaturated: Linoleic (I)	Carbohydrate (J)	Calcium (K)	Phosphorus (L)	Iron (M)	Potassium (N)	Vitamin A Value (O)	Thiamin (P)	Riboflavin (Q)	Niacin (R)	Ascorbic Acid (S)
			Grams	Percent	Calories	Grams	Grams	Grams	Grams	Grams	Grams	Milligrams	Milligrams	Milligrams	Milligrams	I.U.	Milligrams	Milligrams	Milligrams	Milligrams
	FRUIT AND FRUIT PRODUCTS (CONTINUED)																			
	Pears: (cont.)																			
294	Canned, solids and liquid, sirup pack, heavy (halves or slices).	1 cup	255	80	195	1	1	—	—	—	50	13	18	.5	214	10	.03	.05	.3	3
	Pineapple:																			
295	Raw, diced	1 cup	155	85	80	1	Trace	—	—	—	21	26	12	.8	226	110	.14	.05	.3	26
	Canned, heavy sirup pack, solids and liquid:																			
296	Crushed, chunks, tidbits	1 cup	255	80	190	1	Trace	—	—	—	49	28	13	.8	245	130	.20	.05	.5	18
	Slices and liquid:																			
297	Large	1 slice; 2¼ tbsp liquid.	105	80	80	Trace	Trace	—	—	—	20	12	5	.3	101	50	.08	.02	.2	7
298	Medium	1 slice; 1¼ tbsp liquid.	58	80	45	Trace	Trace	—	—	—	11	6	3	.2	56	30	.05	.01	.1	4
299	Pineapple juice, unsweetened, canned.	1 cup	250	86	140	1	Trace	—	—	—	34	38	23	.8	373	130	.13	.05	.5	[27]80
	Plums:																			
	Raw, without pits:																			
300	Japanese and hybrid (2⅛-in diam., about 6½ per lb with pits).	1 plum	66	87	30	Trace	Trace	—	—	—	8	8	12	.3	112	160	.02	.02	.3	4
301	Prune-type (1½-in diam., about 15 per lb with pits).	1 plum	28	79	20	Trace	Trace	—	—	—	6	3	5	.1	48	80	.01	.01	.1	1
	Canned, heavy sirup pack (Italian prunes), with pits and liquid:																			
302	Cup	1 cup[36]	272	77	215	1	Trace	—	—	—	56	23	26	2.3	367	3,130	.05	.05	1.0	5
303	Portion	3 plums; 2¾ tbsp liquid.[36]	140	77	110	1	Trace	—	—	—	29	12	13	1.2	189	1,610	.03	.03	.5	3
	Prunes, dried, "softenized," with pits:																			
304	Uncooked	4 extra large or 5 large prunes.[36]	49	28	110	1	Trace	—	—	—	29	22	34	1.7	298	690	.04	.07	.7	1
305	Cooked, unsweetened, all sizes, fruit and liquid.	1 cup[36]	250	66	255	2	1	—	—	—	67	51	79	3.8	695	1,590	.07	.15	1.5	2
306	Prune juice, canned or bottled	1 cup	256	80	195	1	Trace	—	—	—	49	36	51	1.8	602	—	.03	.03	1.0	5
	Raisins, seedless:																			
307	Cup, not pressed down	1 cup	145	18	420	4	Trace	—	—	—	112	90	146	5.1	1,106	30	.16	.12	.7	1
308	Packet, ½ oz (1½ tbsp)	1 packet	14	18	40	Trace	Trace	—	—	—	11	9	14	.5	107	Trace	.02	.01	.1	Trace
	Raspberries, red:																			
309	Raw, capped, whole	1 cup	123	84	70	1	1	—	—	—	17	27	27	1.1	207	160	.04	.11	1.1	31
310	Frozen, sweetened, 10-oz container	1 container	284	74	280	2	1	—	—	—	70	37	48	1.7	284	200	.06	.17	1.7	60
	Rhubarb, cooked, added sugar:																			
311	From raw	1 cup	270	63	380	1	Trace	—	—	—	97	211	41	1.6	548	220	.05	.14	.8	16
312	From frozen, sweetened	1 cup	270	63	385	1	1	—	—	—	98	211	32	1.9	475	190	.05	.11	.5	16
	Strawberries:																			
313	Raw, whole berries, capped	1 cup	149	90	55	1	1	—	—	—	13	31	31	1.5	244	90	0.04	0.10	0.9	88
	Frozen, sweetened:																			
314	Sliced, 10-oz container	1 container	284	71	310	1	1	—	—	—	79	40	48	2.0	318	90	.06	.17	1.4	151

315	Whole, 1-lb container (about 1¾ cups).	1 container	454	76	415	2	1	—	—	—	107	59	73	2.7	472	140	.09	.27	2.3	249
316	Tangerine, raw, 2⅜-in diam., size 176, without peel (about 4 per lb with peels and seeds).	1 tangerine	86	87	40	1	Trace	—	—	—	10	34	15	.3	108	360	.05	.02	.1	27
317	Tangerine juice, canned, sweetened.	1 cup	249	87	125	1	Trace	—	—	—	30	44	35	.5	440	1,040	.15	.05	.2	54
318	Watermelon, raw, 4 by 8 in wedge with rind and seeds (1/16 of 32⅔-lb melon, 10 by 16 in).	1 wedge with rind and seeds[37]	926	93	110	2	1	—	—	—	27	30	43	2.1	426	2,510	.13	.13	.9	30
	GRAIN PRODUCTS																			
	Bagel, 3-in diam.:																			
319	Egg	1 bagel	55	32	165	6	2	0.5	0.9	0.8	28	9	43	1.2	41	30	.14	.10	1.2	0
320	Water	1 bagel	55	29	165	6	1	.2	.4	.6	30	8	41	1.2	42	0	.15	.11	1.4	0
321	Barley pearled, light uncooked	1 cup	200	11	700	16	2	.3	.2	.8	158	32	378	4.0	320	0	.24	.10	6.2	0
	Biscuits, baking powder, 2-in diam. (enriched flour, vegetable shortening):																			
322	From home recipe	1 biscuit	28	27	105	2	5	1.2	2.0	1.2	13	34	49	.4	33	Trace	.08	.08	.7	Trace
323	From mix	1 biscuit	28	29	90	2	3	.6	1.1	.7	15	19	65	.6	32	Trace	.09	.08	.8	Trace
	Breadcrumbs (enriched):[38]																			
324	Dry, grated	1 cup	100	7	390	13	5	1.0	1.6	1.4	73	122	141	3.6	152	Trace	.35	.35	4.8	Trace
	Soft. See White bread (items 349–350).																			
	Breads:																			
325	Boston brown bread, canned, slice, 3¼ by ½ in.[38]	1 slice	45	45	95	2	1	.1	.2	.2	21	41	72	.9	131	[39]0	.06	.04	.7	0
	Cracked-wheat bread (¾ enriched wheat flour, ¼ cracked wheat):[38]																			
326	Loaf, 1 lb	1 loaf	454	35	1,195	39	10	2.2	3.0	3.9	236	399	581	9.5	608	Trace	1.52	1.13	14.4	Trace
327	Slice (18 per loaf)	1 slice	25	35	65	2	1	.1	.2	.2	13	22	32	.5	34	Trace	.08	.06	.8	Trace
	French or vienna bread, enriched:[38]																			
328	Loaf, 1 lb	1 loaf	454	31	1,315	41	14	3.2	4.7	4.6	251	195	386	10.0	408	Trace	1.80	1.10	15.0	Trace
	Slice:																			
329	French (5 by 2½ by 1 in)	1 slice	35	31	100	3	1	.2	.4	.4	19	15	30	.8	32	Trace	.14	.08	1.2	Trace
330	Vienna (4¾ by 4 by ½ in).	1 slice	25	31	75	2	1	.2	.3	.3	14	11	21	.6	23	Trace	.10	.06	.8	Trace
	Italian bread, enriched:																			
331	Loaf, 1 lb	1 loaf	454	32	1,250	41	4	.6	.3	1.5	256	77	349	10.0	336	0	1.80	1.10	15.0	0
332	Slice, 4½ by 3¼ by ¾ in.	1 slice	30	32	85	3	Trace	Trace	Trace	.1	17	5	23	.7	22	0	.12	.07	1.0	0
	Raisin bread, enriched:[38]																			
333	Loaf, 1 lb	1 loaf	454	35	1,190	30	13	3.0	4.7	3.9	243	322	395	10.0	1,057	Trace	1.70	1.07	10.7	Trace
334	Slice (18 per loaf)	1 slice	25	35	65	2	1	.2	.3	.2	13	18	22	.6	58	Trace	.09	.06	.6	Trace
	Rye Bread:																			
	American, light (⅔ enriched wheat flour, ⅓ rye flour):																			
335	Loaf, 1 lb	1 loaf	454	36	1,100	41	5	0.7	0.5	2.2	236	340	667	9.1	658	0	1.35	0.98	12.9	0
336	Slice (4¾ by 3¾ by 7/16 in).	1 slice	25	36	60	2	Trace	Trace	Trace	.1	13	19	37	.5	36	0	.07	.05	.7	0
	Pumpernickel (⅔ rye flour, ⅓ enriched wheat flour):																			
337	Loaf, 1 lb	1 loaf	454	34	1,115	41	5	.7	.5	2.4	241	381	1,039	11.8	2,059	0	1.30	.93	8.5	0

[36]Weight includes pits. After removal of the pits, the weight of the edible portion is 258 g for item 302, 133 g for item 303, 43 g for item 304, and 213 g for item 305.
[37]Weight includes rind and seeds. Without rind and seeds, weight of the edible portion is 426 g.
[38]Made with vegetable shortening.
[39]Applies to product made with white cornmeal. With yellow cornmeal, value is 30 International Units (I.U.).

Table A-1. **(Continued)**

Item No. (A)	Foods, approximate measures, units, and weight (edible part unless footnotes indicate otherwise) (B)			Water (C)	Food Energy (D)	Protein (E)	Fat (F)	Fatty Acids: Saturated (total) (G)	Fatty Acids: Unsaturated: Oleic (H)	Fatty Acids: Unsaturated: Linoleic (I)	Carbohydrate (J)	Calcium (K)	Phosphorus (L)	Iron (M)	Potassium (N)	Vitamin A Value (O)	Thiamin (P)	Riboflavin (Q)	Niacin (R)	Ascorbic Acid (S)
			Grams	Percent	Calories	Grams	Grams	Grams	Grams	Grams	Grams	Milligrams	Milligrams	Milligrams	Milligrams	I.U.	Milligrams	Milligrams	Milligrams	Milligrams
	GRAIN PRODUCTS (CONTINUED)																			
	Bread: (cont.)																			
	Rye Bread: (cont.)																			
	Pumpernickel: (cont.)																			
338	Slice (5 by 4 by ⅜ in)	1 slice	32	34	80	3	Trace	.1	Trace	.2	17	27	73	.8	145	0	.09	.07	.6	0
	White bread, enriched:[38]																			
	Soft-crumb type:																			
339	Loaf, 1 lb	1 loaf	454	36	1,225	39	15	3.4	5.3	4.6	229	381	440	11.3	476	Trace	1.80	1.10	15.0	Trace
340	Slice (18 per loaf)	1 slice	25	36	70	2	1	.2	.3	.3	13	21	24	.6	26	Trace	.10	.06	.8	Trace
341	Slice, toasted	1 slice	22	25	70	2	1	.2	.3	.3	13	21	24	.6	26	Trace	.08	.06	.8	Trace
342	Slice (22 per loaf)	1 slice	20	36	55	2	1	.2	.2	.2	10	17	19	.5	21	Trace	.08	.05	.7	Trace
343	Slice, toasted	1 slice	17	25	55	2	1	.2	.2	.2	10	17	19	.5	21	Trace	.06	.05	.7	Trace
344	Loaf, 1½ lb	1 loaf	680	36	1,835	59	22	5.2	7.9	6.9	343	571	660	17.0	714	Trace	2.70	1.65	22.5	Trace
345	Slice (24 per loaf)	1 slice	28	36	75	2	1	.2	.3	.3	14	24	27	.7	29	Trace	.11	.07	.9	Trace
346	Slice, toasted	1 slice	24	25	75	2	1	.2	.3	.3	14	24	27	.7	29	Trace	.09	.07	.9	Trace
347	Slice (28 per loaf)	1 slice	24	36	65	2	1	.2	.3	.2	12	20	23	.6	25	Trace	.10	.06	.8	Trace
348	Slice, toasted	1 slice	21	25	65	2	1	.2	.3	.2	12	20	23	.6	25	Trace	.08	.06	.8	Trace
349	Cubes	1 cup	30	36	80	3	1	.2	.3	.3	15	25	29	.8	32	Trace	.12	.07	1.0	Trace
350	Crumbs	1 cup	45	36	120	4	1	.3	.5	.5	23	38	44	1.1	47	Trace	.18	.11	1.5	Trace
	Firm-crumb type:																			
351	Loaf, 1 lb	1 loaf	454	35	1,245	41	17	3.9	5.9	5.2	228	435	463	11.3	549	Trace	1.80	1.10	15.0	Trace
352	Slice (20 per loaf)	1 slice	23	35	65	2	1	.2	.3	.3	12	22	23	.6	28	Trace	.09	.06	.8	Trace
353	Slice, toasted	1 slice	20	24	65	2	1	.2	.3	.3	12	22	23	.6	28	Trace	.07	.06	.8	Trace
354	Loaf, 2 lb	1 loaf	907	35	2,495	82	34	7.7	11.8	10.4	455	871	925	22.7	1,097	Trace	3.60	2.20	30.0	Trace
355	Slice (34 per loaf)	1 slice	27	35	75	2	1	.2	.3	.3	14	26	28	.7	33	Trace	.11	.06	.9	Trace
356	Slice, toasted	1 slice	23	24	75	2	1	.2	.3	.3	14	26	28	.7	33	Trace	.09	.06	.9	Trace
	Whole-wheat bread:																			
	Soft-crumb type:[38]																			
357	Loaf, 1 lb	1 loaf	454	36	1,095	41	12	2.2	2.9	4.2	224	381	1,152	13.6	1,161	Trace	1.37	.45	12.7	Trace
358	Slice (16 per loaf)	1 slice	28	36	65	3	1	.1	.2	.2	14	24	71	.8	72	Trace	.09	.03	.8	Trace
359	Slice, toasted	1 slice	24	24	65	3	1	.1	.2	.2	14	24	71	.8	72	Trace	.07	.03	.8	Trace
	Firm-crumb type:[38]																			
360	Loaf, 1 lb	1 loaf	454	36	1,100	48	14	2.5	3.3	4.9	216	449	1,034	13.6	1,238	Trace	1.17	.54	12.7	Trace
361	Slice (18 per loaf)	1 slice	25	36	60	3	1	.1	.2	.3	12	25	57	.8	68	Trace	.06	.03	.7	Trace
362	Slice, toasted	1 slice	21	24	60	3	1	.1	.2	.3	12	25	57	.8	68	Trace	.05	.03	.7	Trace
	Breakfast, cereals:																			
	Hot type, cooked:																			
	Corn (hominy) grits, degermed:																			
363	Enriched	1 cup	245	87	125	3	Trace	Trace	Trace	.1	27	2	25	.7	27	[40]Trace	.10	.07	1.0	0
364	Unenriched	1 cup	245	87	125	3	Trace	Trace	Trace	.1	27	2	25	.2	27	[40]Trace	.05	.02	.5	0
365	Farina, quick-cooking, enriched.	1 cup	245	89	105	3	Trace	Trace	Trace	.1	22	147	[41]113	([42])	25	0	.12	.07	1.0	0
366	Oatmeal or rolled oats	1 cup	240	87	130	5	2	.4	.8	.9	23	22	137	1.4	146	0	.19	.05	.2	0
367	Wheat, rolled	1 cup	240	80	180	5	1	—	—	—	41	19	182	1.7	202	0	.17	.07	2.2	0
368	Wheat, whole-meal	1 cup	245	88	110	4	1	—	—	—	23	17	127	1.2	118	0	.15	.05	1.5	0
	Ready-to-eat:																			
369	Bran flakes (40% bran), added sugar, salt, iron, vitamins.	1 cup	35	3	105	4	1	—	—	—	28	19	125	12.4	137	1,650	.41	.49	4.1	12
370	Bran flakes with raisins, added sugar, salt, iron, vitamins.	1 cup	50	7	145	4	1	—	—	—	40	28	146	17.7	154	2,350	.58	.71	5.8	18

No.	Food	Measure																		
	Corn flakes:																			
371	Plain, added sugar, salt, iron, vitamins.	1 cup	25	4	95	2	Trace	—	—	—	21	([43])	9	0.6	30	1,180	0.29	0.35	2.9	9
372	Sugar-coated, added salt, iron, vitamins.	1 cup	40	2	155	2	Trace	—	—	—	37	1	10	1.0	27	1,880	.46	.56	4.6	14
373	Corn, puffed, plain, added sugar, salt, iron, vitamins.	1 cup	20	4	80	2	1	—	—	—	16	4	18	2.3	—	940	.23	.28	2.3	7
374	Corn, shredded, added sugar, salt, iron, thiamin, niacin.	1 cup	25	3	95	2	Trace	—	—	—	22	1	10	.6	—	0	.11	.05	.5	0
375	Oats, puffed, added sugar, salt, minerals, vitamins.	1 cup	25	3	100	3	1	—	—	—	19	44	102	2.9	—	1,180	.29	.35	2.9	9
	Rice, puffed:																			
376	Plain, added iron, thiamin, niacin.	1 cup	15	4	60	1	Trace	—	—	—	13	3	14	.3	15	0	.07	.01	.7	0
377	Presweetened, added salt, iron, vitamins.	1 cup	28	3	115	1	0	—	—	—	26	3	14	[44]1.1	43	1,250	.38	.43	5.0	[45]15
378	Wheat flakes, added sugar, salt, iron, vitamins.	1 cup	30	4	105	3	Trace	—	—	—	24	12	83	([43])	81	1,410	.35	.42	3.5	11
	Wheat, puffed:																			
379	Plain, added iron, thiamin, niacin.	1 cup	15	3	55	2	Trace	—	—	—	12	4	48	.6	51	0	.08	.03	1.2	0
380	Presweetened, added salt, iron, vitamins.	1 cup	38	3	140	3	Trace	—	—	—	33	7	52	[44]1.6	63	1,680	.50	.57	6.7	[45]20
381	Wheat, shredded, plain	1 oblong biscuit or ½ cup spoon-size biscuits.	25	7	90	2	1	—	—	—	20	11	97	.9	87	0	.06	.03	1.1	0
382	Wheat germ, without salt and sugar, toasted.	1 tbsp	6	4	25	2	1	—	—	—	3	3	70	.5	57	10	.11	.05	.3	1
383	Buckwheat flour, light, sifted	1 cup	98	12	340	6	1	0.2	0.4	0.4	78	11	86	1.0	314	0	.08	.04	.4	0
384	Bulgur, canned, seasoned	1 cup	135	56	245	8	4	—	—	—	44	27	263	1.9	151	0	.08	.05	4.1	0
	Cake icings. See Sugars and Sweets (items 532–536).																			
	Cakes made from cake mixes with enriched flour:[46]																			
	Angelfood:																			
385	Whole cake (9¾-in diam. tube cake).	1 cake	635	34	1,645	36	1	—	—	—	377	603	756	2.5	381	0	.37	.95	3.6	0
386	Piece, 1/12 of cake	1 piece	53	34	135	3	Trace	—	—	—	32	50	63	.2	32	0	.03	.08	.3	0
	Coffeecake:																			
387	Whole cake (7¾ by 5⅝ by 1¼ in).	1 cake	430	30	1,385	27	41	11.7	16.3	8.8	225	262	748	6.9	469	690	.82	.91	7.7	1
388	Piece, ⅙ of cake	1 piece	72	30	230	5	7	2.0	2.7	1.5	38	44	125	1.2	78	120	.14	.15	1.3	Trace
	Cupcakes, made with egg, milk, 2½-in diam.:																			
389	Without icing	1 cupcake	25	26	90	1	3	.8	1.2	.7	14	40	59	.3	21	40	.05	.05	.4	Trace
390	With chocolate icing	1 cupcake	36	22	130	2	5	2.0	1.6	.6	21	47	71	.4	42	60	.05	.06	.4	Trace
	Devil's food with chocolate icing:																			
391	Whole, 2 layer cake (8- or 9-in diam.).	1 cake	1,107	24	3,755	49	136	50.0	44.9	17.0	645	653	1,162	16.6	1,439	1,660	1.06	1.65	10.1	1
392	Piece, 1/16 of cake	1 piece	69	24	235	3	8	3.1	2.8	1.1	40	41	72	1.0	90	100	.07	.10	.6	Trace
393	Cupcake, 2½-in diam	1 cupcake	35	24	120	2	4	1.6	1.4	.5	20	21	37	.5	46	50	.03	.05	.3	Trace
	Gingerbread:																			
394	Whole cake (8-in square)	1 cake	570	37	1,575	18	39	9.7	16.6	10.0	291	513	570	8.6	1,562	Trace	0.84	1.00	7.4	Trace
395	Piece, 1/9 of cake	1 piece	63	37	175	2	4	1.1	1.8	1.1	32	57	63	.9	173	Trace	.09	.11	.8	Trace
	White, 2 layer with chocolate icing:																			
396	Whole cake (8- or 9-in diam.)	1 cake	1,140	21	4,000	44	122	48.2	46.4	20.0	716	1,129	2,041	11.4	1,322	680	1.50	1.77	12.5	2

[40] Applies to white varieties. For yellow varieties, value is 150 International Units (I.U.).
[41] Applies to products that do not contain di-sodium phosphate. If di-sodium phosphate is an ingredient, value is 162 mg.
[42] Value may range from less than 1 mg to about 8 mg depending on the brand. Consult the label.
[43] Value varies with the brand. Consult the label.
[44] Value varies with the brand. Consult the label.
[45] Applies to product with added ascorbic acid. Without added ascorbic acid, value is trace.
[46] Excepting angelfood cake, cakes were made from mixes containing vegetable shortening; icings, with butter.

Table A-1. (Continued)

Item No. (A)	Foods, approximate measures, units, and weight (edible part unless footnotes indicate otherwise) (B)			Water (C)	Food Energy (D)	Protein (E)	Fat (F)	Saturated (total) (G)	Unsaturated: Oleic (H)	Unsaturated: Linoleic (I)	Carbohydrate (J)	Calcium (K)	Phosphorus (L)	Iron (M)	Potassium (N)	Vitamin A Value (O)	Thiamin (P)	Riboflavin (Q)	Niacin (R)	Ascorbic Acid (S)
			Grams	Percent	Calories	Grams	Grams	Grams	Grams	Grams	Grams	Milligrams	Milligrams	Milligrams	Milligrams	I.U.	Milligrams	Milligrams	Milligrams	Milligrams
	GRAIN PRODUCTS (CONTINUED)																			
	Cakes: (cont.)																			
	White: (cont.)																			
397	Piece, 1/16 of cake	1 piece	71	21	250	3	8	3.0	2.9	1.2	45	70	127	.7	82	40	.09	.11	.8	Trace
	Yellow, 2 layer with chocolate icing:																			
398	Whole cake (8- or 9-in diam.)	1 cake	1,108	26	3,735	45	125	47.8	47.8	20.3	638	1,008	2,017	12.2	1,208	1,550	1.24	1.67	10.6	2
399	Piece, 1/16 of cake	1 piece	69	26	235	3	8	3.0	3.0	1.3	40	63	126	.8	75	100	.08	.10	.7	Trace
	Cakes made from home recipes using enriched flour:[47]																			
	Boston cream pie with custard filling:																			
400	Whole cake (8-in diam.)	1 cake	825	35	2,490	41	78	23.0	30.1	15.2	412	553	833	8.2	[48]734	1,730	1.04	1.27	9.6	2
401	Piece, 1/12 of cake	1 piece	69	35	210	3	6	1.9	2.5	1.3	34	46	70	.7	[48]61	140	.09	.11	.8	Trace
	Fruitcake, dark:																			
402	Loaf, 1-lb (7½ by 2 by 1½ in).	1 loaf	454	18	1,720	22	69	14.4	33.5	14.8	271	327	513	11.8	2,250	540	.72	.73	4.9	2
403	Slice, 1/30 of loaf	1 slice	15	18	55	1	2	.5	1.1	.5	9	11	17	.4	74	20	.02	.02	.2	Trace
	Plain sheet cake:																			
	Without icing:																			
404	Whole cake (9-in square)	1 cake	777	25	2,830	35	108	29.5	44.4	23.9	434	497	793	8.5	[48]614	1,320	1.21	1.40	10.2	2
405	Piece, 1/9 of cake	1 piece	86	25	315	4	12	3.3	4.9	2.6	48	55	88	.9	[48]68	150	.13	.15	1.1	Trace
	With uncooked white icing:																			
406	Whole cake (9-in square)	1 cake	1,096	21	4,020	37	129	42.2	49.5	24.4	694	548	822	8.2	[48]669	2,190	1.22	1.47	10.2	2
407	Piece, 1/9 of cake	1 piece	121	21	445	4	14	4.7	5.5	2.7	77	61	91	.8	[48]74	240	.14	.16	1.1	Trace
	Pound:[49]																			
408	Loaf, 8½ by 3½ by 3¼ in.	1 loaf	565	16	2,725	31	170	42.9	73.1	39.6	273	107	418	7.9	345	1,410	.90	.99	7.3	0
409	Slice, 1/17 of loaf	1 slice	33	16	160	2	10	2.5	4.3	2.3	16	6	24	.5	20	80	.05	.06	.4	0
	Spongecake:																			
410	Whole cake (9¾-in diam. tube cake).	1 cake	790	32	2,345	60	45	13.1	15.8	5.7	427	237	885	13.4	687	3,560	1.10	1.64	7.4	Trace
411	Piece, 1/12 of cake	1 piece	66	32	195	5	4	1.1	1.3	.5	36	20	74	1.1	57	300	.09	.14	.6	Trace
	Cookies made with enriched flour:[50] [51]																			
	Brownies with nuts:																			
	Home-prepared, 1¾ by 1¾ by ⅞ in:																			
412	From home recipe	1 brownie	20	10	95	1	6	1.5	3.0	1.2	10	8	30	.4	38	40	.04	.03	.2	Trace
413	From commercial recipe	1 brownie	20	11	85	1	4	.9	1.4	1.3	13	9	27	.4	34	20	.03	.02	.2	Trace
414	Frozen, with chocolate icing,[52] 1½ by 1¾ by ⅞ in.	1 brownie	25	13	105	1	5	2.0	2.2	.7	15	10	31	.4	44	50	.03	.03	.2	Trace
	Chocolate chip:																			
415	Commercial, 2¼-in diam., ⅜ in thick.	4 cookies	42	3	200	2	9	2.8	2.9	2.2	29	16	48	1.0	56	50	.10	.17	.9	Trace
416	From home recipe, 2⅓-in diam.	4 cookies	40	3	205	2	12	3.5	4.5	2.9	24	14	40	.8	47	40	.06	.06	.5	Trace
417	Fig bars, square (1⅝ by 1⅝ by ⅜ in) or rectangular (1½ by 1¾ by ½ in).	4 cookies	56	14	200	2	3	.8	1.2	.7	42	44	34	1.0	111	60	.04	.14	.9	Trace
418	Gingersnaps, 2-in diam., ¼ in thick.	4 cookies	28	3	90	2	2	.7	1.0	.6	22	20	13	.7	129	20	.08	.06	.7	0

419	Macaroons, 2¾-in diam., ¼ in thick.	2 cookies	38	4	180	2	9	—	—	—	25	10	32	.3	176	0	.02	.06	.2	0
420	Oatmeal with raisins, 2⅝-in diam., ¼ in thick.	4 cookies	52	3	235	3	8	2.0	3.3	2.0	38	11	53	1.4	192	30	.15	.10	1.0	Trace
421	Plain, prepared from commercial chilled dough, 2½-in diam., ¼ in thick.	4 cookies	48	5	240	2	12	3.0	5.2	2.9	31	17	35	0.6	23	30	0.10	0.08	0.9	0
422	Sandwich type (chocolate or vanilla), 1¾-in diam., ⅜ in thick.	4 cookies	40	2	200	2	9	2.2	3.9	2.2	28	10	96	.7	15	0	.06	.10	.7	0
423	Vanilla wafers, 1¾-in diam., ¼ in thick.	10 cookies	40	3	185	2	6	—	—	—	30	16	25	.6	29	50	.10	.09	.8	0
	Cornmeal:																			
424	Whole-ground, unbolted, dry form.	1 cup	122	12	435	11	5	.5	1.0	2.5	90	24	312	2.9	346	[53]620	.46	.13	2.4	0
425	Bolted (nearly whole-grain), dry form.	1 cup	122	12	440	11	4	.5	.9	2.1	91	21	272	2.2	303	[53]590	.37	.10	2.3	0
	Degermed, enriched:																			
426	Dry form	1 cup	138	12	500	11	2	.2	.4	.9	108	8	137	4.0	166	[53]610	.61	.36	4.8	0
427	Cooked	1 cup	240	88	120	3	Trace	Trace	.1	.2	26	2	34	1.0	38	[53]140	.14	.10	1.2	0
	Degermed, unenriched:																			
428	Dry form	1 cup	138	12	500	11	2	.2	.4	.9	108	8	137	1.5	166	[53]610	.19	.07	1.4	0
429	Cooked	1 cup	240	88	120	3	Trace	Trace	.1	.2	26	2	34	.5	38	[53]140	.05	.02	.2	0
	Crackers:[38]																			
430	Graham, plain, 2½-in square		14	6	55	1	1	.3	.5	.3	10	6	21	.5	55	0	.02	.08	.5	0
431	Rye wafers, whole-grain, 1⅞ by 3½ in.	2 wafers	13	6	45	2	Trace	—	—	—	10	7	50	.5	78	0	.04	.03	.2	0
432	Saltines, made with enriched flour.	4 crackers or 1 packet	11	4	50	1	1	.3	.5	.4	8	2	10	.5	13	0	.05	.05	.4	0
	Danish pastry (enriched flour), plain without fruit or nuts:[54]																			
433	Packaged ring, 12 oz	1 ring	340	22	1,435	25	80	24.3	31.7	16.5	155	170	371	6.1	381	1,050	.97	1.01	8.6	Trace
434	Round piece, about 4¼-in diam. by 1 in.	1 pastry	65	22	275	5	15	4.7	6.1	3.2	30	33	71	1.2	73	200	.18	.19	1.7	Trace
435	Ounce	1 oz	28	22	120	2	7	2.0	2.7	1.4	13	14	31	.5	32	90	.08	.08	.7	Trace
	Doughnuts, made with enriched flour:[38]																			
436	Cake type, plain, 2½-in diam., 1 in high.	1 doughnut	25	24	100	1	5	1.2	2.0	1.1	13	10	48	.4	23	20	.05	.05	.4	Trace
437	Yeast-leavened, glazed, 3¾-in diam., 1¼ in high.	1 doughnut	50	26	205	3	11	3.3	5.8	3.3	22	16	33	.6	34	25	.10	.10	.8	0
	Macaroni, enriched, cooked (cut lengths, elbows, shells):																			
438	Firm stage (hot)	1 cup	130	64	190	7	1	—	—	—	39	14	85	1.4	103	0	.23	.13	1.8	0
	Tender stage:																			
439	Cold macaroni	1 cup	105	73	115	4	Trace	—	—	—	24	8	53	.9	64	0	.15	.08	1.2	0
440	Hot macaroni	1 cup	140	73	155	5	1	—	—	—	32	11	70	1.3	85	0	.20	.11	1.5	0
	Macaroni (enriched) and cheese:																			
441	Canned[55]	1 cup	240	80	230	9	10	4.2	3.1	1.4	26	199	182	1.0	139	260	.12	.24	1.0	Trace
442	From home recipe (served hot)[56]	1 cup	200	58	430	17	22	8.9	8.8	2.9	40	362	322	1.8	240	860	.20	.40	1.8	Trace
	Muffins made with enriched flour:[38]																			
	From home recipe:																			
443	Blueberry, 2⅜-in diam., 1½ in high.	1 muffin	40	39	110	3	4	1.1	1.4	.7	17	34	53	.6	46	90	.09	.10	.7	Trace

[47] Excepting spongecake, vegetable shortening used for cake portion; butter, for icing. If butter or margarine used for cake portion, vitamin A values would be higher.

[48] Applies to product made with a sodium aluminum-sulfate type baking powder. With a low-sodium type baking powder containing potassium, value would be about twice the amount shown.

[49] Equal weights of flour, sugar, eggs, and vegetable shortening.

[50] Products are commercial unless otherwise specified.

[51] Made with enriched flour and vegetable shortening except for macaroons which do not contain flour or shortening.

[38] Made with vegetable shortening.

[52] Icing made with butter.

[53] Applies to yellow varieties; white varieties contain only a trace.

[54] Contains vegetable shortening and butter.

[55] Made with corn oil.

[56] Made with regular margarine.

Table A-1. (Continued)

Item No. (A)	Foods, approximate measures, units, and weight (edible part unless footnotes indicate otherwise) (B)			Water (C)	Food Energy (D)	Protein (E)	Fat (F)	Fatty Acids: Saturated (total) (G)	Fatty Acids: Unsaturated: Oleic (H)	Fatty Acids: Unsaturated: Linoleic (I)	Carbohydrate (J)	Calcium (K)	Phosphorus (L)	Iron (M)	Potassium (N)	Vitamin A Value (O)	Thiamin (P)	Riboflavin (Q)	Niacin (R)	Ascorbic Acid (S)
			Grams	*Percent*	*Calories*	*Grams*	*Grams*	*Grams*	*Grams*	*Grams*	*Grams*	*Milligrams*	*Milligrams*	*Milligrams*	*Milligrams*	*I.U.*	*Milligrams*	*Milligrams*	*Milligrams*	*Milligrams*
	GRAIN PRODUCTS (CONTINUED)																			
	Muffins: (cont.)																			
	From home recipe: (cont.)																			
444	Bran	1 muffin	40	35	105	3	4	1.2	1.4	.8	17	57	162	1.5	172	90	.07	.10	1.7	Trace
445	Corn (enriched degermed cornmeal and flour), 2⅜-in diam., 1½ in high.	1 muffin	40	33	125	3	4	1.2	1.6	.9	19	42	68	.7	54	[57]120	.10	.10	.7	Trace
446	Plain, 3-in diam., 1½ in high.	1 muffin	40	38	120	3	4	1.0	1.7	1.0	17	42	60	0.6	50	40	0.09	0.12	0.9	Trace
	From mix, egg, milk:																			
447	Corn, 2⅜-in diam., 1½ in high.[58]	1 muffin	40	30	130	3	4	1.2	1.7	.9	20	96	152	.6	44	[57]100	.08	.09	.7	Trace
448	Noodles (egg noodles), enriched, cooked.	1 cup	160	71	200	7	2	—	—	—	37	16	94	1.4	70	110	.22	.13	1.9	0
449	Noodles, chow mein, canned	1 cup	45	1	220	6	11	—	—	—	26	—	—	—	—	—	—	—	—	—
	Pancakes, (4-in diam.):[38]																			
450	Buckwheat, made from mix (with buckwheat and enriched flours), egg and milk added.	1 cake	27	58	55	2	2	.8	.9	.4	6	59	91	.4	66	60	.04	.05	.2	Trace
	Plain:																			
451	Made from home recipe using enriched flour.	1 cake	27	50	60	2	2	.5	.8	.5	9	27	38	.4	33	30	.06	.07	.5	Trace
452	Made from mix with enriched flour, egg and milk added.	1 cake	27	51	60	2	2	.7	.7	.3	9	58	70	.3	42	70	.04	.06	.2	Trace
	Pies, piecrust made with enriched flour, vegetable shortening (9-in diam.):																			
	Apple:																			
453	Whole	1 pie	945	48	2,420	21	105	27.0	44.5	25.2	360	76	208	6.6	756	280	1.06	.79	9.3	9
454	Sector, ⅐ of pie	1 sector	135	48	345	3	15	3.9	6.4	3.6	51	11	30	.9	108	40	.15	.11	1.3	2
	Banana cream:																			
455	Whole	1 pie	910	54	2,010	41	85	26.7	33.2	16.2	279	601	746	7.3	1,847	2,280	.77	1.51	7.0	9
456	Sector, ⅐ of pie	1 sector	130	54	285	6	12	3.8	4.7	2.3	40	86	107	1.0	264	330	.11	.22	1.0	1
	Blueberry:																			
457	Whole	1 pie	945	51	2,285	23	102	24.8	43.7	25.1	330	104	217	9.5	614	280	1.03	.80	10.0	28
458	Sector, ⅐ of pie	1 sector	135	51	325	3	15	3.5	6.2	3.6	47	15	31	1.4	88	40	.15	.11	1.4	4
	Cherry:																			
459	Whole	1 pie	945	47	2,465	25	107	28.2	45.0	25.3	363	132	236	6.6	992	4,160	1.09	.84	9.8	Trace
460	Sector, ⅐ of pie	1 sector	135	47	350	4	15	4.0	6.4	3.6	52	19	34	.9	142	590	.16	.12	1.4	Trace
	Custard:																			
461	Whole	1 pie	910	58	1,985	56	101	33.9	38.5	17.5	213	874	1,028	8.2	1,247	2,090	.79	1.92	5.6	0
462	Sector, ⅐ of pie	1 sector	130	58	285	8	14	4.8	5.5	2.5	30	125	147	1.2	178	300	.11	.27	.8	0
	Lemon meringue:																			
463	Whole	1 pie	840	47	2,140	31	86	26.1	33.8	16.4	317	118	412	6.7	420	1,430	.61	.84	5.2	25
464	Sector, ⅐ of pie	1 sector	120	47	305	4	12	3.7	4.8	2.3	45	17	59	1.0	60	200	.09	.12	.7	4
	Mince:																			
465	Whole	1 pie	945	43	2,560	24	109	28.0	45.9	25.2	389	265	359	13.3	1,682	20	.96	.86	9.8	9
466	Sector, ⅐ of pie	1 sector	135	43	365	3	16	4.0	6.6	3.6	56	38	51	1.9	240	Trace	.14	.12	1.4	1
	Peach:																			
467	Whole	1 pie	945	48	2,410	24	101	24.8	43.7	25.1	361	95	274	8.5	1,408	6,900	1.04	.97	14.0	28
468	Sector, ⅐ of pie	1 sector	135	48	345	3	14	3.5	6.2	3.6	52	14	39	1.2	201	990	.15	.14	2.0	4

	Pecan:																			
469	Whole	1 pie	825	20	3,450	42	189	27.8	101.0	44.2	423	388	850	25.6	1,015	1,320	1.80	.95	6.9	Trace
470	Sector, 1/7 of pie	1 sector	118	20	495	6	27	4.0	14.4	6.3	61	55	122	3.7	145	190	.26	.14	1.0	Trace
	Pumpkin:																			
471	Whole	1 pie	910	59	1,920	36	102	37.4	37.5	16.6	223	464	628	7.3	1,456	22,480	.78	1.27	7.0	Trace
472	Sector, 1/7 of pie	1 sector	130	59	275	5	15	5.4	5.4	2.4	32	66	90	1.0	208	3,210	.11	.18	1.0	Trace
473	Piecrust (home recipe) made with enriched flour and vegetable shortening, baked.	1 pie shell, 9-in diam.	180	15	900	11	60	14.8	26.1	14.9	79	25	90	3.1	89	0	.47	.40	5.0	0
474	Piecrust mix with enriched flour and vegetable shortening, 10-oz pkg. prepared and baked.	Piecrust for 2-crust pie, 9-in diam.	320	19	1,485	20	93	22.7	39.7	23.4	141	131	272	6.1	179	0	1.07	.79	9.9	0
475	Pizza (cheese) baked, 4¾-in sector; 1/8 of 12-in diam. pie.[19]	1 sector	60	45	145	6	4	1.7	1.5	0.6	22	86	89	1.1	67	230	0.16	0.18	1.6	4
	Popcorn, popped:																			
476	Plain, large kernel	1 cup	6	4	25	1	Trace	Trace	.1	.2	5	1	17	.2	—	—	—	.01	.1	0
477	With oil (coconut) and salt added, large kernel.	1 cup	9	3	40	1	2	1.5	.2	.2	5	1	19	.2	—	—	—	.01	.2	0
478	Sugar coated	1 cup	35	4	135	2	1	.5	.2	.4	30	2	47	.5	—	—	—	.02	.4	0
	Pretzels, made with enriched flour:																			
479	Dutch, twisted, 2¾ by 2⅝ in.	1 pretzel	16	5	60	2	1	—	—	—	12	4	21	.2	21	0	.05	.04	.7	0
480	Thin, twisted, 3¼ by 2¼ by ¼ in.	10 pretzels	60	5	235	6	3	—	—	—	46	13	79	.9	78	0	.20	.15	2.5	0
481	Stick, 2¼ in long	10 pretzels	3	5	10	Trace	Trace	—	—	—	2	1	4	Trace	4	0	.01	.01	.1	0
	Rice, white, enriched:																			
482	Instant, ready-to-serve, hot	1 cup	165	73	180	4	Trace	Trace	Trace	Trace	40	5	31	1.3	—	0	.21	([59])	1.7	0
	Long grain:																			
483	Raw	1 cup	185	12	670	12	1	.2	.2	.2	149	44	174	5.4	170	0	.81	.06	6.5	0
484	Cooked, served hot	1 cup	205	73	225	4	Trace	.1	.1	.1	50	21	57	1.8	57	0	.23	.02	2.1	0
	Parboiled:																			
485	Raw	1 cup	185	10	685	14	1	.2	.1	.2	150	111	370	5.4	278	0	.81	.07	6.5	0
486	Cooked, served hot	1 cup	175	73	185	4	Trace	.1	.1	.1	41	33	100	1.4	75	0	.19	.02	2.1	0
	Rolls, enriched:[38]																			
	Commercial:																			
487	Brown-and-serve (12 per 12-oz pkg.), browned.	1 roll	26	27	85	2	2	.4	.7	.5	14	20	23	.5	25	Trace	.10	.06	.9	Trace
488	Cloverleaf or pan, 2½-in diam., 2 in high.	1 roll	28	31	85	2	2	.4	.6	.4	15	21	24	.5	27	Trace	.11	.07	.9	Trace
489	Frankfurter and hamburger (8 per 11½-oz pkg.).	1 roll	40	31	120	3	2	.5	.8	.6	21	30	34	.8	38	Trace	.16	.10	1.3	Trace
	Hard, 3¾-in diam., 2 in high.	1 roll	50	25	155	5	2	.4	.6	.5	30	24	46	1.2	49	Trace	.20	.12	1.7	Trace
	Hoagie, or submarine, 11½ by 3 by 2½-in.	1 roll	135	31	390	12	4	.9	1.4	1,4	75	58	115	3.0	122	Trace	.54	.32	4.5	Trace
	From home recipe:																			
492	Cloverleaf, 2½-in diam., 2 in high.	1 roll	35	26	120	3	3	.8	1.1	.7	20	16	36	.7	41	30	.12	.12	1.2	Trace
	Spaghetti, enriched, cooked:																			
493	Firm stage, "al dente," served hot.	1 cup	130	64	190	7	1	—	—	—	39	14	85	1.4	103	0	.23	.13	1.8	0
494	Tender stage, served hot	1 cup	140	73	155	5	1	—	—	—	32	11	70	1.3	85	0	.20	.11	1.5	0
	Spaghetti (enriched) in tomato sauce with cheese																			
495	From home recipe	1 cup	250	77	260	9	9	2.0	5.4	.7	37	80	135	2.3	408	1,080	.25	.18	2.3	13
496	Canned	1 cup	250	80	190	6	2	.5	.3	.4	39	40	88	2.8	303	930	.35	.28	4.5	10

[57] Applies to product made with yellow cornmeal.
[58] Made with enriched degermed cornmeal and enriched flour.
[59] Product may or may not be enriched with riboflavin. Consult the label.

Table A-1. (Continued)

Item No. (A)	Foods, approximate measures, units, and weight (edible part unless footnotes indicate otherwise) (B)			Water (C)	Food Energy (D)	Protein (E)	Fat (F)	Fatty Acids: Saturated (total) (G)	Fatty Acids: Unsaturated: Oleic (H)	Fatty Acids: Unsaturated: Linoleic (I)	Carbohydrate (J)	Calcium (K)	Phosphorus (L)	Iron (M)	Potassium (N)	Vitamin A Value (O)	Thiamin (P)	Riboflavin (Q)	Niacin (R)	Ascorbic Acid (S)
			Grams	Per-cent	Cal-ories	Grams	Grams	Grams	Grams	Grams	Grams	Milli-grams	Milli-grams	Milli-grams	Milli-grams	I.U.	Milli-grams	Milli-grams	Milli-grams	Milli-grams
	GRAIN PRODUCTS (CONTINUED)																			
	Spaghetti (enriched) with meat balls and tomato sauce:																			
497	From home recipe	1 cup	248	70	330	19	12	3.3	6.3	.9	39	124	236	3.7	665	1,590	.25	.30	4.0	22
498	Canned	1 cup	250	78	260	12	10	2.2	3.3	3.9	29	53	113	3.3	245	1,000	.15	.18	2.3	5
499	Toaster pastries	1 pastry	50	12	200	3	6	—	—	—	36	[60]54	[60]67	1.9	[60]74	500	.16	.17	2.1	([60])
	Waffles, made with enriched flour, 7-in diam.:[38]																			
500	From home recipe	1 waffle	75	41	210	7	7	2.3	2.8	1.4	28	85	130	1.3	109	250	.17	.23	1.4	Trace
501	From mix, egg and milk added	1 waffle	75	42	205	7	8	2.8	2.9	1.2	27	179	257	1.0	146	170	.14	.22	.9	Trace
	Wheat flours:																			
	All-purpose or family flour, enriched:																			
502	Sifted, spooned	1 cup	115	12	420	12	1	0.2	0.1	0.5	88	18	100	3.3	109	0	0.74	0.46	6.1	0
503	Unsifted, spooned	1 cup	125	12	455	13	1	.2	.1	.5	95	20	109	3.6	119	0	.80	.50	6.6	0
504	Cake or pastry flour, enriched, sifted, spooned.	1 cup	96	12	350	7	1	.1	.1	.3	76	16	70	2.8	91	0	.61	.38	5.1	0
505	Self-rising, enriched, unsifted, spooned.	1 cup	125	12	440	12	1	.2	.1	.5	93	331	583	3.6	—	0	.80	.50	6.6	0
506	Whole-wheat, from hard wheats, stirred.	1 cup	120	12	400	16	2	.4	.2	1.0	85	49	446	4.0	444	0	.66	.14	5.2	0
	LEGUMES (DRY), NUTS, SEEDS; RELATED PRODUCTS																			
	Almonds, shelled:																			
507	Chopped (about 130 almonds)	1 cup	130	5	775	24	70	5.6	47.7	12.8	25	304	655	6.1	1,005	0	.31	1.20	4.6	Trace
508	Slivered, not pressed down (about 115 almonds).	1 cup	115	5	690	21	62	5.0	42.2	11.3	22	269	580	5.4	889	0	.28	1.06	4.0	Trace
	Beans, dry:																			
	Common varieties as Great Northern, navy, and others:																			
	Cooked, drained:																			
509	Great Northern	1 cup	180	69	210	14	1	—	—	—	38	90	266	4.9	749	0	.25	.13	1.3	0
510	Pea (navy)	1 cup	190	69	225	15	1	—	—	—	40	95	281	5.1	790	0	.27	.13	1.3	0
	Canned, solids and liquid:																			
	White with—																			
511	Frankfurters (sliced)	1 cup	255	71	365	19	18	—	—	—	32	94	303	4.8	668	330	.18	.15	3.3	Trace
512	Pork and tomato sauce	1 cup	255	71	310	16	7	2.4	2.8	.6	48	138	235	4.6	536	330	.20	.08	1.5	5
513	Pork and sweet sauce	1 cup	255	66	385	16	12	4.3	5.0	1.1	54	161	291	5.9	—	—	.15	.10	1.3	—
514	Red kidney	1 cup	255	76	230	15	1	—	—	—	42	74	278	4.6	673	10	.13	.10	1.5	—
515	Lima, cooked, drained	1 cup	190	64	260	16	1	—	—	—	49	55	293	5.9	1,163	—	.25	.11	1.3	—
516	Blackeye peas, dry, cooked (with residual cooking liquid).	1 cup	250	80	190	13	1	—	—	—	35	43	238	3.3	573	30	.40	.10	1.0	—
517	Brazil nuts, shelled (6–8 large kernels).	1 oz	28	5	185	4	19	4.8	6.2	7.1	3	53	196	1.0	203	Trace	.27	.03	.5	—
518	Cashew nuts, roasted in oil	1 cup	140	5	785	24	64	12.9	36.8	10.2	41	53	522	5.3	650	140	.60	.35	2.5	—

No.	Food	Measure																		
	Coconut meat, fresh:																			
519	Piece, about 2 by 2 by ½ in	1 piece	45	51	155	2	16	14.0	.9	.3	4	6	43	.8	115	0	.02	.01	.2	1
520	Shredded or grated, not pressed down.	1 cup	80	51	275	3	28	24.8	1.6	.5	8	10	76	1.4	205	0	.04	.02	.4	2
521	Filberts (hazelnuts), chopped (about 80 kernels).	1 cup	115	6	730	14	72	5.1	55.2	7.3	19	240	388	3.9	810	—	.53	—	1.0	Trace
522	Lentils, whole, cooked	1 cup	200	72	210	16	Trace	—	—	—	39	50	238	4.2	498	40	.14	.12	1.2	0
523	Peanuts, roasted in oil, salted (whole, halves, chopped).	1 cup	144	2	840	37	72	13.7	33.0	20.7	27	107	577	3.0	971	—	.46	.19	24.8	0
524	Peanut butter	1 tbsp	16	2	95	4	8	1.5	3.7	2.3	3	9	61	.3	100	—	.02	.02	2.4	0
525	Peas, split, dry, cooked	1 cup	200	70	230	16	1	—	—	—	42	22	178	3.4	592	80	.30	.18	1.8	—
526	Pecans, chopped or pieces (about 120 large halves).	1 cup	118	3	810	11	84	7.2	50.5	20.0	17	86	341	2.8	712	150	1.01	.15	1.1	2
527	Pumpkin and squash kernels, dry, hulled.	1 cup	140	4	775	41	65	11.8	23.5	27.5	21	71	1,602	15.7	1,386	100	.34	.27	3.4	—
528	Sunflower seeds, dry, hulled	1 cup	145	5	810	35	69	8.2	13.7	43.2	29	174	1,214	10.3	1,334	70	2.84	.33	7.8	—
	Walnuts:																			
	Black:																			
529	Chopped or broken kernels	1 cup	125	3	785	26	74	6.3	13.3	45.7	19	Trace	713	7.5	575	380	.28	.14	.9	—
530	Ground (finely)	1 cup	80	3	500	16	47	4.0	8.5	29.2	12	Trace	456	4.8	368	240	.18	.09	.6	—
531	Persian or English, chopped (about 60 halves).	1 cup	120	4	780	18	77	8.4	11.8	42.2	19	119	456	3.7	540	40	.40	.16	1.1	2
	SUGARS AND SWEETS																			
	Cake icings:																			
	Boiled, white:																			
532	Plain	1 cup	94	18	295	1	0	0	0	0	75	2	2	Trace	17	0	Trace	0.03	Trace	0
533	With coconut	1 cup	166	15	605	3	13	11.0	.9	Trace	124	10	50	0.8	277	0	0.02	.07	0.3	0
	Uncooked:																			
534	Chocolate made with milk and butter.	1 cup	275	14	1,035	9	38	23.4	11.7	1.0	185	165	305	3.3	536	580	.06	.28	.6	1
535	Creamy fudge from mix and water.	1 cup	245	15	830	7	16	5.1	6.7	3.1	183	96	218	2.7	238	Trace	.05	.20	.7	Trace
536	White	1 cup	319	11	1,200	2	21	12.7	5.1	.5	260	48	38	Trace	57	860	Trace	.06	Trace	Trace
	Candy:																			
537	Caramels, plain or chocolate	1 oz	28	8	115	1	3	1.6	1.1	.1	22	42	35	.4	54	Trace	.01	.05	.1	Trace
	Chocolate:																			
538	Milk, plain	1 oz	28	1	145	2	9	5.5	3.0	.3	16	65	65	.3	109	80	.02	.10	.1	Trace
539	Semisweet, small pieces (60 per oz).	1 cup or 6-oz pkg	170	1	860	7	61	36.2	19.8	1.7	97	51	255	4.4	553	30	.02	.14	.9	0
540	Chocolate-covered peanuts	1 oz	28	1	160	5	12	4.0	4.7	2.1	11	33	84	.4	143	Trace	.10	.05	2.1	Trace
541	Fondant, uncoated (mints, candy corn, other).	1 oz	28	8	105	Trace	1	.1	.3	.1	25	4	2	.3	1	0	Trace	Trace	Trace	0
542	Fudge, chocolate, plain	1 oz	28	8	115	1	3	1.3	1.4	.6	21	22	24	.3	42	Trace	.01	.03	.1	Trace
543	Gum drops	1 oz	28	12	100	Trace	Trace	—	—	—	25	2	Trace	.1	1	0	0	Trace	Trace	0
544	Hard	1 oz	28	1	110	0	Trace	—	—	—	28	6	2	.5	1	0	0	0	0	0
545	Marshmallows	1 oz	28	17	90	1	Trace	—	—	—	23	5	2	.5	2	0	0	Trace	Trace	0
	Chocolate-flavored beverage powders (about 4 heaping tsp per oz):																			
546	With nonfat dry milk	1 oz	28	2	100	5	1	.5	.3	Trace	20	167	155	.5	227	10	.04	.21	.2	1
547	Without milk	1 oz	28	1	100	1	1	.4	.2	Trace	25	9	48	.6	142	—	.01	.03	.1	0
548	Honey, strained or extracted	1 tbsp	21	17	65	Trace	0	0	0	0	17	1	1	.1	11	0	Trace	.01	.1	Trace
549	Jams and preserves	1 tbsp	20	29	55	Trace	Trace	—	—	—	14	4	2	.2	18	Trace	Trace	.01	Trace	Trace
550		1 packet	14	29	40	Trace	Trace	—	—	—	10	3	1	.1	12	Trace	Trace	Trace	Trace	Trace
551	Jellies	1 tbsp	18	29	50	Trace	Trace	—	—	—	13	4	1	.3	14	Trace	Trace	.01	Trace	1
552		1 packet	14	29	40	Trace	Trace	—	—	—	10	3	1	.2	11	Trace	Trace	Trace	Trace	1
	Sirups:																			
	Chocolate-flavored sirup or topping:																			
553	Thin type	1 fl oz or 2 tbsp	38	32	90	1	1	.5	.3	Trace	24	6	35	.6	106	Trace	.01	.03	.2	0
554	Fudge type	1 fl oz or 2 tbsp	38	25	125	2	5	3.1	1.6	.1	20	48	60	.5	107	60	.02	.08	.2	Trace
	Molasses, cane:																			
555	Light (first extraction)	1 tbsp	20	24	50	—	—	—	—	—	13	33	9	.9	183	—	.01	.01	Trace	—

[60] Value varies with the brand. Consult the label.

Table A-1. (Continued)

Item No. (A)	Foods, approximate measures, units, and weight (edible part unless footnotes indicate otherwise) (B)			Water (C)	Food Energy (D)	Protein (E)	Fat (F)	Fatty Acids: Saturated (total) (G)	Fatty Acids: Unsaturated: Oleic (H)	Fatty Acids: Unsaturated: Linoleic (I)	Carbohydrate (J)	Calcium (K)	Phosphorus (L)	Iron (M)	Potassium (N)	Vitamin A Value (O)	Thiamin (P)	Riboflavin (Q)	Niacin (R)	Ascorbic Acid (S)
			Grams	Percent	Calories	Grams	Grams	Grams	Grams	Grams	Grams	Milligrams	Milligrams	Milligrams	Milligrams	I.U.	Milligrams	Milligrams	Milligrams	Milligrams
	SUGAR AND SWEETS (CONTINUED)																			
	Sirups: (cont.)																			
	Molasses, cane: (cont.)																			
556	Blackstrap (third extraction)	1 tbsp	20	24	45	—	—	—	—	—	11	137	17	3.2	585	—	.02	.04	.4	—
557	Sorghum	1 tbsp	21	23	55	—	—	—	—	—	14	35	5	2.6	—	—	—	.02	Trace	—
558	Table blends, chiefly corn, light and dark.	1 tbsp	21	24	60	0	0	0	0	0	15	9	3	.8	1	0	0	0	0	0
	Sugars:																			
559	Brown, pressed down	1 cup	220	2	820	0	0	0	0	0	212	187	42	7.5	757	0	.02	.07	.4	0
	White:																			
560	Granulated	1 cup	200	1	770	0	0	0	0	0	199	0	0	.2	6	0	0	0	0	0
561		1 tbsp	12	1	45	0	0	0	0	0	12	0	0	Trace	Trace	0	0	0	0	0
562		1 packet	6	1	23	0	0	0	0	0	6	0	0	Trace	Trace	0	0	0	0	0
563	Powdered, sifted, spooned into cup.	1 cup	100	1	385	0	0	0	0	0	100	0	0	.1	3	0	0	0	0	0
	VEGETABLE AND VEGETABLE PRODUCTS																			
	Asparagus, green:																			
	Cooked, drained:																			
	Cuts and tips, 1½- to 2-in lengths:																			
564	From raw	1 cup	145	94	30	3	Trace	—	—	—	5	30	73	0.9	265	1,310	0.23	0.26	2.0	38
565	From frozen	1 cup	180	93	40	6	Trace	—	—	—	6	40	115	2.2	396	1,530	.25	.23	1.8	41
	Spears, ½-in diam. at base:																			
566	From raw	4 spears	60	94	10	1	Trace	—	—	—	2	13	30	.4	110	540	.10	.11	.8	16
567	From frozen	4 spears	60	92	15	2	Trace	—	—	—	2	13	40	.7	143	470	.10	.08	.7	16
568	Canned, spears, ½-in diam. at base.	4 spears	80	93	15	2	Trace	—	—	—	3	15	42	1.5	133	640	.05	.08	.6	12
	Beans:																			
	Lima, immature seeds, frozen, cooked, drained:																			
569	Thick-seeded types (Fordhooks)	1 cup	170	74	170	10	Trace	—	—	—	32	34	153	2.9	724	390	.12	.09	1.7	29
570	Thin-seeded types (baby limas)	1 cup	180	69	210	13	Trace	—	—	—	40	63	227	4.7	709	400	.16	.09	2.2	22
	Snap:																			
	Green:																			
	Cooked, drained:																			
571	From raw (cuts and French style).	1 cup	125	92	30	2	Trace	—	—	—	7	63	46	.8	189	680	.09	.11	.6	15
	From frozen:																			
572	Cuts	1 cup	135	92	35	2	Trace	—	—	—	8	54	43	.9	205	780	.09	.12	.5	7
573	French style	1 cup	130	92	35	2	Trace	—	—	—	8	49	39	1.2	177	690	.08	.10	.4	9
574	Canned, drained solids (cuts).	1 cup	135	92	30	2	Trace	—	—	—	7	61	34	2.0	128	630	.04	.07	.4	5
	Yellow or wax:																			
	Cooked, drained:																			
575	From raw (cuts and French style).	1 cup	125	93	30	2	Trace	—	—	—	6	63	46	.8	189	290	.09	.11	.6	16
576	From frozen (cuts)	1 cup	135	92	35	2	Trace	—	—	—	8	47	42	.9	221	140	.09	.11	.5	8
577	Canned, drained solids (cuts).	1 cup	135	92	30	2	Trace	—	—	—	7	61	34	2.0	128	140	.04	.07	.4	7

	Beans, mature. See Beans, dry (items 509–515) and Blackeye peas, dry (item 516).																			
	Bean sprouts (mung):																			
578	Raw	1 cup	105	89	35	4	Trace	—	—	—	7	20	67	1.4	234	20	.14	.14	.8	20
579	Cooked, drained	1 cup	125	91	35	4	Trace	—	—	—	7	21	60	1.1	195	30	.11	.13	.9	8
	Beets:																			
	Cooked, drained, peeled:																			
580	Whole beets, 2-in diam.	2 beets	100	91	30	1	Trace	—	—	—	7	14	23	.5	208	20	.03	.04	.3	6
581	Diced or sliced	1 cup	170	91	55	2	Trace	—	—	—	12	24	39	.9	354	30	.05	.07	.5	10
	Canned, drained solids:																			
582	Whole beets, small	1 cup	160	89	60	2	Trace	—	—	—	14	30	29	1.1	267	30	.02	.05	.2	5
583	Diced or sliced	1 cup	170	89	65	2	Trace	—	—	—	15	32	31	1.2	284	30	.02	.05	.2	5
584	Beet greens, leaves and stems, cooked, drained.	1 cup	145	94	25	2	Trace	—	—	—	5	144	36	2.8	481	7,400	.10	.22	.4	22
	Blackeye peas, immature seeds, cooked and drained:																			
585	From raw	1 cup	165	72	180	13	1	—	—	—	30	40	241	3.5	625	580	.50	.18	2.3	28
586	From frozen	1 cup	170	66	220	15	1	—	—	—	40	43	286	4.8	573	290	.68	.19	2.4	15
	Broccoli, cooked, drained:																			
	From raw:																			
587	Stalk, medium size	1 stalk	180	91	45	6	1	—	—	—	8	158	112	1.4	481	4,500	.16	.36	1.4	162
588	Stalks, cut into ½-in pieces	1 cup	155	91	40	5	Trace	—	—	—	7	136	96	1.2	414	3,880	.14	.31	1.2	140
	From frozen:																			
589	Stalk, 4½ to 5 in long	1 stalk	30	91	10	1	Trace	—	—	—	1	12	17	.2	66	570	.02	.03	.2	22
590	Chopped	1 cup	185	92	50	5	1	—	—	—	9	100	104	1.3	392	4,810	.11	.22	.9	105
	Brussels sprouts, cooked, drained:																			
591	From raw, 7–8 sprouts (1¼ to 1½-in diam.).	1 cup	155	88	55	7	1	—	—	—	10	50	112	1.7	423	810	.12	.22	1.2	135
592	From frozen	1 cup	155	89	50	5	Trace	—	—	—	10	33	95	1.2	457	880	.12	.16	.9	126
	Cabbage:																			
	Common varieties:																			
	Raw:																			
593	Coarsely shredded or sliced	1 cup	70	92	15	1	Trace	—	—	—	4	34	20	0.3	163	90	0.04	0.04	0.02	33
594	Finely shredded or chopped	1 cup	90	92	20	1	Trace	—	—	—	5	44	26	.4	210	120	.05	.05	.3	42
595	Cooked, drained	1 cup	145	94	30	2	Trace	—	—	—	6	64	29	.4	236	190	.06	.06	.4	48
596	Red, raw, coarsely shredded	1 cup	70	90	20	1	Trace	—	—	—	5	29	25	.6	188	30	.06	.04	.3	43
597	Savoy, raw, coarsely shredded or sliced.	1 cup	70	92	15	2	Trace	—	—	—	3	47	38	.6	188	140	.04	.06	.2	39
598	Cabbage, celery (also called pe-tsai or wongbok), raw, 1-in pieces.	1 cup	75	95	10	1	Trace	—	—	—	2	32	30	.5	190	110	.04	.03	.5	19
599	Cabbage, white mustard (also called bokchoy or pakchoy), cooked, drained.	1 cup	170	95	25	2	Trace	—	—	—	4	252	56	1.0	364	5,270	.07	.14	1.2	26
	Carrots:																			
	Raw, without crowns and tips, scraped:																			
600	Whole, 7½ by 1⅛ in, or strips, 2½ to 3 in long.	1 carrot or 18 strips	72	88	30	1	Trace	—	—	—	7	27	26	.5	246	7,930	.04	.04	.4	6
601	Grated	1 cup	110	88	45	1	Trace	—	—	—	11	41	40	.8	375	12,100	.07	.06	.7	9
602	Cooked (crosswise cuts), drained	1 cup	155	91	50	1	Trace	—	—	—	11	51	48	.9	344	16,280	.08	.08	.8	9
	Canned:																			
603	Sliced, drained solids	1 cup	155	91	45	1	Trace	—	—	—	10	47	34	1.1	186	23,250	.03	.05	.6	3
604	Strained or junior (baby food)	1 oz (1¾ to 2 tbsp)	28	92	10	Trace	Trace	—	—	—	2	7	6	.1	51	3,690	.01	.01	.1	1
	Cauliflower:																			
605	Raw, chopped	1 cup	115	91	31	3	Trace	—	—	—	6	29	64	1.3	339	70	.13	.12	.8	90
	Cooked, drained:																			
606	From raw (flower buds)	1 cup	125	93	30	3	Trace	—	—	—	5	26	53	.9	258	80	.11	.10	.8	69
607	From frozen (flowerets)	1 cup	180	94	30	3	Trace	—	—	—	6	31	68	.9	373	50	.07	.09	.7	74

Table A-1. (Continued)

Item No. (A)	Foods, approximate measures, units, and weight (edible part unless footnotes indicate otherwise) (B)			Water (C)	Food Energy (D)	Protein (E)	Fat (F)	Fatty Acids: Saturated (total) (G)	Unsaturated: Oleic (H)	Unsaturated: Linoleic (I)	Carbohydrate (J)	Calcium (K)	Phosphorus (L)	Iron (M)	Potassium (N)	Vitamin A Value (O)	Thiamin (P)	Riboflavin (Q)	Niacin (R)	Ascorbic Acid (S)
			Grams	Percent	Calories	Grams	Grams	Grams	Grams	Grams	Grams	Milligrams	Milligrams	Milligrams	Milligrams	I.U.	Milligrams	Milligrams	Milligrams	Milligrams
	VEGETABLE AND VEGETABLE PRODUCTS (CONTINUED)																			
	Celery, Pascal type, raw:																			
608	Stalk, large outer, 8 by 1½ in, at root end.	1 stalk	40	94	5	Trace	Trace	—	—	—	2	16	11	.1	136	110	.01	.01	.1	4
609	Pieces, diced	1 cup	120	94	20	1	Trace	—	—	—	5	47	34	.4	409	320	.04	.04	.4	11
	Collards, cooked, drained:																			
610	From raw (leaves without stems)	1 cup	190	90	65	7	1	—	—	—	10	357	99	1.5	498	14,820	.21	.38	2.3	144
611	From frozen (chopped)	1 cup	170	90	50	5	1	—	—	—	10	299	87	1.7	401	11,560	.10	.24	1.0	56
	Corn, sweet:																			
	Cooked, drained:																			
612	From raw, ear 5 by 1¾ in	1 ear[61]	140	74	70	2	1	—	—	—	16	2	69	.5	151	[62]310	.09	.08	1.1	7
	From frozen:																			
613	Ear, 5 in long	1 ear[61]	229	73	120	4	1	—	—	—	27	4	121	1.0	291	[62]440	.18	.10	2.1	9
614	Kernels	1 cup	165	77	130	5	1	—	—	—	31	5	120	1.3	304	[62]580	.15	.10	2.5	8
	Canned:																			
615	Cream style	1 cup	256	76	210	5	2	—	—	—	51	8	143	1.5	248	[62]840	.08	.13	2.6	13
	Whole kernel:																			
616	Vacuum pack	1 cup	210	76	175	5	1	—	—	—	43	6	153	1.1	204	[62]740	.06	.13	2.3	11
617	Wet pack, drained solids	1 cup	165	76	140	4	1	—	—	—	33	8	81	.8	160	[62]580	.05	.08	1.5	7
	Cowpeas. See Blackeye peas. (Items 585–586).																			
	Cucumber slices, ⅛ in thick (large, 2⅛-in diam.; small, 1¾-in diam.):																			
618	With peel	6 large or 8 small slices	28	95	5	Trace	Trace	—	—	—	1	7	8	.3	45	70	.01	.01	.1	3
619	Without peel	6½ large or 9 small pieces.	28	96	5	Trace	Trace	—	—	—	1	5	5	0.1	45	Trace	0.01	0.01	0.1	3
620	Dandelion greens, cooked, drained	1 cup	105	90	35	2	1	—	—	—	7	147	44	1.9	244	12,290	.14	.17	—	19
621	Endive, curly (including escarole), raw, small pieces.	1 cup	50	93	10	1	Trace	—	—	—	2	41	27	.9	147	1,650	.04	.07	.3	5
	Kale, cooked, drained:																			
622	From raw (leaves without stems and midribs).	1 cup	110	88	45	5	1	—	—	—	7	206	64	1.8	243	9,130	.11	.20	1.8	102
623	From frozen (leaf style)	1 cup	130	91	40	4	1	—	—	—	7	157	62	1.3	251	10,660	.08	.20	.9	49
	Lettuce, raw:																			
	Butterhead, as Boston types:																			
624	Head, 5-in diam	1 head[63]	220	95	25	2	Trace	—	—	—	4	57	42	3.3	430	1,580	.10	.10	.5	13
625	Leaves	1 outer or 2 inner or 3 heart leaves.	15	95	Trace	Trace	Trace	—	—	—	Trace	5	4	.3	40	150	.01	.01	Trace	1
	Crisphead, as Iceberg:																			
626	Head, 6-in diam	1 head[64]	567	96	70	5	1	—	—	—	16	108	118	2.7	943	1,780	.32	.32	1.6	32
627	Wedge, ¼ of head	1 wedge	135	96	20	1	Trace	—	—	—	4	27	30	.7	236	450	.08	.08	.4	8
628	Pieces, chopped or shredded	1 cup	55	96	5	Trace	Trace	—	—	—	2	11	12	.3	96	180	.03	.03	.2	3
629	Looseleaf (bunching varieties including romaine or cos), chopped or shredded pieces.	1 cup	55	94	10	1	Trace	—	—	—	2	37	14	.8	145	1,050	.03	.04	.2	10
630	Mushrooms, raw, sliced or chopped	1 cup	70	90	20	2	Trace	—	—	—	3	4	81	.6	290	Trace	.07	.32	2.9	2

631	Mustard greens, without stems and midribs, cooked, drained.	1 cup	140	93	30	3	1	—	—	—	6	193	45	2.5	308	8,120	.11	.20	.8	67
632	Okra pods, 3 by 5/8 in, cooked	10 pods	106	91	30	2	Trace	—	—	—	6	98	43	.5	184	520	.14	.19	1.0	21
	Onions:																			
	Mature:																			
	Raw:																			
633	Chopped	1 cup	170	89	65	3	Trace	—	—	—	15	46	61	.9	267	[65]Trace	.05	.07	.3	17
634	Sliced	1 cup	115	89	45	2	Trace	—	—	—	10	31	41	.6	181	[65]Trace	.03	.05	.2	12
635	Cooked (whole or sliced), drained.	1 cup	210	92	60	3	Trace	—	—	—	14	50	61	.8	231	[65]Trace	.06	.06	.4	15
636	Young green, bulb (3/8 in diam.) and white portion of top.	6 onions	30	88	15	Trace	Trace	—	—	—	3	12	12	.2	69	Trace	.02	.01	.1	8
637	Parsley, raw, chopped	1 tbsp	4	85	Trace	Trace	Trace	—	—	—	Trace	7	2	.2	25	300	Trace	.01	Trace	6
638	Parsnips, cooked (diced or 2-in lengths).	1 cup	155	82	100	2	1	—	—	—	23	70	96	.9	587	50	.11	.12	.2	16
	Peas, green:																			
	Canned:																			
639	Whole, drained solids	1 cup	170	77	150	8	1	—	—	—	29	44	129	3.2	163	1,170	.15	.10	1.4	14
640	Strained (baby food)	1 oz (1 3/4 to 2 tbsp)	28	86	15	1	Trace	—	—	—	3	3	18	.3	28	140	.02	.03	.3	3
641	Frozen, cooked, drained	1 cup	160	82	110	8	Trace	—	—	—	19	30	138	3.0	216	960	.43	.14	2.7	21
642	Peppers, hot, red, without seeds, dried (ground chili powder, added seasonings).	1 tsp	2	9	5	Trace	Trace	—	—	—	1	5	4	.3	20	1,300	Trace	.02	.2	Trace
	Peppers, sweet (about 5 per lb, whole), stems and seeds removed:																			
643	Raw	1 pod	74	93	15	1	Trace	—	—	—	4	7	16	.5	157	310	.06	.06	.4	94
644	Cooked, boiled, drained	1 pod	73	95	15	1	Trace	—	—	—	3	7	12	.4	109	310	.05	.05	.4	70
	Potatoes, cooked:																			
645	Baked, peeled after baking (about 2 per lb, raw).	1 potato	156	75	145	4	Trace	—	—	—	33	14	101	1.1	782	Trace	.15	.07	2.7	31
	Boiled (about 3 per lb, raw):																			
646	Peeled after boiling	1 potato	137	80	105	3	Trace	—	—	—	23	10	72	.8	556	Trace	.12	.05	2.0	22
647	Peeled before boiling	1 potato	135	83	90	3	Trace	—	—	—	20	8	57	.7	385	Trace	.12	.05	1.6	22
	French-fried, strip, 2 to 3 1/2 in long:																			
648	Prepared from raw	10 strips	50	45	135	2	7	1.7	1.2	3.3	18	8	56	.7	427	Trace	.07	.04	1.6	11
649	Frozen, oven heated	10 strips	50	53	110	2	4	1.1	.8	2.1	17	5	43	.9	326	Trace	.07	.01	1.3	11
650	Hashed brown, prepared from frozen.	1 cup	155	56	345	3	18	4.6	3.2	9.0	45	28	78	1.9	439	Trace	.11	.03	1.6	12
	Mashed, prepared from—																			
	Raw:																			
651	Milk added	1 cup	210	83	135	4	2	.7	.4	Trace	27	50	103	.8	548	40	.17	.11	2.1	21
652	Milk and butter added	1 cup	210	80	195	4	9	5.6	2.3	0.2	26	50	101	0.8	525	360	0.17	0.11	2.1	19
653	Dehydrated flakes (without milk), water, milk, butter, and salt added.	1 cup	210	79	195	4	7	3.6	2.1	.2	30	65	99	.6	601	270	.08	.08	1.9	11
654	Potato chips, 1 3/4 by 2 1/2 in oval cross section.	10 chips	20	2	115	1	8	2.1	1.4	4.0	10	8	28	.4	226	Trace	.04	.01	1.0	3
655	Potato salad, made with cooked salad dressing.	1 cup	250	76	250	7	7	2.0	2.7	1.3	41	80	160	1.5	798	350	.20	.18	2.8	28
656	Pumpkin, canned	1 cup	245	90	80	2	1	—	—	—	19	61	64	1.0	588	15,680	.07	.12	1.5	12
657	Radishes, raw (prepackaged) stem ends, rootlets cut off.	4 radishes	18	95	5	Trace	Trace	—	—	—	1	5	6	.2	58	Trace	.01	.01	.1	5
658	Sauerkraut, canned, solids and liquid.	1 cup	235	93	40	2	Trace	—	—	—	9	85	42	1.2	329	120	.07	.09	.5	33
	Southern peas. See Blackeye peas (items 585–586).																			
	Spinach:																			
659	Raw, chopped	1 cup	55	91	15	2	Trace	—	—	—	2	51	28	1.7	259	4,460	.06	.11	.3	28
	Cooked, drained:																			
660	From raw	1 cup	180	92	40	5	1	—	—	—	6	167	68	4.0	583	14,580	.13	.25	.9	50

[61] Weight includes cob. Without cob, weight is 77g for item 612, 126 g for item 613.
[62] Based on yellow varieties. For white varieties, value is trace.
[63] Weight includes refuse of outer leaves and core. Without these parts, weight is 163 g.

[64] Weight includes core. Without core, weight is 539 g.
[65] Value based on white-fleshed varieties. For yellow-fleshed varieties, value in International Units (I.U.) is 70 for item 633, 50 for item 634, and 80 for item 635.

Table A-1. (Continued)

Item No. (A)	Foods, approximate measures, units, and weight (edible part unless footnotes indicate otherwise) (B)			Water (C)	Food Energy (D)	Protein (E)	Fat (F)	Fatty Acids: Saturated (total) (G)	Fatty Acids: Unsaturated: Oleic (H)	Fatty Acids: Unsaturated: Linoleic (I)	Carbohydrate (J)	Calcium (K)	Phosphorus (L)	Iron (M)	Potassium (N)	Vitamin A Value (O)	Thiamin (P)	Riboflavin (Q)	Niacin (R)	Ascorbic Acid (S)
			Grams	Percent	Calories	Grams	Grams	Grams	Grams	Grams	Grams	Milligrams	Milligrams	Milligrams	Milligrams	I.U.	Milligrams	Milligrams	Milligrams	Milligrams
	VEGETABLE AND VEGETABLE PRODUCTS (CONTINUED)																			
	Spinach: (cont.)																			
	Cooked, drained: (cont.)																			
	From frozen:																			
661	Chopped	1 cup	205	92	45	6	1	—	—	—	8	232	90	4.3	683	16,200	.14	.31	.8	39
662	Leaf	1 cup	190	92	45	6	1	—	—	—	7	200	84	4.8	688	15,390	.15	.27	1.0	53
663	Canned, drained solids	1 cup	205	91	50	6	1	—	—	—	7	242	53	5.3	513	16,400	.04	.25	.6	29
	Squash, cooked:																			
664	Summer (all varieties), diced, drained.	1 cup	210	96	30	2	Trace	—	—	—	7	53	53	.8	296	820	.11	.17	1.7	21
655	Winter (all varieties), baked, mashed.	1 cup	205	81	130	4	1	—	—	—	32	57	98	1.6	945	8,610	.10	.27	1.4	27
	Sweetpotatoes:																			
	Cooked (raw, 5 by 2 in; about 2½ per lb):																			
666	Baked in skin, peeled	1 potato	114	64	160	2	1	—	—	—	37	46	66	1.0	342	9,230	.10	.08	.8	25
667	Boiled in skin, peeled	1 potato	151	71	170	3	1	—	—	—	40	48	71	1.1	367	11,940	.14	.09	.9	26
668	Candied, 2½ by 2-in piece	1 piece	105	60	175	1	3	2.0	.8	.1	36	39	45	.9	200	6,620	.06	.04	.4	11
	Canned:																			
669	Solid pack (mashed)	1 cup	255	72	275	5	1	—	—	—	63	64	105	2.0	510	19,890	.13	.10	1.5	36
670	Vacuum pack, piece 2¾ by 1 in.	1 piece	40	72	45	1	Trace	—	—	—	10	10	16	.3	80	3,120	.02	.02	.2	6
	Tomatoes:																			
671	Raw, 2⅗-in diam. (3 per 12 oz pkg.).	1 tomato[66]	135	94	25	1	Trace	—	—	—	6	16	33	.6	300	1,110	.07	.05	.9	[67]28
672	Canned, solids and liquid	1 cup	241	94	50	2	Trace	—	—	—	10	[68]14	46	1.2	523	2,170	.12	.07	1.7	41
673	Tomato catsup	1 cup	273	69	290	5	1	—	—	—	69	60	137	2.2	991	3,820	.25	.19	4.4	41
674		1 tbsp	15	69	15	Trace	Trace	—	—	—	4	3	8	.1	54	210	.01	.01	.2	2
	Tomato juice, canned:																			
675	Cup	1 cup	243	94	45	2	Trace	—	—	—	10	17	44	2.2	552	1,940	.12	.07	1.9	39
676	Glass (6 fl oz)	1 glass	182	94	35	2	Trace	—	—	—	8	13	33	1.6	413	1,460	.09	.05	1.5	29
677	Turnips, cooked, diced	1 cup	155	94	35	1	Trace	—	—	—	8	54	37	.6	291	Trace	.06	.08	.5	34
	Turnip greens, cooked, drained:																			
678	From raw (leaves and stems)	1 cup	145	94	30	3	Trace	—	—	—	5	252	49	1.5	—	8,270	.15	.33	.7	68
679	From frozen (chopped)	1 cup	165	93	40	4	Trace	—	—	—	6	195	64	2.6	246	11,390	.08	.15	.7	31
680	Vegetables, mixed, frozen, cooked	1 cup	182	83	115	6	1	—	—	—	24	46	115	2.4	348	9,010	.22	.13	2.0	15
	MISCELLANEOUS ITEMS																			
	Baking powders for home use:																			
	Sodium aluminum sulfate:																			
681	With monocalcium phosphate monohydrate.	1 tsp	3.0	2	5	Trace	Trace	0	0	0	1	58	87	—	5	0	0	0	0	0
682	With monocalcium phosphate monohydrate, calcium sulfate.	1 tsp	2.9	1	5	Trace	Trace	0	0	0	1	183	45	—	—	0	0	0	0	0
683	Straight phosphate	1 tsp	3.8	2	5	Trace	Trace	0	0	0	1	239	359	—	6	0	0	0	0	0
684	Low sodium	1 tsp	4.3	2	5	Trace	Trace	0	0	0	2	207	314	—	471	0	0	0	0	0
685	Barbecue sauce	1 cup	250	81	230	4	17	2.2	4.3	10.0	20	53	50	2.0	435	900	.03	.03	.8	13

	Beverages, alcoholic:																			
686	Beer	12 fl oz	360	92	150	1	0	0	0	0	14	18	108	Trace	90	—	.01	.11	2.2	—
	Gin, rum, vodka, whisky:																			
687	80-proof	1½-fl oz jigger	42	67	95	—	—	0	0	0	Trace	—	—	—	1	—	—	—	—	—
688	86-proof	1½ fl oz jigger	42	64	105	—	—	0	0	0	Trace	—	—	—	1	—	—	—	—	—
689	90-proof	1½ fl oz jigger	42	62	110	—	—	0	0	0	Trace	—	—	—	1	—	—	—	—	—
	Wines:																			
690	Dessert	3½-fl oz glass	103	77	140	Trace	0	0	0	0	8	8	—	—	77	—	.01	.02	.2	—
691	Table	3½-fl oz glass	102	86	85	Trace	0	0	0	0	4	9	10	.4	94	—	Trace	.01	.1	—
	Beverages, carbonated, sweetened, nonalcoholic:																			
692	Carbonated water	12 fl oz	366	92	115	0	0	0	0	0	29	—	—	—	—	0	0	0	0	0
693	Cola type	12 fl oz	369	90	145	0	0	0	0	0	37	—	—	—	—	0	0	0	0	0
694	Fruit-flavored sodas and Tom Collins mixer.	12 fl oz	372	88	170	0	0	0	0	0	45	—	—	—	—	0	0	0	0	0
695	Ginger ale	12 fl oz	366	92	115	0	0	0	0	0	29	—	—	—	0	0	0	0	0	0
696	Root beer	12 fl oz	370	90	150	0	0	0	0	0	39	—	—	—	0	0	0	0	0	0
	Chili powder. See Peppers, hot, red (item 642).																			
	Chocolate:																			
697	Bitter or baking	1 oz	28	2	145	3	15	8.9	4.9	.4	8	22	109	1.9	235	20	.01	.07	.4	0
	Semisweet, see Candy, chocolate (item 539).																			
698	Gelatin, dry	1,7-g envelope	7	13	25	6	Trace	0	0	0	0	—	—	—	—	—	—	—	—	—
699	Gelatin, dessert prepared with gelatin dessert powder and water.	1 cup	240	84	140	4	0	0	0	0	34	—	—	—	—	—	—	—	—	—
700	Mustard, prepared, yellow	1 tsp or individual serving pouch or cup.	5	80	5	Trace	Trace	—	—	—	Trace	4	4	.1	7	—	—	—	—	—
	Olives, pickled, canned:																			
701	Green	4 medium or 3 extra large or 2 giant.[69]	16	78	15	Trace	2	.2	1.2	.1	Trace	8	2	.2	7	40	—	—	—	—
702	Ripe, Mission	3 small or 2 large[69]	10	73	15	Trace	2	.2	1.2	.1	Trace	9	1	.1	2	10	Trace	Trace	—	—
	Pickles, cucumber:																			
703	Dill, medium, whole, 3¾ in long, 1¼-in diam.	1 pickle	65	93	5	Trace	Trace	—	—	—	1	17	14	.7	130	70	Trace	.01	Trace	4
704	Fresh-pack, slices 1½-in diam., ¼ in thick.	2 slices	15	79	10	Trace	Trace	—	—	—	3	5	4	.3	—	20	Trace	Trace	Trace	1
705	Sweet, gherkin, small, whole, about 2½ in long, ¾-in diam.	1 pickle	15	61	20	Trace	Trace	—	—	—	5	2	2	.2	—	10	Trace	Trace	Trace	1
706	Relish, finely chopped, sweet	1 tbsp	15	63	20	Trace	Trace	—	—	—	5	3	2	.1	—	—	—	—	—	—
	Popcorn. See items 476–478.																			
707	Popsicle, 3-fl oz size	1 popsicle	95	80	70	0	0	0	0	0	18	0	—	Trace	—	0	0	0	0	0
	Soups:																			
	Canned, condensed:																			
	Prepared with equal volume of milk:																			
708	Cream of chicken	1 cup	245	85	180	7	10	4.2	3.6	1.3	15	172	152	0.5	260	610	0.05	0.27	0.7	2
709	Cream of mushroom	1 cup	245	83	215	7	14	5.4	2.9	4.6	16	191	169	.5	279	250	.05	.34	.7	1
710	Tomato	1 cup	250	84	175	7	7	3.4	1.7	1.0	23	168	155	.8	418	1,200	.10	.25	1.3	15
	Prepared with equal volume of water:																			
711	Bean with pork	1 cup	250	84	170	8	6	1.2	1.8	2.4	22	63	128	2.3	395	650	.13	.08	1.0	3
712	Beef broth, bouillon, consomme.	1 cup	240	96	30	5	0	0	0	0	3	Trace	31	.5	130	Trace	Trace	.02	1.2	—
713	Beef noodle	1 cup	240	93	65	4	3	.6	.7	.8	7	7	48	1.0	77	50	.05	.07	1.0	Trace
714	Clam chowder, Manhattan type (with tomatoes, without milk).	1 cup	245	92	80	2	3	.5	.4	1.3	12	34	47	1.0	184	880	.02	.02	1.0	—
715	Cream of chicken	1 cup	240	92	95	3	6	1.6	2.3	1.1	8	24	34	.5	79	410	.02	.05	.5	Trace
716	Cream of mushroom	1 cup	240	90	135	2	10	2.6	1.7	4.5	10	41	50	.5	98	70	.02	.12	.7	Trace

[66] Weight includes cores and stem ends. Without these parts, weight is 123 g.

[67] Based on year-round average. For tomatoes marketed from November through May, value is about 12 mg; from June through October, 32 mg.

[68] Applies to product without calcium salts added. Value for products with calcium salts added may be as much as 63 mg for whole tomatoes, 241 mg for cut forms.

[69] Weight includes pits. Without pits, weight is 13 g for item 701, 9 g for item 702.

Table A-1. (Continued)

Item No. (A)	Foods, approximate measures, units, and weight (edible part unless footnotes indicate otherwise) (B)			Water (C)	Food Energy (D)	Protein (E)	Fat (F)	Fatty Acids: Saturated (total) (G)	Fatty Acids: Unsaturated: Oleic (H)	Fatty Acids: Unsaturated: Linoleic (I)	Carbohydrate (J)	Calcium (K)	Phosphorus (L)	Iron (M)	Potassium (N)	Vitamin A Value (O)	Thiamin (P)	Riboflavin (Q)	Niacin (R)	Ascorbic Acid (S)
			Grams	Percent	Calories	Grams	Grams	Grams	Grams	Grams	Grams	Milligrams	Milligrams	Milligrams	Milligrams	I.U.	Milligrams	Milligrams	Milligrams	Milligrams
	MISCELLANEOUS ITEMS (CONTINUED)																			
	Soups: (cont.)																			
	Canned, condensed: (cont.)																			
	Prepared with equal vol. of water: (cont.)																			
717	Minestrone	1 cup	245	90	105	5	3	.7	.9	1.3	14	37	59	1.0	314	2,350	.07	.05	1.0	—
718	Split pea	1 cup	245	85	145	9	3	1.1	1.2	.4	21	29	149	1.5	270	440	.25	.15	1.5	1
719	Tomato	1 cup	245	91	90	2	3	.5	.5	1.0	16	15	34	.7	230	1,000	.05	.05	1.2	12
720	Vegetable beef	1 cup	245	92	80	5	2	—	—	—	10	12	49	.7	162	2,700	.05	.05	1.0	—
721	Vegetarian	1 cup	245	92	80	2	2	—	—	—	13	20	39	1.0	172	2,940	.05	.05	1.0	—
	Dehydrated:																			
722	Bouillon, cube ½ in	1 cube	4	4	5	1	Trace	—	—	—	Trace	—	—	—	4	—	—	—	—	—
	Mixes:																			
	Unprepared:																			
723	Onion	1½-oz pkg	43	3	150	6	5	1.1	2.3	1.0	23	42	49	.6	238	30	.05	.03	.3	6
	Prepared with water:																			
724	Chicken noodle	1 cup	240	95	55	2	1	—	—	—	8	7	19	.2	19	50	.07	.05	.5	Trace
725	Onion	1 cup	240	96	35	1	1	—	—	—	6	10	12	.2	58	Trace	Trace	Trace	Trace	2
726	Tomato vegetable with noodles.	1 cup	240	93	65	1	1	—	—	—	12	7	19	.2	29	480	.05	.02	.5	5
727	Vinegar, cider	1 tbsp	15	94	Trace	Trace	0	0	0	0	1	1	1	.1	15	—	—	—	—	—
728	White sauce, medium, with enriched flour.	1 cup	250	73	405	10	31	19.3	7.8	.8	22	288	233	.5	348	1,150	.12	.43	.7	2
	Yeast:																			
729	Baker's, dry, active	1 pkg	7	5	20	3	Trace	—	—	—	3	3	90	1.1	140	Trace	.16	.38	2.6	Trace
730	Brewer's, dry	1 tbsp	8	5	25	3	Trace	—	—	—	3	[70]17	140	1.4	152	Trace	1.25	.34	3.0	Trace

[70] Value may vary from 6 to 60 mg.

TABLE A–2. MINERAL AND VITAMIN CONTENT OF FOODS

Explanatory Notes. The data in this table are intended to provide assistance in the planning of diets for sodium content and for some minerals and vitamins for which recommended allowances have been set. The data were derived from many sources listed below.

These values for minerals and vitamins must be regarded as tentative inasmuch as analyses in many instances have included only a small number of food samples. Wide variations for a nutrient in a given kind of food may occur depending upon the variety or breed, the growing conditions, the processing techniques, the storage conditions, the preparation within the home, and the methods used for analyses.

Sodium. The sodium values for commercially canned vegetables assume 0.6 per cent salt concentration in the regular pack. Salt is ordinarily added to canned meats, fish, poultry, soups; cured meats; cheeses; baked products including breads, quick breads, rolls, cakes, cookies, pies; ready-to-eat and cooked breakfast cereals; salad dressings; butter and margarine.

The amount of salt added to some foods is so highly variable that the values listed in the table pertain to the unsalted product. Included are cooked fresh and frozen vegetables; cooked fresh meats, fish, and poultry; cooked legumes; cooked macaroni, spaghetti, and noodles.

Vitamin E. The table lists the values for alpha-tocopherol. Vitamin E activity is shown by eight tocopherols. Of these alpha-tocopherol is the most active. Assuming the alpha-tocopherol activity to be 1.0, the corresponding activity of other tocopherols is as follows: beta-tocopherol, 0.4; gamma-tocopherol, 0.1; delta-tocopherol, 0.01; alpha-tocotrienol, 0.3; beta-tocotrienol, 0.05; and gamma-tocotrienol, 0.01.

The alpha-tocopherol content of a food slightly underestimates the total vitamin E activity. However, for some foods other tocopherols predominate, and hence the total tocopherol value would considerably overestimate the vitamin E activity.

In values for copper, zinc, and vitamin E, two decimal places are used when the value is less than 0.1. This does not imply greater accuracy, but indicates the presence of some of these nutrients in the food.

SOURCES OF DATA FOR TABLE A–2

DONG, M. H. et al.: "Thiamin, Riboflavin, and Vitamin B_6 Contents of Selected Foods, as Served," *J. Am. Diet. Assoc.,* **76**:156–60, 1980.

FREELAND, J. H., and COUSINS, R. J.: "Zinc Content of Selected Foods," *J. Am. Diet. Assoc.,* **68**:526–29, 1976.

GODDARD, M. S. et al.: *Provisional Table on the Nutrient Content of Frozen Vegetables.* U.S. Department of Agriculture, Hyattsville, Md., 1979.

GREGOR, J. L. et al.: "Magnesium Content of Selected Foods," *J. Food Science,* **43**:1610, 1978.

HAEFLEIN, K. A., and RASMUSSEN, A. I.: "Zinc Content of Selected Foods," *J. Am. Diet. Assoc.,* **70**:610–16, 1977.

MCLAUGHLIN, P. J., and WEIHRAUCK, J. L.: "Vitamin E Content of Foods," *J. Am. Diet. Assoc.,* **75**:647–65, 1979.

MEYER, B. H. et al.: "Pantothenic Acid and Vitamin B_6 in Beef," *J. Am. Diet. Assoc.,* **54**:122–25, 1969.

MURPHY, E. W. et al.: "Provisional Tables on the Zinc Content of Foods," *J. Am. Diet. Assoc.,* **66**:345–55, 1975.

ORR, M. L.: *Pantothenic Acid, Vitamin B_6, and Vitamin B_{12} in Foods.* Home Economics

Research Report No. 36, Agricultural Research Service, U.S. Department of Agriculture, Washington, D.C., 1969.

PENNINGTON, J. A.: *Dietary Nutrient Guide.* AVI Publishing Co., Inc., Westport, Conn., 1976.

PENNINGTON, J. T., and CALLOWAY, D. H.: "Copper Content of Foods," *J. Am. Diet Assoc.*, **63**:143–53, 1973.

PERLOFF, B. P., and BUTRUM, R. R.: "Folacin in Selected Foods," *J. Am. Diet. Assoc.*, **70**:161–72, 1977.

POLANSKY, M. M.: "Vitamin B_6 Components in Fresh and Dried Vegetables," *J. Am. Diet. Assoc.*, **54**:118–21, 1969.

POSATI, L. P., and ORR, M. L.: *Composition of Foods: Dairy and Egg Products*, Ag. Handbook 8–1, U.S. Department of Agriculture, Washington, D.C., 1976.

WATT, B. K., and MERRILL, A. L.: *Composition of Foods—Raw, Processed, Prepared*, Ag. Handbook No. 8, U.S. Department of Agriculture, Washington, D.C., 1963.

Table A–2. **Mineral and Vitamin Content of Foods: Sodium, Magnesium, Copper, and Zinc; Folacin, Pantothenic Acid, Vitamin B-6, Vitamin B-12, and Vitamin E (Values for 100 gm food, edible portion)**

Item No.	Food	Sodium mg	Magnesium mg	Copper mg	Zinc mg	Folacin μg	Pantothenic Acid μg	Vitamin B-6 μg	Vitamin B-12 μg	Vitamin E mg
1	Almonds, fried	4	270	0.8[1]	—[2]	96	470	100	0	24.0 R[3]
2	roasted, salted	198	—	—	2.6	—	250	95	0	—
3	Apple, raw, not peeled	1	8	.09	.05	8	105	30	0	0.6
4	Apple juice, bottled	1	4	.2	.03	tr	—	30	0	.01
5	Applesauce, sweetened	2	5	.4	.1	1	85	30	0	.05
6	Apricots, raw	1	12	.1	.04	3	240	70	0	
7	canned	1	7	.05	.04	1	92	54	0	.9
8	dried, uncooked	26	62	.4	.1	14	753[1]	169[1]	0	
9	cooked	7	20	—	—	—	—	—	0	
10	Apricot nectar	tr	6	—	—	—	100	40	0	
11	Asparagus, green, cooked	1	20 R	.1	1.0	60	600	200	0	2.0
12	canned, regular pack	236	—	.2	—	27	195	55	0	.4
13	low sodium	3								
14	frozen, spears, cooked	1	14	.1	.6	109	410	155	0	1.4 R
15	Avocado	4	45	.4	.4	51	1,070	420	0	1.6
16	Bacon, cooked, drained	1,021	25	.5	4.8	—	330 R	125 R	0.7	.5 R
17	Canadian, cooked	2,555	24							
	Baking powder, home use									
18	sodium aluminum phosphate	10,953								
19	straight phosphate	8,220								
20	tartrate	7,300								
21	low sodium, commercial	6								
22	Banana	1	33	0.2	0.2	28	260	510	0	0.3
23	Barley, pearled, light	3	37	.2	—	—	503	224	0	.02
	Beans, immature									
24	Lima, cooked	1	67	.4	—	34	—	—	0	—
25	canned, regular pack	236	—	—	—	13	130	90	0	—
26	low sodium	4								
27	frozen, Fordhook, cooked	101	48 R	.06	.5	31 R	240	150	0	—
28	snap, green, cooked	4	32 R	.1	.3	40	190 R	80 R	0	.02 R
29	canned, regular pack	236	14	.04	.3	12	75	40	0	.03
30	low sodium	2								
31	frozen, cooked	1	21 R	.05	.2	28	135	70	0	.1
32	snap, yellow, cooked	3	—	—	—	32	250 R	—	0	—
33	canned, regular pack	236	—	—	—	—	—	42	0	
34	low sodium	2								
	Beans, mature									
35	Lima, dry	4	180	.7	2.8	113	975	580	0	7.7
36	cooked	2	—	.2	.9	43	—	—	0	—
37	red, dry	10	163	.8	—	133	500	441	0	2.1
38	cooked	3	—	.4	—	37	—	—	0	—
39	soy, dry	—	—	—	—	171	—	—	0	.9
40	cooked	2	—	.3	.7	—	—	670	0	—
41	white, common, dry	19	170	0.9	2.8	129	725	560	0	0.3

[1] Source of data does not indicate whether value is for raw or cooked food; it is assumed that it represents the raw food.

[2] Dashes denote lack of reliable data for a constituent believed to be present in a measurable amount.

[3] The letter "R" following a value indicates that the only available data were on a raw sample of that food.

42	cooked	7	—	—	1.0	—	—	—	0	—
43	canned, pork with tomato sauce	463	37	.2	1.0	24	92	—	0	—
44	Bean sprouts, Mung, cooked	4	—	—	—	10	—	—	0	.06 R
	Beef									
45	all cuts, lean, broiled, roasted, average	60	29	.2	5.8	4	620 R	160	1.8 R	.4 R
46	simmered, average	60	18	—	6.2	—	—	—	—	—
47	corned, cooked	1,740	25	—	1.9	2	560	148	1.8	
48	hash, canned	540	20	—	2.0		—	242	.8	.03
49	dried	4,300	—	—	—	—	—	—	1.8	
50	hamburger	47	21	.06 R	4.4	4	320	48	1.68	.4
51	pot pie, commercial	366								
52	stew, with vegetables, canned	411	—	.02	1.4	3		120	.65	.2
53	home recipe	37	17	—	—	—	—	—	.65	.2
54	Beets, cooked	43	25	.2	.05	78	150 R	55 R	0	.03
55	canned, regular pack	236	15	.1	—	3	100	50	0	.03
56	low-sodium pack	46								
57	Beet greens, cooked	76	106	.1	.5	60	250	100	0	1.5 R
	Beverages, alcoholic									
58	beer	7	10	0.07	0.03		80	60	0	
59	gin	1								
60	wine, table	5	10	.01	.1		30	40	0	
	Beverages, nonalcoholic									
61	cola		2	.04	.02					
62	fruit drinks		3		.02					
63	Biscuits, baking powder, enriched	626	—	.3	1.0	7	330	—	0	
64	self-rising flour[4]	630								
65	Biscuits, dough, commercial, in can	868								.6
66	Blackberries, raw	1	30	.2	.05	14	240	50	0	
67	Blueberries, raw	1	6	.2	.05	6	156	67	0	
68	frozen, sweet	1	4	—	—	8	121	54	0	
69	Bluefish, baked or broiled	104								
70	Bouillon cubes	24,000								
	Bran. See Cereals									
71	Brazil nuts	1	225	1.5	5.1	4	231	170	0	6.5
	Breads									
72	Boston brown	251	—	.3	—	—	—	—		—
73	corn, southern style, degermed meal	591	33	—	—	—	—	81		
74	cracked wheat	529	35	.2	1.2	25	607	92	0	
75	French, Italian, Vienna	580	22	.4	.9	9	378	53	0	
76	Raisin	365	24	.2	1.2	12	400	40	0	
77	rye, American	557	42	0.2	1.6	23	450	100	0	
78	pumpernickel	569	71	—	1.1	—	500	160	0	
79	white, 3–4% milk solids	507	22	.2	.6	39	430	40	tr	0.1
80	whole wheat, 2% nonfat solids	527	78	.2	1.8	58	760	180	tr	.1

[4] Based on use of self-rising flour containing anhydrous monocalcium phosphate.

Table A-2. **(Continued)**

Item No.	Food	Sodium mg	Magnesium mg	Copper mg	Zinc mg	Folacin µg	Pantothenic Acid µg	Vitamin B-6 µg	Vitamin B-12 µg	Vitamin E mg
81	Broccoli spears, cooked	10	24 R	.1	.2	56	448	112	0	.5 R
82	frozen, cooked	12	21	.04	.3	54	525	170	0	
83	Brussels sprouts, cooked	10	29 R	.08	.4	36	420 (frozen)	175 (frozen)	0	.9
84	Butter, salted	826	2	.03	.05	3		3	tr	1.6
85	unsalted	under 10								
86	Cabbage, raw	20	14	.08	.4	66	205	160	0	1.7
87	cooked, small amount water	14	6	.09	.4	18	112	100	0	
88	Cabbage, celery or Chinese	23	14	—	—	83	—	—	0	.1
	Cakes, home recipe									
89	angel food	283	25	.05	.3	3	200	tr	tr	
90	chocolate with icing	235	42	.3	1.0	6	200		0.1	
91	fruit cake, dark	158	—	.1						
92	gingerbread	237								
93	plain with icing	229								
94	plain, without icing	300			.2			40[5]		2.6
95	pound	110	—	.09	—	7	300	22		1.1
96	sponge	167	8			7				
	Candy									
97	caramels	226	—	0.04	—					
98	chocolate, milk, plain	94	58	.5	.5	7	100	tr	0	0.2
99	fudge, plain	190								1.1
100	hard	32	tr	.09						
101	marshmallow	39	4	.2	.03	0	0	0	0	0
102	mint, chocolate coated	52							0	
103	peanut brittle	31	—	—	—	—	—	—	0	
104	Cantaloupe	12	16	.05	.02	30	250	86	0	0.1
105	Carrots, raw	47	23	.1	.4	32	280	150	0	.4
106	cooked	33	13	.08	.3	24	280	28	0	.4
107	canned, regular pack	236	—	—	.3	3	130	30	0	
108	low sodium	39								
109	Cashew nuts, not salted	15	267	.7	4.4	68	1,300	—	0	.2
110	Cauliflower, raw	13	24	.07	.3	55	1,000	210	0	.03
111	cooked	9	—	.06	—	34	835	170	0	
112	frozen, cooked	10	13 R	.02	.2	—	540	190	0	
113	Celery, raw	126	22	.07	.1	12	429	60	0	.4
114	cooked	88	—	.1	—	—	—	—	0	
	Cereals, breakfast									
115	bran, wheat, crude	9	490	1.5	9.8	258	335	—	0	1.5
116	bran flakes (40% bran)	925	—	.6	3.6	—	875	384	0	
117	bran flakes with raisins	800								
118	corn, puffed	1,060					288		0	.09
119	corn, shredded	988							0	.08
120	cornflakes	1,005	16	0.1	0.3	12	185	65	0	0.1
121	cornflakes, sugar coated	775								
122	corn grits, dry, white, degermed	1	20	—	.4	24	—	147	0	.1
123	cooked	—	3	.05	.1	2	165	34	0	.04
124	cornmeal, degermed, dry	1	47	.1	.8	7				

[5] Nature of sample not clearly defined.

125	cooked		7		.1	9				
126	cornmeal, whole ground, dry	1	106	—	1.8		580	250	0	.2
127	farina, regular, dry	2	25	.2	.5	24	515	67	0	
128	cooked, salted	144	3	.03	.06	4	85	15	0	
129	instant cooking, cooked	188	4							
130	oatmeal, dry	2	144	.6	3.4	52	1,500	140	0	1.5
131	cooked, salted	218	21	.03	.5					
132	rice flakes	987	25	.3	1.4	8	340	125	0	.04
133	rice, puffed, no salt	2	—	.4	1.4	23	378	75	0	.06
134	wheat and barley, malted, dry	1	168	.6	3.6	33				1.1
135	cooked	72	31		.5					
136	wheat, rolled, cooked	tr				49				
137	wheat flakes	1,032	102	.4	1.4	47	469	292	0	.4
138	wheat, puffed, no salt	4	—	.4	2.6	—	—	170	0	.7
139	wheat, shredded, plain	3	133	—	2.8	50	706	244	0	.4
140	Chard, Swiss, cooked	86	65 R	—	—	42	172 R	—	0	
	Cheese									
141	Camembert	842	20	—	2.4	62	1,364	227	1.3	
142	cheddar or American	620	28	0.1	3.1	18	413	74	1.0	0.6
143	cheddar, process	1,189[6]	31	.06	3.6	11	558	80	1.1	
144	cottage, creamed	405	5	.02	.4	12	213	67	.6	
145	uncreamed	406	6	—	.4	13	242	76	.7	
146	cream	296	6	.04	.5	13	271	47	.4	
147	Gouda	819	29	—	3.9	21	340	80	—	
148	Mozzarella	373	19	—	2.2	7	64	56	.7	
149	Parmesan	1,862	51	.4	3.2	8	527	105	—	
150	Swiss	260	36	.1	3.9	6	429	83	1.7	
151	Cherries, raw, sweet	2	14	.1	.1	8	261	32	0	0.1
152	canned, syrup	1	9	.06	—	3	—	30	0	
153	Chicken broiled, dark without skin	86	—	.2 R	2.8	7	1,000	325	.4	.4
154	light without skin	64	19	.1 R	.9	4	800	683	.5	
155	Chicken, canned, boneless	—	12	.1	2.0	2	850	300	.8	.3
156	Chicken potpie, frozen, commercial	411	11	—	—	—	—	86	—	—
157	Chickpeas (garbanzos) dry	8	—	—	2.7	199	—	—	—	—
158	boiled, drained	—	—	—	1.4	102	320	160	0	
159	Chicory	7	13	—	—	52	—	45	0	
160	Chili concarne, canned with beans	531	—	—	—	—	140	103	—	
161	Chili powder with seasoning	1,574	169							
162	Chocolate, bitter	4	292	2.7	2.3	14	190	35	0	
163	Chocolate syrup, thin	52	63	.4	.9					
164	Clams, raw, soft, meat only	36	—		1.5	—	300	80		
165	hard, round, meat only	205	—	—	1.5					
166	canned	—	115	—	1.2	2	300	83		0.2
167	Cocoa, breakfast, dry	6	420	3.6	5.6					0.2
168	processed with alkali	717								

[6] Value based on use of 1.5 per cent anhydrous disodium phosphate as the emulsifying agent; if the emulsifying agent does not contain sodium the value is 650 mg.

Table A-2. **(Continued)**

Item No.	Food	Sodium mg	Magnesium mg	Copper mg	Zinc mg	Folacin µg	Pantothenic Acid µg	Vitamin B-6 µg	Vitamin B-12 µg	Vitamin E mg
169	Coconut, fresh, shredded	23	46	.5	—	24	200	44	0	.7
170	dried, sweetened	—	77	.6	—	—	200	33	0	
171	Coffee, instant, dry	72	456	1.0	.6	—	400	32	0	
172	beverage	1	4	.02	.03		4	tr	0	
173	Collards, cooked	25	57	.3	.7	102 R	450 (frozen)	195 (frozen)	0	
174	Cookies, fig bars	252	—	.2	1.2	4	400	100	0	
175	oatmeal	170	—	.1	1.3	4	—	—		
176	plain, assorted	365	15	.07	.3	9	300	60	0	2.6
177	Corn, sweet, cooked	tr	48 R	.07 R	.4	33 R	540 R	161 R	0	1.2
178	canned, whole kernel, regular pack	236	19	.06	.2	8	220	200	0	.01
179	low-sodium pack	2								
180	Cowpeas, dry, cooked	8	230	.2	1.2	133 R	1,050	562	0	
181	Crabmeat, canned	1,000	34	1.5	4.3	20	600	300	10	1.2
182	Crackers, graham	670	51	.2	1.1	25	540	65	0	
183	saltines, soda	1,100	29	.04	.6	20	500	68	0	0.4
184	Cranberry juice	1								
185	Cranberry sauce	1	2					22		
186	Cream, half and half	41	10	.1	.5	2	289	39	.3	
187	light, coffee	40	9	.1	.3	2	276	32	.2	
188	whipping, light	34	7	.1	.3	4	59	28	.2	
189	Cucumber, not peeled	6	11	.06	.2	15	250	42	0	.2
190	Dandelion greens, cooked	44	36 R	—	—	—	—	—	0	2.5 R
191	Dates, domestic	1	58	.2	—	21	780	153	0	
192	Doughnuts, cake type	501	23	.1	.5	8	387[5]	—		0.7
193	Duck, flesh, raw	74	—	.4					2.8	
194	Eggplant, cooked	1	16 R	.1 R	—	16	220 R	81 R	0	.03
195	Egg, whole, raw	138	12	.1	1.4	65	1,727	120	1.5	.7
196	white, raw	152	9	.05	.02	16	241	3	.07	
197	yolk, raw	49	15	.3	3.0	152	4,429	310	3.8	2.1
198	Endive, curly	14	10	—	—	49	90	20	0	
	Fats. See Oils, Shortening									
199	Figs, raw	2	20	.1	—	14	300	113	0	
200	canned	2	—	—	—	—	69	—	0	
201	dried, uncooked	34	71	.3	—	9	435	175	0	
202	Filberts (hazelnuts)			1.3	3.1	72				23.8
203	Flounder, raw	78	—	.2	0.7	—	850	170	1.2	.4
204	Flour, all purpose	2	25	.2	.7	21	465	60	0	0.03
205	cake	2	—	—	.3	5	320	45	0	.04
206	rye, light	1	73	.4	—	78	720	90	0	.4
207	whole wheat	3	113	.5	2.4	38	1,100	340	0	.8
208	Fruit cocktail	5	7	.03	.02	—	—	33	0	
209	Gelatin, dry	—	33	1.1	—	0	0	0	0	
210	sweetened, ready-to-eat	51	3	.02						
211	Grapefruit, fresh	1	12	.04	.05	11	283	34	0	.3
212	canned	1	11	.04		—	120	20	0	
213	Grapefruit juice, canned	1	—	.01	.03	21	130	11	0	.1
214	frozen, diluted	1	9	—	—	—	162	14	0	
215	Grapes, American	3	13	.09	.3	7	126	80[5]	0	

[5] Nature of sample not clearly defined.

No.	Food									
216	Grape juice, bottled	2	12	.01	—	2	40	18	0	
217	Haddock, raw	61	24	.2	.7	10	130	180	1.3	.4
218	fried, (dipped in egg, milk, bread crumbs)	177	24	.2	1.0	5	100	180	1.3	
219	Heart, beef, lean, raw	86	18	.3	—	—	2,500	250	11.0	.6
220	Herring, raw, Pacific	74	—	.2	—	—	—	—	2.0	1.1
221	smoked, hard	6,231	—	—	—	—	500	200	7.0	
222	Honey, strained	5	3	.04	.08	3	200	20	0	
223	Honeydew melon	12	—	.06	.07	5	207	56	0	
224	Ice cream, chocolate	—	23	0.1						
225	vanilla, 10% fat	87	14	.02	1.1	2	492	46	.5	
226	Ice milk, vanilla, hardened	80	14		.4	2	505	65	.7	
227	Jams and preserves	12	5	.3	.04		—	25	0	.09
228	Jellies	17	4	.1						.09
229	Kale, cooked, leaves with stems	43	37	.05	.2	60 R	376 R	185 R	0	
230	Lamb, lean cut, dry heat	70	21	.06 R	4.3	3	550 R	275 R	2.2 R	.2
231	Lard	0	0	.03	.2			20	0	1.2
232	Lasagna	490	25	—	.8	22	—	—	—	
233	Lemon juice, fresh	1	8	.08	.01	12	103	46	0	
234	Lemonade, frozen, diluted	tr	1	.01	.01	5	11	5	0	
235	Lentils, dry, boiled				3.1	36				
236	Lettuce, crisp head	9	11	.09	.4	37	200	55[5]	0	.06
237	loose leaf, romaine	9	—	.09	.4	44	200	60	0	.4
238	Lime juice, fresh or canned	1	—			4	314		0	
	Liver, cooked, fried									
239	beef	184	18	2.80 R	5.1	145	7,700 R	840 R	80 R	.6
240	calf	118	26	7.9 R	6.1		8,000 R	670 R	60 R	.3
241	chicken, simmered	60	—	.3 R	3.4	—	—	—	25	
242	pork	111	24	1.1 R	—	145	6,400 R	650 R	32 R	
243	Lobster, cooked or canned	210	22	1.7 R	2.2	17	1,500 R	—	0.5 R	1.5 R
244	Macaroni, dry	2	48	.1	1.5	12	—	64	0	.02
245	cooked, firm	1	20	.02	.5	4	150	25	0	
246	Macaroni and cheese	543	20	.04	.7	5	200	23	0.4	
247	Margarine, corn oil, stick, salted	987		0.04	0.2	2				12.9
248	safflower, soybean, stick									17.8
249	soybean, stick									3.1
250	Milk, fresh, whole	49	13	.04	.4	5	314	42	0.36	.06
251	fresh, skim	52	11	.02	.4	5	329	40	.38	tr
252	buttermilk	130	14	.03		11	307	36	.22	
253	evaporated, undiluted	106	24	.1	.8	8	638	50	.16	
254	nonfat dry	549	117	.5	4.5	50	3,235	345	4.0	
255	Milk, goat	50	14	.05	.3	1	310	46	.07	
256	Milk, human	17	3	.05	.2	5	223	11	.05	0.9
	Milk beverages									
257	chocolate flavored with skim milk	64	18		.4	6	261	49	.35	
258	malted with whole milk	81	16		.4	8	289	68	.39	
259	Molasses, light	15	46	1.4		10[5]	350[5]	200[5]	0	0.4
260	black strap	96	258	1.4						

[5]Nature of sample not clearly defined.

Table A-2. **(Continued)**

Item No.	Food	Sodium mg	Magnesium mg	Copper mg	Zinc mg	Folacin µg	Pantothenic Acid µg	Vitamin B-6 µg	Vitamin B-12 µg	Vitamin E mg
261	Muffins, plain	441	23	.2	1.2	7	500	19	.2	
262	Mushrooms, raw	15	—	1.0	1.3	24	2,200	125	0	.08
263	canned	400	8	.4		4	1,000	60	0	
264	Mustard, prepared, yellow	1,252	48							1.8
265	Mustard greens, cooked	18	27	.09	.2	60	164 R	133 R	0	2.0
266	Nectarine	6	13	.08		5	—	17	0	
267	Noodles, enriched, dry	5	126	.2			—	88	tr	
268	cooked	2	—		.6	2	200	7	tr	
269	Oil, corn	0	0	0	0	0	0	0	0	14.3[7]
270	Okra, raw	2	41	0.1	—	24	215	45	0	
271	Olives, green	2,400	22	.3	.08		18		0	
272	ripe	813	—	.4	.3	1	15	14	0	
273	Onions, green, raw	5	21	.04	.3	36	144	—	0	
274	mature, raw	10	12	.1	.3	25	130	130	0	0.1
275	cooked	7	—	.07	—	10	100	100	0	
276	Orange, peeled	1	11	.06	.2	46	250	60	0	.2
277	Orange juice, fresh,	1	11	.08	.02	55	190	40	0	.04
278	canned	1			.02		150	35	0	
279	frozen, diluted	1	10	.01	.02	55	164	28	0	
280	Oysters, Eastern, raw	73	32	17.1	74.7	11	250	50	18	.9
281	Pancakes, wheat, home recipe	425	—	.05	.8	(canned) 9	720	20	tr	
282	Papayas, raw	3	—	.01			218	—	0	
283	Parsley	45	41	.5		116	300	164	0	1.7
284	Parsnips, cooked	8	32 R			67	600[1]	90[1]	0	1.0 R
285	Peaches, raw	1	10	.09	.2	8	170	24	0	
286	canned	2	6	.05	.1	1	50	19	0	
287	dried	16	48	—	—	5		100[1]	0	
288	cooked with sugar	4	15							
289	frozen	2	6			4	132	18	0	
290	Peanuts, roasted	5	175	—	3.0	106	2,100	400	0	7.8
291	salted	418	175	1.0	2.9					8.3
292	Peanut butter	607	173	.6	2.9	79	—	330	0	7.0
293	Pears, raw	2	7	.2	—	14	70	17	0	.5
294	canned	1	5	.04	.3		22	14	0	
295	Peas, green, cooked	1	18	.2	.7	25	—	109	0	.1 R
296	canned, regular pack	236	20	.2	.8	10	150	50	0	
297	low-sodium pack	3								
298	frozen, not thawed	129	24	.1	.8	53	315	130	0	.1
299	Peas, dried, split	40	180	—	3.2	51	2,000	130	0	.09
300	cooked	13	—	.3	1.1	20	220	20	0	
301	Pecans	tr	142	1.4	—	24	1,707	183	0	1.2
302	Peppers, sweet, green, raw	13	18	.1	.06	19	230	260	0	.7
303	Perch, Atlantic, raw	79	—	—	—	9				1.2
304	Pickles, dill	1,428	12	.2	.3	4	225	7[5]	0	

[1]Source of data does not indicate whether value is for raw or cooked food; it is assumed that it represents the raw food.

[7]Vitamin E content, as alpha-tocopherol in other oils; coconut, 0.4; cottonseed, 35.3; olive, 11.9; peanut, 11.6; safflower, 34.1; sesame, 1.4; soybean, 11.0; sunflower, 59.5; wheat germ, 149.4.

[5]Nature of sample not clearly defined.

No.	Food									
305	relish, sweet	712	—	.5	.06					
	Pie, home recipe									
306	apple	301	5	.06	.09	4	110	—	0	1.6
307	cherry	304	—	.04	.04				0	
308	custard	287	—	—			946		—	
309	lemon meringue	282	—	—					—	
310	mince	448	—	.09	.05				—	
311	pumpkin	214	—	—	.4		519	57	—	
312	Piecrust, baked	611	—	.1	.5					.5
313	Pike, walleye, raw	51	—	.2						
314	Pineapple, raw	1	13	0.06	0.2	11	160	88	0	0.1
315	canned	1	8	.1	.2	1	100	74	0	
316	Pineapple juice, canned	1	12	.05	.2	1	100	96	0	
317	Pizza, cheese	702	—	.3	1.2	37				
318	Plums, raw	2	9	.1		6	186	52	0	
319	canned, purple	1	5			1	72	27	0	
320	Popcorn, salted, with oil	1,940	—	.4	3.0			204	0	
321	Pork, fresh, lean, roast	65	29	.06	3.1	5	790 R	259	0.7 R	.08 R
322	picnic ham, simmered	65	18		4.0					
323	Pork, cured, ham, light cure	930	20	.03	4.0	11	675 R	400 R	.6 R	.3
324	canned, spiced or unspiced	1,100	—	.09			—	360		.3
325	Potatoes, baked, no skin	4	18	.2	.5	10	400	138	0	.06 R
326	boiled, unsalted	2	—	.1	.3	7	400	174	0	.04
327	french fried	6	17	.3	.3	22	540 (frozen)	180 (frozen)	0	.2
328	mashed, with milk, table fat, salted	331	14	.1	.4	10	200	100	0	
329	Potato chips	variable to 1,000	55	.3	.8	10	500	180	0	4.3
330	Pretzels	1,680 (variable)	24	.2	1.1		540	19		.2
331	Prunes, dried, uncooked		40	.3		4	460	240	0	
332	cooked	4	20	.2	.3					
333	Prune juice, canned	2	10	.02	.01					
	Pudding									
334	bread with raisin	201	—	.08						
335	chocolate	56	19						—	
336	cornstarch (blanc mange)	65	8	0.04					—	
337	custard, baked	79			0.1	4			—	
338	rennin, using mix	46							—	
339	rice with raisin	71	—	.03	.3				—	
340	tapioca cream	156	—	.04					—	
341	Pumpkin, canned, unsalted	2	12 R	.1		19	400	56	0	1.0
342	Radishes	18	15	.09	.3	24	184	75	0	
343	Raisins, dried	27	35	.3	.2	4	45	240	0	.7
344	Raspberries, red, raw	1	20			5	240	60	0	.3
345	frozen	1				5	270	38	0	
346	Rhubarb, cooked	2	13	.1	.1	7 R	70	25	0	.03 R
347	Rice, white, dry	5	24	.2	1.3	—	550	170	0	.1
348	cooked, salted	374	8	.02	.4	16	225	35	0	

Table A-2. **(Continued)**

Item No.	Food	Sodium mg	Magne-sium mg	Copper mg	Zinc mg	Folacin μg	Panto-thenic Acid μg	Vitamin B-6 μg	Vitamin B-12 μg	Vitamin E mg
349	Rolls, commercial, plain	506	21	.2	1.0		310	35	—	.04
350	sweet	389	20							
351	whole wheat	564	—							
352	Rutabagas, cooked	4	15 R			21	160[1]	100[1]	0	
353	Rye wafers	882	—	.3						
354	Salad dressings									
355	blue cheese	1,094			.3					
356	commercial, mayonnaise type	586			.1					
357	French	1,370	10		0.08					
358	home cooked	728								
359	mayonnaise	597	2	0.2	.2	3				
360	Thousand Island	700	6		.1					
361	Salmon, fresh, broiled	64	40	.2	.8	4	220	670	3.9	1.4
362	canned	387	30	.07	.9	20	550	300	6.9	
363	Sardines, Pacific, canned in tomato sauce	400	24	.04	2.6	16	700	160	10.0	
364	Sauerkraut	747	—	.1	.9		93	130	0	
	Sausage									
365	bologna	1,300	14	.02	1.8	5	—	100	—	.06
366	frankfurters	1,100	13	.08	2.0	4	430	140	1.3	
367	liverwurst			3.0	7.3	30	2,660	200	14.0	.4
368	pork links	958	16			14 R	682	165	.5	.2
369	salami		11							.1
370	Scallops	265	—	.1 R	1.3	16 R	132 R		1.2 R	.6
371	Sesame seed		18	1.6		96			0	
372	Shad, raw	54					608			
373	baked with table fat	79								
374	Sherbet, orange	46	8		.7	7	32	13	0.08	
375	Shrimp, raw	140	42	.6 R	1.5		220	100	.9	.4
376	canned, dry pack		51	.2	2.1	15	210	60	—	
	Soup, canned, diluted with equal part water									
377	bean with pork	403	—	—	—					
378	beef bouillon	326	—	0.01	—					
379	beef noodle	382	—	.04	1.4					
380	chicken noodle	408	10							
381	clam chowder, Manhattan	383	—	—	.6	7	—	54		
382	cream (mushroom) prepared with milk	424	5	—	.5	3				
383	minestrone	406	—							
384	pea, green	367	—				80	40		
385	tomato	396	9	.1	.1					
386	vegetable with beef broth	345	11	.04	1.6	6	140	—	0	
387	Spaghetti, dry	2	—	.2	—	12	—	64	0	
388	cooked, tender	1	—							
389	Spaghetti, with meat balls, canned	488	—	.2					.2	
390	Spinach, raw	71	88	.1	.8	193	300	280	0	1.9

[1] Source of data does not indicate whether value is for raw or cooked food; it is assumed that it represents the raw food.

391	cooked	50	—	.1	.7	91	75 (frozen)	130 (frozen)	0	
392	canned, regular pack	236	63	—	.8	49	65	70	0	.02
393	low-sodium pack	32								
394	Squash, summer, cooked	1	16	.08	.2	10	173 (frozen)	63 (frozen)	0	
395	winter, cooked	1	17			12	280 (frozen)	91 (frozen)	0	.1
396	Strawberries, raw	1	12	—	0.08	16	340	55	0	0.1
397	frozen	1	9	—	.07	9	135	43	0	.2
398	Sugar, brown	30	—	0.4					0	
399	granulated	1	tr	.02	.06				0	
400	Sunflower seeds	30	38	1.8			1,420	1,130	0	49.5
401	Sweet potatoes, baked	12	31	.1	.08 R	12	820 R	218 R	0	4.6 R
402	boiled	10	—	.2		18	700	200	0	
403	Syrup, table blend	68		.4						
404	Tangerine, raw	2	—	.07		21	200	67	0	
405	juice, canned	1					—	32	0	
406	Tapioca, dry	3	4	.06		8			0	
407	Tea, instant, powder		395							
408	beverage		22	.5	.02					
409	Tomato, raw	3	14	.1	.2	39	330	100	0	.3
410	canned, regular pack	130	12	.2	.2	4	230	90	0	
411	low-sodium pack	3								
412	Tomato catsup, regular	1,042	21	.6	.3	5	—	107	0	
413	Tomato juice, canned, regular pack	200	10	.07	.04	7	250	192	0	.2
414	low-sodium pack	3								
415	Tongue, beef, braised	61	16 R	.07 R			2,000	100		
416	Tuna, in oil	800	—	.1	1.0	15	320	425	2.2	
417	Turkey, dark, roasted	99	—	0.1	4.4	7	1,128	—	—	0.6
418	light, roasted	82	28	.1	2.1	5	591	—	—	
419	Turnips, cooked	34	7	.04	.09	20 R	200 R	90 R	0	.03
420	Turnip greens, canned, regular pack	236	58 R			95 R	68		0	2.2
421	frozen, not thawed	23	27	.06	.2	—	54	140	0	
422	Veal, lean, roasted	80	19	.1 R	4.1	17	900	345	1.9	.05
423	stewed	80	—	—	4.2	3	1,060 R	400 R	1.8 R	.05
424	Vinegar, cider	1	1	.09	.1			1		
425	Waffles, home recipe	475	28				650	38	—	
426	Walnuts, black	3	190			77			0	
427	English	2	131	1.4	2.3	66	900	730	0	.9
428	Watermelon	1	8	.07		8	300	68	0	
429	Wheat germ	827	336	2.4	14.3	328	1,200	1,150	0	14.1
430	Yeast, compressed	16	59				3,500	600	0	.08
431	dry, active	52	—	5.0		4,090	11,000	2,000	0	.08
432	dry, brewer's	121	231			3,909	12,000	2,500	0	
433	Yogurt, from partially skimmed milk	46	12		.5	11	389	32	.4	

Table A-3. **Dietary Fiber in Selected Plant Foods***

	Measure	Weight gm	Total Dietary Fiber gm	Noncellulosic Polysaccharides gm	Cellulose gm	Lignin gm
Apple, flesh	1 medium	138	1.96	1.29	0.66	0.01
Apple peel only		100	3.71	2.21	1.01	.49
Banana	1 small	119	2.08	1.33	.44	.31
Beans, baked, canned	1 cup	255	18.53	14.45	3.59	.48
Beans, runner, boiled	1 cup	125	4.19	2.31	1.61	.26
Beverages, concentrated						
Cocoa		100	43.27	11.25	4.13	27.9
Chocolate		100	8.20	2.61	1.16	4.43
Coffee and chicory essence		100	.79	.73	.02	.04
Instant coffee		100	16.41	15.55	.53	.33
Brazil nuts	1 ounce	30	2.32	1.08	.65	.59
Bread, white	1 slice	25	.68	.50	.18	tr
whole-meal	1 slice	25	2.13	1.49	.33	.31
Broccoli tops, cooked	1 cup	155	6.36	4.53	1.78	.05
Brussels sprouts, cooked	1 cup	155	4.43	3.08	1.24	.11
Cabbage, cooked	1 cup	145	4.10	2.55	1.00	.55
Carrots, young, cooked	1 cup	155	5.74	3.44	2.29	tr
Cauliflower, cooked	1 cup	125	2.25	.84	1.41	tr
Cereals						
All-Bran	1 ounce	30	8.01	5.35	1.80	.86
Corn flakes	1 cup	25	2.75	1.82	.61	.33
Grapenuts	¼ cup	30	2.10	1.54	.38	.17
Puffed Wheat	1 cup	15	2.31	1.55	0.39	0.37
Rice Krispies	1 cup	30	1.34	1.04	.23	.07
Shredded Wheat	1 biscuit	25	3.07	2.20	.66	.21
Special K	1 cup	30	1.64	1.10	.22	.32
Sugar Puffs	1 cup	30	1.82	1.20	.30	.33
Cherries, flesh and skin	10 cherries	68	.84	.63	.17	.05
Cookies						
Ginger	4 snaps	28	.56	.41	.08	.07
Oatmeal	4 cookies	52	2.08	1.64	.21	.22
Short, sweet	4 cookies	48	.80	.68	.05	.06
Corn, sweet, cooked	1 cup	165	7.82	7.11	.51	.20
canned	1 cup	165	9.39	8.20	1.06	.13
Flour						
bran		100	44.0	32.7	8.05	3.23
white	1 cup	115	3.62	2.90	.69	.03
whole-meal	1 cup	120	11.41	7.50	2.95	.96
Grapefruit, canned, fruit and syrup	½ cup	100	.44	.34	.04	.06

*Adapted from: Southgate, D. A. T. et al: "A Guide to Calculating Intakes of Dietary Fibre," *J. Human Nutr.*, 30: 303–13, 1976.

Household measures and approximate equivalent weights from: Adams, C. F. and Richardson, M.: *Nutritive Value of Foods*, HG 72. U.S. Department of Agriculture, Washington, D.C., 1977 (See Table A-1.)

Table A-3. **(Continued)**

	Measure	Weight gm	Total Dietary Fiber gm	Noncellulosic Polysaccharides gm	Cellulose gm	Lignin gm
Guavas, canned, fruit and syrup	½ cup	100	3.64	1.67	1.17	.80
Jam, strawberry	1 tablespoon	20	.22	.17	.02	.03
Lettuce, raw	⅙ head	100	1.53	.47	1.06	tr
Mangoes, canned, fruit and syrup	½ cup	100	1.00	.65	.32	.03
Marmalade, orange	1 tablespoon	20	.14	.13	.01	tr
Onions, raw	1 cup sliced	100	2.10	1.55	.55	tr
Oranges, mandarin	1 cup	200	0.58	0.44	0.08	0.06
Parsnips, raw	1 cup diced	100	4.90	3.77	1.13	tr
Peanuts	1 ounce	30	2.79	1.92	.51	.36
Peanut butter	1 tablespoon	16	1.21	.90	.31	tr
Peaches, flesh and skin	1 peach	100	2.28	1.46	.20	.62
Pears, flesh only	1 pear	164	4.00	2.16	1.10	.74
peel only		100	8.59	3.72	2.18	2.67
Peas, frozen, raw		100	7.75	5.48	2.09	.18
canned, drained	1 cup	170	13.35	8.84	3.91	.60
Peppers, cooked	1 pod	73	.68	.43	.25	tr
Pickles	1 ounce	30	.46	.27	.15	.04
Plums	1 plum	66	1.00	.65	.15	.20
Potatoes, raw	1 medium	135	4.73	3.36	1.38	tr
canned, drained		100	2.51	2.23	.28	tr
Potato chips	10 chips	20	.64	.41	.22	tr
Raisins, Sultana	1 ounce	30	1.32	.72	.25	.35
Rhubarb, raw		100	1.78	.93	.70	.75
Strawberries, raw	1 cup	149	2.65	1.39	1.04	.22
canned, fruit and syrup	½ cup	100	1.00	.48	.20	.33
Tomatoes, raw	1 medium	135	1.89	.88	.61	.41
canned, drained	1 cup	240	2.04	1.08	.89	.07
Turnips, raw		100	2.20	1.50	.70	tr

Table A-4. **Exchange Lists for Meal Planning***

Food Exchange List	Measure	Carbohydrate gm	Protein gm	Fat gm	Energy kcal
Milk, nonfat, list 1	1 cup	12	8	tr	80
Milk, whole, list 1	1 cup	12	8	10	170
Vegetables, list 2	½ cup	5	2		25
Fruits, list 3	Varies	10			40
Breads, cereals, and starchy vegetables, list 4	Varies	15	2		70
Meat, low fat, list 5	1 ounce		7	3	55
Meat, medium fat, list 5	1 ounce		7	5.5	80
Meat, high fat, list 5	1 ounce		7	8	100
Fat, list 6	1 teaspoon			5	45

*The data from this table and the *exchange lists* in this book are based on materials in *Exchange Lists for Meal Planning* prepared by Committees of the American Diabetes Association, Inc., and The American Dietetic Association in cooperation with The National Institute of Arthritis, Metabolism and Digestive Diseases and the National Heart and Lung Institute, National Institutes of Health, Public Health Service, U.S. Department of Health, Education and Welfare.

List 1. **Milk, Nonfat, Fortified.** Use only this list for diets restricted in saturated fat.

	Amounts to Use
Skim or nonfat milk	1 cup
Powdered (nonfat dry)	⅓ cup
Canned, evaporated, skim	½ cup
Buttermilk made from skim milk	1 cup
Yogurt, made from skimmed milk, plain unflavored	1 cup
Milk, low fat, fortified	
1 per cent fat, fortified (omit ½ fat exchange)	1 cup
2 per cent fat, fortified (omit 1 fat exchange)	1 cup
Yogurt made from 2 per cent fortified, plain, unflavored (omit 1 fat exchange)	1 cup
Milk, whole	
Whole milk	1 cup
Canned evaporated	½ cup
Buttermilk made from whole milk	1 cup
Yogurt made from whole milk (plain, unflavored)	1 cup

List 2. **Vegetables.** One-half cup equals one exchange.

Asparagus*
Bean sprouts
Beets
Broccoli*†
Brussels sprouts*
Cabbage*
Carrots†
Cauliflower*
Celery
Cucumbers
Eggplant
Greens*†
 Beet greens
 Chard
 Collards
 Dandelion greens
 Kale
 Mustard greens
Greens*† *(cont.)*
 Spinach
 Turnip greens
Mushrooms
Okra
Onions
Rhubarb
Rutabaga
Sauerkraut
String beans, green or yellow
Summer squash
Tomatoes*
Tomato juice*
Turnips*
Vegetable juice cocktail
Zucchini

These vegetables can be used as desired: chicory, Chinese cabbage, endive, escarole, lettuce, parsley, radishes, and watercress. See List 4, Bread Exchanges, for starchy vegetables.

*Good sources of ascorbic acid.
†Good sources of vitamin A.

Table A-4. **(Continued)**

List 3. Fruit Exchanges	Amount to Use
Apple	1 small
Apple juice	⅓ cup
Applesauce (unsweetened)	½ cup
Apricots, fresh†	2 medium
Apricots, dried†	4 halves
Bananas	½ small
Berries, blackberries	½ cup
Blueberries	½ cup
Raspberries	½ cup
Strawberries*	¾ cup
Cherries	10 large
Cider	⅓ cup
Dates	2
Figs, fresh	1
Figs, dried	1
Grapefruit*	½
Grapefruit juice*	½ cup
Grapes	12
Grape juice	¼ cup
Mango*†	½ small
Melon	
Cantaloupe*	¼ small
Honeydew*	⅛ medium
Watermelon	1 cup
Nectarine	1 medium
Orange*	1 small
Orange juice*	½ cup
Papaya*†	¾ cup
Peach†	1 medium
Pear	1 small
Persimmon	1 medium
Pineapple	½ cup
Pineapple juice	⅓ cup
Plums	2 medium
Prunes	2 medium
Prune juice	¼ cup
Raisins	2 tablespoons
Tangerine*	1 large

Cranberries may be used as desired if no sugar is added.

List 4. Bread, Cereal, and Starchy Vegetable Exchanges	Amount to Use
Bread	
White (including French and Italian)	1 slice
Whole wheat	1 slice
Rye or pumpernickel	1 slice
Raisin	1 slice
Bagel, small	½
English muffin, small	½
Frankfurt roll	½
Hamburger bun	½
Plain roll (bread)	1
Dry bread crumbs	3 tablespoons
Tortillas, 6 in.	1

Table A-4. **(Continued)**

Cereal	
Bran flakes	½ cup
Other ready-to-eat unsweetened cereal	¾ cup
Puffed cereal, unfrosted	1 cup
Cereal, cooked	½ cup
Grits, cooked	½ cup
Rice or barley, cooked	½ cup
Pastas, cooked; macaroni, noodles, spaghetti	½ cup
Popcorn, popped	3 cups
Cornmeal, dry	2 tablespoons
Flour	2½ tablespoons
Wheat germ	¼ cup
Crackers	
Arrowroot	3
Graham, 2½ in.	2
Matzoth, 4 × 6 in.	½
Oyster	20
Pretzels, 3⅛ in. × ⅛ in.	15
Rye wafers, 2 × 3½ in.	3
Saltines	6
Soda, 2½ in. square	4
Dried Beans, Peas, and Lentils	
Dried beans, peas, and lentils, cooked	½ cup
Baked beans, no pork	¼ cup
Starchy Vegetables	
Corn	⅓ cup
Corn on cob	1 small
Lima beans	½ cup
Parsnips	⅔ cup
Peas, green, fresh, canned, or frozen	½ cup
Potato, white	1 small
Potato, mashed	½ cup
Pumpkin	¾ cup
Winter squash, acorn or butternut	½ cup
Yam or sweet potato	¼ cup
Prepared Foods	
Biscuit, 2 in. diam. (omit 1 fat exchange)	1
Corn bread, 2 × 2 × 1 in. (omit 1 fat exchange)	1
Corn muffin, 2 in. diam. (omit 1 fat exchange)	1
Crackers, round, butter type (omit 1 fat exchange)	5
Muffin, plain, small (omit 1 fat exchange)	1
Pancake, 5 × ½ in. (omit 1 fat exchange)	1
Potatoes, french fried, 2 in. to 3½ in. (omit 1 fat exchange)	8 pieces
Potato or corn chips (omit 2 fat exchanges)	15
Waffle, 5 × ½ in. (omit 1 fat exchange)	1

List 5. Meat and Protein-Rich Exchanges

Lean Meat, Protein-Rich Exchanges. Use only this list for diets low in saturated fat and cholesterol.

	Amount to Use
Beef: baby beef (very lean), chipped beef, chuck, flank steak, tenderloin, plate ribs, plate skirt steak, round (bottom, top), all cuts rump, spare ribs, tripe	1 ounce
Lamb: leg, rib, sirloin, loin (roast and chops), shank shoulder	1 ounce
Pork: leg (whole rump, center shank), smoked ham (center slices)	1 ounce

Table A-4. **(Continued)**

Veal: leg, loin, rib, shank, shoulder, cutlets	1 ounce
Poultry: without skin of chicken, turkey, Cornish hen, Guinea hen, pheasant	1 ounce
Fish; any fresh or frozen	1 ounce
canned crab, lobster, mackerel, salmon, tuna	¼ cup
clams, oysters, scallops, shrimp	5 or 1 ounce
sardines, drained	3
Cheeses; containing less than 5 per cent butterfat	1 ounce
Cottage cheese: dry or 2 per cent butter fat	¼ cup
Dried peas and beans (omit 1 bread exchange)	½ cup
Medium Fat Meat and Protein-Rich Exhchanges	
Beef: ground, 15 per cent fat; corned beef, canned; rib eye; round, ground (commercial)	1 ounce
Pork: loin, all cuts tenderloin; shoulder arm (picnic); shoulder blade; Boston Butt; Canadian bacon; boiled ham	1 ounce
Liver, heart, kidney, and sweetbreads (high in cholesterol)	1 ounce
Cottage cheese, creamed	¼ cup
Cheese: Mozzarella, ricotta, farmer's, Neufchatel,	1 ounce
Parmesan	3 tablespoons
Eggs (high in cholesterol)	1
Peanut butter (omit 2 fat exchanges)	2 tablespoons
High-Fat Meat and Protein-Rich Exchanges	
Beef: brisket; corned beef brisket; ground beef (over 20 per cent fat); hamburger (commercial); chuck, ground (commercial); rib roast; club and rib steak	1 ounce
Lamb: breast	1 ounce
Pork; spare ribs; loin (back ribs); pork, ground; country style ham; deviled ham	1 ounce
Veal: breast	1 ounce
Poultry; capon, duck (domestic), goose	1 ounce
Cheese; cheddar type	1 ounce
Cold cuts, $4\frac{1}{2} \times \frac{1}{8}$ in.	1 slice
Frankfurter	1 small

List 6. Fat Exchanges

For a diet low in saturated fat and higher in polyunsaturated fat select only from this list.

	Amount to Use
Margarine: soft, tub, or stick (made with corn, cottonseed, safflower, soy, or sunflower oil)	1 teaspoon
Avocado, 4 in. diam.	⅛
Nuts	
Almonds*	10 whole
Peanuts*	
Spanish	20 whole
Virginia	10 whole
Pecans*	2 large, whole
Walnuts	6 small
Other nuts*	6 small
Oil, corn, cottonseed, safflower, soy, sunflower	1 teaspoon
Oil, olive or peanut*	1 teaspoon
Olives*	5 small
Salad dressings, if made with corn, cottonseed, safflower, or soy oil	
French dressing	1 tablespoon

*Fat content is primarily monounsaturated.

Table A-4. **(Continued)**

Italian dressing	1 tablespoon
Mayonnaise	1 teaspoon
Salad dressing, mayonnaise type	2 teaspoons

The following fats should not be used on a diet low in saturated fat.

Margarine, regular stick	1 teaspoon
Butter	1 teaspoon
Bacon fat	1 teaspoon
Bacon, crisp	1 strip
Cream, light	2 tablespoons
Cream, sour	2 tablespoons
Cream, heavy	1 tablespoon
Cream cheese	1 tablespoon
Lard	1 teaspoon
Salad dressings (permitted on restricted diets only if made with allowed oils)	
French dressing	1 tablespoon
Italian dressing	1 tablespoon
Mayonnaise	1 teaspoon
Salad dressing, mayonnaise type	2 teaspoons
Salt pork	¾ in. cube

Table A-5. Cholesterol Content of the Edible Portion of Food*

Food	Household Measure	Weight gm	Cholesterol mg
Beef, lean, trimmed of separable fat, cooked	3 ounces	85	(77)†
Beef-vegetable stew			
Home recipe	1 cup	245	63
Canned	1 cup	245	36
Beef potpie			
Home prepared, baked	1/3 9-in. pie	210	44
Commercial, frozen, unheated	1 pie	216	38
Brains, raw		100	> 2,000
Butter	1 tablespoon	14	35
Buttermilk, from nonfat milk	1 cup	245	5
Cakes, home recipes			
Chocolate, chocolate frosting	1/16 9-in. diam.	75	32
Fruitcake, dark	1/30 8-in. loaf	15	7
Sponge	1/12 10-in. diam.	66	162
Yellow, chocolate frosting	1/16 9-in. diam.	75	33
Baked from mixes			
Angel food	1/12 10-in. diam.	53	0
Chocolate, with eggs, chocolate frosting	1/16 9-in. diam.	69	33
	cupcake, small	36	17
Gingerbread	1/9 8-in. square	63	trace
White, 2 layer, chocolate frosting	1/16 9-in. diam.	71	1
Yellow, 2 layer, with eggs, chocolate frosting	1/16 9-in. diam.	75	36
Caviar, sturgeon, granular	1 tablespoon	16	> 48
Cheeses, natural			
Blue	1 ounce	28	(24)
Camembert	triangular wedge	38	(35)
Cheddar, mild or sharp	1 ounce	28	28
Cottage, creamed, 1% fat	1 cup	267	23
4% fat	1 cup	245	48
Uncreamed	1 cup	200	13
Cream cheese	1 tablespoon	14	16
Edam	1 ounce	28	(29)
Mozzarella, part skim	1 ounce	28	18
Muenster	1 ounce	28	(25)
Parmesan, grated	1 cup	100	(113)
Provolone	1 ounce	28	(28)
Ricotta, part skim	1 ounce	28	(14)
Swiss	slice, rectangular	35	35
Pasteurized process, American	1 ounce	28	(25)
Swiss	1 ounce	28	(26)
Pasteurized process spread	1 tablespoon	14	(9)
Cheese soufflé, home recipe	1/4 of 7-in. diam.	110	184
Chicken, breast, cooked meat and skin	1/2 breast	92	74
meat only	1/2 breast	80	63
Drumstick, meat and skin	1 drumstick	52	47
meat only	1 drumstick	43	39
Chicken à la king, home recipe	1 cup	245	185
Chicken fricassee, home recipe	1 cup	240	96
Chicken potpie, home recipe	1/3 9-in. diam.	232	71
Commercial, frozen, unheated	1 pie	227	29

*Adapted from Feeley, R. M. et al.: "Cholesterol Content of Foods," *J. Am. Diet. Assoc.*, **61**:134–49, 1972.

†Numbers in parentheses indicate imputed values.

Table A-5. **(Continued)**

Food	Household Measure	Weight gm	Cholesterol mg
Chop suey with meat, home recipe	1 cup	250	64
Canned	3 ounces	85	10
Chow mein, without noodles, home recipe	1 cup	250	77
Clams, ‡ raw, meat only	1 cup (19 large soft or 7 round chowders)	227	114
Cod, raw, flesh only	3½ ounces	100	50
Cookies			
Brownies with nuts, home recipe	1 brownie 1¾ in. square	20	17
Ladyfingers	4 ladyfingers	44	157
Corn pudding	1 cup	245	102
Corn bread, home recipe	piece, 2½ in. square	83	58
Baked from mix	piece	55	38
	muffin	40	28
Crab, steamed, meat only	1 cup	125	100
Canned, meat only	1 cup	160	(161)
Cream, half and half	1 tablespoon	15	6
Light, coffee	1 tablespoon	15	10
Sour	1 tablespoon	12	8
Whipped topping (pressurized)	1 cup	60	51
Heavy whipping (unwhipped)	1 tablespoon	15	20
Cream puff, custard filling	1 cream puff	130	188
Custard, baked	½ cup	133	139
Egg, whole	1 large	50	252
White	one	33	0
Yolk	one	17	252
Flounder, raw, flesh only	3½ ounces	100	50
Frog legs, raw (refuse: 35%)	3½ ounces	100	50
Gizzard, chicken, cooked	3 ounces	85	(166)
Turkey, cooked	3 ounces	85	196
Haddock, raw, flesh only	3½ ounces	100	60
Halibut, cooked, flesh only	piece, 6½ × 2½ × ⅝ in.	125	(60)
Heart, beef, cooked	1 cup chopped	145	(398)
Herring, raw, flesh only	3½ ounces	100	85
Ice cream, 10% fat	1 cup	133	53
Frozen custard or French	1 cup	133	97
Ice milk, hardened	1 cup	131	26
Soft-serve	1 cup	175	36
Kidneys, all kinds, cooked	1 cup sliced	140	(1,125)
Lamb, lean, trimmed, cooked	3 ounces	85	(85)
Lard	1 cup	205	195
Liver, including beef, calf, hog, lamb, cooked	3 ounces	85	(372)
Chicken, cooked	1 liver	25	(187)
Turkey, cooked	1 cup chopped	140	839
Lobster, cooked, meat only	1 cup cubed	145	123
Lobster Newburg, with butter, egg yolks, sherry, cream	1 cup	250	456
Macaroni and cheese, home recipe	1 cup	200	42
Mackerel, broiled	piece 8½ × 2½ × ½ in.	105	(106)
Margarine			
All vegetable fat			0
⅔ animal fat, ½ vegetable fat	1 tablespoon	14	7

‡Cholesterol accounts for about 40 per cent of the total sterol content of clams.

Table A-5. **(Continued)**

Food	Household Measure	Weight gm	Cholesterol mg
Milk, whole	1 cup	244	34
Low fat, 1% with 1 to 2% nonfat milk solids	1 cup	246	14
2% fat with 1 to 2% nonfat milk solids	1 cup	246	22
Nonfat, skim	1 cup	245	5
Canned, undiluted evaporated	1 cup	252	79
Condensed sweetened	1 cup	306	105
Dry, to make 1 quart diluted	1 ⅓ cups	91	20
Chocolate beverage, commercial flavored milk drink with 2% added butterfat	1 cup	250	20
Flavored milk	1 cup	250	32
Cocoa, homemade	1 cup	250	35
Muffins, plain, home recipe	1 muffin	40	21
Noodles, whole egg, dry	8-ounce package	227	213
Cooked	1 cup	160	50
Chow mein, canned	1 cup	45	5
Oysters, § meat only, raw	1 cup, 13–19 medium; 19–31 small; 4–6 Pacific medium	240	120
Canned, solids and liquid	3 ounces	85	(38)
Oyster stew, home prepared, 1 part oysters, 2 parts milk	1 cup	240	63
Pancakes, mix, with eggs, milk	cake 6-in. diam.	73	54
Pepper, stuffed with beef and crumbs	pepper with 1 ⅛ cup stuffing	185	56
Pies, baked			
Apple			0
Custard	⅛ of 9-in. diam.	114	120
Lemon chiffon	⅛ of 9 in. diam.	81	137
Lemon meringue	⅛ of 9-in. diam.	105	98
Peach			0
Pumpkin	⅛ of 9-in. diam.	114	70
Popovers, home recipe	1 popover (from ¼ cup batter)	40	59
Pork, lean, trimmed, cooked	3 ounces	85	(75)
Potatoes, au gratin, milk, cheese	1 cup	245	36
Scalloped, milk	1 cup	245	14
Salad, mayonnaise, hard-cooked egg	1 cup	250	162
Pudding, chocolate, mix	1 cup	260	30
Vanilla, home recipe (blanc mange)	1 cup	255	35
Rabbit, domesticated, cooked	1 cup diced	140	(127)
Rice pudding with raisins	1 cup	265	29
Roe, salmon, raw	1 ounce	28	101
Salad dressing			
Mayonnaise, commercial	1 tablespoon	14	10
Salad dressing, home recipe	1 tablespoon	16	12
Mayonnaise-type, commercial	1 tablespoon	15	8
Salmon, red, broiled steak (refuse: 12%)	6¾ × 2½ × 1 in.	145	(59)
Canned, solids and liquid	3 ounces	85	30
Sardines, drained solids	can—3¼ ounces	92	129
Sausage, frankfurter, all meat	1 frank	56	(34)
Scallops, ‖ muscle only, steamed	3 ounces	85	(45)

§Cholesterol accounts for about 40 per cent of the total sterol of oysters.
‖Cholesterol accounts for about 30 per cent of total sterol of scallops.

Table A-5. **(Continued)**

Food	Household Measure	Weight gm	Cholesterol mg
Shrimp, raw, flesh only	3½ ounces	100	150
Canned, drained solids	1 cup—22 large or 76 small	128	192
Spaghetti with meatballs in tomato sauce			
Home recipe	1 cup	248	75
Canned	1 cup	250	39
Sweetbreads (thymus), cooked	3 ounces	85	(396)
Tapioca cream pudding	1 cup	165	159
Tartar sauce, regular	1 tablespoon	14	7
Trout, raw, flesh only	3½ ounces	100	55
Tuna, canned in oil, drained	can (No. ½); 5½ ounces	157	102
Canned in water, solids and liquid	can (No. ½); 6½ ounces	184	(116)
Turkey, cooked, light meat, without skin	3 ounces	85	65
Dark meat, without skin	3 ounces	85	86
Turkey potpie, home prepared	⅓ 9-in. diam.	232	71
Commercial, frozen	1 pie	227	20
Veal, lean, cooked	3 ounces	85	(84)
Waffles, mix, egg, milk	1 waffle 9 × 9 in.	200	119
Welsh rarebit	1 cup	232	71
White sauce, thin	1 cup	250	36
Medium	1 cup	250	33
Thick	1 cup	250	30
Yogurt, nonfat, plain or vanilla	carton; 8 ounces	227	17
Fruit flavored	carton; 8 ounces	227	15

Table A–6. Physical Growth NCHS Percentiles: Girls, Birth to 36 Months*

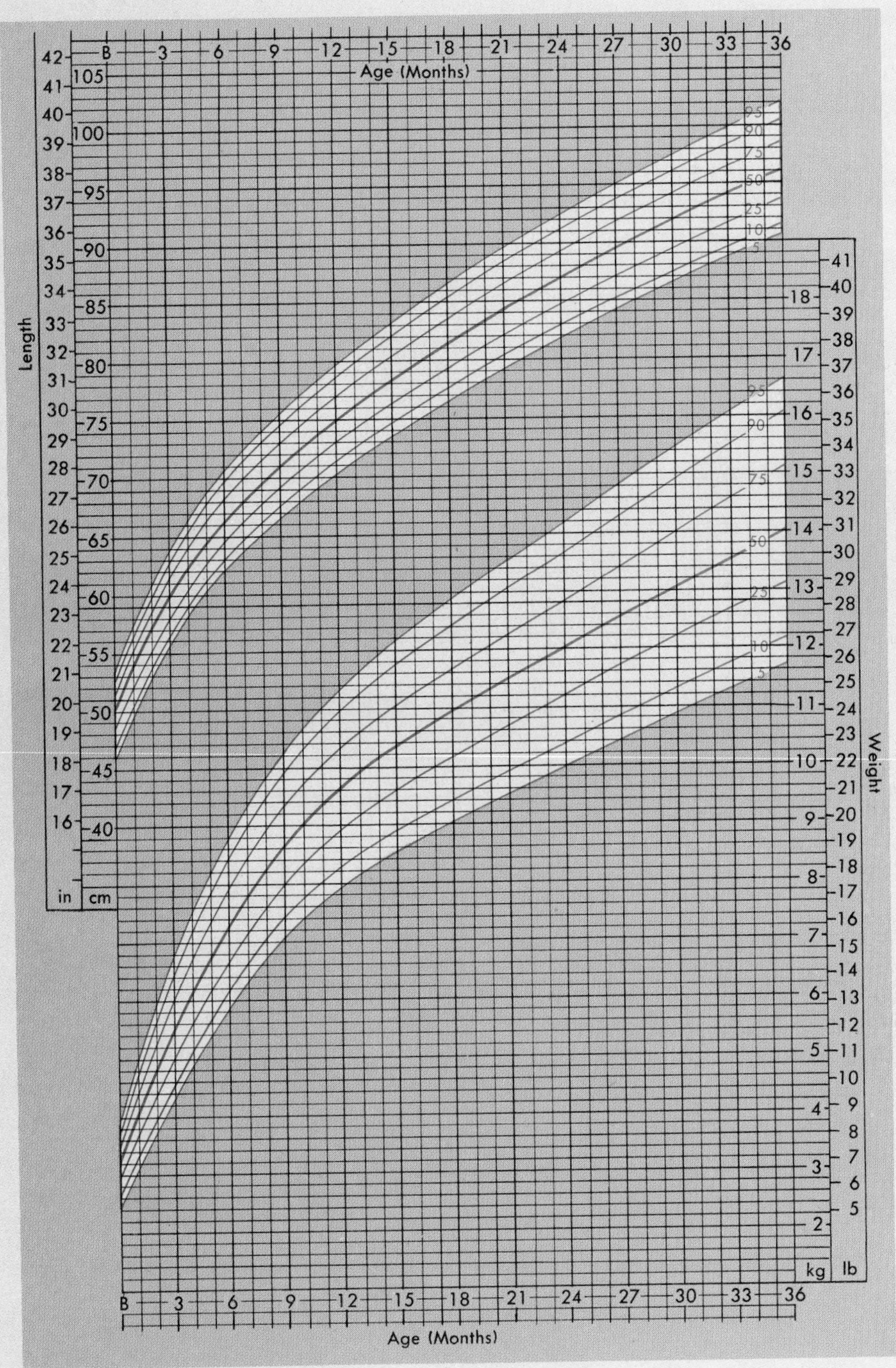

* Charts prepared by Ross Laboratories, Columbus, Ohio. Adapted from: National Center for Health Statistics; *NCHS Growth Charts, 1976*. Monthly Vital Statistics Report. Vol. 25, No. 3, Supp. (HRA) 76–1120. Health Resources Administration, Rockville, Maryland, June 1976. Data from the Fels Research Institute, Yellow Springs, Ohio. Copyright by Ross Laboratories.

Table A–7. Physical Growth NCHS Percentiles: Girls, 2 to 18 Years*

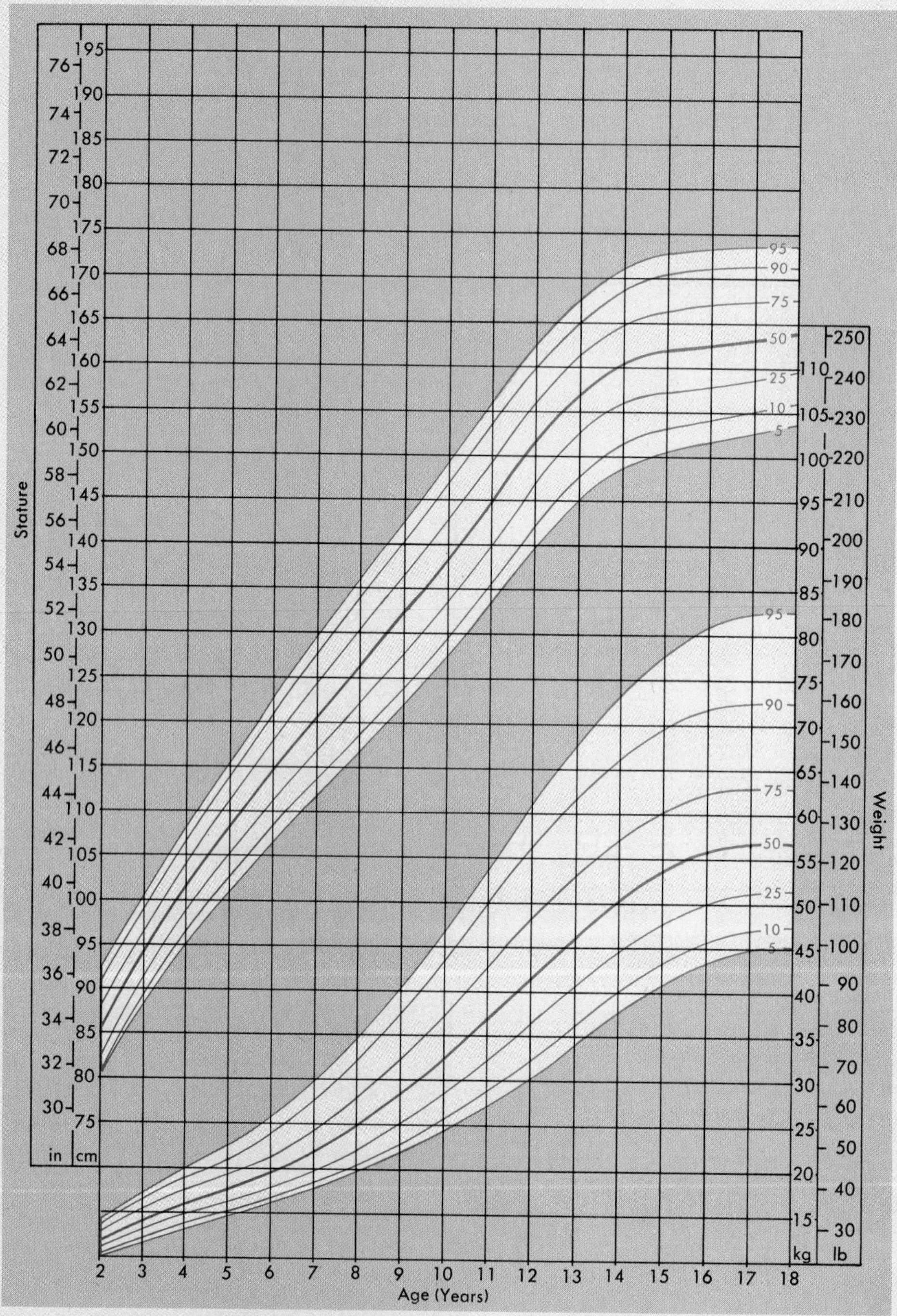

* Charts prepared by Ross Laboratories, Columbus, Ohio. Adapted from: National Center for Health Statistics: *NCHS Growth Charts, 1976.* Monthly Vital Statistics Report. Vol. 25, No. 3, Supp. (HRA) 76–1120. Health Resources Administration, Rockville, Maryland, June 1976. Data from National Center for Health Statistics. Copyright by 1976 Ross Laboratories.

Table A–8. Physical Growth NCHS Percentiles: Boys, Birth to 36 Months*

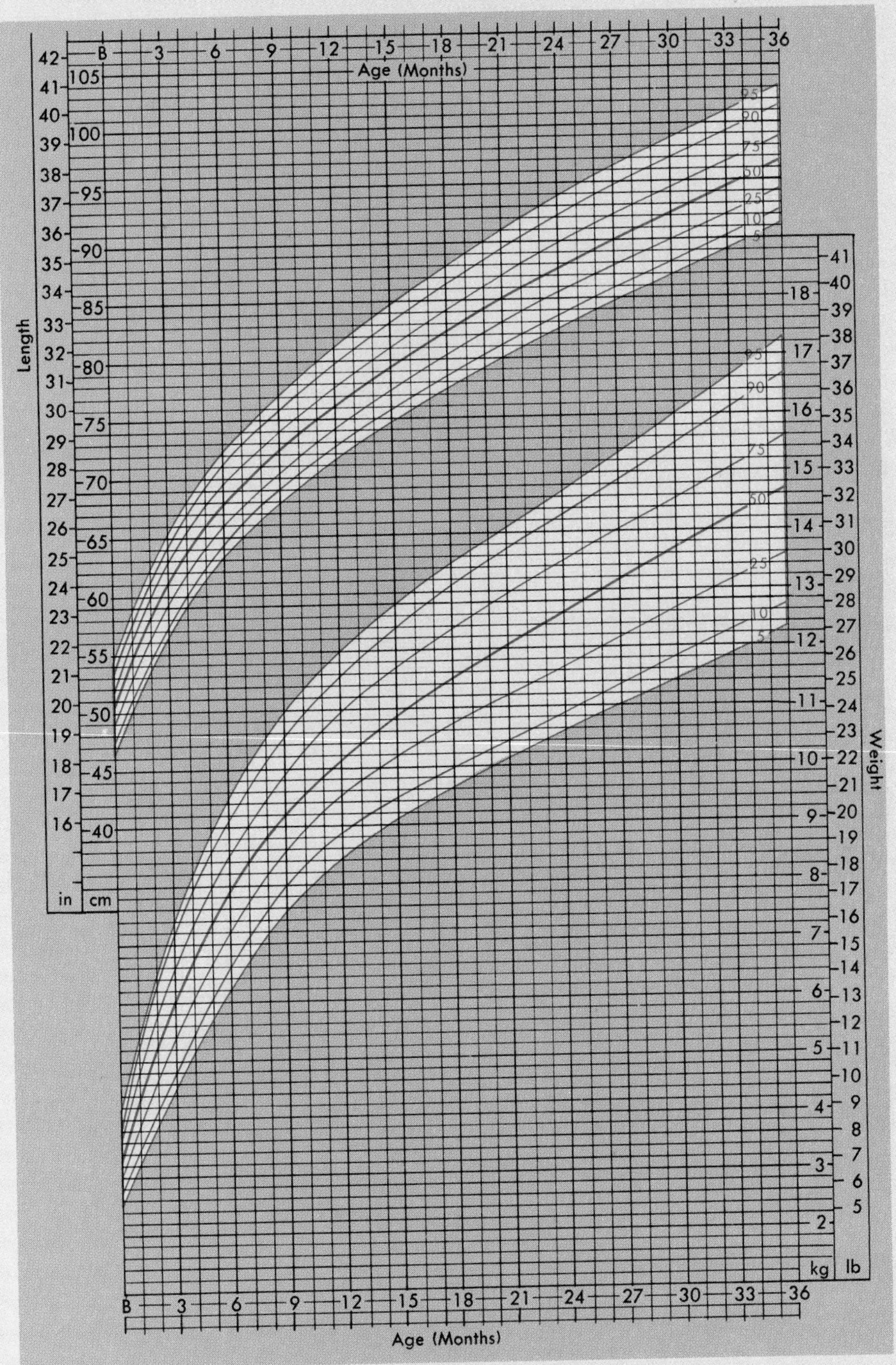

* Charts prepared by Ross Laboratories, Columbus, Ohio. Adapted from: National Center for Health Statistics: *NCHS Growth Charts, 1976.* Monthly Vital Statistics Report. Vol. 25, No. 3, Supp. (HRA) 76–1120. Health Resources Administration, Rockville, Maryland, June 1976. Data from The Fels Research Institute, Yellow Springs, Ohio. Copyright by 1976 Ross Laboratories.

Table A–9. Physical Growth NCHS Percentiles: Boys, 2 to 18 Years*

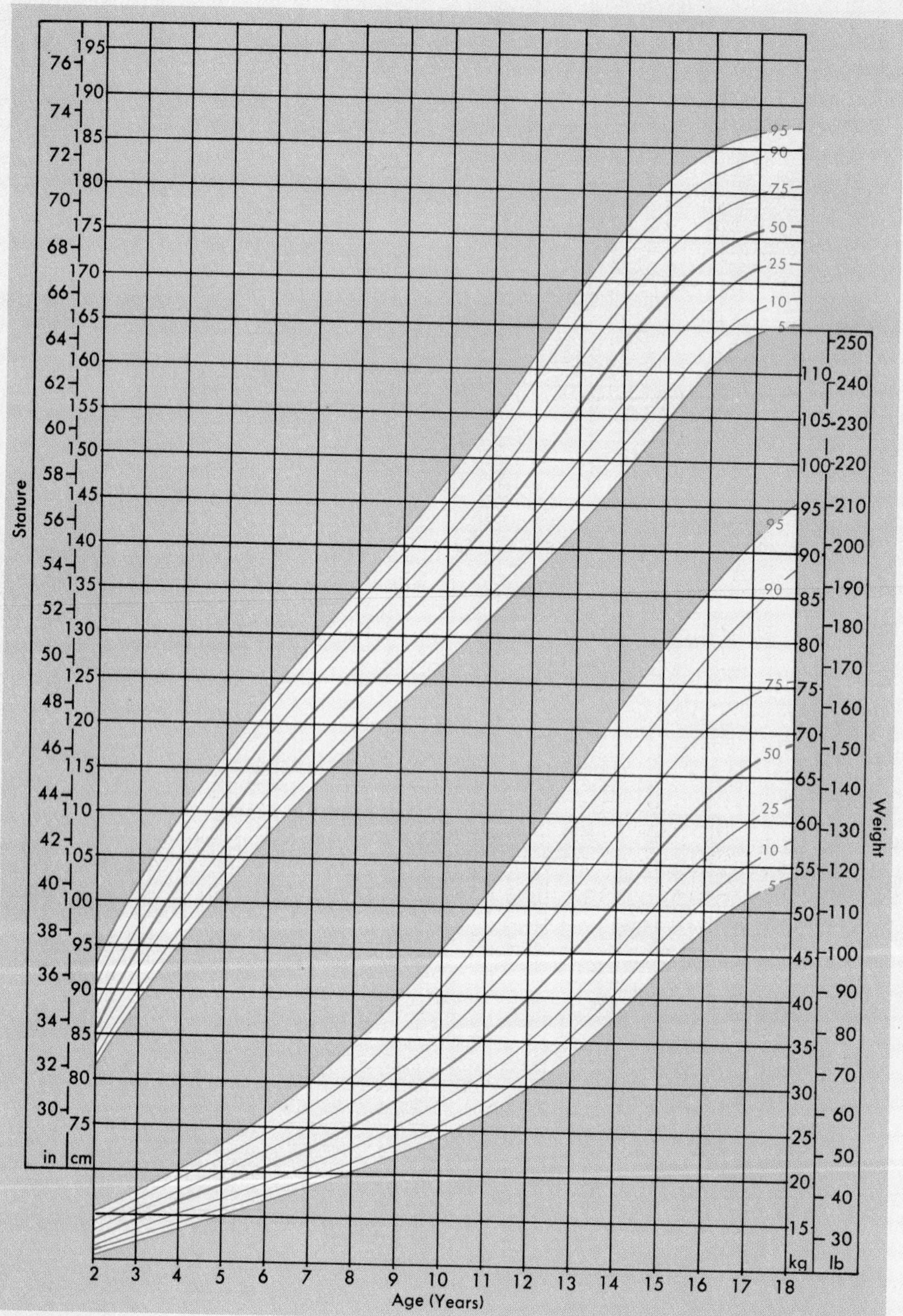

* Charts prepared by Ross Laboratories, Columbus, Ohio. Adapted from: National Center for Health Statistics: *NCHS Growth Charts, 1976.* Monthly Vital Statistics Report, Vol. 25, No. 3, supp. (HRA) 76–1120. Health Resources Administration, Rockville, Maryland, June 1976. Data from National Center for Health Statistics. Copyright by 1976 Ross Laboratories.

Table A-10. **Suggested Weights for Heights for Men and Women***

Height (without shoes) inches	Weight (without clothing) Low	Median pounds	High	Height centimeters	Low	Weight Median kilograms	High
Men							
63	118	129	141	160	54	59	64
64	122	133	145	163	55	60	66
65	126	137	149	165	57	62	68
66	130	142	155	167	59	65	70
67	134	147	161	170	61	67	73
68	139	151	166	173	63	69	75
69	143	155	170	175	65	70	77
70	147	159	174	178	67	72	80
71	150	163	178	180	68	74	81
72	154	167	183	183	70	76	83
73	158	171	188	185	72	77	85
74	162	175	192	188	74	80	87
75	165	178	195	191	75	81	89
Women							
60	100	109	118	152	45	50	54
61	104	112	121	155	47	51	55
62	107	115	125	157	49	52	57
63	110	118	128	160	50	54	58
64	113	122	132	163	51	55	60
65	116	125	135	165	53	57	61
66	120	129	139	167	55	59	63
67	123	132	142	170	56	60	65
68	126	136	146	173	57	62	66
69	130	140	151	175	59	64	69
70	133	144	156	178	60	65	71
71	137	148	161	180	62	67	73
72	141	152	166	183	64	69	75

*Data for heights in inches and weights in pounds taken from: Hathaway, M. L., and Foard, E. D.: *Heights and Weights of Adults in the United States.* Home Economics Research Report No. 10, U.S. Department of Agriculture, Washington, D.C., Table 80, p. 111.

Conversions to centimeters and kilograms were rounded off to the nearest whole number.

Table A-11. **Percentiles for Upper Arm Circumference and Triceps Skinfolds for Whites of the Ten-State Nutrition Survey of 1968–1970***

Age Group	Age Midpoint, years	Arm Circumference Percentiles, mm					Triceps Skinfold Percentiles, mm				
		5th	15th	50th	85th	95th	5th	15th	50th	85th	95th
Males											
0.0–0.4	0.3	113	120	134	147	153	4	5	8	12	15
0.5–1.4	1	128	137	152	168	175	5	7	9	13	15
1.5–2.4	2	141	147	157	170	180	5	7	10	13	14
2.5–3.4	3	144	150	161	175	182	6	7	9	12	14
3.5–4.4	4	143	150	165	180	190	5	6	9	12	14
4.5–5.4	5	146	155	169	185	199	5	6	8	12	16
5.5–6.4	6	151	159	172	188	198	5	6	8	11	15
6.5–7.4	7	154	162	176	194	212	4	6	8	11	14
7.5–8.4	8	161	168	185	205	233	5	6	8	12	17
8.5–9.4	9	165	174	190	217	262	5	6	9	14	19
9.5–10.4	10	170	180	200	228	255	5	6	10	16	22
10.5–11.4	11	177	186	208	240	276	6	7	10	17	25
11.5–12.4	12	184	194	216	253	291	5	7	11	19	26
12.5–13.4	13	186	198	230	270	297	5	6	10	18	25
13.5–14.4	14	198	211	243	279	321	5	6	10	17	22
14.5–15.4	15	202	220	253	302	320	4	6	9	19	26
15.5–16.4	16	217	232	262	300	335	4	5	9	20	27
16.5–17.4	17	230	238	275	306	326	4	5	8	14	20
17.5–24.4	21	250	264	292	330	354	4	5	10	18	25
24.5–34.4	30	260	280	310	344	366	4	6	11	21	28
34.5–44.4	40	259	280	312	345	371	4	6	12	22	28
Females											
0.0–0.4	0.3	107	118	127	145	150	4	5	8	12	13
0.5–1.4	1	125	134	146	162	170	6	7	9	12	15
1.5–2.4	2	136	143	155	171	180	6	7	10	13	15
2.5–3.4	3	137	145	157	169	176	6	7	10	12	14
3.5–4.4	4	145	150	162	176	184	5	7	10	12	14
4.5–5.4	5	149	155	169	185	195	6	7	10	13	16
5.5–6.4	6	148	158	170	187	202	6	7	10	12	15
6.5–7.4	7	153	162	178	199	216	6	7	10	13	17
7.5–8.4	8	158	166	183	207	231	6	7	10	15	19
8.5–9.4	9	166	175	192	222	255	6	7	11	17	24
9.5–10.4	10	170	181	203	236	263	6	8	12	19	24
10.5–11.4	11	173	186	210	251	280	7	8	12	20	29
11.5–12.4	12	185	196	220	256	275	6	9	13	20	25
12.5–13.4	13	186	204	230	270	294	7	9	14	23	30
13.5–14.4	14	201	214	240	284	306	8	10	15	22	28
14.5–15.4	15	205	216	245	281	310	8	11	16	24	30
15.5–16.4	16	211	224	249	286	322	8	10	15	23	27
16.5–17.4	17	207	224	250	291	328	9	12	16	26	31
17.5–24.4	21	215	233	260	297	329	9	12	17	25	31
24.5–34.4	30	230	243	275	324	361	9	12	19	29	36
34.5–44.4	40	232	250	286	340	374	10	14	22	32	39

*Source: Frisancho, A. R.: "Triceps Skin Fold and Upper Arm Muscle Size Norms for Assessment of Nutritional Status," *Am. J. Clin. Nutr.*, 27: 1052–58, 1974.

Table A-12. **Percentiles for Upper Arm Diameter and Upper Arm Circumference for Whites of the Ten-State Nutrition Survey of 1968-1970***

Age Midpoint, years†	Arm Muscle									
	Diameter Percentiles, mm					Circumference Percentiles, mm				
	5th	15th	50th	85th	95th	5th	15th	50th	85th	95th
Males										
0.3	26	30	34	40	42	81	94	106	125	133
1	32	34	39	44	46	100	108	123	137	146
2	35	37	40	44	46	111	117	127	138	146
3	36	38	42	46	48	114	121	132	145	152
4	38	39	43	48	50	118	124	135	151	157
5	39	41	45	50	53	121	130	141	156	166
6	40	43	47	51	53	127	134	146	159	167
7	41	43	48	52	55	130	137	151	164	173
8	44	46	50	55	59	138	144	158	174	185
9	44	46	51	58	64	138	143	161	182	200
10	45	48	53	59	64	142	152	168	186	202
11	48	50	55	62	67	150	158	174	194	211
12	49	52	58	66	70	153	163	181	207	221
13	51	54	62	71	77	159	169	195	224	242
14	53	58	67	74	84	167	182	211	234	265
15	55	59	70	80	86	173	185	220	252	271
16	59	65	73	83	89	186	205	229	260	281
17	66	69	78	86	92	206	217	245	271	290
21	69	74	82	91	97	217	232	258	286	305
30	70	77	86	94	100	220	241	270	295	315
40	71	76	86	96	101	222	239	270	300	318
Females										
0.3	27	29	33	37	40	86	92	104	115	126
1	31	32	37	41	43	97	102	117	128	135
2	34	36	40	44	46	105	112	125	140	146
3	34	37	41	44	46	108	116	128	138	143
4	36	38	42	46	48	114	120	132	146	152
5	38	40	44	48	51	119	124	138	151	160
6	38	41	45	49	53	121	129	140	155	165
7	39	42	47	52	56	123	132	146	162	175
8	41	44	48	53	59	129	138	151	168	186
9	43	45	50	56	62	136	143	157	176	193
10	44	47	52	58	62	139	147	163	182	196
11	44	48	55	62	67	140	152	171	195	209
12	48	51	57	64	68	150	161	179	200	212
13	49	53	59	66	71	155	165	185	206	225
14	53	56	61	70	74	166	175	193	221	234
15	52	55	62	70	74	163	173	195	220	232
16	54	57	64	72	83	171	178	200	227	260
17	54	56	62	71	77	171	177	196	223	241
21	54	58	65	73	80	170	183	205	229	253
30	56	60	68	78	87	177	189	213	245	272
40	57	61	69	80	89	180	192	216	250	279

*Source: Frisancho, A. R.: "Triceps Skin Fold and Upper Arm Muscle Size Norms for Assessment of Nutritional Status," *Am. J. Clin. Nutr.*, 27: 1052-58, 1974.

†The age groups are the same as in Table A-11.

Table A–13. Arm Anthropometry Nomogram for Adults*

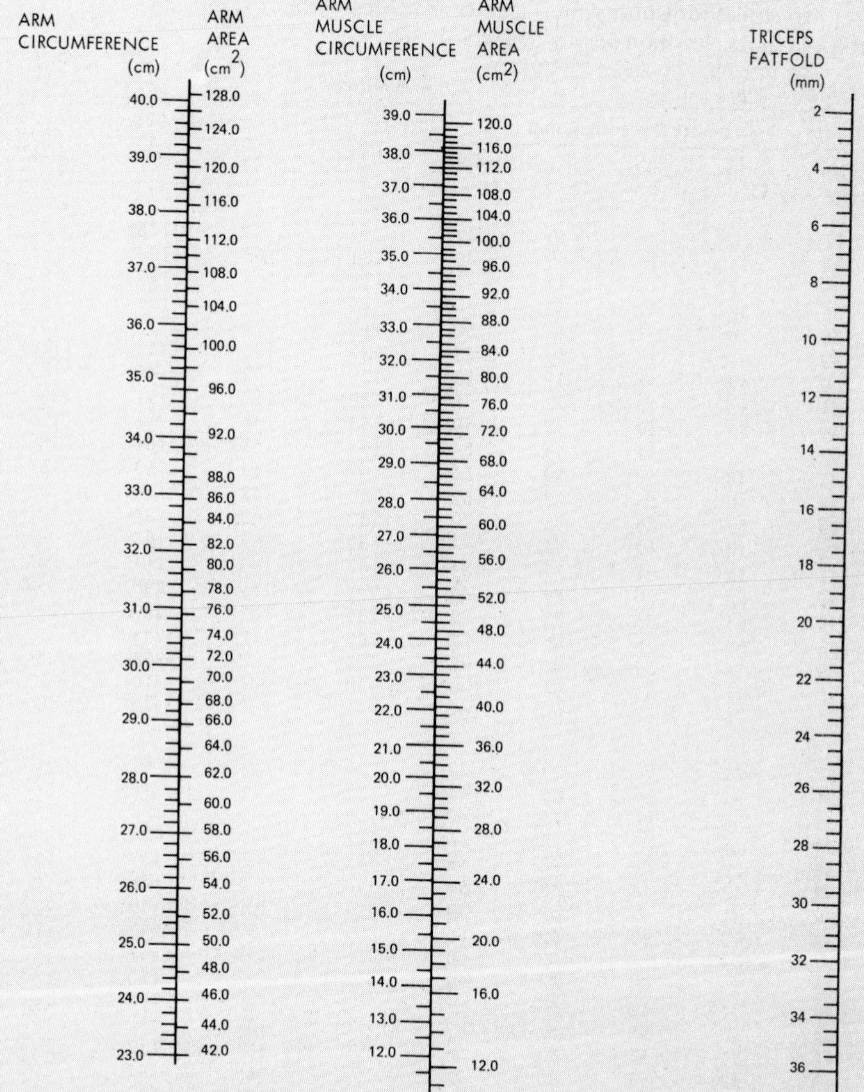

TO OBTAIN MUSCLE CIRCUMFERENCE:

1. LAY RULER BETWEEN VALUE OF ARM CIRCUMFERENCE AND FATFOLD
2. READ OFF MUSCLE CIRCUMFERENCE ON MIDDLE LINE

TO OBTAIN TISSUE AREAS:

1. THE ARM AREA AND MUSCLE AREA ARE ALONGSIDE THEIR RESPECTIVE CIRCUMFERENCES
2. FAT AREA = ARM AREA-MUSCLE AREA

* Source: Gurney, J. M., and Jelliffe, D. B.: "Arm Anthropometry in Nutritional Assessment: Nomogram for Rapid Calculation of Muscle Circumference and Cross-Sectional Muscle and Fat Areas," *Am. J. Clin. Nutr.*, **26**:912–15, 1973.

Table A–14. Arm Anthropometry Nomogram for Children*

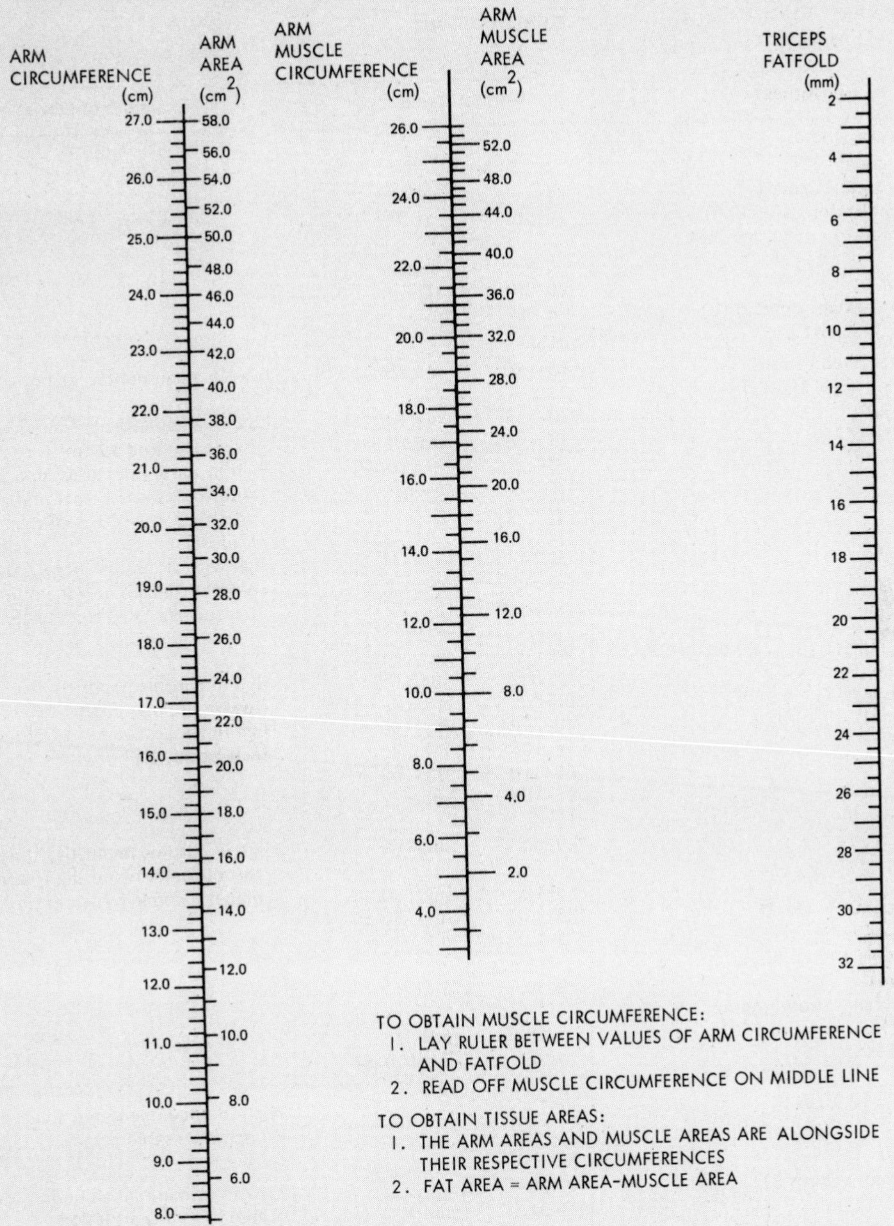

TO OBTAIN MUSCLE CIRCUMFERENCE:

1. LAY RULER BETWEEN VALUES OF ARM CIRCUMFERENCE AND FATFOLD
2. READ OFF MUSCLE CIRCUMFERENCE ON MIDDLE LINE

TO OBTAIN TISSUE AREAS:

1. THE ARM AREAS AND MUSCLE AREAS ARE ALONGSIDE THEIR RESPECTIVE CIRCUMFERENCES
2. FAT AREA = ARM AREA–MUSCLE AREA

* Source: Gurney, J. M., and Jelliffe, D. B.: "Arm Anthropometry in Nutritional Assessment: Nomogram for Rapid Calculation of Muscle Circumference and Cross-Sectional Muscle and Fat Areas," *Am. J. Clin. Nutr.*, **26**:912–15, 1973.

Table A-15. **Normal Constituents of Human Blood**
(B = whole blood; P = plasma; S = serum)

Constituent	Normal Range		Examples of Deviations
Physical Measurements			
Specific gravity (S)	1.025-1.029		
Bleeding time, capillary	1-3	min	
Prothrombin time (Quick, P)	10-20	sec	
Sedimentation rate (Wintrobe)			
Men	0-9	mm/hr	
Women	0-20	mm/hr	
Viscosity (water as unity) (B)	4.5-5.5		
Acid-Base Constituents			
Base, total fixed cations (Na + K + Ca + Mg) (S)	143-150	mEq/L	Low in alkali deficit; diabetic acidosis
Sodium (S)	320-335 139-146	mg/100 ml mEq/L	Low in alkali deficit; diabetic acidosis, excessive fluid administration
Potassium (S)	16-22 4.1-5.6	mg/100 ml mEq/L	High in acute infections, pneumonia, Addison's disease; low in diarrhea, vomiting, correction of diabetic acidosis
Calcium (S)	9-11 4.5-5.5	mg/100 ml mEq/L	High with excessive vitamin D, hyperparathyroidism; low in infantile tetany, steatorrhea, severe nephritis, defective vitamin D absorption
Calcium, ionized (S)	50-60	per cent	
Magnesium (S)	2-3 1.65-2.5	mg/100 ml mEq/L	High in chronic nephritis, liver disease; low in uremia, tetany, severe diarrhea
Chloride (S)	340-372 96-105	mg/100 ml mEq/L	High in congestive heart failure, eclampsia, nephritis
As NaCL (S)	560-614 96-105	mg/100 ml mEq/L	
Phosphorus, inorganic as P (S)			
Child	4.0-6.5	mg/100 ml	High in chronic nephritis, hypoparathyroidism; low during treatment of diabetic coma, hyperparathyroidism
Adult	2.5-4.5	mg/100 ml	
Sulfates as SO_4^{--} (S)	2.5-5.0 0.5-1.0	mg/100 ml mEq/L	
Bicarbonate cation-binding power (S)	19-30	mEq/L	
Serum protein cation-binding power (S)	15.5-18.0	mEq/L	
Lactic acid (S)	10-20 1.1-2.2	mg/100 ml mEq/L	
pH at 38°C (B, P, or S)	7.30-7.45		High in uncompensated alkalosis; low in uncompensated acidosis
Blood Gases			
CO_2 content (venous S)	45-70 20.3-31.5	vol % mM/L	Low in primary alkali deficit, diarrhea; high in hypoventilation
CO_2 content (venous B)	40-60 18-27	vol % mM/L	
CO_2 tension (pCO_2) arterial blood	35-45	mm Hg	pCO_2 in venous blood is about 6 mm higher than arterial or capillary blood
Oxygen content (arterial B)	15-22	vol %	High in polycythemia; low in emphysema
Oxygen content (venous B)	11-16	vol %	
Oxygen capacity (B)	16-24	vol %	
Oxygen tension (pO_2)	85-100	mm Hg	

Table A-15. **(Continued)**

Constituent	Normal Range		Examples of Deviations
Carbohydrates			
Glucose			
Reducing substances (B)	90–120	mg/100 ml	High in diabetes mellitus; low in hyperinsulinism
"True"	60–85	mg/100 ml	
Glucose tolerance			
Fasting sugar	90–120	mg/100 ml	
Highest value	130–140	mg/100 ml	
Highest value reached in	45–60	minutes	
Return to fasting in	1.5–2.5	hr	
Lactose tolerance			
Fasting blood glucose (B)	90–120	mg/100 ml	In lactase deficiency the rise in blood glucose after test dose of lactose is less than 20 mg in 1 hour
Increase in blood glucose after test dose lactose	20	mg/100 ml	
Citric acid (B)	1.3–2.3	mg/100 ml	
(P)	1.6–2.7	mg/100 ml	
Lactic acid (see acid-base constituents)			
Pyruvic acid, fasting (B)	0.7–1.2	mg/100 ml	
Enzymes			
Amylase (Somogyi) (S)	60–180	units/100 ml	High in acute pancreatitis, acute appendicitis
Lactic dehydrogenase (S)	25–100	units/ml	High in myocardial infarction
Lipase (S)	0.2–1.5	units/ml	High in pancreatitis
Leucine-aminopeptidase (S)	1–3.5	units/ml	High in hemolytic anemias
Phosphatase, alkaline (Bodansky) (S) Child	5–14	units/100 ml	High in rickets, bone cancer, Paget's disease, hyperparathyroidism, vitamin D inadequacy; indicates rapid bone growth in young
Adult	1–4		
Transaminases			
Glutamic-oxalacetic (SGOT) (Karmen) (S)	10–40	units/ml	Increased within 24 hours in myocardial infarction; normal after 6 to 7 days
Glutamic-pyruvic (SGPT) (Karmen) (S)	5–35	units/ml	High in hepatic disease, and trauma after surgery
Hematologic Studies			
Cell volume	39–50	per cent	High in polycythemia; low in anemia, prolonged iron deficiency
Red blood cells	4.25–5.25	million per cu mm	High in polycythemia, dehydration; low in anemia, hemorrhage
White blood cells	5,000–9,000	per cu mm	Increased in acute infections, leukemias
Lymphocytes	25–30	per cent	
Neutrophils	60–65	per cent	
Monocytes	4–8	per cent	
Eosinophils	0.5–4	per cent	
Basophils	0–1.5	per cent	
Platelets	125,000–300,000	per cu mm	
Lipids			
Acetone (S)	0.3–2.0	mg/100 ml	High in uncontrolled diabetes and starvation

Table A-15. **(Continued)**

Constituent	Normal Range		Examples of Deviations
Cholesterol, total (S)	125–225	mg/100 ml	High in uncontrolled diabetes mellitus, nephrosis, hypothyroidism, hyperlipidemias
esters	50–67	per cent	
free	33–50	per cent	
Fatty acids, unesterified (P)	8–31	mg/100 ml	
17-Hydroxycorticosteroids (P)	10–13.5	mcg/100 ml	
Lipids, total (P)	570–820	mg/100 ml	
Phospholipid (S)	150–300	mg/100 ml	
Triglycerides (S)	30–140	mg/100 ml	Increased in hyperlipidemias
Nitrogenous Constituents			
Alpha-amino acid nitrogen (S)	3.5–5.5	mg/100 ml	High in severe liver disease; low in nephrosis
Ammonia (B)	40–70	µg/100 ml	High in liver disease
Creatinine (S)	0.5–1.2	mg/100 ml	Increased in renal insufficiency
Creatinine clearance endogenous (B)	120±20	ml	Blood cleared per min by kidney; measure of glomerular filtration
Nonprotein N (NPN) (B)	25–35	mg/100 ml	High in acute glomerulonephritis, dehydration, metallic poisoning, intestinal obstruction, renal failure
Phenylalanine (S)	0.7–4	mg/100 ml	Increased in phenylketonuria
Urea nitrogen (BUN) (B)	8–18	mg/100 ml	High in renal failure, acute glomerulonephritis, mercury poisoning, dehydration; low in hepatic failure
Urea clearance (B)	75	ml/min C_m	C_m = maximal clearance
	54	ml/min C_s	C_s = standard clearance
Uric acid (S)	2–6	mg/100 ml	High in gout, nephritis, arthritis
Proteins			
Total protein (S)	6.5–7.5	gm/100 ml	High in dehydration; low in liver disease, nephrosis
Albumin (S)	3.9–4.5	gm/100 ml	Low in starvation, cirrhosis, proteinuria
Globulin (S)	2.3–3.5	gm/100 ml	High in infections, liver disease, multiple myeloma
Albumin : globulin ratio	1.2–1.9		Low in liver disease, nephrosis
Fibrinogen (P)	0.2–0.5	gm/100 ml	High in infections; low in severe liver disease
Ceruloplasmin (S)	16–33	mg/100 ml	
Gamma globulin (S)	0.7–1.2	gm/100 ml	
Hemoglobin (B)			High in polycythemia; low in prolonged dietary deficiency of iron, anemia
Males	14–17	gm/100 ml	
Females	12–16	gm/100 ml	
Vitamins			
Ascorbic acid (S)	0.3–1.4	mg/100 ml	
Folic acid (*L.casei*) (S)	6–10	µµg/ml	
(*L. casei*) (B)	100–220	µµg/ml	
Niacin (S)	30–150	µg/100 ml	
Riboflavin (S)	2.3–3.7	µg/100 ml	
Thiamin (B)	5.5–9.5	µg/100 ml	
Tocopherol (S)	0.6–2.0	mg/100 ml	
Vitamin A (S)	25–90	µg/100 ml	
Carotene (S)	40–125	µg/100 ml	
Vitamin B-6 (B)	1–18	µg/100 ml	
Vitamin B-12 (S)	10–90	µg/100 ml	

Table A-15. **(Continued)**

Constituent	Normal Range		Examples of Deviations
Miscellaneous			
Bilirubin (S)	0–1.5	mg/100 ml	High in red cell destruction, liver disease
Icterus index	4–6	units	High in jaundice
Copper (S)	80–240	μg/100 ml	Low in anemia, Wilson's disease
Iron (S)			
Men	80–165	μg/100 ml	High in hemochromatosis, liver disease, transfusion hemosiderosis; low in iron-deficiency anemia
Women	65–130	μg/100 ml	
Iron-binding capacity (S)			
Men	250–430	μg/100 ml	High in anemia
Women	220–415	μg/100 ml	
Serum ferritin	10	μg/100 ml or higher	
Transferrin saturation	15	per cent or more	
Lead (S)	1–3	μg/100 ml	
Manganese (S)	2–5	μg/100 ml	
Protein-bound iodine (PBI) (S)	3–8	μg/100 ml	High in hyperthyroidism; low in hypothyroidism
Zinc (S)	100–140	μg/100 ml	

ml = milliliters
mg = milligrams
μg = micrograms
mEq = milliequivalents
gm = grams
cu mm = cubic millimeters

$$\text{mEq per liter} = \frac{\text{mg per liter}}{\text{equivalent weight}}$$

$$\text{mM (millimoles) per liter} = \frac{\text{mg per liter}}{\text{molecular weight}}$$

$$\text{equivalent weight} = \frac{\text{atomic weight}}{\text{valence of element}}$$

volumes per cent = mM per liter × 2.24

Sources of Data:

Oser, B. L., ed.: *Hawk's Physiological Chemistry*, 14th ed. McGraw-Hill Book Company, New York, 1965, pp. 977–79.

Robinson, H. W.: "Biochemistry," in *Rypins' Medical Licensure Examinations*, 11th ed., A. W. Wright, ed. J. B. Lippincott Company, Philadelphia, 1970, pp. 202-5.

Table A-16. **Normal Constituents of the Urine of the Adult**

Specific gravity		1.010-1.025
Reaction	pH	5.5-8.0
Volume	ml per 24 hr	800-1600
		gm per 24 hr
Total solids		55-70
Nitrogenous constituents		
Total nitrogen		10-17
Ammonia		0.5-1.0
Amino acid N		0.4-1
Creatine		None
Creatinine		1-1.5
Protein		None
Purine bases		0.016-0.060
Urea		20-35
Uric acid		0.5-0.7
Acetone bodies		0.003-0.015
Bile		None
Calcium		0.2-0.4
Chloride (as NaCl)		10-15
Glucose		None
Indican		0-0.030
Iron		0.001-0.005
Magnesium (as MgO)		0.15-0.30
Phosphate, total (as phosphoric acid)		2.5-3.5
Potassium (as K_2O)		2.0-3.0
Sodium (as Na_2O)		4.0-5.0
Sulfates, total (as sulfuric acid)		1.5-3.0

Table A-17. **Conversions to and from Metric Measures**

If Measure Is In	Multiply By	To Find
Length		
inches	25.4	millimeters
inches	2.54	centimeters
feet	30.48	centimeters
feet	0.305	meters
centimeters	0.394	inches
meters	3.281	feet
Weight		
grains	64.799	milligrams
ounces (Av.)	28.35	grams
pounds (Av.)	454	grams
pounds	0.454	kilograms
grams	15.432	grains
grams	0.035	ounces (Av.)
grams	0.0022	pounds (Av.)
kilograms	2.205	pounds
Capacity (liquid)		
teaspoons	4.7	milliliters
tablespoons	14.1	milliliters
fluid ounces	29.573	milliliters
cups (8 ounces)	238	milliliters
pints	0.473	liters
quarts	0.946	liters
milliliters	0.034	fluid ounces
liters	1.057	quarts
Energy units		
kilocalories	4.184	kilojoules
kilojoules	0.239	kilocalories
Temperature		
Fahrenheit	subtract 32; then multiply by 5/9	Celsius (Centigrade)
Celsius	multiply by 9/5; then add 32	Fahrenheit

Metric equivalents
- 1 kilogram (kg) = 1,000 grams
- 1 gram (gm) = 1,000 milligrams
- 1 milligram (mg) = 1,000 micrograms
- 1 microgram (mcg, μg, γ) = 1,000 nanograms
- 1 nanogram (ng) = 1,000 picograms (pg)

Multiples
- deca- 10
- hecto- 10^2 (100)
- kilo- 10^3 (1,000)
- mega- 10^6 (1,000,000)

Submultiples
- deci- = one tenth 10^{-1} (0.1)
- centi- = one hundredth 10^{-2} (0.01)
- milli- = one thousandth 10^{-3} (0.001)
- micro-= one millionth 10^{-6} (0.000,001)
- nano- = one billionth 10^{-9} (0.000,000,001)
- pico- = one trillionth 10^{-12} (0.000,000,000,001)

Table A–18. **Recommended Daily Nutrient Intakes—Canada, Revised 1974**
Committee for Revision of the Canadian Dietary Standard, Bureau of Nutritional Sciences, Health and Welfare, Ottawa, Canada

Age years	Sex	Weight kg	Height cm	Energy[a] kcal	Protein gm	Water-Soluble Vitamins: Thiamin mg	Niacin[e] mg	Riboflavin gm	Vitamin B-6[f] mg	Folate[g] μg	Vitamin B-12 μg	Ascorbic Acid[h] mg
0–6 mos	Both	6		kg × 117	kg × 2.2(2.0)[d]	0.3	5	0.4	0.3	40	0.3	20
1–11 mos	Both	9		kg × 108	kg × 1.4	0.5	6	0.6	0.4	60	0.3	20
1–3	Both	13	90	1,400	22	0.7	9	0.8	0.8	100	0.9	20
4–6	Both	19	110	1,800	27	0.9	12	1.1	1.3	100	1.5	20
7–9	M	27	129	2,200	33	1.1	14	1.3	1.6	100	1.5	30
	F	27	128	2,000	33	1.0	13	1.2	1.4	100	1.5	30
10–12	M	36	144	2,500	41	1.2	17	1.5	1.8	100	3.0	30
	F	38	145	2,300	40	1.1	15	1.4	1.5	100	3.0	30
13–15	M	51	162	2,800	52	1.4	19	1.7	2.0	200	3.0	30
	F	49	159	2,200	43	1.1	15	1.4	1.5	200	3.0	30
16–18	M	64	172	3,200	54	1.6	21	2.0	2.0	200	3.0	30
	F	54	161	2,100	43	1.1	14	1.3	1.5	200	3.0	30
19–35	M	70	176	3,000	56	1.5	20	1.8	2.0	200	3.0	30
	F	56	161	2,100	41	1.1	14	1.3	1.5	200	3.0	30
36–50	M	70	176	2,700	56	1.4	18	1.7	2.0	200	3.0	30
	F	56	161	1,900	41	1.0	13	1.2	1.5	200	3.0	30
51+	M	70	176	2,300[b]	56	1.4	18	1.7	2.0	200	3.0	30
	F	56	161	1,800[b]	41	1.0	13	1.2	1.5	200	3.0	30
Pregnant				+300[c]	+20	+0.2	+2	+0.3	+0.5	+50	+1.0	+20
Lactating				+500	+24	+0.4	+7	+0.6	+0.6	+50	+0.5	+30

[a] Recommendations assume characteristic activity pattern for each age group.

[b] Recommended energy allowance for age 66+ years reduced to 2,000 for men and 1,500 for women.

[c] Increased energy allowance recommended during second and third trimesters. An increase of 100 kcal per day is recommended during the first trimester.

[d] Recommended protein allowance of 2.2 gm per kilogram body weight for infants aged 0 to 2 months, and 2.0 gm per kilogram body weight for those aged 3 to 5 months. Protein recommendations for infants, 0 to 11 months, assumes consumption of breast milk or protein of equivalent quality.

[e] Approximately 1 mg of niacin is derived from each 60 mg of dietary tryptophan.

[f] Recommendations are based on the estimated average daily protein intake of Canadians.

[g] Recommendations given in terms of free folate.

[h] Considerably higher levels may be prudent for infants during the first week of life to guard against neonatal tyrosinemia.

Table A-18. (Continued)

Fat-Soluble Vitamins			Minerals							
Vitamin A[i] µg RE	Vitamin D µg cholecalciferol[j]	Vitamin E mg α-tocopherol	Calcium mg	Phosphorus mg	Magnesium mg	Iodine µg	Iron mg	Zinc mg	Age years
400	10	3	500[l]	250[l]	50[l]	35[l]	7[l]	4[l]	0–6 mos
400	10	3	500	400	50	50	7	5	7–11 mos
400	10	4	500	500	75	70	8	5	1–3
500	5	5	500	500	100	90	9	6	4–6
700	2.5[k]	6	700	700	150	110	10	7	7–9 M
700	2.5[k]	6	700	700	150	100	10	7	7–9 F
800	2.5[k]	7	900	900	175	130	11	8	10–12 M
800	2.5[k]	7	1,000	1,000	200	120	11	9	10–12 F
1,000	2.5[k]	9	1,200	1,200	250	140	13	10	13–15 M
800	2.6[k]	7	800	800	250	110	14	10	13–15 F
1,000	2.5[k]	10	1,000	1,000	300	160	14	12	16–18 M
800	2.5[k]	6	700	700	250	110	14	11	16–18 F
1,000	2.5[k]	9	800	800	300	150	10	10	19–35 M
800	2.5[k]	6	700	700	250	110	14	9	19–35 F
1,000	2.5[k]	8	800	800	300	140	10	10	36–50 M
800	2.5[k]	6	700	700	250	100	14	9	36–50 F
1,000	2.5[k]	8	800	800	300	140	10	10	51+ M
800	2.5[k]	6	700	700	250	100	9	9	51+ F
+100	+2.5[k]	+1	+500	+500	+25	+15	+1[m]	+3[m]	Pregnant
+400	+2.5[k]	+2	+500	+500	+75	+25	+1[m]	+7	Lactating

[i]One microgram retinol equivalent (1 µg RE) corresponds to a biologic activity in humans equal to 1 µg retinol (3.33 IU) and 6 µg β-carotene (10 IU).

[j]One microgram cholecalciferol is equivalent to 40 IU vitamin D activity.

[k]Most older children and adults receive enough vitamin D from irradiation but 2.5 µg daily is recommended. This recommended allowance increases to 5.0 µg daily for pregnant and lactating women and for those who are confined indoors or otherwise deprived of sunlight for extended periods.

[l]The intake of breast-fed infants may be less than the recommendation but is considered to be adequate.

[m]A recommended total intake of 15 mg daily during pregnancy and lactation assumes the presence of adequate stores of iron. If stores are suspected of being inadequate, additional iron as a supplement is recommended.

Common Abbreviations

AcCoA: acetyl coenzyme A
ACTH: adrenocorticotropic hormone
ADH: antidiuretic hormone
ADP: adenosine-5′-diphosphate
AMP: adenosine-5′-phosphate
ATP: adenosine-5′-triphosphate
ATPase: adenosine triphosphatase
BMR: basal metabolic rate
BUN: blood urea nitrogen
BV: biologic value
cal: calorie
cc: cubic centimeter
Co I: coenzyme I (NAD)
Co II: coenzyme II (NADP)
DNA: deoxyribonucleic acid
Dopa: dioxy-or dihydroxyphenylalanine
EAA: essential amino acid
EF: extrinsic factor
EFA: essential fatty acid
FAD: flavin adenine dinucleotide, oxidized form
FADH: flavin adenine dinucleotide, reduced form
FAO: Food and Agriculture Organization
FDA: Food and Drug Administration
FFA: free fatty acid
FMN: flavin mononucleotide
FSH: follicle-stimulating hormone
GFR: glomerular filtration rate
gm: gram(s)
GOT: glutamate oxalacetate transaminase
GTF: glucose tolerance factor
HANES: Health and Nutrition Examination Survey
Hb: hemoglobin
HbO_2: oxyhemoglobin
HMP shunt: hexose monophosphate shunt
IF: intrinsic factor
INH: isonicotinic acid hydrazide
INQ: index of nutritional quality
IU: international unit
J: joule
kcal: kilocalorie(s)
kg: kilogram
kJ: kilojoule
L: liter
lb: pound
LCT: long-chain triglyceride
LH: luteinizing hormone
μg: microgram(s)
MCT: medium-chain triglyceride
mEq: milliequivalent(s)
mg: milligram(s)
mJ: megajoule
ml: milliliter(s)
mm: millimeter(s)
mRNA: messenger ribonucleic acid
NAD: nicotinamide adenine dinucleotide
NADP: nicotinamide adenine dinucleotide phosphate
NE: niacin equivalent
NEFA: nonesterified fatty acid
ng: nanogram(s)
NPN: nonprotein nitrogen
NPU: net protein utilization
NRC: National Research Council
oz: ounce
PABA: para-amino benzoic acid
PBI: protein-bound iodine
PCBs: polychlorinated biphenyls
PER: protein efficiency ratio
pg: picogram(s)
pH: hydrogen ion concentration
PKU: phenylketonuria
ppm: parts per million
PTH: parathyroid hormone
RDA: recommended dietary allowances
RE: retinol equivalent
RNA: ribonucleic acid
RNAse: ribonuclease
RQ: respiratory quotient
SH: sulfhydryl
TCA: tricarboxylic acid cycle
αTE: alpha-tocopherol equivalent
TPP: thiamin pyrophosphate

tRNA: transfer ribonucleic acid
TSH: thyroid-stimulating hormone
UNESCO: United Nations Educational Scientific, and Cultural Organization
UNICEF: United Nations Children's Fund
USDA: United States Department of Agriculture
USDHHS: United States Department of Health and Human Services
USP: United States Pharmacopeia
USRDA: United States Recommended Dietary Allowances
WHO: World Health Organization

Glossary

absorption (ab-sorp′shun): the transfer of nutrients across cell membranes; following digestion, nutrients are transferred from the intestinal lumen across the mucosa and into the blood and lymph circulation

acetoacetic acid (as′et-o-as-e′tik): a 4-carbon keto acid; one of the acetone bodies in diabetic urine

acetone (as′et-ōn); dimethyl ketone; accumulates in the blood and excretions when fats are incompletely oxidized as in diabetes mellitus; gives fruity odor to the breath

acetylcholine (as′et-il-kō′lēn): an acetic acid ester of choline; involved in nerve transmission, and other important physiologic functions.

acetyl coenzyme A (as′et-il co-en′zīm); condensation product of acetic acid and coenzyme A; form by which 2-carbon fragment enters the tricarboxylic acid cycle

achlorhydria (a-klor-hi′drĭ-ah): absence of hydrochloric acid in gastric juice

acid: a substance that gives off or donates protons (H + ions)

acidosis (as-ĭd-o′sis): condition caused by accumulation of an excess of acids (anions) in the body, or by excessive loss of base (mineral cations) from the body

acrolein (ak-ro′le-in): an irritating volatile decomposition product of glycerol that results from overheating fat

active transport: the movement of substances across cell membranes by pumping against a concentration gradient; requires source of energy

adenine (ad′en-in): one of the purines (bases) that are constituents of nucleic acid

adenosine triphosphate (ad-en′o-sin tri-fos′fāt): a compound consisting of 1 molecule each of adenine and ribose and 3 molecules of phosphoric acid; two of the phosphate groups are held by high-energy bonds; ATP

adipose (ad′ip-ōs): fat; fatty

aerobic (a-er-o′bik): living in presence of air

agar (ah′gar): an indigestible polysaccharide prepared from moss and seaweed; has property of holding water and is often used to relieve constipation

alanine (al′an-in): a nonessential amino acid occurring widely in foods

albumin (al-bu′min): a protein in tissues and body fluids soluble in water and coagulated by heat; principal protein in blood regulating osmotic pressure; lactalbumin of milk

aldehyde (al′de-hīd): any of a large group of compounds containing the grouping -CHO

aldohexose (al-dō-hex′ōs): a 6-carbon sugar containing a -CHO grouping; glucose, galactose

aldosterone (al-dos′ter-ōn): a steroid hormone produced by the adrenal cortex; increases sodium retention and potassium loss

alkalosis (al-kah-lo′sis): increased alkali reserve (blood bicarbonate) of the blood and other body fluids; caused by excessive ingestion of sodium bicarbonate, persistent vomiting, or hyperventilation; pH of blood is usually increased

allergen (al′ler-jen): substance (usually protein) capable of producing altered response of cell, resulting in manifestation of allergy

amino acid (am′in-o as′id): an organic acid containing an amino (NH_2) group; the building blocks of protein molecules

amylase (am′ilās): salivary or pancreatic enzyme that hydrolyzes starch; ptyalin, amylopsin

amylopectin (am′il-o-pek′tin): polysaccharide found in starch consisting of branched chains of glucose

amylose (am′il-ōs): polysaccharide of starch consisting of unbranched chains of glucose

anabolism (an-ab′oh-lizm): processes for building complex substances from simple substances

anaerobic (an-aer-oh′bik): living in the absence of oxygen

androgen (an′dro-jen): a substance such as testosterone that produces male sex characteristics

anemia (an-e′me-ah): deficiency in the circulating hemoglobin, red blood cells, or packed cell volume

anion (an′i-on): an ion that contains a negative charge of electricity and therefore goes to a positively charged anode

anorexia (an-o-rek′se-ah): loss of appetite

antagonist (an-tag′on-ist): a substance that opposes or neutralizes the action of another substance, e.g., a vitamin antagonist

anthropometry (an-thro-pom′et-re): branch of anthropology dealing with comparative measurements of the parts of the human body.

anti-: a prefix meaning against or opposing; e.g., antiscorbutic means preventing scurvy

antibiotic (an′ti-bi-ot′ik): a substance that inhibits the growth of bacteria

antibody (an′te-bod-e): a protein substance produced in an organism as a response to the presence of an antigen

antigen (an′ti-jen): any substance such as bacteria or foreign protein that, as a result of contact with tissues of the animal body, produces an immune response; an increased reaction such as hypersensitivity may result

antiketogenesis (an-ti-ke-tō-jen′es-is): the prevention of ketosis by stimulating the tricarboxylic acid cycle and thus bringing about oxidation of the ketone bodies

antioxidant (an-te-ok′sid-ant): a substance that prevents deterioration by hindering oxidation, e.g., tocopherols prevent oxidation and rancidity of fats

anuria (au-u′re-ah): lack of urinary secretion

apathy (ap′ath-e): indifference; lack of interest or concern

apatite (ap′ah-tīt): complex calcium phosphate salt giving strength to bones

apoenzyme (ap-o-en′zīm): the protein part of an enzyme

arachidonic acid (ar-ak-id-on′ik): a 20-carbon fatty acid with four double bonds; the physiologically functioning essential fatty acid

arginase (ar′jin-ās): enzyme that splits arginine to urea and ornithine

arginine (ar′jin-in): a diamino acid; required for growth but not required by adults

arteriosclerosis (ar-te-re-o-skle-ro′sis): thickening and hardening of the inner walls of the arteries

ascites (a-si′tēz): accumulation of fluid in the abdominal cavity

ascorbic acid (a-skor′bik): water-soluble vitamin required for collagenous intercellular substance; prevents scurvy; also known as vitamin C

-ase: suffix that is used in naming an enzyme; for example, peptidase

aspartic acid (as-par′tik): a nonessential dibasic amino acid

asymptomatic (a-sim-tō-mat′ik): without symptoms

ataxia (a-tak′se-ah): loss of ability of muscular coordination

atherosclerosis (ath-er-o-skle-ro′sis): thickening of the walls of blood vessels by deposits of fatty materials, including cholesterol

atony (at′o-ne): a lack of normal tone or strength

atrophy (at′ro-fe): a wasting away of cell, tissue, or organ

autosome (aw′tō-sōm): any chromosome other than a sex chromosome

avidin (av′id-in): protein substance in raw egg white which binds biotin and prevents its absorption from the digestive tract

azotemia (a-zo-te′me-ah): elevated levels of nitrogenous constituents in the blood; uremia

basal metabolism (ba′zal me-tab′o-lizm): energy expenditure of the body at rest in the postabsorptive state

base (bās): substance that combines with an acid to form a salt; any molecule or ion that will add on a hydrogen ion

benign (bi-nīn′): mild nature of an illness; with reference to a neoplasm, not malignant

beriberi (ber′ē-ber′ē): a deficiency disease caused by lack of thiamin and characterized by extreme weakness, polyneuritis, emaciation, edema, and cardiac failure

beta-hydroxybutyric acid (ba-tah-hi-drox′e-butir′-ik): a 4-carbon intermediate in oxidation of fatty acids; one of the acetone bodies excreted in the urine in uncontrolled diabetes

bio- (bi-o-): prefix denoting life

bioassay (bi′-o-as-say): testing of activity or potency, as of a vitamin or hormone, on an animal or microorganism

biologic value: a measure of the effectiveness of a nutrient, such as protein, to the living organism

biopsy (bi′op-sē): examination of a piece of tissue removed from a living subject

biotin (bi′o-tin): a vitamin of the B complex; participates in fixation of carbon dioxide in fatty acid synthesis

Bitot's spots (be′tōz): gray, shiny spots on the conjunctiva resulting from malnutrition, especially vitamin A deficiency

botulism (bot′u-lizm): frequently fatal poisoning caused by toxin produced in inadequately sterilized canned food by the *Clostridium botulinum*

buffer (buf′er): a mixture of an acid and its conjugate base that is capable of neutralizing either an acid or a base without appreciably changing the original acidity or alkalinity, e.g., H_2CO_3/HCO_3—

calciferol (kal-sif′er-ol): vitamin D_2; fat-soluble vitamin of plant origin formed by irradiation of ergosterol; prevents rickets

calcification (kal-sif-ik-a′shun): hardening of tissue by a deposit of calcium and also magnesium salts

calcitonin (kal-sit-oh′-nin): hormone secreted by the thyroid gland; hypocalcemic effect; opposes action of parathormone

calculus (kal′ku-lus): an abnormal concretion occurring in any part of the body; usually consists of mineral salts around an organic nucleus

calorie (kal′o-rē): a unit of heat measurement; in nutrition, the kilocalorie is the amount of heat required to raise the temperature of 1 kg water 1°C

calorimetry (kal-or-im′et-rē): measurement of heat produced by the body, or from a food; *direct:* measure of heat produced by a subject in a closed chamber; *indirect:* measurement of heat by determining consumption of oxygen and sometimes carbon dioxide and calculating the amount of heat produced

carbonic acid (kar-bon′ik): the acid formed when carbon dioxide is dissolved in water; H_2CO_3

carboxylase (kar-bok′sil-ās): a thiamin-containing enzyme that catalyzes the removal of the carboxyl group of alpha keto acids, e.g., decarboxylation of pyruvic acid

carboxypeptidase (kar-box-e-pep′tid-ās): an intestinal enzyme which catalyzes the splitting of peptides

carotene (kar′o-tēn): precursor of vitamin A; yellow plant pigments occurring abundantly in dark green leafy and deep yellow vegetables

casein (ka′se-in): principal protein in milk; a phosphoprotein

catabolism (kat-ab′o-lizm): process for breaking down complex substances to simpler substances; usually yields energy

catalyst (kat′ah-list): a substance which in minute amounts initiates or modifies the speed of a chemical or physical change without itself being changed

cation (kat′i-on): an ion that carries a positive charge and migrates to the negatively charged pole

cellulose (sel′u-lōs): the structural fibers of plants; an indigestible polysaccharide

cephalin (sef′al-in): a phospholipid in brain and nervous tissue

ceruloplasmin (ser-ul′o-plaz-min): copper-containing protein in blood plasma

cheilosis (ki-lo′sis): lesions of the lips and the angles of the mouth; characteristic of riboflavin deficiency

chelation (ke-la′shun): formation of a bond between a metal ion and two or more polar groupings of a single molecule

cholecalciferol (ko-le-kal-sif′er-ol): vitamin D_3 formed from 7-dehydrocholesterol

cholecystitis (ko-le-sis-ti′tis): inflammation of the gallbladder

cholecystokinin (ko-le-sis-tō-kin′in): hormone produced in duodenum in presence of fat; stimulates contraction of gallbladder and release of bile

cholelithiasis (ko-le-lith-i′a-sis): gallstones in the gallbladder

cholesterol (ko-les′ter-ol): the commonest member of the sterol group; found in animal foods and made within the body; a constituent of gallstones and of atheroma

choline (ko′lēn): a nitrogenous base that donates methyl groups; a component of lecithin and acetylcholine; sometimes classed as a B-complex vitamin

chondroitin sulfate (kon-droi′tin): a mucopolysaccharide widely distributed in skin and cartilage

chylomicrons (ki′lo-mi′krons): large molecules of fat occurring in lymph and plasma after a fat-rich meal; consist of triglycerides attached to a small amount of protein

chymotrypsin (ki-mo-trip′sin): enzyme produced in pancreas for the hydrolysis of protein

citric acid (sit′rik): an organic acid containing three carboxyl groups; one of compounds in the Krebs or citric acid cycle; a constituent of citrus fruits

citrovorum factor (sit-ro-vor′um): folinic acid, the active form of folic acid

citrulline (sit-rul′in): an amino acid formed from ornithine in the urea cycle

Clostridium (klos-trid′i-um): a genus of bacteria,

chiefly anaerobic, found in soils and in the intestinal tract, e.g., *botulinum, perfringens*

coagulation (ko-ag-u-la′shun): process of changing into a clot, as in heating of an egg, curdling of milk

cobalamine (ko-bal′ah-min): compound containing cobalt grouping found in vitamin B-12

cocarboxylase (ko-kar-box′il-ās): thiamin-containing coenzyme of carboxylase

coenzyme (ko-en′zīm): the prosthetic group of an enzyme; a substance, for example, a vitamin, that conjugates with a protein molecule to form an active enzyme

coenzyme A: a complex nucleotide containing pantothenic acid; combines with acetyl groups to yield active acetate which can enter the Krebs cycle; involved in fatty acid oxidation and synthesis and cholesterol synthesis

coenzyme Q: involved in transfer of electrons in cytochrome chain

colitis (ko-li′tis): inflammation of the colon

collagen (kol′aj-in): widely distributed protein that makes up the matrix of bone, cartilage, and connective tissue

colloid (kol′oid): matter dispersed through another medium; particles are larger than crystalline molecules but not large enough to settle out; do not pass through an animal membrane

colostrum (ko-los′trum): milk secreted during the first few days after the birth of a baby

coma (ko′mah): state of unconsciousness

complementarity: the ability of one substance to supply a missing substance in another; e.g., one food supplies amino acids lacking in another, thus providing a "complete" amino acid mixture

congenital (kon-jen′it-al): existing at or before birth with reference to certain physical or mental traits

coronary (kor′o-na-re): like a crown; related to blood vessels supplied to the heart muscle

cortex (kor′tex): outer layers of an organ, e.g., adrenal cortex

cortisone (kor′ti-sōn): hormone of the adrenal cortex; influences carbohydrate metabolism

creatine (kre′at-in): a nitrogenous constituent of muscle; phosphorylated form essential for muscle contraction

creatinine (kre-at′in-in): a nitrogen-containing substance derived from catabolism of creatine and present in the urine

crude fiber: plant fiber that remains after sample has been treated with sulfuric acid and sodium hydroxide; chiefly cellulose and lignin

cryptoxanthine (kript-o-zan′thin): a yellow pigment present in some foods; precursor of vitamin A

cystine (sis′tin): sulfur-containing nonessential amino acid

-cyte: suffix meaning cell; for example, adipocyte

cytochrome (si′tō-krom): a respiratory enzyme; consists of a number of hemochromogens; undergoes alternate reduction and oxidation

cytology (si-tol′oh-je): the anatomy, chemistry, physiology, and pathology of the cell

cytoplasm (si′to-plazm): substance within the cell exclusive of the nucleus

cytosine (si′tō-sin): one of the nitrogenous bases in nucleic acid

deamination, deaminization (de-am-in-a′shun): removal of the amino (NH_2) group from an amino acid

debility (de-bil′i-te): weakness

dehydrocholesterol, 7- (de-hi-dro-ko-les′ter-ol): cholesterol derivative in the skin that is converted to vitamin D

dehydrogenases (de-hi-dro′jen-ās-es): enzymes that catalyze oxidation by transferring hydrogen to a hydrogen acceptor

denaturation (de-na-tur-a′shun): the alteration of the natural properties of a substance by physical or chemical means; e.g., heat coagulation of protein

deoxypyridoxine (de-ok′se-pir-id-oks′in): a compound similar in structure to pyridoxine that is antagonistic to the action of pyridoxine

deoxyribonucleic acid (DNA) (de-ok′se-ri-bo-nu-kla′ik): giant molecule in cell nucleus which determines hereditary traits; consists of four bases attached to ribose and phosphate

dermatitis (der-mat-i′tis): inflammation of the surface of the skin

dextrin (dex′trin): intermediate product in breakdown of starches; a polysaccharide

dicoumarin (di-koo′mah-rin): antiprothrombin; anticlotting factor first isolated from sweet clover

diffuse (dif-ūs′): not localized

diffusion: the movement of particles from an area of higher concentration to one of lower concentration

digestion (di-jes′chun): the hydrolysis of foods in the digestive tract to simpler substances so they can be used by the body

diglyceride (di-glis′er-id): a fat containing 2 fatty acid molecules
disaccharidase (di-sak′ar-id-ās): enzyme which hydrolyzes disaccharides
disaccharide (di-sak′ar-id): a carbohydrate that yields two simple sugars upon hydrolysis; sucrose, maltose, lactose
distal (dis′tal): part of structure farthest from the point of attachment
diuresis (di-u-re′sis): increased secretion of urine
duodenum (du-o-de′num): first portion of the small intestine, extending from the pylorus to the jejunum
dys-: prefix meaning bad
dysgeusia (dis-goo′-se-ah): perverted sense of taste; "bad" taste
dysosmia (dis-ahs′-me-ah): impaired sense of smell; obnoxious odor
dyspepsia (dis-pep′se-ah): indigestion or upset stomach
dysphagia (dis-fa′je-ah): difficulty in swallowing
dyspnea (disp′ne-ah): difficulty or distress in breathing

eclampsia (ĕ-klamp′se-ah): convulsions occurring during pregnancy and associated with edema, hypertension, and proteinuria
edema (ĕ-de′mah): presence of abnormal amounts of fluid in intercellular spaces
elastin (ĕ-las′tin): insoluble yellow elastic protein in connective tissue
electrolyte (el-ek′tro-līt): any substance which dissociates into ions when dissolved and thus conducts an electric current
emaciation (e-ma-se-a′shun): wasting of the body; excessive leanness
-emia: suffix that denotes a condition of the blood; for example, hypoglycemia
emulsion (e-mul′shun): a system of two immiscible liquids in which one is finely divided and held in suspension by another
endemic (en-dem′ik): prevalence of a disease in a given region
endo-: prefix meaning inner or within
endocrine (en′do-krin): pertaining to glands that secrete substances into the blood for control of metabolic processes
endogenous (en-doj′en-us): originating in the cells or tissues of the body
endoplasmic reticulum (en′do-plaz-mik ret-ic′u-lum): the system of membranes within the cell that permits communication between cellular, nuclear, and extracellular environment
endosperm (en′do-sperm): reserve food material of the plant; the starchy center of the cereal grain
enter-: combining term denoting intestine
enteritis (en-ter-i′tis): inflammation of the intestine
enterocrinin (en-ter-o-krī′nin): hormone of small intestine that stimulates secretion of intestinal juice
enterogastrone (en-ter-o-gas′trōn): hormone secreted by duodenal mucosa upon stimulation by fat; inhibits secretion of gastric juice and reduces motility
enterokinase (en-ter-o-kīn′ās): enzyme of intestinal juice that converts trypsinogen to trypsin
enteropathy (en-ter-op′ath-e): any disease of the intestine
enzyme (en′zīm): an organic compound of protein nature produced by living tissue to accelerate metabolic reactions; hydrolases, oxidases, transferases, dehydrogenases, peptidases, and others
epidemiology (ep-i-dem′-e-ol-o-ji): the science of epidemic diseases; factors that influence frequency and distribution of disease
epinephrine (ep-in-ef′rin): secretion of the medulla of the adrenal gland that stimulates energy metabolism; adrenaline
epithelium (ep-ith-e′le-um): the covering layer of the skin and mucous membranes
ergosterol (er-gos′ter-ol): a sterol found chiefly in plants; when exposed to ultraviolet light becomes vitamin D
erythrocyte (er-ith′ro-sīt): mature red blood cell
erythropoieses (er-ith-ro-po-e′sis): formation of red blood cells
essential amino acid: an amino acid that must be supplied in the diet to provide the body's need for it
essential fatty acid: a fatty acid that must be present in the diet and that prevents certain deficiencies of the skin and blood capillaries; linoleic acid, arachidonic acid
estrogen (es′tro-jen): hormone secreted by the ovary
etiology (e-te-ol′o-je): cause of a disease
exacerbation (ex-as-er-ba′shun): increase in severity of symptoms
exogenous (ex-oj′en-us): originating or produced from the outside
extracellular (extra-sel′u-lar): situated or occurring outside the cells
extrinsic factor (ex-trin′sik): vitamin B-12; term used by Castle prior to identification of the nature of the compound

exudate (ex′u-dāt): a fluid discharged into the tissues or any cavity

familial (fam-il′e-al): common to a family

fatty acids (fat′e): open-chain monocarboxylic acids containing only carbon, hydrogen, and oxygen

favism (fa′vism): condition caused by eating certain species of beans, e.g., *Vicia faba;* symptoms include fever, abdominal pain, headache, anemia, coma

febrile (feb′ril): feverish; having a fever

ferritin (fer′it-in): water-soluble storage form of iron in the body; composed of protein (apoferritin) and colloidal ferric iron

fetor hepaticus (fe′tor hep-at′ik-us): offensive odor to the breath present in persons with severe liver disease

fibrosis (fi-bro′sis): formation of fibrous tissue in repair processes

fistula (fis′tu-lah): a tubelike ulcer leading from an abscess cavity or organ to the surface, or from one abscess cavity to another

flatulence (flat′u-lens): distention of stomach or intestines with gases

flavin adenine dinucleotide, FAD (fla′vin ad′en-in di-nu′kle-o-tīd): a coenzyme consisting of riboflavin and adenosine diphosphate required for the action of various dehydrogenases

flavin mononucleotide, FMN (fla′vin mon-o-nu′kle-o-tīd): a riboflavin-containing coenzyme involved in the action of dehydrogenases

flavoprotein (fla-vo-pro′te-in): a conjugated protein that contains a flavin and is involved in tissue respiration

fluoridation (floo-or-id-a′shun): the use of fluoride, as in water, to reduce the incidence of tooth decay

folacin (fo′lah-sin): folic acid, a vitamin of the B complex

folic acid (fo′lik): a vitamin of the B complex necessary for the maturation of red blood cells and synthesis of nucleoproteins; also known as folacin and pteroylglutamic acid

folinic acid (fo-lin′ik): the active form of folacin; citrovorum factor

follicle (fol′ikl): small excretory sac or gland, e.g., hair follicle, ovarian follicle

fortification (for-ti-fik-a′shun): the addition of one or more nutrients to a food to make it richer than the unprocessed food, e.g., vitamin D milk

fructose (fruk′tōs): a 6-carbon sugar found in fruits and honey; also obtained from the hydrolysis of sucrose; fruit sugar, levulose

galactose (gal-ak′tōs): a single sugar resulting from the hydrolysis of lactose

galactosemia (gal-ak′tō-se′me-ah): accumulation of galactose in the blood owing to a hereditary lack of an enzyme to convert galactose to glucose; accompanied by severe mental retardation

gastrectomy (gas-trek′tō-me): surgical removal of part or all of the stomach

gastrin (gas′trin): hormone secreted by pyloric mucosa that stimulates secretion of hydrochloric acid by parietal cells

genetic (jen-et′ik): congenital or inherited

-genic: suffix meaning to produce or give rise to; for example, ketogenic

gingivitis (jin-jĭ-vi′tis): inflammation of the gums

gliadin (gli′ad-in): a protein fraction of wheat gluten

globulin (glob′u-lin): a class of proteins insoluble in water and alcohol; serum globulin, lactoglobulin, myosin

glomerulus (glom-er′u-lus): the tuft of capillaries at the beginning of each tubule in the kidney

glossitis (glos-i′tis): inflammation of the tongue

glucagon (gloo′kag-on): hormone produced by the alpha cells of the islets of Langerhans; raises blood sugar by increasing glycogen breakdown

glucocorticoid (glu′ko-kor-tĭ-koid): hormone produced by the adrenal cortex that influences glucose metabolism

glucogenic (glu-ko-jen′ik): glucose forming

gluconeogenesis (glu′ko-ne-o-jen′e-sis): formation of glucose from noncarbohydrate sources, namely, certain amino acids and the glycerol fraction of fats

glucose (glu′kōs): a single sugar occurring in fruits and honey; also obtained by the hydrolysis of starch, sucrose, maltose, and lactose; the sugar found in the blood; dextrose, grape sugar

glutamic acid (glu-tam′ik): a dibasic nonessential amino acid widely distributed in proteins

glutathione (glu-ta-thi′ōn): a tripeptide of glycine, glutamic acid, and cystine; can act as hydrogen acceptor and hydrogen donor

glutathione peroxidase (glu-ta-thī′ōn per-ok′si-dās): a selenium-containing enzyme believed to deactivate lipid peroxides

gluten (glu′ten): protein in wheat and other cereals that gives elastic quality to a dough

glyceride (glis′er-id): organic ester of glycerol; fats are esters of fatty acids and glycerol

glycerol (glis′er-ol): a 3-carbon alcohol derived from the hydrolysis of fats

glycine (gli′sin): aminoacetic acid; a nonessential amino acid

glycogen (gli′ko-jen): polysaccharide produced from glucose by the liver or the muscle; "animal" starch

glycogenesis (gli′ko-jen-ĭ-sis): formation of glycogen from glucose by the liver or muscle

glycogenolysis (gli-ko-jen-ol′ĭ-sis): enzymatic breakdown of glycogen to glucose

glycolysis (gli-kol′ĭ-sis): the anaerobic conversion of glucose to pyruvic and lactic acids, an energy-yielding process

glycosuria (gli-ko-su′re-ah): presence of sugar in the urine

goiter (goi′ter): enlargement of the thyroid gland

goitrogen (goi′tro-jen): a substance that leads to goiter

guanine (gwan′in): one of the nitrogenous bases in nucleic acids

hem-, hema-, hemo-: prefixes referring to blood

hematocrit (he-mat′o-krit): separation of red cells from the plasma

hematuria (he-mat-u′re-ah): condition in which urine contains blood

heme (hēm): deep red pigment consisting of ferrous iron linked to protoporphyrin

heme iron: form of iron in hemoglobin and in myoglobin which is absorbed intact

hemicellulose (hem-i-sel′u-lōs): a class of indigestible polysaccharides that form the cell wall of plants

hemochromatosis (hem-o-kro-ma-to′sis): a condition in which excessive iron absorption leads to skin pigmentation and deposits of hemosiderin in the liver and other organs

hemoglobin (he-mo-glo′bin): the iron-protein pigment in the red blood cells; carries oxygen to the tissues

hemolytic (he-mo-lit′ik): causing separation of hemoglobin from the red blood cells

hemopoietic, hematopoietic (he-mo-poi-et′ik): concerned with the formation of blood

hemorrhage (hem′or-ej): loss of blood from the vessels; bleeding

hemosiderin (he′mo-sid′er-in): water-insoluble storage form of iron in the body

heparin (hep′ar-in): a mucopolysaccharide that prevents clotting of blood

hepatic (hep-at′ik): pertaining to the liver

hepatomegaly (hep-at-o-meg′ah-le): enlargement of the liver

heterozygous (het-er-o-zi′gus): possessing dissimilar pairs of genes for any hereditary trait

hexose (heks′ōs): a 6-carbon sugar; glucose, fructose, galactose

histidine (his′tid-in): an essential amino acid

homeostasis (ho-me-o-sta′sis): tendency to maintain equilibrium in normal body states

homogenize (ho-moj′en-īz): to make of uniform quality throughout

homozygous (ho-mo-zi′gus): having identical pairs of genes for any given pair of hereditary traits

hormone (hor′mōn): substance produced by an organ to produce a specific effect in another organ

hydrogenation (hi′dro-jen-a′shun): the addition of hydrogen to a compound, such as an unsaturated fatty acid to produce a solid fat

hydrolysate (hi-drol′is-āt): the product of hydrolysis; e.g., protein hydrolysate is a mixture of the constituent amino acids when the protein molecule is split by acids, alkalies, or enzymes

hydrolysis (hi-drol′is-is): the splitting up of a product by the addition of water

hydroxyapatite (hī-drok′sē-ap′a tīt): a naturally occurring mineral crystal containing calcium, phosphorus, hydrogen, and oxygen.

hydroxyproline (hi′drok-se-pro′lin): a nonessential amino acid occurring abundantly in collagen

hyper-: a prefix meaning above, beyond, or excessive

hypercalcemia (hi-per-kal-se′me-ah): abnormally high calcium level in the blood

hypercalciuria (hi-per-kal-se-u′re-ah): abnormal calcium excretion in the urine

hyperchlorhydria (hi-per-klor-hi′dre-ah): increased hydrochloric acid secretion by stomach cells

hyperchromic (hi-per-krōm′ik): abnormally high color

hyperemia (hi-per-e′me-ah): excess of blood in any part of the body

hyperesthesia (hi-per-es-the′zĭ-ah): increased sensitivity to touch or pain

hyperglycemia (hi-per-glī-se′me-ah): an excess of sugar in the blood

hyperkalemia (hi-per-kah-le′me-ah): an increased level of potassium in the blood

hyperlipoproteinemia (hi-per-lipo-pro-te-ne′mi-ah): increased concentration of lipoproteins in the blood

hyperplasia (hi-per-pla′se-ah): abnormal multiplication of normal cells

hypertriglyceridemia (hi-per-tri-glis-er-id-e′me-ah): increased levels of triglycerides in the blood

hypertrophic (hi-per-tro′fik): pertaining to enlargement of an organ due to increase in size of its constituent cells

hyperuricemia (hi-per-u-ris-e′me-ah): excess of uric acid in the blood; one of the characteristics of gout

hypervitaminosis (hi-per-vi-tah-min-o′sis): condition produced by excessive ingestion of vitamins, especially vitamins A and D

hypo-: prefix meaning lack or deficiency

hypoalbuminemia (hi-po-al-bu-min-e′me-ah): low albumin level of the blood

hypochlorhydria (hi-po-klor-hid′re-ah): decreased secretion of hydrochloric acid by the cells of the stomach

hypochromic (hi-po-krom′ik): below normal color; e.g., pale red blood cells lacking hemoglobin

hypogeusia: diminished sense of taste

hypoglycemia (hi-po-gli-se′me-ah): a lower than normal level of glucose in the blood

hypokalemia (hi-po-kal-e′me-ah): decreased potassium level in the blood

hyposmia (hi-pos′mi-ah): diminished sense of smell

hypothalamus (hi-po-thal′am-us): a group of nuclei at the base of the brain; includes centers of appetite control, cells that produce antidiuretic hormone

idiopathic (id-e-o-path′ik): pertaining to a disease of unknown origin

idiosyncrasy (id-e-o-sin′kra-se): a susceptibility to action of food or drugs that is characteristic or peculiar to an individual person

ileum (il′e-um): lower portion of the small intestine extending from the jejunum to the cecum

ileus (il′e-us): obstruction of the bowel

infarction (in-fark′shun): the formation of an area of dead tissue resulting from obstruction of blood vessels supplying the part

ingest (in-jest′): to take food into the body

inositol (in-os′it-ol): a 6-carbon alcohol found especially in cereal grains; combines with phosphate to form phytic acid

insidious (in-sid′e-us): pertaining to the progress of a disease with few if any symptoms to indicate its seriousness

insulin (in′su-lin): hormone secreted by beta cells of the islets of Langerhans of the pancreas; promotes utilization of glucose and lowers blood sugar

interstitial (in-ter-stish′al): situated in spaces between tissues

intra-: prefix meaning within

intracellular (in-trah-sel′u-lar): within the cell

intravenous (in-trah-ve′nus): into or from within a vein

intrinsic factor (in-trin′sik): mucoprotein in gastric juice which facilitates absorption of vitamin B-12; deficient in patients with pernicious anemia

iodopsin (i-o-dop′sin): pigment found in cones of the retina; visual violet

ion (i′on): an atom or group of atoms carrying a charge of electricity; e.g., cations, anions

ionize (i′on-īz): to separate molecules into electrically charged atoms or group of atoms; the number of negative charges exactly equals the number of positive charges

ischemia (is-ke′me-ah): a local deficiency of blood, chiefly from narrowing of the arteries

isocaloric (i-sō-kal-or′ik): containing an equal number of calories

isoleucine (i-sō-lu′sin): an essential amino acid

isotopes (i′so-tōps): atoms of the same element having the same atomic numbers and chemical properties but differing in the nuclear masses

-itis: suffix denoting inflammation; for example, colitis

jaundice (jon′dis): condition characterized by elevated bilirubin level of the blood and deposit of bile pigments in skin and mucous membranes

jejunum (je-joo′num): middle portion of small intestine; extends from duodenum to ileum

joule (jool): the unit of energy in the metric system; 1 calorie equals 4.184 joules (J)

keratin (ker′at-in): an insoluble sulfur-containing protein found in the skin, nails, hair

keratomalacia (ker′at-o-mal-a′shah): dryness and ulceration of the cornea resulting from vitamin A deficiency

keto-: a prefix denoting the presence of the carbonyl (CO) group

ketogenesis (ke-to-jen′es-is): formation of ketones from fatty acids and some amino acids

α-ketoglutaric acid (ke-tō-gloo-tar′ik): one of the intermediates in the tricarboxylic acid cycle; also the product of oxidative deamination of glutamic acid

ketone (ke′tōn): any compound containing a ketone (CO) grouping; ketone bodies include acetone, beta-hydroxybutyric acid, and acetoacetic acid

ketosis (ke-tō′sis): condition resulting from incomplete oxidation of fatty acids, and the consequent accumulation of ketone bodies

kilocalorie (kil′o-ka′lo-re): the unit of heat used in nutrition; the amount of heat required to raise 1,000 gm water 1°C (from 15.5 to 16.5°C); also known as the large calorie

kwashiorkor (kwash-e-or′kor): deficiency disease related principally to protein lack and seen in severely malnourished children; characterized by growth failure, edema, pigment changes in the skin

labile (la′bil): chemically unstable

lactalbumin (lak-tal-bu′min): a protein in milk

lactic acid (lak′tik): 3-carbon acid produced in milk by bacterial fementation of lactose; also produced during muscle contraction by anaerobic glycolysis

lactose (lak′tōs): a disaccharide composed of glucose and galactose; the form of carbohydrate in milk

lamina propria (lam′in-ah pro′pre-ah): connective-tissue structure that supports the epithelial cells of the intestinal mucosa

lecithin (les′ith-in): a phospholipid occurring in nervous and organ tissues, and in egg yolk; effective emulsifer

leucine (lu′sin): an essential amino acid

lignin (lig′nin): woody part of plants; a noncarbohydrate component of dietary fiber

linoleic acid (lin-o-le′ic): an 18-carbon fatty acid with two double bonds; essential for growth and skin health

linolenic acid (lin-o-len′ik): an 18-carbon fatty acid with three double bonds; not an essential fatty acid

lipase (lip′ās): an enzyme that hydrolyzes fat

lipid (lip′id): a term for fats including neutral fats, oils, fatty acids, phospholipids, cholesterol

lipogenesis (lip-o-jen′es-is): formation of fat

lipoic acid (lip-o′ik): thioctic acid; protogen; a factor that functions with thiamin pyrophosphate in removing the carboxyl group from alpha keto acids such as pyruvic acid

lipolysis (lip-ol′is-is): the splitting up of fat

lipoprotein (li-po-pro′te-in): a conjugated protein that incorporates lipids to facilitate transportation of the lipids in an aqueous medium

lipotropic (lip-o-trop′ik): pertaining to substances that prevent accumulation of fat in the liver

lithiasis (li-thi′a-sis): the formation of calculi of any kind

low-density lipoproteins: complexes of triglycerides, cholesterol, and phospholipids with proteins in the blood; account for about three fourths of the cholesterol in the blood

lysine (li′sēn): a diamino essential amino acid

lysosomes (li′so-sōms): structures of cell cytoplasm that contain digestive enzymes

macrocyte (mak′ro-sīt): an abnormally large red blood cell

malaise (mal-āz′): discomfort, distress, or uneasiness

malignant (mal-ig′nant): occurring in severe form, frequently fatal; in tumors refers to uncontrollable growth as in cancer

maltose (mawl′tōs): a disaccharide resulting from starch hydrolysis; yields 2 molecules glucose on further hydrolysis

maramus (mar-az′mus): extreme protein-calorie malnutrition marked by emaciation, especially severe in young children who receive insufficient amounts of food

matrix (ma′trix): the groundwork in which something is cast; for example, protein is the bone matrix into which mineral salts are deposited

megaloblast (meg′al-o-blast): primitive red blood cell of large size with large nucleus; present in blood when there is deficiency of vitamin B-12 and/or folic acid

menadione (men-a-di′on): synthetic compound with vitamin K activity

metabolic pool (met-ah-bol′ik): the assortment of nutrients available at any given moment of time for the metabolic activities of the body, e.g., amino acid pool, calcium pool

metabolism (me-tab′o-lism): physical and chemical changes occurring within the organism; includes synthesis of biologic materials and breakdown of substances to yield energy

metabolite (me-tab′oh-līt): any substance that results from physical and chemical changes within the organism

methionine (meth-i′o-nin): an essential sulfur-containing amino acid; supplies labile methyl groups

micelle (mis-el′): a microscopic particle of lipids and bile salts
microcyte (mi′kro-sīt): small red blood cell
microvilli (mi′kro-vil′li): minute structures visible by electron microscope, present on surface of mucosal epithelium; the "brush border"
milliequivalent, mEq (mil′lĭ-e-kwiv′ah-lent): concentration of a substance per liter of solution; obtained by dividing the milligrams per liter by the equivalent weight
mitochondria (mit-o-kon′dre-ah): rod-shaped or round structures in cell that trap energy-rich ATP
monoglyceride (mono-glis′er-id): an ester of glycerol with one fatty acid
monosaccharide (mon-o-sak′ar-id): a single sugar not affected by hydrolysis; includes glucose, fructose, galactose
monounsaturated (mon-o-un-sat′u-ra-ted): having a single double bond as in a fatty acid, e.g., oleic acid
morbidity (mor-bid′it-e): the proportion of disease to health in a community
motility (mo-til′it-e): ability to move spontaneously
mucin (mu′sin): a substance containing mucopolysaccharides secreted by goblet cells of the intestine and other glandular cells; has a protective and lubricating action
mucopolysaccharide (mu′ko-pol-e-sak′er-id): any of a group of polysaccharides combined with other groups such as protein
mucoprotein (mu′ko-pro′te-in): a conjugated protein containing a carbohydrate group such as chondroitin sulfuric acid
mucosa (mu-ko′sah): membrane lining the gastrointestinal, respiratory, and genitourinary tracts
myo-: prefix meaning muscle
myocardium (mi-o-kar′de-um): the heart muscle
myoglobin (mi-o-glo′bin): an iron-protein complex in muscle that transports oxygen; somewhat similar to hemoglobin
myosin (mi′o-sin): a soluble protein in muscle; combines with actin to form actomyosin, an enzyme that catalyzes the dephosphorylation of ATP during muscle contraction

nausea (naw′se-ah): sickness at the stomach; inclination to vomit
necrosis (ne-kro′sis): death of a cell or cells or of a portion of tissue
neonatal (ne-o-na′tal): pertaining to the newborn
neoplasm (ne′o-plasm): new or abnormal, uncontrolled growth, such as a tumor
nephron (nef′ron): the functional unit of the kidney consisting of a tuft of capillaries known as the glomerulus attached to the renal tubule
neuritic (nu-rit′ik): pertaining to inflammation of a nerve
neuropathy (nu-rop′ath-e): disease of the nervous system
niacin (ni′ah-sin): one of the water-soluble B complex vitamins which functions as a coenzyme in cell respiration; antipellagra factor
niacin equivalent: the total niacin available from the diet including preformed niacin plus that derived from the metabolism of tryptophan; 60 mg tryptophan = 1 mg niacin
niacinamide (ni′ah-sin-am′id): biologically active form of niacin occurring in the tissues
nicotinamide adenine dinucleotide, NAD (nik′o-tin-am′id ad′en-in di-nu′kle-o-tid): coenzyme for a number of enzymes, chiefly dehydrogenases
nicotinic acid (nik-o-tin′ik): niacin
nocturia (nok-tu′re-ah): excessive urination at night
nonheme iron: the form of iron in fruits, vegetables, cereals, eggs, and dairy products as well as the iron in meat, poultry, and fish not associated with hemoglobin or myoglobin
nucleic acid (nu-kle′ik): complex organic acid containing four bases—adenine, guanine, cytosine, and thymine—attached to ribose and phosphate
nucleoprotein (nu-kle-o-pro′te-in): conjugated protein found in the nuclei of cells; yields a protein fraction and nucleic acid
nucleotide (nu′kle-o-tid): a hydrolytic product of nucleic acid; contains one purine or pyrimidine base and a sugar phosphate
nutrient (nu′tre-ent): chemical substance in foods which nourishes, e.g., amino acid, fat, calcium
nutrient density: the ratio of the nutritive value of a food or diet to its caloric contribution
nyctalopia (nik-tal-o′pe-ah): night blindness
nystagmus (nis-tag′mus): rhythmic rapid movement of the eyeball

oleic acid (o-le′ik): an 18-carbon fatty acid containing one double bond; widely distributed in foods
oliguria (ol-ig-u′re-ah): scanty secretion of urine
-ology: suffix meaning science of, study of

ophthalmia (of-thal′me-ah): severe inflammation of the eye

organelles (or-gan-elz′): the various structures of the cell such as lysosomes, mitochondria

ornithine (or′nith-in): an amino acid formed from arginine when urea is split off

osmosis (oz-mo′sis): passage of a solvent from the lesser to the greater concentration when two solutions are separated by a membrane

ossification (os-if-ik-a′shun): formation of bone

osteo-: prefix meaning bone

osteomalacia (os-te-o-mal-a′se-ah): softening of the bone, chiefly in adults

osteoporosis (os-te-o-po-ro′sis): reduction of the quantity of bone, occurring principally in women after middle age; the remaining bone is normally mineralized

oxalic acid (oks-al′ik): a dicarboxylic acid present in foods such as spinach, chard, rhubarb; forms insoluble salts with calcium

oxaloacetic acid (oks-al-o-as-e′tik): a 3-carbon ketodicarboxylic acid; an intermediate in the tricarboxylic acid cycle

oxidation (oks-id-a′shun): increase in positive charges on an atom or loss of negative charges

palmitic acid (pal-mit′ik): a 16-carbon saturated fatty acid widespread in foods

pancreozymin (pan′kre-o-zi′min): hormone produced in duodenal mucosa that stimulates secretion of pancreatic enzymes

pantothenic acid (pan-to-then′ik): one of the B-complex vitamins; a constituent of coenzyme A

parathormone (par-at-hor-mōn): secretion of parathyroid gland that regulates calcium and phosphorus metabolism

parenchyma (par-en′ki-mah): functional tissue of an organ or gland as distinct from its supporting framework

parenteral (par-en′ter-al): by other means than through the gastrointestinal tract; introduction of nutrients by vein or into subcutaneous tissues

paresthesia (par-es-the′zi-ah): abnormal sensation such as numbness, burning, pricking

parturition (par-tu-rish′un): giving birth to a child

path-, patho-, -pathy: combining forms meaning disease, e.g., *patho*genic, nephro*pathy*

pathology (path-ol′o-je): science dealing with disease; structural and functional changes caused by disease

pectin (pek′tin): a polysaccharide found in many fruits and having gelling properties

pellagra (pel-lah′gra): a deficiency disease of the skin, gastrointestinal tract, and nervous system caused by lack of niacin and associated with other nutritional deficiencies

pentose (pen′tōs): a simple sugar containing 5 carbon atoms; ribose, arabinose, xylose

peptide linkage (pep′tid): the CO-NH linkage of two amino acids by condensation of the amino group of one amino acid with the carboxyl group of another amino acid

peptone (pep′tone): an intermediate product of protein digestion

perinatal (per-ĭ-na′tal): pertaining to before, during, or after the time of birth

peristalsis (per-is-tal′sis): the rhythmic, wavelike movement produced by muscles of the small intestine to move food forward

phagocyte (fag′o-sīt): a cell capable of ingesting bacteria or other foreign material

phenylalanine (fen-il-al′ah-nin): an essential amino acid; consists of a phenyl group attached to alanine

phenylketonuria (fe-nil-ke-to-nu′re-ah): excretion of phenylpyruvic acid and other phenyl compounds in urine because of congenital lack of an enzyme required for conversion of phenylalanine to tyrosine; characterized by mental retardation

phospholipid (fos′fo-lip′id): a fatlike compound that contains a phosphate and another group such as a nitrogen base in addition to glycerol and fatty acids, e.g., lecithin, cephalin

phosphoprotein (fos-fo-pro′te-in): a conjugated protein that contains phosphorus, e.g., nucleoprotein, casein

phosphorylate (fos-fo′ril-ate): to introduce a phosphate grouping into an organic compound, e.g., glucose monophosphate produced by action of enzyme *phosphorylase*

photosynthesis (fo-to-sin′the-sis): the process whereby the chlorophyll in green plants utilizes the energy from the sun to synthesize carbohydrate from carbon dioxide and water

phylloquinone (fil′o-kwin-ōn): vitamin K

phytic acid (fi′tik): a phosphoric acid ester of inositol found in seeds; interferes with absorption of calcium, magnesium, iron, zinc

pica (pi′kah): a hunger for substances not fit for food

pinocytosis (pin-o-si-to′sis): the taking up of droplets (for example, fat) by a cell by surrounding the liquid with part of the membrane

plaque (plak): any patch or flat area; atherosclerotic plaque is a deposit of lipid material in the blood vessel

plasma (plaz′mah): fluid portion of the blood before clotting has taken place

poly-: prefix meaning much or many

polyneuritis (pol-e-nu-ri′tis): inflammation of a number of nerves

polypeptide (pol-e-pep′tid): a compound consisting of more than three amino acids; an intermediate stage in protein digestion

polyphagia (pol-e-fa′je-ah): excessive eating

polysaccharide (pol-e-sak′ar-id): a class of carbohydrates containing many single sugars; includes starch, glycogen, dextrins, pectins, cellulose, and others

polyunsaturated fatty acid: fatty acids containing two or more double bonds; linoleic, linolenic, and arachidonic acids

porphyrin (por′fir-in): a pigmented compound containing four pyrrole nuclei joined in a ring structure; combines with iron in hemoglobin

precursor: anything that precedes another or from which another is derived; for example, carotene is a precursor to vitamin A

prenatal (prē-na′tal): preceding birth

proenzyme (pro-en′zīm): inactive form of an enzyme, e.g., pepsinogen

progesterone (prō-jes′ter-ōn): hormone of corpus luteum which prepares endometrium for reception and development of the fertilized ovum

prognosis (prog-no′sis): forecast of probable result from attack of disease

proline (pro′lēn): a nonessential amino acid

prophylaxis (pro-fil-ak′sis): prevention of disease

prosthetic group (pros-thet′ik): chemical group attached to a molecule such as protein; nonprotein part of an enzyme

protease (pro′te-ās): an enzyme that digests protein

protein efficiency ratio: a measure of the quality of a protein by calculating the weight gain of an experimental animal per gram of protein fed

proteinuria (pro′te-in-u′ri-ah): excretion of protein in the urine

proteolytic (pro′te-o-lit′ik): effecting the hydrolysis of protein

proteose (pro′te-ōs): a derivative of protein formed during digestion

prothrombin (pro-throm′bin): factor in blood plasma for blood clotting; precursor of thrombin

protoplasm (pro′to-plazm): form of living matter in all cells

protoporphyrin (pro′tō-por′fir-in): a porphyrin combined with iron and globin forming hemoglobin

provitamin (pro-vi′tah-min): precursor of a vitamin

proximal (prok′sim-al): nearest to the head or point of attachment

pteroylglutamic acid (ter′o-il-glu-tam′ik): folic acid

puerperium (pur-pe′ri-um): the period after labor until involution of the uterus

purine (pu′rin): organic compounds containing heterocyclic nitrogen structures that are catabolized to uric acid; supplied especially by flesh foods and synthesized in the body

pyridoxal phosphate (pir-ī-dok′sal fos′fate): a coenzyme that contains vitamin B-6

pyridoxine (pi-ri-dox′in): one of the forms of vitamin B-6

pyruvic acid (pi-ru′vik): a 3-carbon keto acid; an intermediate in glucose metabolism

rancid (ran′sid): term that describes rank taste or smell that results from decomposition of fatty acids

regurgitation (re-gur-jit-a′shun): the backward flow of food; casting up of undigested food

relapsing (re-laps′ing): return of symptoms

remission (re-mish′un): a lessening of the severity or temporary abatement of symptoms

renal (re′nal): pertaining to the kidney

renal threshold: the level of concentration of a substance in the blood beyond which it is excreted in the urine

renin: enzyme produced by the kidney; pressor substance

rennin (ren′in): enzyme in gastric juice that coagulates milk protein

repletion (rep-le′shun): to fill up; to restore

resection (re-sek′shun): removal of part of an organ

residue (rez′i-du): remainder; the contents remaining in the intestinal tract after digestion of food; includes fiber and other unabsorbed products

resorption (re-sorp′shun): a loss of substance, e.g., loss of mineral salts from bone

reticulocyte (re-tik′u-lo-sīt): a young red blood cell occurring during active blood regeneration

reticuloendothelium (re-tik′u-lo-en-dō-the′le-um): a system of macrophages concerned with phagocytosis; present in spleen, liver, bone marrow, connective tissues, and lymph nodes

retinene (ret′in-ēn): vitamin A aldehyde; intermediate step in bleaching of visual purple

retinol (ret′in-ol): vitamin A alcohol

retinopathy (ret-in-op′ath-e): degenerative disease of the retina

rhodopsin (ro-dop′sin): visual purple; pigment of the rods of the retina bleached by light; vitamin A required for regeneration

riboflavin (ri′bo-fla′vin): heat-stable B-complex vitamin and a constituent of flavin enzymes; vitamin B-12

ribonucleic acid, RNA (ri-bo-nu-kle′ik): molecules in cytoplasm which serve for transfer of amino acid code from nucleus and the synthesis of protein

ribose (ri′bōs): 5-carbon sugar; a constituent of nucleic acid

ribosomes (ri′bo-sōms): dense particles in cell cytoplasm that are the site of protein synthesis

rickets (rik′ets): a deficiency disease of the skeletal system caused by a lack of vitamin D or calcium or both, and often resulting in bone deformities

saccharin (sak′ah-rin): a sweetening agent that is 300 to 500 times as sweet as sugar; yields no calories

Salmonella (sal-mo-nel′ah): group of bacteria causing intestinal infection; frequently contaminates foods

saponification (sap-on′if-ik-a′shun): the action of alkali on a fat to form a soap

satiety (sat-i′et-e): feeling of satisfaction following meals

saturated (sat′u-ra-ted): a state in which a substance holds the most of another substance that it can

scurvy (skur′vē): a deficiency disease caused by lack of ascorbic acid and leading to swollen bleeding gums, hemorrhages of the skin and mucous membranes, and anemia

secretin (se-kre′tin): a hormone secreted by the epithelium of the duodenum upon stimulation by the acid chyme; stimulates secretion of pancreatic juice and bile

serine (se′rin): one of the amino acids occurring in protein; nonessential

serosa (ser-o′sah): the membranes lining the peritoneal, pericardial, and pleural cavities and covering their contents

serum (se′rum): the fluid portion of the blood that separates from the blood cells after clotting

siderophilin (sid′er-o-fil′in): an iron-transferring protein; transferrin

sorbitol (sor′bit-ol): a 6-carbon sugar alcohol with a sweet taste; used commercially to maintain moisture and inhibit crystal formation

sphincter (sfink′ter): a muscle surrounding and closing an orifice

sphingomyelin (sfing-go-mi′el-in): a phospholipid found in the brain, spinal cord, and kidney

stasis (sta′sis): retardation or cessation of flow of blood in the vessels; congestion

steapsin (ste-ap′sin): a hormone in pancreatic juice that hydrolyzes fat; lipase

stearic acid (ste′rik): a saturated fatty acid containing 18 carbon atoms

steatorrhea (ste-at-o-re′ah): excessive amount of fat in the feces

stenosis (sten-o′sis): narrowing of a passage

steroid (ste′roid): a group of compounds similar in structure to cholesterol; includes bile acids, sterols, sex hormones

sterol (ste′rol): an alcohol of high molecular weight; cholesterol, ergosterol

stomatitis (sto-ma-ti′tis): inflammation of the mucous membranes of the mouth

sub-: prefix denoting beneath, or less than normal

substrate (sub′strāt): substance upon which an enzyme acts

succinic acid (suk-sen′ik): a 3-carbon dicarboxylic acid that is an intermediate in the tricarboxylic acid cycle

sucrose (su′krōs): cane or beet sugar; a disaccharide that yields glucose and fructose when hydrolyzed

syn-: prefix meaning with, together

syndrome (sin′drōm): a set of symptoms occurring together

synergism (sin′er-jizm): the joint action of agents which when taken together increases each other's effectiveness

synthesis (sin′thes-is): process of building up a compound

systemic (sis-tem′ik): pertaining to the body as a whole

tachycardia (tak-e-kar′de-ah): rapid beating of the heart

testosterone (tes-tos′ter-ōn): testicular hormone responsible for male secondary sex characteristics

tetany (tet′an-e): a condition marked by intermittent muscular contraction accompanied by fibrillar tremors and muscular pains; seen in hypocalcemia, alkalosis.

thiamin (thi′am-in): a B-complex vitamin; with

phosphate forms coenzymes of decarboxylases; essential for carbohydrate metabolism

thio-: prefix meaning sulfur containing

threonine (thre′o-nin): an essential amino acid

thrombus (throm′bus): a clot in a blood vessel formed by coagulation of blood

thymine (thi′min): one of the four nitrogenous bases in nucleic acid

thyroxine (thī-rok′sin): iodine-containing hormone produced by the thyroid gland; regulates the rate of energy metabolism

tocopherol (tok-of′er-ōl): vitamin E; antioxidant alcohol occurring in vegetable germ oils; alpha-, beta-, gamma-, delta-tocopherol

-tomy: suffix meaning to cut into, e.g., gastrectomy

tophi (to′fi): sodium urate deposits in fibrous tissues near the joints; present in gout

tox-: prefix meaning poison

toxemia of pregnancy (tok-se′me-ah): a disorder of pregnancy characterized by hypertension, edema, albuminuria

transamination (trans′am-in-a′shun): transfer of an amino group to another molecule, e.g., transfer to a keto acid, thus forming another amino acid

transferase (trans′fer-ās): an enzyme that transfers a chemical grouping from one compound to another, for example, transaminase, transphosphorylase

transferrin (trans-fer′in): iron-binding protein for transport of iron in blood; siderophilin

trauma (traw-mah): wound or injury usually inflicted suddenly

trichinosis (trik-in-o′sis): illness caused by eating raw pork that is infested by *Trichinella spiralis,* a worm

triglyceride (tri-glis′er-id): an ester of glycerol and three fatty acids

trypsin (trip′sin): a protein-digesting enzyme secreted by the pancreas and released into the small intestine

trypsinogen (trip-sin′o-jen): inactive form of trypsin

tryptophan (trip′tō-fan): an essential amino acid that contains the indole ring; a precursor of niacin

tyramine (tir′am-en): a pressor amine that has an action similar to epinephrine; produced by decarboxylation of tyrosine; found especially in cheeses and some wines

tyrosine (ti′ro-sin): semiessential amino acid; spares phenylalanine; the amino acid in thyroxine

urea (u-re′ah): chief nitrogenous consistent of the urine; formed by the liver when amino acids are deaminized

uremia (u-re′me-ah): presence of urinary constituents in the blood resulting from deficient secretion of urine

uric acid (u-rik): a nitrogenous constituent formed in the metabolism of purines; excreted in the urine; blood levels increased in gout

valine (va′lin): an essential amino acid

vegan (ve-gan): one who excludes all animal foods from his or her diet

vegetarian: one who excludes one or more classes of animal foods from his or her diet; thus, vegans, lactovegetarian, lacto-ovo-vegetarian

villus (vil′us): fingerlike projection of the intestinal mucosa

viosterol (vi-os′ter-ol): vitamin D formed by irradiation of ergosterol

visual purple: photosensitive pigment found in the rods of the retina; rhodopsin

vitamin (vi′tah-min): organic compound occurring in minute amounts in foods and essential for numerous metabolic reactions; fat-soluble A, D, E, and K; water-soluble ascorbic acid and B complex including thiamin, riboflavin, niacin, pantothenic acid, biotin, vitamin B-6, vitamin B-12, folacin, and others

xanthine (zan′thin): an intermediate in the metabolism of purines; related to uric acid

xanthomatosis (zan-thō-mat-o′sis): accumulation of lipids in the form of tumors in various parts of the body

xerophthalmia (zer-of-thal′me-ah): dry infected eye condition caused by lack of vitamin A

xerosis (ze-ro′sis): abnormal dryness of skin and eye

xylose (zi′lōs): a 5-carbon aldehyde sugar that is not metabolized by the body

zein (za′in): a protein of low biologic value present in corn

zymogen (zi′mo-jen): the inactive form of an enzyme

Index

References to illustrations are printed in boldface type. Footnotes are indicated by the letter *"n,"* tables by the letter *"t."*

CRITERIA FOR NUTRITIONAL ASSESSMENT

Anthropometric Measurements

$$\text{\% Desirable Body Weight} = \frac{\text{Actual weight}}{\text{Desirable body weight}} \times 100$$

(See Tables A-6 to A-10)

$$\text{\% Weight Change} = \frac{\text{Usual weight}-\text{Current weight}}{\text{Usual weight}} \times 100$$

Triceps Skinfold (TSF), in mm: See Table A-11.

Mid-Arm Circumference (MAC), in cm: See Table A-11.

Mid-Arm Muscle Circumference (MAMC), in cm = MAC(cm)–[0.314 × TSF(mm)]

Biochemical Measurements

$$\text{Creatinine Height Index (CHI)} = \frac{\text{Measured Urinary Creatinine}}{\text{Ideal Urinary Creatinine}} \times 100$$

Ideal Urinary Creatinine Values

Men*		Women†	
Height (cm)	Ideal Creatinine (mg)	Height (cm)	Ideal Creatinine (mg)
157.5	1288	147.3	830
160.0	1325	149.9	851
162.6	1359	152.4	875
165.1	1386	154.9	900
167.6	1426	157.5	925
170.2	1467	160.0	949
172.7	1513	162.6	977
175.3	1555	165.1	1006
177.8	1596	167.6	1044
180.3	1642	170.2	1076
182.9	1691	172.7	1109
185.4	1739	175.3	1141
188.0	1785	177.8	1174
190.5	1831	180.3	1206
193.0	1891	182.9	1240

*Creatinine coefficient (men) = 23 mg/kg of ideal body weight.
†Creatinine coefficient (women) = 18 mg/kg of ideal body weight.

Serum Proteins	**Albumin** (gm/dl)	**Transferrin** (mg/dl)
adequate	⩾ 3.5	> 200
mild depletion	3.0–3.5	150–175
moderate depletion	2.1–3.0	100–150
severe depletion	< 2.1	< 100

$$\text{Apparent Nitrogen Balance} = \frac{\text{Protein Intake}}{6.25} = (\text{Urinary Urea Nitrogen} + 4)$$

Serum Transferrin (TFN) = (0.8 × T.I.B.C.) – 43